HARRISON'S
ADVANCES *in*
CARDIOLOGY

HARRISON'S ADVANCES *in* CARDIOLOGY

Eugene Braunwald, MD, MD (HON), ScD (HON)

Distinguished Hersey Professor of Medicine, Faculty Dean for Academic
Programs at Brigham and Women's Hospital and Massachusetts
General Hospital, Harvard Medical School; Chief Academic
Officer, Partners HealthCare System
Boston, Massachusetts

McGRAW-HILL
Medical Publishing Division

New York   Chicago   San Francisco   Lisbon   London   Madrid
Mexico City   Milan   New Delhi   San Juan   Seoul   Singapore
Sydney   Toronto

McGraw-Hill

A Division of The **McGraw·Hill** *Companies*

Harrison's Advances in Cardiology

1234567890 DOC/DOC 098765432

ISBN 0-07-137088-9

This book was set in Times Roman by Progressive Information Technologies.
The editors were Martin Wonsiewicz and Barbara Holton.
The production supervisor was Catherine H. Saggese.
The cover designer was John Vairo, Jr.
The text designer was Marsha Cohen/Parallelogram.

RR Donnelley was printer and binder.

This book is printed on acid-free paper.

Library of Congress Cataloging-in-Publication Data

Harrison's advances in cardiology/[edited by] Eugene Braunwald.
    p. cm.
Includes bibliographical references and index.
ISBN 0-07-137088-9
1. Cardiology. 2. Cardiovascular system—Diseases—Treatment. I. Braunwald, Eugene,
   1929–

RC667 .H355 2002
616.1'2—dc21
                                                         2002026546

616.12 HAR   X

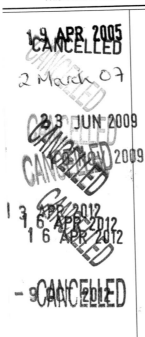

Contents

SECTION I
Atherosclerosis/Lipids

SECTION II
Hypertension

SECTION III
Acute Coronary Syndromes/Myocardial Infarction

SECTION IV
Coronary Artery Disease

SECTION VI
Arrhythmias

SECTION VII
Ventricular Dysfunction and Heart Failure

SECTION VIII
Vascular Disease

SECTION IX
Other

Contributors

Elliott M. Antman, MD
Associate Professor of Medicine
Harvard Medical School
Director, Samuel A. Levine Cardiac Unit
Brigham and Women's Hospital
Boston, Massachusetts
Chapter 25

Piero Anversa, MD
Professor of Medicine
Director, Cardiovascular Research Institute
New York Medical College
Valhalla, New York
Chapter 70

Lawrence J. Appel, MD, MPH
Associate Professor of Medicine
Johns Hopkins University School of Medicine
Baltimore, Maryland
Chapter 12

William F. Armstrong, MD
Professor of Internal Medicine
Director, Echocardiography Laboratory
Associate Clinical Chief, Division of Cardiology
Department of Internal Medicine
The University of Michigan Health System
Ann Arbor, Michigan
Chapter 31

Richard Baffour, PhD
Senior Scientist
Cardiovascular Research Institute
MedStar Research Institute
Washington Hospital Center
Washington, DC
Chapter 38

Helmut Baumgartner, MD
Department of Cardiology
Vienna General Hospital
University of Vienna
Vienna, Austria
Chapter 52

John Beltrame, MD
Cardiology Unit
North Western Adelaide Health Service
Adelaide University, Adelaide, Australia
Chapter 46

Alan K. Berger, MD
Assistant Professor
Division of Cardiology and
Division of Epidemiology
University of Minnesota
Minneapolis, Minnesota
Chapter 27

Bradford C. Berk, MD, PhD
Paul N. Yu Professor of Cardiology
Chairman, Department of Medicine
The University of Rochester
Chief, Cardiology Unit
Director, Center for Cardiovascular Research
The University of Rochester Medical School
Rochester, New York
Chapter 2

David B. Bharucha, MD, PhD
Assistant Professor of Medicine
Attending Electrophysiologist
Mount Sinai Medical Center
New York, New York
Chapter 64

Robert O. Bonow, MD
Goldberg Distinguished Professor of Cardiology
Northwestern University Feinberg School
    of Medicine
Chief, Division of Cardiology
Northwestern Memorial Hospital
Chicago, Illinois
Chapter 55

Nancy D. Bridges, MD
Professor of Pediatrics
Associate Chief of Pediatric Cardiology
Director, Pediatric Pulmonary Hypertension
    Program
Mount Sinai Medical Center
New York, New York
Chapter 99

Maria Mori Brooks, PhD
Assistant Professor of Epidemiology
University of Pittsburgh
Graduate School of Public Health
Pittsburgh, Pennsylvania
Chapter 42

Robert C. Brooks, MD, PhD
Assistant Professor of Medicine
University of Pittsburgh
Staff Physician
Pittsburgh VA Healthcare System
Pittsburgh, Pennsylvania
Chapter 42

Charles J. Bruce, MB, ChB
Senior Associate Consultant
Mayo Clinic and Mayo Foundation
Assistant Professor of Medicine
Division of Cardiovascular Diseases and
    Internal Medicine
Mayo Medical School
Rochester, Minnesota
Chapter 50

Ramon Brugada, MD
Director, Molecular Genetics Program
    Masonic Medical Research Laboratory
Utica, New York
Chapter 57

Grant H. Burch, MD
Assistant Professor of Pediatrics
Interventional Cardiologist
    Doembecher Children's Hospital
Oregon Health Science University
Portland, Oregon
Chapter 48

Alfred E. Buxton, MD
Professor of Medicine
Brown University
Director, Arrhythmia Services
Rhode Island Hospital
Providence, Rhode Island
Chapter 69

Hugh Calkins, MD
Associate Professor of Medicine
Johns Hopkins University School of Medicine
Baltimore, Maryland
Chapter 59

Tracy Q. Callister, MD
President, EBT Research Foundation
Hendersonville, Tennessee
Chapter 36

Mark D. Carlson, MD
Professor and Vice Chairman of Medicine
University Hospitals of Cleveland and
Case Western Reserve University
Cleveland, Ohio
Chapter 79

Bernard R. Chaitman, MD
Professor of Medicine
Saint Louis University Health Science Center
St. Louis, Missouri
Chapter 58

Ray C-J Chiu, MD, PhD
Professor of Surgery
Division of Cardiac Surgery
McGill University
Montreal, Quebec, Canada
Chapter 87

Dorothea Collins, ScD
Department of Veterans Affairs Cooperative
  Studies
Program Coordinating Center
West Haven, Connecticut
Chapter 7

Jack G. Copeland III, MD
Professor and Chief, Cardiothoracic Surgery
Co-Director, Sarver Heart Center
University of Arizona, University Medical Center
Tucson, Arizona
Chapter 85

Roberto Corrocher, MD
Professor of Internal Medicine
University of Verona
Verona, Italy
Chapter 18

Maria Rosa Costanzo, MD
Midwest Heart Specialists
Naperville, Illinois
Chapter 83

James J. Crowley, MD
Associate in Medicine
Interventional Cardiovascular Program
Duke University Medical Center
Durham, North Carolina
Chapter 17

David L. Dawson, MD
Associate Professor, Department of Surgery
Uniformed Services University of the Health
  Sciences
Staff Vascular Surgeon, Wilford Hall Medical
  Center
Lackland Air Force Base, Lackland, Texas
Chapter 91

Teresa De Marco, MD
Associate Professor of Medicine
University of California, San Francisco,
  Medical Center
San Francisco, California
Chapter 78

Katherine M. Detre, MD, DrPH
Professor of Epidemiology
University of Pittsburgh
Graduate School of Public Health
Director, Epidemiology Data Center
Pittsburgh, Pennsylvania
Chapter 42

Vasken Dilsizian, MD
Professor of Medicine and Radiology
Director of Cardiovascular Nuclear Medicine
University of Maryland Medical Center
Baltimore, Maryland
Chapter 34

Donald B. Doty, MD
Chief, Department of Surgery
LDS Hospital
Salt Lake City, Utah
Chapter 53

John R. Doty, MD
Resident, Cardiothoracic Surgery
The Johns Hopkins Hospital
Baltimore, Maryland
Chapter 53

Janice G. Douglas, MD
Professor of Medicine and Physiology and
    Biophysics and Pharmacology
Case Western Reserve University School of
    Medicine
Chief, Division of Hypertension
University Hospitals of Cleveland
Cleveland, Ohio
Chapter 14

Robert D. Dowling, MD
Associate Professor of Surgery
University of Louisville
Louisville, Kentucky
Chapter 86

Carolyn M. Dresler, MD
Director
Medical Affairs Smoking Control
GlaxoSmithKline Consumer Healthcare
Parsippany, New Jersey
Chapter 98

William D. Edwards, MD
Professor of Pathology
Mayo Medical School and
Mayo Graduate School of Medicine
Consultant in Pathology
Department of Laboratory Medicine and Pathology
Mayo Clinic
Rochester, Minnesota
Chapter 49

Stephen G. Ellis, MD
Sones Cardiac Catheterization Laboratory
The Cleveland Clinic Foundation
Cleveland, Ohio
Chapter 32

Stephen E. Epstein, MD
Executive Director, Cardiovascular Research Institute
Director, Vascular Biology Research
MedStar Research Institute
Washington Hospital Center
Washington, DC
Chapter 38

Nathan R. Every, MD
Department of Veterans Affairs
Department of Medicine
University of Washington
Seattle, Washington
Chapter 43

Zahi A. Fayad, PhD
Associate Professor, Department of Radiology and
    Medicine (Cardiology)
Director, Cardiovascular Imaging Research
Mount Sinai Medical Center
New York, New York
Chapter 35

James J. Ferguson, MD
Associate Director, Cardiology Research
Texas Heart Institute at St. Luke's Episcopal Hospital
Assistant Professor
Baylor College of Medicine
Clinical Assistant Professor
The University of Texas Health Science Center
    at Houston
Houston, Texas
Chapter 24

Robert E. Fowles, MD
Clinical Professor of Medicine
University of Utah
Consulting Cardiologist
LDS Hospital
Salt Lake City, Utah
Chapter 26

Shmuel Fuchs, MD
Director, Interventional Myocardial Angiogenesis
Cardiovascular Research Institute
MedStar Research Institute
Washington Hospital Center
Washington, DC
Chapter 38

Valentin Fuster, MD, PhD
Professor of Medicine
Director, The Zena and Michael A. Wiener
    Cardiovascular Institute
Mount Sinai School of Medicine
New York, New York
Chapter 35

Haralambos Gavras, MD, FRCP
Professor of Medicine
Boston University School of Medicine
Chief, Hypertension and Atherosclerosis
Boston Medical Center
Boston, Massachusetts
Chapter 13

Irene Gavras, MD
Professor of Medicine
Boston University School of Medicine
Attending Physician
Boston Medical Center
Boston Massachusetts
Chapter 13

Bartolomeo Giannattasio, MD, PhD
Division of Cardiology
University Hospitals of Cleveland
Cleveland, Ohio
Chapter 79

Jeffrey S. Ginsberg, MD
McMaster University Medical Centre
Hamilton, Ontario, Canada
Chapter 88

Domenico Girelli, MD, PhD
Assistant
Department of Clinical and Experimental Medicine
University of Verona
Verona, Italy
Chapter 18

Michael K. Gould, MD, MS
Research Associate and Staff Physician
VA Palo Alto Health Care System
Assistant Professor of Medicine and of Health
    Research and Policy
Stanford University Medical Center
Stanford, California
Chapter 89

Laman A. Gray, Jr., MD
Professor of Surgery
Director, Division of Thoracic and
    Cardiovascular Surgery
University of Louisville
Louisville, Kentucky
Chapter 86

Ihor Gussak, MD PhD
Associate Director
Cardiovascular Research and Development
Associate Global Clinical Manager
Aventis Pharmaceuticals, Inc.
Bridgewater, New Jersey
Chapter 58

Patrick Hanly, MD
Department of Medicine
Respiratory Division
St. Michael's Hospital
Center of Sleep and Chronobiology
University of Toronto
Toronto, Canada
Chapter 11

Judith S. Hochman, MD
Director, Cardiac Care and Stepdown Units
Director of Cardiac Research
St. Luke's–Roosevelt Hospital Center
Professor of Medicine
Columbia University
New York, New York
Chapter 29

Katherine J. Hoercher, RN
Director of Research, Kaufman Center
    for Heart Failure
The Cleveland Clinic Foundation
Cleveland, Ohio
Chapter 82

Victor Hoffstein, PhD, MD
Professor
Department of Medicine
University of Toronto
Staff Respirologist
St. Michael's Hospital
Toronto, Ontario, Canada
Chapter 11

Adrian Iania, MD
Associate Professor of Medicine
Head, Department of Nephrology
Tel Aviv Medical Center
Ichilov Hospital
University Tel Aviv Medical School
Tel Aviv, Israel
Chapter 73

Jeffrey M. Isner, MD †
Departments of Medicine and Surgery
St. Elizabeth's Medical Center and
    Tufts University School of Medicine
Boston, Massachusetts
Chapter 40

Allan S. Jaffe, MD
Consultant in Cardiology and Laboratory Medicine
Professor of Medicine
Mayo Clinic and Medical School
Rochester, Minnesota
Chapter 19

Mark E. Josephson, MD
Professor of Medicine
Harvard Medical School
Director, Cardiology Division
Beth Israel Deaconess Medical Center
Boston, Massachusetts
Chapter 63

Samir R. Kapadia, MD
Assistant Professor of Medicine
University of Washington
Seattle, Washington
Chapter 45

David A. Kass, MD
Professor of Medicine and Biomedical Engineering
Johns Hopkins University School of Medicine
Baltimore, Maryland
Chapter 80

Vineet Kaushik, MD
Department of Cardiac Electrophysiology
University of California, San Francisco,
    Medical Center
San Francisco, California
Chapter 78

Clive Kearon, MD, PhD
McMaster Medical Unit
Henderson General Hospital
McMaster University
Hamilton, Ontario, Canada
Chapter 88

J. Ward Kennedy, MD
Professor of Medicine
University of Washington
Seattle, Washington
Chapter 1

† Deceased

Karl B. Kern, MD
Professor of Medicine
Associate Director
Cardiac Catheterization Laboratories
Sarver Heart Center
University Medical Center
Tucson, Arizona
Chapter 68

Scott Kinlay, MBBS
Instructor, Department of Medicine
Harvard Medical School
Director, Intravascular Imaging
Brigham and Women's Hospital
Boston, Massachusetts
Chapter 30

Robert A. Kloner, MD, PhD
Professor of Medicine
Keck School of Medicine at the University
   of Southern California
Director of Research
Heart Institute
Good Samaritan Hospital
Los Angeles, California
Chapter 33

Theodore J. Kolias, MD
Clinical Assistant Professor of Internal Medicine
Division of Cardiology
University of Michigan Health System
Ann Arbor, Michigan
Chapter 31

Peter R. Kowey, MD
Professor of Medicine
Jefferson Medical College
Philadelphia, Pennsylvania
Chief of Cardiology
Main Line Health System
Wynnewood, Pennsylvania
Chapter 64

Zvonimir Krajcer, MD
Clinical Professor of Medicine
Baylor College of Medicine and
The University of Texas Health Science
   Center at Houston
Director, Peripheral Vascular Intervention
St. Luke's Episcopal Hospital
Texas Heart Institute
Houston, Texas
Chapter 96

Harlan M. Krumholz, MD
Sections of Cardiology and Epidemiology
Yale–New Haven Hospital Center for Outcomes
   Research and Evaluation
Department of Epidemiology and Public Health
Yale University School of Medicine
New Haven, Connecticut
Chapter 27

Roger J. Laham, MD
Division of Cardiology
Department of Medicine
Harvard Medical School and Beth Israel Deaconess
   Medical Center
Boston, Massachusetts
Chapter 39

Carl V. Leier, MD
Overstreet Professor of Medicine and Pharmacology
Division of Cardiology
Heart–Lung Research Institute
The Ohio State University Medical Center
Columbus, Ohio
Chapter 77

William C. Little, MD
Professor of Internal Medicine
Chief of Cardiology
Wake Forest University School of Medicine
Winston-Salem, North Carolina
Chapter 75

Peter Liu, MD
Director, Heart and Stroke
Lewar Center of Excellence in Cardiovascular
    Research,
Toronto General Hospital
Toronto, Canada
Chapter 76

Douglas W. Losordo, MD
Chief of Cardiovascular Research
St. Elizabeth's Medical Center
Associate Professor of Medicine
Tufts University School of Medicine
Boston, Massachusetts
Chapter 40

Russell V. Luepker, MD
Mayo Professor and Head
Division of Epidemiology
School of Public Health
University of Minnesota
Minneapolis, Minnesota
Chapter 22

Gordon Mack, MD
Division of Pediatric Cardiology
Department of Pediatrics
University of Saskatchewan
Royal University Hospital
Saskatoon, Saskatchewan, Canada
Chapter 48

Alan Maisel, MD
Professor of Medicine
Director, Coronary Care Unit, Heart Failure
    Research Unit,
Division of Cardiology, Department of Medicine
VA San Diego Health Care System
University of California, San Diego
San Diego, California,
Chapter 74

Douglas L. Mann, MD
Gordon Cain Chair and Professor of Medicine
Baylor College of Medicine
Staff Physician, Veteran's Affairs Medical Center
Houston, Texas
Chapter 71

Warren J. Manning, MD
Associate Professor of Medicine and Radiology
Harvard Medical School
Chief, Non-invasive Cardiac Imaging
Beth Israel Deaconess Medical Center
Boston, Massachusetts
Chapter 67

Frank I. Marcus, MD
Professor of Medicine
University of Arizona Sarver Heart Center
Tucson, Arizona
Chapter 59

Barry J. Maron, MD
Director, The Hypertrophic Cardiomyopathy
    Center
Minneapolis Heart Institute Foundation
Minneapolis, Minnesota
Chapter 60

Steven P. Marso, MD
Assistant Professor
University of Missouri — Kansas City
Saint Luke's Hospital
Mid-America Heart Institute
Kansas City, Missouri
Chapter 32

J.J.M. Marx, MD
University Medical Center Utrecht
Utrecht, The Netherlands
Chapter 100

Charles Maynard, PhD
Health Services Research and Development
Department of Veterans Affairs
Department of Health Services
University of Washington
Seattle, Washington
Chapter 43

Patrick M. McCarthy, MD
Surgical Director, Kaufman Center for Heart Failure
Cleveland Clinic Foundation
Cleveland, Ohio
Chapter 82

Peter A. McCullough, MD, MPH
Associate Professor
University of Missouri — Kansas City
School of Medicine
Chief, Cardiology Section
Truman Medical Center
Kansas City, Missouri
Chapter 21

Mary McGrae McDermott, MD
Assistant Professor
Department of Preventive Medicine
Northwestern University Medical School,
Chicago, Illinois
Chapter 90

Luisa Mestroni, MD
Director, Adult Medical Genetics Program
Director, Molecular Genetics
University of Colorado Cardiovascular Institute
University of Colorado Health Sciences Center,
Denver, Colorado
Chapter 72

Andrew D. Michaels, MD
Assistant Professor of Medicine
Cardiovascular Research Institute
University of California San Francisco
   Medical Center
San Francisco, California
Chapter 54

Fred Morady, MD
Professor of Medicine
Director, Clinical Electrophysiology Laboratory
University of Michigan Medical Center
Ann Arbor, Michigan
Chapter 62

David A. Morrow, MD
Instructor in Medicine
Harvard Medical School
Associate Physician, Cardiovascular Division
Brigham and Women's Hospital
Boston, Massachusetts
Chapter 25

Charles J. Mullany, MB, MS
Consultant, Division of Cardiovascular Surgery
Professor of Surgery
Mayo Medical School
Mayo Clinic
Rochester, Minnesota
Chapter 56

James E. Muller, MD
Division of Cardiology
Massachusetts General Hospital
Boston, Massachusetts
Chapter 20

Christoph A. Nienaber, MD
Professor of Internal Medicine and Cardiology
Director, Division of Cardiology and Angiology
The University of Rostock
Rostock, Germany
Chapter 94

Hakan Oral, MD
Assistant Professor of Medicine
Cardiac Electrophysiology
University of Michigan,
Ann Arbor, Michigan
Chapter 62

Dean Ornish, MD
Founder and President
Preventive Medicine Research Institute
Clinical Professor of Medicine
University of California, San Francisco
San Francisco, California
Chapter 8

Catherine M. Otto, MD
Professor of Medicine
Director, Cardiology Fellowship Program
Acting Director, Division of Cardiology
University of Washington
Seattle, Washington
Chapter 5

Kenneth Ouriel, MD
Professor of Surgery
The Ohio State University
Chairman, Department of Vascular Surgery
The Cleveland Clinic Foundation
Cleveland, Ohio
Chapter 92

Nilesh U. Patel, MD
Attending Surgeon
Lenox Hill Hospital
New York, New York
Chapter 44

Bertram Pitt, MD
Professor of Medicine
University of Michigan Medical School
Ann Arbor, Michigan
Chapter 76

Thomas A. Ports, MD
Professor of Medicine
Interventional Cardiology
Cardiovascular Research Institute
University of California at San Francisco
    Medical Center
San Francisco, California
Chapter 54

Mark J. Post, MD
Angiogenesis Research Center
Section of Cardiology
Dartmouth Medical School and
    Dartmouth-Hitchcock Medical Center
Hanover, New Hampshire
Chapter 39

Silvia G. Priori, MD, PhD
Associate Professor of Cardiology
Director of Molecular Cardiology
Fondazione Salvatore Maugeri
Pavia, Italy
Chapter 61

Paolo Raggi, MD
Associate Professor,
Tulane University School of Medicine,
New Orleans, Louisiana
Chapter 36

Charanjit S. Rihal, MD
Division of Cardiovascular Diseases and Internal
    Medicine and the Section of Biostatistics, Mayo
    Clinic and Mayo Foundation,
Rochester, Minnesota
Chapter 50

James L. Ritchie, MD
Professor of Medicine
University of Washington
Seattle, Washington
Chapter 43

Robert Roberts, MD
Chief of Cardiology
Don W. Chapman Professor of Medicine
Professor of Cell Biology, Molecular Physiology &
    Biophysics
Baylor College of Medicine
Houston, Texas
Chapter 57

Sander J. Robins, MD
Department of Medicine
Boston University School of Medicine
Boston, Massachusetts
Chapter 7

Mark Roest, PhD
Investigator
Research Laboratory Clinical Chemistry
University Medical Center Utrecht
Utrecht, The Netherlands
Chapter 100

Raphael Rosenhek, MD
Department of Cardiology
University of Vienna
Vienna, Austria
Chapter 52

Allan M. Ross, MD
The Cardiovascular Research Institute
George Washington University School of Medicine,
Washington, DC
Chapter 28

Abraham Rothman, MD
Professor of Pediatrics
Chief of Pediatric Cardiology
University of California, San Diego
San Diego, California
Chapter 47

Hanna Bloomfield Rubins, MD, MPH
Director, Center for Chronic Disease
  Outcomes Research
Minneapolis VA Medical Center
Professor of Medicine
University of Minnesota
Minneapolis, Minnesota
Chapter 7

David J. Sahn, MD
Professor of Pediatrics
Director, Pediatric Cardiology,
Oregon Health Sciences University Hospital
Portland, Oregon
Chapter 48

Takayuki Saito, MD, PhD
Department of Cardiovascular Surgery
Nagoya City University Graduate School
  of Medical Sciences
Nagoya, Japan
Chapter 87

Leslie A. Saxon, MD
Associate Professor of Medicine
Director, EP Laboratory and Implantable
  Device Service
University of California, San Francisco,
  Medical Center
San Francisco, California
Chapter 78

Peter J. Schwartz, MD
Professor and Chairman
Department of Cardiology
Policlinico S. Matteo IRCCS and University of Pavia
Pavia, Italy
Chapter 61

John E. Scoble, MD
Clinical Director, Renal Services
Guy's and St Thomas' Trust
Guy's Hospital
London, England
Chapter 97

Frank W. Sellke, MD
Department of Surgery
Harvard Medical School and Beth Israel Deaconess
  Medical Center
Boston, Massachusetts
Chapter 39

Saul Shiffman, PhD
Professor of Psychology, Psychiatry and
    Pharmaceutical Science
University of Pittsburgh
Senior Scientific Advisor
Pinney Associates
Pittsburgh, Pennsylvania
Chapter 98

Donald S. Silverberg, MD
Associate Professor of Medicine
Department of Nephrology
Tel Aviv Medical Center
Ichilov Hospital
University Tel Aviv Medical School
Tel Aviv, Israel
Chapter 73

Michael Simons, MD
Section of Cardiology and Angiogenesis
    Research Center
Dartmouth Medical School and
    Dartmouth-Hitchcock Medical Center
Hanover, New Hampshire
Chapter 39

Peter Sleight, MD
Professor Emeritus of Cardiovascular Medicine
Hon. Consultant Physician
University of Oxford, John Radcliffe Hospital,
Oxford, United Kingdom
Chapter 37

Nicholas G. Smedira, MD
Co-Director, Cardiothoracic Residency Program
Attending Staff, Heart & Lung Transplant Surgeon
Department of Thoracic & Cardiovascular Surgery
The Cleveland Clinic Foundation
Cleveland, Ohio
Chapter 84

Thomas L. Spray, MD
Alice Langdon Warner Professor of Surgery
University of Pennsylvania
Chief, Division of Cardiothoracic Surgery
Children's Hospital of Philadelphia
Philadelphia, Pennsylvania
Chapter 99

Dennis L. Sprecher, MD
Section Head, Preventive Cardiology
    and Rehabilitation
The Cleveland Clinic Foundation
Cleveland, Ohio
Chapter 6

Eugenio Stabile, MD
Research Fellow, Vascular Biology Laboratory
Cardiovascular Research Institute
MedStar Research Institute
Washington Hospital Center
Washington, DC
Chapter 38

Richard S. Stack, MD
Professor of Medicine, Director of Interventional
    Cardiovascular Program,
Duke University Medical Center
Durham, North Carolina
Chapter 17

Jan A. Staessen, MD, PhD
Hypertension and Cardiovascular Rehabilitation
    Unit
Department of Molecular and Cardiovascular
    Research
University of Leuven
Leuven, Belgium
Chapter 15

William G. Stevenson, MD
Associate Professor of Medicine
Harvard Medical School
Director, Clinical Electrophysiology Program
Brigham and Women's Hospital
Boston, Massachusetts
Chapter 66

Allan D. Struthers, MD
Professor of Cardiovascular Medicine
  and Therapeutics
Ninewells Hospital and Medical School
Dundee, Scotland, United Kingdom
Chapter 3

Valavanur A. Subramanian, MD
Director, Department of Surgery
Lenox Hill Hospital
New York, New York
Chapter 44

James F. Symes, MD
Departments of Medicine and Surgery
St. Elizabeth's Medical Center and Tufts University
  School of Medicine
Boston, Massachusetts
Chapter 40

Matthew R.G. Taylor, MD
Director, Adult Clinical Genetics
University of Colorado Health Sciences Center
Attending Staff, University of Colorado Hospital
Denver, Colorado
Chapter 72

Paul S. Teirstein, MD
Director, Interventional Cardiology
Scripps Clinic
La Jolla, California
Chapter 41

Andrew M. Tonkin, MD
Director, Health, Medical, and Scientific Affairs
National Heart Foundation of Australia
Adjunct Professor, Department of Epidemiology
  and Preventive Medicine
Monash University
Victoria, Australia
Chapter 9

Zoltan G. Turi, MD
Professor of Medicine
Director, Invasive Cardiology
MCP Hahnemann University
Philadelphia, Pennsylvania
Chapter 51

E. Murat Tuzcu, MD
Professor of Medicine
Staff Cardiologist
Director of Intravascular Ultrasound
The Cleveland Clinic Foundation
Cleveland, Ohio
Chapter 45

James E. Udelson, MD
Associate Chief, Division of Cardiology
Director, Nuclear Cardiology
Co-Director, Heart Failure and Transplant Center
New England Medical Center
Associate Professor of Medicine
Tufts University School of Medicine
Boston, Massachusetts
Chapter 23

Yvonne T. van der Schouw, PhD
Julius Center for General Practice and Patient
  Oriented Research,
University Medical Center Utrecht,
Utrecht, The Netherlands
Chapter 100

Peter R. Vale, MD
Departments of Medicine and Surgery
St. Elizabeth's Medical Center and Tufts University
  School of Medicine
Boston, Massachusetts
Chapter 40

Nosratolaf D. Vaziri, MD
Professor of Medicine, Physiology and Biophysics
Chief, Division of Nephrology and Hypertension
University of California, Irvine
Irvine, California
Chapter 10

Gus J. Vlahakes, MD
Associate Professor of Surgery
Harvard Medical School
Visiting Surgeon
Massachusetts General Hospital
Boston, Massachusetts
Chapter 95

Jih Shiun Wang, MD
Division of Cardiovascular Surgery
Yang-Ming University/Veterans General Hospital
Taipei, Taiwan
Chapter 87

Gretchen Wells, MD, PhD
Assistant Professor of Internal Medicine
Internal Medicine-Cardiology
Wake Forest University School of Medicine
Winston-Salem, North Carolina
Chapter 75

Dov Wexler, MD
Department of Cardiology
Tel Aviv Medical Center
Tel Aviv, Israel
Chapter 73

Harvey White, ScD, MBBS
Clinical Professor and Director
Cardiovascular Research Unit
Green Lane Hospital
Auckland, New Zealand
Chapter 29

Peter W.F. Wilson, MD
Professor of Medicine
Director of Laboratories
Framingham Heart Study
Boston University School of Medicine
Boston, Massachusetts
Chapter 4

D. George Wyse, MD, PhD
Professor, Department of Medicine (Cardiology)
University of Calgary, Faculty of Medicine
Cardiac Electrophysiologist,
Calgary Regional Health Authority,
Calgary Alberta, Canada
Chapter 65

Alberto Zanchetti, MD
Professor of Medicine
Centre of Clinical Physiology and Hypertension
University of Milan, Maggiore Hospital
Milan, Italy
Chapter 16

Kenton J. Zehr, MD
Assistant Professor of Surgery, Mayo Medical
  School
Consultant, Division of Cardiovascular Surgery
Mayo Clinic
Rochester, Minnesota
Chapter 93

William A. Zoghbi, MD
Professor of Medicine
Director, Echocardiography Research
Baylor College of Medicine
Houston, Texas
Chapter 81

Preface

Disorders of the cardiovascular system are the most common causes of death and serious morbidity in the industrialized world. In 2001, more than 40% of all deaths in the United States were attributed to cardiac and vascular diseases. These conditions accounted for almost 5 millions years of potential life lost.

Despite these sobering statistics, progress in cardiovascular medicine has been immense, and is, in fact, accelerating. Our understanding of the pathobiology of most forms of heart disease has advanced steadily and there have been enormous advances in the diagnosis, treatment, and prevention of cardiovascular disorders. For example, during the decade from 1990 to 2000, the age-adjusted death rates from cardiovascular disease declined by one fifth and death rates from acute myocardial infarction and stroke declined by one-third. Similar progress has been made in other major cardiovascular disorders, including hypertension, valvular and congenital heart disease, congestive heart failure, and the arrhythmias. Given the breathtaking pace of the advances in cardiology, it is more important than ever for physicians responsible for the care of patients with cardiovascular disease to remain up-to-date.

Harrison's Online is an internet version of *Harrison's Principles of Internal Medicine,* with frequent updates so as to make it a living textbook. These updates include solicited reviews. The most interesting 100 of these in cardiology have been further updated and revised, and are presented in this volume.

Advances in Cardiology is divided into nine sections. An attempt has been made to include advances in the understanding of the pathobiology of disease, diagnosis, and therapy. Summaries of a number of key clinical trials are also included. Given the enormous breadth and depth of clinical cardiovascular research, it is not intended that this volume cover all or even most of the important advances in this field. This inability to be complete is one of the difficulties with print publishing. For additional information on advances in cardiology, the reader is referred to *www.harrisonsonline.com.* An additional advantage of on-line publication is that it can be updated on a weekly, and indeed if necessary, a daily, basis.

During the last few years, a large amount of medical information has been reformatted from print to electronic publication. *Advances in Cardiology* represents an early example of the opposite. It is designed for the reader who still wishes to "hold and hug" a book and prefers reading and studying a subject in print.

The editor thanks the authors for their efforts and cooperation. Martin Wonsiewicz, Publisher, and Barbara Holton, Editing Supervisor, McGraw-Hill, and Kathryn Saxon, my Editorial Associate, deserve appreciation for their substantial contribution to the production of this book.

Eugene Braunwald, M.D.
Boston, Massachusetts

HARRISON'S ADVANCES *in* CARDIOLOGY

CHAPTER

1

CHLAMYDIA PNEUMONIAE AND CORONARY ARTERY DISEASE

J. Ward Kennedy

Introduction

In recent years there has been increasing interest in the relationship between infection, inflammation, and the development of atherosclerosis. The first association of infection with the development of experimental atherosclerosis was reported in 1978 in germ-free chickens infected with an avian herpesvirus (Fabricant et al., 1978). Since then, many observations have been published on the association between coronary artery disease (CAD) and *Helicobacter pylori, Chlamydia pneumoniae,* and cytomegalovirus (CMV) infections.

The attention of many clinical cardiologists was drawn to the potential importance of inflammation in the development of CAD by the publication of a subset analysis of the U.S. Physicians' Health Study investigators. That randomized

controlled trial of aspirin and/or β-carotene vs. placebo for the primary prevention of new coronary events demonstrated that aspirin effectively reduced the number of new ischemic events, while β-carotene was shown to be ineffective (Steering Committee, 1989). Then, in 1997, these investigators reported that the benefits of aspirin were greatest in those subjects who had elevated baseline levels of C-reactive protein (Ridker et al., 1997). This suggested that aspirin may have exerted some or all of its beneficial effect through its anti-inflammatory, rather than its antiplatelet, activity.

The role of infection in the development of CAD was reviewed by Danesh and colleagues. They compiled the seropositivity data from 20 studies of *H. pylori,* 18 studies of *C. pneumoniae,* and 18 studies of CMV and evaluated the presence of antibody to these organisms and the presence of CAD (Danesh et al., 1947). They concluded that the evidence relating *C. pneumoniae* to CAD is much stronger than it is for the other two organisms.

Recently, investigators from the Cardiovascular Heath Study have reported the results of a nested case-control study of serologic evidence of prior infection with *C. pneumoniae,* herpes simplex virus type 1 (HSV-1), and CMV with the development of myocardial infection (MI) or death from CAD (Siscovick et al., 2000). They concluded that elderly patients with IgG antibodies to HSV-1 had a two-fold increase in the incidence of MI or death from CAD. Antibodies to CMV were not associated with an increased risk of MI or CAD death, while only high titers of IgG antibodies to *C. pneumoniae* (1:1034) were associated with MI and CAD death. Since these observations were limited to individuals $\geq$ 65 years of age, they may not apply to younger individuals.

Characteristics of *C. pneumoniae*

Grayston and colleagues isolated *C. pneumoniae* in 1965. In 1986 it was determined that *C. pneumoniae* was the cause of some upper respiratory infections, and in 1988 the organism was established as the third species of *Chlamydia* and named *pneumoniae.* Currently it is believed to be the cause of about 10% of community-acquired pneumonias and 5% of episodes of bronchitis and sinusitis in adults. *C. pneumoniae* infection is global in its distribution, and a majority of individuals will become infected sometime during their lifetime. Half of individuals will have been infected by age 20, and 80% of men and 70% of women are seropositive by age 70 years. The high prevalence of antibody in males over the age of 20 has not been explained, but some have suggested that this may be related to the higher prevalence of atherosclerosis in men. *C. pneumoniae* antibodies resolve in about 3 to 5 years following infection, although individuals who still harbor the organism may have no detectable antibody.

C. pneumoniae and Atherosclerosis

C. pneumoniae has a clear affinity for atherosclerotic plaques. The organism can frequently be identified in atherosclerotic lesions in the aorta and coronary and carotid arteries but can almost never be found in the normal portions of these vessels (Kuo et al., 1993). In a recent study of tissues from autopsies on 38 individuals, polymerase chain reaction and immunochemistry techniques identified *C. pneumoniae* protein in 47% of samples from the cardiovascular system, while it was present in only 5 to 13% of the samples of lungs, liver, spleen, and bone marrow (Jackson et al., 1997). Seropositivity for *C. pneumoniae* has clearly been associated with the presence of CAD (Danesh et al., 1997). It has also been reported that in patients with unstable CAD, elevated levels of C-reactive protein and *C. pneumoniae* antibody titers are both predictive of the development of recurrent unstable angina and acute MI (Biasucci et al., 1999).

Experimental data also support a role for *C. pneumoniae* in the development of atherosclerosis. In rabbits fed a cholesterol-enhanced diet, intranasal inoculation of *C. pneumoniae* greatly increased the development of intimal thickening of the aorta in the infected animals as compared to the controls. This effect was markedly reduced in rabbits that received injections of azithromycin (Muhlestein et al., 1998). The same group of investigators had earlier demonstrated that a high proportion of patients undergoing atherectomy of coronary lesions for the treatment of symptomatic CAD had *C. pneumoniae* bacterial protein identified in the plaque material removed during these procedures (Muhlestein et al., 1996).

Antibiotic Therapy and Coronary Artery Disease

Several small trials of antibiotic therapy directed toward *C. pneumoniae* in patients with CAD have now been reported, and several larger trials have been initiated or are about to begin enrollment.

Gupta and colleagues screened 220 patients with prior MI for *C. pneumoniae* antibodies. Those with high titers (> 1:64) were randomized to azithromycin or placebo therapy. After 18 months of follow-up, the incidence of cardiovascular events including cardiovascular death, unstable angina, or MI was much higher in untreated patients with high antibody titers as compared to those with negative or low titers (Gupta et al., 1997). Surprisingly, the patients with high baseline titers who received azithromycin therapy had a marked reduction in cardiovascular events when compared to the untreated patients with high baseline antibody titers, suggesting that antibiotic therapy had a major beneficial effect on their clinical course.

In another antibiotic trial, Gurfinkel and colleagues randomized 202 patients with unstable angina to 30 days of roxithromycin therapy or placebo. These investigators found a marked reduction in a composite end-point of recurrent angina, acute MI, or ischemic death at 31 days in those receiving antibiotic therapy as compared to the controls ($p = .036$) (Gurfinkel et al., 1997). These two positive trials of antibiotic therapy directed toward *C. pneumoniae* in patients with CAD have greatly spurred interest in the potential utility of antibiotic therapy in patients with or at risk of developing CAD. Several large randomized trials are now planned or are under way to examine this therapy further. WIZARD is an industry-sponsored randomized controlled trial that has enrolled 3500 patients with prior MI and positive antibodies to *C. pneumoniae* to 3 months of azithromycin therapy or placebo. Few side effects of the therapy were encountered during the initial phase of the trial, and the patients are now in long-term follow-up. Grayston and colleagues at the University of Washington, Seattle, have initiated ACES, an NIH- and industry-supported randomized controlled trial of azithromycin in 4000 patients with chronic CAD. The patients enrolled in this study are receiving 600 mg of azithromycin or placebo once a week for 1 year and are being followed for a mean of 3.5 years.

Muhlestein and colleagues have reported the results of the ACADEMIC trial (Muhlestein et al., 2000). In this study 302 patients with positive anti-bodies for *C. pneumoniae* were randomized to azithromycin, 500 mg per week for 3 months, and followed for 24 months. No benefit was seen during the first 6 months, but there was a trend for a reduction in cardiovascular events in treated patients vs. controls between 6 and 24 months.

The Azithromycin in Acute Coronary Syndromes (AZACS) is a 1400-patient trial carried out by investigators at Cedars Sinai Medical Center in Los Angeles. This trial includes patients with and without positive antibodies for *C. pneumoniae*. This is the largest antibiotic trial to date to be carried out in patients with acute coronary artery syndromes and is very near completion (Shaw, 2001). A unique trial that has just started enrolling patients is PROVE-IT. This will evaluate the outcome in 4000 patients of lipid-lowering therapy with pravastatin, 40 mg/d, vs. atorvastatin, 80 mg/d, with antibiotic therapy with gatifloxacin vs. placebo (Cannon CP et al., 2002).

Because of the results of these early antibiotic trials, other investigators have looked at the relationship of prior antibiotic therapy to the subsequent development of CAD. Meier and colleagues evaluated 3315 patients included in the U.K. General Practice Research Database with a diagnosis of acute MI and 13,139 patients without a history of acute MI. They demonstrated that patients with acute MI were significantly less likely to have received tetracycline or quinolone antibiotics in the 3 years prior to their infarction than those individuals who did not have an acute MI (Meier et al., 1999). This suggests that antibiotic therapy that is known to be effective against *C. pneumoniae* reduces the likelihood of the subsequent development of acute MI. It is equally interesting to note that commonly used antibiotics that are not effective against *C. pneumoniae*, including penicillin, sulfonamides, and the cephalosporins, had no relationship to the incidence of acute MI.

In addition to efforts to prevent MI and the development of CAD with antibiotic therapy directed toward *C. pneumoniae*, a trial of roxithromycin therapy to prevent restenosis following coronary artery stenting has been reported (Neumann et al., 2001). This double-blind trial randomized 1010 patients immediately following stenting to roxithromycin,

300 mg daily for 28 days, or placebo. Restenosis of $\geq 50\%$ was present at the 6-month follow-up angiograms in 31% of the antibiotic-treated patients and in 29% of the controls ($p = .43$). At 1 year, the rate of death and MI were slightly but insignificantly higher in the patients randomized to antibiotic therapy. There was, however, a significant benefit of antibiotic therapy in patients with high antibody titers in both a reduction in restenosis and the need for revascularization in the first year of follow-up. In patients with negative or low antibody titers, however, the placebo patients had less restenosis and required fewer revascularization procedures than those receiving antibiotic therapy.

SUMMARY

There is a growing body of evidence that infection with *C. pneumoniae* plays a role in the development and/or the progression of CAD. If this is true, it is likely that the presence of the bacteria in the atherosclerotic plaque increases the inflammatory response in that tissue and thereby increases the likelihood of plaque rupture and the subsequent development of unstable angina or acute MI. The findings of two small trials of antibiotic therapy in patients with known CAD suggest that antibiotic therapy against *C. pneumoniae* may reduce the incidence of new ischemic events. Despite these interesting results, there is not yet enough evidence to justify the use of antibiotic therapy in the management of patients with CAD. It is possible that the larger trials that are now just beginning will demonstrate that antibiotic therapy reduces the occurrence of new ischemic events. If this does occur, it will then be necessary to determine if this effect is specifically related to antibiotic effect on the *C. pneumoniae* organism, a generalized and nonspecific anti-inflammatory effect of the therapy; or an antibiotic effect against multiple organisms located in the mouth, gastrointestinal tract, and/or coronary arteries. Whatever the outcome of these trials, the results will be of great interest. As we await the outcome of these ongoing investigations, it is the author's practice to preferentially select antibiotics

that are effective against *C. pneumoniae* when they are also appropriate agents for treating intercurrent illnesses such as bronchitis and bacterial pneumonia in patients who are also at risk of developing or are known to have CAD.

REFERENCES

Biasucci AM et al: Elevated levels of C-reactive protein at discharge in patients with unstable angina predict recurrent instability. Circulation 99:855, 1999

Cannon CP et al: Design of the Pravastatin or Atovastatin Evaluation and Infection Therapy (PROVE IT)-TIMI 22 trial. Am J Cardiol 89:860, 2002

Danesh C et al: Chronic infections and coronary artery disease: Is there a link? Lancet 350:430, 1997

Fabricant CG et al: Virus-induced atherosclerosis. J Exp Med 148:335, 1978

Gupta S et al: Elevated *Chlamydia pneumoniae* antibodies, cardiovascular events, and azithromycin in male survivors of myocardial infarction. Circulation 96:404, 1997

Gurfinkel E et al: Randomized trial of roxithromycin in non-Q-wave coronary syndromes: ROXIS Pilot Study. Lancet 350:404, 1997

Jackson LA et al: Specificity of detection of *C. pneumoniae* in cardiovascular atheroma: Evaluation of the innocent bystander hypothesis. Am J Pathol 150:1785, 1997

Kuo CC et al: Demonstration of *Chlamydia pneumoniae* in atherosclerotic lesions of coronary arteries. J Infect Dis 167:841, 1993

Meier CR et al: Antibiotics and risk of subsequent first-time acute myocardial infarction. JAMA 281:427, 1999

Muhlestein JB et al: Increased incidence of *Chlamydia* species within the coronary arteries of patients with symptomatic atherosclerosis versus other forms of cardiovascular disease. J Am Coll Cardiol 27:1555, 1996

Muhlestein JB et al: Infection with *Chlamydia pneumoniae* accelerates the development of atherosclerosis and treatment with azithromycin prevents it in a rabbit model. Circulation 97:633, 1998

Muhlestein JB et al: Randomized secondary prevention trial of azithromycin in patients with coronary artery disease: Primary clinical results of the ACADEMIC study. Circulation 102:1755, 2000

Neumann F-J et al: Treatment of *C. pneumoniae* infection with roxithromycin and effect of neointima and proliferation after coronary stent placement (ISAR-3): A randomized, double blind, placebo controlled trial. Lancet 357: 2085, 2001

Ridker PM et al: Inflammation, aspirin, and the risk of cardiovascular disease in apparently healthy men. N Engl J Med 336:973, 1997

Shaw PK: Link between infection and atherosclerosis. Circulation 103:5, 2001

Siscovick et al: *Chlamydia pneumoniae,* herpes simplex virus type 1, and cytomegalovirus and incident myocardial infarction and coronary heart disease death in older adults. Circulation 102:2335, 2000

Steering Committee of the Physicians' Health Study Research Group: Final report of the aspirin component of the ongoing Physicians' Health Study. N Engl J Med 321:129, 1989

2

ANGIOTENSIN II, OXIDATIVE STRESS, AND ATHEROSCLEROSIS

Bradford C. Berk

Introduction

Many risk factors that promote atherosclerosis have been identified. These include hypertension, hyper-cholesterolemia, diabetes, decreased estrogen in postmenopausal women, increased homocysteine, and cigarette smoking. Recently, it has become clear that a mechanism common to these risk factors is oxidative stress. In this chapter, oxidative stress refers to increased generation of reactive oxygen species, which include H_2O_2, O_2^-, and OH^-. Another recent finding is that angiotensin II, which has been associated with atherosclerosis progression (Hayek et al., 1998; Keidar et al., 1997) and myocardial infarction (SOLVD Investigators, 1992), also increases reactive oxygen species (Fukui et al., 1995; Rajagopalan et al., 1996). Thus this chapter will present information that links oxidative stress induced by angiotensin II with atherosclerosis. Several of the cellular pathways by which angiotensin II mediates the clinical events associated with atherosclerosis, such as coagulation, inflammation, and plaque progression, will be discussed.

Evidence to support a role for reactive oxygen species in atherosclerosis received strong support initially from the finding that oxidized low-density lipoprotein (LDL) was more atherogenic than native LDL. It became clear that most of the oxidation occurred within the vessel wall rather than in the circulating blood, indicating that reactive oxygen species were being generated in the wall. Observations that suggest a chronic oxidative stress among cells in the vessel wall include the appearance in atherosclerotic plaque of protein and lipid modifications unique to reactive oxygen species such as nitrotyrosine and 4-hydroxynonenol (Leeuwenburgh et al., 1997). In fact, circulating byproducts of these oxidative events have been shown to correlate with risk factors. For example, isoprostanes formed by a nonenzymatic process of lipid peroxidation are increased in patients with ischemic heart disease and are transiently elevated by cigarette smoking (Patrono and FitzGerald, 1997). An important role for angiotensin II in promoting vessel wall oxidative stress was suggested by the following findings: (1) it stimulates reactive oxygen species production by human macrophages, endothelial cells, and vascular smooth-muscle cells; (2) it increases oxidative modification of LDL (Scheidegger et al., 1997); and (3) it induces expression of cytokines (tumor necrosis factor, interleukins, and platelet-derived growth factor) that stimulate production of reactive oxygen species. In fact, angiotensin II is currently the most potent stimulus identified for generation of reactive oxygen species by vascular smooth-muscle cells. Thus, multiple biochemical and epidemiologic data suggest that increased reactive oxygen species generation, mediated in part by angiotensin II, contributes to the pathogenesis of atherosclerosis.

Angiotensin II has been shown to play a critical role in the pathogenesis of hypertension, inflammation, atherosclerosis, and congestive heart failure (Table 2–1). Several studies suggest that increased activity of the renin-angiotensin system contributes to these diseases. One early study showed that patients with inappropriately elevated levels of renin (relative to sodium excretion) were at significantly greater risk for myocardial infarction (Alderman et al., 1991). Polymorphisms of the angiotensin-converting enzyme (ACE) gene have been correlated with increased circulating levels of ACE, higher angiotensin II, and in some populations increased myocardial infarction. Conversely, inhibiting the renin-angiotensin system with ACE inhibitors appears to decrease the risk of myocardial infarction in patients with congestive heart failure, as shown in the SAVE and SOLVD trials. Previous animal studies have shown that (1) angiotensin II increases atherosclerosis in hypercholesterolemia, and (2) inhibitors of the renin-angiotensin system (both ACE inhibitors and AT1R blockers) decrease atheroscle-

rosis (Hayek et al., 1998; Keidar et al., 1997). Long-term trials of ACE inhibitors to limit atherosclerosis and cardiovascular events have yielded positive results. Both the SAVE and HOPE trials showed decreased myocardial infarction and need for coronary artery interventions. These results provide strong evidence of the role of angiotensin II in atherosclerosis.

Angiotensin II–Mediated Events: Specificity Determined by Receptor Type, Tissue, and Second Messengers

Angiotensin II is the primary mediator of the renin-angiotensin system and regulates physiologic responses, including salt and water balance, blood pressure, and vascular tone. These effects are mediated by stimulation of salt and water transport in the kidney, stimulation of adrenal aldosterone release, increased central nervous system sympathetic output, and direct effects on vascular smooth-muscle cell contractility. A key question is how can angiotensin II elicit so many diverse effects. Three explanations are supported by the literature: (1) different receptor types, (2) tissue-specific events, and (3) second messengers. Angiotensin II can bind to

TABLE 2-1

ANGIOTENSIN II, OXIDATIVE STRESS, AND ATHEROSCLEROSIS

Proatherogenic effect	Mechanism
Vascular smooth-muscle cell growth	Intracellular reactive oxygen species and p38
Generation of superoxide	Increased expression of NAD(P)H oxidase
Activation of adhesion molecules	NF-κB induction by reactive oxygen species
Monocyte/macrophage activation	Direct effect on macrophages
Abdominal aortic aneursysms	Inflammation and matrix metalloprotease activity
Oxidation of LDL	Stimulates 12-lipoxygenase in macrophages
Procoagulant	Stimulates platelet aggregation (decreased NO); stimulates PAI-1

ABBREVIATIONS: NF-κB, nuclear factor-κB; LDL, low-density lipoprotein; NO, nitric oxide; PAI-1, plasminogen activator inhibitor 1.

high-affinity receptors of at least three types, termed *AT1R, AT2R,* and *AT4R,* which are highly regulated in a developmental, tissue-specific, and disease-specific context. The AT1R is the dominant receptor expressed in the adult and appears to mediate most of the actions of angiotensin II. However, the AT2R has been shown to mediate *apoptosis* (programmed cell death) induced by angiotensin II in endothelial cells and, in animal models, to promote vascular smooth-muscle cell apoptosis after arterial injury. In addition, AT4R, expressed primarily in endothelial cells, may be very important in expression of procoagulant molecules such as plasminogen activator inhibitor (PAI) 1. Because the AT1R is the dominant receptor in adults, this discussion will focus on the AT1R. The relative expression of these receptors among different tissues may be important in the biologic effects of angiotensin II. For example, vascular smooth-muscle cells express high levels of AT1R, and during chronic treatment with AT1R blockers there is a decrease in AT1R expression due to the high circulating angiotensin II levels. As a consequence, when a patient discontinues treatment with an AT1R blocker there is no rebound increase in blood pressure, despite high circulating levels of angiotensin II, because of low AT1R expression.

Direct Effects of Angiotensin II on Vascular Smooth-Muscle Cells

Angiotensin II stimulates many responses in vascular smooth-muscle cells that are proatherogenic. These include (1) direct increases in vascular smooth-muscle cell growth (Berk et al., 1989; Geisterfer et al., 1988) and autocrine growth factors; (2) expression of enzymes that produce mediators of inflammation such as phospholipase A_2 and the reduced form of nicotinamide adenine dinucleotide (NAD(P)H) oxidase (Griendling et al., 1994; Schlondorff et al., 1987); (3) stimulation of inflammatory gene expression such as the signal transducers and activators of transcription (STAT) pathway (Marrero et al., 1995); and (4) induction of gene transcription for proto-oncogenes such as c-*fos* (Taubman et al., 1989). As discussed below, a com-

mon theme for these proatherogenic effects is generation of reactive oxygen species.

Reactive Oxygen Species as Mediators of Angiotensin II Signal Events

Reactive oxygen species are generated by a variety of extracellular and intracellular mechanisms. While extracellular generation of reactive oxygen species by tissue macrophages in the atherosclerotic plaque may be important for oxidation of LDL, generation of reactive oxygen species by angiotensin II in vascular smooth-muscle cells is primarily intracellular. In vascular smooth-muscle cells, the predominant source of agonist-stimulated 0_2^- formation is a plasma membrane NAD(P)H oxidase (Griendling et al., 1994), which accounts for > 90% of 0_2^- formation in vessels (Mohazzab et al., 1994). Several features of the vascular smooth-muscle cell NAD(P)H oxidase differentiate it from the neutrophil oxidase: The two most important are that the vascular smooth-muscle cell oxidase is highly regulated and that its production of superoxide is continuous. Angiotensin II is a powerful inducer of the oxidase and may increase superoxide production in vascular smooth-muscle cells by 800%. Recent molecular cloning has shown that the unique vascular isoform is a protein called *Nox1* (for non-neutrophil oxidase), which is a member of a multigene family (Suh et al., 1999). This enzyme is required for the growth-promoting effects of angiotensin II in vascular smooth-muscle cells.

It has become clear that intracellular reactive oxygen species generated in response to hormonal stimuli may act as second messengers (Griendling et al., 2000). Three lines of evidence support this concept:

1. Stimulation of vascular smooth-muscle cells with platelet-derived growth factor or angiotensin II increases production of reactive oxygen species (Griendling et al., 1994; Sundaresan et al., 1995).
2. Most of the 0_2^- generated in vascular smooth-muscle cells appears to be produced intracellularly (Griendling et al., 1994).

3. Inhibiting O_2^- production with antioxidants blocks signal transduction by platelet-derived growth factor (Sundaresan et al., 1995).

Signal pathways that are redox sensitive and hence regulated by reactive oxygen species may be defined by specific activation of upstream mediators, which include phospholipases, small G proteins, and tyrosine kinases (Abe and Berk, 1998). Final effectors include serine/threonine kinases such as the mitogen-activated protein (MAP) kinases, which activate specific transcription factors. Inflammatory cytokines and growth factors activate many of these second messengers, suggesting important similarities between reactive oxygen species and inflammation. Specific mediators for redox-sensitive angiotensin II activation of vascular smooth-muscle cells include epidermal growth factor receptor transactivation, p38 MAP kinase, and Akt—another serine/threonine kinase (Ushio-Fukai et al., 1999a; Ushio-Fukai et al., 1999b). As a consequence of increased production of superoxide and hydrogen peroxide, a new pattern of gene expression occurs. In an experiment in which Nox1 was overexpressed to increase intracellular oxidative stress selectively, more than 200 genes were upregulated including genes predominantly related to cell cycle, growth, and cancer (Arnold et al., 2001). These results suggest the importance of angiotensin II–mediated reactive oxygen species in cell growth.

Endothelial Cell Dysfunction is a Consequence of Angiotensin II–Mediated Reactive Oxygen Species Generation

A pathogenic mechanism that links angiotensin II, oxidative stress, and atherosclerosis is endothelial dysfunction. Endothelial dysfunction is measured experimentally by the physiologic increase in vessel diameter that occurs in response to blood flow (e.g., after ischemia) or hormonal stimulation (e.g., bradykinin or acetylcholine). These endothelium-dependent vasodilators work by stimulating endothelial cell production of nitric oxide (NO). Because NO is itself a reactive oxygen species, it can undergo a chemical reaction with O_2^- to generate peroxynitrite

($ONOO^-$). This molecule no longer has the vasodilating properties of NO. As a result, NO produced in the presence of reactive oxygen species exhibits less biologic effect. Endothelial dysfunction is a surrogate for atherosclerosis because it is associated with cardiovascular risk factors and because NO exerts multiple effects that are antiatherogenic. Specifically, NO decreases platelet aggregation, inhibits endothelial cell expression of receptors for monocytes, inhibits vascular smooth-muscle cell proliferation, and inhibits LDL uptake (Harrison, 1997a).

Several studies suggest that excessive angiotensin II is associated with endothelial cell dysfunction by virtue of increased reactive oxygen species. The TREND study evaluated the ability of the ACE inhibitor quinapril to alter endothelial cell dysfunction associated with atherosclerosis (Mancini et al., 1996). Patients with angiographically proven coronary artery disease treated with quinapril for 6 months showed significant improvement in endothelial cell vasodilation. This study suggests that decreasing angiotensin II formation may prevent the endothelial cell dysfunction observed in atherosclerosis. Because ACE inhibitors also increase bradykinin formation, it is possible that increased bradykinin resulted in increase NO production. However, it appears more likely that the effect of quinapril was primarily mediated by decreased angiotensin II since AT1R blockers (which have no effect on bradykinin) also improve angiotensin II–induced endothelial cell dysfunction and limit diet-induced atherosclerosis.

The strongest data that link angiotensin II, oxidative stress, and endothelial cell dysfunction are animal studies of angiotensin II–induced hypertension. In a series of studies from the laboratories of Griendling and Harrison, rats were made hypertensive to ~200 mmHg by infusion of either angiotensin II or norepinephrine (Harrison, 1997b; Laursen et al., 1997; Rajagopalan et al., 1996). Endothelial cell dysfunction was observed only with angiotensin II; endothelial cell dysfunction and hypertension correlated with increased superoxide production by rat arteries. The mechanism was shown to be related to increased production of reactive oxygen species by several approaches. First, there was an excellent temporal correlation between the rise in blood pressure and increased superoxide formation by vessels. Second, the increase in superoxide formation was correlated with increased activity of NAD(P)H oxidase and increased expression of p22phox, a component of the NAD(P)H oxidase. Finally, blood pressure and endothelial cell dysfunction were normalized by infusion of an antioxidant enzyme or the AT1R blocker, losartan. Recent clinical trials in patients with hypertension support this mechanism (Schiffrin et al., 2000). In a study by Schiffrin and colleagues, 19 untreated patients with mild essential hypertension were randomly assigned to losartan or atenolol treatment for 1 year. While both treatments reduced blood pressure to a comparable degree, after 1 year the ratio of the width of the media to the diameter of the lumen of arteries from losartan-treated patients was significantly reduced, whereas atenolol-treated patients exhibited no significant change. Endothelium-dependent relaxation (acetylcholine-induced) was normalized by losartan but not by atenolol. Endothelium-independent relaxation (by sodium nitroprusside) was unchanged after treatment. These studies suggest that human essential hypertension is associated with oxidative stress and endothelial cell dysfunction mediated by the AT1R.

Other Proatherogenic Effects of Angiotensin II Associated with Oxidative Stress

In addition to effects on reactive oxygen species, angiotensin II exerts proinflammatory and procoagulant effects on platelets, monocytes, endothelial cells, and vascular smooth-muscle cells. For example, angiotensin II promotes platelet aggregation by both decreasing an anticoagulant (nitric oxide) and by increasing a procoagulant (PAI-1). Similarly, angiotensin II promotes endothelial cell apoptosis and adhesion of monocytes to endothelial cells. Importantly, induction of vascular cell adhesion molecule 1 is mediated by reactive oxygen species (Marui et al., 1993), further demonstrating the role of reactive oxygen species in angiotensin II–mediated proatherogenic events. Angiotensin II also

stimulates the expression and activity of matrix metalloproteases, which may alter vascular structure. A potentially novel role for angiotensin II is to promote abdominal aortic aneurysm (AAA) formation. Recently, Daugherty and co-workers provided exciting insights into potential relationships between angiotensin II, atherosclerosis, and AAA formation (Daugherty et al., 2000). These authors studied the effects of Ang II in $apoE^{-/-}$ mice, which have increased total cholesterol and very low density lipoprotein and LDL levels and develop spontaneous atherosclerosis even when fed a low fat/low cholesterol diet (Plump et al., 1992). Angiotensin II infusion dramatically promoted vascular pathology, including an increase in the extent of atherosclerosis, a change in the nature of lesions and surrounding adventitial tissue, and formation of large AAAs. This is of potential clinical relevance since the HOPE trial showed a 16% decrease in appearance of AAAs in patients on the ACE inhibitor ramipril.

SUMMARY

Angiotensin II is a multifaceted hormone. Recent data suggest an important role for angiotensin II in atherosclerosis, essential hypertension, and AAA formation. These effects are mediated, in part, by generation of oxidative stress via angiotensin II induction of NADH oxidase (specifically, Nox1). The increase in reactive oxygen species results in endothelial cell dysfunction and loss of the atheroprotective effects of NO derived from endothelial cells. In addition, there are proatherogenic effects of angiotensin II on vessel cells related to induction of procoagulant and proinflammatory mediators. The increase in angiotensin II–dependent oxidative stress is a new finding that correlates with many of these proatherogenic effects.

REFERENCES

Abe J. Berk BC: Reactive oxygen species as mediators of signal transduction in cardiovascular disease. Trends Cardiovasc Med 8:59, 1998

Alderman MH et al: Association of the renin sodium profile with the risk of myocardial infarction in patients with hypertension. N Engl J Med 324:1098, 1991

Arnold RS et al: Hydrogen peroxide mediates the cell growth and transformation caused by the mitogenic oxidase Nox1. Proc Natl Acad Sci USA 98:5550, 2001

Berk BC et al: Angiotensin II-stimulated protein synthesis in cultured vascular smooth muscle cells. Hypertension 13:305, 1989

Daugherty A et al: Angiotensin II promotes atherosclerotic lesions and aneurysms in apolipoprotein E-deficient mice. J clin Invest 105:1605, 2000

Fukui T et al: NADPH oxidase activity and cytochrome b558 α-subunit mRNA expression are increased in aortas from hypertensive rats. Circulation 92:I-231, 1995

Geisterfer AAT et al: Angiotensin II induces hypertrophy, not hyperplasia, of cultured rat aortic smooth muscle cells. Circ Res 62:749, 1988

Griendling KK et al: Angiotensin II stimulates NADH and NADPH oxidase activation in cultured vascular smooth muscle cells. Circ Res 74:1141, 1994

Griendling KK et al: Modulation of protein kinase activity and gene expression by reactive oxygen species and their role in vascular physiology and pathophysiology. Arterioscler Thromb Vasc Biol 20:2175, 2000

Harrison DG: Cellular and molecular mechanisms of endothelial cell dysfunction. J Clin Invest 100:2153, 1997a

Harrison DG: Endothelial function and oxidant stress. Clin Cardiol 20:II-11, 1997b

Hayek T et al: Antiatherosclerotic and antioxidative effects of captopril in apolipoprotein E-deficient mice. J Cardiovasc Pharmacol 31:540, 1998

Keidar S et al: The angiotensin-II receptor antagonist, losartan, inhibits LDL lipid peroxidation and atherosclerosis in apolipoprotein E-deficient mice. Biochem Biophys Res Commun 236:622, 1997

Laursen JB et al: Role of superoxide in angiotensin II-induced but not catecholamine-induced hypertension. Circulation 95:588, 1997

Leeuwenburgh C et al: Mass spectrometric quantification of markers for protein oxidation by tyrosyl radical, copper, and hydroxyl radical in low density lipoprotein isolated from human atherosclerotic plaques. J Biol Chem 272:3520, 1997

Mancini GB et al: Angiotensin-converting enzyme inhibition with quinapril improves endothelial vasomotor dysfunction in patients with coronary artery disease. The TREND (Trial on Reversing ENdothelial Dysfunction) Study. Circulation 94:258, 1996

Marrero MB et al: Direct stimulation of Jak/STAT pathway by the angiotensin II AT1 receptor. Nature 375:247, 1995

Marui N et al: Vascular cell adhesion molecule-1 (VCAM-1) gene transcription and expression are regulated through an antioxidant-sensitive mechanism in human vascular endothelial cells. J Clin Invest 92:1866, 1993

Mohazzab KM et al: NADH oxidoreductase is a major source of superoxide anion in bovine coronary artery endothelium. Am J Physiol 266:H2568, 1994

Patrono C, FitzGerald GA: Isoprostanes: Potential markers of oxidant stress in atherothrombotic disease. Arterioscler Thromb Vasc Biol 17:2309, 1997

Plump AS et al: Severe hypercholesterolemia and atherosclerosis in apolipoprotein E-deficient mice created by homologous recombination in ES cells. Cell 71:343, 1992

Rajagopalan S et al: Angiotensin II-mediated hypertension in the rat increases vascular superoxide production via membrane NADH/NADPH oxidase activation. Contribution to alterations of vasomotor tone. J Clin Invest 97:1916, 1996

Scheidegger KJ et al: Angiotensin II increases macrophage-mediated modification of low density lipoprotein via a lipoxygenase-dependent pathway. J Biol Chem 272:21609, 1997

Schiffrin EL et al: Correction of arterial structure and endothelial dysfunction in human essential hypertension by the angiotensin receptor antagonist losartan. Circulation 101:1653, 2000

Schlondorff D et al: Angiotensin II stimulates phospholipases C and A_2 in cultured rat mesangial cells. Am J Physiol (Cell Physiol) 253:C113, 1987

SOLVD Investigators: Effect of enalapril on mortality and the development of heart failure in asymptomatic patients with reduced left ventricular ejection fractions. N Engl J Med 327:685, 1992

Suh YA et al: Cell transformation by the superoxide-generating oxidase Mox1. Nature 401:79, 1999

Sundaresan M et al: Requirement for generation of H_2O_2 for platelet-derived growth factor signal transduction. Science 270:296, 1995

Taubman MB et al: Angiotensin II induces c-*fos* mRNA in aortic smooth muscle. Role of Ca^{2+} mobilization and protein kinase C activation. J Biol Chem 264:526, 1989

Ushio-Fukai M et al: Reactive oxygen species mediate the activation of Akt/protein kinase B by angiotensin II in vascular smooth muscle cells. J Biol Chem 274:22699, 1999a

Ushio-Fukai M et al: Role of reactive oxygen species in angiotensin II-induced transactivation of epidermal growth factor receptor in vascular smooth muscle cells. Circulation 100:I-263, 1999b

3

EFFECT OF ALDOSTERONE ON THE VASCULAR BED: INTRODUCING THE ALDOSTERONE-INDUCED VASCULOPATHY

Allan D. Struthers

Introduction

The traditional view is that angiotensin II is the principal culprit in the renin-angiotensin-aldosterone system. However, it is now appreciated that aldosterone is a second culprit and that the harmful effects of aldosterone are additional to the harmful effects of angiotensin II. In fact there is more escape of aldosterone than there is of angiotensin II in heart failure patients taking chronic angiotensin-converting enzyme (ACE) inhibitor therapy. This is because ACE inhibitors increase plasma potassium, and potassium is a strong secretagogue for aldosterone. The important clinical point is that there is plenty of residual aldosterone around for this to be a potential problem, even in the presence of an ACE inhibitor.

Indeed the RALES trial showed clearly that despite ACE inhibitor therapy, aldosterone amplifies cardiac death in patients with congestive heart failure. This leads to the question: What are the mecha-

nisms whereby aldosterone amplifies cardiac death? Three key processes are now thought to contribute:

1. A specific aldosterone vasculopathy
2. Aldosterone-induced myocardial fibrosis
3. Aldosterone-induced sympathovagal imbalance

Each of these will be discussed in turn, although it is possible that the latter two are in part manifestations of the aldosterone-induced vasculopathy.

Aldosterone Vasculopathy

The first important finding is that aldosterone is now known to be synthesized by human vascular cells (Takeda et al., 1996). Furthermore, aldosterone is now recognized to produce a number of different adverse effects on the vasculature. The most important one is that aldosterone reduces and spironolactone increases endothelial nitric oxide (NO) bioactivity

(Ikeda et al., 1995; Farquharson and Struthers, 2000). What is particularly striking about this effect is that aldosterone blockade increases endothelial NO activity by the large margin of 94% (Farquharson and Struthers, 2000), which is much greater than any other therapy (Figure 3-1); For example, ACE inhibitors and statins usually reduce endothelial dysfunction by only 25 to 35%. Reducing endothelial dysfunction is important because it is very likely to be associated with a reduced future incidence of cardiovascular events. This idea is based on two observations. First, four studies show clearly that endothelial dysfunction at baseline is indeed associated with future cardiovascular events. Second, there are three treatments (statins, ACE inhibitors in the HOPE trial, and spironolactone in the RALES trial) that in parallel improve brachial artery endothelial function and reduce cardiovascular events and mortality in large trials. (The data for the effects of Vitamin E on endothelial dysfunction and on cardiovascular events are equally mixed for both end-points, which could be said to make Vitamin E a fourth therapy where treatment-induced changes in endothelial dysfunction correspond with treatment-induced changes in cardiovascular events.)

How, therefore, does aldosterone produce endothelial dysfunction? One distinct possibility is that aldosterone might be causing an increase in superoxide radicals, which degrade endogenous NO. This possibility arises because angiotensin II is well known to generate superoxide anions, and angiotensin II–induced generation of oxygen free radicals is a key process in angiotensin II–induced endothelial dysfunction: the importance of this mechanism was proven by the fact that Vitamin C virtually negates angiotensin II–induced endothelial dysfunction. The relevance of this is that one of the lessons of the past 10 years is that aldosterone now appears to have virtually the same biologic effects as angiotensin II. Furthermore, since angiotensin II and aldosterone both cause reduced NO bioactivity, it would be surprising if their mechanisms producing such an effect were to be different. Therefore, there is a strong possibility that aldosterone-induced impairment of vascular NO arises because aldosterone induces oxidative stress in the endothelium. If so, the implications would be enormous,

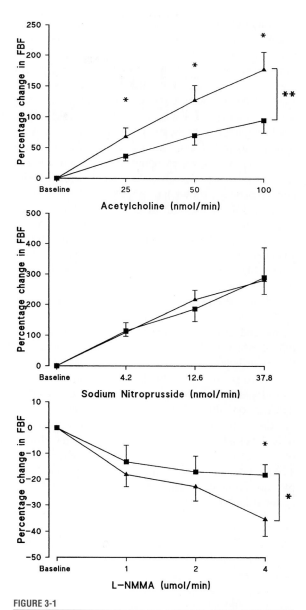

FIGURE 3-1

Forearm blood flow responses to 3 doses of acetylcholine, sodium nitroprusside and L-NMMA after placebo (■) or spironolactone (▲) therapy for one month

since oxidative stress is now regarded as a universal mechanism contributing to tissue injury in many different diseases and in many different organs.

Although aldosterone does appear to have definite effects on vascular NO, it remains distinctly possible that aldosterone-induced impairment of endothelial function is also due to other non-NO mechanisms. In this regard, it may be particularly relevant that spironolactone increases total-body Potassium and Magnesium. The relevance of this is threefold: (1) it has been suggested that K^+ is an endothelial-derived hyperpolarising factor in its own right causing endothelial-dependent vasodilatation; (2) oral magnesium therapy per se improves endothelial function in anginal patients, although it is not known whether this is by an NO or non-NO mechanism; and (3) it has been shown in hypertension that ouabain as a Na/K inhibitor specifically inhibits bradykinin-induced vasodilatation, whereas L-N-Monomethyl arginine (L-NMMA) does not, which again supports the idea that K^+ could in itself be an endothelial-derived vasodilator contributing to endothelial function or dysfunction. Thus the possibility arises that aldosterone reduces the "independent" endothelial vasodilator effect of Potassium (or Magnesium) and that this contributes to aldosterone-induced vasculopathy.

There is even more to aldosterone producing its vasculopathy than aldosterone-induced endothelial dysfunction, although admittedly the latter is probably the main influence; aldosterone also appears to reduce vessel compliance by reducing distensibility of the vascular smooth-muscle layer (Duprez et al., 1998). It is unknown whether this is a primary effect of aldosterone or whether it is secondary to reduced endothelial NO activity.

In addition to aldosterone-induced vasculopathy, aldosterone has potentially harmful effects within the blood vessel lumen, where it promotes blood clotting by inhibiting fibrinolysis. It does this by increasing plasminogen activator inhibitor 1 (Brown et al., 2000).

Therefore, aldosterone has harmful effects on all three layers of the blood vessel, i.e., the lumen, the endothelium, and the smooth muscle (Figure. 3-2). Clearly, the combination of these three harmful vascular effects of aldosterone would be expected to lead to microthrombi and tissue infarction and injury, and this has been demonstrated (Rocha et al., 1998, Rocha & Stier 2001). Indeed, in the animal models of spontaneously hypertensive rats, spironolactone reduced tissue injury (brain, kidney) by 60 to 70% at a dose of spironolactone that did not alter the blood pressure (Rocha et al., 1998). Similarly in the LNAME model of rat hypertension, aldosterone blockade and adrenalectomy both totally blocked myocardial necrosis at doses that did not alter the blood pressure at all. Therefore in both of these animal models, endogenous aldosterone is mediating severe tissue infarction/injury that is very likely to be caused at least in part by aldosterone-induced vasculopathy.

Another completely separate vascular effect of aldosterone has come to light. It appears that aldosterone can activate vascular angiotensin responses. Aldosterone can enhance the binding of angiotensin II to its receptors and amplify angiotensin II responses. Aldosterone significantly increases the

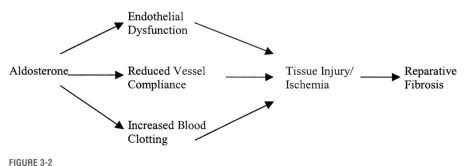

FIGURE 3-2

Aldosterone vasculopathy

binding density of both ACE and angiotensin II receptors in animal experiments. In tissue culture, aldosterone increases ACE mRNA 23-fold (Harada et al., 2001). In order to explore this phenomenon in humans, Farquharson and Struthers (2000) showed that spironolactone reduced vascular tissue ACE activity, since spironolactone reduced the vascular response to exogenous angiotensin I but had no effect on the response to angiotensin II. In this experimental model, infused angiotensin I does not have any vascular effects until it is converted into angiotensin II, which is why the differential infusion of angiotensin I and II can be used to assess vascular ACE activity. This raises a new possibility that aldosterone may exert a positive feedback loop on vascular ACE (Figure 3-3). In that sense, aldosterone blockade may exert "extra ACE inhibition" over and above traditional ACE inhibitor therapy.

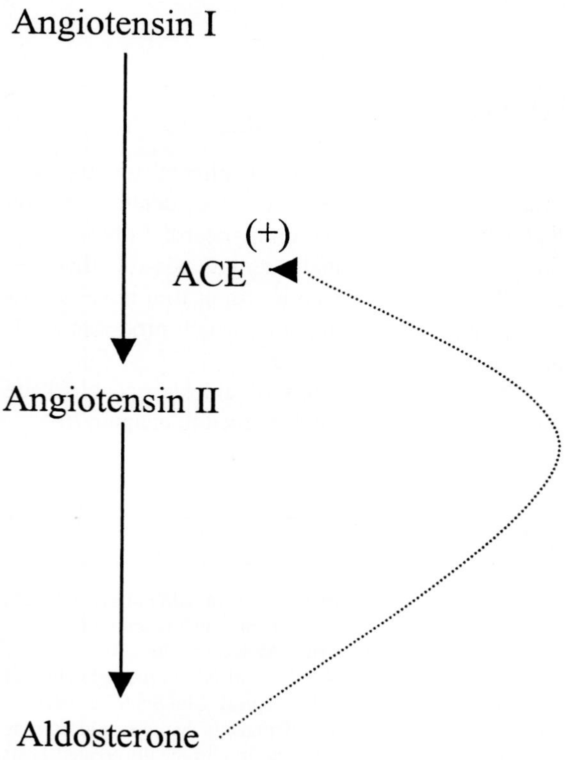

Aldosterone-Induced Myocardial Fibrosis

A wealth of data from Weber and colleagues has accumulated over the past 10 years to show that aldosterone also promotes myocardial fibrosis (Weber and Brilla, 1991). This was first shown in experimental animals and has been confirmed in humans, using plasma collagen markers such as procollagen type III aminoterminal peptide (MacFadyen et al., 1997). However, we do not know at this stage whether aldosterone promotes myocardial fibrosis as a primary effect or whether aldosterone vasculopathy together with aldosterone-induced increase in blood clotting leads to tissue microinfarcts, which are then repaired by fibrosis. In truth, it is likely to be a combination of both processes.

Aldosterone-Induced Sympathovagal Imbalance

Spironolactone has been shown to have important autonomic effects; for example, spironolactone reduces cardiac adrenergic activity but, perhaps more importantly, increases parasympathetic activity (MacFadyen et al., 1997). The importance of a parasympathomimetic effect can be illustrated by animal studies of coronary artery ligation, where coincidental vagal stimulation dramatically improved survival and reduced the incidence of reperfusion arrhythmias. Such an effect of aldosterone blockade boosting parasympathetic activity is particularly prominent in the 6 A.M. to 10 A.M. period of the day when endogenous aldosterone is high (Yee et al., 2001). Indeed, the early morning surge of aldosterone may produce an autonomic imbalance acutely, which promotes the well-known early morning peak in cardiac deaths.

Angiotensin I

ACE (+)

Angiotensin II

Aldosterone

FIGURE 3-3

Feedback Amplification of Aldosterone on ACE activity

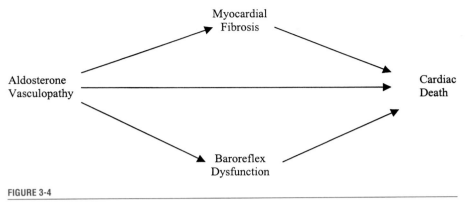

FIGURE 3-4

Hypothesis linking aldosterone vasculopathy with cardiac death

The link between aldosterone and the autonomic nervous system can be demonstrated in yet another way. Baroreflex sensitivity is a further way of assessing autonomic balance (or imbalance). Animal and human studies have clearly shown that aldosterone per se inhibits baroreflex activity. The importance of a blunted baroreflex activity has been clearly demonstrated by numerous studies showing that baroreflex insensitivity is an independent predictor of mortality, as is poor heart rate variability, which are two standard techniques for assessing autonomic balance. Thus the fact that aldosterone has adverse effects on autonomic balance could well be pivotal in the role of aldosterone in promoting cardiac death.

However, there is a whole new twist to this concept. Recently it has become apparent that NO is a key regulator of autonomic function in humans (Chowdhary and Townend, 1999). Thus the probability arises that vascular NO is a key determinant of autonomic balance, and thus therapies that increase vascular NO will produce the knock-on effect of also improving autonomic imbalance (Spiker et al., 2000).

Arising from this is the idea that the key culprit mechanism with regard to aldosterone may well be its ability to produce a vasculopathy characterized by NO deficit, and that aldosterone-induced fibrosis and aldosterone-induced autonomic imbalance could be a consequence of aldosterone vasculopathy (Figure 3-4).

SUMMARY

Aldosterone exerts harmful effects on the key processes that promote cardiac death, i.e., on endothelial dysfunction, on myocardial fibrosis, and on sympathovagal imbalance. It is possible that they are all attributable to some extent to a novel aldosterone-induced vasculopathy, which produces a relative deficit of vascular NO.

The beneficial effects of aldosterone blockade with spironolactone are described in chapter 76.

REFERENCES

Brown NJ et al: Synergistic effect of adrenal steroids and angiotensin II on plasminogen activator inhibitor-1 production. J Clin Endocrinol Metab 85:336, 2000

Chowdhary S, Townend JN: Role of NO in the regulation of cardiovascular autonomic control. Clin Sci 97:5, 1999

Duprez DA et al: Inverse relationship between aldosterone and large artery compliance in chronically treated heart failure patients. Eur Heart J 19:1371, 1998

Farquharson C, Struthers AD: Spironolactone increases NO bioactivity, improves endothelial dysfunction and suppresses vascular AI/AII conversion in chronic heart failure. Circulation 101:594, 2000

Harada E et al: Aldosterone induces ACE gene expression in cultured neonatal rat cardiocytes. Circulation 104:137, 2001

Ideka U et al: Aldosterone inhibits nitric oxide synthesis in rat vascular smooth muscle cells induced by interleukin-1 β. Eur J Pharmacol 290:69, 1995

MacFadyen RJ et al: Aldosterone blockade reduces vascular collagen turnover, improves heart rate variability and reduces early morning rise in heart rate in heart failure patients. Cardiovasc Res 35:30, 1997

Rocha R et al: Mineralocorticoid blockade reduces vascular injury in stroke prone hypertensive rats. Hypertension 31 [part 2]:451, 1998

Rocha R, Stier CT, Pathophysiological effects of aldosterone in cardiovascular tissue. Trends in Endocrinology of Metabolism 12:308,2001

Spiker LE et al: Baroreceptor dysfunction induced by NO synthase inhibition in humans. J Am Coll Cardiol 36:213, 2000

Takeda Y et al: Regulation of aldosterone synthase in human vascular cells by AII and ACTH. J Clin Endocrinol Metab 81:2797, 1996

Weber K, Brilla CG: Pathological hypertrophy and cardiac interstitium: Fibrosis and renin angiotensin aldosterone system. Circulation 83:1849, 1991

Yee KM et al: Circadian influence of aldosterone blockade on QT dispersion and heart rate variability in chronic heart failure. J Am Coll Cardiol 37:1800, 2001

4

HOMOCYSTEINE, VITAMINS, AND CARDIOVASCULAR DISEASE

Peter W.F. Wilson

The presence of homocysteine in the urine was noted to be a rare pediatric condition, associated with musculoskeletal abnormalities and the development of venous thromboembolism and arterial disease in adolescence. With the advent of improved tests to assay homocysteine concentrations in the 1960s, it was noted that increased levels of homocysteine in the blood were associated with premature vascular arterial disease in persons without obvious genetic defects. More recent research has demonstrated that elevated homocysteine levels are common and may increase the risk for cardiovascular disease (Bostom et al., 1999; Boushey et al., 1995; Ridker et al., 1999), although some studies have not observed an alteration in vascular risk (Evans et al., 1997).

Relations Between Homocysteine Levels and Vitamins

Subclinical deficiencies of vitamin B_6 (pyridoxine), vitamin B_{12}, or folate are relatively common, and approximately 25 to 30% of the adult population is affected. Moderately elevated homocysteine levels frequently accompany these subclinical deficien-

cies. Fasting homocysteine concentrations are typically greater in the elderly compared with middle-aged adults and are higher in men than in women. The prevalence of elevated homocysteine (>14 μmol/L) increases with age in both sexes. Plasma homocysteine levels are inversely correlated with vitamin intake.

The relations of vitamins B_1, B_2, B_6, B_{12}, folate, niacin, retinol, vitamin C, and vitamin E to homocysteine levels have all been studied, but the greatest interest has been shown for vitamins B_6 and B_{12} and folate, as they have been closely linked to key metabolic pathways. The two lowest deciles of folate, the lowest decile of vitamin B_{12} and the lowest decile of pyridoxal phosphate were associated with higher mean levels of homocysteine in older Framingham Study participants (Selhub et al., 1993; Table 4-1). Similarly, homocysteine concentrations were elevated among participants in the Health Professionals Study who consumed less than 280 μg/d of folate. It is now believed that suboptimal vitamin status, assessed by dietary intake or blood levels, is relatively common and may provide the primary explanation for elevated homocysteine levels in the population.

TABLE 4-1

MEAN HOMOCYSTEINE LEVELS IN ELDERLY FRAMINGHAM COHORT PARTICIPANTS

	Age	n	Mean homocysteine, μmol/L	Homocysteine 14 μmol/L, %
Men				
	65–74	239	11.8	25.3
	75–79	110	11.9	26.7
	80+	108	14.1	48.3
p(for trend by age)			<.001	<.001
Women				
	65–74	310	10.7	19.5
	75–79	204	11.9	28.9
	80+	189	13.2	41.4
p(for trend by age)			<.001	<.001
p(sex)			.003	.09

SOURCE: After J Selhub et al., JAMA 270:2693, 1993.

Naturally occurring sources of folate in the diet include orange juice and green, leafy vegetables. Cold breakfast cereals often include folate, and recently this food item has become an increasingly important source of dietary folate. There are strong positive associations between cereal consumption and plasma folate levels, but the relation plateaus near five to six servings per week of cereal. Approximately a quarter of the adult population in the United States consumes vitamin supplements that contain folate (and often vitamin B_6 and vitamin B_{12}), and these persons tend to have lower homocysteine levels.

Low vitamin B_{12} status can also account for elevated homocysteine levels, as this vitamin is a necessary cofactor in several homocysteine metabolic steps. Inadequate production of intrinsic factor in the stomach can result in a severe vitamin B_{12} deficiency with substantially elevated homocysteine concentrations, but this etiology has been thought to be an infrequent cause of low vitamin B_{12} status

in older vitamin B_{12}–deficient Framingham participants. Gastric hypochlorhydria and achlorhydria are more common than inadequate intrinsic factor, especially in older individuals, and can lead to impaired absorption of vitamin B_{12} because low pH is needed to dissociate vitamin B_{12} from food.

Studies of nutrient intake and surveys of the association of homocysteine levels with vascular disease led to the conclusion that increasing folate intake in the population at large would benefit homocysteine levels and reduce vascular disease incidence. Nutritional education, supplements, and food fortification of cereal and flour products were all thought to be possible, and the experience of observational studies of coronary heart disease, homocysteine, and nutrient status were used to estimate the effects (Tucker et al., 1996).

Inadequate folate intake in the early stages of pregnancy has been associated with fetal abnormalities such as spina bifida and anencephaly, and in

1996 the U.S. Food and Drug Administration mandated folate fortification of American flour and cereal grains on or before January 1, 1998. The effect of fortification was evaluated in the Framingham Offspring population sample. Among persons not taking folate supplements, the prevalence of low plasma folate levels fell from 22% to 2% and elevated homocysteine (>13 μmol/L) declined from 19% to 10% after folate fortification (Table 4-2; Jacques et al., 1999). The adequacy of dietary folate in the United States is still being debated, however, and excess folate intake may be detrimental, masking the megaloblastic anemia associated with vitamin B_{12} deficiency and pernicious anemia (Mills, 2000).

A variety of enzymatic defects and variants have been associated with elevated homocysteine levels, including cystathionine beta synthase, methylene tetrahydrofolate reductase (thermolabile and nonthermolabile variants), and methionine synthase. As some of these enzymes have vitamins as cofactors, there is a newly realized potential for gene-environmental interactions and consideration of heterozygotic and homozygotic variants. For instance, the allele for the thermolabile form of methylene tetrahydrofolate reductase is present in approximately 15 to 25% of Americans; persons who are homozygotic for the variant are more likely to have elevated homocysteine levels, provided they have suboptimal folate status. If folate status determined by diet or plasma levels is adequate in these individuals, the plasma homocysteine concentrations tend to be normal (Jacques et al., 1996).

TABLE 4-2

PLASMA FOLATE AND HOMOCYSTEINE CONCENTRATIONS BEFORE AND AFTER FOLIC ACID FORTIFICATION[a]

Characteristic	Study group	Control group
Mean plasma folate, ng/mL		
Baseline	4.6	4.6
Follow-up	10.0	4.8
	($p < .001$)	
Plasma folate <3 ng/mL, %		
Baseline	22.0	25.3
Follow-up	1.7	20.7
	($p < .001$)	
Mean fasting total homocysteine, μmol/L		
Baseline	10.1	10.0
Follow-up	9.4	10.2
	($p < .001$)	
Fasting total homocysteine >13 μmol/L, %		
Baseline	18.7	17.6
Follow-up	9.8	21.0
	($p < .001$)	

[a] Before and after folic acid (study group) versus before folate fortification alone (control group). Significant statistical comparisons for baseline and follow-up within study groups are shown.
SOURCE: After PF Jacques, N Engl J Med 340:1449, 1999.

Homocysteine Levels and Vascular Disease

Elevated homocysteine levels are more common in persons who develop atherosclerotic vascular disease (Dennis et al., 1997; Welch and Loscalzo, 1998). Although the pathogenic mechanisms are not definite, it is thought that elevated homocysteine levels impair thrombolysis and are directly toxic to the endothelial and vascular smooth-muscle cells (Welch and Loscalzo, 1998). Recent research has suggested that increased antioxidant effects accompany elevated homocysteine levels, including enhanced in vivo lipid peroxidation (Voutilainen et al., 1999) and elevated superoxide dismutase levels (Wilcken et al., 2000), and experts have suggested that "homocysteine-induced oxidant stress is responsible for vascular injury and dysfunction" (Jacobsen, 2000). The impaired endothelial function often noted with elevated homocysteine levels may be improved by pretreatment with oral folic acid or antioxidants such as vitamin C and vitamin E (Nappo et al., 1999; Wilmink et al., 2000).

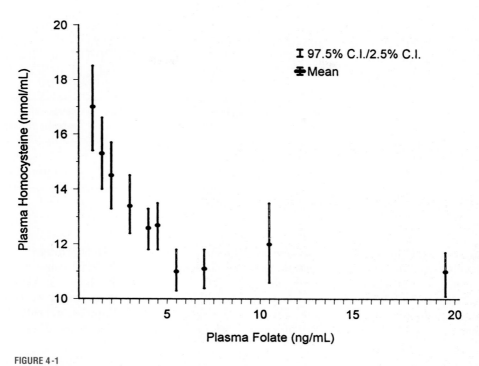

FIGURE 4-1

Mean plasma homocysteine concentrations (and 95% confidence intervals) by deciles of plasma folate. Means are adjusted for age, sex, and other plasma vitamins. (After Selhub et al., 1993.)

Observational studies have reported relatively consistent associations between elevated homocysteine levels and risk for cardiovascular disease outcomes, including coronary artery disease, carotid stenosis, stroke, and peripheral vascular disease (Boushey et al., 1995). Some major studies have not reported significant associations (Evans et al., 1997). Data from a recently published large case-control study (European Concerted Action Project, or COMAC), involving 750 European men and women with vascular disease and a similar number of controls, are shown in Table 4-3. In this report, homocysteine levels >12 μmol/L (the top 20% of the homocysteine distribution for controls) were associated with a significantly elevated odds ratios for all vascular disease, coronary heart disease, cerebrovascular disease, and peripheral vascular disease (Graham et al., 1997). Universal screening of homocysteine levels for persons without heart disease or those with existing atherosclerotic disease is not recommended. The American Heart Association recommends that homocysteine levels be screened only when the etiology of atherosclerotic disease is not easily attributable to more commonly measured risk factors (Malinow et al., 1999).

A meta-analysis concerning homocysteine levels and atherosclerotic disease concluded that a 5-μmol/L increment in homocysteine levels is associated with a 1.6-fold risk for coronary artery disease in men and a 1.8-fold risk in women. The authors attributed 10% of coronary artery disease risk to homocysteine elevations (Boushey et al., 1995). The role of folate therapy to reduce homocysteine levels and coronary disease risk is largely unanswered at the present, but the efficacy of vitamin supplements is being tested in vascular prevention trials

TABLE 4-3

ADJUSTED RELATIVE RISK AND 95% CONFIDENCE INTERVALS (CI) FOR VASCU-
LAR DISEASE IN THE EUROPEAN CONCERTED ACTION PROJECT ACCORDING
TO PRESENCE OF ELEVATED HOMOCYSTEINE (>12 μmol/L) IN CASES AND
CONTROLS

	All vascular disease	Coronary heart disease	Cerebrovascular disease	Peripheral vascular disease
Odds ratio	1.9	2.0	1.7	1.7
95% CI	(1.4 to 2.8)	(1.4 to 2.8)	(1.1 to 2.7)	(1.0 to 2.9)

SOURCE: After IM Graham et al., JAMA 277:1775, 1997.

that are under way. The premise of most of these trials is that combinations of folic acid, vitamin B_6, and vitamin B_{12} will reduce the risk of clinical atherosclerotic disease (Dennis et al., 1997).

An intriguing new area for research is the role of homocysteine levels and atherosclerotic disease among persons with kidney disease, as coronary heart disease is an important cause of debility and death in patients with impaired kidney function or kidney failure. Mean levels of homocysteine are approximately 10 μmol/L in healthy adults and 14 to 15 μmol/L in coronary disease cases, but

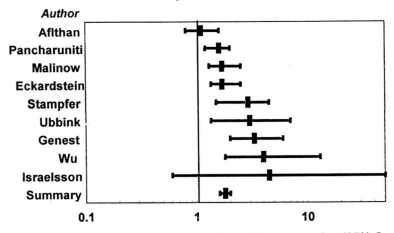

Fasting Homocysteine and Coronary Artery Disease Summary and Meta-Analysis

FIGURE 4-2

Estimated overall odds ratios for coronary heart disease and stroke associated with elevated homocysteine. (After Boushey et al., 1995.)

higher levels are commonly observed in patients with end-stage kidney disease, in whom levels typically range from 20 to 30 μmol/L (Dennis et al., 1997). These elevations are often present despite regular use of folate supplementation and demonstration of normal folate levels in the plasma. In particular, it has been proposed that renal transplant recipients are excellent candidates for a clinical trial of high-dose B vitamins to prevent cardiovascular outcomes (Bostom et al., 2001). These planned trials, and those already in progress, should add valuable information concerning the utility of folate supplementation to prevent atherosclerotic disease in persons with and without kidney disease.

From the National Heart, Lung, and Blood Institute's Framingham Heart Study, supported by NIH/NHLBI contract N01-HC-38038

REFERENCES

Bostom AG et al: Nonfasting plasma total homocysteine levels and all-cause and cardiovascular disease mortality in elderly Framingham men and women. Arch Intern Med 159:1077, 1999

Bostom AG et al: Power shortage: Clinical trials testing the "homocysteine hypothesis" against a background of folic acid–fortified cereal grain flour. Ann Intern Med 135:133, 2001

Boushey CJ et al: A quantitative assessment of plasma homocysteine as a risk factor for vascular disease: Probable benefits of increasing folic acid intakes. JAMA 274:1049, 1995

Dennis VW et al: Hyperhomocysteinemia: Detection, risk assessment, and treatment. Curr Opin Nephrol Hypertens 6:483, 1997

Evans RW et al: Homocyst(e)ine and risk of cardiovascular disease in the Multiple Risk Factor Intervention Trial. Arterioscler Thromb Vasc Biol 17:1947, 1997

Graham IM et al: Plasma homocysteine as a risk factor for vascular disease. The European Concerted Action Project. JAMA 277:1775, 1997

Jacobsen DW: Hyperhomocysteinemia and oxidative stress: Time for a reality check? Arterioscler Thromb Vasc Biol 20:1182, 2000

Jacques PF et al: Relation between folate status, a common mutation in methylenetetrahydrofolate reductase, and plasma homocysteine concentrations. Circulation 93:7, 1996

Jacques PF et al: The effect of folic acid fortification on plasma folate and total homocysteine concentrations. N Engl J Med 340:1449, 1999

Malinow MR et al: Homocyst(e)ine, diet, and cardiovascular diseases: A statement for healthcare professionals from the Nutrition Committee, American Heart Association. Circulation 99:178, 1999

Mills JL: Fortification of foods with folic acid—how much is enough? N Engl J Med 342:1442, 2000

Nappo F et al: Impairment of endothelial functions by acute hyperhomocysteinemia and reversal by antioxidant vitamins. JAMA 281:2113, 1999

Ridker PM et al: Homocysteine and risk of cardiovascular disease among postmenopausal women. JAMA 281:1817, 1999

Selhub J et al: Vitamin status and intake as primary determinants of homocysteinemia in the elderly. JAMA 270:2693, 1993

Tucker KL et al: Folic acid fortification of the food supply. Potential benefits and risks for the elderly population. JAMA 276:1879, 1996

Voutilainen S et al: Enhanced in vivo lipid peroxidation at elevated plasma total homocysteine levels. Arterioscler Thromb Vasc Biol 19:1263, 1999

Welch GN, Loscalzo J: Homocysteine and atherothrombosis. N Engl J Med 338:1042, 1998

Wilcken DE et al: Relationship between homocysteine and superoxide dismutase in homocystinuria: Possible relevance to cardiovascular risk. Arterioscler Thromb Vasc Biol 20:1199, 2000

Wilmink HW et al: Influence of folic acid on postprandial endothelial dysfunction. Arterioscler Thromb Vasc Biol 20:185, 2000

THE LINK BETWEEN AORTIC SCLEROSIS AND ATHEROSCLEROSIS

Catherine M. Otto

Calcific aortic valve disease encompasses a range from sclerosis to severe stenosis. Aortic valve sclerosis, defined as focal areas of thickening on the aortic valve leaflets in the absence of obstruction to left ventricular (LV) outflow, is present in about 25% of adults over 65 years of age (Stewart et al., 1997). More severe valve thickening results in increased leaflet stiffness and obstruction to LV ejection with an increased transvalvular flow velocity and a decreased valve area. Although there is wide individual variability, in adults with initially mild stenosis (transvalvular velocity $\geq$ 2.5 m/s), disease progression is predictable with an average increase in jet velocity of 0.33 $\pm$ 0.34 m/s per year, an increase in mean gradient of 7 $\pm$ 7 mmHg/year and a decrease in valve area of 0.12 $\pm$ 0.19 cm^2/year (Otto et al., 1997).

Clinical outcome in adults with asymptomatic aortic stenosis is similar to that in age-matched controls, with a risk of sudden death <1% per year. In contrast, once clinical symptoms supervene, outcome is poor unless surgical valve replacement is performed. The rate of symptom onset is 8% per year for adults with mild stenosis (transvalvular velocity < 3.0 m/s), 17% per year for those with moderate stenosis (velocity, 3 to 4 m/s), and 40% per year for those with severe valve stenosis (velocity > 4 m/s) (Otto et al., 1997).

The adverse clinical outcomes associated with aortic valve stenosis have long been recognized. It is also clear that some patients with aortic sclerosis will have progressive disease resulting in stenosis and the eventual need for valve replacement. Until recently, however, valve sclerosis in the absence of outflow obstruction was considered a benign incidental finding on echocardiography. This chapter will discuss the recent studies elucidating the disease process at the tissue level of calcific aortic valve disease, associated clinical factors, and the adverse outcomes associated with aortic valve sclerosis. Aortic sclerosis has many similarities to atherosclerosis, but important differences in these two disease processes are present as well.

Molecular and Cellular Mechanisms of Disease

The normal aortic valve leaflet consists of three layers, with an endothelial covering on both sides of the leaflet. Tensile strength is provided by the fibrosa, with dense collagen bundles arranged circumferentially relative to the leaflet edge. In the ventricularis, elastic fibers are oriented perpendicular to the leaflet edge along the ventricular aspect of the leaflet. The spongiosa is a layer of loose connective and adipose tissue, often confined to the basal third of the leaflet, but often becoming more prominent with age. Aortic valve leaflets are avascular and have few smooth-muscle cells.

The early lesion of calcific aortic valve disease is characterized by a subendothelial lesion on the aortic side of the leaflet, with displacement of the elastic lamina (Otto et al., 1994; Figure 5-1, See Color Plate 1). Endothelial disruption is postulated to occur, although it is difficult to demonstrate in surgical or autopsy valve tissue. Factors that may increase endothelial disruption include increased tensile stress and decreased shear stress—factors that may account for the earlier age at presentation of patients with calcified bicuspid valves.

The subendothelial lesion contains large amounts of neutral lipid, with immunohistochemical studies demonstrating the presence of low-density lipoprotein (LDL) and lipoprotein (a) [Lp(a)] with evidence for oxidization of LDL in these areas (O'Brien et al., 1996; Olsson et al., 1999). Standard histologic stains indicate the presence of large amounts of extracellular protein, which has not yet been characterized.

The early lesions of calcific aortic valve disease have a prominent cellular infiltrate consisting predominantly of macrophages, with lesser numbers of T lymphocytes. Smooth-muscle cells are not seen; even in normal valves, only rare smooth-muscle cells are seen, located at the leaflet base on the ventricular side of the valve. Activation of macrophages is evident with foam cells and with production of proteins that mediate calcification, such as osteopontin (O'Brien et al., 1995). The role of valve fibroblasts in the disease process remains unclear, with recent studies showing isolation of calcifying cells from aortic valve tissue.

Recent studies from the author's laboratory have also demonstrated angiotensin-converting enzyme (ACE) activity and production in early lesions and the presence of AT1 and AT2 receptors in aortic valves, colocalizing with areas of lipid infiltration.

Other studies have demonstrated increased matrix metalloproteinase activity and upregulation of adhesion molecules by endothelial cells.

An important difference between atherosclerosis and aortic stenosis is the mechanism of clinical events. Most clinical events due to atherosclerosis are related to plaque instability and thrombosis with vessel occlusion. In contrast, calcific aortic valve disease becomes clinically evident when the sheer bulk of the lesion increases leaflet stiffness, resulting in a pressure gradient across the aortic valve. To date, there is no evidence that valvular lesions become unstable or are associated with thrombosis.

Associated Clinical and Genetic Factors

The similarities between aortic sclerosis and atherosclerosis at the tissue level suggest that these diseases may be related clinically as well. The Cardiovascular Health Study offered an opportunity to examine the association between clinical factors and an abnormal valve on echocardiography in a large population-based sample of adults over age 65 years (Stewart et al., 1997). Aortic sclerosis was present in 26% and aortic stenosis in 2% of the 5210 subjects over 65 years of age. Using multivariate Cox regression analysis, the clinical factors associated with an abnormal valve on echocardiography were age (twofold increased risk for each 10-year increase in age), male gender (twofold increased risk), smoking (35% increase in risk), hypertension (20% increase in risk), and elevated LDL and Lp(a) levels (Table 5-1).

The magnitude of risk due to these clinical factors was similar to that seen for coronary artery disease (CAD) risk factors in the elderly. The postulated mechanisms for the increased risk associated with these clinical factors are similar to those proposed for atherosclerosis. Hypertension might result in abnormally high tensile stress on the leaflets or high flow rates might lead to low shear stress, resulting in endothelial injury and disruption. Elevated levels of LDL and Lp(a) might

TABLE 5-1

FACTORS ASSOCIATED WITH AORTIC SCLEROSIS OR STENOSIS BY STEPWISE MULTIPLE LOGISTIC REGRESSION

Clinical factor	Odds ratio	95% Confidence limits
Age	2.18[a]	2.15–2.20
Male gender	2.03	1.7–2.5
Lp(a)	1.23[b]	1.14–1.32
Height (cm)	0.84[c]	0.75–0.93
History of hypertension	1.23	1.1–1.4
Present smoking	1.35	1.1–1.7
LDL cholesterol (mg/dL)	1.12[b]	1.03–1.23
Glucose (mg/dL)	1.04[b]	1.01–1.07

[a] ±10-year increase
[b] ±75th vs. 25th percentile
[c] ±10-unit increase
SOURCE: BF Stewart et al., J Am Coll Cardiol 29:630, 1997, with permission.

facilitate lipid deposition in the leaflets in the presence of endothelial injury from any cause. Smoking may increase risk through mechanisms analogous to those proposed for atherosclerosis, including adverse effects on endothelial permeability and lipoprotein oxidation.

However, because not all patients with CAD have aortic sclerosis—and because about 50% of patients with severe aortic stenosis have no significant CAD—there must be other clinical factors, as yet not understood, that account for differences in the prevalence and clinical presentation of these two disease processes. For example, the relative importance of systemic calcium metabolism versus local tissue factors in the deposition of calcium in the aortic valve leaflets requires further study.

It is also possible that genetic factors play a significant role. The apparent inverse relationship between degenerative valve disease and osteoporosis is intriguing in this regard. A recent small study of adults undergoing cardiac catheterization found a higher prevalence of the vitamin D receptor B allele (compared to b allele) in those with aortic stenosis compared to those undergoing catheterization for CAD alone (Ortlepp et al., 2001). The authors speculate that the B allele may be associated with extraosseous calcification via adaptive mechanisms that also have negative effects on bone density. Alternatively, the B allele may be in linkage disequilibrium with another, unidentified gene involved in calcium metabolism. The apparent association between the vitamin D receptor B allele and calcific aortic valve disease needs confirmation in additional studies, and the possible mechanisms of this association require further study.

Clinical Outcome

Until recently, aortic valve sclerosis was thought to be a benign incidental finding on echocardiography in the elderly, as LV outflow is not obstructed. However, given the early tissue changes seen in the sclerotic aortic valve and the clinical factors associated with aortic sclerosis, it has been hypothesized that the presence of aortic sclerosis would be associated with adverse cardiovascular outcomes.

In the Cardiovascular Health Study (Otto et al., 1999), clinical outcome was compared in subjects with a normal aortic valve versus those with aortic sclerosis on echocardiography. Subjects were followed for a mean interval of 5 years to assess the risk of death from any cause and from cardiovascular causes. Cardiovascular morbidity was defined as the new onset of myocardial infarction (MI), angina, congestive heart failure, or stroke. In order to account for underlying disease, the relative risk for death was assessed in subjects without known CAD at baseline and the relative risk for cardiovascular morbidity was assessed in subjects without known cardiovascular disease at baseline. The Cox regression models also were adjusted for baseline factors associated with aortic sclerosis (age, gender, hypertension, current smoking, shorter height, elevated LDL cholesterol levels, and presence of diabetes).

TABLE 5-2

EVENT RATES AND RELATIVE RISK FOR TOTAL AND CARDIOVASCULAR MORTALITY IN THOSE WITH NO CORONARY HEART DISEASE[a] AT STUDY ENTRY AND CARDIO-VASCULAR EVENTS IN THOSE WITH NO PREVALENT CARDIOVASCULAR DISEASE[b] AT STUDY ENTRY

| | Event rate per 1000 person-yrs | | | |
	NORMAL	SCLEROSIS	Relative risk[c]	95% CI
All deaths	19	37	1.35	1.12–1.61
Cardiovascular deaths	6	14	1.52	1.12–2.05
Myocardial infarction	9	16	1.40	1.07–1.83
Angina	19	26	1.17	0.95–1.43
Congestive heart failure	12	20	1.28	1.01–1.63
Stroke	10	16	1.25	0.96–1.64

[a]Coronary heart disease indicates participants with a history of myocardial infarction, angina, coronary bypass surgery, or angioplasty prior to entry into the Cardiovascular Health Study.
[b]Cardiovascular disease was defined as a validated history of myocardial infarction, angina, congestive heart failure, or stroke.
[c]Cox regression adjusted for age, gender, and baseline-associated factors [Lp(a) levels, height, hypertension, present smoking, LDL levels, and diabetes]; $n = 4271$.
SOURCE: CM Otto et al., N Engl J Med 341:142, 1999, with permission.

As shown in Table 5-2, elderly adults with aortic sclerosis have an approximately 50% increased risk of cardiovascular death compared to adults with a normal aortic valve on echocardiography. In addition, aortic sclerosis was associated with a 40% increased risk for MI and a trend toward an increased risk of congestive heart failure. At first glance, these results seem surprising. Aortic sclerosis is only mild irregular valve thickening without obstruction to outflow, so it is unlikely that the valve thickening itself led to these adverse clinical outcomes. It also is unlikely that these subjects had progressive disease with development of severe stenosis, given our understanding of the expected rate of hemodynamic progression and the time frame of the study. Although the pathophysiologic mechanism of the association between aortic sclerosis and clinical outcome cannot be deduced from this study, it is likely that aortic sclerosis is a marker of subclinical atherosclerosis, rather than a direct influence on clinical outcome.

Comparison with Atherosclerosis

Aortic sclerosis and atherosclerosis have many similarities, with three lines of evidence suggesting a link between these disease processes (Table 5-3). First, at the tissue level, the cellular and molecular mechanisms of disease appear congruent, although aortic sclerosis is associated with greater tissue calcification and lacks smooth-muscle cell proliferation compared to atherosclerosis. Further studies elucidating the similarities and differences between aortic sclerosis and atherosclerosis may improve our understanding of both disease processes. Second, the same clinical factors are associated with both aortic sclerosis and

TABLE 5-3

COMPARISON OF AORTIC SCLEROSIS AND ATHEROSCLEROSIS

	Aortic Sclerosis	Atherosclerosis
Tissue changes		
Inflammatory cells	+ + + +	+ + + +
Lipid infiltration	+ + + +	+ + + +
Calcification	+ + + +	+
Smooth-muscle cell proliferation	−	+ +
Associated clinical factors	+ + +	+ + + +
Genetic factors	?	+ + + +
Clinical outcome		
Risk of cardiovascular death	+ +	+ + + +
Risk of myocardial infarction	+ +	+ + + +
Progression to valve obstruction	+ + + +	−
Mechanism of clinical events	Leaflet stiffness	Plaque instability

atherosclerosis at a comparable magnitude of risk. Third, the presence of aortic sclerosis is associated with an increased risk of MI and cardiovascular death.

However, several unanswered questions remain. Why is there a disparity between coronary artery and aortic leaflet disease severity? In adults with severe aortic stenosis, only 50% have significant coronary artery luminal narrowings. Conversely, most adults with coronary disease undergoing revascularization do not have significant aortic leaflet thickening. What factors predict the rate of progression in an individual patient? It is clear that not all patients with aortic sclerosis develop severe aortic stenosis; factors that predict progression in an individual patient have not been established. Most importantly, we do not yet know if there are interventions to slow or prevent the disease process in the aortic valve leaflets. Although the similarities between atherosclerosis and aortic sclerosis suggest that therapies directed toward the underlying disease process (such as lipid-lowering medications) might be effective, randomized clinical trials are needed before such therapy can be widely recommended.

In the meantime, when aortic sclerosis is seen on echocardiography, the clinician should perform a careful cardiac risk factor assessment and intervene to decrease risk factors, following current guidelines for CAD prevention.

REFERENCES

O'Brien KD et al: Osteopontin is expressed in human aortic valvular lesions. Circulation 92:2163, 1995

O'Brien KD et al: Apolipoproteins B, (a) and E accumulate in the morphologically early lesion of "degenerative" valvular aortic stenosis. Arterioscler Thromb Vasc Biol 16:523, 1996

Olsson M et al: Presence of oxidized low density lipoprotein in nonrheumatic stenotic aortic valves. Arterioscler Thromb Vasc Biol 19:1218, 1999

Ortlepp: The vitamin D receptor genotype predisposes to the development of calcific aortic valve stenosis. Heart 85:635, 2001

Otto CM et al: Characterization of the early lesion of "degenerative" valvular aortic stenosis: Histologic and immunohistochemical studies. Circulation 90:844, 1994

Otto CM et al: A prospective study of asymptomatic valvular aortic stenosis: Clinical, echocardiographic, and exercise predictors of outcome. Circulation 95:2262, 1997

Otto CM et al: Association of aortic-valve sclerosis with cardiovascular mortality and morbidity in the elderly. N Engl J Med 341:142, 1999

Stewart BF et al: Clinical factors associated with calcific aortic valve disease. J Am Coll Cardiol 29:630, 1997

TRIGLYCERIDES AND LOW HDL IN CORONARY RISK ASSESSMENT

Dennis L. Sprecher

Introduction

Landmark studies during the 1950s prompted numerous cross-sectional and longitudinal investigations revealing triglyceride (TG) elevation and high-density lipoprotein cholesterol (HDL) reduction in patients with atherosclerotic disease (Miller, 1987). In the Framingham cohort, cardiovascular risk increases with the level of TG, notably in women (Castelli, 1992). Each lower HDL cholesterol tertile is associated with progressively higher risk for coronary artery disease (CAD), while within each HDL cholesterol tertile, women reveal a more dramatic modification of risk with increasing TG than men. The objective of this chapter is to target new concepts related to TG, HDL, and related lipoprotein particles as cardiovascular risk parameters.

While the independence of HDL cholesterol as a cardiovascular risk factor has been well established [CAD risk increases 2 to 3% for every 1-mg/dL reduction (Gordon et al., 1989)], the risk associated with TG alone, independent of HDL cholesterol, has been controversial (TG, HDL, and CAD—NIH Consensus Development Conference Statement-1992). A meta-analysis incorporating

17 studies in both men (46,413) and women (10,864), published in 1996, argues most persuasively for TG's independent effect beyond HDL. The relative risk in women was 1.78 vs. 1.35 in men, lower but remaining dichotomous by gender when adjustment is made for HDL cholesterol (1.37 and 1.14, respectively, both significant). A representative study in this meta-analysis was the Collaborative Heart Disease Study, which incorporated a total of 5000 initially healthy men from two sites in the United Kingdom (age 45 to 60 years). With 251 events over a 3- to 5-year follow-up, those in the upper 20% for TG values had over twice the risk compared to those in the bottom 20% of the baseline distribution, after adjustment for HDL and total cholesterol. TG values were, in fact, more predictive than total cholesterol (Sprecher, 1998).

The degree of risk associated with HDL and TG appears interactive, with the greatest risk in those with high TG/low HDL cholesterol along with an elevated LDL cholesterol. Specifically, in the setting of TG values a >2.26 mmol/L (>200 mg/dL) an LDL/HDL cholesterol ratio of >5 is associated with a five-fold increase in cardiovascular events, compared to those with normal lipid values. CAD severity has been shown to be far greater in those with both high LDL and TG, rather than high LDL alone.

The recent guidelines of the National Cholesterol Education Program (NCEP Expert Panel, 2001) have suggested HDL cholesterol values of 1.03 mmol/L (40 mg/dL) as the cutpoint below which patients of both genders should be considered at risk for CAD, while Framingham recommend levels <1.03 mmol/L (<40 mg/dL) in men and 1.16 mmol/L (45 mg/dL) in women. It remains unclear what level of TG is associated with cardiovascular risk, even though TG values >2.26 mmol/L (>200 mg/dL) are discussed as "too high" in the NCEP Adult Treatment Panel guidelines (NCEP Expert Panel, 2001). In one study, men in Copenhagen were followed for 8 years, and TG levels predicted CAD events within HDL cholesterol quartiles. Compared to a TG range of 0.44 to 1.09 mmol/L (39 to 97 mg/dL), a range of 1.10 to 1.59 mmol/L (97 to 141 mg/dL) represented a 50% greater risk for incipient CAD, while values >1.6 mmol/L (>142 mg/dL) resulted in a greater than two fold risk.

In the 14-year Baltimore Follow-up Study, an increase in the combined outcome of cardiac events and mortality was evident in CAD patients with TG values >1.13 mmol/L (>100 mg/dL) compared to those < 1.13 mmol/L (<100 mg/dL). A study of patients following coronary artery bypass grafting (CABG) from the Cleveland Clinic Foundation surgical registry (Sprecher et al., 1999) suggested TG values >2.60 mmol/L (>230 mg/dL) were associated with decreased survival among women and a decrease in event-free survival in men. While children and adult athletes often have TG values <1.13 mmol/L (<100 mg/dL), in contrast to subjects with values >1.70 mmol/L (>150 mg/dL) who progressively present with the metabolic syndrome of insulin resistance and associated enhanced density of LDL, a cutpoint in this continuum has not been defined. Many would consider 1.70 mmol/L (150 mg/dL) a better point beyond which risk accrues and for which treatment may be valuable, consistent with the most recent NCEP guidelines (NCEP expert panel, 2001).

Triglyceride values are commonly elevated in the diabetic or insulin-resistant state and as such may simply reflect this endocrinopathy. Analyses of the impact of TG on cardiovascular risk in the Lipid Research Clinic data suggested elimination of the TG effect when adjustment was made for glucose levels (Criqui, 1998). This does not uniformly appear to be the case, however, as elevated TG values appear to portend enhanced cardiovascular risk in those with non-insulin-dependent diabetes mellitus, as demonstrated in the Paris Prospective population, the World Health Organization population, and the author's own cohort of post-CABG patients (Sprecher et al., 2000). TG is probably not simply a surrogate for glucose control, in that the value of such control in protection from macrovascular disease remains controversial and at best modest.

TG and HDL Risk During Lipid-Lowering Treatment

Baseline TG and HDL cholesterol levels have been found to be risk factors for cardiac events in the placebo groups of multiple statin trials (WOSCOPS, 4S, and post-CABG study), in contrast to the treatment groups where these levels lost virtually all of their predictive potential. In the treatment arm of the 4S trial, baseline HDL cholesterol remained modestly relevant, while the increase in HDL cholesterol during the trial contributed to the positive outcome. This suggests that the risk associated with TG and, to some degree, HDL cholesterol can be ameliorated by the use of HMG-CoA reductase inhibitors. Average TG values in these trials approximated 1.70 mmol/L (150 mg/dL). Further, 4S results [mean LDL = 4.91 mmol/L (190 mg/dL)] were enhanced in those with high TG, in contrast to results from the CARE trial [mean LDL = 3.59 mmol/L (139 mg/dL)], where best event reduction was observed in those with lower TG values.

TG- and HDL-related particles appear to be relevant to progression of disease in those already on lipid-lowering treatment (Hodis and Mack, 1998).

This further supports the value of HDL and TG in explaining disease progression, and suggests that we still do not have the correct dose, agent, or combination of agent(s) to adequately deal with these lipoprotein elements.

Triglyceride and HDL levels result from a culmination of events that occur while and after the liver secretes diverse lipoprotein particles, a majority of which float in the very low density lipoprotein (VLDL) density range upon ultracentrifugation (Breslow, 1995; Tall, 1998; Table 6-1). VLDL is typically 80% triglyceride. Numerous environmental factors (e.g., sugar and fat intake, exercise) in addition to metabolic disturbances (e.g., obesity, insulin resistance, or diabetes, resulting in excess free fatty acids) affect both the composition and size of the VLDL (TG-rich) particle. The larger VLDL particles have apolipoprotein (apo) E exposed, and after brief hydrolysis by lipoprotein lipase (LpL), can be recognized by receptors for lipoprotein receptor–related protein and exit the plasma space. Alternatively, processed VLDL (i.e., VLDL remnants) can continue down the cascade catalyzed by hepatic lipase (HTgL) to LDL. Smaller VLDL are not as amenable to hydrolysis by LpL and interact through an exposed apo B protein on their surface, facilitating egress through the apo B/apo E LDL-receptor. Apo CIII compromises LpL activity, is pivotal in VLDL catabolism by delaying clearance, and is thereby relevant to TG serum levels. Elevated apo CIII in VLDL is associated with disease progession. Cholesteryl ester and fatty acids processed off VLDL and remnants by LpL contribute to the maturation of HDL, from dense lipid-accepting HDL_3 particles to the cholesteryl ester–enriched HDL_2 particles. HDL_3 may also accept material from the vasculature resulting in cardiovascular protection, as suggested in the STARS and LOCAT trials. Larger TG and cholesteryl ester–enriched VLDL particles are particularly good substrates for cholesteryl ester transfer protein (CETP) activity, which catalyzes the transfer of VLDL-TG, as well as TG on smaller intermediate forms, to HDL and LDL, with coordinated transfer of cholesteryl ester in

the opposite directions. Such particle modifications lessen the cholesterol moiety, i.e., decrease HDL cholesterol levels, and to some extent LDL cholesterol levels, due to the replacement by TG, and predispose both HDL_2 and LDL to processing by hepatic lipase, the former towards HDL_3 and the latter towards denser forms of LDL. Overall, these metabolic processes provide the backdrop for a variable vascular exposure to cholesterol-rich apo B–related particles represented grossly by TG serum values along with potential protective mechanisms related to HDL. This chapter makes it clear that the risk associated with TG is intricately involved with the cardiovascular risk associated with HDL and LDL.

While TG lowering generally decreases the impact of CETP activity, the vascular benefits are unclear (Tall, 1998). A genetic polymorphism in CETP, leading to higher CETP activities, results in greater disease progression and a greater angiographic response to statin therapy. In contrast, among Japanese-American men, intron 14 and 15 mutations have been related to lower CETP activities, higher HDL cholesterol values, and about 40% greater incidence of CAD. In the former study, CETP activity was atherogenic, and in the latter, protective. Transgenic mice experiments have suggested that CETP activity is protective from vascular lesions in the setting of hypertriglyceridemia and atherogenic in the absence of high TG values.

Increases in LpL activity chemically produced in mice have resulted in less diet-induced atherosclerosis. A recent study has demonstrated lower LpL activity and a higher incidence of common LpL gene defects in humans with previous myocardial infarction. Neither statins nor resins are noted to alter the level of this enzyme. However, both niacin and fibric acid derivatives augment LpL activity. Fibrates also reduce apo CIII levels, thereby also enhancing LpL activity and allowing more rapid intermediate particle flux, with less opportunity for conversion to dense LDL. These data again suggest that intermediate particle processing contributes significantly to vascular disease (Sprecher, 1998; Hodis and Mack, 1998).

TABLE 6-1

PREDOMINANTLY TRIGLYCERIDE/HDL ALTERING STUDIES

	Rx n/total n gender	Time, years	Drug	TC, mg/dL (mmol/L)	LDL, mg/dL (mmol/L)	TG, mg/dL (mmol/L)	HDL, mg/dL (mmol/L)	MLD	% in CHD events
Angiography Trials									
FATS 1°	36/120 Men	2.5	NA/CME	271 (6.99) −23%	191 (4.92) −32%	194 (2.19) −29%	39 (1.01) 41%	0.04% p = .003	—
BECAIT 2°	47/92 Men post-MI	5	Bezafibrate	267 (6.87) −14%	181 (4.66) −4%	216 (2.44) −31%	35 (0.89) 9%	0.13 mm p = .05	(11 vs. 3 events) p = .02
LOCAT 2°	197/395 Post-CABG men	2.5	Gemfibrozil	199 (5.14) −5.5%	139 (3.58) −4.5%	146 (1.65) −36%	31.4 (0.81) 21%	0.05 mm p = .002	—
DAIS 2°	207/418 Men and Women	3	Fenofibrate	215 (5.56) −10%[a]	131 (3.38) −5%[a]	230 (2.59) −28%[a]	42 (1.09) 8%[a]	0.04 mm	(Not powered for clinical end-points)

TABLE 6-1

PREDOMINANTLY TRIGLYCERIDE/HDL ALTERING STUDIES *(Continued)*

	Rx *n*/total *n* gender	Time, years	Drug	TC, mg/dL (mmol/L)	LDL, mg/dL (mmol/L)	TG, mg/dL (mmol/L)	HDL, mg/dL (mmol/L)	MLD	% in CHD events
Outcome Trials									
LRC-CDPT 2°	1119/3908 Men	5	NA	253 (6.52) −10%	UK	189 (2.13) −26%	UK	NA	↓ 13% (*p* < .05)
Stockholm 2°	279/555 Post-MI Men and Women	5	Clofibrate and NA	246 (6.35) −13%	160 (4.13) UK	209 (2.36) −19%	48 (1.24) UK	NA	↓ 36% (CHD mortality) (*p* < .05)
Helsinki 1°	2051/4081 Men	5	Gemfibrozil	267 (6.87) −11%	190 (4.9) 10%	178 (2.01) −35%	47 (1.22) 11%	NA	↓ 34% (*p* = .02)
BIP 2°	[a]1561/3122 Men and Women	5	Bezafibrate	212 (5.46) −4%	148 (3.81) −5%	149 (1.68) −22%	34.6 (0.89) 12%	NA	↓ 9% (*p* = .27)
VA-HIT 2°	[a]1265/2531 Men	4.6	Gemfibrozil	175 (4.51) −5%	111 (2.86) −10.4%	161 (1.82) −33%	33 (0.85) 6%	NA	↓22% (*p* = .006)

[a] Estimates.

ABBREVIATIONS: HDL, high-density lipoprotein; TC, total cholesterol; LDL, low-density lipoprotein; TG, triglyceride; MLD, minimal luminal diameter; CHD, coronary heart disease; 1°, primary prevention; 2°, secondary prevention; NA, nicotinic acid; CME, cholestyramine; MI, myocardial infarction; CABG, coronary artery bypass graft; UK, unknown.

TG Clinical Studies (Table 1)

The lack of vascular benefit from LDL lowering in subjects with CAD and baseline values <3.23 mmol/L (<125 mg/dL) in the CARE and LIPID trials, along with the clear benefit resulting from gemfibrozil use in CAD subjects with mean LDL values of 2.87 mmol/L (111 mg/dL), suggest that TG-related risk is particularly present in the low-LDL setting, and that it is a risk responsive to fibrates and not statins. Further, when LDL values are particularly high, e.g., >4.14 mmol/L (>160 mg/dL), then both statins and fibric acid derivatives are effective in reducing events (Helsinki Heart Study (Manninen, 1992) and WOSCOPS, both primary prevention trials). This occurs regardless of LDL lowering (9% vs. >20%, respectively) in the setting of very contrasting TG effects. A reduction in coronary mortality has been reported in two predominately TG-lowering studies: the Stockholm Ischemic Study and a 15-year follow-up of the Lipid Research Clinics Coronary Drug Project Trial (LRC-CDPT) niacin arm (11% reduction) (The Coronary Drug Project research group, 1975). An association between the degree of TG reduction and events has been reported thus far only in the Stockholm trial (Carlson and Rosenhamer, 1988). Total TG values were not associated with cardiovascular outcomes in the VA HDL Intervention Trial, while HDL cholesterol and various TG-related particles were (Rubins, 1999).

A contrast between angiographic outcomes in two groups of patients, one on a niacin/resin combination and the other on a statin/resin combination (FATS), suggested some minor relative benefit to the niacin group (average change in % stenosis (−0.3 vs. −1.1, respectively; Brown et al., 1990). While LDL of 4.91 mmol/L (190 mg/dL) was decreased equally in both groups [to 3.36 vs. 2.84 mmol/L (130 vs. 110 mg/dL)], TG values decreased more [2.26 mmol/L (200 mg/dL) to 1.55 vs. 2.03 mmol/L (137 vs. 180 mg/dL)], and HDL cholesterol increased more [1.01 to 1.42 vs. 1.06 mmol/L (39 to 55 vs. 41 mg/dL)] in the niacin group. Perhaps the impact of niacin on intermediate metabolism (i.e., LpL activity), over simply the decrease in hepatic synthesis and receptor activity contributes to some vascular improvements (Criqui, 1998).

Two trials using fibric acid derivatives (BECAIT (Ericsson, 1996) and LOCAT (Frick, 1997), resulting in virtually no LDL change, revealed angiographic benefits in the high LDL/TG setting [4.65/2.44 mmol/L (180/216 mg/dL)] and average LDL/TG setting [3.62/1.65 mmol/L (140/ 146 mg/dL)]. In type 2 diabetic patients [DAIS, $n = 418$; LDL/TG = 3.36/2.60 mmol/L (130/230 mg/dL)], fenofibrate producing as little as a 6% LDL cholesterol lowering, proved beneficial to patients with CAD (Diabetes Atherosclerosis Intervention Study Investigators, 2001). This was based on angiographic evidence and a trend towards fewer events over an average 3-year follow-up. Further, the use of gemfibrozil produced a reduction in cardiac events over 5 years in two additional cohorts, one with LDL values of 4.91 mmol/L (190 mg/dL), (Helsinki) (Manninen, 1992) and the other of 2.87 mmol/L (111 mg/dL) (VA-HIT) (Rubins, 1999 [see also Rubins, Chapter 7, this volume]), along with comparable TG values [1.81 to 2.03 mmol/L (160 to 180 mg/dL)]. Bezafibrate reduced events in a sub-cohort of the BIP trial with TG levels >2.26 mmol/L (>200 mg/dL), but did not significantly reduce events overall. The VA-HIT cohort was profoundly obese (body-mass index of 29 compared to 26.7 in BIP), suggesting a relatively greater insulin-resistant population enriched with fibrate-responsive intermediate particles (Sprecher, 1998).

Risk/Treatment Recommendations

The story of triglycerides and HDL perhaps parallels, but predates, the status of LDL in the early 1980s, when the LRC-CPPT was positive, but the conviction of practitioners towards treatment (i.e., acceptance of the efficacy of lipid lowering) was not widespread. Further, the current modalities towards LDL lowering with HMG-CoA reductase inhibitors, known to remove not only LDL but also cholesterol-rich particles higher in the lipoprotein metabolic cascade, may partially if not totally coincide with the benefits of other more TG-directed approaches, e.g., niacin or fibric acid derivatives. In the average LDL setting 3.36 to 4.14 mmol/L (130 to 160 mg/dL), as HDL drifts below 1.03 mmol/L (40 mg/dL) in men or 1.16 to 1.23 mmol/L (45 to 50 mg/dL) in women, along with a progressive increase in TG above 1.69 mmol/L (150 mg/dL), the patient's risk for CAD or progression of ongoing CAD increases. For LDL cholesterol values <3.23 mmol/L (<125 mg/dL), TG/HDL values more dramatically influence risk since they mark the presence of intermediate particles and/or modifications in HDL.

The Adult Treatment Panel III suggests a non-HDL cholesterol (TC − HDL cholesterol) target 0.76 mmol/L (30 mg/dL) above the LDL cholesterol goal when TG >2.26 mmol/L (>200 mg/dL) (NCEP Expert Panel, 2001). No HDL cholesterol treatment target is provided. The bias toward TG treatment (relative to HDL cholesterol) rests more firmly on pathophysiologic grounds than clinical outcomes, in that HDL cholesterol elevation has correlated more significantly with a decrease in cardiovascular events. However, our current pharmacologic treatment strategies influence both TG and HDL cholesterol, making it difficult to determine their respective individual contributions. Perhaps the focus on non-HDL treatment, if accepted by the practitioner, will better parallel improved patient-event reduction.

It seems therefore reasonable to consider the addition of niacin (in the nondiabetic) and/or fibric acid derivatives (gemfibrozil or fenofibrate) in the setting of abnormal HDL/TG. This is particularly the case when LDL is low or normal and the patient is at high risk or already has CAD. The treatment route should still be LDL lowering first, particularly in the case where the baseline value is >3.23 mmol/L (>125 mg/dL), to which other agents can be added. This is based on the extensive literature on statins and their efficacy. Dietary regimens, along with combination therapy which critically influences these intermediate particles, will inevitably become more important in future health care.

REFERENCES

Breslow J: Familial disorders of high-density lipoprotein metabolism, In *The Metabolic and Molecular Bases of Inherited Disease,* 7th ed, CR Scriver et al (eds). New York, McGraw-Hill, 1995, pp 2031–2052

Brown G, et al: Regression of coronary artery disease as a result of intensive lipid-lowering therapy in men with high levels of apolipoprotein B. N Engl J Med 323:1289, 1990

Carlson LA, Rosenhamer G: Reduction of mortality in the Stockholm Ischemic Heart Disease Secondary Prevention Study by combined treatment with clofibrate and nicotinic acid. Acta Med Scand 223:405, 1988

Castelli WP: Epidemiology of triglycerides: A view from Framingham. Am J Cardiol 70:3H, 1992

Criqui MH: Triglycerides and cardiovascular disease. A focus on clinical trials. Eur Heart J 19:A36, 1998

Diabetes Atherosclerosis Intervention Study Investigators: Effect of fenofibrate on progession of coronary-artery disease in type 2 diabetes: The Diabetes Atherosclerosis Intervention Study, a randomised study. Lancet 357:905, 2001

Ericsson C et al: Angiographic assessment of effects of bezafibrate on progression of coronary artery disease in young male postinfarction patients. Lancet 347:849, 1996

Frick M et al: Prevention of the angiographic progression of coronary and vein graft atherosclerosis by gemfibrozil after coronary bypass surgery in men with low levels of HDL cholesterol. Circulation 96:2137, 1997

Gordon DJ et al: High-density lipoprotein cholesterol and cardiovascular disease. Four prospective American studies. Circulation 79:8, 1989

Hodis HN, Mack WJ: Triglyceride-rich lipoproteins and progression of atherosclerosis. Eur Heart J 19:A40, 1998

Manninen V et al: Joint effects of serum triglycerides and LDL cholesterol and HDL cholesterol concentrations on coronary heart disease risk in the Helsinki Heart Study—implications for treatment. Circulation 85:37, 1992

Miller NE: Associations of high-density lipoprotein subclasses and apolipoproteins with ischemic heart disease and coronary atherosclerosis. Am Heart J 113:589, 1987

NCEP Expert Panel: Executive summary of the third report of the National Cholesterol Education Program (NCEP) Expert Panel on Detection, Evaluation, and Treatment of High Blood Cholesterol in Adults. (Adult Treatment Panel III). JAMA 285:2486, 2001

Rubins HB et al: Gemfibrozil for the secondary prevention of coronary heart disease in men with low levels of high-density lipoprotein cholesterol. NEJM 341:410, 1999

Sprecher DL: Triglycerides as a risk factor for coronary artery disease. Am J Cardiol 82:49U, discussion 85U, 1998

Sprecher DL et al: Triglycerides, HDL-c and diabetes: Prediction of post-coronary artery bypass grafting survival in women. American College of Cardiology, 48th Annual Scientific Session. J Am Coll Cardiol 33(Suppl A):272A, 1999

Sprecher DL et al: Preoperative triglycerides predict post-CABG survival in diabetic patients: A sex analysis. Diabetes Care 23:1648, 2000

Tall AR: An overview of reverse cholesterol transport. Eur Heart J 19:A31, 1998

The Coronary Drug Project Research Group: Clofibrate and niacin in coronary heart disease. JAMA 231:360, 1975

Abbreviation List

Enzymes:
Cholesterol ester transfer protein (CETP)
Hepatic triglyceride lipase (HTgL)
Lipoprotein lipase (LpL)
Lecithin cholesteryl acetyl transferase (LCAT)

Lipoprotein particles:
High density lipoprotein (HDL)
intermediate density lipoprotein (IDL)
Low density lipoprotein (LDL)
Very low density lipoprotein (VLDL)

Other:
Apolipoprotein CIII (Apo CIII)
Coronary Artery Disease (CAD)
Triglyceride (TG)

Trials:
MARS – The Monitored Atherosclerosis Regression Study
CLAS – The Cholesterol-Lowering Atherosclerosis Study
STARS – The St. Thomas Atherosclerosis regression Study
FATS – The Familial Atherosclerosis Treatment Study
CCAIT – The Canadian Coronary Atherosclerosis Intervention Trial
LOCAT – Lopid Coronary Angiography Trial
BECAIT – Bezafibrate Coronary Atherosclerosis Intervention Trial
CDP – Coronary Drug Project
Stockholm Ischemic Study
Helsinki – Helskinki Heart Study
BIP – Bezofibrate Infarction Prevention Trial
VA-HIT – VA-HDL Intervention Trial
DAIS – Diabetes Atherosclerosis Intervention Study
WOSCOPS – West of Scotland Coronary Prevention Study
4S – Scandinavian Simvastatin Survival Study
CARE – Cholesterol and Recurrent Events trial
LIPID – Long-term Intervention with Pravastatin in Ischemic Disease

GEMFIBROZIL IN THE SECONDARY PREVENTION OF CORONARY HEART DISEASE: THE VA-HIT TRIAL

Hanna Bloomfield Rubins, Dorothea Collins, Sander J. Robins

Although most patients with established coronary heart disease (CHD) have an elevated level of low-density lipoprotein (LDL) cholesterol, a substantial minority (about 20 to 30%) have low-risk LDL cholesterol in association with low levels of high-density lipoprotein (HDL) cholesterol (Rubins et al., 1995). A low level of HDL cholesterol [i.e.,$<$0.91 mmol/L ($<$35 mg/dL)], with or without an elevated LDL cholesterol [i.e.,$<$3.36 mmol/L ($<$130 mg/dL)], is an independent risk factor for new or recurrent CHD events. However, until the recent publication of the Department of Veterans Affairs HDL Intervention Trial (VA-HIT), there were no clinical trial data to guide decisions about lipid therapy for this population (Rubins et al., 1999). In this chapter we summarize and discuss the results of VA-HIT.

Methods

This study was a randomized, placebo-controlled clinical trial conducted at 20 VA medical centers throughout the United States. The hypothesis of the study was that therapy aimed at raising HDL cholesterol and lowering triglycerides would reduce the incidence of major coronary events in men with established CHD, low levels of HDL cholesterol, and low levels of LDL cholesterol. Gemfibrozil was chosen as the intervention because it was the agent considered most likely to raise HDL cholesterol and lower triglycerides while having the least effect on LDL cholesterol concentrations.

*VA-HIT was supported by the Cooperative Studies Program of the Department of Veterans Affairs Office of Research and Development and by a supplemental grant from Parke-Davis, a division of Warner Lambert.

The views expressed in this article are those of the authors and do not necessarily represent the Department of Veterans Affairs.

The following were the major entrance criteria:

1. Age < 74 years
2. Established CHD, defined by the presence of one of the following:
    a. History of myocardial infarction (MI)
    b. Angina corroborated by objective evidence of ischemia
    c. History of coronary revascularization
    d. >50% stenosis of more than one major epicardial coronary artery by angiography
3. Absence of serious comorbid conditions
4. HDL cholesterol ≤1.30 mmol/L (≤40 mg/dL), LDL cholesterol ≤ 3.62 mmol/L (≤140 mg/dL), and triglycerides ≤3.39 mmol/L (≤300 mg/dL).

Patients were randomized to either gemfibrozil, 1200 mg/d, or matching placebo. A study coordinator saw patients 1 month after randomization and then every 3 months for the duration of the study. The staff provided instruction in the American Heart Association Step 1 diet and advised each patient to consult with his primary physician regarding an appropriate exercise regimen. All patients were expected to attend regular follow-up visits whether or not they were still taking study medication and were followed until death, refusal of further visits, or the conclusion of the study.

The primary end-point was the combined incidence of nonfatal MI or CHD death, as determined by the end-points committee, which was blinded to treatment assignment and lipid results. Clinically silent MIs were included, defined as the occurrence on routine annual electrocardiogram of new diagnostic Q waves. All electrocardiograms were read at a central electrocardiographic coding center using the Minnesota code. Secondary outcomes included other cardiovascular and cerebrovascular events and procedures, cancer, and total mortality. A stroke adjudication committee composed of three neurologists blinded to treatment assignment and lipid levels used predefined criteria to adjudicate strokes, a secondary outcome, on the basis of clinical and radiographic data.

All analyses used an intent-to-treat approach. The study was not designed to have adequate power to detect differences in total mortality.

Results

2531 patients were recruited from September 1991 through December 1993 and were followed for an average of 5 years. The baseline characteristics of the enrolled patients are shown in Table 7-1.

TABLE 7-1

BASELINE CHARACTERISTICS IN THE VA HDL INTERVENTION TRIAL (VA-HIT), N = 2531

Age (yrs.)	64 ± 7
Male (%)	100
Current Smoker (%)	21
Hypertension (%)	57
Diabetes (%)	25
Prior myocardial infarction (%)	61
Medication use (%)	
Aspirin	82
Calcium channel blockers	53
ACE inhibitors	21
Beta blockers	43
Waist circumference (cm)	103 ± 12
Body mass index (kg/m^2)	29 ± 5
Plasma lipids [mmol/L (mg/dL)]	
Total cholesterol	4.53 ± 0.65 (175 ± 25)
LDL cholesterol	2.87 ± 0.59 (111 ± 23)
HDL cholesterol	0.83 ± 0.13 (32 ± 5)
Triglycerides	1.82 ± 0.77 (161 ± 68)

NOTE: Numbers with ± indicate mean and standard deviation; diabetes and hypertension are defined by clinical history; ACE, angiotensin-converting enzyme.

Two-thirds of the patients were over the age of 65. There was a high prevalence of diabetes (25%), hypertension (57%), and overweight (mean body mass index 29 kg/m^2). The average LDL cholesterol was 2.9 mmol/L (111 mg/dL), and the average HDL cholesterol was 0.83 mmol/L (32 mg/dL).

As compared with placebo, at 1 year patients in the gemfibrozil group had an average HDL cholesterol increase of 6%, a triglyceride reduction of 31%, and a total cholesterol reduction of 4%; all these changes were statistically significant. In contrast, the on-trial LDL cholesterol did not differ between the two groups.

As shown in Table 7-2, gemfibrozil was associated with a highly significant 22% relative risk reduction for the primary end-point, nonfatal MI and CHD death. While cardiac revascularization procedures were less common in the gemfibrozil group, the difference in rates was not statistically significant. Cerebrovascular events, including strokes, transient ischemic attacks, and carotid endarterectomies, were also significantly reduced in the gemfibrozil group.

TABLE 7-2

MAJOR EVENTS IN VA-HIT BY TREATMENT GROUP

Event	Placebo ($n = 1267$) No. (%)	Gemfibrozil ($n = 1264$) No. (%)	Risk reduction, %[a] (95% CI)	p Value[a]
Nonfatal myocardial infarction or CHD death	275 (21.7)	219 (17.3)	22 (7 to 35)	.006
Nonfatal myocardial infarction, CHD death, or confirmed stroke	330 (26)	258 (20.4)	24 (11 to 36)	<.001
Nonfatal myocardial infarction	184 (14.5)	146 (11.6)	23 (4 to 38)	.02
CHD death	118 (9.3)	93 (7.4)	22 (−2 to 41)	.07
Total deaths	220 (17.4)	198 (15.7)	11 (−8 to 27)	.23
Investigator-designated stroke	88 (7.0)	64 (5.1)	29 (2 to 48)	.04
Confirmed stroke	76 (6)	58 (4.6)	25 (−6 to 47)	.10
Transient ischemic attack	53 (4.2)	22 (1.7)	59 (33 to 75)	<.001
CABG or PTCA	287 (22.7)	266 (21)	9 (−8 to 23)	.29
Peripheral vascular surgery	28 (2.2)	19 (1.5)	33 (−20 to 63)	.18
Carotid endarterectomy	44 (3.5)	16 (1.3)	65 (37 to 80)	<.001
Hospitalization for unstable angina	453 (35.8)	457 (36.2)	−0.4 (−14 to 12)	.95
Hospitalization for congestive heart failure	168 (13.3)	134 (10.6)	22 (2 to 38)	.04

[a] Relative risk reductions, 95% confidence intervals, and p values are derived from Cox models.
ABBREVIATIONS: CABG, coronary artery bypass graft; PTCA, percutaneous transluminal coronary angioplasty; CHD, coronary heart disease; CI, confidence interval.

For confirmed strokes ($n = 134$), the vast majority of which were ischemic, the relative risk reduction with gemfibrozil was 25% (Rubins et al., 2001).

In order to determine whether there were any differences in treatment response among patient subgroups, an exploratory analysis was conducted using the expanded end-point of nonfatal MI, coronary death, or stroke. As shown in the Figure 7-1, gemfibrozil was associated with a relative risk reduction in all subgroups examined, with the

exception of current cigarette smokers. Thus diabetics and nondiabetics, older and younger patients, patients with and without hypertension, patients on and not on aspirin, and patients with lipids above and below the median values all appeared to derive a clinical benefit from the therapy.

Gemfibrozil was well tolerated in this population of predominantly older men with multiple comorbidities. The rate of medication discontinuation was the same in the treatment and control groups—30% at the end of the trial. The only symptom reported significantly more often in the gemfibrozil group was stomach upset. Overall, there were fewer deaths and fewer incident cancers in the gemfibrozil group.

A secondary analysis of the VA-HIT data explored the relationship between the major lipid fractions, both at baseline and during the trial, and the occurrence of CHD events (Robins et al., 2001). In multivariate analysis, among the three major lipids, only the on-trial level of HDL cholesterol was significantly associated with the development of CHD events. Nevertheless, taken together, on-trial levels of HDL cholesterol, LDL cholesterol, and triglyceride accounted for less than 25% of the treatment benefit associated with gemfibrozil. It is likely therefore that other effects of the drug, discussed below, play a role in its clinical effectiveness.

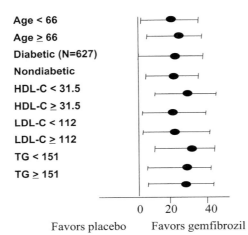

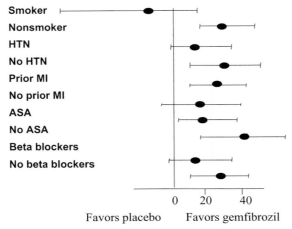

FIGURE 7-1

Relative risk reductions (%) and 95% confidence intervals for coronary heart disease death, myocardial infarction, and adjudicated stroke in subgroups in VA-HIT

Implications

This is the first large-scale trial to show that lipid therapy that did not lower the concentration of LDL cholesterol was effective for the prevention of major cardiovascular events in patients with established CHD. This suggests that, in addition to the well-known benefits of lowering elevated LDL cholesterol, therapy aimed at HDL cholesterol and triglycerides may also be a useful therapeutic approach for prevention of CHD.

Mechanisms

As is the case for all clinical drug trials, we can only speculate on the mechanisms responsible for the observed clinical benefit. Gemfibrozil is known to have favorable effects on lipid metabolism (e.g., increase in HDL cholesterol; improvements in triglyceride metabolism; change in the composition, size, or density of LDL particles) and on other processes that may affect the development or manifestations of atherothrombotic disease (e.g., endothelial function, coagulation, and inflammation). Gemfibrozil and other fibrates lower plasma triglycerides by stimulating intravascular lipolysis. This process liberates excess apoproteins and lipids for use in the formation of new HDL particles. Fibrates also increase HDL by stimulating the hepatic synthesis of apo AI and apo AII, the major protein constituents of HDL. HDL is thought to exert its antiatherogenic effect principally by serving as the acceptor particle for peripherally derived cholesterol, which it transports to the liver for excretion from the body, a process known as *reverse cholesterol transport* (Hill and McQueen, 1997). The decrease in triglyceride level observed with fibrates is accompanied by a decrease in LDL density and an increase in LDL particle size; larger, more buoyant LDL particles are thought to be less atherogenic than smaller, denser particles. Fibrates also have antiinflammatory effects and direct effects on endothelial function that can result in atherosclerotic plaques that are less likely to rupture and cause clinical sequelae. These agents are also known to alter various hemostatic parameters, including clotting factor VII and plasminogen activator inhibitor 1, leading to a less prothrombotic state.

Other Clinical Trials

Previous clinical trials of lipid therapy have all focused on LDL cholesterol reduction, although some have used regimens designed to lower LDL cholesterol as well as to raise HDL cholesterol and lower triglycerides. More important, no other major clinical trial has enrolled patients with as low a level of LDL cholesterol as were enrolled in VA-HIT. Therefore, there is little information on whether other interventions, such as statins, niacin, or drug combinations, would be as beneficial as gemfibrozil in CHD patients with low LDL cholesterol. With respect to statins, the best information comes from subgroup analyses from two large clinical trials that included patients with a wide range of baseline LDL cholesterol (Sacks et al., 1996; LIPID Study Group, 1998; Sacks et al., 2000). In these studies, pravastatin was not associated with a reduction in major cardiovascular events in the subgroup of patients with LDL cholesterol <3.23 mmol/L (<125 mg/dL). Clinical trials specifically designed to assess the efficacy of statins or statin/fibrate combinations in persons with low levels of LDL cholesterol are currently underway.

Approach to the Patient with Low HDL Cholesterol

Lifestyle intervention, as well as treatment for concomitant risk factors (e.g., diabetes and hypertension), is recommended for all patients with low HDL cholesterol. Lifestyle interventions (weight loss, increased physical activity, and smoking cessation, as applicable) are particularly important in patients with the metabolic syndrome, as emphasized in the recent treatment recommendations of the National Cholesterol Education Program (NCEP Expert Panel, 2001). The metabolic syndrome is diagnosed when three or more of the following risk factors are present: abdominal obesity, high triglycerides, low HDL cholesterol, hypertension, and glucose intolerance.

Routine pharmacologic therapy to raise HDL cholesterol is not currently supported by clinical trial evidence, with the exception of two groups. For those in whom low HDL cholesterol is accompanied by high LDL cholesterol [>3.36 mmol/L (>130 mg/dL)], pharmacologic management directed towards lowering the LDL cholesterol with statins is indicated in patients with established CHD and may also be appropriate for those at high risk of CHD, based on the results of the Air Force/Texas Coronary Atherosclerosis Prevention Study (Downs et al., 1998). For CHD patients with low HDL cholesterol and low levels of LDL cholesterol [<3.36 mmol/L (<130 mg/dL)], VA-HIT shows that gemfibrozil is effective for prevention of recurrent cardiac events.

REFERENCES

Downs JR et al: Primary prevention of acute coronary events with lovastatin in men and women with average cholesterol levels. Results of AFCAPS/TexCAPS. JAMA 279:1615, 1998

Hill SA, McQueen MJ: Reverse cholesterol transport— a review of the process and its clinical implications. Clin Biochem 30:517, 1997

The Long-term Intervention with Pravastatin in Ischaemic Disease (LIPID) Study Group: Prevention of cardiovascular events and death with pravastatin in patients with coronary heart disease and a broad range of initial cholesterol levels. N Engl J Med 339:1349, 1998

NCEP Expert Panel: Executive summary of the third report of the National Cholesterol Education Program (NCEP) Expert Panel on Detection, Evaluation, and Treatment of High Blood Cholesterol in Adults (Adult Treatment Panel III). JAMA 285:2486, 2001

Robins SJ et al: Relation of events to baseline and on-trial lipids with gemfibrozil in the VA HDL Intervention Trial (VA-HIT). JAMA 285:1585, 2001

Rubins HB et al: Distribution of lipids in 8,500 men with coronary artery disease. Am J Cardiol 75:1196, 1995

Rubins HB et al: Gemfibrozil for the secondary prevention of coronary heart disease in men with low levels of high-density lipoprotein cholesterol. N Engl J Med 341:410, 1999

Rubins HB et al: Reduction in stroke with gemfibrozil in men with coronary heart disease and low HDL-cholesterol: The VA HDL Intervention trial (VA-HIT). Circulation 103:2828, 2001

Sacks FM et al: The effect of pravastatin on coronary events after myocardial infarction in patients with average cholesterol levels. N Engl J Med 335:1001, 1996

Sacks FM et al: Effect of pravastatin in subgroups defined by coronary risk factors: The Prospective Pravastatin Pooling Project. Circulation 102:1893, 2000

INTENSIVE LIFE-STYLE CHANGES IN THE MANAGEMENT OF CORONARY HEART DISEASE

Dean Ornish

During the past 10 years, increasing evidence has provided a more complete understanding of the mechanisms of coronary heart disease (CHD). This understanding provides increasing justification for using intensive life-style changes in managing CHD. While coronary atherosclerosis contributes to myocardial ischemia, so do other mechanisms that may change rapidly—for better and for worse. These include variations in coronary artery vasomotor tone, platelet aggregability, blood viscosity, endothelial stability, inflammation, and collateral circulation.

Each of these mechanisms may be directly influenced by life-style factors, including cigarette smoking, diet, emotional stress, depression, and exercise. The most common cause of myocardial infarction, sudden cardiac death, or unstable angina is rupture of an atherosclerotic plaque, often associated with localized coronary thrombosis and/or coronary artery spasm. Research publications since 1990 have shown consistently that intensive risk factor modification can reduce cardiac events quite rapidly by stabilizing the endothelium within a relatively short period of time, whether via comprehensive changes in diet and life-style or with lipid-lowering drugs, or both, even before there is time for meaningful regression in coronary atherosclerosis.

In this chapter, some of these mechanisms are discussed; the evidence from life-style intervention trials is described; and strategies that may be helpful in motivating patients to make and to maintain beneficial changes in diet and life-style are summarized (Ornish, 1992).

Life-Style Factors
Smoking

Although smoking contributes to the progression of coronary atherosclerosis, nicotine is also a powerful stimulant of vasoconstriction and platelet aggregation. Changes in these more dynamic mechanisms help to explain why smoking cessation may quickly reduce the risk of myocardial infarction. Male and female ex-smokers have about the same mortality rate from heart disease as nonsmokers only 2 to 3 years after quitting.

The evidence that smoking cessation will reduce the rate of CHD comes from a large set of epidemiologic and pathophysiologic studies (Atherosclerosis Study Group, 1984). In the Coronary Artery Surgery Study, patients undergoing coronary artery bypass surgery who continued to smoke had an almost twofold relative risk of death. After 10 years of follow-up, smokers were more likely to have angina, to be unemployed, to have greater limitation of activity, and to have more hospital admissions (Cavender et al., 1992).

Diet

Dietary intake of saturated fat and cholesterol has been linked with coronary atherosclerosis in a large number of epidemiologic studies, animal research, and randomized controlled trials in humans. Less well known is how quickly dietary fat and cholesterol may affect myocardial perfusion via changes in platelet aggregation and coronary vasomotor tone. For example, dietary fat intake increases plasma levels of factor VII coagulant activity (VIIa) and thus coagulability. The effect is rapid, so that much of the benefit of dietary fat reduction on thrombogenic risk in CHD is likely to occur within a short time. Changing to a low-fat, low-cholesterol diet may decrease plasma levels of factor VII coagulant activity. Collateral vessels are smaller in diameter than epicardial coronary arteries, so the coronary microcirculation may be particularly affected by these changes. Even a single high-fat meal transiently impairs endothelial function and blood flow within only 1 h, whereas this does not occur on a low-fat diet.

Although patients often receive conflicting information about what constitutes an optimal diet, increasing scientific evidence indicates that a meat-based diet is high in disease-causing substances and low in protective ones, whereas a plant-based diet is low in harmful substances and high in protective ones. For example, dietary cholesterol is found only in meat and animal products, which tend to be high in both total fat and in saturated fat. A plant-based diet has no cholesterol and, with few exceptions, is low in total fat and in saturated fat. Meat is rich in oxidants such as iron [which may oxidize low-density lipoprotein (LDL) cholesterol to a more atherogenic form] yet low in antioxidants, whereas a plant-based diet is low in oxidants and high in antioxidants. Meat has virtually no dietary fiber, which is rich in a plant-based diet.

In other words, what we *include* in our diets is as important as what we *exclude*. There is growing interest in what are known as "functional foods," i.e., foods containing substances that are disease-preventing and health-promoting beyond the traditional nutrients such as the amount of fat, protein, and carbohydrates that they contain. There are many other substances in a plant-based diet that may be protective, including phytochemicals, isoflavonoids, lignans, carotenoids, retinols, lycopene, geninstein, and others.

The step 1 and step 2 diets recommended by the American Heart Association and the National Cholesterol Education Program, as well as the "TLC" (Therapeutic Lifestyle Changes) diet described in the more recent Adult Treatment Panel III (ATP III) guidelines (Expert Panel, 2001) do not go far enough to stop the progression of coronary atherosclerosis in the majority of patients with coronary heart disease as assessed by serial coronary arteriography (Ornish, 1994). Why not?

The level of plasma LDL is regulated by the LDL receptor, a cell-surface glycoprotein that removes LDL from plasma by receptor-mediated endocytosis. Most patients with coronary atherosclerosis have plasma LDL cholesterol levels that are many times higher than the level necessary to saturate the LDL receptor system. For them, a step 1 or step 2 diet may still saturate and suppress the LDL receptor system, thereby leading to further progression of coronary atherosclerosis and little fall in plasma cholesterol levels. However, further reduction of dietary fat and cholesterol may be sufficient to cause significant reductions in plasma LDL cholesterol and regression of coronary atherosclerosis.

In clinical practice, patients with hypercholesterolemia are often prescribed a step 2 or TLC diet. When they return on their next visit, their LDL cholesterol usually has not declined very much. Patients are then often told that they "failed diet," when, in actuality, they just didn't go far enough.

Many patients, perhaps most, can achieve the therapeutic goal of LDL < 2.6 Mmol/L (<100 mg/dL) without lipid-lowering drugs if they make changes in diet and life-style that are more intensive than the NCEP panel recommended. After 1 year, these intensive changes in diet and life-style reduced LDL cholesterol by 40% [from an average LDL of 3.7 to 2.2 Mmol/L (143.3 to 86.6 mg/dL)] in ambulatory patients who were not taking cholesterol-lowering drugs (Ornish et al., 1998). In Asia, where a very low fat diet is the norm, the average LDL in the entire population is < 2.5 Mmol/L (<95 mg/dL) (Campbell et al., 1998). It has been estimated that nearly $30 billion a year are spent each year in the United States on cholesterol-lowering drugs, yet much of this could be avoided by making comprehensive life-style changes that go beyond the conventional guidelines.

There is a spectrum of dietary changes based on a patient's diagnosis and the ability to metabolize dietary saturated fat and cholesterol. The "reversal diet" is designed for those who have been diagnosed with CHD. This is a whole-foods vegetarian diet high in complex carbohydrates, low in simple carbohydrates (e.g., sugar, concentrated sweeteners, alcohol, white flour), and very low in fat (approximately 10% of calories). The diet consists primarily of fruits, vegetables, grains, and beans (including soy-based foods) supplemented by moderate amounts of non fat dairy and egg whites. Overweight patients or those with high triglyceride levels are especially encouraged to limit their intake of simple sugars and alcohol, since these may provoke an insulin response. Insulin increases the conversion of calories into triglycerides and stimulates HMG CoA reductase. In contrast, the fiber in whole foods slows absorption of food and prevents an excessive insulin response. High-protein diets are not recommended.

The "prevention diet" is customized to meet the needs of an individual. As discussed above, there is a genetic variability in how efficiently (or inefficiently) someone can metabolize dietary saturated fat and cholesterol based in part on the number of LDL receptors. Since it is difficult to measure the number of LDL receptors in the general population, one can use the ratio of total cholesterol to high-density lipoprotein (HDL) cholesterol as a surrogate marker. If a person's total cholesterol is consistently <3.9 Mmol/L (<150 mg/dL) or if the ratio of total cholesterol to HDL is consistently less than 4.0, then either that person is not eating very much saturated fat and cholesterol or the person is very efficient at metabolizing it (due in part to the number of LDL receptors); either way, their risk of coronary atherosclerosis is low. If not, then the person can begin making moderate changes (e.g., a step 1 or step 2 or TLC diet); if that is enough to bring their lipid values into this range, then that may be all they need to do.

For most people, however, a step 1 or step 2 diet does not go far enough to achieve these lipid goals. Patients then have a choice: to go on the reversal diet or to begin a lifetime of cholesterol-lowering drugs. Patients should be supported in whatever choice they make as long as they understand the full range of therapeutic options.

A Mediterranean diet is better than the American diet but not as healthful as an Asian diet. Heart attacks and deaths from heart disease are lower in Mediterranean countries than in the United States but are even lower in Asian countries such as Japan and China, where the dietary intake of fat, cholesterol, and olive oil is lower than in Mediterranean countries. In terms of their postprandial effect on endothelial function, the beneficial components of the Mediterranean and Lyon Diet Heart Study diets appear to be antioxidant-rich foods (including vegetables, fruits, and their derivatives such as vinegar) and omega-3-rich fish and canola oils, but not olive oil, which may reduce blood flow.

The supplements in Table 8-1 are recommended for most men and postmenopausal women. Patients on statin drugs should first consult with their physician before taking antioxidant vitamins.

Emotional Stress and Hostility

Emotional stress may lead to myocardial ischemia both via coronary artery spasm and by increased platelet aggregation within coronary arteries. Stress may lead to coronary spasm mediated either by direct α-adrenergic stimulation or secondary to the

TABLE 8-1

RECOMMENDED SUPPLEMENTS FOR MOST ADULTS

Vitamin C	1000 mg/d (1 g/d)
Vitamin E	400 I.U. per day
Folate	1 mg/d (to reduce homocysteine levels, a risk factor for coronary heart disease)
Fish oil	3 g/d (provides omega-3 fatty acids)
Selenium	100–200 µg/d

Multivitamin without iron for men and postmenopausal women (adjust above amounts as needed); premenopausal women may benefit from a multivitamin with iron.

Replace animal or dairy protein with soy protein when possible.

release of thromboxane A_2 from platelets, perhaps via increasing circulating catecholamines or other mediators. Both thromboxane A_2 and catecholamines are potent constrictors of arterial smooth muscle and powerful endogenous stimulators of platelet aggregation.

Personally relevant mental stress may be an important precipitant of myocardial ischemia—often silent—in patients with coronary artery disease. Acute mental stress may be a frequent trigger of transient myocardial ischemia, myocardial infarction, and sudden cardiac death (Bairey et al., 1990). Postmenopausal women may have greater cardiovascular responses to stress than men or premenopausal women. Atherosclerotic monkeys with chronic psychosocial disruption had coronary artery *constriction* in response to acetylcholine, whereas atherosclerotic monkeys living in a stable social setting had coronary artery *vasodilation* in response to acetylcholine, even though both groups of monkeys were consuming a cholesterol-lowering diet (Williams et al., 1991).

In an analysis of over 45 studies, hostility has emerged as one of the most important personality variables in CHD (Miller et al., 1996). The effects of hostility are equal to or greater in magnitude than the traditional risk factors for heart disease. Hostility appears to be a primary toxic component of the type A behavioral pattern.

Depression

Several studies have shown that depression significantly increases the risk of developing CHD. One study of 1551 people in the Baltimore area who were free of heart disease in 1981 found that those who were depressed were more than four times as likely to have a heart attack in the next 14 years. Depression increased risk as much as did hypercholesterolemia (Pratt et al., 1996). Depression also increases the risk of subsequent myocardial infarction in patients with existing CHD. Unfortunately, depression often goes untreated.

One study examined the survival of elderly men and women hospitalized for an acute myocardial infarction who had emotional support compared with those patients who lacked such support. More than three times as many men and women died in the hospital who had no source of emotional support compared with those with two or more sources of support. Among those who survived and were discharged from the hospital, after 6 months 53% of those with no source of support had died compared with 36% of those with one source and 23% of those with two or more sources of support. These figures did not change significantly after 1 year. When controlled for other factors that might have influenced survival (such as severity of the infarction, age, gender, other illnesses, depression), men and women who reported no emotional support had almost three times the mortality risk compared with those who had at least one source of support (Berkman et al., 1992). In another study, investigators followed 222 patients who had suffered myocardial infarction and found that those who were depressed were four times as likely to die in the next 6 months as those who were not depressed (Lesperance et al., 1996).

Many depressed patients are, paradoxically, in a constant state of hyperarousal, causing sustained hyperactivity of the two principal effectors of the stress response: the corticotropin-releasing hormone (CRH) system and the locus coeruleus–norepinephrine (LC-NE) system. Norepinephrine may precipitate vasoconstriction, platelet aggregation, and arrhythmias. Cortisol may accelerate atherosclerosis. When patients are treated for depression, these changes in CRH and LC-NE may return to normal. Beta blockers help blunt the hyperarousal state but may exacerbate depression, whereas meditation may reduce hyper reactivity without causing depression.

Social factors, including social support, play an important role in adherence to comprehensive life-style changes and may have powerful effects on morbidity and mortality independent of influences on known risk factors. An increasing number of studies have shown that those who feel socially isolated have three to five times the risk of premature death, not only from CHD but also from all causes, when compared to those who have a sense of connection and community (House et al., 1988). For example, investigators at Duke University studied almost 1400 men and women who underwent coronary angiography and were found to have had at least one severe coronary artery stenosis. After 5 years, men and women who were unmarried and who did not have a close confidant—someone to talk with on a regular basis—were over three times as likely to have died than those who were married, had a confidant, or both. These differences were independent of any other known medical prognostic risk factors (Williams et al., 1992).

Exercise

The role of exercise in the prevention and treatment of CHD is well known and is supported by several reviews of the literature. Two meta-analyses indicated that the risk of death was doubled in those who were physically inactive when compared with more active individuals (Berlin and Colditz, 1990). Rehabilitation programs incorporating exercise also show modest benefits of exercise in preventing recurrent CHD events. None of 22 individual randomized trials in the meta-analysis had the power to show a significant treatment effect, but in a meta-analysis employing the intention-to-treat analysis, there was a significant reduction of 25% in 1- to 3-year rates of CHD and total mortality in the patients receiving cardiac rehabilitation when compared with control patients.

Moderate exercise provides most of the improvement in longevity (compared to more intensive exercise) while minimizing the risks of exercising. In one study, investigators performed treadmill testing on 10,224 men and 3120 women who were apparently healthy (Blair et al., 1989). Based on their fitness level, these participants were divided into five categories, ranging from least fit (group 1) to most fit (group 5). The researchers followed this population to determine how their level of physical fitness related to their death rates. After 8 years, the least fit had a death rate more than three times greater than the most fit. More important, though, was the finding that most of the benefits of physical fitness occurred between groups 1 and 2. However, even substantial decreases in cardiovascular fitness resulting from decades of inactivity can be substantially reversed with modest endurance training.

Can Intensive Life-style Changes Reverse Coronary Heart Disease?

The Lifestyle Heart Trial was the first randomized, clinical trial to investigate whether ambulatory patients could be motivated to make and sustain comprehensive life-style changes and, if so, whether the progression of coronary atherosclerosis could be stopped or reversed (without using lipid-lowering drugs), as measured by computer-assisted quantitative coronary arteriography (Ornish et al., 1998). This study derived from earlier studies that used noninvasive measures such as exercise thallium scintigraphy and radionuclide ventriculography (Ornish et al., 1983).

Experimental-group patients made and maintained comprehensive life-style changes for 5 years, whereas control-group patients made more moderate changes. In the experimental group, the average percent diameter stenosis, as measured by quantitative coronary arteriography, showed even more improvement in percent diameter stenosis after 5 years than after 1 year, whereas in the control group the average stenosis worsened after 1 year and continued to progress after 5 years (Fig. 8-1).

The risk ratio of total cardiac events was 2.5 times greater in the control group than in the experimental group ($p = .0002$).

Changes in stenosis were strongly associated with adherence to the life-style intervention and with changes in lipids. Older patients improved as much as younger ones. On average, the more participants changed their diet and life-style, the more they improved (Fig. 8-2). The risks of revascularization increase with age, but the benefits of intensive life-style changes do not seem to be age-related.

These moderate changes in coronary atherosclerosis were accompanied by substantial improvements in myocardial perfusion as measured by cardiac positron emission tomography (PET) scans (Gould et al., 1995) (Fig. 8-3).

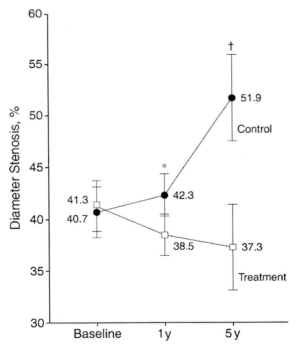

FIGURE 8-1.

Mean percentage diameter stenosis in treatment and control groups at baseline, 1 year, and 5 years. Error bars represent SEM; *, $p = .02$ by between-group 2-tailed test; †, $p = .001$ by between-group 2-tailed test (From Ornish, D et al., JAMA 280:2001, 1998).

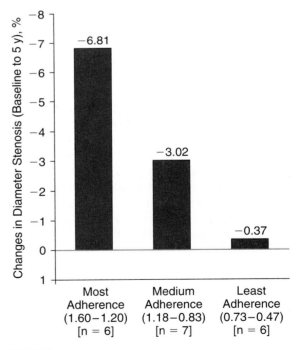

FIGURE 8-2.

Changes in percentage diameter stenosis by 5-year adherence tertiles for the experimental group (From Ornish, D et al., JAMA 280:2001, 1998).

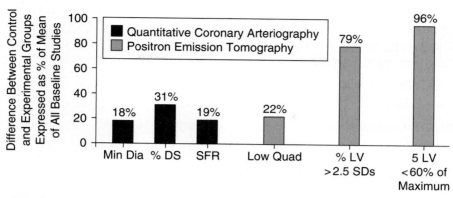

FIGURE 8-3.

Comparison of changes by positron emission tomography (PET) and quantitative coronary arteriography (QCA). The PET measures were myocardial quadrant with the lowest average activity (Low Quad), percentage of left ventricle (LV) outside 2 SDs of normals, and percentage of LV activity less than 60% of maximal activity. Measurements by QCA were minimum absolute lumen diameter (Min Dia); percent diameter stenosis (percent DS) and stenosis flow reserve (SFR) derived from the integrated effects of lumen diameter, percent DS, and cumulative length effects based on fluid dynamic equations, all as previously validated and reported. The absolute difference in changes between the control and experimental groups (without the minus or plus sign for direction of change) was expressed as a percentage of the mean of each measurement at baseline for all patients (From Gould, KL, JAMA 274:894, 1995).

These findings also have particular significance for women. Women have less access to bypass surgery and angioplasty. When women undergo these operations, they have higher morbidity and mortality rates than men. However, women may be able to reverse heart disease even more easily than men when they make comprehensive life-style changes or when they take lipid-lowering drugs.

Multicenter Life-style Demonstration Project

The next research question was: how practical and cost-effective are intensive life-style changes? The Multicenter Life-style Demonstration Project was designed to determine if comprehensive life-style changes can be a direct alternative to revascularization for selected patients without increasing cardiac events.

In the past, insurance companies, managed care organizations, and Medicare were reluctant to pay for intensive life-style interventions, in part because these were viewed only as prevention: increasing costs in the short run for a possible savings years later. Also, since approximately 20 to 30% of patients change insurers each year, even if cost savings result from life-style interventions, they may accrue to another company. However, a program of comprehensive life-style changes may be offered as a much less costly alternative treatment to revascularization for selected patients who are eligible for coronary artery bypass surgery (CABG) or percutaneous transluminal coronary angioplasty (PTCA) (under the supervision of the referring physician), thereby resulting in immediate and substantial cost savings.

Is it safe to offer intensive life-style changes as an alternative to revascularization? CABG is effective in reducing angina and improving cardiac function. However, when compared with medical therapy and followed for 16 years, CABG improved survival in only a very small subgroup of patients: those with reduced left ventricular function and stenotic lesions of the left main coronary artery of

TABLE 8-2

COMPARISON OF INTENSIVE LIFE-STYLE CHANGES (ILC), ANGIOPLASTY (PTCA), AND BYPASS SURGERY (CABG)

	ILC	PTCA	CABG
Rapid ↓ angina	x	x	x
Rapid ↑ myocardial perfusion	x	x	x
↓ Cardiac events	x		x (subset)
Continued ↓ in stenosis over time	x		
Continued ↑ in perfusion over time	x		
Improvements in nondilated lesions	x		
Improvements in nonbypassed lesions	x		
Costs	+	+++	+++++

>59%. Median survival was not prolonged in patients with left main disease <60% and normal left ventricular function, even if a significant right coronary artery stenosis >70% was also present (Alderman et al., 1990). Varnauskas, 1998).

PTCA was developed with the hope of providing a less invasive, lower risk approach to the management of coronary artery disease and its symptoms. In low-risk patients with stable disease, aggressive lipid-lowering therapy is at least as effective as angioplasty and usual care in reducing the incidence of ischemic events (Pitt et al., 1999).

The majority of adverse events related to coronary artery disease, myocardial infarction, sudden death, and unstable angina are due to the rupture of an atherosclerotic plaque of less than 40 to 50% stenosis. This often occurs in the setting of vessel spasm and results in thrombosis and occlusion of the vessel (Fuster et al., 1992). CABG and PTCA are usually not performed on lesions <50% stenosed and do not affect nonbypassed or nondilated lesions, whereas comprehensive life-style changes (or lipid-lowering drugs) may help stabilize all lesions, including mild lesions (<50% stenosis). Also, mild lesions that undergo catastrophic progression usually have a less well-developed network of collateral circulation to protect the myocardium than do more severe stenoses.

Bypass surgery and angioplasty have risks of morbidity and mortality associated with them, whereas there are no significant risks from eating a well-balanced low-fat, low-cholesterol diet; stopping smoking; or engaging in moderate walking, stress management techniques, and psychosocial support (Table 8-2).

A total of 333 patients completed the Multicenter Life-style Demonstration Project (194 in the experimental group and 139 in the control group). It was found that experimental group patients were able to avoid revascularization for at least 3 years by making comprehensive life-style changes at substantially lower cost without increasing cardiac morbidity and mortality (Ornish, 1998). These patients reported reductions in angina comparable to what can be achieved with revascularization. The average savings per patient were $29,529.

Practical Considerations

Life-style factors such as diet, smoking, and emotional stress often interact. For example, people are often more likely to overeat, smoke, work too hard, or abuse drugs and alcohol when they feel lonely, depressed, or isolated. Thus, stress management techniques and group support may address some of these deeper concerns, thereby making it easier for patients to change diet and quit smoking (Ornish and Hart, 1998). Sometimes, patients may also benefit from referral to a psychotherapist for treatment of depression with counseling and/or antidepressants.

The conventional medical thinking is that taking a statin drug is easy and most patients will comply but that making comprehensive life-style changes is virtually impossible for almost everyone. In fact, fewer than 50% of patients who are prescribed statin drugs are taking them as prescribed just 1 year later (Rogers and Bullman, 1995). One might think that compliance to lipid-lowering drugs would always be much higher than to comprehensive diet and life-style changes, since taking pills is relatively easy and the side effects are minimal for most patients. However, cholesterol-lowering drugs do not make most patients feel better. They are taken today in hopes that there may be a long-term benefit by reducing the risk of a myocardial infarction or sudden cardiac death.

To many patients, concepts such as "risk factor modification" and "prevention" are considered boring, and they do not initiate or sustain the levels of motivation needed to make intensive life-style changes. "Am I going to live longer, or is it just going to *seem* longer?" Also, the prospects of a myocardial infarction or death are so frightening for many patients that their denial often keeps them from thinking about them at all. Because of this, adherence becomes difficult. (Patients will often adhere to a risk factor reduction program very well for a few weeks after a heart attack until the denial returns.) Fear is a powerful motivator in the short but not in the long term.

While fear of dying may not be a sustainable motivator, joy of living often is. Paradoxically, it may be easier for some patients to make comprehensive changes all at once than to make small, gradual changes or even to take a cholesterol-lowering drug. For example, when patients follow a step 2 diet, they often have a sense of deprivation but not much apparent benefit. LDL cholesterol is reduced by an average of only 5%, frequency of angina does not improve much, lost weight is usually regained, and coronary artery lesions tend to progress. However, patients who make comprehensive life-style changes often experience significant and sustained reductions in frequency of angina, LDL cholesterol, and weight; also, coronary artery lesions tend to regress rather than progress. Patients usually report rapid decreases in angina and often describe other improvements within weeks; these rapid improvements in angina, well-being, and quality of life sustain motivation and help to explain the high levels of adherence in these patients. Instead of viewing life-style changes solely in terms of risk factor reduction in hopes of future benefit, patients begin to experience more immediate benefits, thereby reframing the reason for making these changes in behavior from fear of dying to joy of living.

This is a particularly rewarding and emotionally fulfilling way to practice medicine, both for patients and the physicians and other health professionals who work with them. Much more time is available to spend with patients addressing the underlying life-style factors that influence the progression of CHD, yet costs are substantially lower. The major reason that most stable patients undergo CABG or PTCA is to reduce the frequency of angina, and comparable results may be obtained by making comprehensive life-style changes alone. Instead of pressuring physicians to see more patients in less time, this is a different approach to reducing medical costs that is caring and compassionate as well as cost-effective and competent.

The physician, who is often pressed for time, need not provide all of the training in changing diet and life-style. He or she can act as the "quarterback," providing direction and supervision. The author and colleagues at the non profit Preventive Medicine Research Institute have trained teams of health professionals at clinical sites around the country in this program of comprehensive life-style changes. The professionals include cardiologists, registered dietitians, exercise physiologists, psychologists, chefs, stress management specialists, registered nurses, and administrative support personnel. These teams, in turn, work with their patients to motivate them to make and maintain comprehensive life-style changes.

In practice, patients with CHD should be offered a range of therapeutic options, including comprehensive life-style changes, medications (including lipid-lowering drugs), angioplasty, and bypass surgery. The physician should explain the relative risks, benefits, costs, and side effects of each approach and then support whatever the patient decides. Whether or not a patient chooses to make intensive life-style changes is a personal decision, but he or she should have all the facts in order to make an informed choice.

REFERENCES

Alderman EL et al: Ten year follow up of survival and myocardial infarction in the randomized Coronary Artery Surgical Study. Circulation 82:1629, 1990

Atherosclerosis Study Group: Optimal resource for primary prevention of atherosclerosis diseases. Circulation 157A, 1984

Bairey CN et al: Mental stress as an acute trigger of ischemic left ventricular dysfunction and blood pressure elevation in coronary artery disease. Am J Cardiol, 66: 28G, 1990

Berkman LF et al: Emotional support and survival after myocardial infarction. A prospective, population-based study of the elderly. Ann Intern Med 117:1003, 1992

Berlin, JA, Colditz GA: A meta-analysis of physical activity in the prevention of coronary heart disease. Am J Epidemiol 132,612, 1990

Blair SN et al: Physical fitness and all-cause mortality. JAMA 262:2395, 1989

Campbell TC et al: Diet, lifestyle, and the etiology of coronary artery disease: The Cornell China Study. Am J Cardiol 82:18T, 1998

Cavender JB et al, for the CASS Investigators: Effects of smoking on survival and morbidity in patients randomized to medical or surgical therapy in the Coronary Artery Surgery Study (CASS): 10-year follow-up. J Am Coll Cardiol 20:287, 1992

Expert Panel on Detection, Evaluation, and Treatment of High Blood Cholesterol in Adults: Executive summary of the third report of the National Cholesterol Education Program (NCEP) expert panel on detection, evaluation,

and treatment of high blood cholesterol in adults. JAMA 285:2486, 2001

Fuster V et al: The pathogenesis of coronary artery disease and the acute coronary syndromes. N Eng J Med 326:242, 1992

Gould KL et al: Changes in myocardial perfusion abnormalities by positron emission tomography after long-term, intense risk factor modification. JAMA 274:894, 1995

House JS et al: Social relationships and health. Science 241:540, 1988

Lesperance F et al: Major depression before and after myocardial infarction: Its nature and consequences. Psychosom Med 58:99, 1996

Miller TQ et al: A meta-analytic review of research on hostility and physical health. Psychol Bull 119:322, 1996

Ornish D: *Dr. Dean Ornish's Program for Reversing Heart Disease.* New York: Random House, 1990; Ballantine Books, 1992

Ornish D: Dietary treatment of hyperlipidemia. J Cardiovasc Risk 1:283, 1994

Ornish D: Avoiding revascularization with lifestyle changes: The Multicenter Lifestyle Demonstration Project. Am J Cardiol 82:72T, 1998

Ornish D, Hart J: Intensive risk factor modification, in *Clinical Trials in Cardiovascular Disease,* C. Hennekens, J. Manson (eds). Boston, Saunders, 1998

Ornish D et al: Effects of stress management training and dietary changes in treating ischemic heart disease. JAMA 249:54, 1983

Ornish D et al: Can intensive lifestyle changes reverse coronary heart disease? Five-year follow-up of the Lifestyle Heart Trial. JAMA 280:2001, 1998

Pitt B et al: Aggressive lipid-lowering therapy compared with angioplasty in stable coronary artery disease. Atorvastatin versus Revascularization Treatment Investigators. N Engl J Med 341:70, 1999

Pratt LA et al: Depression, psychotropic medication, and risk of myocardial infarction. Circulation 94:3123, 1996

Rogers PG, Bullman WR: Prescription medication compliance: A review of the baseline of knowledge. A report of the National Council on Patient Information and Education. J Pharmacoepidemiol 2:3, 1995

Varnauskas E, for the European Coronary Surgery Study Group: Twelve-year follow-up of survival in the randomized European Coronary Surgery Study. N Eng J Med 319:332, 1998

Williams JK et al: Psychosocial factors impair vascular responses of coronary arteries. Circulation 84:2201, 1991

Williams RB et al: Prognostic importance of social and economic resources among medically treated patients with angiographically documented coronary artery disease. JAMA 267:520, 1992

9

THE LONG-TERM INTERVENTION WITH PRAVASTATIN IN ISCHAEMIC DISEASE (LIPID) STUDY

Andrew Tonkin, on behalf of the LIPID Study Group

Cardiovascular disease represents the major public health burden in developed countries and is projected to become the major global public health problem. In many countries, coronary heart disease (CHD) is the most common cause of premature death, and stroke is the major cause of serious, long-term disability.

Epidemiologic studies have established conclusively that serum cholesterol level is a major risk factor for CHD and possibly also for ischemic stroke. Until the past 5 to 10 years, however, data on the relative benefits and risks of lipid-modifying therapy were controversial. That lipid-lowering therapy prevented CHD events had already been established; whether the benefit extended to prevention of stroke and total mortality had not been shown before the recent trials. There was also concern that lipid-lowering therapy might increase non-cardiovascular mortality.

The availability of more potent lipid-modifying agents, the 3-hydroxy-3-methylglutaryl-coenzyme A (HMG-CoA) reductase inhibitors, has allowed treatment effects to be tested more stringently, in large-scale trials. The Long-Term Intervention with Pravastatin in Ischaemic Disease (LIPID) study was the largest published trial (LIPID Study Group 1995; 1998). In particular, the study was designed to test the effects of treatment in the group of CHD patients who are most representative of those seen in practice: those with an average range of serum cholesterol levels. The effects of pravastatin were tested on a background of usual care of such patients.

Study Design

The design and baseline characteristics of patients in the LIPID study have been described in detail (LIPID Study Group, 1995). In all, 9014 patients aged 31 to 75 years, from virtually all (87) major hospitals in Australia and New Zealand, were recruited to the study between June 1990 and December 1992. They had had either acute myocardial infarction (MI) (64%) or hospitalization for unstable angina (36%) between 3 months and 3 years previously. After a period of standard dietary advice, they were required to have a total serum cholesterol in the range of 4.0 to 7.0 mmol/L (155 to 271 mg/dL), and triglyceride <5.0 mmol/L (<445 mg/dL). After their informed consent, they were randomly allocated to receive either pravastatin, 40 mg once a day at bedtime, or matching placebo.

During follow-up, their doctors managed patients as they considered appropriate. This included the possibility of starting lipid-modifying therapy, if this was considered indicated on the basis of new scientific evidence and the result of local lipid testing. The primary prespecified outcome of the study was CHD mortality. All analyses were on an intention-to-treat basis.

Results and Principal Outcomes

Full results have been published (LIPID Study Group, 1998). The pravastatin-assigned and placebo-assigned patient groups were very well matched in terms of baseline characteristics. Median age was 62 years, but 39% were older than 65 years; 83% of the cohort were male, 82% were taking aspirin, 47% were taking beta blockers, 36% were receiving chronic nitrate therapy, and 41% had had prior revascularisation—either coronary artery bypass grafting, coronary angioplasty or both (Table 9-1).

Final patient visits took place between June and September 1997, when the mean duration of follow-up was 6.0 years, after notification from the independent Data and Safety Monitoring Committee that the prespecified boundary rule for stopping, a difference of 3 SD in total mortality between the two groups, had been exceeded. At the end of follow-up, 19% of patients assigned to pravastatin had stopped the trial drug and 24% of those assigned to placebo had begun open-label therapy with a lipid-modifying drug.

Averaging the changes in lipid fractions over 5 years, treatment with pravastatin resulted in a decrease in plasma total cholesterol of 1.0 mmol/L (39 mg/dL) from the median 5.6 mmol/L (218 mg/dL) (an 18% reduction when compared with placebo); a decrease in LDL cholesterol of 25% from 3.9 mmol/L (150 mg/dL); a decrease in triglycerides of 11% from 1.6 mmol/L (142 mg/dL); and

TABLE 9-1

BASELINE CHARACTERISTICS OF PATIENTS RANDOMLY ASSIGNED TO RECEIVE PRAVASTATIN OR PLACEBO IN THE LIPID TRIAL

Characteristic	Pravastatin group, % $n = 4052$	Placebo group, % $n = 4512$
Age, years		
Median	62	62
> 65	39	39
Sex		
Female	17	17
Qualifying event		
Myocardial infarction	64	64
Unstable angina	36	36
Medication		
Aspirin	83	82
Beta blocker	46	48
Nitrate	35	36
Median lipid levels, mmol/L (mg/dL)		
Total cholesterol	5.6 (218)	5.6 (218)
LDL cholesterol	3.9 (150)	3.9 (150)
HDL cholesterol	0.9 (36)	0.9 (36)
Triglycerides	1.6 (142)	1.6 (138)

an increase in HDL cholesterol of 5% from 0.9 mmol/L (36 mg/dL) ($p <. 001$ for all comparisons).

The effects of treatment on the prespecified cardiovascular outcomes are shown in Kaplan-Meier estimates of the incidence of major outcomes (Fig. 9-1).

There was a highly significant difference in the rate of death from CHD (the primary study endpoint) from 8.3% in the placebo group to 6.4% in the pravastatin group ($p = .0004$). Rates of all prespecified cardiovascular events were also significantly lower in the pravastatin treatment group. Overall mortality was significantly lower in the pravastatin group (11.0%) than in the placebo group (14.1%, $p = .00002$) (Table 9-2).

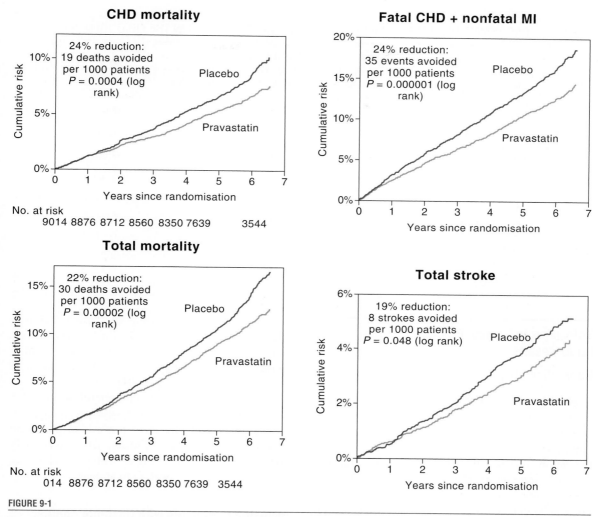

FIGURE 9-1

For every 1000 patients assigned to pravastatin, over the entire study period, death from coronary heart disease was avoided in 19 patients (death from any cause in 30, myocardial infarction in 35, and stroke in 8).

There were fewer deaths from cancer in those assigned to pravastatin (128 cancers) than in those assigned placebo (141) (not significant), and fewer deaths from trauma and suicide in the pravastatin-treated group, although numbers were small (6 and 11, respectively).

Treatment with pravastatin was very safe. A total of 403 newly diagnosed cancers occurred in 379 patients assigned to receive pravastatin, compared with 417 cancers in 399 patients assigned to placebo ($p = .43$). There were no differences in other serious adverse events. Also, there was no significant difference in major liver enzyme abnormalities, nor in other laboratory results, particularly in creatine kinase levels.

The LIPID cohort trial, which will further assess the long-term safety and cost-effectiveness of open-label pravastatin over an even more prolonged period of follow-up, is currently proceeding.

TABLE 9-2

CARDIOVASCULAR EVENTS ACCORDING TO TREATMENT GROUP IN THE LIPID TRIAL

Event	Pravastatin group, % n = 4512	Placebo group, % n = 4502	Relative risk reduction (%)	p
CHD death	6.4	8.3	24	<.0004
Cardiovascular death	7.3	9.6	25	<.0001
Death from any cause	11.0	14.1	22	<.00002
Any myocardial infarction	7.4	10.3	29	<.000001
Revascularisation (bypass surgery or angioplasty)	13.0	15.7	20	<.0001
Hospitalisation for unstable angina	22.3	24.6	12	.005
Any stroke	3.7	4.5	19	.048

Relevance to Clinical Practice: Other Results

Generalizability of the Findings

The results of the LIPID study have major implications for clinical management of patients who are known to have CHD. Not only is the data set the largest available on the effects of lipid-modifying therapy in such patients, but the patients enrolled in this study were representative of the patients currently seen in usual practice. The "average" cholesterol range at baseline most closely reflected levels of typical patients, and benefits of pravastatin were demonstrated on a background of therapy such as aspirin, beta blockers, and revascularization, which represent usual practice in management of CHD patients.

Furthermore, beneficial effects were consistent across all prespecified subgroups. The LIPID study was not designed to have adequate power to demonstrate reliably the effects in such subgroups. However, coronary events (fatal CHD and non-fatal MI), the prespecified end-point for subgroup analyses, were reduced consistently in all subgroups predefined according to age, sex, qualifying diagnosis, other coronary risk factors, and baseline lipid parameters, with no evidence of any statistical hetero-geneity in effects according to these subgroups. This is illustrated in Fig. 9-2. Similar relative risk reductions then translate to greater overall benefit in those at highest absolute risk of further events, such as the elderly (Hunt et al., 2001).

Among patients with cholesterol levels <5.5 mmol/L (<215 mg/dL), there were separately, significant beneficial effects of pravastatin that were consistent with the overall result. The results apply equally to this group, many of whom are often not considered for lipid-lowering treatment.

Inclusion of Patients with Unstable Angina.

In many hospitals, unstable angina is a more frequent indication for admission than acute MI. Because of this, LIPID deliberately included patients with either acute coronary syndrome, stratified according to this diagnosis at the time of randomization. Survival over 6 years was no different according to whether patients qualified with MI or unstable angina. Similar significant reductions in the risk of CHD events, including MI, unstable angina, and revascularization, and also in mortality were observed in both groups (Tonkin et al., 2000). The inclusion in the LIPID study of patients with unstable angina and delay in random allocation of patients until at least 3 months after their acute

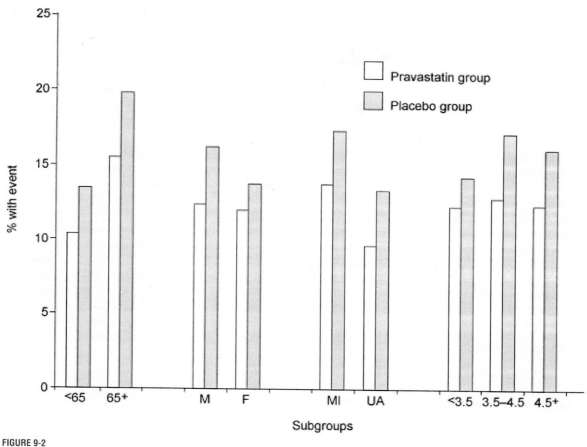

FIGURE 9-2

Prevalence of fatal coronary heart disease or nonfatal myocardial infarction (MI) within subgroups defined in the LIPID trial protocol. Subgroups: age, under 65 years or 65 years and over; sex, male or female; qualifying event, MI or hospitalization for unstable angina (UA), baseline total cholesterol, <3.5 mmol/L, 3.5-4.5 mmol/L, or ≥4.5 mmol/L.

coronary syndrome (when risk of further CHD events approximates that in patients with stable angina) allow further generalization of the results beyond survivors of acute coronary syndromes to all patients with known CHD. As patients were started on pravastatin therapy at least 3 months after the qualifying event, the study provides no data on what benefit might have accrued had treatment been started earlier.

Stroke as an End-Point

The etiology of stroke is multifactorial. There have been concerns that while rates of nonhemor-

rhagic or ischemic stroke are greater with increased plasma cholesterol levels, hemorrhagic stroke (for which the major risk factor is hypertension) might be increased in those with low cholesterol levels. The incidence of stroke is also closely related to age, doubling each decade after 55 years. The LIPID study included 1316 patients over the age of 70 years at baseline. An expert committee (including neurologists) reviewed all available data, including data from imaging and autopsy, to verify stroke outcomes and classify subtypes according to prespecified definitions. The background use of aspirin by 82% of patients and their average range of cholesterol levels at baseline make the findings of the LIPID study more important.

A total of 419 strokes were verified, similar to the total number of strokes reported in meta-analyses of all previous trials of HMG-CoA reductase inhibitors. In LIPID, total strokes generally were significantly reduced by 19% by pravastatin (3.7% in the pravastatin group and 4.5% in the placebo group, $p = .048$) (White et al., 2000). There was a 23% reduction in nonhemorrhagic stroke (3.4% in the pravastatin group and 4.4% in the placebo group, $p = .022$), which was consistent across the different types of ischemic stroke.

Many factors may have contributed to stroke reduction with pravastatin, including the reduction in cardiac events (decrease in acute MI and consequent left ventricular thrombus and heart failure, less need for coronary bypass surgery, and percutaneous intervention) as well as effects of pravastatin on the cerebral circulation and aortic arch atheroma.

Mechanism of Benefit

The benefits observed in the LIPID trial were associated with evidence of delay in the rate of progression of atherosclerosis documented in a substudy of 522 patients who were representative of the whole study and who had serial evaluations of their carotid wall thickness (MacMahon et al., 1998). At 4 years, the mean carotid wall thickness was significantly less in the pravastatin group than in the placebo group ($p < .001$). This independent evidence confirms that the reduction in cardiovascular end-points was associated with delayed progression of atherosclerosis. The possible contribution to treatment effects of other potential actions of pravastatin is being investigated in other substudies.

The Need to Consider Absolute Risk of Patients

The LIPID study provides the most compelling body of data so far about the effects of lipid-modifying therapy in patients with CHD. Pravastatin, on a background of usual dietary advice and other usual therapy, was shown to decrease total mortality and to prevent MI, stroke, subsequent need for myocardial revascularisation, and occurrence of unstable angina. In absolute terms, treatment of only 21 patients with pravastatin over 6 years prevented, in one patient, death, non-fatal MI, and/or non-fatal stroke. As analysis was on an intention-to-treat basis, benefit for compliant patients would probably be even greater.

Because the benefits (without adverse effects) were obtained in a cohort that was very representative of typical patients in usual practice with baseline cholesterol levels in the range 4.0 to 7.0 mmol/L (155 to 271 mg/dL), virtually all CHD patients should now be considered for lipid-modifying therapy. Analyses have shown that treatment with pravastatin in the LIPID study was very cost effective. The trial showed that the relative reduction in risk was similar across clinical subgroups, although absolute risk and benefit varied. Lipid lowering should now be among the first-line therapies for secondary prevention, along with aspirin, beta blockers, and angiotensin-converting enzyme inhibitors.

REFERENCES

Hunt D et al: Benefit of pravastatin on cardiovascular events and mortality in older patients with coronary heart disease equal or exceed those seen in younger patients. Ann Intern Med 134:831, 2001

LIPID Study Group: Design features and baseline characteristics of the LIPID (Long-Term Intervention with Pravastatin in Ischaemic Disease) Study: A randomized trial in patients with previous acute myocardial infarction and/or unstable angina pectoris. Am J Cardiol 76:474, 1995

LIPID Study Group: Prevention of cardiovascular events and death with pravastatin in patients with coronary heart disease and a broad range of initial cholesterol levels. N Engl J Med 339:1349, 1998

MacMahon S et al: Effects of lowering average or below-average cholesterol levels on the progression of carotid atherosclerosis: Results of the LIPID atherosclerosis substudy. On behalf of the LIPID Trial Research Group. Circulation 97:1784, 1998

Tonkin A et al: Beneficial effects of pravastatin in 3260 patients with unstable angina: Results from the LIPID study. Lancet 356:1871, 2000

White H et al: Pravastatin therapy and the risk of stroke. N Engl J Med 343:317, 2000

CHAPTER

10

EFFECTS OF ERYTHROPOIETIN THERAPY AND ANEMIA CORRECTION ON BLOOD PRESSURE AND LEFT VENTRICULAR FUNCTION AND STRUCTURE

Nosratola D. Vaziri

The kidney is the principal site of production of erythropoietin, a 30.5-kDa glycoprotein hormone, which is essential for survival, proliferation, and differentiation of erythroid progenitor cells. Chronic renal failure results in a predictable decline in erythropoietin production that frequently leads to severe, often disabling, anemia. The associated anemia can contribute to left ventricular (LV) hypertrophy and dilation, compounding the effects of hypervolemia and hypertension, which are prevalent in this population. Maintenance replacement therapy with recombinant human erythropoietin (rEPO) ameliorates anemia of chronic renal failure, improves patients' physical and mental performances, and mitigates LV enlargement. Early in the course of phase I and II clinical trials, it became apparent that rEPO therapy frequently results in a significant rise in arterial blood pressure (Buckner et al., 1990). This phenomenon was subsequently confirmed in numerous clinical and laboratory investigations and described in several recent reviews (Vaziri, 1999, 2000; Maschio, 1995). The present chapter is intended to provide an overview of the effects of rEPO therapy and anemia correction on arterial pressure and LV function and structure in patients with advanced renal failure.

rEPO-Induced Hypertension

Incidence

In one of the initial multicenter clinical trials of rEPO, 70% of the study patients exhibited a rise in mean arterial blood pressure exceeding 10 mmHg (Buckner et al., 1990). Analysis of the published studies has revealed that following the institution of regular rEPO therapy 40% of patients with end-state renal disease (ESRD) develop clinically significant de novo hypertension or exacerbation of preexisting hypertension (Maschio, 1995).

Clinical Course

Hypertension is a delayed and time-dependent complication of rEPO therapy and usually occurs from 2 weeks to 6 months after the onset of therapy (Buckner et al., 1990; Vaziri, 2000; Maschio, 1995). The associated hypertension is generally mild to moderate and can be readily controlled by intensification of fluid removal during dialysis (ultrafiltration), initiation of antihypertensive agents, or augmentation of the existing antihypertensive regimens. However, on rare occasions, rEPO therapy results in severe hypertension, leading to encephalopathy and convulsions necessitating intensive antihypertensive therapy and at least temporary cessation of rEPO usage. rEPO-induced hypertension is usually marked by a greater rise in systolic blood pressure during the day and a greater elevation in diastolic blood pressure during the night (Maschio, 1995). A search for risk factors predisposing to rEPO-induced hypertension has yielded contradictory results. Preexisting hypertension, severe pretreatment anemia, the presence of native kidneys (as opposed to the anephric state),

and a very high dosage of rEPO have been considered as potential risk factors for rEPO-induced hypertension by some but not all authors (Buckner et al., 1990; Maschio, 1995). In addition, chronic intravenous administration of rEPO has been shown to cause a greater rise in arterial pressure as compared to that seen with the subcutaneous route.

In addition to raising blood pressure in dialysis-dependent patients with ESRD, maintenance rEPO therapy causes hypertension in predialysis patients with chronic renal insufficiency. rEPO therapy has been shown to exacerbate hypertension and proteinuria and accelerate the loss of nephrons in rats with chronic renal failure produced by 5/6 nephrectomy. Since uncontrolled hypertension is a known risk factor for the progression of renal disease, the deleterious effect of rEPO therapy in animals with experimental renal insufficiency must be largely due to the associated hypertension. Studies of the effect of rEPO therapy on the progression of renal disease in predialysis patients with chronic renal failure are limited and have yielded contradictory results. Large-scale clinical studies are needed to address this issue. In the meantime, caution should be exercised in the use of rEPO in the treatment of anemia in as-yet dialysis-independent patients with chronic renal failure. Particular attention should be given to hypertension control to avoid potential acceleration of nephron loss in such patients (Levin, 1999). It should be noted that prolonged and severe anemia during the predialysis period has been shown to contribute to LV hypertrophy (LVH) and cardiac damage in patients with chronic renal insufficiency. Thus, amelioration of anemia with rEPO therapy together with strict control of the associated hypertension may mitigate cardiac damage without adversely affecting the course of the renal disease.

In addition to its routine use in the treatment of anemia of renal failure, rEPO is often used in the management of anemia associated with cancer, chemotherapy, AIDS, chronic inflammatory disorders (e.g., rheumatoid arthritis), and several other conditions in patients with normal kidney function. rEPO therapy does not usually cause clinically significant hypertension in such patients. This is because intact kidneys can mount counterregulatory responses to mitigate the effects of rEPO on blood pressure in these settings.

Pathogenesis

Despite expanding blood volume by increasing erythrocyte mass, rEPO therapy frequently results in a net reduction of cardiac output by reversing the anemia-induced high-output state. Thus, rEPO therapy does not usually cause volume-dependent hypertension. Instead, rEPO-induced hypertension is associated with and primarily due to increased systemic vascular resistance (Buckner et al., 1990; Vaziri, 1999, 2000; Maschio, 1995). Several factors have been implicated in the pathogenesis of the rEPO-induced rise in vascular resistance and arterial pressure:

Correction of Anemia

The rise in hematocrit from subnormal values towards normal values was originally thought to raise systemic vascular resistance by increasing blood viscosity (Buckner et al., 1990). In addition, increased erythrocyte mass was considered to promote diversion of endothelium-derived nitric oxide (NO) by hemoglobin away from the underlying vascular smooth muscle and, hence, diminish vasodilatory tone (Buckner et al., 1990). It should be noted, however, that changes in hematocrit from subnormal to near-normal values fall within the flat segment of the hematocrit-viscosity curve and as such have minimal impact on blood viscosity and vascular resistance. Additionally, unlike free hemoglobin that serves as a potent scavenger of NO, hemoglobin contained in circulating erythrocytes can actually function as a NO transporter by forming S-nitroso-hemoglobin in the presence of high P_{O_2} (e.g., in the lungs) and releasing NO in the presence of low P_{O_2} in the peripheral tissues. Thus, contrary to the original views, normal levels of hemoglobin contained in erythrocytes appear to facilitate and not hinder tissue perfusion.

In an attempt to dissect the role of anemia correction from that of rEPO per se, subgroups of 5/6 nephrectomized rats were treated for 6 weeks with either rEPO or multiple small packed red blood cell transfusions gauged to mimic the effect of rEPO on hematocrit. A third group of animals was rendered iron deficient prior to initiation of rEPO therapy so as to prevent anemia correction despite rEPO administration. The study revealed a marked rise in blood pressure of equal severity in both iron-sufficient and iron-deficient animals despite anemia correction in the former but not in the latter group. Moreover, multiple small transfusions did not change blood pressure despite successful anemia correction. These experiments clearly demonstrated that maintenance rEPO therapy rather than anemia correction is responsible for the associated hypertension (Vaziri et al., 1996). It was further found that by raising basal and stimulated cytosolic ionized calcium concentration, which is the final pathway for vascular smooth-muscle tone and contraction, rEPO elevates blood pressure and confers resistance to the vasodilatory action of nitric oxide, otherwise known as endothelium-derived relaxing factor (Vaziri et al., 1996). Dissociation of erythropoietic from pressor actions of rEPO was convincingly demonstrated in subsequent studies of patients with ESRD. (Kaupke et al., 1994).

Modification of Endogenous Vasoconstrictive Factors

Although rEPO therapy does not usually change plasma renin activity or angiotensin II concentration, it has been shown to augment gene expressions of renin and angiotensinogen in the kidney and vascular tissues (Eggena et al., 1991). Thus, up-regulation of the tissue renin-angiotensin system may, in part, contribute to the pathogenesis of rEPO-induced hypertension.

Several in vivo and in vitro studies have demonstrated a significant rise in endothelin 1 production with rEPO administration. Based on these observations, increased production of this potent vasopressor is thought to play a role in the pathogenesis of hypertension associated with rEPO therapy. Results of these studies have been summarized in a recent review (Vaziri, 1999).

The available studies of the effect of rEPO on production of prostaglandins are limited. These studies suggest that rEPO promotes production of vasoconstrictive and inhibits production of vasodilatory prostaglandins. If true, this phenomenon can contribute to rEPO-induced hypertension.

Several studies have shown that rEPO does not directly affect plasma catecholamine concentrations. However, by restoring normal oxygen-carrying capacity, correction of anemia with rEPO can actually alleviate the hyperadrenergic state associated with severe anemia. Conversely, uncontrolled rEPO-induced hypertension can contribute to congestive heart failure, which is a hyperadrenergic state. The studies of the effect of rEPO therapy on vasoconstrictive response to α_1-adrenergic stimulation have yielded contradictory results. While some have shown enhanced vasoconstrictive response following rEPO administration, others have found no such effect (Vaziri, 1999).

Elevation of Cytoplasmic [Ca^{2+}]

Long-term administration of rEPO to humans and animals with chronic renal failure has been shown to raise resting cytoplasmic [Ca^{2+}], which is the ultimate determinant of vascular smooth-muscle tone (Vaziri, 1999; Vaziri et al., 1996). In addition, rEPO therapy augments the magnitude of the agonist-stimulated rise in cytoplasmic [Ca^{2+}], which is the final pathway of vascular smooth-muscle contraction (Vaziri, 1999; Vaziri et al., 1996). Thus, by raising the resting and stimulated cytoplasmic [Ca^{2+}], rEPO therapy can raise systemic vascular resistance, which is the primary feature of rEPO-induced hypertension.

Direct Vasoconstrictor Action

At high concentrations rEPO causes contraction in isolated vascular tissues in vitro (Vaziri et al., 1995). However, single-dose administration of rEPO does not change the blood pressure in either animals or humans (Vaziri, 1999; Vaziri et al., 1995).

Impaired Vasodilator Tone

Long-term rEPO therapy has been shown to diminish the magnitude of the hypotensive response to intravenous administration of NO donors, nitro-prusside and S-nitroso-penicillamine, in rats with chronic renal failure (Vaziri et al., 1996). Moreover, vasorelaxation response to the above NO donors is significantly impaired in vascular tissue preparations obtained from the rEPO-treated animals (Vaziri et al., 1996). These observations point to the occurrence of a rEPO-induced resistance to the vasodilatory action of exogenous and presumably endogenous NO. Given the well-known contribution of endothelium-derived NO in the regulation of vascular resistance and blood pressure, induction of NO resistance by rEPO therapy must play a major role in the pathogenesis of the associated hypertension. The vasodilatory action of NO is due to a cyclic guanosine monophosphate (cGMP)—mediated lowering of cytoplasmic [Ca^{2+}]. Thus, rEPO-induced elevation of cytoplasmic [Ca^{2+}] in vascular smooth muscle may account for the associated NO resistance. In fact, restoration of normal cytoplasmic [Ca^{2+}] by concurrent administration of the long-acting dihydropyridine calcium channel blocker, felodipine, has been shown to reverse rEPO-induced hypertension and improve NO metabolism in animals with chronic renal failure (Ni et al., 1998).

Treatment

Mild forms of rEPO-induced hypertension in dialysis-dependent patients can frequently be controlled by increasing the rate of fluid removal by ultrafiltration during dialysis. However, in many instances, volume reduction alone is insufficient and antihypertensive medications are required. Several classes of antihypertensive agents are commonly used in the treatment of rEPO-induced hypertension. For instance, long-acting dihydropyridine or benzothiazepine calcium channel blockers are frequently used with favorable results. Likewise, angiotensin-converting enzyme inhibitors, angiotensin II type I receptor blockers, and α_1-adrenergic receptor blockers have been used successfully. In severe cases, a combination of ultrafiltration and multiple antihypertensive agents may be required. On rare occasions when other measures have failed, the potent direct vasodilator, minoxidil, has been used with some success. Malignant or accelerated hypertension is an extremely uncommon consequence of rEPO therapy. However, when present, it may require temporary withholding of rEPO usage together with vigorous antihypertensive therapy to control hypertension and protect target organs.

Cardiac Effects of rEPO Therapy and Anemia Correction

Left ventricular abnormalities, including LVH and dilation (LVD) as well as congestive heart failure (CHF), are extremely common in the end-stage renal disease (ESRD) population. For instance, 80% of ESRD patients have evidence of LV enlargement (London et al., 1987; Silberberg et al., 1989; Parfrey et al., 1996), which is primarily due to the associated hypertension and hypervolemia. In addition, anemia, which is a nearly constant feature of renal failure, and surgically created arteriovenous blood access necessary for hemodialysis procedure, contribute to development of LVH, LVD, and CHF by augmenting cardiac output and LV workload. Consequently, anemia is an independent risk factor for clinical cardiac disease, echocardiographically demonstrable cardiac abnormalities, and mortality in patients with ESRD (Foley et al., 1996).

Several studies have shown that partial correction of anemia with rEPO therapy can improve LVH (London et al., 1989; Macdougall et al., 1990). However, available studies conducted to explore the effect of normalization of hematocrit have yielded inconclusive results. For example, complete correction of anemia by rEPO therapy has been reported to cause partial regression of LVH in small groups of dialysis-dependent (Jeren-Strugic et al., 2000) and as-yet dialysis-independent patients (Hayashi et al., 2000) with advanced renal disease. In another study, normalization of hematocrit improved the sense of well being and quality-of-life indices but failed to halt progression of LVH/LVD in a group of ESRD patients with preexisting asymptomatic LVH or LVD

(Foley et al., 2000). Finally, a large multicenter study intended to assess the effect of normalization of hematocrit in ESRD patients with moderate to severe symptomatic heart disease showed a trend for higher mortality in patients assigned to the high hematocrit group (Besarab et al., 1998). It should be noted, however, that assignment to the high hematocrit group did not ensure attainment of normal hematocrit in all patients. In fact, hematocrit values were significantly lower in patients who ultimately died than those who survived. Consequently, greater mortality in the high hematocrit group could not be attributed to anemia correction with certainty. Further examination of the data showed that individuals who died had received more frequent dosages of intravenous iron preparation and less adequate dialysis than the surviving patients. Thus, anemia correction, per se, does not appear to have been responsible for the observed trend for higher mortality in this study.

CHF is frequently associated with a fall in hematocrit (Anand et al., 1993; Haber et al., 1991; Rich et al., 1996). In fact, deterioration of CHF has been shown to result in a parallel reduction in hematocrit (Silverberg et al., 2000). Conversely, anemia has been shown to be an independent risk factor for CHF in the general population (Kannel, 1987). Thus, CHF can lead to anemia, and anemia can exacerbate CHF. Based on these observations, correction of the mild to moderate anemia associated with CHF may ameliorate cardiac function in patients with CHF. In fact, correction of the mild anemia by subcutaneous rEPO therapy in a group of patients with moderate to severe CHF was recently shown to significantly increase LV ejection fraction, improve New York Heart Association score, reduce mortality, and lower the diuretic requirement as compared with the untreated group (Silverberg et al., 2001).

Taken together, the available data suggest that amelioration of anemia may be useful in prevention of LV dysfunction and treatment of preexisting heart disease. However, it is important to carefully monitor patients for development of rEPO-induced hypertension and control blood pressure in all instances to maximize the benefit of anemia correction.

REFERENCES

Anand IS et al: Pathogenesis of edema in chronic severe anemia: Studies of body water and sodium, renal function, haemodynamic variables, and plasma hormones. Br Heart J 70:357, 1993

Besarab A et al: The effects of normal as compared with low hematocrit in patients with cardiac disease who are receiving hemodialysis and epoetin. N Engl J Med 339:584, 1998

Buckner FS et al: Hypertension following erythropoietin therapy in anemic hemodialysis patients. Am J Hypertens 3:947, 1990

Eggena P et al: Influence of recombinant human erythropoietin on blood pressure and tissue renin-angiotensin systems. Am J Physiol 261:E642, 1991

Foley RN et al: The impact of anemia on cardiomyopathy, morbidity and mortality in end-stage renal disease. Am J Kidney Dis 28:53, 1996

Foley RN et al: Effect of hemoglobin levels in hemodialysis patients with asymptomatic cardiomyopathy. Kidney Int 58:1325, 2000

Haber HL et al: The erythrocyte sedimentation rate in congestive heart failure. N Engl J Med 324:353, 1991

Hayashi T et al: Cardiovascular effect of normalizing the hematocrit level during erythropoietin therapy in predialysis patients with chronic renal failure. Am J Kidney Dis 35:250, 2000

Jeren-Strugic B et al: Morphologic and functional changes of left ventricle in dialyzed patients after treatment with recombinant human erythropoietin. Angiology 51:131, 2000

Kannel WB: Epidemiology and prevention of cardiac failure: Framingham Study insights. Eur Heart J 8(Suppl F):23, 1987

Kaupke CJ et al: Effect of erythrocyte mass on arterial blood pressure in dialysis patients receiving maintenance erythropoietin therapy. J Am Soc Nephrol 4:1874, 1994

Levin A: How should anemia be managed in pre-dialysis patients? Nephrol Dial Transplant 14:66, 1999

London GM et al: Uremic cardiomyopathy: An inadequate left ventricular hypertrophy. Kidney Int 31:973, 1987

London GM et al: Vascular changes in hemodialysis patients in response to recombinant human erythropoietin. Kidney Int 36:878, 1989

Macdougall IC et al: Long-term cardiorespiratory effects of amelioration of renal anemia by erythropoietin. Lancet 335:489, 1990

Maschio G: Erythropoietin and systemic hypertension. Nephrol Dial Transplant 10:74, 1995

Ni Z et al: Nitric oxide metabolism in erythropoietin-induced hypertension: Effect of calcium channel blockade. Hypertension 32:724, 1998

Parfrey PS et al: Outcome and risk factors for left ventricular disorders in chronic uremia. Nephrol Dial Transplant 11:1277, 1996

Rich MW et al: Iatrogenic congestive heart failure in older adults: Clinical course and prognosis. J Am Geriatr Soc 44:638, 1996

Silberberg JS et al: Impact of left ventricular hypertrophy on survival in end-stage renal disease. Kidney Int 36:286, 1989

Silverberg DS et al: The use of subcutaneous erythropoietin and intravenous iron for the treatment of the anemia of severe, resistant congestive heart failure improves cardiac and renal function and functional cardiac class, and markedly reduces hospitalizations. J Am Coll Cardiol 35:1737, 2000

Silverberg DS et al: The effect of correction of mild anemia in severe, resistant congestive heart failure using subcutaneous erythropoietin and intravenous iron: A randomized controlled study. J Am Coll Cardiol 37:1775, 2001

Vaziri ND: Mechanism of erythropoietin-induced hypertension. Am J Kidney Dis 33:821, 1999

Vaziri ND: Vascular effects of erythropoietin and anemia correction. Semin Nephrol 20:356, 2000

Vaziri ND et al: In vivo and in vitro pressor effects of erythropoietin in rats. Am J Physiol 269:F838, 1995

Vaziri ND et al: Role of nitric oxide resistance in erythropoietin-induced hypertension in rats with chronic renal failure. Am J Physiol 271:E113, 1996

11

HYPERTENSION AND SLEEP APNEA

V. Hoffstein, P. Hanly

Introduction

Obstructive sleep apnea (OSA) is characterized by repetitive episodes of airway occlusion during sleep. By definition, these occlusions must last longer than 10 s; generally they last 20 to 40 s. In the most severe cases they can occur as frequently as every 30 s and may last over a minute. Sometimes airway occlusion is not complete but is sufficient to reduce the airflow by >50% of baseline. Such episodes are termed *hypopneas*. They are accompanied by qualitatively similar physiologic events and are thought to have similar clinical consequences as apneas. The number of apneas and hypopneas per hour of sleep is termed the *apnea/hypopnea index* (AHI).

There is virtually no disagreement regarding the acute effect of apneas on blood pressure. Virtually all studies demonstrate surges in blood pressure following apneic episodes. However, the precise mechanisms responsible for these rises in blood pressure are complex. As summarized in a recent review (Fletcher, 2000), they include direct effects of intermittent hypoxemia and hypercapnea on chemoreceptors and sympathetic activity, resetting in the baroreceptor function, changes in the fluid–atrial natriuretic peptide balance in response to intrathoracic pressure fluctuations during obstructive episodes, overstressed

sympathetic nervous system from sleep disruption and arousals, changes in endothelial cells, and vascular remodeling. These mechanisms are not independent but interact in a complex fashion, leading to hypertension. Some patients have surges in blood pressure that far exceed their normal blood pressure. However, whether these nocturnal episodes of hypertension carry into wakefulness, leading to sustained daytime hypertension, is still very much a matter of debate. Considering that sleep apnea is a common problem, affecting 5 to 10% of the adult population (Young et al., 1993); it is important to determine whether OSA is an independent risk factor for hypertension.

The controversy is well illustrated by the following statements taken from two recent reviews. In one, Silverberg and co-workers examined 36 studies dealing with sleep-disordered breathing and hypertension and concluded that " . . . the accumulated data obtained by many different researchers support the hypothesis that essential hypertension is mainly due to increased upper airway resistance during sleep," even when various confounding factors are taken into account (Silverberg and Oksenberg, 1997). In the other, the Conference on Health Outcomes of Sleep Apnea issued a statement that " . . . none of these studies has been large enough or long enough to firmly establish that treatment of

OSA contributes to long-term control of blood pressure" (American Thoracic Society/ American Sleep Disorders Association, 1998). Stradling and Davies, having reviewed the evidence linking blood pressure and sleep apnea concluded—" . . . what a mess!" (Stradling and Davies, 1997).

In this chapter we point out the reasons for controversy and address two questions that describe the nature of the OSA-hypertension: (1) is sleep apnea an independent risk factor for hypertension? and (2) does treatment of sleep apnea normalize blood pressure?

Is Sleep Apnea an Independent Risk Factor for Hypertension?

There are a number of studies comparing blood pressures between apneic and nonapneic individuals, as well as examining (using various forms of regression analysis) whether sleep apnea is an independent determinant of blood pressure. The results are not uniform for several reasons. We know that both conditions (hypertension and sleep apnea) are influenced by the same common factors—obesity, age, gender, alcohol, smoking, and others. Consequently, it is to be expected that the relationship between blood pressure and sleep apnea will be attenuated, sometimes losing statistical significance when these factors together with the AHI are used as "independent" variables in regression analysis with blood pressure as the dependent variable. This is well illustrated by the results of one study that examined 1504 randomly selected residents of Copenhagen, Denmark, of whom 748 had measurements of blood pressure and nocturnal respiration (Jennum and Sjøl, 1993). Although there was a significant difference in blood pressure between subjects with and without sleep apnea, this difference disappeared and the relationship between blood pressure and sleep apnea became nonsignificant when age, gender, body mass index (BMI), and alcohol and tobacco consumption were included in the statistical analysis.

Sometimes the reasons for discordant results between different investigations are obvious. In several early investigations, important confounding factors listed above were either not taken into account or multivariate analysis was not performed. In other studies blood pressure was not measured, but instead the subjects were classified as being hypertensive or not, based on self-reports. In many other investigations, sleep studies were not performed consistently in all subjects but only in selected subsamples.

Many of these obvious shortcomings, particularly treatment of confounding factors, were overcome in later investigations, but the disagreement between various studies as to whether sleep apnea is an independent risk factor for hypertension persisted. The reasons for this are more subtle and are due to the differences in methodology—data accumulation, type of population (sleep clinic vs. general) examined, definition of hypertension, definition and identification of respiratory events, (particularly hypopneas), and interpretation. Consequently, it is important that the results be interpreted in the context of the study design.

Recent On-Going Trials

The longest large-scale trial designed to study the relationship between sleep apnea and blood pressure in community population is the Wisconsin Sleep Cohort Study (Young et al., 1997). It included 1060 men and women, all of whom had in-laboratory nocturnal polysomnography; standardized and consistent measurements of evening and morning blood pressure; anthropometric measurements, i.e., age, weight, height, and body circumferences (neck, hip, waist); and information regarding use of antihypertensive medications, tobacco, and alcohol. The authors concluded that "there is a dose-response relationship between sleep-disordered breathing and hypertension, independently of the known confounding factors." The difference in blood pressure between nonapneic individual (AHI = 0) and equally obese apneic individual (AHI = 30) was modest, approximately 7/4 mmHg (systolic/diastolic). The odds ratio for hypertension associated with sleep apnea was 2. The longitudinal nature of this study has already allowed prospective analysis of the data (Peppard et al., 2000). The authors found that there was a dose-response relationship for development of hypertension. The highest odds ratio for hypertension at 4 years' follow-up was 2.9 for those with AHI > 15 at baseline, compared to the reference category of AHI = 0 at baseline.

Another large-scale, on-going community-based study is the Sleep Heart Health Study (Nieto et al., 2000). More than 11,000 participants were recruited from other on-going studies dealing with cardiovascular disease; almost 7000 were enrolled, and eventually almost 6500 subjects (≥40 years) were analyzed. All had in-home nocturnal polysomnography, recording of anthropometric data, and measurement of blood pressure performed by a trained interviewer during a home visit. After adjustment for age, sex, ethnicity, BMI, neck circumference, waist/hip ratio, alcohol use, and smoking, the investigators found that the highest odds ratio for hypertension (in those with AHI > 30 as compared to those with AHI < 2) was 1.4. The most recent results from the same cohort indicate that sleep-disordered breathing is associated not only with hypertension but also with other manifestations of cardiovascular disease, such as heart failure, stroke, and coronary artery disease (Shahar et al., 2001). The odds ratios ranged between 1.3 and 2.4, depending on the particular manifestation of cardiovascular disease.

In another large-scale community study, almost 17,000 men and women living in two counties in southern Pennsylvania were contacted by phone (Bixler et al., 2000). Eventually 1741 of them (1000 women and 741 men) had in-laboratory polysomnography. Blood pressure was measured on the evening of sleep study. Similar to the previous studies, the authors found a dose-response relationship between the severity of sleep-disordered breathing and hypertension. The odds ratio for hypertension, relative to the reference group of non-snoring subjects with AHI = 0, were as high as 6.8 for those with AHI > 15.

In addition to the community-based studies, there are now several studies based on the cohort of patients referred to sleep laboratories for investigation of possible sleep apnea. Sleep apnea was found to be an independent risk factor for hypertension, as it was in the community population. In a large sample of almost 3000 patients, each apneic event per hour of sleep above AHI = 10 was associated with approximately 1% increase in the odds for hypertension (Lavie et al., 2000). In another study, the authors found that the probability of uncontrolled hypertension increased by almost 2% for each apneic event per hour of sleep (Grote et al., 2000). In a very careful case-controlled study of 24-h ambulatory blood pressure in patients with sleep apnea and normal controls matched for age, BMI, alcohol, smoking, treated hypertension, and ischemic heart disease, the authors found that patients with sleep apnea had higher systolic blood pressure at night and higher diastolic blood pressure during the day and night than normal controls; the differences in blood pressure ranged between 5 and 9 mmHg (Davies et al., 2000).

The main and consistent outcome of the above studies is confirmation that sleep apnea is an independent risk factor for hypertension. Its significance is attenuated by inclusion of other factors that can influence blood pressure, so that the resulting odds ratio for sleep apnea and hypertension is approximately 2. The effect of the confounding factors, particularly age, gender, and obesity, is complex and significantly alters the relationship between sleep apnea and hypertension

Do Hypertensives have more Sleep Apnea?

Considerably fewer studies examined the relationship between OSA and hypertension from a different viewpoint—not prevalence of hypertension in sleep apnea, but prevalence of sleep apnea in a hypertensive population. Many, but not all, investigations found a significantly higher prevalence of sleep apnea among hypertensives, ranging between 12 and 83% (Worsnop et al., 1998). However, all of the studies are limited by small sample size. Whereas epidemiologic studies of blood pressure in sleep apnea usually involve thousands of patients, these studies are generally limited to fewer than 100 patients. Furthermore, some studies did not have a control group of healthy nonhypertensives, and others did not control for intake of antihypertensive medications. It is not possible to correct or adjust the results to take into account these limitations, but the overall result to date is in favor of increased prevalence of sleep apnea among patients with essential hypertension.

Does Treatment of Sleep Apnea Normalize Blood Pressure?

What happens to blood pressure in hypertensive apneic patients when their sleep apnea is treated, usually with continuous positive airway pressure (CPAP)? Acute effects of CPAP on blood pressure during sleep are indisputable: application of CPAP —provided the pressure is sufficient to abolish apneas, hypopneas, and hypoxemia—reduces or completely eliminates cyclical elevations in blood pressure.

However, chronic effects of CPAP on daytime hypertension have not been conclusively ascertained. A review of 22 studies dealing with the effect of treatment of OSA on blood pressure concluded that successful treatment of sleep apnea reduces blood pressure (Silverberg and Oksenberg, 1997). However, methodologic constraints of all studies limit their generalizability and do not permit drawing a definitive conclusion regarding the effect of CPAP on blood pressure (Fletcher, 1996, 2000; Stradling and Davies, 1997). The most common confounding factor with significant influence on the final conclusions is the lack of proper untreated controls matched to the treated group by age, gender, BMI, severity of hypertension, and severity of apnea. Other important factors that limit the power of treatment studies include effect of medications, small numbers of patients, short follow-up time, and quantification of compliance with CPAP.

Some of these concerns were addressed in a recent randomized, placebo-controlled study of the effect of CPAP on blood pressure (Faccenda et al., 2001). Ambulatory blood pressure was recorded con-tinuously for 48 hours at the end of each treatment arm (CPAP and placebo). The authors found only trivial reductions in blood pressure (<2 mmHg) in blood pressure after CPAP. However, follow-up time was very short, and there remains a possibility that a much longer treatment time is necessary to demonstrate a clinically significant reduction in blood pressure.

Despite the methodologic difficulties inherent in all of the investigations, their contribution to our understanding of the complexity of the linkage between OSA and hypertension is of great significance. These studies have heightened our awareness of the fact that hypertensive apneic patients constitute a highly heterogeneous population. Some patients exhibit normal nocturnal reduction in blood pressure ("dippers"), while others do not ("non-dippers"). There is preliminary evidence indicating that non-dippers have higher vascular morbidity and poorer response to treatment of blood pressure than dippers. Severity of hypertension can affect the response to treatment: mildly hypertensive apneics may not demonstrate a significant reduction in blood pressure as compared to those with more severe hypertension. Length of follow-up and compliance with CPAP are important: patients may exhibit a reduction in blood pressure after several weeks of treatment that is not sustained after several months. Only a large, randomized clinical trial can determine the usefulness of CPAP in treatment of hypertension. No such trial exists at present, although the accumulated cross-sectional and some longitudinal data are sufficient to justify such a trial.

Conclusion

Apneic events stress the cardiovascular system by several mechanisms, causing nocturnal elevations in blood pressure. That these cyclical elevations in blood pressure lead to sustained daytime hypertension in humans remains to be proven. Epidemiologic studies indicate that sleep apnea has an independent effect on blood pressure, which remains significant, although weakened, even after taking into account the effect of common confounding factors. However, this association between the two common disorders (OSA and hypertension) does not imply causality. Successful treatment of sleep apnea with CPAP eliminates nocturnal surges of blood pressure, but whether it also reduces daytime blood pressure in hypertensive individuals is not clear.

REFERENCES

American Thoracic Society/American Sleep Disorders Association: Statement on health outcomes research in sleep apnea. Am J Respir Crit Care Med 157:335, 1998

Bixler EO et al: Association of hypertension and sleep-disordered breathing. Arch Intern Med 160:2289, 2000

Davies CWH et al: Case-control study of 24 hour ambulatory blood pressure in patients with obstructive sleep apnea and normal matched control subjects. Thorax 55:736, 2000

Faccenda JF et al: Randomized placebo-controlled trial of continuous positive airway pressure on blood pressure in the sleep apnea-hypopnea syndrome. Am J Respir Crit Care Med 163:344, 2001

Fletcher EC: Can the treatment of sleep apnea syndrome prevent the cardiovascular consequences? Sleep 19:S67, 1996

Fletcher EC: Hypertension in patients with sleep apnea, a combined effect? Thorax 55:726, 2000

Grote L et al: Sleep-related breathing disorder is an independent risk factor for uncontrolled hypertension. J Hypertens 19:679, 2000

Jennum P, Sjøl A: Snoring, sleep apnea and cardiovascular risk factors: The MONICA II study. Int J Epidemiol 22:439, 1993

Lavie P et al: Obstructive sleep apnea syndrome as a risk factor for hypertension: Population study. BMJ 320:479, 2000

Nieto FJ et al, for the Sleep Heart Health Study: Association of sleep-disordered breathing, sleep apnea, and hypertension in a large community-based study. JAMA 283:1829, 2000

Peppard PE et al: Prospective study of the association between sleep-disordered breathing and hypertension. N Engl J Med 342:1378, 2000

Shahar E et al, for the Sleep Heart Health Study Research Group: Sleep-disordered breathing and cardiovascular disease: Cross-sectional results of the Sleep Heart Health Study. Am J Respir Crit Care Med 163:19, 2001

Silverberg DS, Oksenberg A: Essential hypertension and abnormal upper airway resistance during sleep. Sleep 20:794, 1997

Stradling J, Davies RJO: Sleep apnea and hypertension—what a mess! Sleep 20:789, 1997

Worsnop CJ et al: The prevalence of obstructive sleep apnea in hypertensives. Am J Respir Crit Care Med 157:111, 1998

Young T et al: The occurrence of sleep-disordered breathing among middle-aged adults. N Engl J Med 328:1230, 1993

Young T et al: Population-based study of sleep-disordered breathing as a risk factor for hypertension. Arch Intern Med 157:1746, 1997

12

THE EFFECT OF DIET ON BLOOD PRESSURE

Lawrence J. Appel

Elevated blood pressure is a complex phenotype that results from environmental and genetic factors and their interactions. Of the environmental factors that affect blood pressure (e.g., diet, physical inactivity, toxins, and psychosocial factors), dietary factors have a prominent, and likely predominant, role in blood pressure homeostasis. In observational studies, elevated blood pressure has been associated with numerous dietary factors, including excess weight; high dietary intakes of sodium, alcohol, caffeine, fat, and cholesterol; and low dietary intakes of potassium, calcium, magnesium, and fiber. However, the potential for confounding limits the ability of observational studies to draw firm inferences about causality, especially for dietary factors.

To isolate the effects of individual nutrients or dietary factors, investigators have conducted controlled trials that test the effects of just one dietary factor or nutrient at a time. Results from such trials, in conjunction with evidence from observational studies and from animal studies, have implicated high salt (sodium chloride) intake, high weight, and excessive alcohol consumption as the primary dietary determinants of elevated blood pressure. Recent investigations have expanded our understanding of the impact of diet, specifically, the beneficial effects of a desirable dietary pattern, of increased potassium intake, and of reduced sodium intake to levels below current recommendations. Other trials have elucidated the role of dietary factors in the prevention of hypertension and the effects of dietary interventions in the elderly.

Clinical Trials

The Trials of Hypertension Prevention, Phase I (TOHP I)

TOHP I was a randomized, controlled trial that assessed the effects of three lifestyle interventions (sodium reduction, weight loss, and stress management over 18 months) and four pill supplement interventions (potassium, calcium, magnesium, and fish oil over 6 months) in 2182 individuals with a diastolic blood pressure of 80 to 89 mmHg (The Trials of Hypertension Prevention Collaborative Research Group, 1992). The weight loss intervention led to a mean, net weight loss of 3.9 kg (8.5 lb) and significant reductions in systolic and diastolic blood pressures of 2.9 and 2.3 mmHg, respectively. The reduced sodium intervention significantly lowered urinary sodium excretion by 44 mmol/d and systolic and diastolic blood pressures by 1.7 and 0.9 mmHg, respectively. For both weight loss and sodium reduction, there were significant dose-response relationships. In contrast, neither the stress management nor pill supplement interventions significantly reduced blood pressure. By simultaneously evaluating several nonpharmacologic therapies in the same study population, TOHP I provided valuable information on the comparative effects of several nonpharmacologic therapies.

The Trials of Hypertension Prevention, Phase II (TOHP II)

TOHP II was a randomized, controlled trial that tested the effects of three lifestyle interventions (sodium reduction, weight loss, and combined weight loss and sodium reduction) on blood pressure and incident hypertension over 3 to 4 years of follow-up in overweight individuals with a diastolic blood pressure of 83 to 89 mmHg and a systolic blood pressure <140 mmHg (The Trials of Hypertension Prevention Collaborative Research Group, 1997). At 6 months, the height of intervention adherence, the incidence of hypertension was lowest in the combined group (2.7%), intermediate in the weight loss (4.2%) and sodium reduction (4.5%) groups, and highest in the control group (7.3%). At 18 months, the pattern persisted. By the end of follow-up, the incidence of hypertension was 18 to 22% less in each lifestyle group ($p < .05$ compared to control) but not different from each other. Results of this trial indicate that lifestyle interventions can prevent hypertension over the long term. Also, the pattern of incident hypertension at 6 and 18 months suggests that the effects of weight loss and reduced sodium intake, under optimal conditions of adherence, may be additive.

The Trials of Nonpharmacologic Interventions in the Elderly (TONE)

TONE was a randomized, controlled trial that tested the effects of three lifestyle interventions (sodium reduction, weight loss, and combined weight loss and sodium reduction) on blood pressure control in the elderly over 18 to 30 months (Whelton et al.,

1998). Participants were 975 older-aged persons with a systolic blood pressure <145 mmHg and a diastolic blood pressure <85 mmHg on one medication. Medication withdrawal was attempted 3 months after the start of interventions. The primary outcome variable was a composite end-point defined by the occurrence after medication withdrawal of an average blood pressure >150/90 mmHg, resumption of medication, or a cardiovascular event. Those assigned to a sodium reduction intervention achieved and sustained an average reduction in sodium intake of nearly 40 mmol/d. Likewise, those assigned to a weight loss intervention achieved and sustained an average reduction in weight of nearly 4.5 kg (10 lb). Among the 585 obese participants, the hazard ratio of developing an end-point relative to control was 0.60 for reduced sodium intake alone, 0.64 for weight loss alone, and 0.47 for combined reduced sodium and weight loss (each $p < .05$). Among the 390 nonobese participants, the hazard ratio of developing an end-point relative to control was 0.75 for reduced sodium intake alone ($p < .05$). The frequency of cardiovascular events during follow-up was similar in each group. Results from this trial indicate that reduced sodium intake and weight loss are feasible, effective, and safe nonpharmacologic interventions in older persons. Furthermore, in the context of an older-aged population with high adherence, these results indicate that weight loss and sodium reduction, together, have substantially greater effects than either intervention alone.

Dietary Approaches to Stop Hypertension (DASH) Trial

DASH was a randomized feeding study that assessed the effects of modifying dietary patterns on blood pressure in 459 adults with a systolic blood pressure <160 mmHg and diastolic blood pressure 80 to 95 mmHg (Appel et al., 1997). For 3 weeks, participants were fed a control diet low in fruits, vegetables, and dairy products but with fat content typical of U.S. consumption. Participants were then randomized to receive for 8 weeks: (1) the control diet, (2) a diet rich in fruits and vegetables but otherwise similar to control, or (3) a "combination" diet that emphasized fruits, vegetables, and low-fat dairy products. The combination diet also included whole grains, poultry, fish, and nuts but reduced levels of fat, red meat, sweets, and sugar-containing beverages. In each diet, sodium and weight were held constant. Compared to control, the combination diet reduced systolic and diastolic blood pressure by 5.5 and 3.0 mmHg, respectively (each $p < .001$); the fruits and vegetables diet reduced systolic blood pressure by 2.8 mmHg ($p < .001$) and diastolic blood pressure by 1.1 mmHg ($p = .07$). The reductions in blood pressure were achieved within 2 weeks and then sustained for 6 more weeks (Figure 12-1). Among 133 hypertensive participants, the combination diet reduced systolic and diastolic blood pressure by 11.4 and 5.5 mmHg, respectively (each $p < .001$);

in 326 nonhypertensive participants, corresponding reductions were 3.5 mmHg ($p < .001$) and 2.1 mmHg ($p = .003$). African Americans tended to have greater blood pressure reductions than non-African Americans. Results from this trial provide strong evidence that in addition to salt, weight, and alcohol, other dietary factors can substantially affect blood pressure. Furthermore, the impressive results from DASH have both public health and clinical significance. A population-wide reduction in systolic blood pressure of the magnitude observed in DASH normotensives could substantially reduce the occurrence of cardiovascular disease in the general population. The blood pressure reductions observed in hypertensives have obvious clinical significance and are similar in magnitude to the blood pressure reductions from drug monotherapy.

The DASH-Sodium (DASH-Na) Trial

The DASH-Na trial was a randomized feeding study that tested the effects on blood pressure of three levels of sodium reduction in two distinct diets (Sacks et al., 2001). The three sodium levels were "higher" (target of 150 mmol/d, reflecting typical U.S. consumption), "intermediate" (target of 100 mmol/d, reflecting the upper limit of current U.S. recommendations), and "lower" (target of 50 mmol/d, reflecting a level that could produce additional lowering of blood pressure). A total of 412 participants were assigned at random to eat a control diet typical of U.S. intake or the DASH diet. Within their assigned diet, participants ate higher, intermediate, and lower sodium levels, each for 30 days in random order. The eligibility criteria in the DASH and DASH-Na trials were similar.

Main results are displayed in Figure 12-2. In the control diet, reducing sodium intake from the higher to the intermediate level reduced systolic blood pressure by 2.1 mmHg ($p < .001$); reducing sodium intake from intermediate to lower further reduced systolic blood pressure by 4.6 mmHg ($p < .001$). In the DASH diet, corresponding changes in systolic blood pressure were -1.3 ($p < .05$) and -1.7 mmHg ($p < .01$), respectively. The effects of sodium reduction were significant in nonhypertensives and

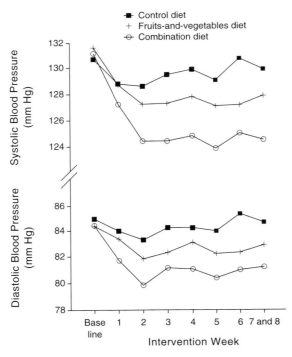

FIGURE 12-1

Mean systolic and diastolic blood pressure at baseline and during each intervention week in the DASH trial. (Reproduced from LJ Appel et al: N Engl J Med 336:1117, 1997, with permission.)

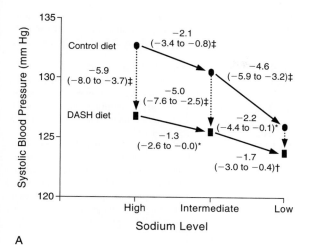

A

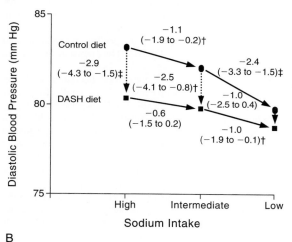

B

FIGURE 12-2

The effect on systolic blood pressure (panel *A*) and diastolic blood pressure (panel *B*) of reduced sodium intake and the DASH diet. * $p < .05$; † $p < .01$; ‡ $p < .001$. (Reproduced from FM Sacks et al: N Engl J Med 344:3, 2001, with permission.)

7.1 mmHg in nonhypertensive persons and by 11.5 mmHg in hypertensives. The pattern of results was similar for diastolic blood pressure.

Results from the DASH-Na trial support population-wide recommendations to reduce sodium intake. These data also document the benefit of sodium reduction to levels below the currently recommended upper limit of 100 mmol/d and the benefit both of consuming the DASH diet and of reducing sodium intake. Long-term health benefits will depend on the ability of individuals to make long-lasting dietary changes and the increased availability of lower sodium foods.

The Prevention and Treatment of Hypertension Study (PATHS)

PATHS was a randomized, controlled trial that tested the effects of an alcohol reduction behavioral intervention in 641 nondependent moderate to heavy drinkers with diastolic blood pressure of 80 to 99 mmHg (Cushman et al.; 1998). From a baseline intake of approximately 6 drinks per day, the average change from the cognitive-behavioral intervention was a net reduction of 1.3 drinks per day. The average changes in blood pressure, net of control, were systolic and diastolic blood pressure reductions of 1.2 mmHg ($p = .17$) and 0.7 mmHg ($p = .18$), respectively. Overall, these results do not support alcohol reduction interventions as the sole means to reduce blood pressure in nondependant moderate to heavy drinkers. Still, attaining a moderate intake of alcohol (≤ 2 drinks per day among those who drink) is a reasonable component of a multifactorial lifestyle intervention.

Conclusion

In aggregate, these trials support the hypothesis that multiple dietary factors influence blood pressure and that modification of diet can have powerful and beneficial effects, even in older persons. The dietary strategies that have the greatest impact on blood pressure rely on life-style modifications (i.e., weight loss,

hypertensives, whites and African Americans, and women and men. The DASH diet reduced systolic blood pressure significantly at each sodium level, more so with higher than lower sodium. Compared to the control diet with higher sodium, the DASH diet with lower sodium reduced systolic blood pressure by

sodium reduction, alcohol moderation, and a desirable dietary pattern) rather than pill supplementation with individual nutrients (e.g., calcium or magnesium). It is noteworthy that achieving and sustaining life-style modification have been demonstrated in the setting of clinical trials, some of which lasted 3 or more years.

These trials also demonstrate that life-style modification can have important roles in both normotensive and hypertensive individuals. In normotensive individuals, lifestyle modifications have the potential to prevent the onset of hypertension and, more broadly, to reduce blood pressure and thereby lower the risk of vascular disease in the general population. In hypertensives, life-style modifications can serve as initial therapy in stage 1 hypertension before the addition of medication and as an adjunct to medication in persons already on drug therapy. In hypertensives with controlled blood pressure, such therapies can facilitate medication step down or even withdrawal in certain individuals. In view of such benefits, physicians should be strong advocates of life-style modification in all of their patients.

REFERENCES

Appel LJ et al: The effect of dietary patterns on blood pressure: Results from the Dietary Approaches to Stop Hypertension (DASH) Clinical Trial. N Engl J Med 336:1117, 1997

Cushman WC et al: Prevention and Treatment of Hypertension Study (PATHS): Effects of an alcohol treatment program on blood pressure. Arch Intern Med 158:1197, 1998

DASH Web Page, http://dash.bwh.harvard.edu

Joint National Committee on Prevention, Detection, Evaluation, and Treatment of High Blood Pressure: The Sixth Report of the Joint National Committee on the Prevention, Detection, Evaluation, and Treatment of High Blood Pressure. Arch Intern Med 157:2413, 1997

Sacks FM et al, for the DASH-Sodium collaborative research group. A clinical trial of the effects on blood pressure of reduced dietary sodium and the DASH dietary pattern (The DASH-Sodium Trial). N Engl J Med 344:3, 2001

The Trials of Hypertension Prevention Collaborative Research Group: The effects of nonpharmacologic interventions on blood pressure of persons with high normal levels. JAMA 267:1213, 1992

The Trials of Hypertension Prevention Collaborative Research Group: Effects of weight loss and sodium reduction intervention on blood pressure and hypertension incidence in overweight people with high-normal blood pressure. The Trials of Hypertension Prevention, Phase II. Arch Intern Med 157:657, 1997

Whelton PK et al: The effects of oral potassium on blood pressure: A quantitative overview of randomized, controlled clinical trials. JAMA 227:1624, 1997

Whelton PK et al, for the TONE Collaborative Research Group: Efficacy of sodium reduction and weight loss in the treatment of hypertension in older persons: Main results of the randomized, controlled trial of nonpharmacologic interventions in the elderly (TONE). JAMA 279:839, 1998

Working Group on Primary Prevention of Hypertension, National High Blood Pressure Education Program: Working Group report on primary prevention of hypertension. Arch Intern Med 153:186, 1993

13

ANGIOTENSIN RECEPTOR BLOCKERS IN THE TREATMENT OF HYPERTENSION

Irene Gavras & Haralambos Gavras

Interruption of the Renin-Angiotensin Cascade

Research in the field of the renin-angiotensin system over the past decades has culminated in the development of two new classes of antihypertensive drugs: the angiotensin-converting enzyme (ACE) inhibitors and the selective angiotensin II receptor blockers (ARBs). Both classes of drugs lower the blood pressure by interrupting the actions of angiotensin II. Figure 13-1 shows a simplified representation of the renin-angiotensin cascade, illustrating the steps that lead from the renin-substrate interaction to the formation of the effector hormone angiotensin II. It should be noted that the ACE acts also on substrates other than angiotensin I, and another of its important activities is the degradation of bradykinin. Therefore ACE inhibition results in (1) partial interruption of the formation of angiotensin II (partial because angiotensin II can also be generated by alternative, though less efficient, enzymatic pathways); and (2) diminished degradation—and therefore potentiation—of bradykinin. The latter

accounts for some of the desirable and most of the undesirable effects of ACE inhibition. The alternative, non-renin non-ACE enzymatic pathways may assume a more important role if the generation of angiotensin II is chronically curtailed by blockade of the main pathway (i.e., by renin inhibitors or ACE inhibitors, respectively). Therefore, complete withdrawal of the effects of angiotensin II would be achieved only via blockade of its receptors.

Angiotensin II can be viewed both as a hormone circulating systemically and acting on various target organs and as a paracrine/autocrine/intracrine factor generated within certain tissues and acting locally on adjacent cells or on the same cells that produce it. Systemically, angiotensin II is a potent vasopressor and steroidogenic (aldosterone-stimulating) hormone. Its local actions are mostly determined by the cell types of the target tissues and include trophic/mitogenic effects; alterations in ion transport across cell membranes; and alterations in intracellular signaling pathways, which favor cell growth and proliferation, enhanced electrical stimulation, etc. Table 13-1 lists some of the known systemic and tissue-specific

RENIN-ANGIOTENSIN CASCADE

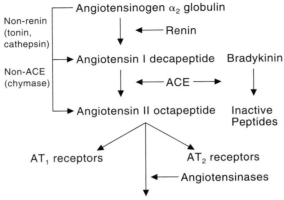

FIGURE 13-1

TABLE 13-1

ACTIONS OF ANGIOTENSIN II VIA AT_1 RECEPTOR STIMULATION

Systemic (endocrine) effects of circulating angiotensin II

Vasoconstrictive (preferentially coronary, renal, cerebral)

Steroidogenic (aldosterone)

Dipsogenic (CNS effect)

Renin-suppressing (negative feedback)

Tissue-specific effects of angiotensin II as local hormone

Trophic/mitogenic (cardiac and vascular myocytes, fibroblasts)

Inotropic/contractile (cardiomyocytes)

Chronotropic/arrhythmogenic (cardiomyocytes)

Thrombogenic (plasminogen activator inhibitor)

Oxidative (generation of reactive oxygen species)

Ion transport channels (myocytes, renal cells)

Neuroexcitation (sympathetic nerve terminals)

Endothelin stimulation (endothelial cells)

Vasopressin stimulation (CNS)

Note: CNS, central nervous system.

effects of angiotensin II. Angiotensin II acts via two main subtypes of receptors: the AT_1 and AT_2(Goodfriend et al, 1996). All of the physiologically important actions are mediated by the AT_1 subtype. The AT_2 receptors are important for fetal development, but their numbers diminish in the postnatal period, although they may increase in case of tissue injury, such as in myocardial cells during decompensation of heart failure. Currently their exact physiologic role is still poorly understood. A major advance in cardiovascular pharmacotherapy 10 years ago was the development of selective AT_1 receptor antagonists that effectively block all systemic and local actions of angiotensin II without affecting other vasoactive systems (e.g., kinins) (Timmerman et al., 1991). Unlike the polypeptide angiotensin II antagonist analogues used in clinical research in the early 1970s, the new ARBs are nonpeptide, orally active, highly selective blockers of the AT_1 receptors and have no effects on other neurohormonal systems, except those regulated by angiotensin II itself.

Pharmacology of the ARBs

The first agent to be introduced from this new class was losartan. In the United States, there are now six ARBs that have already been introduced or have gained approval of the U.S. Food and Drug Administration. All ARBs have the same general pharmacodynamic effects resulting from inhibition of angiotensin II. However, they differ in pharmocokinetic characteristics (Csajka et al., 1997), such as competitive or insurmountable binding to the AT_1 receptor, potency, percentage of renal or hepatic clearance, degradation into active or inactive metabolites, and duration of action (Table 13-2). Whether these characteristics translate into clinically significant differences remains to be seen. Some agents may also have additional unique pharmacologic effects because of their particular chemical structure, other than those resulting from angiotensin II blockade; for example, losartan has a unique uricosuric

TABLE 13-2

PHARMACOKINETICS OF SOME ORAL AT$_1$ RECEPTOR BLOCKERS

Drug	Active metabolite	Bioavailability, %	Food effect	Half life, h	%Protein bound	Daily dose, mg	Excretion, %	
							Urinary	Fecal
Losartan	EXP 3174	33	Minimal	2 (6−9)	98.7 (99.8)	25−100	35	60
Valsartan	None	25	↓ 40−50	6	95	80−320	13	
Irbesartan	None	60−80	None	11−15	90	75−300	20	60
Candesartan	CV-11974	42	None	3 (11)	99.5	8−32	60	40
Telmisartan	None	30−60	Minimal	24	>98	40−80	1.5	>98
Eprosartan	None	13	Minimal	5−9	98	300−600	7	90

property that is not seen with valsartan or irbesartan and that is attributable only to the parent compound, not to the active metabolite (although the latter is responsible for the prolonged AT$_1$ receptor blocking effect of the agent) (van den Meiracker et al., 1995).

Inhibition of angiotensin II results in lowering of blood pressure due to a reduction in systemic vascular resistance. Vasodilation occurs preferentially in the vital organs (heart, kidney, brain, adrenals), whose vasculature is more sensitive to the pressor effect of angiotensin than the vasculature of abdominal viscera and musculocutaneous tissues. This leads to redistribution of blood flow with enhanced perfusion of vital organs in the face of falling systemic blood pressure (Liang et al., 1978). As a result, coronary blood flow increases even in the absence of increased myocardial oxygen demand. Angiotensin blockade can also cause redistribution of regional blood flow within organs, according to local vascular sensitivity. In the kidney it increases effective renal blood flow and alters the intrarenal hemodynamics by dilating the afferent more than the efferent arterioles; this causes a fall in intraglomerular pressure, which accounts for the antiproteinuric and nephroprotective effects of angiotensin blockade, above and beyond those attributable to blood pressure lowering per se. This also accounts for the fall in glomerular filtration rate, which, in case of bilateral renal artery stenoses

or stenosis of the main artery to a solitary kidney, can lead to a functional (reversible) renal insufficiency.

Blockade of AT$_1$ receptors results in decreased secretion of aldosterone and increased circulating levels of plasma renin and angiotensin II (due to interruption of the negative-feedback control of renin release). Whether these higher levels of angiotensin II exert additional effects mediated via the non-blocked AT$_2$ receptors remains to be demonstrated.

At the tissue level, chronic ARB treatment causes reversal of left ventricular hypertrophy and arterial wall thickening, diminished proliferation of fibroblasts in the interstitium of myocardial, renal, and other tissues; and attenuation of locally generated humoral factors (such as endothelin, norepinephrine, various enzymes, growth factors, and oncogenes), whose release is controlled by the AT$_1$ receptor of angiotensin II.

Use of ARBs in Hypertension

ARBs are effective antihypertensive agents, with an efficacy profile similar to that of other common antihypertensives and a side-effect profile similar to placebo (Gavras, 1997). As monotherapy, ARBs are effective in 60 to 70% of patients with mild to moderate hypertension, and addition of a diuretic increases the response rate to over 80%. Several controlled clinical trials have compared the efficacy and tolerability of different ARBs against those of hydrochlorothiazide, the ACE inhibitors enalapril or lisinopril, and the β-adrenergic blocker atenolol. In all cases, the efficacy of the ARB was no different from the standard agent, whereas the side-effect profile was significantly better. This was particularly evident in patients known to be intolerant to ACE inhibitors because of cough. ARBs are equally effective in young and older hypertensives, in males and females; however, like ACE inhibitors and β-adrenergic blockers, ARBs as monotherapy tend to be less effective in African-American patients, who seem to require higher doses and/or addition of a diuretic for optimal response.

Experimental studies in animals and early clinical trials suggest that ARBs have the same cardioprotective and nephroprotective properties demonstrated by ACE inhibitors. Indeed, they usually reverse left ventricular hypertrophy and arterial wall thickening, attenuate myocardial ischemia, and may suppress cardiac arrhythmias as well as or better than ACE inhibitors. They also correct proteinuria to the same extent as ACE inhibitors. As a result, they diminish the rate of progression of chronic renal failure in diabetic nephropathy or other renal parenchymal diseases. Most of the clinical trials published so far have used losartan, but limited studies with other ARBs suggest that, as with ACE inhibitors, these are most probably class effects (Mimran and Ribstein, 1999). So far there are no publications of large outcome trials to definitively show improvement in the incidence of clinical end-points, such as stroke, cardiovascular events, or renal failure.

However, the first trials with losartan and irbesartan in diabetic nephropathy have recently been completed, and their results were published in September 2001. In summary, the Reduction of Endpoints in Non-insulin Dependent Diabetes Mellitus with the Angiotensin II Antagonist Losartan (RENAAL) study (Brenner et al., 2001) found a significant reduction in the rate of progression of various renal parameters over the 3.5 years of average follow-up: the progression to end-stage renal disease (ESRD) was reduced by 28%, the doubling of serum creatinine decreased by 25%, and the protein-uria decreased by 35%. There was a 20% reduction in the combined end-points of ESRD or death, which was not statistically significant, but there was a significant decrease by 32% in the rate of hospitalization for heart failure and a decrease by 28% in the occurrence of heart attacks. The benefits were more pronounced with the 100-mg daily dose than with 50 mg daily.

Similar results were reported in the two trials using irbesartan. The Irbesartan in Type 2 Diabetes with Microalbuminuria (IRMA) trial (Parving et al., 2001) found a 24% decrease in microalbuminuria with the 150-mg daily dose of irbesartan and a 46% decrease with 300 mg daily. The progression to diabetic nephropathy was reduced significantly by 68% with the higher dose, whereas with the lower dose it was reduced by 44%, which was not statistically significant. The companion Irbesartan Diabetic Nephropathy Trial (IDNT) (Lewis et al., 2001) compared the effects of irbesartan with those of amlodipine over an average period of 2.6 years in patients with equally good blood pressure control. Compared to amlodipine, irbesartan showed a 37% risk reduction in doubling serum creatinine and a 23% risk reduction in reaching ESRD. As with losartan, there was no significant difference in overall rate of combined fatal and nonfatal cardiovascular and cerebrovascular events, but the amlodipine group had a significantly higher rate of heart failure. These findings are consistent with the results of various meta-analyses comparing calcium blockers with other antihypertensive classes (Pahor et al., 2001).

Currently, there are several other ongoing controlled clinical trials with various ARBs designed to document diminished morbidity and mortality in subpopulations of patients with diabetes mellitus, heart disease, or kidney disease in comparison to standard antihypertensive treatment with diuretics, beta blockers, or calcium channel blockers. They are designated by a variety of acronyms (LIFE, VALIANT, CHARM, OPTIMAAL, etc.) and are expected to run for several years before significant differences between groups can be demonstrated. The first such study was the ELITE trial, comparing the ARB losartan versus the ACE inhibitor captopril in older patients with chronic congestive heart failure (Pitt et al., 1997). The results indicated a 46% decrease in mortality in the losartan-treated patients, due to reduced incidence of sudden death, attributable most likely to a significant difference in QT dispersion resulting in diminished incidence of arrhythmias (Brooksby et al., 1999). However, a larger study specifically designed to make this comparison, the ELITE II trial, found that losartan was not superior to captopril in terms of survival but was significantly better tolerated (Pitt et al., 2000).

Conclusions

What is the place of ARBs among the other classes of antihypertensive agents at this time? On the basis of their efficacy profile in terms of blood pressure lowering, they are at least as suitable as the currently recommended "first choice" agents (beta blockers and thiazides) for the unselected, generally healthy hypertensive population. The favorable side-effect profile should be balanced against the higher cost. For selected populations in whom ACE inhibition is considered mandatory, such as in those with postmyocardial infarct, chronic heart failure, diabetic nephropathy, and other progressive renal parenchymal diseases, ARBs currently should be considered to be a reasonable substitute only for patients unable to tolerate ACE inhibitors due to cough or angioedema. These recommendations may change if the ongoing multicenter trials mentioned above demonstrate superiority of ARBs over other classes of drugs, in which case they would become the treatment of choice. Patients unable to tolerate ACE inhibition because of orthostatic hypotension or functional renal insufficiency would most likely develop the same problems with ARBs. Finally, like ACE inhibitors, ARBs are absolutely contraindicated in pregnancy, as they may adversely affect fetal development.

REFERENCES

Brenner BM et al: Effects of losartan on renal and cardiovascular outcomes in patients with type 2 diabetes and nephropathy. N Eng J Med 345:861, 2001

Brooksby P et al: Effects of losartan and captopril on QT dispersion in elderly patients with heart failure. ELITE study group. Lancet 354:395, 1999

Csajka C et al: Pharmacokinetic-pharmacodynamic profile of angiotensin II receptor antagonists. Clin Pharmacol 32:1, 1997

Gavras H: Angiotensin II antagonism: A new avenue of hypertension management. Blood Pressure 6 (Suppl 1):42, 1997

Goodfiend TL et al: Angiotensin receptors and their antagonists. N Engl J Med 334:1649, 1996

Lewis EJ et al: Renoprotective effect of the angiotensin-receptor antagonist irbesartan in patients with nephropathy due to type 2 diabetes. N Eng J Med 345:851, 2001

Liang C et al: Renin-angiotensin system inhibition in conscious sodium-depleted dogs: Effects on systemic and coronary hemodynamics. J Clin Invest 61:874, 1978

Mimran A, Ribstein J: Angiotensin receptor blockers: Pharmacology and clinical significance. J Am Soc Nephrol 10 (Suppl 12):S273, 1999

Pahor M et al: Blood pressure lowering treatment. Lancet 358:156, 2001

Parving HH et al: The effect of irbesartan on the development of diabetic nephropathy in patients with type 2 diabetes. N Eng J Med 345:870, 2001

Pitts B et al: Randomized trial of losartan versus captopril in patients over 65 with heart failure (Evaluation of Losartan In The Elderly Study, ELITE). Lancet 349:747, 1997

Pitt B et al: Effect of losartan compared with captopril on mortality in patients with symptomatic heart failure: randomised trial—the Losartan Heart Failure Survival Study ELITE II. Lancet 355:1582, 2000

Timmerman PBMWM et al: The discovery of a new class of highly specific nonpeptide angiotensin II receptor antagonists. Am J Hypertens 4 (Suppl 4, pt 2):275S, 1991

Van den Meiracker AH et al: Hemodynamic and biochemical effects of the AT$_1$ receptor antagonist irbesartan in hypertension. Hypertension 25:22, 1995

EFFECT OF RAMIPRIL VERSUS AMLODIPINE ON RENAL OUTCOMES IN HYPERTENSIVE NEPHROSCLEROSIS: THE AFRICAN AMERICAN STUDY OF KIDNEY DISEASE AND HYPERTENSION TRIAL

Janice G. Douglas

Background

Mortality from cerebrovascular and coronary artery disease has declined substantially during the past two decades in the United States due in great part to blood pressure control, while the prevalence of end-stage renal disease (ESRD) due to hypertension has increased progressively. African Americans have a greater prevalence and more severe hypertension and more significant target organ damage than other racial ethnic groups in the United States. Despite the observation that diabetes mellitus is the leading cause of ESRD in the United States, among African Americans, uncontrolled or poorly controlled hypertension has been the leading cause. The U.S. Renal Data System (USRDS) reports that African Americans have a 4.5-fold greater likelihood of developing ESRD than whites, with hypertension as a major contributor (US Renal Data System USRDS 1999 Annual Data Report, 1999). The risk of ESRD secondary to hypertension in African Americans has been reported to be as high as 20-fold greater than in whites. The optimal strategy to retard the progressive increment in hypertensive ESRD, which has increased by 50% between 1990 and 1998 in African Americans, remains to be determined. Promising among the recent interventions that have been implicated in slowing the progression of renal disease and prevention of ESRD are arterial blood pressure reduction and the use of angiotensin-converting enzyme (ACE) inhibitors.

Unfortunately, no definitive data are available on the efficacy of this class of antihypertensive agents and/or levels of blood pressure control for African Americans with progressive renal disease, primarily due to low enrollment in randomized controlled trials.

Study Design

The African American Study of Kidney Diseases and Hypertension (AASK) trial is an ongoing multicenter randomized prospective trial sponsored by the National Institute of Diabetes and Digestive and Kidney Diseases (NIDDK). This trial is a 2 × 3 factorial design involving 21 clinical centers in the United States, a central data coordinating center, and a data and safety monitoring board. There were 1094 African Americans with hypertensive kidney disease of mild to moderate severity [glomerular filtration rates (GFR) between 20 and 65 mL/min per 1.73 m^2] who were enrolled and randomized between February 1995 and September 1998. The blinded observation period was completed at the end of September 2001.

AASK was designed to evaluate the efficacy of two different levels of blood pressure control (low versus usual) and one of three antihypertensive agents: a beta blocker, metoprolol (50 to 200 mg/d, Toprolol XL), versus an ACE inhibitor, ramipril (2.5 to 10 mg/d, Altase), versus a dihydropyridine calcium channel blocker (DHP-CCB), amlodipine (5 to 10 mg/d Norvasc. The treatment goals include mean arterial blood pressure (MAP) of <92 mmHg (125/75), or 102 to 107 mmHg (<140/90). Patients were randomly assigned to amlodipine ($n = 217$), ramipril ($n = 436$), or metoprolol ($n = 441$), with doses increased to the maximum as needed to achieve goal blood pressure. If maximum-tolerated doses of the blinded drug failed to reach the assigned blood pressure goal, furosemide, a diuretic, and other agents (doxazosin, clonidine, and hydralazine or minoxidil) were added sequentially to the primary agent. Diabetic participants and participants with >2.5 g of urinary protein excretion per 24 h at baseline were specifically excluded.

The primary end-points of this study include the rate decline of GFR as determined using iothalamate clearance (both chronic, starting 3 months after initiation of therapy, and total GFR change over the entire follow-up period). The main secondary end-point is a composite including the time from randomization to (1) a 50% decline in GFR or an absolute decline of 25 mL/min per 1.73 m^2, (2) ESRD, or (3) death. Proteinuria (urinary protein to creatinine ratio) represented another secondary end-point. The decision for an early halt of the amlodipine arm was announced at the 33rd Annual Meeting of the American Society of Nephrology (Toronto, Canada, October 13 to 16, 2000), and the results of an interim analysis of the comparison of the amlodipine to ramipril arms were presented.

In September 2000, the NIDDK of the National Institutes of Health (NIH) called an early halt to the amlodipine arm of the AASK trial after careful deliberation by an independent data safety monitoring board (DSMB). It was observed that patients with proteinuria >1 g/d demonstrated renoprotection with the use of either ramipril (the ACE inhibitor) or metoprolol (the beta blocker) as compared to amlodipine, the DHP-CCB. A separate analysis of data in patients with baseline proteinuria >1 g/d was not included in the original primary or secondary end-point analysis plans. However, after the onset of the study, results of several clinical trials and meta-analyses revealed the renoprotective effects of ACE inhibition on proteinuric diabetic and nondiabetic renal disease with >1 g of proteinuria (Levey, 1999). Moreover, at the initiation of the study, there were no data concerning any differences between DHP-CCBs and non-DHP-CCBs on their effect on renal function, i.e., proteinuria and changes in GFR, in patients with nondiabetic renal disease.

The ramipril and metoprolol arms of AASK continued until completion of the study in September 2001. The AASK interim analysis of the amlodipine-ramipril comparison was published earlier [The African American Study of Kidney Disease (AASK) Study Group, 2001].

Observations

Randomization resulted in baseline demographics that were not significantly different between the amlodipine and ramipril groups. In these two groups combined, at baseline mean age was 54 years, 61% were men, mean blood pressure was 151/96 mmHg, and mean GFR was 46 mL/min per 1.73m². The median urinary protein/creatinine ratio was 0.11, and this ratio exceeded 0.22 in approximately one-third of patients. At entry to baseline, 62% were taking a CCB, 40% an ACE inhibitor, and 27% a beta blocker. At the time of the interim analysis, median follow-up of GFR was 37 and 36 months in the ramipril and amlodipine groups, respectively. After 3 months, an average of 57% of patients in both groups received the highest dose of their randomized study drug, approximately 75% of patients were on a diuretic, and in both groups, patients took a mean of 1.75 antihypertensive drugs in addition to their randomized drug.

After the 3-month visit, mean blood pressures did not differ significantly between the ramipril and amlodipine groups (mean blood pressure, 134.5/82.2 mmHg and 132.9/81.4 mmHg, respectively). However, among the one-third of patients with baseline urinary protein to creatinine ratio >0.22 (corresponding to urine protein excretion of about 300 mg/d, a value identifying clinically significant proteinuria), the mean rate of GFR decline was 40% slower in the ramipril than the amlodipine group after 3 months (chronic phase) and was 36% slower in the ramipril than the amlodipine group from baseline to 3 years (total slope). Consistent with a strong inverse association between GFR and proteinuria at baseline, similar results were obtained in the subgroup with baseline GFR <40 mL/min per 1.73 m².

Due to an acute increase in GFR among the two-thirds of patients without frank proteinuria (urinary protein (<300 mg/d), the mean total GFR change from baseline to 3 years did not differ significantly between the ramipril and amlodipine groups for the entire study cohort. However, for the entire cohort, the ramipril group had a 36% slower mean GFR decline after 3 months. Additional obser-

vations were that the risk of the clinical composite outcome, including large declines in GFR, ESRD, or death, was reduced by 38% for the entire ramipril group (Fig. 14-1). Moreover, the relative risk for ESRD or death was reduced by 41% with ramipril while the mean decline in GFR event or ESRD was reduced by 38% (Fig. 14-1). Of interest is the fact that the amlodipine group experienced a significant increase in urinary protein excretion compared to the ramipril group for patients in both baseline urine protein/creatinine strata. In the entire cohort, the geometric mean urine protein/creatinine ratio increased by 58% in the amlodipine group and decreased by 20% in the ramipril group from baseline to 6 months. From baseline to 36 months the mean changes were an increase of 8.7% for ramipril and 108% for amlodipine (Fig. 14-2). In addition, among the two-thirds of patients without proteinuria at baseline, amlodipine was associated with a 56% more rapid progression to overt proteinuria (>300 mg/d) as compared to ramipril.

Discussion

This interim analysis clearly demonstrates a renoprotective effect of ramipril as compared to amlodipine in hypertensive nephrosclerosis in participants beyond the threshold of clinically significant "dipstick positive" proteinuria (>300 mg/d or urinary protein/creatinine ratio of >0.22). Observations that support this conclusion include a significant reduction in the risk of the clinical composite outcome, a slower decline in GFR, and a reduction in urinary protein excretion with ramipril as compared to amlodipine. Moreover, a renoprotective effect of ramipril is also suggested in the nonproteinuria participants because randomization to ramipril significantly reduced proteinuria compared to amlodipine in the subgroup without clinically significant proteinuria at baseline, and because the ramipril group experienced a significant reduced rate of the composite clinical event outcome compared to amlodipine in the full cohort. The subgroup without proteinuria at baseline also experienced a slowed progression (56%) to clinically significant proteinuria on

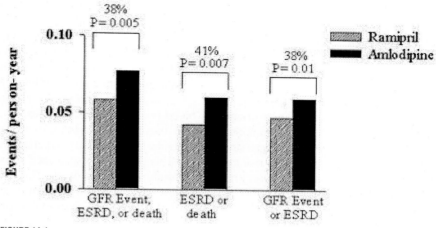

FIGURE 14-1

Relative risk reduction for patients randomized to ramipril ($n = 436$) as compared to those assigned to amlodipine ($n = 217$). GFR, glomerular filtration rate; ESRD, end-stage renal disease.

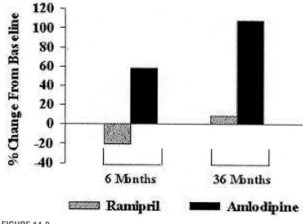

FIGURE 14-2

Change in urinary protein excretion from baseline.

ramipril as compared to amlodipine. It is of interest that prior recommendations as to a beneficial effect of ACE inhibition in both diabetic and nondiabetic renal insufficiency targeted higher levels of protein per day as the threshold where a renoprotective effect is demonstrated. This AASK interim analysis suggests a significantly lower threshold but cannot define the specific cut point. Prior observations on the use of ACE inhibitors in diabetic and nondiabetic renal disease are described by Levey (1999).

This interim analysis is important as it is the first outcome trial to demonstrate a significant beneficial effect of ACE inhibition in African Americans and emphasizes the importance of this class of drugs on prevention of target organ damage that extends beyond blood pressure control. Angiotensin II has been documented to augment growth factor production, oxidative stress, matrix production, etc., all of which have the potential to facilitate disease progression. The ability of ACE inhibitors to lower urinary protein excretion has been suggested as an additional mechanism that retards renal disease progression. Microalbuminuria and frank proteinuria are risk factors for cardiovascular as well as renal disease. Prior observations that suggested that ACE inhibitors are not effective in African Americans were based on the use of this class of drugs as monotherapy for blood pressure control (Rahman et al., 1997). However, as AASK demonstrates, when an ACE inhibitor is used in combination with a diuretic and other agents, blood pressure control is achieved and the renoprotection is apparent. Moreover, AASK demonstrated that the number of drugs, the percent of participants on diuretics, and the achieved blood pressure (133/82 mmHg) were similar for participants randomized to amlodipine and ramipril. This strengthens the argument that the renoprotective effect of ramipril as compared to amlodipine is independent of the achieved blood pressures.

SUMMARY

An interim analysis of the AASK trial at 3 years demonstrates a renoprotective effect (slower decline in GFR; delayed onset of significant decrease in GFR, ESRD, or death; and a decrease in urinary protein excretion) of the ACE inhibitor ramipril as compared to the dihydropyridine calcium channel blocker (DHP-CCB) amlodipine in patients with mild to moderate renal insufficiency. The beneficial effect occurred in the presence of similar levels of blood pressure control and was apparent in proteinuric (beyond the threshold of "dipstick positive" proteinuria, 300 mg/d) hypertensive nephrosclerosis. This benefit was suggested to extend to nonproteinuric patients as well. The data suggest that DHP-CCBs should be used with caution in the presence of mild to moderate renal insufficiency.

REFERENCES

Levey AS: Concise review: Angiotensin-converting enzyme inhibitors in nondiabetic renal disease, May 21, 1999; http://www.harrisonsonline.com

Rahman M et al: Pathophysiology and treatment implications of hypertension in the African American population. Endocrinol Metab Clin North Am 26:125, 1997

The African-American Study of Kidney Disease and Hypertension (AASK) Study Group: Effect of ramipril versus amlodipine on renal outcomes in hypertensive nephrosclerosis: A randomized controlled trial. JAMA 285:2719, 2001

US Renal Data System, USRDS 1999 Annual Data Report. Bethesda MD: National Institutes of Health, National Institute of Digestive and Kidney Diseases, 1999

TREATMENT OF SYSTOLIC HYPERTENSION IN THE ELDERLY—RESULTS OF THE SYSTOLIC HYPERTENSION IN EUROPE TRIAL

Jan A. Staessen

Isolated systolic hypertension occurs in approximately 15% of men and women aged ≥60 years (Staessen et al., 1990). In 1989, the European Working Party on High Blood Pressure in the Elderly initiated the double-blind placebo-controlled SYST-EUR (Systolic Hypertension in Europe) trial in order to investigate whether active treatment could reduce the cardiovascular complications of this disorder. Fatal and nonfatal stroke combined constituted the primary end-point. The SYST-EUR trial stopped after the second of four planned interim analyses, when predefined stopping rules revealed that active treatment diminished the incidence of stroke (Amery et al., 1991).

Methods

As described in detail elsewhere, patients were recruited from 198 centers in 23 eastern and western European countries (Amery et al., 1991; Staessen et al., 1991a). Each center maintained a register of

screened patients, and eligible patients were at least 60 years old. In the sitting position, systolic blood pressure was 160 to 219 mmHg, with diastolic blood pressure <95 mmHg. In the standing position, systolic blood pressure was ≥140 mmHg. These blood pressure criteria were based on the means of six readings, two in each position at three baseline visits 1 month apart. Patients could not be enrolled if systolic hypertension was secondary to a condition for which specific medical or surgical treatment was indicated. The other exclusion criteria included retinal hemorrhage or papilledema, congestive heart failure, dissecting aortic aneurysm, a serum creatinine concentration at presentation of ≥180 μmol/L (≥2 mg/dL) a history of stroke or myocardial infarction (MI) within 1 year before possible randomization, dementia or substance abuse, any condition prohibiting a sitting or standing position, and any severe concomitant cardiovascular or noncardiovascular disorder.

After stratification by center, gender, and previous cardiovascular complications, the patients were randomized to double-blind treatment with active medication or placebo. Active treatment was started with nitrendipine (10 to 40 mg/d). If necessary, the calcium channel blocker was combined with or replaced by enalapril (5 to 20 mg/d), hydrochlorothiazide (12.5 to 25 mg/d), or both. In the control group matching placebo pills were employed similarly. The study drugs were stepwise titrated and combined to reduce sitting systolic blood pressure by ≥20 mmHg to <150 mmHg (Amery et al., 1991). Death, stroke, retinal hemorrhage or exudates, MI, congestive heart failure, dissecting aortic aneurysm, and renal insufficiency were the predefined end-points. The blinded End-Point Committee ascertained all major events by reviewing the local patient files or other source documents, by requesting detailed written information from the investigators, or by both approaches.

Statistical analysis was performed with SAS software (SAS Institute, Inc.), using 2-sided tests. Comparisons of means, proportions, and rates relied on the standard normal z-test, the χ^2-statistic, and the log-rank test, respectively. Net blood pressure differences after randomization were calculated by subtracting the mean change from baseline during active treatment from the corresponding change in the control group (Staessen et al., 1997b). Cox regression was used to calculate relative hazard rates adjusted for covariables and confounders.

Morbidity and Mortality Results in the Intention-to-Treat Analysis

Patients Characteristics at Randomization

Of 8926 patients entered in the registers of screened patients, 6403 (71.7%) were enrolled in the run-in period and 4695 (52.6%) were randomized (Staessen et al., 1997a) (Figure 15-1). Eastern European centers recruited 1994 patients (42.5%).

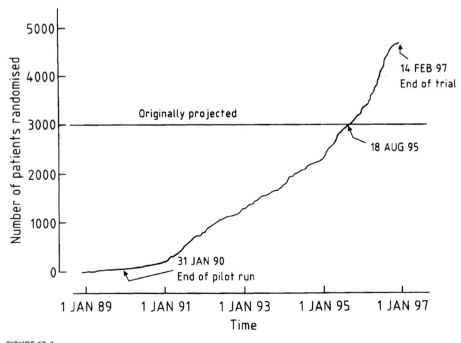

FIGURE 15-1

Flow of patients. (From JA Staessen et al., Arch Intern Med 158:1681, 1998, with permission.)

At randomization, the patients in the placebo ($n = 2297$) and active-treatment ($n = 2398$) groups were similar in sex ratio, age, blood pressure, pulse rate, body mass index, serum cholesterol, the use of tobacco and alcohol, the prevalence of diabetes mellitus, previous cardiovascular complications, and antihypertensive treatment (Table 15-1).

Treatment and Blood Pressure Control

At median follow-up (2 years), 866 of the patients randomized to placebo and 1014 of those randomized to active treatment remained in double-blind follow-up (70.1% versus 78.9% $p < .001$). Of the actively treated patients, 856 (84.4%) were taking nitrendipine (mean daily dose, 28.2 mg), 330 (32.5%) enalapril (13.8 mg/d), 164 (16.2%) hydrochlorothiazide (21.2 mg/d), and 10 (1.0%) other antihypertensive drugs. For the matching placebos in the control group, these numbers were 800 (92.4%), 477 (55.1%), 297 (34.3%), and 8 (0.9%), respectively. At 2 years, the sitting systolic/diastolic blood pressure had fallen by 13/2 mmHg in the placebo group and by 23/7 mmHg in the active-treatment group. The between-group differences averaged 10.1 mmHg systolic (95% CI: 8.8

TABLE 15-1

CLINICAL FEATURES OF TREATMENT GROUPS AT RANDOMIZATION

Characteristic	Placebo ($n = 2297$)	Active treatment ($n = 2398$)
Mean (SD) age, y	70.2 (6.7)	70.3 (6.7)
Mean (SD) blood pressure, mmHg[a]		
Sitting systolic, mmHg	173.9 (10.1)	173.8 (9.9)
Sitting diastolic, mmHg	85.5 (5.9)	85.5 (5.8)
Mean (SD) sitting heart rate, beats/min	73.0 (8.1)	73.3 (7.9)
Mean (SD) body mass index, kg/m^2		
Men	26.3 (3.1)	26.6 (3.5)
Women	27.5 (4.4)	27.2 (4.5)
Mean (SD) serum cholesterol, mmol/L		
Total cholesterol	6.0 (1.2)	6.0 (1.2)
High-density lipoprotein cholesterol	1.4 (0.5)	1.4 (0.5)
Characteristic present at baseline, no. (%)		
Female	1520 (66.2%)	1618 (67.5%)
Previous antihypertensive medication	1083 (47.1%)	1104 (46.0%)
Cardiovascular complications	697 (30.3%)	705 (29.4%)
Diabetes mellitus[b]	240 (10.4%)	252 (10.5%)
Current smokers	164 (7.1%)	179 (7.5%)
Abstaining from alcohol	1674 (72.9%)	1724 (71.9%)
Drinking ≥ 1 unit alcohol per day	267 (11.6%)	258 (10.8%)

[a]The blood pressure of individual patients was the mean of six readings (two at three baseline visits 1 month apart).
[b]Defined according to the 1994 criteria of the World Health Organization.

to 11.4 mmHg) and 4.5 mmHg diastolic (95% CI: 3.9 to 5.1 mmHg) (Staessen et al., 1997a).

Outcome Results in the Intention-to-Treat Analysis

Active treatment reduced the total stroke rate from 13.7 to 7.9 events per 1000 patient-years (Table 15-2) (Staessen et al., 1997a). Nonfatal stroke alone decreased by 44% ($p = .007$). In the active treatment group, all fatal and nonfatal cardiac end-points, including sudden death, declined by 26% ($p = .03$). Nonfatal cardiac end-points decreased by 33% ($p = .03$). A similar trend was observed for nonfatal heart failure (-36%; $p = .06$), for all cases of heart failure (-29%; $p = .12$), and for fatal and

nonfatal MI (-30%; $p = .12$). Active treatment reduced all fatal and nonfatal cardiovascular end-points by 31% ($p <. 001$). Cardiovascular mortality tended to be less on active treatment (-27%; $p = .07$), but all-cause mortality was not influenced (-14%; $p = .22$). In terms of absolute benefit, at the rates observed in the placebo group, treating 1000 older patients with isolated systolic hypertension for 5 years would prevent 29 strokes or 53 major cardiovascular events (Staessen et al., 1997a).

Fatal and nonfatal cancer (change with active treatment: -15%; 95% CI: -38 to 16%; $p = .29$) and hemorrhages other than cerebral or retinal (-10%; 95% CI: -52 to 69%; $p = .74$) occurred with similar frequency in both treatment groups (Staessen et al., 1997a).

TABLE 15-2

MAJOR END-POINTS IN THE INTENTION-TO-TREAT ANALYSIS

Nature of end-point	Rate per 1000 patient-years (number of end-points)		Relative difference with rate in placebo group	
	Placebo ($n = 2297$)	Active ($n = 2398$)	% rate (95% CI)	p
Mortality				
Total	24.0 (137)	20.5 (123)	-14 (-33 to 9)	.22
Cardiovascular	13.5 (77)	9.8 (59)	-27 (-48 to 2)	.07
Noncardiovascular	10.2 (58)	10.0 (60)	-1 (-31 to 41)	.95
Nonfatal end-points				
Stroke	10.1 (57)	5.7 (34)	-44 (-63 to -14)	.007
Cardiac end-points	12.6 (70)	8.5 (50)	-33 (-53 to -3)	.03
Fatal and nonfatal end-points				
Stroke	13.7 (77)	7.9 (47)	-42 (-60 to -17)	.003
Cardiac end-points[a]	20.5 (114)	15.1 (89)	-26 (-44 to -3)	.03
Heart failure	8.7 (49)	6.2 (37)	-29 (-53 to 10)	.12
Myocardial infarction	8.0 (45)	5.5 (33)	-30 (-56 to 9)	.12
All fatal and nonfatal cardiovascular end-points	33.9 (186)	23.3 (137)	-31 (-45 to -14)	<.001

[a]Nonfatal and fatal cardiac end-points included fatal and nonfatal heart failure, fatal and nonfatal myocardial infarction, and sudden death.

Other Findings

Subgroup and Per-Protocol Analysis

In the intention-to-treat analysis, male sex, previous cardiovascular complications, older age, higher systolic blood pressure, and smoking at randomization were positively and independently correlated with cardiovascular risk (Staessen et al., 1998a). Furthermore, for total ($p = .009$) and cardiovascular ($p = .09$) mortality, the benefit of antihypertensive drug treatment weakened with higher age. For total mortality ($p = .05$), the benefit of treatment increased with higher systolic blood pressure at entry, and for stroke ($p = .01$) it was most evident in nonsmokers (92.7% of all patients). Otherwise, the relative benefit of therapy was similar in all subgroups.

In the per-protocol analysis, active treatment reduced total mortality by 26% ($p = .05$); all fatal and nonfatal cardiovascular end-points by 32% ($p < .001$); all strokes by 44% ($p = .004$); nonfatal stroke by 48% ($p = 0.005$); and all cardiac end-points, including sudden death, by 26% ($p = 0.05$) (Staessen et al., 1998a).

Calcium Channel Blockade and Cardiovascular Prognosis

The full relative benefit of treatment was observed as early as 6 months after randomization, when most patients of the active-treatment group were still on monotherapy with nitrendipine (Staessen et al., 1998b). To verify that treatment with the dihydropyridine provided protection against cardiovascular complications, the 1327 patients who throughout the whole follow-up remained on monotherapy with nitrendipine were matched by sex, age, previous cardiovascular complications, and systolic blood pressure at entry with an equal number of placebo patients. In this analysis, nitrendipine reduced cardiovascular mortality by 41% ($p \leq .05$), all cardiovascular end-points by 33%, and fatal and nonfatal cardiac end-points by 33% (Staessen et al., 1998b).

Outcome in Diabetic and Nondiabetic Patients

At randomization, 492 patients (10.5%) had diabetes (Table 15-1). At median follow-up, the net differences in blood pressure between the placebo and active-treatment groups were 8.6 mmHg systolic and 3.9 mmHg diastolic in the diabetic patients and 10.3 mmHg and 4.6 mmHg, respectively, in the 4203 nondiabetic patients (Tuomilehto et al., 1999).

In diabetic patients, with adjustments for possible confounders applied, active treatment reduced all-cause mortality by 55%, cardiovascular mortality by 76%, all cardiovascular end-points by 69%, fatal and nonfatal stroke by 73%, and all cardiac end-points by 63% (Figure 15-2). In the nondiabetic patients, active treatment decreased all cardiovascular end-points by 26% and fatal and nonfatal stroke by 38%. Active treatment reduced total mortality ($p = .04$), cardiovascular mortality ($p = .02$), and all cardiovascular end-points ($p = .01$) significantly more in the diabetic than in the nondiabetic patients (Tuomilehto et al., 1999).

Prevention of Dementia

The Vascular Dementia Project investigated whether antihypertensive drug treatment could reduce the incidence of dementia (Forette et al., 1991, 1998; Seux et al., 1998). At baseline and follow-up, cognitive function was assessed by the mini-mental status examination; if the score was ≤ 23, the diagnosis of dementia was established based on the *Diagnostic and Statistical Manual of Mental Disorders,* third edition, revised (DSM-III-R).

In total, 2418 patients were enrolled in the dementia study. Median follow-up by intention to treat was 2.0 years. Among the 32 incident cases of dementia, 23 were Alzheimer's disease, 7 had a mixed etiology, and only 2 were vascular. Compared with placebo ($n = 1180$), active treatment ($n = 1238$) reduced the incidence of dementia by 50% ($p = .05$), from 7.7 to 3.8 cases per 1000 patient-years (Figure 15-3). In the per-protocol analysis, active treatment decreased the rate by 60% ($p = .03$). Active treatment prevented mainly degenerative dementia.

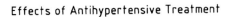

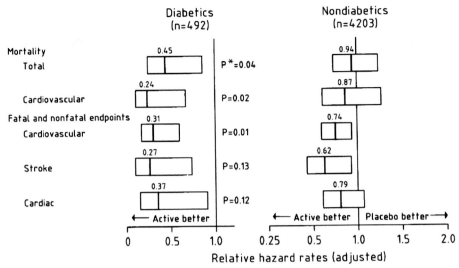

FIGURE 15-2

Relative hazard rates of active treatment versus placebo in diabetic and nondiabetic patients with cumulative adjustments for sex, age, previous cardiovascular complications, systolic blood pressure at entry, smoking, and residence in western Europe. The p-values refer to the treatment-by-diabetes interaction and indicate whether the treatment effect was significantly different according to the presence of diabetes at randomization. (From J Tuomilehto et al., N Engl J Med 340:677, 1999; with permission.)

After termination of the placebo-controlled phase of the SYST-EUR trial in February 1997, all patients were offered active trial medication for a further period of observation (Syst-Eur 2) (Gasowski et al., 1999). Median follow-up increased from 2.0 to 3.9 years, and the number of incident cases of dementia from 32 to 64. Systolic/diastolic pressure in the former placebo group drifted gradually towards the level in the active treatment group but at 8 years of follow-up remained 3.3/3.9 mmHg above the level in the active-treatment group ($p < .001$). Long-term active-treatment ($n = 1485$), compared to control ($n = 1417$), reduced the incidence of dementia by 55% from 7.4 to 3.3 cases per 1000 patient-years (43 v. 21 patients; $p = .0008$). By inference, treatment of 1000 patients for 5 years could prevent 20 cases of dementia (95% CI: 7 to 33 cases).

Renal Function

The long-term changes in renal function were studied in 2258 treated and 2148 untreated patients, of whom 455 had diabetes mellitus and 390 had proteinuria. Serum creatinine concentration at randomization was <176.8 μmol/L (<2.0 mg/dL), averaging 88 μmol/L (Voyaki et al., 2001).

At the time of the last serum creatinine measurement, the blood pressure difference ($p < .001$) between the two groups was 11.6/4.1 mmHg. In the intention-to-treat analysis (11427 patient-years), serum creatinine and the calculated creatinine clearance were not influenced by active treatment. However, in the patients randomized to active treatment, the incidence of mild renal dysfunction [serum creatinine ≥ 176.8 μmol/L (≥ 2.0 mg/dL)] decreased

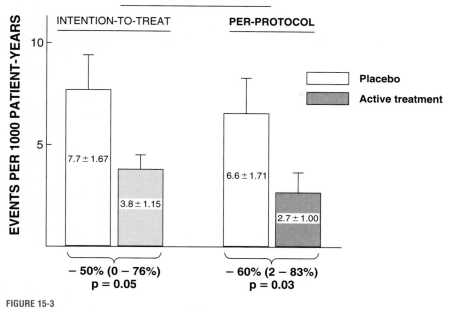

FIGURE 15-3

Incidence of dementia by treatment group in the intention-to-treat and per-protocol analyses.

by 64% (p = .04) and that of proteinuria by 33% (p = 0.03) (Voyaki et al., 2001). Active treatment reduced the risk of proteinuria more (p = .04) in diabetic than in nondiabetic patients: 71 v. 20% (Figure 15-4). In nonproteinuric patients active treatment did not influence serum creatinine (+0.84 μmol/L; p = .13), whereas in patients with proteinuria at entry serum creatinine decreased on active treatment (−6.52 μmol/L; p = 0.02). The p-value for interaction was .001.

Prognostic Stratification Based on Ambulatory Blood Pressure Monitoring

Within the framework of the SYST-EUR trial, the Study on Ambulatory Blood Pressure Monitoring was set up to compare the prognostic accuracy of conventional and ambulatory blood pressure measurements (Staessen et al., 1992, 1999; Emelianov et al., 1998; Fagard et al., 2000). Of 198 SYST-EUR centers, 46 opted to enroll their patients. Progress

reports showed that: (1) the daytime systolic blood pressure decreased by 2 to 3 mmHg on long-term placebo treatment (Staessen et al., 1996); (2) in parallel-group trials or in clinical experiments focusing on blood pressure profiles, ambulatory monitoring does not allow economizing on sample size (Staessen et al., 1994); and (3) it is possible to calculate the trough-to-peak ratio in parallel-group trials while fully accounting for placebo effects as well as interindividual variability (Staessen et al., 1997b).

At randomization (n = 808), blood pressure was on average 22.0/2.0 mmHg higher (p < .001) on conventional than on daytime (from 10 A.M. to 8 P.M) ambulatory measurement. In the placebo group (n = 393), the 24-h daytime and nighttime (from midnight to 6 A.M.) systolic ambulatory blood pressures predicted the incidence of cardiovascular complications over and beyond the conventional blood pressure (Staessen et al., 1999). The 24-h level and the night-to-day ratio of systolic pressure were significantly and independently correlated with the

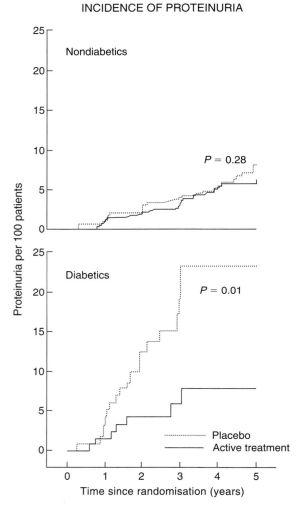

FIGURE 15-4

Kaplan-Meier estimates modeling the incidence of proteinuria in nondiabetic (top) and diabetic (bottom) patients. P-values (log-rank test) refer to the difference between placebo and active treatment. (From SM Voyaki et al., J Hypertens 19:511, 2001, with permission.)

pressure at randomization did not significantly predict cardiovascular risk, regardless of the technique of blood pressure measurement (Staessen et al., 1999). This observation confirmed that nitrendipine-based treatment substantially reduced the excess risk conferred by the increased systolic pressure at randomization.

Further analyses showed that patients with sustained hypertension (clinic and daytime systolic pressure $\geq$ 160 mmHg) had higher electrocardiographic voltages and rates of cardiovascular complications than did patients with nonsustained hypertension (clinic systolic pressure $\geq$ 160 mmHg and daytime systolic pressure $<$ 140 mmHg) (Fagard et al., 2000). The favorable effect of active treatment on these outcomes was significant only in patients with sustained hypertension.

Conclusions

In summing up the SYST-EUR trial, four conclusions emerge. First, the trial confirmed the findings of the Systolic Hypertension in the Elderly Program (SHEP Cooperative Research Group, 1991) in that older subjects with isolated systolic hypertension should be treated to prevent or postpone stroke and other cardiovascular complications (Staessen et al., 1997a, 1998a). Second, long-acting dihydropyridines constitute a valid alternative to diuretics and beta blockers in the primary prevention of cardiovascular disorders in older hypertensive patients. Third, calcium channel blockade may be particularly indicated in diabetic patients with isolated systolic hypertension whose renal function is normal (Tuomilehto et al., 1999) and in patients at risk of dementia (Forette et al., 1998). Finally, the circumstantial evidence for the potentially dangerous side effects of calcium channel blockers was not borne out, when put to the test of a double-blind placebo-controlled clinical trial.

Acknowledgements

This chapter is dedicated to the memory of Professor Antoon Amery, who died on November 2, 1994. The

incidence of all cardiovascular end-points in the placebo group (Figure 15-5). The hazard rates associated with a 10-mmHg increase in the 24-h systolic pressure and with a 10% higher systolic night-to-day ratio were 1.23 (95% CI: 1.03 to 1.46; p = .02) and 1.41 (95% CI: 1.03 to 1.94; p = .03), respectively. In the active-treatment group (n = 415), systolic

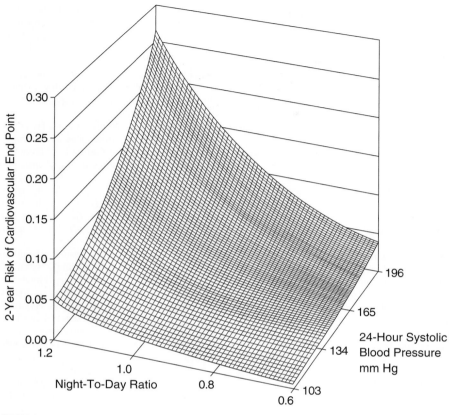

FIGURE 15-5

Whole-day level and night-to-day ratio of systolic blood pressure at randomization as independent predictors of the 2-year incidence of cardiovascular end-points in the placebo group. The event rate was standardized to female sex, 69.6 years (mean age), no previous cardiovascular complications, nonsmoking, and residence in western Europe. (From JA Staessen et al., JAMA 282:539, 1999, with permission.)

Syst-Eur trial was a concerted action of the BIO-MED Research Program sponsored by the European Union. The trial was carried out in consultation with the World Health Organization, the International Society of Hypertension, the European Society of Hypertension, and the World Hypertension League. The trial was sponsored by Bayer (Wuppertal, Germany). The National Fund for Scientific Research (Brussels, Belgium) provided additional support. Study medication was donated by Bayer and Merck Sharpe and Dohme (West Point, PA). A list of the investigators participating in this trial appears in Staessen et al.; 1997a and 1998a.

REFERENCES

Amery A et al: Syst-Eur. A multicentre trial on the treatment of isolated systolic hypertension in the elderly: Objectives, protocol, and organization. Aging Clin Exp Res 3:287, 1991

Emelianov D et al, on behalf of the Syst-Eur Investigators: Conventional and ambulatory blood pressure measurement in older patients with isolated systolic hypertension: Baseline observations in the Syst-Eur trial. Blood Press Monit 3:173, 1998

Fagard RH et al, for the Systolic Hypertension in Europe (Syst-Eur) Trial Investigators: Response to antihypertensive therapy in older patients with sustained and nonsustained systolic hypertension. Circulation 102:1139, 2000

Forette F et al: Is prevention of vascular dementia possible? The Syst-Eur Vascular Dementia Project. Aging Clin Exp Res 3:373, 1991

Forette F et al, on behalf of the Syst-Eur Investigators: Prevention of dementia in randomised double-blind placebo-controlled Systolic Hypertension in Europe (Syst-Eur) trial. Lancet 352:1347, 1998

Gasowski J et al, on behalf of the Systolic Hypertension in Europe Investigators: Systolic Hypertension in Europe (Syst-Eur) Trial Phase 2: Objectives, protocol and initial progress. J Hum Hypertens 13:135, 1999

Seux ML et al: Correlates of cognitive status of old patients with isolated systolic hypertension: The Syst-Eur Vascular Dementia Project. J Hypertens 16:963, 1998

SHEP Cooperative Research Group: Prevention of stroke by antihypertensive drug treatment in older persons with isolated systolic hypertension. Final results of the Systolic Hypertension in the Elderly Program (SHEP). JAMA 265:3255, 1991

Staessen J et al: Editorial review. Isolated systolic hypertension in the elderly. J Hypertens 8:393, 1990

Staessen J et al: Twenty-four hour blood pressure monitoring in the Syst-Eur trial. Aging Clin Exp Res 4:85, 1992

Staessen JA et al, on behalf of the Syst-Eur Investigators: Clinical trials with ambulatory blood pressure monitoring: Fewer patients needed? Lancet 344:1552, 1994

Staessen JA et al, on behalf of the Systolic Hypertension in Europe (SYST-EUR) Trial Investigators: Ambulatory monitoring uncorrected for placebo overestimates long-term antihypertensive action. Hypertension 27:414, 1996

Staessen JA et al, for the Systolic Hypertension in Europe (Syst-Eur) Trial Investigators: Randomised double-blind comparison of placebo and active treatment for older patients with isolated systolic hypertension. Lancet 350:757, 1997a

Staessen JA et al, on behalf of the Systolic Hypertension in Europe (SYST-EUR) Trial Investigators: Determining the trough-to-peak ratio in parallel-group trials. Hypertension 29:659, 1997b

Staessen JA et al, for the Systolic Hypertension in Europe (Syst-Eur) Trial Investigators: Subgroup and per-protocol analysis of the randomized European trial on isolated systolic hypertension in the elderly. Arch Intern Med 158:1681, 1998a

Staessen JA et al, for the Systolic Hypertension in Europe (Syst-Eur) Trial Investigators: Calcium channel blockade and cardiovascular prognosis in the European trial on isolated systolic hypertension. Hypertension 32:410, 1998b

Staessen JA et al, for the Systolic Hypertension in Europe Trial Investigators: Predicting cardiovascular risk using conventional and ambulatory blood pressure in older patients with systolic hypertension. JAMA 282:539, 1999

Tuomilehto J et al, for the Systolic Hypertension in Europe (Syst-Eur) Trial Investigators: Effects of calcium-channel blockade in older patients with diabetes and systolic hypertension. N Engl J Med 340:677, 1999

Voyaki SM et al, for the Systolic Hypertension in Europe (Syst-Eur) Trial Investigators: Follow-up of renal function in treated and untreated older patients with isolated systolic hypertension. J Hypertens 19:511, 2001

16

THE INTENSITY OF TREATMENT OF HYPERTENSION: THE HYPERTENSION OPTIMAL TREATMENT (HOT) STUDY

Alberto Zanchetti

It is well documented that treatment of hypertension reduces cardiovascular morbidity and mortality (Collins and Peto, 1994). However, patients treated for hypertension remain at a greater risk of cardiovascular complications than normotensive individuals (Isles et al., 1986). One possible explanation is that the blood pressure of hypertensive patients is seldom lowered by treatment to strictly normotensive levels. On the other hand, concerns have been expressed that too vigorous a reduction in blood pressure may be associated with increased cardiovascular risk, the so-called J-curve concept (Cruickshank et al., 1987). The issue of how far blood pressure should be lowered to achieve the greatest reduction of cardiovascular morbidity and mortality, and in particular the question of whether there are additional benefits (or risks) in lowering blood pressure of hypertensive patients to fully normotensive levels (70 to 85 mmHg diastolic blood pressure), had not been approached by any of the previous randomized and prospective trials of antihypertensive therapy. This was the main reason for conducting the Hypertension Optimal Treatment (HOT) study (Hansson and Zanchetti, 1993).

Study Design

The principal aims of this study were as follows:

1. To assess the association between major cardiovascular events (nonfatal myocardial infarction, nonfatal stroke, and cardiovascular death) and three different target diastolic blood pressures (DBP) to which the patients had been randomized
2. To assess the association between major cardiovascular events and the DBP actually achieved during treatment
3. To determine whether the addition of a low dose of acetylsalicylic acid (75 mg/d) to antihypertensive treatment reduces the rate of major cardiovascular events (this part of the study is not reported here).

Altogether, 18,790 hypertensive patients were randomized to achieve three different DBP targets ($\leq$90 mmHg, $\leq$85 mmHg, $\leq$80 mmHg). The patients were from 26 countries (mostly in Europe and North America) and aged 50 to 80 years (mean

61.5 years), 53% were males, and their baseline DBP was 100 to 115 mmHg (mean 105 mmHg). The study was conducted according to the Prospective, Randomized, Open with Blinded End-point evaluation (PROBE) design. Randomization was computer-generated and stratified for age, sex, previous antihypertensive therapy, smoking, previous myocardial infarction, previous coronary heart disease, previous stroke, and diabetes.

Treatment consisted of five successive steps in order to achieve the randomized target: (1) administration of the calcium antagonist felodipine at a low dose of 5 mg/d; (2) addition of a low dose of either an angiotensin-converting enzyme (ACE) inhibitor or a beta blocker; (3) increase of the felodipine dose to 10 mg/d; (4) increase of the ACE inhibitor or beta-blocker dose; and (5) addition of a diuretic or of another antihypertensive drug. Randomized treatment was continued for an average of 3.8 years, and only 2.6% of the randomized patients were lost to follow-up. All events were validated by an Independent Clinical Event Committee according to criteria set in the study protocol (Hansson et al., 1998).

Results

Effects on Blood Pressure

A major achievement of the HOT study was the marked reduction in both diastolic and systolic blood pressures (SBP) achieved with the stepped therapeutic regimen. Compared with blood pressure at randomization, diastolic values were reduced by an average of 22.3 mmHg and systolic values by 28.0 mmHg, with a DBP ≤ 90 mmHg being achieved in as many as 91.5% of the patients. In previous trials of antihypertensive therapy, a similar DBP target was reached in only 65 to 77% of patients.

In the three randomized groups, DBP was reduced by 20.3 mmHg, 22.3 mmHg, and 24.3 mmHg and SBP by 26.2 mmHg, 28.0 mmHg, and 29.9 mmHg, respectively. DBP was reduced from a mean of 105 mmHg to a mean of 85.2 mmHg in the group whose target was ≤ 90 mmHg, 83.2 mmHg in the group

whose target was ≤ 85 mmHg, and 81.1 mmHg in the group whose target was ≤ 80 mmHg. The average DBP difference between randomized groups was only 2 mmHg, instead of the expected 5 mmHg.

Effects on Mortality and Morbidity

Differences in event rates between target groups were rather small, as were the between-group blood pressure differences. Table 16-1 shows only the trend for the rate of myocardial infarction to be lower at the lower target DBP, and this was of borderline significance (a 25% reduction in the group whose target was ≤ 85 mmHg and 28% reduction in the group whose target was ≤ 80 mmHg as compared with the group whose target was ≤ 90 mmHg).

When the incidence of various types of event was related to the DBP and SBP achieved throughout the study, confidence intervals were narrowest in the DBP range of 75 to 95 mmHg and in the SBP range of 130 to 140 mmHg, suggesting adequate precision of the estimated risk within these limits. As illustrated in Fig. 16-1, the lowest risk for major cardiovascular events was at a mean achieved DBP of 82.6 mmHg and at a mean SBP of 138.5 mmHg, suggesting that the "optimal" blood pressures for minimizing the risk of major cardiovascular events are between 80 and 85 mmHg for DBP and between 135 and 140 mmHg for SBP. There was no evidence, however, of a significant increase of risk for any type of events at blood pressures lower than these "optimal" levels (down to 70 mmHg DBP and 120 mmHg SBP).

Effects in Hypertensive Patients with Diabetes Mellitus

There were 1501 patients in the HOT study who had diabetes mellitus at baseline, equally distributed in the three target DBP groups (diabetes was a factor used in randomization). A statistically significant decline in the rate of major cardiovascular events ($p = .005$) and in cardiovascular mortality rate ($p = .016$) was seen in relation to the target DBP groups. As illustrated in Fig. 16-2, in the group randomized to ≤ 80 mmHg, the risk of

TABLE 16-1

EVENTS IN RELATION TO TARGET BLOOD PRESSURE GROUPS

Event	Number of events	Events/1000 patient-years	p for trend	Comparison	Relative risk (95% CI)
Major cardiovascular events					
≤90 mmHg	232	9.9		90 vs 85	0.99 (0.83–1.19)
≤85 mmHg	234	10.0		85 vs 80	1.08 (0.89–1.29)
≤80 mmHg	217	9.3	.50	90 vs 80	1.07 (0.89–1.28)
All myocardial infarction					
≤90 mmHg	84	3.6		90 vs 85	1.32 (0.95–1.82)
≤85 mmHg	64	2.7		85 vs 80	1.05 (0.74–1.48)
≤80 mmHg	61	2.6	.05	90 vs 80	1.37 (0.99–1.91)
All stroke					
≤90 mmHg	94	4.0		90 vs 85	0.85 (0.64–1.11)
≤85 mmHg	111	4.7		85 vs 80	1.24 (0.94–1.64)
≤80 mmHg	89	3.8	.74	90 vs 80	1.05 (0.79–1.41)
Cardiovascular mortality					
≤90 mmHg	87	3.7		90 vs 85	0.97 (0.72–1.30)
≤85 mmHg	90	3.8		85 vs 80	0.93 (0.70–1.24)
≤80 mmHg	96	4.1	.49	90 vs 80	0.90 (0.68–1.21)
Total mortality					
≤90 mmHg	188	7.9		90 vs 85	0.97 (0.79–1.19)
≤85 mmHg	194	8.2		85 vs 80	0.93 (0.77–1.14)
≤80 mmHg	207	8.8	.32	90 vs 80	0.91 (0.74–1.10)

NOTE: $n = 6264$, 6264 and 6262 in the target groups ≤90 mmHg, ≤85 mmHg, and ≤80 mmHg, respectively.

SOURCE: From L Hansson et al: Lancet 351:1755, 1998, by courtesy of The Lancet.

major cardiovascular events was halved in comparison with that of the group whose target was ≤90 mmHg. The approximate halving of the risk was also observed for myocardial infarction, although the small number of events made it statistically nonsignificant; all stroke also showed a nonsignificant 30% decrease at the lowest target blood pressure. Cardiovascular mortality in the ≤80 mmHg target group was significantly reduced to one-third of that occurring in the group randomized to ≤90 mmHg, and total mortality was reduced by 45%, a change close to statistical significance.

Effects in Hypertensive Patients with Ischemic Heart Disease (IHD)

There were 3080 patients with IHD at baseline, defined as patients with previous myocardial infarction, other previous coronary heart disease, or baseline electrocardiograms with Minnesota codes 1:1 or 1:2 (signs of myocardial infarction) or 4:1–2 or 5:1–2 (signs of ischemia). The rate of major cardiovascular events declined nonsignificantly in relation to the target DBP groups to which the patients had been randomized (77, 68, and 62/1000 patient-years, respectively, in the

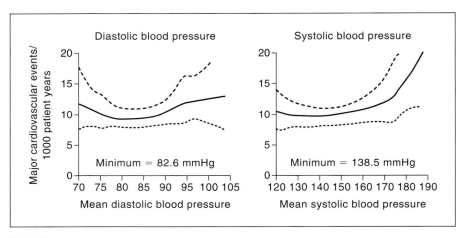

FIGURE 16-1

Estimated incidence (continuous curves) and 95% confidence intervals (dashed curves) of major cardio-vascular events in relation to achieved mean diastolic and systolic blood pressure (averages of all mea-surements from entry to event). Minimum, indicates the blood pressure at the lowest point of the curves. (Modified from L Hansson et al: Lancet 351: 1755, 1998, by courtesy of The Lancet.)

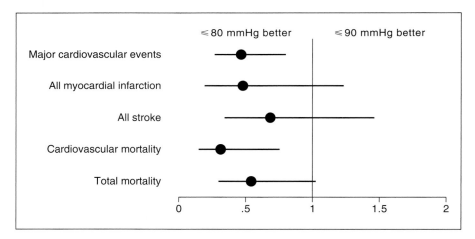

FIGURE 16-2

Effect of intensive lowering of diastolic blood pressure in the diabetic patients of the HOT study. Relative risk (filled circles) and 95% confidence limits (horizontal bars) of being randomized to ≤80 mmHg DBP rather than to ≤90 mmHg.

target groups ≤90 mmHg, ≤85 mmHg, and ≤80 mmHg), and the decline became significant after exclusion of smokers (unpublished observations). The stroke rate also showed a significant reduction from 35 to 30 and 20/1000 patient-years in relation to the target DBP groups (p for trend, .046), with a 43% reduction in the group randomized to the low-est DBP target compared with the group random-ized to the highest DBP target. Even in patients with IHD there was no significant trend for any type of event to increase in the group with the lowest DBP target.

Effects According to Gender and Age

The beneficial effects of more pronounced lowering of DBP both on major cardiovascular events and on myocardial infarction were more marked in women than in men; in particular, women had a significant reduction in myocardial infarction rate (44%) when randomized to ≤80 mmHg DBP rather than to ≤90 mmHg DBP ($p = .034$), while men had an insignificant reduction of only 17%. Patients younger than 65 years and patients aged 65 years or older had similar trends toward a reduction of myocardial infarction (28 and 27%, respectively), but in both age groups the trends did not reach statistical significance (Kjeldsen et al., 2000).

Effects on Renal Function

Among the HOT study patients, 470 had baseline serum creatinine >133 μmol/L (>1.5 mg/dL) and 1367 had serum creatinine >115 μmol/L (>1.3 mg/dL). These patients with renal impairment had significantly higher incidences of all types of cardiovascular event (adjusted relative risks between 1.4 and 2.8). This indicates that elevation in serum creatinine is a powerful predictor of cardiovascular events and death. However, patients with elevated baseline serum creatinine achieved SBP and DBP values no different from those of patients with lower baseline creatinine, though at the cost of more intensive antihypertensive treatment (Ruilope et al., 2001; Zanchetti et al., 2001b). No significant changes in serum creatinine concentration were seen at the end of the 3.8-year treatment period in the great majority of patients, independently of their baseline creatinine values and of the DBP target to which they had been randomized. However, there was a small group of 120 patients whose serum creatinine rose to ≥177 μmol/L (≥2.0 mg/dL) at the end of the study: this worsening of renal function occurred

in 17.9% of patients with baseline creatinine >133 μmol/L (>1.5 mg/dL) and in only 0.4% of patients with baseline creatinine ≤133 μmol/L (≤1.5 mg/dL) (Ruilope et al., 2001).

Effects on Quality of Life

The HOT study has demonstrated that substantial reductions in both systolic and diastolic blood pressures can be obtained, and DBP ≤90 mmHg can be achieved in more than 90% of hypertensive patients with an intensive treatment regimen, based on a long-acting calcium antagonist, felodipine, and the combination of two or more drugs in about two-thirds of the patients. The medications administered were well tolerated, and a careful study of patients' well-being showed an overall improvement as compared with baseline; this improvement was better in the ≤80-mmHg target group than in the other target groups. Overall, well-being was also better the lower the achieved blood pressure, and complaints of headache were fewer (Wikland et al., 1997).

Conclusions

The analyses of event rates in the groups randomized to different DBP targets together with the analyses of event rates in relation to achieved blood pressure demonstrate the benefits of intensive lowering of blood pressure in patients with hypertension, down to 140 mmHg systolic and 85 mmHg diastolic, or lower. Pronounced lowering of blood pressure was particularly beneficial in the subgroup of patients with diabetes mellitus, in whom the risk of major cardiovascular events and that of cardiovascular mortality was reduced by about 50 and 66%, respectively, in patients randomized to ≤80 mmHg DBP. This is in line with recent observations in the diabetic patients of the United Kingdom Prospective Diabetes Study (UKPDS; 1998). Efforts to achieve pronounced lowering of blood pressure was not associated with any significant additional risk even in patients with IHD, for whom caution had been

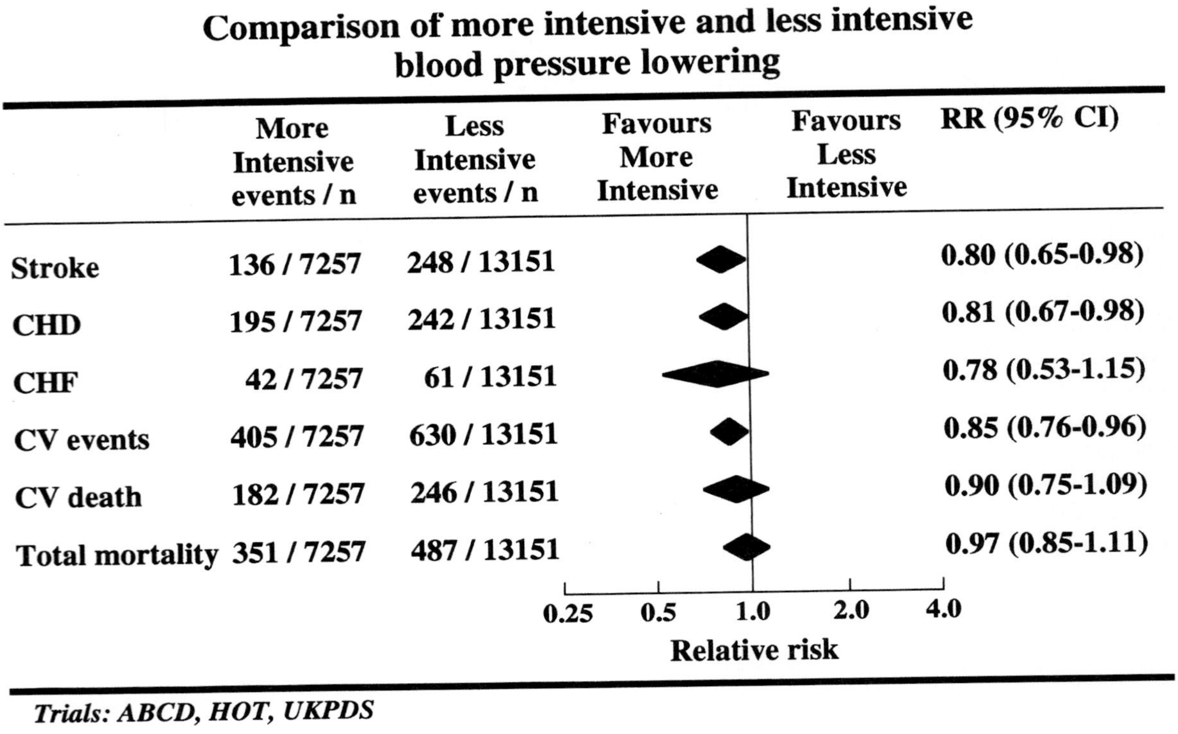

Comparison of more intensive and less intensive blood pressure lowering

	More Intensive events / n	Less Intensive events / n	Favours More Intensive	Favours Less Intensive	RR (95% CI)
Stroke	136 / 7257	248 / 13151			0.80 (0.65-0.98)
CHD	195 / 7257	242 / 13151			0.81 (0.67-0.98)
CHF	42 / 7257	61 / 13151			0.78 (0.53-1.15)
CV events	405 / 7257	630 / 13151			0.85 (0.76-0.96)
CV death	182 / 7257	246 / 13151			0.90 (0.75-1.09)
Total mortality	351 / 7257	487 / 13151			0.97 (0.85-1.11)

0.25   0.5   1.0   2.0   4.0

Relative risk

Trials: ABCD, HOT, UKPDS

FIGURE 16-3

Comparisons of more intensive blood pressure lowering strategies with less intensive strategies. Diamonds represent the 95% confidence intervals (CI) for pooled estimates of effect and are centred on pooled relative risk. (Modified from Blood Pressure Lowering Treatment Trialists' Collaboration: Lancet 355:1955, 2000.)

TABLE 16-2

COMPARISON OF EVENT INCIDENCE[a] IN THE HOT STUDY AND IN PREVIOUS TRIALS OF ANTIHYPERTENSIVE TREATMENT.[b]

	HOT study (Mean age, 61 years)	Previous trials (Mean age, 56 years)
Total mortality	8.3	12.3
Cardiovascular mortality	3.8	6.5
All stroke	4.2	4.4
All myocardial infarction	3.0	7.8

[a] Event incidence is expressed as events/1000 patient-years.
[b] Data from previous trials calculated from meta-analysis by R Collins and R Peto, in JD Swales (ed): *Textbook of Hypertension.* Oxford, Blackwell Scientific, 1994.

recommended by the proposers of the J-shaped curve concept (Cruickshank et al., 1987).

A recent meta-analysis (Blood Pressure Lowering Treatment Trialists' Collaboration, 2000), largely based on the HOT study but also including the smaller UKPDS (1998) and ABCD studies (Estacio et al., 1998), has confirmed a significant reduction of the incidences of stroke, coronary events, and major cardiovascular events with more intensive blood pressure lowering strategies (Fig. 16-3).

On the whole, there was a very low event rate in the HOT study. In Table 16-2, event rates in the HOT study are compared with those in actively treated patients in the meta-analysis of all previous trials of

antihypertensive treatment calculated by Collins and Peto (1994). In the HOT study, patients' total mortality was 67%, cardiovascular mortality 58%, and myocardial infarction rate only 38% of the respective rates in actively treated patients of all previous studies, despite a higher mean age in the HOT study than in patients of the meta-analysis (61.5 years versus 56 years, respectively). Furthermore, a recent analysis of the baseline characteristics of the HOT study patients (Zanchetti et al., 2001a) has shown that they were by no means low-risk patients at baseline: 50% of them were classified as at high or very high risk according to World Health Organization/ International Society of Hypertension guidelines

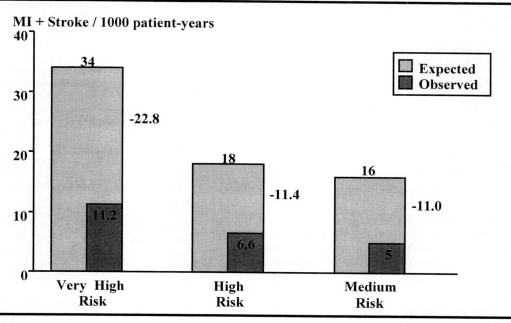

Observed Versus Expected Rates of MI and Strokes in HOT Study Patients Stratified by Baseline Risk

FIGURE 16-4

Expected (shaded columns) and observed (black columns) rates of myocardial infarction and stroke in HOT study patients classified as at very high, high, or medium initial risk of cardiovascular disease. Presumptive benefit is the difference between expected and observed rates. (From data of Zanchetti et al: J Hypertens 19: 819, 2001a).

(Guidelines Subcommittee, 1999). It is therefore likely that the particularly low event rate found in the HOT study is due to the very effective blood pressure control achieved in this study, with only 8.5% of treated patients remaining at DBP >90 mmHg (versus 23 to 35% in the previous studies included in the meta-analysis).

Stratification of HOT study patients according to their baseline risk also made it clear that, despite their excellent blood pressure control, their incidence of cardiovascular events remained proportional to their pretreatment risk. The relative risk of very high versus medium risk strata was between two and three (Zanchetti et al., 2001a). However, the rates of myocardial infarction and stroke observed during prolonged and intensive treatment were much lower than those expected on the basis of baseline risk. Figure 16-4 shows that for every 1000 patients intensively treated for 1 year, approximately 23 myocardial infarctions and strokes can presumably be avoided in very high risk patients, and 11 in medium-risk patients. Figure 16-4 also illustrates the fact that the greater absolute benefit of treating very high risk patients should not obscure the fact that the higher the risk stratum to which a patient initially belongs, the higher the residual risk of cardiovascular morbidity and mortality. Some of this residual risk may be irreversible and may only be avoided by earlier initiation of treatment.

In conclusion, the various analyses so far completed of the HOT study data strengthen the recommendation that the intensity of antihypertensive treatment should be such as to bring blood pressure down to at least 140 mmHg SBP and 85 mmHg DBP, with efforts to achieving even lower values in diabetic patients. The HOT study observations should also be considered as an argument to improve physicians' performance in the early control of high blood pressure, and to envisage more aggressive strategies on the other reversible cardiovascular risk factors, especially smoking, diabetes, and lipid abnormalities, in addition to the control of blood pressure in hypertensive patients.

REFERENCES

Blood Pressure Lowering Treatment Trialists' Collaboration: Effects of ACE inhibitors, calcium antagonists, and other blood-pressure-lowering drugs: Results of prospectively designed overviews of randomised trials. Lancet 355: 1955, 2000

Collins R, Peto R: Antihypertensive drug therapy: Effects on stroke and coronary heart disease, in Textbook of Hypertension, JD Swales (ed). Oxford, Blackwell Scientific, 1994, pp 1156–1164

Cruickshank JM et al: Benefits and potential harm of lowering high blood pressure. Lancet 1: 581, 1987

Estacio RO et al: The effect of nisoldipine as compared with enabafril on cardiovascular outcomes in patients with non-insulin dependent diabetes and hypertension. N Engl J Med 338:645, 1998.

Guidelines Subcommittee: 1999 World Health Organization–International Society of Hypertension guidelines for the management of hypertension. J Hypertens 17:151, 1999

Hansson L et al: Effects of intensive blood-pressure lowering and low-dose aspirin in patients with hypertension: Principal results of the Hypertension Optimal Treatment (HOT) randomized trial. Lancet 351:1755, 1998

Hansson L, Zanchetti A: The Hypertension Optimal Treatment Study (the HOT Study). Blood Press 2:62, 1993

Isles CG et al: Mortality in patients of the Glasgow Blood Pressure Clinic. J Hypertens 4:141, 1986

Kjeldsen SE et al: Influence of gender and age on preventing cardiovascular disease by antihypertensive treatment and acetylsalicylic acid. The HOT Study. J Hypertens 18:629, 2000

Ruilope LM et al: Renal function and intensive lowering of blood pressure in hypertensive participants of the Hypertension Optimal Treatment (HOT) Study. J Am Soc Nephrol 12:218, 2001

United Kingdom Prospective Diabetes Study Group: Tight blood pressure control and risk of macrovascular and microvascular complications in type 2 diabetes: UKPDS 38. BMJ 317:703, 1998

Wiklund I et al: Does lowering the blood pressure improve the mood? Quality of life results from the Hypertension Optimal Treatment (HOT) Study. Blood Press 6:357, 1997

Zanchetti A et al: Risk assessment and treatment benefit in intensively treated hypertensive patients of the Hypertension Optimal Treatment (HOT) study. J Hypertens 19:819, 2001a

Zanchetti A et al: Effects of individual risk factors on the incidence of cardiovascular events in the treated hypertensive patients of the Hypertension Optimal Treatment (HOT) Study. J Hypertens 19:1149, 2001b

17

RENAL ARTERY STENTING: INDICATIONS AND RESULTS

James J. Crowley & Richard S. Stack

Renal Artery Angioplasty

Although the long-term results of percutaneous angioplasty of renal artery stenosis were not as good as those from surgery, the technique gained widespread acceptance because of its relative ease of performance, the low risk of serious complications, and the rapid return of patients to normal daily life. Deployment of renal artery stents during angioplasty has overcome many of the shortfalls of angioplasty alone, so that this technique has become the mainstay of therapy in patients with atherosclerotic renal artery stenosis.

The initial reports of angioplasty alone for atherosclerotic renal artery stenosis showed wide variation in outcomes. It is clear that different patient and lesion characteristics influence overall results. Factors that adversely affect success include longer lesions, small vessel size, ostial involvement with atherosclerosis, older age, and occluded vessels. Perhaps the most important factor is the location of the lesion. When plaque does not involve the ostium of the artery, the technical success of angioplasty alone is 80% and restenosis occurs in 20 to 30%. However, only 20% of atherosclerotic lesions are truly nonostial. The technical success rate for ostial lesions is only 25 to 60% with restenosis as the primary cause of failure in these patients due to intimal hyperplasia, elastic recoil of the dilated artery, or recurrent atherosclerosis.

Renal Artery Stenting

Stenting provides a scaffold that buttresses the arterial wall; it prevents plaque from repositioning itself across the lumen or a dissection from causing abrupt vessel closure. There are now a number of studies that report the preliminary results with stents for treatment of atherosclerotic renal artery stenosis. In these studies, the most common indications for stent use have been an inadequate angioplasty result, the presence of dissection, and an ostial lesion or restenosis after previous angioplasty (Blum et al., 1997; Dorros et al., 1998; Lederman et al., 1999; White et al., 1997). Therefore, these patients represent a group that has failed conventional angioplasty or is known to have a poor outcome. Despite this, the technical success of stent procedures was usually greater than 90%. In most cases, it was possible to deploy the stent satisfactorily without leaving residual stenosis or dissection. In one randomized study, which compared stenting of ostial lesions to angioplasty alone, results were clearly better with stenting (van de Ven et al., 1999). The technical success was 57% for angioplasty compared to 88% after stenting. Restenosis after successful primary stenting was 14% compared to 48% after angioplasty alone.

Atherosclerotic Renal Artery Disease

The overall effect on blood pressure and renal function after stenting for atherosclerotic renal artery stenosis is similar to that of *successful* balloon angioplasty: 60% of patients have clinical improvement in blood pressure, and 15 to 40% have improved renal function. There is also evidence that even in those patients without improvement or with continued deterioration in serum creatinine, the rate of deterioration is slowed (Harden et al., 1997). The incidence of restenosis, which is 8 to 15%, has improved with greater experience of this technique. Restenosis is more common in smaller caliber arteries (Lederman et al., 1999).

Fibromuscular Dysplasia

In patients with the less common condition of fibromuscular dysplasia, angioplasty alone is recognized as the treatment of choice because complications are unusual and results are excellent. Successful dilatation of the lesions occurs in >85% of patients. Restenosis occurs in 10% and usually responds to redilatation (Martin et al., 1994). In many cases, recurrence is probably due to incomplete dilatation at the first attempt. After a successful procedure, the arteries tend to smooth out and lose their beaded appearance. Clinical improvement in hypertension occurs in up to 80% of patients, and 25 to 58% are cured.

Complications

For most patients, renal artery angioplasty or stenting is a relatively straightforward procedure and they can be discharged the following day. Serious complications such as renal artery perforation, retroperitoneal hemorrhage, or renal artery thrombosis are rare. Acute contrast-induced renal failure may occur in 15% but is usually transient, and creatinine returns to preprocedural levels. These patients usually have pre-existing renal failure. Other complications such as femoral artery pseudoaneurysm and arteriovenous fistula can occur at the site of the femoral artery sheath. Rarely, thromboembolic complications such as distal cholesterol embolization may occur.

Current Indications for Renal Artery Angioplasty and Stenting

Because percutaneous procedures are less invasive than surgery, they have the potential to benefit a wider spectrum of patients. There is a need for greater understanding of the pathophysiology of renal failure and hypertension, particularly in patients with atherosclerotic disease who may have a number of different mechanisms leading to the development of symptoms. However, there are a number of patient groups for whom treatment can be recommended.

Patients with global renal ischemia (i.e., those with bilateral significant renal artery stenosis or with unilateral renal artery stenosis of a single functioning kidney) are at risk of progression to occlusion and development of renal failure and should undergo revascularization. Surgical data indicate that in those with renal failure, improvement can be expected in 50 to 85% (Dean et al., 1991; Novick et al., 1987).

Patients with severe uncontrolled hypertension and either unilateral or bilateral stenoses should undergo angioplasty and/or stenting. Improvement can be expected in 60% of patients with atherosclerotic disease and in >85% of patients with fibromuscular dysplasia.

In patients with renal failure and unilateral renal artery stenosis, the most appropriate management is unclear. The presence of an elevated creatinine indicates bilateral parenchymal disease, suggesting that the stenosis is not the primary cause of renal dysfunction. However, it is also possible that restoration of normal blood flow to the affected side may cause some improvement in renal function. Functional studies may not be helpful for determining the contribution of the stenosis to renal failure. It would seem prudent to consider angioplasty or stenting when there is clear evidence of disease progression in order to minimize the rate of deterioration.

Finally, patients who have unilateral renal artery stenosis without renal failure or hypertension probably do not require intervention. However, the incidence of progression of these lesions to occlusion is high and may be unpredictable (Crowley et al., 1998). It is therefore important to follow patients with significant disease to prevent loss of kidney function.

REFERENCES

Blum U et al: Treatment of ostial renal artery stenoses with vascular endoprostheses after unsuccessful balloon angioplasty. N Engl J Med 336:459, 1997

Crowley JJ et al: Progression of renal artery stenosis in patients undergoing cardiac catheterization. Am Heart J 136:913, 1998

Dean RH et al: Evolution of renal insufficiency in ischemic nephropathy. Ann Surg 213:446, 1991

Dorros G et al: Four-year follow-up of Palmaz-Schatz stent revascularization as treatment for atherosclerotic renal artery stenosis. Circulation 98:642, 1998

Harden PN et al: Effect of renal-artery stenting on progression of renovascular renal failure. Lancet 349:1133, 1997

Lederman RJ et al: Renal artery stents: Characteristics and outcomes after 369 procedures. J Am Coll Cardiol 33(Suppl A):22A, 1999

Martin LG et al: Percutaneous angioplasty of the renal arteries, in *Vascular Disease: Surgical and Interventional Therapy,* DE Strandness, A van Breda (eds). New York, Churchill Livingstone, 1994, pp 721–41

Novick AC et al: Trends in surgical revascularization for renal artery disease. Ten years' experience. JAMA 257:498, 1987

van de Ven PJG et al: Arterial stenting and balloon angioplasty in ostial atherosclerotic renovascular disease: A randomised trial. Lancet 353:282, 1999

White CJ et al: Renal artery stent placement: Utility in lesions difficult to treat with balloon angioplasty. J Am Coll Cardiol 30:1445, 1997

CHAPTER

18

POLYMORPHISMS IN THE FACTOR VII GENE AND THE RISK OF MYOCARDIAL INFARCTION

Domenico Girelli & Roberto Corrocher

Coagulation factor VII, a vitamin K–dependent serine protease, plays a pivotal role in initiating thrombosis, which underlies most acute manifestations of coronary atherosclerotic disease (CAD), including myocardial infarction (MI). The major event triggering MI is disruption of the atherosclerotic plaque, with exposure of flowing blood to tissue factor, a glycoprotein elaborated by all the major cells infiltrating the plaque (smooth-muscle cells, macrophages) and accumulated especially in the lipid-rich core. Tissue factor binds 1:1 with high affinity to factor VII, which circulates mainly as a 50-kDa inactive single-chain zymogen. On contact with tissue factor, factor VII is converted to the fully active two-chain form (factor VIIa), with subsequent activation of factors IX and X, leading to thrombin generation. Factor VIIa has some peculiarities in terms of kinetics and regulation properties, underscoring its role in initiating arterial thrombosis. Factor VIIa persists in the circulation with a half-life of 2.4 h, which is surprisingly long compared to the half-lives of other activated vitamin K–dependent coagulation proteins. Moreover, unlike most of the coagulation enzymes, which are rapidly inhibited in plasma by antithrombin III in the presence of heparin, factor VIIa is inhibited only slowly under these conditions. Recently, however, a role in inhibiting the factor VIIa/tissue factor–mediated activation of factor X has been attributed to the so-called tissue factor pathway inhibitor (TFPI).

Plasma Levels of Factor VII and the Risk of Myocardial Infarction

Interest in the relationship between factor VII and CAD was stimulated by the finding from the Northwick Park Heart Study that elevated factor VII levels were related to fatal MI (Meade et al., 1986). In this classic prospective study on 1511 males 40 to 64 years of age at the time of recruitment, elevation of 1 SD in plasma factor VII was associated with a 62% increase in risk over the first 5 years of the study. A similar trend was observed by some (Heinrich et al., 1994; Redondo et al., 1999) but not all population-based studies (Folsom et al., 1997; Smith et al., 1997). Differences in the methodology of factor VII assay have been suggested as an explanation for these discrepancies. Indeed, the assay used in the Northwick Park Heart Study was reported as particularly sensitive.

Determinants of Plasma Factor VII Levels

Many environmental factors influence plasma factor VII levels. They increase with age and obesity. Sex hormones play a role; it has been observed that postmenopausal women have higher factor VII levels than premenopausal women of the same age, and that oral contraceptives as well as hormone replacement therapy are associated with a moderate increase of factor VII levels. Dietary fats and plasma triglycerides are also important determinants of factor VII levels, although their effects seem to be strongly dependent on postprandial or fasting status. It is noteworthy that these factors explain only a relatively small variation of factor VII levels. By contrast, studies on twin pairs have shown that genetic influences account for 57 to 63% of variation in factor VII levels (de Lange et al., 2001).

Genetics of Factor VII

The human factor VII gene spans 12.8 kb and is located on chromosome 13q34-qter, just 2.8 kb upstream of the factor X gene. Several polymorphic sites have been identified (Fig. 18-1; Table 18-1) to have implications in modulating the plasma levels of the gene product. Three common polymorphisms that have been more extensively studied are (1) a decamer insertion at position −323 in the 5′ promoter region (where allele A1 corresponds to the absence of the decamer and allele A2 to its insertion); (2) the substitution of glutamine (Q) for arginine (R) at codon 353 (R353Q) in the catalytic domain (exon 8); and (3) a variable number (five

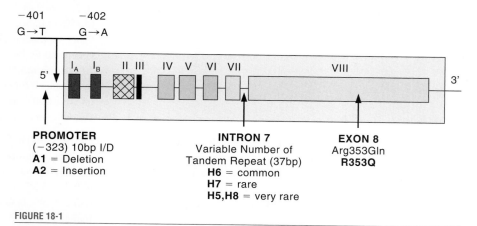

FIGURE 18-1

Factor VII gene common polymorphisms.

TABLE 18-1

POLYMORPHISMS IN THE FACTOR VII GENE

Nomenclature	Gene localization	Mutation	Proposed functional mechanism	Allele frequency
−323 A1/A2	Promoter	Absence (A1 allele) or presence (A2 allele) of a decamer (10 bp) insertion, at position −323 from the start of translation	Reduced promoter activity by 33% in the A2 allele compared to A1 allele	**A2** allele: North to South gradient in Europe (from 9.5% in Norway to 16% in Italy); 24.4% in Gujarati Indians; 32% in Greenland Inuits; 33% in Afrocaribbeans
−401G/T	Promoter	G to T substitution at position −401	Altered binding of nuclear proteins to the promoter; reduced transcriptional activity associated with the T allele	−401**T** allele: 9% in Sweden
−402G/A	Promoter	G to A substitution at position −402	Altered binding of nuclear proteins to the promoter; increased transcriptional activity associated to the A allele	−402**A** allele: 29% in Sweden
IVS7	Hypervariable region 4 of intron 7	A variable number of 37-bp tandem repeats (VNTR): 5 repeats (H5); 6 repeats (H6); 7 repeats (H7); 8 repeats (H8).	Differential efficiency of mRNA splicing	North to South gradient in Europe. (**H6:** from 73% in Norway to 62% in Italy). (**H7:** from 24% in Norway to 35% in Italy). Other populations: **H6:** 38% Greenland Inuits; 72% Afrocaribbeans;**H7:** 62% in Greenland Inuits; 28% in Afrocaribbeans **H5, H8:** very rare alleles.
R353Q	Exon 8	Replacement of arginine (R) by glutamine (Q) in the codon 353, caused by a G to A substitution	Reduced secretion of factor VII associated to the Q allele	**Q** allele: North to South gradient in Europe: from 8.5% in Norway to 15% in Italy. 25.8% in Gujarati Indians; 29% in Greenland Inuits; 8.5% in Afrocaribbeans

to eight) of 37-bp repeats in the hypervariable region 4 of intron 7 (IVS7), where allele *a* (also called H7) corresponds to the presence of seven monomers, *b* (H6) corresponds to the presence of six monomers, *c* (H5) corresponds to the presence of five monomers, and *d* (H8) corresponds to the presence of eight monomers. Two additional promoter polymorphisms arise at positions −401 (G to T) and −402 (G to A).

Influence of Factor VII Gene Polymorphisms on Plasma Factor VII Levels

Population studies have indicated that the A1/A2, R535Q, and IVS7 polymorphisms are responsible for up to 30% of the variation in factor VII levels

(Bernardi et al., 1997). It is noteworthy that several genotype-phenotype correlation studies have clearly documented that the rare alleles of each polymorphism (i.e., A2, Q, and H7) are associated with decreased levels of factor VII, suggesting a potential protection against MI. In a recent study (Girelli et al., 2000), the mean level of factor VIIa was 66% lower in A2A2 than in A1A1 subjects, and 72% lower in QQ than in RR subjects, with intermediate levels in heterozygotes. With respect to the IVS7 polymorphism, subjects with the H7H7 genotype had mean factor VIIa levels 34% lower than subjects with the more frequent H6H6 genotype (Fig. 18-2).

Substantial geographic differences in factor VII genotypes have been described; and the frequency of alleles associated with low factor VII levels seems to vary according to the different risk of MI

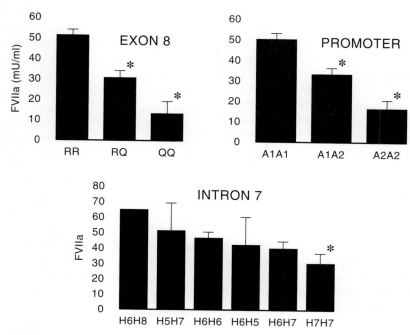

FIGURE 18-2

Plasma levels of FVIIa in 396 subjects, according to FVII gene polymorphisms. *$p < .05$ by ANOVA and Tukey post-hoc test. (*Data extrapolated from Girelli et al, 2000.*)

in populations. For example, the frequency of the A2 allele in the promoter is lower (near 9%) in northern Europe, where the incidence of MI is high, as compared to that in southern Europe (near 15%), where the risk of MI is relatively low.

The relative influence of the above-mentioned polymorphisms on factor VII levels has yet to be fully resolved, as none of them has been definitely proved to be functional. Studies in transfected COS cells found a similar expression of factor VII 353R and factor VII 353Q in cell lysates, but lower levels of factor VII 353Q in the medium, suggesting that the point mutation in exon 8 may reduce the efficiency of protein secretion. Others showed that the A1/A2 polymorphism in the promoter reduced the rate of transcription, with ensuing reduction in the synthesis of factor VII. The evaluation of the contribution of the Q and A2 alleles to the variation in factor VII levels is complicated by the presence of a strong linkage disequilibrium between these two polymorphisms, with a degree of allelic association of >80%. On the other hand, the phenotype analysis of subjects in which A2 and Q were not coupled suggested an independent contribution of each allele in lowering factor VII. Recently, an independent contribution has been suggested for the IVS7 polymorphism, mediated by differential mRNA splicing efficiency (Pinotti et al., 2000). Returning to the promoter polymorphisms, both the −401 and −402 polymorphisms have been found to strongly influence the binding properties of nuclear proteins and alter transcriptional activity in vitro. The rare −401T allele, which exhibited complete linkage with the A2 allele, was associated with reduced transcription and reduced plasma factor VII levels. The rare −402A allele, in contrast, conferred increased transcriptional activity and was associated with elevated factor VII levels in plasma.

Gene-environmental interactions have been reported—i.e., a genotype-specific effect of triglycerides on factor VII levels being the correlation restricted to the carriers of the R allele of the R353Q polymorphism. However, these findings have not been confirmed by other studies.

Factor VII Gene Polymorphisms and Cardiovascular Risk

The established association of certain factor VII gene alleles with decreased levels of factor VII points them out as possible *protective* factors against MI. Up to now, this issue remains a matter of discussion because of the different results from published studies. This is not at all surprising; it is the rule for most of the polymorphisms in candidate genes for CAD. Several reasons account for these discrepancies. CAD is a complex disease in which myriad genetic and environmental factors are involved and with many different clinical phenotypes. Indeed, the heterogeneity of selection criteria for patients and controls, as well as that of clinical end-points (e.g., MI; stable or unstable angina; coronary atherosclerosis, either angiographically proven or not; progression of disease), often makes the comparison among different studies unfeasible. The documented difference in the frequencies of factor VII gene polymorphisms among different ethnic groups is another possible explanation. Finally, the predictive power of individual polymorphisms may also vary among populations according to differences in the overall prevalence of classic risk factors and differences in gene-environment interactions.

A first Italian study of 165 subjects with *familial* MI and 225 controls found that homozygosity for the Q allele was associated with a strong and significant protection against MI [odds ratio (OR), 0.08; 95% confidence interval (CI), 0.01 to 0.9)] (Iacoviello et al., 1998). Other studies in patients from northern Europe failed to detect an influence of the R353Q polymorphism on the risk of MI (Doggen et al., 1998; Lane et al., 1996). Furthermore, an Australian study (Wang et al., 1997) found no association between the R353Q polymorphism and the angiographically documented severity of coronary atherosclerosis. On the other hand, it is biologically plausible that factor VII does not influence the development of coronary atherosclerosis—only its thrombotic complications, e.g., MI. A more recent study (Girelli et al., 2000) investigated three factor VII gene polymorphisms (A1A2, R353Q, and IVS7) in 444 Italian subjects with coronary angiography documentation. When a comparison was made between patients with or without coronary disease (CAD vs. CAD free), none of the polymorphisms was associated with the atherosclerotic phenotype. On the other hand, this study focused on a specific question that is not uncommon in clinical practice: Why does MI not occur in some patients despite the presence of angiographically documented severe CAD? Indeed, in the CAD group with severe, multivessel disease, there were significantly more heterozygotes and homozygotes for the A2 and Q alleles among those who had not had MI than among those who had had MI. The adjusted OR for MI among the patients with the A1A2 or RQ genotype was 0.47 (95% CI, 0.27 to 0.81) (Fig. 18-3). In other words, each of these two alleles was associated with a decrease of about 50% in the risk of MI.

Another recent study found a reduced procedural risk for coronary catheter intervention in carriers of the Q allele from a population of 666 patients with angiographically documented CAD

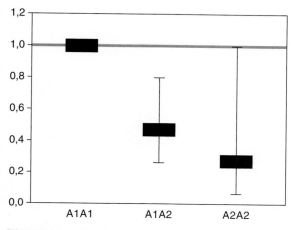

FIGURE 18-3

Risk of myocardial infarction in patients with severe, multivessel CAD, stratified by the factor VII promoter genotype. A graded effect is evident: homozygosity and heterozygosity for A2 allele decreased the risk of MI by 71% and 53%, respectively. Odds ratios (95% CIs) adjusted for sex, smoking, etc., by multiple logistic regression.

(Mrozikiewicz et al., 2000). Taken together, the data available so far suggest that, at least in certain well-characterized subgroups of CAD patients, e.g., with angiographically documented multivessel disease and/or homogeneous ethnic background, factor VII gene markers may help to predict the risk of thrombotic complications. On the other hand, it should be kept in mind that all the literature available so far deals with association studies, which are limited by the case-control design. The results need to be confirmed in prospective cohort studies.

Conclusion

Up to now, any practical implication in the management of CAD patients is premature. However, it is noteworthy that there is increasing evidence of a potential benefit from low-dose regimens of oral anticoagulants in certain categories of subjects at high cardiovascular risk. For example, the Thrombosis Prevention Trial showed that low-dose warfarin (mean INR, 1.47) independently reduced the rate of death due to CAD in high-risk men (The Medical Research Council's General Practice Research Framework Investigators, 1998). Remarkably, the low-normal factor VII levels resulting from low-dose warfarin treatment substantially overlap those associated with the protective factor VII genotypes. Such a pharmacologic approach could be effectively restricted to persons with unfavorable genotypes (i.e., A1A1 or RR); those with the protective genotypes could be excluded because of the low probability of benefit and increased risk of bleeding. Thus, in a future pharmacogenetic scenario, genotyping for factor VII genetic markers may help identify subgroups of CAD patients who might benefit from various therapies.

REFERENCES

Bernardi F et al: Contribution of factor VII genotype to activated FVII levels: Differences in genotype frequencies between northern and southern European populations. Arterioscler Thromb Vasc Biol 17:2548, 1997 de Lange M et al: The genetics of haemostasis: A twin study. Lancet 357:101, 2001

Doggen CJM et al: A genetic propensity to high factor VII is not associated with the risk of myocardial infarction in men. Thromb Haemost 80:281, 1998

Folsom AR et al: Prospective study of hemostatic factors and incidence of coronary heart disease: The Atherosclerosis Risk in Communities (ARIC) Study. Circulation 96:1102, 1997

Girelli D et al: Polymorphisms in the factor VII gene and the risk of myocardial infarction in patients with coronary artery disease. N Engl J Med 343:774, 2000

Heinrich J et al: Fibrinogen and factor VII in the prediction of coronary risk: Results from the PROCAM study in healthy men. Arterioscler Thromb 14:54, 1994

Iacoviello L et al: Polymorphisms in the coagulation factor VII gene and the risk of myocardial infarction. N Engl J Med 338:79, 1998

Lane A et al: Factor VII Arg/Gln353 polymorphism determines factor VII coagulant activity in patients with myocardial infarction (MI) and control subjects in Belfast and in France but is not a strong indicator of MI risk in the ECTIM study. Atherosclerosis 119:119, 1996

Meade TW et al: Haemostatic function and ischaemic heart disease: Principal results of the Northwick Park Heart Study. Lancet 2:533, 1986

The Medical Research Council's General Practice Research Framework. Thrombosis Prevention Trial: Randomised trial of low-intensity oral anticoagulation with warfarin and low-dose aspirin in the primary prevention of ischaemic heart disease in men at increased risk. Lancet 351:233, 1998

Mrozikiewicz PM et al: Reduced procedural risk for coronary catheter interventions in carriers of the coagulation factor VII-Gln353 gene. J Am Coll Cardiol 36:1520, 2000

Pinotti M et al: Modulation of factor VII levels by intron 7 polymorphisms: Population and in vitro studies. Blood 95:3423, 2000

Redondo M et al: Coagulation factors II, V, VII, and X, prothrombin gene 20210G-to-A transition, and factor V Leiden in coronary artery disease: High factor V clotting activity is an independent risk factor for myocardial infarction. Arterioscler Thromb Vasc Biol 19:1020, 1999

Smith FB et al: Hemostatic factors as predictors of ischemic heart disease and stroke in the Edinburgh Artery Study. Arterioscler Thromb Vasc Biol 17:3321, 1997

Wang XL et al: Polymorphisms of factor V, factor VII, and fibrinogen genes: Relevance to severity of coronary artery disease. Arterioscler Thromb Vasc Biol 17:246, 1997

TROPONINS IN CARDIOVASCULAR DIAGNOSIS AND ASSESSMENT OF PROGNOSIS

Allan S. Jaffe

The use of biochemical tests to evaluate possible myocardial injury has been part of the diagnostic armamentarium for 50 years. The development of the troponin markers has markedly improved abilities in this area. The paradigm that was used for years with less sensitive short-lived markers is now undergoing rapid change. Add to this the enhanced specificity of the troponin markers, and the result is a revolution in how patients with cardiovascular disease are evaluated. Soon, the troponin markers will replace creatine kinase isoenzyme containing M and B subunits (MB-CK) as the markers of choice for the evaluation of possible cardiac injury.

Basic Biology of the Troponins

There are three cardiac troponins: troponins I (cTnI), T (cTnT), and C (cTnC); cTnC lacks cardiac specificity, and cTnI and cTnT are the end products of unique cardiac-specific genes and, therefore, have a high level of cardiac specificity.

Issues of Specificity

Tissue specificity is well proven for cTnI; cTnI is not found in any tissue but myocardium, including tissues evaluated during neonatal development. This latter observation is important as proteins expressed during neonatal development are frequently reexpressed in response to tissue injury. When severely damaged skeletal muscle is probed with specific antibodies to cTnI, no evidence of this cardiac form is found. These data support clinical studies that fail to find cTnI in the blood of patients with severe, acute, or chronic skeletal muscle injury in the absence of concomitant cardiac disease.

The cTnT is more complex. The cardiac isoform is expressed in skeletal muscle during neonatal development and reexpressed with tissue injury.

Fortuitously, the isoforms that are reexpressed are not detected with the monoclonal antibodies used in the present clinical assay. (Ricchiuti V et al., 1998)

Issues of Sensitivity

Troponins exist in two pools. There is an early releasable pool that has been labeled "cytosolic," which contributes about 5% of the cTnT and 3% of the cTnI. This is roughly equivalent to the amount of MB-CK in the cytosol. The major fraction of troponin is complexed to the contractile apparatus. Overall amounts of troponin range from thirteen- to fifteenfold greater than the amount of MB-CK.

The release pattern of troponin is related to these pools. Early release occurs with the same time course as MB-CK from the early releasable pool. Despite the fact that this pool is equivalent to the pool for MB-CK, higher levels and greater percentage increments of change—and thus higher levels of sensitivity—have been observed. Thus, the troponin markers are more sensitive for the diagnosis of cardiac injury.

The pool of troponin complexed to the contractile apparatus is released more slowly. Thus, elevations of troponin after cardiac injury persist for prolonged periods of time, despite rapid clearance, because of continuing release as the injured area remodels. Elevations of troponin persist for at least 6 to 8 days and often much longer. There does not appear to be a relationship between the persistence of elevations and infarct size, the type of infarction (Q wave or non-Q wave), or the type of therapy.

The combination of increased sensitivity and prolonged elevations explains why elevations of the troponins are far more apt to be detected, not only in patients with ischemic heart disease but also in patients with a variety of other insults as well.

Assay Issues

For cTnT, the initial assay employed an antibody in the so-called tagged position that had some minor degrees of cross-reactivity with skeletal muscle. This led to false-positive increases. A new assay with more specific antibodies has reduced the number of elevations observed.

Assay problems with cTnI recently have emerged as an issue. Much of the troponin is released from myocardium as complexes. Thus, the configuration of antibodies and their ability to detect these complexes in addition to any free cTnI are critical. Some antibody configurations do not optimize detection of all forms, leading to variable results. Furthermore, it is not clear whether it is in blood or in myocardium that the epitopes detected by some of these antibodies can be degraded. Heterotopic antibodies (antibodies to the proteins used to make the monoclonal antibodies used for detection) have been reported, and technical issues related to fibrin strands have also led to concerns about false-positive analytic results.

A large number of values have been used to define the reference ranges; cTnT assays started using the limit of detectability as abnormal and have stayed with that value despite the development of more sensitive methods. The cTnI assays have used the initial limit of detectability, a putative normal range, or values that correlate with MB-CK elevations. In fact, in the absence of cardiac injury, troponin values should be undetectable with most clinical assays. Thus, any elevation is abnormal. Using this criterion finds abnormalities in substantial numbers of patients that are difficult to explain. However, using higher values blunts sensitivity.

Point-of-care assays are available for both cTnT and cTnI if laboratory turnaround times are inadequate.

Clinical Use of The Troponins
(See Table 19-1)

Acute Ischemic Heart Disease

Elevations of biomarkers in the past have been considered by some to be synonymous with an ischemic mechanism of injury. This is obviously not the case. An important issue in this area is whether to diagnose patients who present with ischemic symptoms, electrocardiograph (ECG) changes, and

TABLE 19-1

INDICATIONS FOR THE MEASUREMENT OF TROPONINS FOR DIAGNOSIS AND PROGNOSIS

Indication	Comment
To determine if cardiac injury is present when concomitant skeletal muscle injury is present (e.g., postoperatively, after trauma, in the critically ill)	Takes advantage of the improved specificity of troponin measurements
To diagnose acute myocardial infarction	Should be more accurate, is more sensitive; especially valuable late after the event
To define a high-risk group with myocardial infarction	Elevations in the first sample presage an adverse in-hospital and long-term prognosis.
To define a high-risk group with unstable angina pectoris	Elevations on admission or during the first 8–12 h define a high-risk group.
To diagnose myocardial infarction in patients who present with chest pain and nondiagnostic ECGs	Clearly effective; major issue is the proper reference value. With low cutoffs, markers have high accuracy early, but there are more elevations that are difficult to explain.
Patients after cardioversion or ablations, with pericarditis or cardiac contusion	Any cardiac injury will cause elevations.
Congestive heart failure	Elevations may not be due to coronary artery disease.
Hypertension	Elevations may not be due to coronary artery disease.
Myocarditis	Test of choice if disease is active
Renal failure	Elevations are cardiac in etiology; many are likely secondary to the abnormal metabolic milieu of renal failure.
Extreme exercise (ultra excercise)	Mixed data

elevations of troponin but not MB-CK as having infarction or unstable angina with some degree of necrosis. Because the mechanism of injury is similar, it is likely that over time all of these patients will be designated as having some degree of ischemic-mediated cardiac injury. Clinical information will then be used to ascertain prognosis.

Acute Myocardial Infarction

With the assays for the troponins that are currently available, troponin values exceed the upper bound of the normal range at about the same time as values of MB-CK (beginning at 4 to 6 h). All patients have elevations by 8 to 12 h. The data suggest that cTnT, although it is slightly heavier than cTnI (molecular weights of 33,500 and 23,500 respectively), is released slightly earlier. Values peak at approximately 24 h, and, for cTnT, a second peak has been described in some patients (Katus HA et al., 1991). Increases persist in most patients for at least 6 to 8 days and can be present for as long as 2 to 3 weeks. This allows one to make what has been termed the *retrospective diagnosis* of acute infarction as well. The troponins replace LD isoenzymes for this purpose.

With recanalization, troponin egress into plasma is accentuated. It appears that the persistence of elevations is not influenced.

The integrated values under the troponin curve are related to measures such as ejection fraction. Given the perturbations caused by differences in therapy (recanalization vs. the lack thereof), the ability to use peak values to assess infarct size, as with MB-CK, is subjective at best.

There is prognostic significance to early elevations of troponin levels in patients with acute infarction. This is related in part to the fact that elevations of troponin take time to develop, and patients who present late benefit less from aggressive acute intervention. However, it has been difficult to totally ascribe the nearly doubling of mortality to this phenomenon alone. (Ohman EM et al., 1996)

These patients also seem to be at greater risk over time. Mortality and event rates after acute infarction are different in patients with initial elevations of troponin and in those who did not manifest elevations. (Stubbs P et al., 1996)

Troponin markers are especially useful in complex clinical situations where increases in MB-CK could be attributable to skeletal muscle injury. Thus, elevations improve the ability to diagnose perioperative cardiac injury (Adams JE et al., 1994, 1996) and cardiac injury in patients who are critically ill (Guest TM 1995). In the latter group, evidence of cardiac injury is often occult and heralds an adverse short-term prognosis.

Unstable Angina

It is now clear that a substantial number of patients with unstable angina but no increases in MB-CK have elevations of troponin levels either on presentation or during the initial 8 to 12 h of hospitalization. Some of these elevations reflect events that occurred days prior to presentation, but most reflect the enhanced sensitivity of the troponins. Roughly 30% of patients with unstable angina manifest this pattern. Elevations of troponin presage an increased risk of subsequent events, including mortality (Antman EM et al., 1996; Galvani M 1997; Hamm CW et al., 1992).

In general, the greater the elevation, the higher the risk (Antman EM et al., 1996).

Individuals are more prone to have troponin elevations if they have unstable angina and ST-segment change. ST-segment change has been suggested to be a surrogate for increased procoagulant activity. In addition, there is anatomic evidence and an enhanced response to agents such as low-molecular-weight heparin and abciximab that support this association.

Screening of Patients with Chest Pain for Myocardial Infarction

This is a controversial area because the event rates in patients with noncardiac chest pain are so low that even elevations of troponins in a small subset may not presage a large effect in the short term. However, detection of patients at risk for subsequent events is clearly achievable with the troponin markers. Hamm and colleagues evaluated >700 patients presenting with chest pain in the absence of definitive ECG changes (Hamm et al., 1992). Values over the level of detectability (a sensitive criterion) were considered abnormal. All patients at risk for subsequent events were detected by elevations (Hamm CW et al., 1997). In addition, utilizing this sensitive cutoff, troponin elevations were comparable to early markers of cardiac injury (e.g., myoglobin and MB-CK isoforms) and could include or exclude cardiac injury within 6 h. The problem with this strategy is that there are individuals with minor elevations who are difficult to triage because of the lack of an understandable pathophysiology for cardiac injury. The proper cutoff values for routine use require additional investigation.

Other Elevations of the Cardiac Troponins

Because of the increased sensitivity of troponins and the persistence of elevations for so long after events, a large number of minor elevations are detected. Some of these are due to assay problems that will be improved by newer iterations of the assays. However, given the increased sensitivity of the troponins, it is likely that substantial numbers of individuals will have cardiac injury more sensitively detected than ever before, and care must be taken not to exclude such individuals from clinical evaluation and/or care.

Cardiac Injury of a Nonischemic Nature Should Result in Elevated Levels

Both cardioversion and cardiac ablation procedures increase troponin values modestly. Similarly, patients with severe pericarditis, toxic reactions to chemotherapeutic agents (e.g., 5-Fluorouracil), and cardiac contusion—and patients after cardiac surgery—will all have elevations.

Occult Coronary Artery Disease

The lack of sensitivity of the coronary angiogram for detection of coronary atherosclerosis has been known for many years. Thus, it is conceivable that some patients who present clinically as if ischemic injury were present could have such injury, despite normal coronary angiography. Furthermore, because the troponins are more sensitive, elevations of troponin substantiated by the findings of necrosis at autopsy can occur in the absence of ECG changes, new regional dysfunction, or increases in other biomarkers. Thus, exclusion of an ischemic etiology for elevations predicated on normal coronary arteriography should be taken with some degree of caution.

Congestive Heart Failure

Patients with congestive heart failure can have elevations of troponin if acutely decompensated and sometimes even during chronic decompensation. Elevations could represent events related to concomitant coronary artery disease. On the other hand, there is adequate information suggesting that increased wall stress and a vulnerable subendocardium could also be responsible for cardiac injury in these patients. [Hence the idea that, because coronary abnormalities are not diagnosed in such patients, elevations may be spurious.]

Severe Hypertension

This is another circumstance in which elevations of troponin have been observed. The subendocardium is known to be vulnerable to ischemic injury, especially in patients with left ventricular hypertrophy. Given the high intracavitary pressures, increased wall stress, and reduced blood flow per gram of myocardium to the subendocardium, marked increases in blood pressure could damage the subendocardium. The pathophysiologic significance of these elevations remains to be discovered, but, again, elevations may not be false-positive.

Myocarditis

Myocarditis has been an extremely difficult entity to diagnose in the past because of the frequent lack of detection of necrosis, which could be missed on biopsy. When elevations of cTnT are used to detect necrosis and immunohistochemistry is used to look for abnormal lymphocyte pools, a much more substantial incidence of a lymphocytic myocarditis is documented. (Lauer B et al., 1997)

Patients with Renal Failure

Initially, patients with renal failure were thought to have spurious elevations of the troponins, especially cTnT. Recent immunohistochemical data confirm that these elevations are likely of a cardiac etiology. This is consistent with the high frequency of coronary heart disease in patients with renal failure and the known effects of the abnormal metabolic milieu of renal failure on the turnover of muscle proteins.

Extreme Exercise

Data after extreme exertion have yielded conflicting results. Elevations in troponin are not observed after marathon runs, but some elevations have been reported in some studies with ultra exercise (triathlons). Elevations are usually reported in association with regional wall motion abnormalities, suggesting a cardiac etiology. These are only a few examples of how increases in troponin markers may be positive rather than false positive. Cardiotoxins not appreciated previously, transient viral infections, cardiac contusion, and the like may all be detectable by elevations of the troponins. Calling these increases false positive misses a chance to define new pathophysiology and to understand their significance.

Future Directions

New, more sensitive iterations of the troponin assays have been developed. These assays detect even minor increases in the troponins. With these assays, normal subjects have very low levels of cTnT and cTnI. However, elevations that are well below the limit of detection of present assays are common in patients with congestive heart failure, those treated with adriamycin, and some patients with tumors. Thus, it is likely that with more sensitive assays, we will be able to begin to understand the subtle chronic disease states that can injure myocardium slowly over time.

REFERENCES

Adams JE et al: Diagnosis of perioperative myocardial infarction with measurement of cardiac troponin I. N Engl J Med 330:670, 1994

Adams JE et al: Improved detection of cardiac contusion with cardiac troponin I. Am Heart J 131:308, 1996

Antman EM et al: Cardiac-specific troponin I levels to predict the risk of mortality in patients with acute coronary syndromes. N Engl J Med 335:1342, 1996

Galvani M: Prognostic influence of elevated values of cardiac troponin I in patients with unstable angina. Circulation 95:2053, 1997

Guest TM: Myocardial injury in critically ill medical patients: A surprisingly frequent complication. JAMA 273:1945, 1995

Hamm CW et al: The prognostic value of serum troponin T in unstable angina. N Engl J Med 327:146, 1992

Hamm CW et al: Emergency room triage of patients with acute chest pain by means of rapid testing for cardiac troponin T or troponin I. N Engl J Med 337:1648, 1997

Katus HA et al: Diagnostic efficiency of troponin T measurements in acute myocardial infarction. Circulation 83:902, 1991

Lauer B et al: Cardiac troponin T in patients with clinically suspected myocarditis. J Am Coll Cardiol 30:1354, 1997

Ohman EM et al: Cardiac troponin T levels for risk stratification in acute myocardial ischemia. GUSTO IIA Investigators. N Engl J Med 335:1333, 1996

Ricchiuti V et al: Cardiac troponin T isoforms expressed in renal diseased skeletal muscle will not cause false-positive results by the second generation cardiac troponin T assay by Boehringer Mannheim. Clin Chem 44:1919, 1998

Stubbs P et al: Prognostic significance of admission troponin T concentrations in patients with myocardial infarction. Circulation 94:1291, 1996

CARDIOVASCULAR RISKS OF SEXUAL ACTIVITY

James E. Muller

Anecdotal reports that sexual activity may cause myocardial infarction (MI) have led to concerns among the public and, in particular, among cardiac patients and their spouses about the safety of such activity (Trimble, 1970; Nalbangtil et al., 1976). This concern was heightened in 1998 with the introduction of sildenafil (Viagra) and other agents for the treatment of male erectile dysfunction.

The fear that sexual activity may lead to a cardiovascular event is considered to be a major contributor to the failure of many patients to resume sexual relations following a MI (Hellerstein and Friedman, 1970). In the past, clinicians had few data with which to reassure patients. They were forced to rely on the "physiologic equivalence" argument in which they reassured patients that sexual activity was safe if the patient could climb two flights of stairs (Tardif, 1989). Fortunately, new data are available that more precisely quantify the risks of sexual activity in the general population

and in cardiac patients (Muller et al., 1996). In addition, new data are now available documenting the safety of sildenafil therapy (Morales et al., 1998; Zusman et al., 1999; Kloner, 2000; Olsson et al., 2000).

Data from the Myocardial Infarction Onset Study

The National Heart, Lung and Blood Institute sponsored a multicenter study in which over 1700 patients with MI were interviewed soon after their event to identify triggers. The case-crossover method, a new epidemiologic technique, was developed for this study to account for the potential chance occurrence of a possible trigger prior to the event. The method has been used successfully to quantitate the risks of potential triggers such as heavy exertion, anger, and (of importance for the present discussion) sexual activity (Muller et al., 1996).

Among the population interviewed there were 858 patients who were sexually active in the year

* Dr. Muller is a consultant to Pfizer, the manufacturer of sildenafil

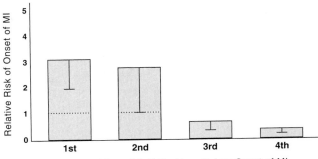

FIGURE 20-1

Induction time of onset of myocardial infarction (MI) after sexual activity. Each of the 4 h prior to MI onset was assessed as an independent hazard period, and sexual activity in each hour was compared with the control intervals. Only the two 1-h periods immediately prior to MI onset were associated with an increased risk, suggesting an induction time of less than 2 h. Error bars indicate 95% confidence intervals. The dotted line represents baseline risk. *(Adapted from JE Muller et al., JAMA 275:1405, 1996, with permission.)*

prior to MI. Only 3% of these reported sexual activity in the 2 h prior to MI, the period generally found to account for triggering. When chance occurrence was eliminated, sexual activity was found to account for only 0.9 % of cases. The relative risk of

MI in 2 h following sexual activity was 2.5 (95% CI, 1.7 to 3.7) (Fig. 20-1).

The data on the subset of patients who had known cardiac disease prior to their MI are of particular value for counseling. Among patients with

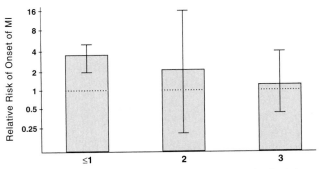

FIGURE 20-2

Modification by regular exertion of the risk that sexual activity might trigger myocardial infarction. Error bars indicate 95% confidence intervals. The dotted line represents baseline risk. MET, metabolic equivalents of oxygen consumption; $p_{trend} = .01$. *(Adapted from JE Muller et al., JAMA 275:1405, 1996, with permission.)*

prior angina, the relative risk was 2.1 (95% CI, 0.8 to 5.8), while among those with prior MI, it was 2.9 (95% CI, 1.3 to 6.5). Thus, the relative risk that sexual activity would trigger a MI was not greater in cardiac patients than among the general population. It was also found that regular exertion conferred protection against triggering by sexual activity, as it had for other triggers. The risk decreased from 3.0 to 1.9 to 1.2 for patients who exercised [>6 METs (metabolic equivalent of O_2 consumption)] once or not at all, twice, and three or more times per week, respectively ($p_{trend} = .01$) (Fig. 20-2).

Counseling Regarding the Cardiovascular Risks of Sexual Activity

The Public

While a relative risk of 2 can serve as the basis for the alarming statement that "sexual activity doubles the risk of infarction," the public is best served by an emphasis on the minuscule increase in *absolute* risk that sexual activity produces. Data from the Framingham Heart Study indicate that a nondiabetic, nonsmoking male has an hourly risk of myocardial infarction of one chance in a million (Anderson et al., 1991). If that individual engages in sexual activity, the risk doubles to two chances in a million and then reverts to baseline within 2 h. This low level of absolute risk indicates that fear of a MI should not be a factor in the decision by a healthy individual to engage in sexual activity.

Patients with Known Cardiovascular Disease

Similar considerations apply to most cardiac patients. Following a MI, patients should undergo some form of stress test to identify those in whom exertion produces significant myocardial ischemia and/or heart failure. Such patients should be cautioned against sexual activity until appropriate therapy is initiated.

Patients who pass a stress test, and their partners, should be told that sexual activity produces

only a small increase in absolute risk. The baseline hourly risk that such an individual will experience MI is approximately 10 chances in 1 million (Moss and Benhorin, 1990). Sexual activity in patients with angina, which is associated with a relative risk of 2.1, would only increase the risk to 21 chances in 1 million and only for the subsequent 2 h.

The risks quoted above apply only to nonfatal MI, for which the most precise data are available; individuals also face risks of sudden death and stroke. However, there are no data to suggest selective triggering of these events, and their occurrence is less frequent in population studies than nonfatal MI. Hence, the risk of any major cardiac event (nonfatal MI, death, and stroke) is likely to be less than double the risk of nonfatal MI—a multiple that produces only a low level of absolute risk.

These data form the basis for counseling by the physician that, although sexual activity can trigger a cardiovascular event, the risk is too small to be a deterrent in most patients.

Cardiovascular Risk and Treatment of Sexual Dysfunction

The introduction of sildenafil in 1998 as an effective treatment for erectile dysfunction led to considerable concern over the level of cardiovascular risk in patients taking the agent and engaging in sexual activity. The U.S. Food and Drug Administration established a web site to monitor spontaneous reports of cardiovascular events in patients receiving sildenafil treatment. Over 100 deaths were reported in the millions of patients taking the drug. These reports led to numerous studies, which have, in general, failed to document any excess risk due to sildenafil except when it is used in combination with nitrates (Morales et al., 1998; Kloner, 2000; Olsson et al., 2000).

In addition, as noted above, sexual activity is associated with a small increase in absolute risk of MI. By making sexual activity possible, sildenafil would be expected to be indirectly responsible for a small number of events. A combined committee of the American College of Cardiology and the American Heart Association published an expert consensus document for sildenafil use in cardiac patients (Cheitlin et al., 1999). The committee stressed that sildenafil is absolutely contraindicated in patients receiving nitrates or any NO donor since extreme hypotension can result. It was noted that exercise testing to determine if the patient can tolerate approximately 6 METs of exertion is useful for providing guidance to patients with known cardiac disease.

Recommendations for Treatment of Sexual Dysfunction in Patients with Cardiovascular Disease

A conference was held to permit experts in cardiovascular disease and the treatment of sexual dysfunction to form consensus recommendations (DeBusk et al., 2000). The recommendations are as follows:

- For *low-risk* patients (i.e., those with controlled hypertension or stable angina), treatment for sexual dysfunction can be initiated without further testing.
- For *high-risk* patients (i.e., those with uncontrolled hypertension, unstable angina, or recent MI), specific cardiac treatment is required prior to treatment of sexual dysfunction.
- For *intermediate- or indeterminant-risk* patients (i.e., those with class II congestive heart failure or more than two risk factors for coronary artery disease), further cardiac testing is required prior to treatment for sexual dysfunction.

SUMMARY

While sexual activity can trigger a major cardiovascular event, the absolute risk is low, even for cardiac patients, providing they can pass a stress test. The availability of sildenafil and other effective therapy for sexual dysfunction is likely to enhance the ability of cardiac patients, many of whom have erectile dysfunction, to engage in sexual activity. While the use of sildenafil must be avoided in those taking nitrate therapy, concerns over its safe use have been greatly diminished by the availability of new information from scientific studies.

REFERENCES

Anderson KM et al: An updated coronary risk profile: A statement for health professionals. American Heart Association Scientific Statement. Circulation 83:356, 1991

Cheitlin MD et al: American College of Cardiology/American Heart Association Expert Consensus Document. J Am Coll Cardiol 33:273, 1999

DeBusk R et al: Management of sexual dysfunction in patients with cardiovascular disease: Recommendations of the Princeton Consensus Panel. Am J Cardiol 86:175, 2000

Hellerstein HK, Friedman EH: Sexual activity and the postcoronary patient. Arch Intern Med 125:987, 1970

Kloner RA: Cardiovascular risk and sildenafil. Am J Cardiol 86(Suppl):57F, 2000

Morales A et al: Clinical safety of oral sildenafil citrate (Viagra) in the treatment of erectile dysfunction. Int J Impot Res 10:69, 1998

Moss AJ, Benhorin J: Prognosis and management after a first myocardial infarction. N Engl J Med 322:743, 1990

Muller JE et al: Triggering of myocardial infarction by sexual activity. Low absolute risk and prevention by regular physical exertion. JAMA 275:1405, 1996

Nalbangtil I et al: Sudden death in sexual activity. Am Heart J 91:405, 1976

Olsson AM, Persson CA, for the Swedish sildenafil investigators group: Efficacy and safety of Viagra (sildenafil citrate) in men with cardiovascular disease and erectile dysfunction. J Am Coll Cardiol 35:A1202, 2000

Tardif GS: Sexual activity after a myocardial infarction. Arch Phys Med Rehabil 70:763, 1989

Trimble GX: The coital coronary. Med Aspects Hum Sex 5:64, 1970

Zusman RM et al: Overall cardiovascular profile of sildenafil citrate. Am J Cardiol 83:35C, 1999

OUTCOME OF MYOCARDIAL INFARCTION IN PATIENTS WITH RENAL FAILURE

Peter A. McCullough

For the purposes of this chapter, chronic renal disease (CRD) refers to patients with a calculated creatinine clearance (CrCl) <1.0 mL/s (<60 mL/min), with a corrected CrCl <0.75 mL/s (<45 mL/min) per 72 kg, and not on any form of renal replacement therapy. This population, in general, is composed of men with baseline serum creatinine (Cr) >124 μmol/L (>1.4 mg/dL), and women with Cr >150 μmol/L (>1.7 mg/dL). End-stage renal disease (ESRD) refers to patients on renal replacement therapy, which, in the majority of studies cited, will be hemodialysis. Acute myocardial infarction (AMI) refers to both ST-segment elevation and non-ST-segment elevation types unless otherwise specified.

Renal Dysfunction as a Prognostic Factor in Myocardial Infarction

In the past several decades, considerable advances have been made in the diagnosis and treatment of AMI in the general population. These advances include early paramedic response and defibrillation; coronary care units; and pharmacotherapy including antiplatelet agents, antithrombotics, beta receptor-blocking agents, angiotensin-converting enzyme (ACE) inhibitors, and intravenous thrombolytic agents. In addition, in recent years, primary angioplasty for ST-segment-elevation AMI has become a well-accepted mode of treatment. These advances, however, have not been tested in patients with CRD or ESRD, primarily because such patients are commonly excluded from randomized treatment trials. Retrospective studies of coronary care unit patients have identified renal dysfunction as the most significant prognostic factor for long-term mortality when adjusting for other clinical factors including age, gender, and comorbidities (McCullough et al., 2000). In addition, retrospective studies of patients with AMI consistently find renal dysfunction as an independent predictor of death, with a greater impact on mortality than baseline demographics or therapies received (Hannen et al., 2000). Patients with ESRD have the highest mortality after AMI of any large, chronic disease population (Fig. 21-1) (Herzog et al., 2000). It has been postulated that there are four categories of reasons why patients with renal dysfunction have poor cardiovascular outcomes in a variety of settings: (1) excess comorbidities associated with CRD and ESRD, particularly diabetes and heart

Outcome of Myocardial Infarction in Patients with Renal Failure

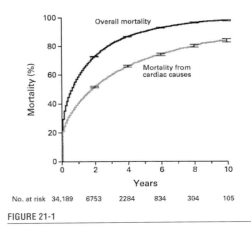

FIGURE 21-1

Cumulative mortality after myocardial infarction in patients with end-stage renal disease from the U.S. Renal Data System.

failure; (2) therapeutic nihilism; (3) toxicity of therapies; and (4) special biologic and pathophysiologic factors in renal dysfunction that cause worsened outcomes.

Reasons for Poor Outcomes in Patients with Renal Dysfunction

In one study (Beattie et al., 2001), the comorbidities of patients with ST-segment-elevation AMI and CRD [mean Cr, 239 μmol/L (2.7 mg/dL)] included older age (mean, 70.2 years), diabetes (38.1%), and prior heart failure (23.2%). In the same study, those with ESRD had similar rates of comorbidities, including age (mean 64.9 years), diabetes (40.4%), and prior heart failure (31.7%). This study also confirmed that among the CRD and ESRD groups, there were lower rates of use of reperfusion therapy (thrombolysis or primary angioplasty) and beta blockers, suggesting some contribution to poor outcomes from underutilization of proven therapies. It is possible that patients with renal dysfunction may present later in their course, have more

contraindications, or have other aspects about their presentations that prompt clinicians to use fewer therapies.

Data on the toxicity of treatments for AMI due to renal dysfunction have not been reported in many studies, primarily due to the fact that CRD patients have been excluded from these trials. It is known that the risks of bleeding are elevated in patients with renal dysfunction with aspirin, unfractionated heparin, low-molecular-weight heparin, thrombolytics, glycoprotein IIb/IIIa receptor antagonists, and thienopyridine antiplatelet agents. This is primarily due to the fact that uremia causes platelet dysfunction by a mechanism that is independent of and, hence, additive to pharmacologically induced platelet antagonism or antithrombosis (Weigert and Schafer, 1998). In patients with renal dysfunction, the best measure of bleeding risk is bleeding time (Weigert and Schafer, 1998). However, it is unlikely that bleeding complications account for the large differences seen in mortality between CRD and ESRD patients with AMI and those with AMI with preserved renal function.

Another special risk to patients with CRD is radiocontrast-induced nephropathy. McCullough and colleagues demonstrated the risks of acute renal failure requiring dialysis in patients with CRD who underwent percutaneous coronary intervention (PCI) (Fig. 21-2) (McCullough et al., 1997). In this study, patients who developed acute renal failure requiring dialysis after PCI suffered a 35.7% in-hospital mortality rate and had a 2-year survival of only 18.8%. Hence, it can be anticipated that the risks of acute renal failure potentially outweigh the benefits of angiography and PCI in patients with AMI when the CrCl is <0.5 mL/s (<30 mL/min).

The last explanation for poor outcomes in patients with AMI and CRD or ESRD is that there are special biologic processes at play promoting acceleration of atherosclerosis, thrombosis, heart failure, mechanical complications, arrhythmias, and death. The odds ratios for the complications of AMI have all been demonstrated to be significantly elevated in patients with CRD and ESRD compared to those with normal renal function (Table 21-1) (Beattie et al., 2001).

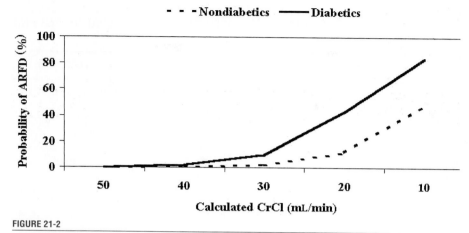

FIGURE 21-2

Risks of acute renal failure requiring dialysis in patients with chronic renal disease undergoing angiography and percutaneous intervention. ARFD = acute renal failure requiring dialysis. CrCl = creatinine clearance

Basic science studies have suggested potential mechanisms for accelerated atherosclerosis that include enhanced oxidation of low-density lipoprotein cholesterol; elevations in homocysteine resulting in reduced function of nitric oxide, leading to endothelial dysfunction and thrombosis; and pathogenic arterial calcification. In addition, the characteristic atherogenic dyslipidemia that develops in renal dysfunction includes low levels of high-density lipoprotein cholesterol, elevated triglycerides, and elevated lipoprotein(a).

Left ventricular hypertrophy (LVH) has been shown to increase the risk of death with AMI and is present in over 80% of patients with CRD and ESRD (Foley et al., 1998). Mechanisms for worsened AMI complications related to LVH include changes in the intercellular matrix of the myocardium resulting in decreased compliance, leading to diastolic dysfunction heart failure, higher left ventricular end-diastolic pressure, and mitral regurgitation, and potentially contributing to higher rates of cardiogenic shock. Higher rates of arrhythmias may be related to the underlying substrate of LVH or reduced left ventricular function, uremic myocyte dysfunction, electrolyte disturbances, or higher rates of adverse drug interactions related to renal dysfunction.

Treatment of Acute Myocardial Infarction in Patients with Renal Dysfunction

The clinician faced with the highest risk populations, patients with CRD and ESRD, has little evidence on which to base treatment decisions in AMI, as indicated above. Table 21-2 provides some general strategies based on the risks and benefits to the CRD and ESRD populations. This table lists treatments that have proved to reduce recurrent myocardial infarction and cardiovascular death in randomized trials in the general population. It lists agents that are either metabolized by the liver or have recommendations for dose adjustment based on CrCl; the latter include low-molecular-weight heparins and glycoprotein IIb/IIIa receptor antagonists. The major bleeding risks include older age, low body weight, and renal dysfunction. Table 21-2 also lists agents that are approved in a weight-adjusted dose form. In general, therapies that have proved successful in the general population should be extended to the CRD and ESRD populations when possible (Levey et al., 1998). It is possible that greater utilization of proven therapies, despite the heightened risk for

TABLE 21-1

RISKS OF COMPLICATIONS IN PATIENTS WITH ST-SEGMENT-ELEVATION AMI AND CRD OR ESRD

	CRD,(OR),p^a	ESRD, (OR), p^a
Sustained ventricular tachycardia	2.21 (1.11–4.43) .02	2.31 (0.65–8.30) .18
Ventricular fibrillation	4.17 (2.27–7.65) .0001	2.95 (0.95–9.22) .07
Complete heart block	5.64 (2.23–14.27) .0001	5.88 (1.42–24.34) .03
Asystole	15.23 (4.56–50.90) .0001	11.84 (2.32–60.41) .009
Pulmonary edema	3.36 (2.41–4.67) .0001	4.41 (2.37–8.23) .0001
Acute mitral regurgitation	3.81 (1.31–11.10) .02	7.08 (1.64–30.60) .02
Cardiogenic shock	3.57 (2.15–5.93) .0001	4.09 (1.73–9.68) .003

^{a} OR, odds ratio given with 95% confidence limits; p values in comparison to patients with normal renal function.
ABBREVIATIONS: AMI, acute myocardial infarction; CRD, chronic renal disease; ESRD, end-stage renal disease.
SOURCE: Adapted from JN Beattie et al: Am J Kidney Dis 37:1191, 2001, with permission

complications, will lead to reductions in the high mortality rates reported in the CRD and ESRD populations.

SUMMARY

Renal dysfunction confers the highest risk state for poor outcomes after AMI, mediated in part by excess comorbidities including high rates of diabetes and congestive heart failure. Further research is needed into the unique pathogenic mechanisms in the renal failure state that promote accelerated atherosclerosis, lead to AMI complications, and promote the development of heart failure and arrhythmias. Outcomes can potentially be improved by extension of proven therapies in the general population to patients with CRD and ESRD with proper dose adjustment and heightened surveillance for drug interactions and medical complications.

TABLE 21-2

THERAPEUTIC STRATEGIES FOR PATIENTS WITH AMI AND CRD OR ESRD

	ST-segment-elevation AMI	Non-ST-segment-elevation AMI
Aspirin (at least 160 mg soluble per day)	+++	+++
Clopidogrel (300 mg oral load, then 75 mg orally per day)	+++ In conjunction with coronary stenting	+++
Beta blockers (intravenous and/or oral, hepatic metabolism) Atenolol Propranolol Carvedilol Timolol	+++	+++
Unfractionated heparin (intravenous with weight-based nomogram)	+++ In conjunction with thrombolysis	++ In conjunction with glyco-proteinIIb/IIIa inhibitors
Peptide and nonpeptide glycoprotein IIb/IIIa inhibitors [intravenous, dose adjusted for CrCl <0.5 mL/s (<30 mL/min)] Eptifibatide (heptapeptide) Tirofiban (nonpeptide mimetic)	—	+++
Monoclonal Fab fragment glycoprotein IIb/IIIa inhibitor Abciximab	+ In conjunction with percutaneous coronary intervention	+ In conjunction with percutaneous coronary intervention
Low-molecular-weight heparin [subcutaneous, dose adjusted for CrCl <0.5 mL/s (<30 mL/min)] Enoxaparin	—	+++
Thrombolysis (weight-adjusted dosing) Tissue plasminogen activator (tPA) Tenecteplase	+++	—
Early angiography and percutaneous coronary intervention	++ CRD when CrCl >0.5 mL/s (>30 mL/min) or ESRD	+ CRD when CrCl >0.5 mL/s (>30 mL/min) or ESRD

TABLE 21-2

THERAPEUTIC STRATEGIES FOR PATIENTS WITH AMI AND CRD OR ESRD *(CONTINUED)*

	ST-segment-elevation AMI	Non-ST-segment-elevation AMI
Angiotensin-converting enzyme inhibitors (in cases where LV ejection fraction <40% or heart failure) Captopril Enalapril Lisinopril Ramipril Trandolapril	++ Caveats: hyperkalemia and hypotension	+ Caveats: hyperkalemia and hypotension

NOTE: +++ , Data are supportive; ++ , data are somewhat supportive; + , risks outweigh benefits, data are marginally supportive, or studies not available; — , not recommended

ABBREVIATIONS: AMI, acute myocardial infarction; CRD, chronic renal disease; ESRD, end-stage renal disease.

REFERENCES

Beattie JN et al: Determinants of mortality after myocardial infarction in patients with advanced renal dysfunction. Am J Kidney Dis 37:1191, 2001

Foley RN et al: Clinical epidemiology of cardiovascular disease in chronic renal disease. Am J Kidney Dis 32(5 Suppl 3):S112, 1998

Hannan EL et al: Short- and long-term mortality for patients undergoing primary angioplasty for acute myocardial infarction. J Am Coll Cardiol 36:1194, 2000

Herzog CA et al: Long-term survival of renal transplant recipients in the United States after acute myocardial infarction. Am J Kidney Dis 36:145, 2000

Levey AS et al: Controlling the epidemic of cardiovascular disease in chronic renal disease: What do we know? What do we need to learn? Where do we go from here? National Kidney Foundation Task Force on Cardiovascular Disease. Am J Kidney Dis 32:853, 1998

McCullough PA et al: Acute renal failure after coronary intervention: Incidence, risk factors, and relationship to mortality. Am J Med 103:368, 1997

McCullough PA et al: Risks associated with renal dysfunction in coronary care unit patients. J Am Coll Cardiol 36:679, 2000

Weigert AL, Schafer AI: Uremic bleeding: Pathogenesis and therapy. Am J Med Sci 316:94, 1998

22

EFFORTS TO SHORTEN DELAY TIME IN TREATMENT OF ACUTE MYOCARDIAL INFARCTION

Russell V. Luepker

Introduction

Coronary heart disease (CHD) is the most common cause of death in American men and women, accounting for 529,659 fatalities in 1999 (American Heart Association, 2002). An estimated 1,100,000 Americans annually experience a first (650,000) or recurrent (450,000) acute myocardial infarction (AMI) due to CHD, and more than one-third of them will die during that event (American Heart Association, 2002). Approximately 250,000 individuals will die within hours of the onset of symptoms and before they reach the hospital. This out-of-hospital sudden death is due to cardiac arrest, most commonly from ventricular fibrillation. Out-of-hospital deaths account for more than half of all CHD mortality. Approximately 12.6 million Americans have a history of CHD with previous MI, angina pectoris, or both (American Heart Association, 2002). They are at significantly increased risk for events, including out-of-hospital death. Survivors of AMI face chronic disability from heart failure, angina pectoris, and functional limitations based on the amount of myocardial damage resulting from the AMI.

Among the striking findings of the recent era is the dramatic decline in age-adjusted CHD mortality that began in the mid-1960s and continues today. From 1965 to 1994, the average age-adjusted CHD decline was 2.8% per year (National Institutes of Health, 2000). This decrease was observed in both genders and in all racial groups. A part of this improvement is derived from declining AMI incidence (new cases). The remainder has come from improving case fatality or a decline in mortality among those hospitalized for AMI. The result of these trends has been a significant increase in the life span of Americans—and an increase in the number of patients with chronic CHD as well (National Institutes of Health, 2000). Less recognized, but also significant, is the observation that absolute mortality has fallen only slightly as people still succumb to CHD, but at older ages.

The postulated reasons for these age-adjusted declines in incidence, case fatality, and CHD mortality are many and debated. However, it is clear that traditional risk factor–based prevention has played an important role, particularly in the 1970s and 1980s, with falling rates of cigarette smoking, declining blood cholesterol levels, and improved treatment of hypertension. Of equal importance are advances in medical therapy for AMI, which play an increasing role in the decline, particularly in the 1990s (McGovern et al., 2001). The advent of the coronary care unit with intensive monitoring, control over arrhythmias, and drug treatment is implicated along with the advent of acute reperfusion therapy, including thrombolysis, percutaneous transluminal coronary angioplasty, and coronary artery bypass grafting. The results are falling case fatality and survival with less myocardial damage. Follow-up monitoring, rehabilitation, reperfusion, and pharmacologic treatment for chronic CHD also contribute to the improved survival.

Among the more important observations in acute CHD care is making these effective treatments available to patients in a timely fashion. This is obvious in cardiac arrest but is also critical in reperfusion and other therapies where outcomes are best when treatment is delivered early (Gruppo Italiano, 1986). In recent years, there has been considerable focus on the need to treat patients with acute myocardial ischemia rapidly to limit infarct size and improve survival. Several sources of delay inhibit application of therapies known to be beneficial. Widespread availability of these treatments and recognition of the importance of their timely application has led to greater scrutiny of these sources of delay and the development of programs to reduce delay in to appropriate treatment.

Sources of Delay

The time period from onset of symptoms of AMI to definitive therapy (usually reperfusion) is referred to as *delay time* and is commonly divided into three periods. The first period comprises symptom onset to patient action to seek treatment, such as going to the hospital or calling the emergency medical system (EMS). This is the longest period of delay and constitutes 59 to 75% of the total time. The second period is from the decision to obtain medical care to arrival at the hospital. This is transport time, whether by ambulance, auto, or other methods. It is routinely 3 to 8% of total delay time and is a function of method of transport, availability and quality of transport services, and distance from the health care facility. Finally, the period from arrival at the hospital to definitive therapy is the third element. Hospital assessment time and implementation of a treatment decision constitute 22 to 33% of total delay time and depend on the organization of the emergency room, the availability of skilled physicians to make treatment decisions, and the ability to implement those decisions quickly.

It is apparent that most delay takes place in the initial phase when patient symptom recognition and decision-making occur. This delay period has undergone considerable study in recent years (Simons-Morton et al., 1998). In summary, a number of individual characteristics are associated with longer delay, including older age, female gender, African-American race, low socioeconomic group, and lack of health insurance. One important characteristic surprisingly associated with prolonged delay is a previous history of CHD or AMI. Those with known cardiovascular disease take at least as long as patients with first attacks. Individual factors associated with decreased delay include increased symptom severity, typicality of symptoms, and belief that CHD is preventable. External factors associated with increased delay include symptom presentation at home, travelling home during symptom onset, having a spouse at home, being with family members, and attempting to contact a physician.

These associations may operate through a variety of individual factors, including knowledge, belief, attribution, and practical barriers to taking action. A patient with AMI must recognize the presence of abnormal symptomatology, attribute it to a condition requiring medical attention, decide to seek care, arrange transportation, and travel to the hospital. Barriers to this process can arise at each one of these steps. Patients may have inadequate knowledge of heart attack symptoms, maladaptive coping strategies, misattribution of the symptoms to noncardiac causes, denial, fear, or other characteristics. There is considerable literature on the time period for prehospital delay. A review of data from 12 U.S. and European studies published between 1969 and 1987 found median prehospital delay times ranging from 2.5 to 7.0 h (Bolte, 1987). One group described a 6-h median delay time for African Americans in 1983/1984, and the same group reported a 2.6-h median delay time in King County, Washington, in 1986/1987. The Minnesota Heart Survey found a median delay time of 2.5 h in 1991. It is apparent from these studies that prehospital delay is substantial, but trends in the United States suggest recent declines despite different populations and case definitions.

Transportation time is a relatively minor fraction of overall delay. It depends on both environmental and individual factors. Availability of qualified emergency medical services and distance to the health care facility are important components. However, more important for the patient is the mode of transportation. The minority of individuals (20 to 40%) call 911 for emergency medical transport. The majority use their personal car, are driven by a friend, take a taxi, or use public transportation. This method of transportation is of particular concern as it denies the patient the benefits of skilled emergency care and rapid transport. It places others at risk as patients drive themselves to the hospital. Until recently, relatively little work had been done to improve use of the EMS to reduce transport time or to optimize medical therapy during transport.

Time delays from arrival at the hospital to definitive treatment were significantly prolonged, with an average time of 153 min reported in 1989 (Sharkey et al., 1989). It was noted then that thrombolysis administered in the emergency department significantly reduced the average delay time. In response, most hospitals have developed protocols to assure rapid diagnosis and treatment of patients with suspected AMI. Delay times within hospitals have fallen significantly in the past decade, although some hospitals fail to have a well-organized, systematic team approach to this important problem.

Public and Patient Education Programs

Observations of prolonged patient delay and the potential for significant benefits have led to attempts to reduce this time in patients with known CHD and in the general population. These programs focus on mass media strategies supplemented by small media and direct patient education. Most of these studies have been pre-post design without controls, and many have been in Europe. Among the notable well-designed studies is that of Ho and colleagues, who utilized a 2-month mass media campaign with television, radio, and newspaper in Washington state (Ho et al., 1989). Median delay time decreased from 2.6 to 2.3 h, which was not statistically significant. Herlitz and colleagues described a 1-year campaign of mass and specialized media in Sweden using newspaper, printed patient materials, and radio (Herlitz et al., 1991). All patients admitted to the coronary care unit had a significant decline in median delay from 3.0 to 2.6 h. Those with confirmed AMI had a median delay decrease from 3.0 to 2.3 h. A 1-year mass and local media campaign with television, radio, newspapers, and printed brochures in Switzerland demonstrated a decrease in median delay time from 3.0 to 2.7 h, which was significant (Gaspoz et al., 1996).

There are numerous other studies available that failed to show any effect on delay time. Although each of these studies sought to increase use of the EMS, none was effective in that objective. Despite the observation that these community studies were not ideal in design, much has been learned from them. It is clear that a mass media campaign that is sustained and supported by other forms of communication can reduce delay time. This is particularly true in communities where the delay time is prolonged at baseline. It is also apparent that campaigns that lack a high intensity are unlikely to produce any changes.

The REACT Trial

The Rapid Early Action for Coronary Treatment (REACT) trial attempted to improve on these designs with a randomized study of 20 U.S. cities of approximately 100,000 population each in a sustained campaign of over 1 year. The design of the REACT trial is described in detail elsewhere (Simons-Morton et al., 1998).

The REACT trial intervention utilized several education strategies to reduce delay time and improve the use of the EMS:

1. Organization of community health professionals and community leaders in each city, forming a local advisory group. These groups organized speaker bureaus and performed other volunteer activities, distributing information throughout the community.
2. Public education, including a mass media campaign aimed at potential heart attack victims and bystanders who might facilitate health care seeking.
3. Professional education of physicians, nurses, rehabilitation staff, emergency department staff, and ambulance staff. This was aimed specifically at enlisting these professionals to deliver appropriate messages to their patients and act quickly when suspecting AMI.
4. Patient education for those with known CHD or elevated CHD risk factors.

The baseline median delay time was 2.3 h, much lower than observed in previous studies. Although the median delay time declined modestly over the 18-month intervention, similar changes were observed in the comparison communities. The differences between the intervention and control were not significant. However, there were increases in the number of patients presenting to the emergency room with chest pain (13%) and the number of patients who called the 911/EMS (20%). In addition, reperfusion within 1 h of presentation improved in the first 6 months of the study, favoring the intervention communities (Luepker et al., 2000).

SUMMARY

Delay time to the treatment of AMI remains a significant problem. However, some elements of delay have improved—particularly organization of hospitals for timely diagnosis and treatment. Transport and patient delay remain a problem, as do the behaviors of high-risk patients with known CHD. The majority of individuals do not use appropriate 911/EMS services during their AMI. Patient delay time, while declining somewhat, still results in many patients presenting long after the onset of symptoms when the benefits of reperfusion are limited. Others delay and never come to medical assistance, presenting as "sudden" out-of-hospital death, or so-called silent myocardial infarctions. Patients with CHD are not receiving adequate instructions from health providers, and those at high risk rarely are taught how to respond. Directed and sustained mass and individual education has the potential to improve delay time and bring more patients to effective treatment, but health professionals must also add their support with direct education of their patients.

REFERENCES

American Heart Association: *Heart and Stroke Facts: 2002 Heart and Stroke Statistical update.* Dallas, American Heart Association, 2002

Bolte HD: Coronary heart disease: New therapeutic developments. Heartbeat 4:4, 1987

Gaspoz JM et al: Impact of a public campaign on pre-hospital delay in patients reporting chest pain. Heart 76:150, 1996

Gruppo Italiano per lo Studio Streptochinasi nell'Infarcto Miocardico (GISSI): Effectiveness of intravenous thrombolytic treatment in acute myocardial infarction. Lancet 1:397, 1986

Herlitz J et al: Effect of a media campaign to reduce delay times for acute myocardial infarction on the burden of chest pain patients in the emergency department. Cardiology 79:127, 1991

Ho MT et al: Delay between onset of chest pain and seeking medical care: The effect of public education. Ann Emerg Med 18:727, 1989

Luepker RV et al, for the REACT Study Group: Effect of a community intervention on patient delay and emergency medical service use in acute coronary heart disease: The Rapid Early Action for Coronary Treatment (REACT) Trial. JAMA 284:60, 2000

McGovern PG et al: Trends in acute coronary heart disease mortality, morbidity, and medical care from 1985 through 1997: The Minnesota Heart Survey. Circulation 104:19, 2001

National Institutes of Health, National Heart, Lung, and Blood Diseases: *Morbidity and Mortality: 2000 Chart-book on Cardiovascular, Lung, and Blood Diseases.* Bethesda, MD, U.S. Department of Health and Human Services, National Institutes of Health, May 2000

Sharkey SW et al: An analysis of time delays preceding thrombolysis for acute myocardial infarction. JAMA 262:3171, 1989

Simons-Morton DG et al: Rapid early action for coronary treatment: Rationale, design, and baseline characteristics. Acad Emerg Med 5:726, 1998

23

EMERGENCY DEPARTMENT IMAGING FOR SUSPECTED CORONARY ARTERY DISEASE

James E. Udelson

Introduction

Each year in the United States, between 5 and 7 million visits occur to Emergency Departments (EDs) for patients with chest pain or other symptoms suggestive of acute cardiac ischemia (Selker and Zalenski, 1997). The majority of such patients do not have diagnostic electrocardiograms (ECGs) and present an important diagnostic challenge for the internist, cardiologist, or ED physician. The goals in evaluating such patients are not only to rapidly identify patients *with* an acute coronary syndrome for aggressive reperfusion therapy but also, if possible, to rapidly identify patients *without* an acute coronary syndrome, as the majority of these patients may be safely discharged home for outpatient follow-up and not consume hospital-based resources. It is apparent from studies that follow up patients after initial presentation to an ED for chest pain or other symptoms suggestive of acute ischemia that many patients are hospitalized unnecessarily (i.e., are hospitalized but ultimately found to not have an acute coronary syndrome), and

a small but important number are mistakenly discharged from an ED and are later found to have had an infarct (McCarthy et al., 1990; Lee et al., 1987; Pope et al., 2000).

For patients with symptoms suggestive of acute ischemia but a nondiagnostic ECG, a contemporary evidence-based approach involves admitting such patients to a telemetry or chest pain observation unit, obtaining serial enzyme studies over 12 to 18 h, and then, if serial ECG and enzyme studies are negative, performing a stress test with or without imaging. This approach is based on two randomized prospective controlled trials demonstrating that such a "chest pain unit" protocol results in similar event rates at lower resource utilization than does a traditional hospital admission to rule out a myocardial infarction (MI) (Roberts et al., 1997; Farkouh et al., 1998). However, in these studies the vast majority of patients admitted to the observation units and evaluated with such a protocol have completely negative studies and are discharged to home (Roberts et al., 1997; Farkouh et al., 1998). Ideally, the majority of patients who do not have an acute coronary syndrome could potentially be identified much earlier in the process, obviating even the 16- to 24-h observation and testing period.

The Role of Perfusion Imaging

As the primary pathophysiologic abnormality in patients with acute coronary syndromes is an abnormality in myocardial blood flow, noninvasive imaging of myocardial perfusion in this setting is conceptually attractive. The feasibility of imaging myocardial perfusion in the ED setting was demonstrated over 20 years ago, using planar thallium 201 techniques (Wackers et al., 1979). These studies demonstrated that (1) it was feasible to perform perfusion imaging in this manner, and (2) the performance characteristics of the imaging data for identifying patients with acute myocardial infarction were acceptable. However, despite these promising early reports, the use of thallium 201 in this setting was impractical. The "redistribution" characteristics of thallium 201 mandate that imaging the initial distribution take place relatively quickly; thus, a portable camera system is needed. These are not widely available, nor does such an approach lend itself to contemporary single-photon emission computed tomography (SPECT) imaging. Moreover, thallium 201 is generator produced and thus is not always readily available for acute use in the ED setting.

These hurdles have been overcome with the introduction of technetium 99m–based agents in the 1990s, such as sestamibi and tetrofosmin, based on their relative lack of redistribution (Beller, 1995). Thus, even if images are acquired 45 to 60 min after the time of injection, the perfusion pattern will reflect myocardial blood flow at the time of injection rather than at the time of imaging. This characteristic makes these agents more ideal for perfusion imaging of patients in the ED setting, as injection can be done at rest in the ED, and the patient then transported to the Nuclear Medicine department for high-quality SPECT imaging. This protocol is analogous to that often employed in the ED setting for patients with suspected pulmonary embolus. These patients are often sent directly for a ventilation/perfusion scan, then returned to the ED while the results are incorporated into the information base available to the evaluating ED physician, who makes a subsequent triage decision (admit or discharge).

Relation Between Imaging Results and Outcomes

There is now a substantial body of literature evaluating the performance of rest SPECT perfusion imaging in the ED setting. In one of the first studies, Bilodeau and colleagues performed rest SPECT sestamibi imaging in patients who were already hospitalized for suspected unstable angina, and injected them with the tracer at the time of an episode of spontaneous chest pain while also obtaining an ECG (Bilodeau et al., 1991). The sensitivity of the SPECT sestamibi images for determining the presence of a severe coronary stenosis on subsequent angiography was 96%, while the sensitivity of the ECG was only 35%. In the setting of acute MI, Christian and co-workers described a series of patients with no ST elevations who were nonetheless having an acute MI with coronary occlusion (Christian et al., 1991). Despite the absence of obvious ECG abnormalities, acute rest sestamibi studies demonstrated that these patients had perfusion defects, which quantitatively involved an average of 20% of the left ventricular myocardium. Thus, in these early reports, acute perfusion imaging detected abnormalities in patients with acute coronary syndromes more often than the ECG.

Varetto and colleagues were the first to report on the performance of acute perfusion imaging brought directly into the ED setting. In 64 ED patients with suspected acute ischemia, the SPECT sestamibi images provided important discriminatory information regarding the presence or absence of an acute MI or unstable angina (Varetto et al., 1993). This study represented an important step forward, as it was the first to report follow-up of patients who had a normal resting SPECT sestamibi study in the ED. Among that group of patients, none ruled in for an MI, none had coronary artery disease by angiography or stress testing, and over the 18-month follow-up, none had untoward cardiac events. Thus the negative predictive value for ruling out an acute coronary syndrome or long-term follow-up cardiac events was extremely high. This study laid the foundation for establishing both a diagnostic and a prognostic use for the perfusion imaging information.

Since that publication, several other studies have followed involving larger numbers of patients but with similar results (Hilton et al., 1994; Tatum et al., 1997; Heller et al., 1998). When one examines the published observational series regarding the relationship between SPECT perfusion imaging results in the ED setting and patient outcomes, the negative predictive value for ruling out an MI in the ED setting is 99–100%, and the negative predictive value for ruling out an MI or any follow-up cardiac event is approximately 97% (Table 23-1). Patients with positive results have a substantially higher risk of untoward cardiac events during the index hospitalization as well as during follow-up (Figs. 23-1 (see Color Plate 2) and 23-2).

TABLE 23-1

MYOCARDIAL PERFUSION IMAGING TO DETECT MYOCARDIAL INFARCTION IN ACUTE CHEST PAIN STUDIES

Author	n	Sens	Spec	Ppv	Npv
Wackers	203	100	63	55	100
Varetto	64	100	67	43	100
Hilton	102	100	78	38	99
Tatum	438	100	78	7	100
Kontos	532	93	71	15	99
Heller	357	90	60	12	99

ABBREVIATIONS: PPV, positive predictive value; NPV, negative predictive value; Sens, sensitivity; Spec, specificity.

Comparison with Biomarkers of Acute Coronary Syndromes

There are several distinctions between the information provided by SPECT myocardial perfusion imaging in this setting and that provided by serial cardiac enzyme analysis. The various cardiac enzymes that are generally evaluated mark the presence of myocardial necrosis and will be positive in the vast majority of patients with acute MI (Adams et al., 1993). Recent data also suggest that among patients with what is traditionally regarded as an unstable anginal syndrome, approximately 30% will have positive troponin markers (Antman et al., 1996). This subgroup of patients with unstable angina is at higher risk for adverse cardiac events over time compared to patients with an unstable angina syndrome but normal troponin results (Antman et al., 1996, Hamm et al., 1999). Moreover, the subset of unstable angina patients with elevated troponin markers appears to be the group of patients who gain the most benefit from aggressive antiplatelet therapy with platelet glycoprotein IIb/IIIa inhibitors (Hamm et al., 1999, Heeschen et al., 1999). However, the majority of patients with unstable angina will have enzyme marker levels within the normal range. In contrast, myocardial perfusion imaging should theoretically be abnormal in any patient with an abnormality in myocardial blood flow, including patients with both an acute MI and unstable angina. The high sensitivity and negative predictive value of the published studies support the concept that perfusion imaging can provide powerful discriminatory value in this setting.

Another important distinction between the results of perfusion imaging and biomarker testing is the significant difference in the time course during which results are abnormal in patients with acute coronary syndromes. Perfusion imaging data should be abnormal almost immediately after an abnormality in myocardial blood flow is established. Cardiac enzyme markers, and particularly the troponins, may begin to show abnormal results 4 to 8 h after symptom onset, with the peak abnormality being evident

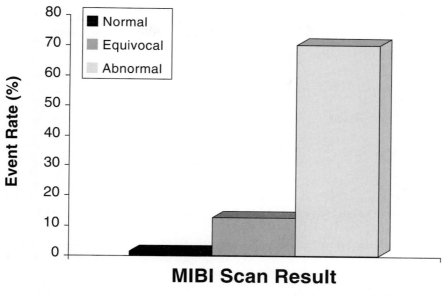

MIBI Scan Result

Hilton et al, JACC 1994

FIGURE 23–2

Cardiac event rate (*y*-axis) as a function of results of resting ^{99m}Tc sestamibi imaging (*x*-axis) in emergency department patients with suspected ischemia. Patients with a normal scan had a very low event rate, and patients with an abnormal scan a very high event rate. Patients with an "equivocal" scan had an intermediate event rate, likely reflecting some patients whose scans were influenced by artifacts, while others had small areas of ischemia or infarct. MIBI, ^{99m}Tc sestamibi. (Adapted from TC Hilton et al: J Am Coll Cardiol 23:1016, 1994.

12 to 18 h after symptom onset. In a multicenter study of cardiac enzyme markers, optimal sensitivity for troponins T or I to detect acute MI occurred at 18 h after symptom onset (Zimmerman et al., 1999). Similarly, the most powerful prognostic value for adverse cardiac events using troponin assays also occurs at approximately 18 h after symptom onset (Newby et al., 1998).

Consistent with these data is a study from Kontos and colleagues of a large group of patients seen in the Chest Pain ED at the Medical College of Virginia (Kontos et al., 1999). In this study, SPECT sestamibi imaging performed in the ED was 92% sensitive for detecting acute MI, while cardiac troponin I values drawn at the same time had a sensitivity of only 30%.

Subsequently, the maximum troponin I value over the first 24 h had sensitivity similar to that of the acute rest sestamibi imaging, but at a distinctly later time. Thus, acute perfusion imaging has the potential to identify acute coronary syndromes *much earlier* in their evolution than enzyme markers. This could potentially translate into earlier application of aggressive reperfusion or antiplatelet therapies in the appropriate setting.

Moreover, data from a multicenter trial of perfusion imaging in the ED setting has demonstrated that even once enzyme results are available, SPECT perfusion imaging data provided incremental, independent value for predicting unfavorable cardiac events (Fig. 23-3) (Heller et al., 1998).

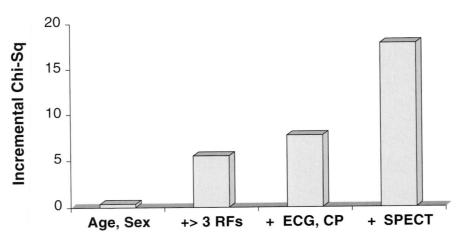

FIGURE 23–3

Analysis of the incremental value of resting perfusion imaging data to predict cardiac events in emergency department patients with suspected ischemia. The incremental Chi-square value (*y*-axis) measures the strength of the association between individual factors added to the knowledge base in incremental fashion (*x*-axis) and unfavorable cardiac events. Addition of SPECT perfusion imaging data (SPECT) adds high statistically significant value even with knowledge of age, sex, risk factors (RFs) for coronary artery disease, ECG changes, and presence/absence of chest pain (CP). (Adapted from GV Heller et al: J Am Coll Cardiol 31:1011, 1998.)

Cost Effectiveness

While the incorporation of myocardial perfusion imaging into an ED strategy engenders an added cost, the potential for reduction of inappropriate hospital or observation unit admissions might more than offset the additional costs of imaging. Weissman and co-workers found that over 50% of the physicians' decisions were affected by the perfusion imaging results and estimated a potential cost saving of approximately $900 per patient (Weissman et al., 1996). Similar results were calculated in another decision analytic model (Radensky et al., 1997).

In a study of several thousand patients evaluated in a chest pain center incorporating myocardial perfusion imaging, it was reported that following incorporation of perfusion imaging into the algorithm, the "missed MI" rate (i.e., the proportion of patients sent directly home from the ED but who were actually having an MI) dropped from 1.8% to 0.1%, while unnecessary hospital admissions were also reduced (Ziffer et al., 1998). Estimated savings (charges) were approximately $1900 per patient.

Unanswered Questions

The observational data on the relation between perfusion imaging results in the ED setting and outcomes were strong, and several studies suggested that perfusion imaging in this setting might be cost effective. However, important unanswered questions remained in place despite this robust literature. In none of these studies were the perfusion imaging results allowed to actually affect clinicians' decision-making in the ED. Thus, it was unclear whether ED or other physicians evaluating such patients could confidently incorporate the imaging data into their own decision-making and actually reduce unnecessary admissions in practice. Moreover, the cost-effectiveness data were uncontrolled and often based on modeling or assumptions regarding decisions that might be made given the perfusion data.

A review by the National Heart Attack Alert Program Technology Assessment Working Group of the various technologies available to aid ED physicians in this setting to help optimize the detection of acute ischemia found that very few diagnostic modalities in this setting have been subject to rigorous evaluation in a randomized prospective clinical trial format (Selker et al., 1997). Thus, there was a need for a more rigorous evaluation of perfusion imaging in this setting before such policy- and guideline-setting groups could recommend widespread application.

Randomized Trials Involving ED Patients with Acute Chest Pain and Myocardial Perfusion Imaging

There is a large body of observational studies involving the use of technetium 99 m-based imaging in ED patients presenting with chest pain, which have been consistent in showing that perfusion imaging has a higher sensitivity for detecting myocardial ischemia than either the ECG or initial values of cardiac enzymes and a very high negative predictive value for ruling out an MI or cardiac events in ED patients with suspected ischemia. None of these studies evaluated the impact of incorporating imaging data into the decision-making process, however. There are now two trials in which patients have been randomly assigned to have or not to have imaging data influence subsequent management. These two randomized studies evaluated the benefit of using this modality on health care costs and length of hospital stay and for its ability to influence ED physicians triage decision-making.

Stowers and colleagues evaluated 46 patients presenting to the ED with ongoing chest pain and a nondiagnostic ECG, who underwent ^{99m}Tc tetrofosmin imaging before being randomly assigned to a conventional arm (physicians blinded from imaging

results) or perfusion imaging–guided arm (imaging results were unblinded to the physician) (Stowers et al., 2000). The study's primary analyses focused on assessing the differences in total in-hospital costs and average lengths of stay between the two study arms. They found that median hospital costs were $1843 less for patients in perfusion-guided strategy compared with costs with conventional management. In addition to these cost differences, the conventional arm had a 2.0-day longer median hospital stay and a 1.0-day longer median stay in the intensive care unit. This study also demonstrated that physicians provided with imaging results ordered fewer cardiac catheterizations, without any difference in outcomes by hospital discharge or by 30 days of follow-up. Thus, while the study population was small, there appears to be a cost benefit and shorter lengths of stay for intermediate-risk chest pain patients admitted from the ED when myocardial perfusion imaging results are made available as part of the diagnostic strategy.

The ERASE Chest Pain Study

To address the issue in a larger context and to evaluate whether perfusion imaging has an impact on clinical decision-making, a prospective, multicenter, randomized, controlled clinical trial of perfusion imaging in patients with suspected acute ischemia in the ED setting was performed. The Emergency Room Assessment of Sestamibi for Evaluating Chest Pain (ERASE Chest Pain) trial took place at a diverse group of seven hospital EDs (Udelson, 1999). This study was designed specifically to reflect real-life practice, i.e., as an "effectiveness" trial. Over 2500 patients with symptoms suggestive of acute cardiac ischemia to the evaluating ED physician but with a nondiagnostic ECG for acute ischemia or infarction were randomized to one of two evaluation strategies. The control strategy was the usual ED strategy for evaluating such patients, which generally included enzyme analysis. The second strategy was the usual ED strategy supplemented by information from acute rest SPECT sestamibi imaging. Patients randomized to the scan strategy were injected with sestamibi in the ED and then transported to the Nuclear Medicine department for SPECT imaging. The results were called immediately to the ED physician, who incorporated the imaging information into his or her triage decision. The primary end-point of the trial was the appropriateness of the decision to hospitalize or discharge home directly from the ED. All patients, whether admitted or discharged directly from the ED, were followed up with subsequent enzyme analysis and stress testing, and all information (including catheterization when performed) was used to partition the study subjects into those with an acute cardiac ischemic syndrome (positive enzymes, positive stress test, or catheterization evidence of significant coronary disease) or those without acute coronary ischemia (all negative follow-up studies with negative stress testing and no events at 30 days).

Among patients with an acute ischemic syndrome, both the scan and no scan randomization groups had a very high and appropriate admission rate to the hospital from the ED. However, among patients ultimately found to *not* have an acute ischemic syndrome, those initially randomized to the scan strategy had a highly significant reduction in unnecessary hospitalizations. There was a 20% reduction in the relative risk of being hospitalized among those randomized to the scan strategy who were ultimately found to be free of acute cardiac ischemia ($p < .001$). This reduction in the unnecessary hospitalization rate was seen in all age groups, in the presence or absence of risk factors, in men and in women, in hospitals with high- or low-volume EDs, and in hospitals with or without previous experience with imaging in this setting. In a multivariate analysis, the imaging data were among the most powerful factors associated with the decision to appropriately discharge the patient from the ED. Thus the data were robust and potentially generalizable to a much wider setting.

Image Interpretation in Suspected Acute Ischemia Patients

An important goal in the triage of patients with suspected acute ischemia seen in the ED setting is the optimal identification of those who do have an acute ischemic syndrome. To this end, in the interpretation of resting myocardial perfusion images in this setting, it is important to aim for high sensitivity, i.e., when confronted with a study that is equivocal for abnormality, to err on the side of interpreting as abnormal. This is supported by one study that reported the prognostic significance of resting perfusion imaging in ED patients with suspected ischemia but that also categorized imaging results as normal, equivocal, or abnormal (Hilton et al., 1994). Patients who had a normal resting sestamibi study had an extremely low risk, while patients with an abnormal study had a substantially higher risk. Patients with a study read as "equivocal," however, had an intermediate (i.e., not low) risk (Fig. 23-2). These latter studies likely represent a subgroup of patients whose scans have artifacts such as diaphragm or breast attenuation and another subgroup of patients with small territories of ischemia at the time of injection. Given these results, interpretation of perfusion images in this setting should be "aggressive," in order to optimize sensitivity for detecting acute ischemia.

Image interpreters use several methodologies in an attempt to better classify "equivocal" images as truly normal or abnormal. These include incorporating information from gated SPECT imaging of regional function, attenuation correction algorithms, and prone imaging.

In standard stress/rest imaging, fixed defects, possibly representing diaphragm or breast attenuation artifact, can often be interpreted more correctly as infarct or artifact by incorporating gated SPECT information (Taillefer et al., 1997). Theoretically in ED imaging, this may not be as helpful as there is only one image set, the resting perfusion image. An area of mildly abnormal uptake such as a mild infero-basal defect, which may represent diaphragm attenuation artifact or a small area of ischemia with preserved regional function, may not only represent artifact but also be an area that was ischemic at the time of injection and that has recovered wall motion by the time of imaging. In this setting, attenuation correction may theoretically be more helpful.

There are as yet few data addressing this point. In a preliminary study, Hendel and colleagues examined the ERASE Chest Pain trial database in which some centers routinely used attenuation correction and gated SPECT imaging (Hendel et al., 2000). In 319 patients, the use of both attenuation correction and gating reduced the number of equivocal scans and increased reader confidence in interpretation. By segmental scoring, scores were more normal in patients ultimately found to not have an acute ischemic syndrome, by both methods. However, attenuation correction slightly reduced the scores of patients with an acute ischemic syndrome (inappropriately). From these data it appears that either method has the potential to be useful, though gating perhaps more so. The comparative usefulness of these modalities will need to be reevaluated as attenuation correction techniques continue to evolve.

Prone imaging can also be used to assist in the determination of the presence or absence of a true abnormality in the inferior wall, discriminating from diaphragmatic attenuation (Kiat et al., 1992; Perault et al., 1995). While this has not been systematically studied in the ED setting, the experience in the author's laboratory has been that in selected situations prone imaging may be quite effective in this regard (Fig. 23-4 (see Color Plate 3)).

Setting Up an ED Imaging Service

Setting up an ED perfusion imaging protocol requires significant contribution and cooperation from many "stakeholders," including ED physicians and support personnel; cardiologists, who are often called upon to assist in the decision-making; and nuclear medicine and/or nuclear cardiology physicians, who must perform and interpret the imaging with confidence and quality. While a reduction in unnecessary hospitalization with potential associated cost savings is a worthy goal and outcome, in some provider settings there are paradoxical incentives that may work against such a program. For instance, short observation or telemetry unit admissions to rule out MI can in some settings be profitable for hospitals, based on the local payment system. Thus, sending such patients home directly from the ED

may be an important source of lost income for an institution. Adoption of this proven technology into such a setting will often require re-aligning incentives among payers and providers to allow incorporation of such a potential cost-effective algorithm into the ED setting. When used properly and with expertise, a reduction in unnecessary hospitalization is obviously favorable for patients and for the health care system.

It is also important to define the ideal patients eligible for an imaging protocol. Patients who report to the ED with symptoms consistent with an acute coronary syndrome and an ECG diagnostic for acute ischemia or infarction do not benefit from acute imaging. Such patients are triaged based on the presence of ST-segment elevation or depression into appropriate algorithms for acute MI or unstable angina/non-ST-segment elevation infarction, respectively (Braunwald et al., 2000). Ideal patients for imaging are those with nondiagnostic or normal ECGs and symptoms suspicious for acute ischemia. Ideal patients also have no prior history of infarction or significant Q waves on the ECG; those patients who do will often have a perfusion defect representative of the old infarction, and thus the data will not be as helpful for discrimination of a new acute ischemic syndrome.

Future Directions

While the data from the ERASE Chest Pain trial provide compelling evidence for incorporation of acute SPECT myocardial perfusion imaging into ED evaluation strategies for patients with suspected acute ischemia, future studies will refine the patient population likely to benefit most from such a procedure. There are likely certain clinical characteristics of such patients, which may on a larger scale be identified by ECG predictive instruments, for example, in which the pretest probability of acute ischemia is so low that imaging is not beneficial. The optimal combination of imaging data, enzyme data, and stress testing and the temporal distribution of such testing also need to be better defined.

However, given the difficulty that many physicians have evaluating such patients with confidence, reflected by the very high rate of admission for observation or evaluation from the ED, the incorporation of perfusion imaging has the potential to reduce unnecessary hospitalizations significantly, with potential associated cost savings.

REFERENCES

Adams JE III et al: Cardiac troponin I: A marker with high specificity for cardiac injury. Circulation 88:101, 1993

Antman EM et al: Cardiac-specific troponin I levels to predict the risk of mortality in patients with acute coronary syndromes. N Engl J Med 335:1342, 1996

Beller GA: Radiopharmaceuticals in nuclear cardiology, in *Clinical Nuclear Cardiology,* GA Beller (ed) Philadelphia, Saunders, 1995, pp 37–81

Bilodeau L et al: Technetium-99m sestamibi tomography in patients with spontaneous chest pain: Correlations with clinical, electrocardiographic and angiographic findings. J Am Coll Cardiol 18:1684, 1991

Braunwald E et al: ACC/AHA guidelines for the management of patients with unstable angina and non-ST-segment elevation myocardial infarction. A report of the American College of Cardiology/American Heart Association Task Force on Practice Guidelines (Committee on the Management of Patients With Unstable Angina). J Am Coll Cardiol 36:970, 2000

Christian TF et al: Noninvasive identification of myocardium at risk in patients with acute myocardial infarction and nondiagnostic electrocardiograms with technetium-99m-Sestamibi. Circulation 83:1615, 1991

Farkouh ME et al: A clinical trial of a chest pain observation unit for patients with unstable angina. N Engl J Med 339:1882, 1998

Hamm CW et al: Benefit of abciximab in patients with refractory unstable angina in relation to serum troponin T levels. c7E3 Fab Antiplatelet Therapy in Unstable Refractory Angina (CAPTURE) Study Investigators. N Engl J Med 340:1623, 1999

Heeschen C et al: Troponin concentrations for stratification of patients with acute coronary syndromes in relation to therapeutic efficacy of tirofiban. PRISM Study Investigators. Platelet Receptor Inhibition in Ischemic Syndrome Management. Lancet 354:1757, 1999

Heller GV et al: Clinical value of acute rest technetium-99m tetrofosmin tomographic myocardial perfusion imaging in patients with acute chest pain and nondiagnostic electrocardiograms. J Am Coll Cardiol 31:1011, 1998

Hendel RC et al: The impact of attenuation correction and gating on SPECT perfusion imaging in patients presenting to the emergency department with chest pain (abstr.). Circulation 102:II-543, 2000

Hilton TC et al: Technetium-99m sestamibi myocardial perfusion imaging in the emergency room evaluation of chest pain. J Am Coll Cardiol 23:1016, 1994

Kiat H et al: Quantitative stress-redistribution thallium-201 SPECT using prone imaging: Methodologic development and validation. J Nucl Med 33:1509, 1992

Kontos MC et al: Comparison of myocardial perfusion imaging and cardiac troponin I in patients admitted to the emergency department with chest pain. Circulation 99:2073, 1999

Lee TH et al: Clinical characteristics and natural history of patients sent home from the emergency room. Am J Cardiol 60:220, 1987

McCarthy BD et al: Detecting acute cardiac ischemia in the emergency department: A review of the literature. J Gen Intern Med 5:365, 1990

Newby LK et al: Value of serial troponin T measures for early and late risk stratification in patients with acute coronary syndromes. Circulation 98:1853, 1998

Perault C et al: Quantitative comparison of prone and supine myocardial SPECT MIBI images. Clin Nucl Med 20:678, 1995

Pope JH et al: Missed diagnoses of acute cardiac ischemia in the emergency department. N Engl J Med 342:1163, 2000

Radensky PW et al: Potential cost effectiveness of initial myocardial perfusion imaging for assessment of emergency department patients with chest pain. Am J Cardiol 79:595, 1997

Roberts RR et al: Costs of an emergency department-based accelerated diagnostic protocol vs. hospitalization in patients with chest pain: A randomized controlled trial. JAMA 278:1670, 1997

Selker HP, Zalenski RJ: An evaluation of technologies for detecting acute cardiac ischemia in the emergency department: A report of the NIH national heart attack alert program. Ann Emerg Med 29:1, 1997

Stowers SA et al: An economic analysis of an aggressive diagnostic strategy with single photon emission computed tomography myocardial perfusion imaging and early exercise stress testing in emergency department patients who present with chest pain but nondiagnostic electrocardiograms: Results from a randomized trial. Ann Emerg Med 35:17, 2000

Taillefer R et al: Comparative diagnostic accuracy of Tl-201 and Tc-99m sestamibi SPECT imaging (perfusion and ECG-gated SPECT) in detecting coronary artery disease in women. J Am Coll Cardiol 29:69, 1997

Tatum JL et al: Comprehensive strategy for the evaluation and triage of the chest pain patient. Ann Emerg Med 29:116, 1997

Udelson JE: The ERASE Chest Pain trial. Presented at "Special Session: Clinical Trials" at the 72nd Scientific Sessions of the American Heart Association: November, 1999; Atlanta, GA

Varetto T et al: Emergency room technetium-99m sestamibi imaging to rule out acute myocardial ischemic events in patients with nondiagnostic electrocardiography. J Am Coll Cardiol 22:1804, 1993

Wackers FJT et al: Potential value of thallium-201 scintigraphy as a means of selecting patients for the coronary care unit. Br Heart J 41:111, 1979

Weissman IA et al: Cost-effectiveness of myocardial perfusion imaging with SPECT in the emergency department evaluation of patients with unexplained chest pain. Radiology 199:353, 1996

Ziffer J et al: Improved patient outcomes and cost-effectiveness of utilizing nuclear cardiology protocols in an Emergency Department chest pain center. J Nucl Med 39:139P, 1998

Zimmerman J et al: Diagnostic marker cooperative study for the diagnosis of myocardial infarction. Circulation 99:1671, 1999

CLOPIDOGREL

James J. Ferguson

Aspirin is the most common form of antiplatelet therapy used in the United States, but, despite its widespread clinical use, it is not universally protective and can be associated with a number of significant adverse side effects. Up until recently, the thienopyridine ticlopidine was the first-line alternative in patients who could not tolerate aspirin. However, ticlopidine has its own risks for major adverse events, including neutropenia (which occurs in 0.5 to 2% of patients after 4 weeks of use and is almost always reversible) and thrombotic thrombocytopenic purpura (which is rare but nevertheless a known potential risk). As a result, blood counts are recommended every 2 to 4 weeks during the first few months of ticlopidine therapy. Clopidogrel, another thienopyridine that is an analogue of ticlopidine, was approved in 1997 for use in the United States, and since then has largely replaced ticlopidine for cardiovascular applications. This chapter describes the pharmacology and pharmacodynamics of clopidogrel and summarizes the currently available clinical data in cardiology.

Pharmacology and Pharmacodynamics

Clopidogrel bisulfate is a thienopyridine, similar to ticlopidine. It is the active dextrorotatory enantiomer of the racemic mixture resulting from substitution of the benzyl carbon of ticlopidine (Fig. 24-1). Formally known as methyl(s)-a-(2-chlorophenyl)-6,7-dihydrothie1no[3,2-C] pyridine-5(4H)-acetate sulfate, clopidogrel has an empiric formula of $C_{16}H_{16}ClNO_2S \cdot H_2SO_4$ and a molecular weight of 419.9. (Schror, 1993; Quinn/Fitzgerald, 1999).

Clopidogrel does not inhibit ADP-induced platelet activation in platelet-rich plasma in vitro but does inhibit it significantly after oral administration, a mechanism of action that is completely distinct from that of aspirin, which blocks cyclooxygenase and the formation of thromboxane (Fig. 24-2) (Schafer, 1996). It is generally believed that clopidogrel is biotransformed and activated in the liver; biotransformation of the thienopyridines by the hepatic cytochrome P450 system has been well documented, and plasma levels of the parent drug are not detectable 2 h after oral administration. However, the precise active metabolite(s) of ticlopidine and clopidogrel have not been precisely identified. It has been proposed that this metabolite is highly reactive and labile and binds quickly and irreversibly to platelets, altering certain receptors, interfering with the binding of ADP, and blocking further ADP-induced signaling. Recent data have also suggested that both ticlopidine and clopidogrel can interfere with in vitro ADP-induced aggregation of washed human platelets; thus, biotransformation may not be a necessary step. This effect was *not*

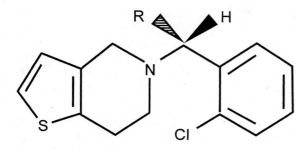

Ticlopidine   R = H

Clopidogrel   R = CO$_2$CH$_3$

FIGURE 24-1

The structure of ticlopidine and clopidogrel. For ticlopidine R = H; for clopidogrel R = CO$_2$CH$_3$

noted when either plasma or albumin was present. Regardless of the exact mechanism, thienopyridines produce a permanent inhibition of the low-affinity ADP receptor, and platelets exposed to clopidogrel are irreversibly inhibited for their lifetime. (Geiger et al., 1998; Savi et al., 1996; Herbert et al., 1993a,1993b.)

Clopidogrel is rapidly absorbed after oral administration, reaching peak plasma concentrations approximately 1 h after an oral dose. Steady-state concentrations are reached after approximately 3 days of consecutive dosing. Food or antacids do not appear to interfere with its absorption or bioavailability. Both clopidogrel and its primary metabolite (a carboxylic acid derivative) are highly protein-bound (in vitro binding to albumin of 98% and 94%, respectively). The elimination half-life of the main circulatory

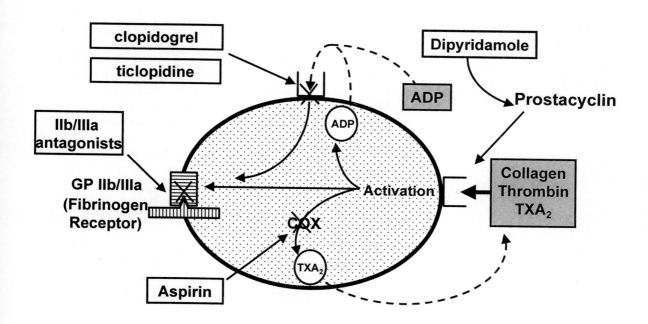

ADP = adenosine diphosphate, TXA$_2$ = thromboxane A$_2$, COX = cyclooxygenase.

FIGURE 24-2

The mechanism of action of antiplatelet agents. (Modified from Al Schafer: Am J Med 101:199, 1996.)

metabolite is 8 h. Approximately one-half of an oral dose of clopidogrel is excreted in the urine, and 46% is excreted in the feces within 5 days. There are no significant differences in men and women of the primary metabolite. The drug is well absorbed in the elderly and has comparable pharmacodynamic effects in the elderly to those in younger patients. Evaluation of the pharmacodynamic effects of clopidogrel has shown significant inhibition of platelet function within 2 h to of a 400-mg dose, an effect that persists for up to 48 h. With repeated oral daily doses of 50 to 100 mg, a significant antiplatelet effect is measurable at 48 h and reaches steady state 4 to 7 days after initiating therapy. Platelet function returns to normal (as measured by platelet aggregation and bleeding time) by 1 week after stopping therapy. Dose-ranging studies have shown that a clopidogrel dose of 75 mg/d provides a similar degree of platelet inhibition to that achieved with 250 mg bid of ticlopidine. (Schror, 1993; Quinn/Fitzgerald, 1999; Boneau/Destelle, 1996).

Clinical Data

At the present time there have been two large-scale prospective randomized controlled clinical trials of clopidogrel: the CAPRIE trial and the CURE trial. Two additional studies have prospectively compared clopidogrel with ticlopidine in interventional cardiology, and a fifth study, CREDO (investigating the role of oral loading prior to intervention and the role of prolonged aspirin/clopidogrel combination therapy following coronary intervention), will be available shortly.

The CAPRIE Trial

The CAPRIE trial (Clopidogrel versus Aspirin in Patients at Risk of Ischemic Events) was a large-scale randomized trial of the safety and efficacy of clopidogrel (75 mg/d) versus aspirin (325 mg/d) in 19,185 patients with atherosclerotic vascular disease followed for up to 3 years (CAPRIE Steering Comm. 1996). The study population included patients with recent ischemic stroke (within 6 months), recent myocardial infarction (MI) (within 35 days), or symptomatic

peripheral arterial disease. The primary end-point was the composite incidence of stroke (fatal and non-fatal), MI (fatal and nonfatal), and other vascular death. At a mean follow-up of 1.9 years, the clopidogrel group had significantly fewer composite first events (5.32% per year risk vs. 5.83% per year with aspirin; relative risk reduction, 8.7%; $p = .043$; Fig. 24-3). The individual events by treatment group and by outcome end-point are shown in Table 24-1. The outcome event most dramatically reduced by clopidogrel therapy was MI. The greatest relative risk reduction [23.8% was noted in patients with peripheral arterial disease, in whom the annual event rate was reduced from 4.86% with aspirin to 3.71% with clopidogrel ($p = .0028$).] There were no major differences between the aspirin and clopidogrel groups in terms of safety. The incidence of significant neutropenia was 0.10% in the clopidogrel group and 0.17% in the aspirin group.

Despite the fact that there was a nonsignificant trend favoring aspirin in patients enrolled with recent MI, when the entire cohort of patients with *any* history of MI was examined, there was a trend favoring clopidogrel similar to that seen in the overall population (relative risk reduction, 7.4%). Moreover, when patients with coronary disease and either concomitant cerebrovascular disease or concomitant peripheral vascular disease were examined, there was striking superiority of clopidogrel in reducing outcome events in this population (relative risk reduction, 22.7%). Mechanistically, an important factor may be the key role that ADP plays in shear-induced platelet aggregation. In peripheral vascular disease and coronary artery disease plus disease in other vascular beds, there is a greater atherosclerotic burden, more shear forces, and, probanly, a more important role for ADP-induced platelet activation/aggregation. Recent additional analyses of the CAPRIE cohort have documented the significant benefit of clopidogrel over aspirin in patients with a prior history of coronary astery bypass graft (CABG) and in patients with diabetes and the benefits of clopidogrel over aspirin in preventing not only intial events (the primary CAPRIE analysis) but also recurrent and total vascular events. (Bhatt et al., 2001; Ferguson et al., 2001).

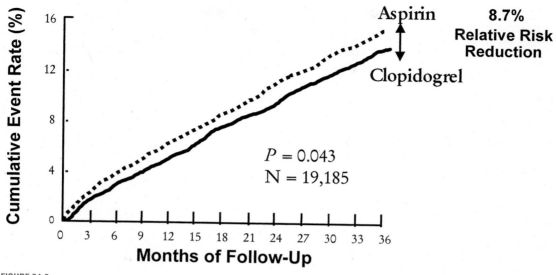

FIGURE 24-3

Primary outcome endpoints in the CAPRIE trial.

The CURE Trial

The CURE trial (clopidogrel in Unstable Angina to Prevent Recurrent Ischemic Events) was a multicenter, randomized, double-blind, placebo-controlled study comparing combination therapy with aspirin and clopidogrel vs. aspirin alone in patients with acute coronary syndromes. A total of 12,562 patients with unstable angina or non-Q-wave MI (within 24 h of their last episode of pain) received aspirin 75 to 325 mg and then were randomized to clopidogrel (300-mg load followed by 75 mg daily) or placebo for 3 months to 1 year. The primary end-point was a composite of cardiovascular death, MI, or stroke. The main safety end-points were major bleeding (disabling or symptomatic intracranial or intraocular bleeding; or transfusion of more than two units). Life-threatening bleeding was defined as a hemoglobin decline of >50 g/L (5 g/dL), hypotension requiring inotropes, bleeding requiring surgery or more than four units of blood, or intracranial bleeding.

Seventy-five percent of the patients enrolled in the CURE trial had unstable angina, 25% had

an elevated enzyme or troponin level, 94% had an abnormal electrocardiogram, and half had ST-segment deviation. Approximately 30% of the patients underwent revascularization. Mean follow-up was 9 months. Treatment with clopidogrel and aspirin was associated with a 20% relative reduction in the primary end-point of cardiovascular death, MI, or stroke (Table 24-2, Fig. 24-4), largely driven by a 23% relative reduction in the incidence of MI. Differences in the other components of the primary end-point (cardiovascular death, stroke, non-cardiovascular death) failed to reach statistical significance. There was a 31% reduction in in-hospital refractory ischemia (2.06% to 1.42%, $p = .001$) and a 25% reduction in severe ischemia (5.03% to 3.83%, $p = .001$). The curves for the primary end-point began to diverge very early, favoring clopidogrel (within the first few hours). At 24 h, a 20% relative reduction in the composite death, MI, and stroke was also noted. The benefits of clopidogrel were present across all major subgroups: patients with and without major ST-segment deviation, enzyme or troponin eleva-

TABLE 24-1

INDIVIDUAL AND COMPOSITE FIRST-OUTCOME EVENTS IN CAPRIE

| Subgroup and treatment group | Individual first-outcome events | | | | Other vascular death | Total | Event rate per year, % | Relative risk reduction, % (95% CI) | p |
| | Stroke | | MI | | | | | | |
	Non-fatal	Fatal	Non-fatal	Fatal					
Stroke									
Clopidogrel (n = 6054[a])	298	17	33	11	74	433	7.15	7.3 (−5.7 to 18.7)	.26
Aspirin (n = 5979)	322	16	37	14	72	461	7.71		
MI									
Clopidogrel (n = 5787)	37	5	143	20	86	291	5.03	−3.7	.66
Aspirin (n = 5843)	34	8	152	22	67	283	4.84		
PAD									
Clopidogrel (n = 5795)	70	11	50	18	66	215	3.71	23.8	.0028
Aspirin (n = 5797)	74	8	81	27	87	277	4.86		
All patients									
Clopidogrel (n = 17636)	405	33	226	49	226	939	5.32	8.7	.043
Aspirin (n = 17619)	430	32	270	63	226	1021	5.83		

[a] Patient years at risk.

ABBREVIATIONS: MI, myocardial infarction; PAD, peripheral arterial disease.

tion, prior and subsequent revascularization (Table 24-3). Benefits were also noted in composite events with long-term therapy in addition to inhospital benefit (Table 24-4). Although there was a 34% excess of major bleeding in the clopidogrel arm, there was no significant excess of life-threatening bleeding with combination therapy. Additional analyses of the subset of patients undergoing revascularization (Mehta et al., 2001) have also shown that there was substantial clinical benefit in CURE patients undergoing PCI who were pretreated (prior to PCI) with clopidogrel (added to existing aspirin therapy) and subsequently treated with long-term aspirin/clopidogrel therapy.

CLOPIDOGREL IN CORONARY STENTING

The most common area of application for thienopyridines in cardiology is following stent placement. Initially, ticlopidine plus aspirin supplanted chronic

TABLE 24-2

MAJOR ENDPOINTS IN CURE

	Aspirin, % ($n = 6303$)	Aspirin/ clopidogrel, % ($n = 6259$)	Relative risk	p
Death				
Cardiovascular death	5.4	5.1	0.92	–
Myocardial infarction	6.7	5.2	0.77	<.001
Stroke	1.4	1.2	0.85	–
Composite	11.5	9.3	0.80	.00005
Non cardiovascular death	0.7	0.7	0.96	–
Major bleeding	2.7	3.6	1.34	.003
Life-threatening bleeding	1.8	2.1	1.15	–
Minor bleeding	8.6	15.3	1.78	<.001
Transfusions	2.2	2.8	1.28	.03

coumadin anticoagulation in stent patients. Since then, given the favorable safety profile of clopidogrel over ticlopidine, clopidogrel has largely replaced ticlopidine in patients undergoing coronary intervention. A number of retrospective, historically controlled clinical trials have suggested that clopidogrel plus aspirin may be at least as good as ticlopidine plus aspirin in patients undergoing coronary stent placement. Two additional trials have examined this prospectively.

The CLASSICS trial (Bertand, 2000) was a multicenter, randomized, controlled trial of clopidogrel plus aspirin vs. ticlopidine plus aspirin in 1020 patients undergoing coronary stent implantation at 48 European centers. The three treatment groups included aspirin (325 mg/d) plus ticlopidine (250 mg bid; $n = 340$), aspirin plus clopidogrel (75 mg/d; $n = 335$), or aspirin plus front-loaded clopidogrel (300 mg oral loading followed by 75 mg/d; $n = 345$). Therapy was initiated within 6 h of the stent procedure and continued for 28 days afterward. The trial was primarily designed

as a safety study. Patients requiring the use of glycoprotein (GP) IIb/IIIa antagonists were excluded from the study. The primary end-point of the study was the composite of bleeding, neutropenia, thrombocytopenia, and early drug discontinuation for noncardiac adverse events. A secondary end-point was clinical efficacy, assessed as the composite of cardiovascular death, MI, and target vessel revascularization at 30 days. The primary safety end-point was significantly reduced with clopidogrel, occurring in 9.1% of the ticlopidine group, 6.3% of the 75-mg clopidogrel group, 2.9% of the 300/75-mg clopidogrel group, and 4.6% in the two clopidogrel groups combined. There were no instances of thrombocytopenia with clopidogrel. The major contribution to the primary end-point came from a much higher percentage of early drug discontinuation for noncardiac adverse events (primarily allergic reactions, gastrointestinal disorders, and skin rashes) with ticlopidine (8.2%) compared to 5.1% in the 75-mg clopidogrel group, 20% in the 300/75-mg clopidogrel group, and 3.5% in the two

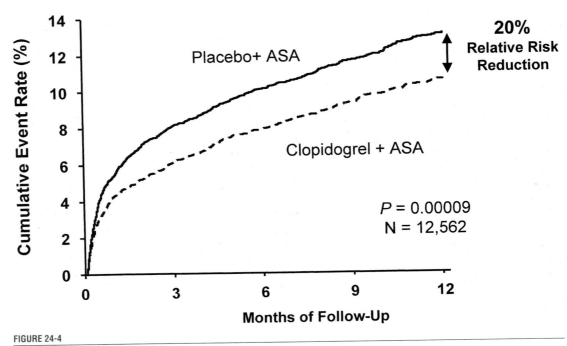

FIGURE 24-4

Primary outcome endpoints in the CURE trial.

clopidogrel groups combined. The secondary end-point of composite adverse cardiac events was not significantly different among the groups—0.9%, 1.5%, 1.2%, in the respective treatment arms; 1.3% in the two clopidogrel groups combined.

In another recent study by Muller and colleagues, (2000); 700 patients (899 lesions) were randomized to receive either a 4 week course of ticlopidine (500 mg/d) or clopidogrel (75 mg/d) in addition to 100 mg of aspirin following elective or emergent percutaneous coronary intervention (Muller et al., 2000). Oral loading therapy was not utilized in this study. The primary cardiac end-point was the composite of cardiac death, urgent target vessel revascularization, angiographically documented thrombotic stent occlusion, or nonfatal MI within 30 days. The primary noncardiac end-point was the composite of noncardiac death, stroke, severe peripheral vascular or hemorrhagic events, or any adverse event requiring discontinuation of study medication. Primary cardiac events occurred in 17 patients [11 (3.1%) with clopidogrel and 6 (1.7%) with ticlopidine ($p = .24$)]; primary noncardiac events occurred in 49 patients [16 (4.5%) with clopidogrel and 33 (9.6%) with ticlopidine ($p = .01$)]

The forthcoming CREDO trial will further examine the use of clopidogrel in patients undergoing coronary stenting. This factorially designed trial will first assess the potential advantages of acute preprocedural loading with clopidogrel and then go on to explore the potential benefits of short- vs. long-term combination therapy with aspirin and clopidogrel in secondary prevention of recurrent events in this population. Other future studies of clopidogrel in patients with cardiovascular disease include WATCH (a three-arm study in the United States, Britain, and Canada of aspirin vs. clopidogrel vs. coumadin in patients with heart failure), COMMIT (a large-scale, 30,000-patient study in China comparing aspirin vs. aspirin plus clopidogrel

TABLE 24-3

OUTCOMES IN CLINICAL SUBGROUPS IN CURE

	Aspirin, %	Aspirin/ clopidogrel, %	Relative risk
ST ↓ (n = 6723)	14.3	11.5	0.79
No ST ↓ (n = 6288)	8.7	7.0	0.80
(+) Enzymes (n = 3174)	13.1	10.7	0.81
(−) Enzymes (n = 9385)	10.9	8.8	0.79
Hx prev. revascularization (n = 2246)	14.6	8.4	0.55
No Hx prev. revascularization (n = 10316)	10.8	9.5	0.87
(+) Study revascularization (n = 4582)	13.9	11.4	0.81
(−) Study revascularization (n = 7900)	10.1	8.1	0.79

TABLE 24-4

EARLY VS. LATE OUTCOMES IN CURE

	<30 Days			>30 Days		
	Aspirin,%	Aspirin + Clopidogrel,%	RR[a]	Aspirin,%	Aspirin + Clopidogrel,%	RR
Primary end-point	5.4	4.2	0.79	6.4	5.2	0.81
Primary end-point + refractory ischemia	9.3	7.3	0.83	10.7	9.7	0.89
Major bleed	1.6	2.0	1.26	1.2	1.7	1.46
Life-threatening bleed	1.0	1.2	1.23	0.8	0.9	1.05

[a]RR, relative risk.

in patients with acute MI), and a study evaluating the utility of aspirin plus clopidogrel in preserving dialysis shunt access. Trials of combined aspirin/clopidogrel therapy in patients with atrial fibrillation and stroke are also under way.

Neutropenia and TTP

Some concerns have been raised recently (Bennett et al., 2000) about the adverse side effect of neutropenia and TTP. While these are known side effects of the thienopyridines, their incidence appears to be substantially lower with clopidogrel than with ticlopidine. Routine monitoring of blood counts is not felt to be necessary with clopidogrel, but a low level risk should be recognized.

CURRENT ROLE

Given the large-scale clinical data from CAPRIE and CURE, and the favorable safety profile of clopidogrel, there are a number of clinical scenarios where clopidogrel should be considered (Table 24-5) that fall into two general categories: monotherapy and combination therapy.

Monotherapy

First of all, as monotherapy, clopidogrel can serve as a substitute for aspirin in aspirin-allergic or intolerant patients or in patients with significant gastrointestinal pathology in whom aspirin may be relatively contraindicated. It should be considered as a slightly (but significantly) superior alternative to aspirin in patients with peripheral vascular disease, multibed vascular disease, previous bypass surgery, or diabetes. Clopidogrel should also be used as a general substitute for ticlopidine in patients who require new thienopyridine therapy (such as stent patients). Clopidogrel is better tolerated, has a faster onset of action, is a once-a-day drug, does not require hematologic monitoring, and (in the United States) is actually cheaper than ticlopidine. All of these

TABLE 24-5

POTENTIAL CLINICAL APPLICATIONS OF CLOPIDOGREL

Monotherapy
  Substitute for ticlopidine
  Aspirin allergy
  Aspirin intolerance
  ? Peripheral artery disease
  ? Multibed vascular disease
  ? Diabetes
  ? Prior coronary artery bypass graft
  ? Events despite aspirin Rx

Combination therapy (with aspirin)
  Coronary stents (4 weeks Rx)
  Brachytherapy for in-stent restenosis (6–12 months)
  Acute Coronary Syndromes—acute Rx
  Acute Coronary Syndromes—chronic Rx
  High-risk atrial fibrillation and patient unable to take warfarin
  ? Peripheral arterial disease
  ? Multibed vascular disease
  ? Diabetes
  ? Prior coronary artery bypass graft
  ? Events despite aspirin Rx
  ? High-risk coronary stents (long-term Rx)
  ? High-risk coronary intervention (long-term Rx)
  ? Prior vascular events
  ? Multiple risk factors
  ? Aspirin "resistance"
  ? Hypercoagulable states

strongly favor clopidogrel as a broad replacement for ticlopidine in clinical practice. A more difficult question is whether patients who are already on chronic ticlopidine therapy and tolerating it well should be switched to clopidogrel. Since most of the risk for blood dyscrasias with ticlopidine comes in the first 6 months, a switch after this time may not be absolutely necessary. However, given the ever-decreasing clinical role of ticlopidine in cardiovascular disease (at least in the United States), this is becoming less and less of an issue.

Combination Therapy

The second general area of potential clinical application is as combination therapy with aspirin. For cornary stenting, short-term therapy (4 weeks) with clopidogrel and aspirin should be regarded as the standard of care. In patients undergoing vascular brachytherapy for in-stent restenosis, prolonged combination therapy (6 to 12 months) is an emerging standard. In patients with acute coronary syndromes, the CURE trial demonstrated convincing benefit of combination therapy for both initial management and for long-term secondary prevention. Logistical issues have emerged as this strategy is implemented (particularly with aggressive invasive management) with the addition of GPIIb/IIIa antagonists and concerns about the safety of emergency CABG surgery in patients on combination therapy, and widespread acute use will probably await the availability of additional data on acute intervention, GPIIb/IIIa antagonists (that were excluded from CURE), and emergency CABG. Combination therapy should also be considered in patients requiring more than aspirin therapy alone (such as high-risk patients with atrial fibrillation who, for whatever reason, are unable to take warfarin). Also, patients who present with new cardiovascular events while already on aspirin therapy may be expressing clinical manifestations of aspirin "failure." Given the recent awareness of a substantial group of patients in whom aspirin therapy may not provide adequate antiplatelet protection, clopidogrel could be considered as adjunctive therapy in this group of patients as a whole. An additional group of patients who might benefit from the combination of clopidogrel and aspirin are those patients felt to be at high risk for recurrent events, such as patients with a previous MI, stroke, or transient ischemic attack; patients with diabetes; patients with multibed vascular disease; or even patients with multiple risk factors or recurrent vascular events. There may even be a role (to be better defined in the CREDO trial) for more prolonged use of combination therapy in "higher risk" patients undergoing coronary intervention. Finally, the general group of patients with hypercoagulable states may also benefit from the clopidogrel-aspirin combination. While at first glance all of these potential applications of combination therapy might appear somewhat confusing, all of them represent situations in which aspirin monotherapy may simply not be adequate.

SUMMARY

In the United States, clopidogrel has largely displaced ticlopidine for cardiovascular applications, largely on the basis of its superior safety profile. As monotherapy, clopidogrel is the first-line alternative in patients unable to take aspirin and may be considered in other high-risk circumstances (peripheral artery disease; multibed vascular disease, diabetes, etc.). Combination therapy with aspirin plus clopidogrel is the standard of care (short-term) in patients undergoing coronary stent placement and (long-term) patients treated with intracoronary brachytherapy for in-stent restenosis. The utility of combination therapy for nonstent coronary interventions or for more general long-term therapy remains unclear at this point. The combination of clopidogrel with aspirin in the broader treatment of patients with atherosclerotic disease has tremendous potential as a multitargeted approach to antiplatelet therapy. There was substantial benefit to combination therapy in patients with acute coronary syndromes in the large-scale CURE, both in-hospital and long-term, but logistical concerns (at least for acute therapy) surrounding an aggressive invasive approach, GPIIb/IIIa antagonists, and emergency CABG surgery still need to be addressed. There is an emerging role for the clopidogrel/aspirin combination therapy in the broader group of patients who require more intensive antithrombotic therapy and in whom aspirin alone may not be adequate. Clopidogrel is a substantial addition to the antiplatelet armamentarium, and, in all likelihood, in years to come will play an increasingly important role in the antithrombotic therapy of patients with cardiovascular disease.

REFERENCES

Bennett CL et al: Thrombotic thrombocytopenic purpura associated with clopidogrel. N Engl J Med 342:1773, 2000

Bertrand ME et al: Double-blind study of the safety of clopidogrel with and without a loading dose in combination with aspirin after coronary stenting. Circulation 102:624, 2000

Bhatt DL et al: Superiority of clopidogrel versus aspirin in patients with prior cardiac surgery. Circulation 103:363, 2001

Boneau B, Destelle G: Platelet anti-aggregating activity and tolerance of clopidogrel in atherosclerotic patients. Thromb Haemost 76:939, 1996

CAPRIE Steering Committee: A randomised, blinded, trial of clopidogrel versus aspirin in patients at risk of ischemic events. Lancet 348:1329, 1996

Ferguson JJ et al: The effect of clopidogrel versus aspirin on recurrent clinical events and total vascular mortality: Results from the CAPRIE trial. J Am Coll Cardiol 37 (Suppl A):336A, 2001

Geiger J et al: Ligand specificity and ticlopidine effects distinguish three human platelet ADP receptors. Eur J Pharmacol 351:235, 1998

Herbert JM et al: Clopidogrel, a novel antiplatelet and antithrombotic agent. Cardiovasc Drug Rev 11:180, 1993a

Herbert JM et al: Inhibitory effect of clopidogrel on platelet adhesion and intimal proliferation following arterial injury. Arterioscler Thromb 13:1171, 1993b

Mehta SR et al; for the Clopidogrel in Unstable Angina to Prevent Recurrent Events Trial (CURE) Investigators: Effects of pretreatment with clopidogrel and aspirin followed by long-term therapy in patients undergoing percutaneous coronary intervention: the PCI-CURE study. Lancet 358:527, 2001

Muller C et al: A randomized comparison of clopidogrel and aspirin versus ticlopidine and aspirin after the placement of coronary artery stents. Circulation 101:590, 2000

Quinn MJ, Fitzgerald DJ: Ticlopidine and clopidogrel. Circulation 100:1667, 1999

Savi P et al: Clopidogrel, an antithrombotic drug acting on the ADP-dependent activation pathway of human platelets. Clin Appl Thromb/Hemost 2:35, 1996

Schafer AI: Antiplatelet therapy. Am J Med 101:199, 1996

Schror K: The basic pharmacology of ticlopidine and clopidogrel. Platelets 4:252, 1993

The Clopidogrel in Unstable Angina to Prevent Recurrent Events (CURE) Trial Investigators: Effects of clopidogrel in addition to aspirin in patients with acute coronary syndromes without ST-segment elevation. N Engl J Med 345:494, 2001

25

LOW-MOLECULAR-WEIGHT HEPARIN IN NON-ST ELEVATION ACUTE CORONARY SYNDROMES

David A. Morrow & Elliott M. Antman

The onset of unstable coronary artery disease is typically marked by rupture or erosion of an atherosclerotic plaque with ensuing formation of intravascular thrombus (Lee and Libby, 1997). A breach in the protective fibrous cap exposes the highly procoagulant contents of the atheroma core to the circulating bloodstream. Concomitant activation of the coagulation cascade and platelet aggregation culminate in the formation of a flow-limiting thrombus in the coronary artery. In non-ST elevation acute coronary syndromes, the thrombus is usually partially obstructive or only transiently occlusive. Thus, antithrombin and antiplatelet therapies directed at halting the propagation of unstable thrombus have become fundamental to the early management of unstable angina (UA) and non-ST elevation myocardial infarction (MI) (Braunwald et al., 2000).

Inhibiting Thrombogenesis: The Role of Heparins

The Coagulation Cascade as a Target for Therapy

Upon exposure to circulating blood, tissue factor within the atheroma core interacts with factor VII to activate the extrinsic coagulation pathway and generate activated factor X (Xa) (Figure 25-1). Factor Xa converts prothrombin to thrombin (IIa), the key enzyme that generates fibrin. In addition, factors Xa and IIa both exert feedback interactions, which stimulate further production of Xa as well as promote platelet activation and aggregation (Dahlback, 2000). In particular, the activation of factor IX to IXa leads to further Xa generation and perpetuates activation of the coagulation cascade. This cascade

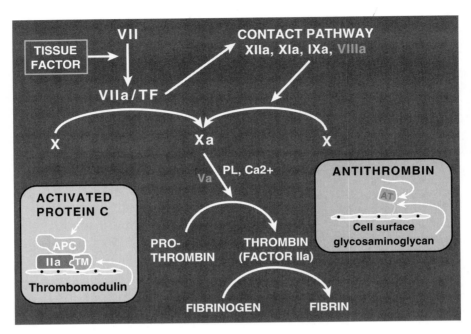

FIGURE 25-1

Summary of key participants in the coagulation cascade and its regulation. Coagulation factors XIIa, XIa, Xa, IXa, IIa, are inhibited by antithrombin. Factors VIIIa and Va are inhibited by activated protein C. TF, tissue factor; PL, phospholipid; Ca^{2+}, calcium; AT, antithrombin; APC, activated protein C; TM, thrombomoldulin.

of coagulation proteins is controlled by several mechanisms, including the protein C system, tissue factor pathway inhibitor, and the serine protease inhibitor antithrombin (Figure 25-1). Catalyzed by endothelial cell proteoglycans, antithrombin inactivates factors XIIa, XIa, IXa, Xa, and thrombin. This action of endothelial proteoglycans is reproduced by the anticoagulant drug heparin.

Mechanisms of Action: Unfractionated and Low-Molecular-Weight Heparins

Unfractionated heparin (UFH) is a mixture of complex mucopolysaccharide chains of widely varying length and molecular mass (3000 to 30,000 Da). Low-molecular-weight heparin (LMWH) is manufactured by controlled enzymatic or chemical depolymerization of long glycosaminoglycans to produce a more homogeneous mixture of smaller

chains with an average molecular weight of near 5000 (Weitz, 1997). With heparins of either type, activation of antithrombin is mediated by binding to a unique pentasaccharide sequence on the heparin molecule (Figure 25-2). An additional 13 saccharide residues are necessary for binding of the heparin-antithrombin complex to the heparin-binding domain of thrombin. In contrast, inhibition of factor Xa requires binding only to antithrombin activated by the specific pentasaccharide. In UFH the majority of chains containing the pentasaccharide sequence are composed of at least 18 residues. However, in LMWH preparations, <50% of such chains are of adequate length to form the ternary heparin-antithrombin-thrombin complex. As a result, LMWHs have greater relative activity against factor Xa, i.e., a higher anti-Xa:anti-IIa activity ratio, compared to UFH, which has an anti-Xa:anti-IIa ratio of 1.0.

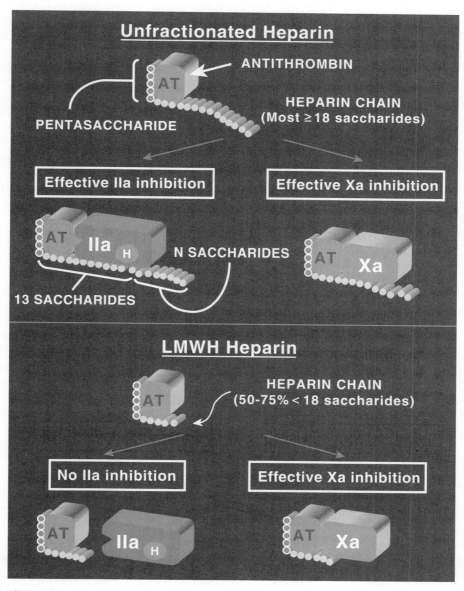

FIGURE 25-2

Activation of antithrombin (AT) and inhibition of factor Xa and thrombin (factor IIa) by unfractionated and low-molecular-weight-heparins (LMWH) (see text for details). While the majority of chains in unfractionated heparin are composed of at least 18 residues, in LMWH preparations, <50% of such chains are of adequate length to form a heparin-antithrombin-thrombin complex. Top and bottom panels depict representative heparin chains of >18 and <18 saccharides in length, respectively. H, heparin binding domain of thrombin.

Advantages of LMWH

Though UFH has been a mainstay of anticoagulant therapy, it has a number of important disadvantages (Antman, 2001). Due to extensive nonspecific binding to serum proteins, macrophages, and endothelial cells, UFH has a relatively low and variable bioavailability. The resulting fluctuation in anticoagulant effect necessitates frequent hematologic monitoring and poses a challenge to maintaining levels within the therapeutic target range. In addition, UFH has been associated with a "rebound" increase in thrombotic events upon discontinuation and carries an appreciable risk of heparin-associated thrombocytopenia and thrombosis.

The LMWHs overcome each of these deficiencies as well as offer several additional theoretical advantages (Table 25-1). Foremost, by virtue of their enhanced anti-Xa activity, LMWHs achieve greater "upstream" inhibition of the coagulation cascade. Because each molecule of Xa generates many molecules of thrombin, inhibition of coagula-

tion at this higher level enables LMWH to significantly reduce the production of new thrombin, in addition to inhibiting previously formed active thrombin. Further, LMWH has less susceptibility to inhibition by platelet factor 4, a greater capacity to release tissue factor-pathway inhibitor, and less nonspecific binding by plasma proteins. Each of these factors contributes to a greater stability of anticoagulant effect. Moreover, LMWHs may also have less propensity to stimulate, and may even act to suppress, platelet activation and aggregation. Finally, with uniform high degrees of bioavailability, LMWH may be administered subcutaneously, yielding a predictable level of anticoagulation without the need for an infusion pump or monitoring of the activated partial thromboplastin time.

Differences between LMWHs

Variation in the molecular weight and average length of the glycosaminoglycan chains distinguishes available preparations of LMWH and confers diversity in the level of relative anti-Xa:anti-IIa activity (Table 25-2). In addition, the LMWHs differ with respect to their ionic form, release profile of tissue factor-pathway inhibitor, and potential to cause bleeding in experimental models (Weitz, 1997). Together, these differences in structure and function may be of clinical importance and should caution against the assumption of a uniform effect across the entire drug class.

TABLE 25-1

COMPARISON OF UNFRACTIONATED VERSUS LOW-MOLECULAR WEIGHT HEPARINS

	Unfractionated heparin	Low-molecular-weight heparin
Anti-Xa:anti-IIa activity ratio	1	>1
Inhibits activated thrombin	Yes	Yes
Inhibits thrombin production	+	+++
Bioavailability	Low	High
Requires monitoring of aPTT	Yes	No
Neutralized by platelet factor 4	Yes	No

NOTE: aPTT, activated partial thromboplastin time.

Clinical Evaluation of LMWH

UFH has been embraced in expert guidelines and by clinicians for the treatment of non-ST elevation acute coronary syndromes largely on the basis of data from six clinical trials showing a directionally consistent trend toward the reduction of death or MI among patients with UA treated with UFH and aspirin compared with aspirin alone. These studies were summarized in a meta-analysis suggesting a 33% reduction in clinical events with combined antithrombotic and antiplatelet therapy (RR, 0.67;

TABLE 25-2

COMPARISON OF LOW-MOLECULAR-WEIGHT HEPARIN PREPARATIONS

Preparation	Mean molecular weight	Anti-Xa:anti-IIa ratio
Ardeparin (Normiflo)	6000	1.9
Dalteparin (Fragmin)	6000	2.7
Enoxaparin (Lovenox)	4200	3.8
Nadroparin (Fraxiparine)	4500	3.6
Reviparin (Clivarine)	4000	3.5
Tinzaparin (Inohep)	4500	1.9

SOURCE: (Adapted from JI Weitz: N Engl J Med 3:688, 1997, with permission. ©1997 Massachusetts Medical Society. All rights reserved.)

95% CI, 0.44 to 1.02) (Oler et al., 1996). In spite of the widespread clinical acceptance of UFH, its multiple practical and therapeutic limitations render appealing the introduction of alternative antithrombotic therapies with even an equivalent profile of efficacy and safety.

LMWH in the Acute Management of Unstable Coronary Disease

Several of the LMWHs have been compared with aspirin alone or with UFH and aspirin for the management of UA and non-Q-wave MI. In the first such studies, the combination of aspirin and nadroparin was compared with aspirin and intravenous UFH or with aspirin alone for treatment of patients with UA (Gurfinkel et al., 1995). In this single-blind, randomized trial, treatment with nadroparin was associated with a significant reduc-

tion in cardiovascular or major bleeding events compared with UFH (Table 25-3). Subsequent trials have expanded on these initial promising results with nadroparin as well as other LMWHs.

In separate double-blind, randomized protocols of similar general design and entry criteria but different control therapy, the Fragmin during Instability in Coronary Artery Disease (FRISC) and Fragmin in Unstable Coronary Artery Disease (FRIC) investigators evaluated the safety and efficacy of dalteparin in combination with aspirin for the acute and chronic management of UA and non-Q-wave MI (FRISC Study Group, 1996; Klein et al., 1997). The chronic phase results will be detailed subsequently. In the acute phase, FRISC compared dalteparin (120 IU/kg subcutaneously twice daily) for 6 days to placebo among patients within 72 h of ischemic symptoms and demonstrated a 63% reduction in the rate of death or nonfatal MI. In contrast, when evaluated in FRIC against an active control in the form of UFH, dalteparin showed no advantage. There were very few episodes of major bleeding in either trial, and no difference was seen in minor bleeding between dalteparin and UFH in FRIC. Based on the results of these two studies, the FRIC investigators concluded that dalteparin was a safe alternative to UFH in the acute management of UA and non-ST elevation MI. Similar to these findings with dalteparin but in distinction to prior work with nadroparin, the Fraxiparine in Ischemic Syndromes (FRAXIS) trial demonstrated comparable but not superior efficacy to UFH when nadroparin was studied among nearly 3500 patients in a double-blinded fashion (The FRAXIS Study Group, 1999).

Two randomized, double-blind, parallel group trials have evaluated enoxaparin for the acute management of non-ST elevation acute coronary syndromes. In the Efficacy and Safety of Subcutaneous Enoxaparin in Non-Q-Wave Coronary Events (ESSENCE) trial, patients with rest symptoms in the prior 24 h were treated with aspirin and allocated to either enoxaparin, 1 mg/kg subcutaneously daily, or intravenous UFH (Cohen et al., 1997). At 14 days, patients treated with enoxaparin were at significantly lower risk of

TABLE 25-3

RANDOMIZED CLINICAL TRIALS EVALUATING THE EFFICACY OF LOW-MOLECULAR-WEIGHT HEPARINS IN THE ACUTE AND CHRONIC PHASE MANAGEMENT OF PATIENTS WITH UNSTABLE ANGINA AND NON-Q-WAVE MYOCARDIAL INFARCTION

Investigator/Trial	Patients	Size	LMWH	Comparator	Duration of phase, days	End-point	Time-point, days	Event rates (LMWH vs. comparator)
Trials of Acute Phase LMWH Therapy								
Gurfinkel, 1997	UA	219	Nadroparin	UFH	5–7	MI, RA, UR, or major bleed	7	22 vs. 63%, $p = .0001$
FRISC Studsy Group, 1996	UA/NSTEMI	1506	Dalteparin	Placebo	6	Death or MI	6	1.8 vs. 4.8%, $p = .001$
Klein, 1997 (FRIC)	UA/NSTEMI	1482	Dalteparin	UFH	6	Death or MI	6	3.9 vs. 3.6%, $p = $ NS
Cohen, 1997 (ESSENCE)	UA/NSTEMI	3171	Enoxaparin	UFH	2–8	Death, MI, or UR	14	16.6 vs. 19.8%, $p = .019$
Antman, 1999 (TIMI 11B)	UA/NSTEMI	3910	Enoxaparin	UFH	3–8	Death, MI, or UR	8	12.4 vs. 14.5%, $p = .048$
FRAXIS Investig, 1999	UA/NSTEMI	3468	Nadroparin	UFH	6	Death, MI, RA, UA	6	14.8 vs. 14.9%, $p = $ NS

TABLE 25-3

RANDOMIZED CLINICAL TRIALS EVALUATING THE EFFICACY OF LOW-MOLECULAR-WEIGHT HEPARINS IN THE ACUTE AND CHRONIC PHASE MANAGEMENT OF PATIENTS WITH UNSTABLE ANGINA AND NON-Q-WAVE MYOCARDIAL INFARCTION (Continued)

Investigator/Trial	Patients	Size	LMWH	Comparator	Duration of phase, days	End-point	Time-point, days	Event rates (LMWH vs. comparator)
Trials of Extended (Chronic) LMWH Therapy								
FRISC Study Group, 1996	UA/NSTEMI	1506	Dalteparin	Placebo	40	Death or MI	40	8.0 and 10.7%, $p = .07$
Klein, 1997 (FRIC)	UA/NSTEMI	1482	Dalteparin	Placebo	45	Death, MI, or UR	45	12.3 vs. 12.3%, $p = $ NS
Antman, 1999 (TIMI 11B)	UA/NSTEMI	3910	Enoxaparin	Placebo	43	Death, MI, or UR	43	17.3 vs. 19.7%, $p = .048$
FRISC II, 1999	UA/NSTEMI	2267	Dalteparin	Placebo	90	Death or MI	30	3.1 vs. 5.9%, $p = .002$
FRAXIS Investig, 1999	UA/NSTEMI	3468	Nadrop × 14 d Nadrop × 14 d	UFH × 6 d Nadrop × 6 d	14	Death, MI, RA, UA	14	20.0 vs. 18.1%, $p = $ NS 20.0 vs. 17.8%, $p = $ NS

ABBREVIATION: LMWH, low-molecular-weight heparin; UA, unstable angina; NSTEMI, non-ST elevation myocardial infarction; UFH, unfractionated heparin; MI, myocardial infarction; RA, refractory angina; UR, urgent revascularization; Nadrop, Nadroparin.

death, MI, or recurrent angina. This benefit was sustained at 30 days and 1 year (13% relative risk reduction, $p = .022$). The Thrombolysis in Myocardial Infarction (TIMI) 11B trial supported and extended these findings during the early phase of therapy with the addition of an intravenous bolus of enoxaparin (30 mg) immediately prior to starting 1 mg/kg subcutaneously every 12 h (Antman et al., 1999a). As such, TIMI 11B showed a 24% reduction in the composite of death, nonfatal MI, or urgent revascularization at 48 h (Figure 25-3), with a persistent advantage at 8 days (Table 25-3) and similar rates of major bleeding compared with UFH. This very early advantage of enoxaparin was not detected in the ESSENCE trial and may be related to the administration of the intravenous bolus and the higher risk profile of patients in TIMI 11B.

A meta-analysis combining data from the ESSENCE and TIMI 11B trials demonstrated a consistent reduction of ~20% in the composite of death or MI by 8 days, with a persistent benefit of enoxaparin at 6 weeks after presentation (Antman et al., 1999b). This durable benefit of enoxaparin contrasts with the progressive convergence of event rates with dalteparin in the FRISC and FRIC trials. One potential explanation is that enoxaparin, with its higher relative anti-Xa:anti-IIa activity, achieved a greater early reduction in thrombus burden that translated into fewer clinical events during the chronic phase. Together, data from the ESSENCE and TIMI 11B trials establish the superiority of enoxaparin over UFH for the acute management of patients with non-ST elevation acute coronary syndromes. In addition, data from TIMI 11B suggest that an intravenous bolus of 30 mg enoxaparin should be considered for high-risk

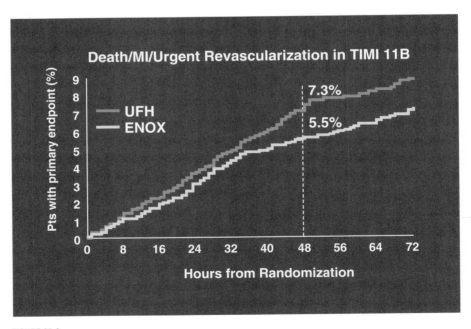

FIGURE 25-3

Kaplan-Meier plots of time to first event of the primary end-point of death, myocardial infarction (MI), or urgent revascularization over the first few days of treatment with enoxaparin (ENOX) and unfractionated heparin (UFH) in TIMI 11B. Pts, patients. (From EM Antman et al: Circulation 100:1593, 1999, with permission.)

patients (e.g., ST-segment depression or elevated serum markers) with rest symptoms in the prior 24 h.

Evaluation of Prolonged Treatment with LMWH

Patients with unstable ischemic heart disease appropriately managed at presentation remain at particular risk for recurrent events in the next 6 to 12 weeks. Persistent activation of the coagulation cascade has been documented up to several months after an index coronary event. Such clinical and experimental observations, together with the "rebound" increase in thrombotic events after discontinuation of UFH, have led investigators to explore the benefits of prolonged antithrombotic therapy. Given the ease and reliability of subcutaneous dosing of the LMWHs, they are particularly appealing for this purpose and have been assessed as chronic therapy in several randomized double-blind trials (Table 25-3).

Both the FRISC and FRIC trials were configured with a placebo-controlled chronic phase in which dalteparin was continued after 6 days at reduced dosing (7500 IU subcutaneously daily). Results were similar in both studies, with loss of the initial benefit in FRISC by 40 days and no benefit from 6 to 45 days in FRIC but with an increased risk of minor bleeding (e.g., 5.1 vs. 2.8% in FRIC). The TIMI 11B investigators also tested the efficacy of extended treatment with LMWH and detected no additional benefit from therapy through 43 days. However, chronic treatment with enoxaparin did carry an excess risk in major bleeding (2.9 vs. 1.5%, $p = .021$).

Though no advantage of prolonged dalteparin was seen in the FRISC or FRIC trials, investigators raised the possibility that more frequent dosing might have resulted in a benefit. The Long-term Low-Molecular-Mass Heparin in Unstable Coronary Artery Disease Trial was thus implemented by the FRISC II investigators to assess the efficacy of 3 months of dalteparin dosed twice daily in two tiers based on body weight (5000 IU or 7500 IU) for high-risk patients with non-ST elevation acute coronary syndromes (FRISC II Investigators, 1999a). Over 2000 patients with symptoms in the prior 48 h and ST-T wave

changes or elevated serum cardiac markers were treated with open-label dalteparin and randomized in a 2 × 2 factorial design to prolonged dalteparin or placebo and an invasive or noninvasive strategy. Among patients in the noninvasive arm, dalteparin conferred a 2.8% absolute reduction in the risk of death or MI by 30 days, which was sustained at 60 but not 90 days after randomization (Figure 25-4). Patients randomized to the invasive arm had no benefit from continuation of dalteparin after revascularization. These results suggest that with more frequent dosing, sustained therapy with dalteparin may reduce recurrent events during the first month among patients managed with a conservative strategy or who are awaiting delayed invasive therapy or evaluation. These data also raise the possibility that the absence of additional benefit with chronic enoxaparin in the TIMI 11B trial may be explained in part by high rates of early revascularization in the study.

Targeting LMWH Therapy

Though none of the clinical trials with LMWHs were configured with power to detect significant differences in individual subgroups, trends in favor of a LMWH for acute management were evident among the majority of important subgroups examined. Additional analyses from several of these trials have also revealed subgroups that may derive particular benefit from the use LMWHs. For example, in the TIMI 11B trial patients with clinical indicators of high risk such as changes in the electrocardiogram or prior aspirin use appeared to derive greater benefit from enoxaparin (Antman et al., 1999a). When such risk markers are combined into a simple clinical score for risk assessment (TIMI Risk Score for Unstable Angina/Non-ST Elevation MI), an increasing gradient of benefit of enoxaparin compared with UFH is revealed with rising risk score (Figure 25-5) (Antman et al., 2000).

Cardiac markers of necrosis have also proven useful for recognizing patients who are likely to benefit most from treatment with LMWHs. Analyses from FRISC and FRISC II suggest that prolonged treatment with dalteparin reduces the risk of

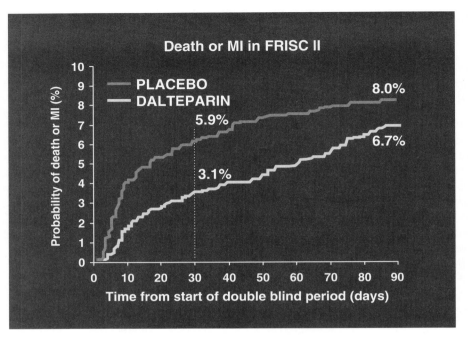

FIGURE 25-4

Probability of death or myocardial infarction (MI) over 3 months of therapy with dalteparin or placebo during the blinded treatment phase of the FRISC II trial. Relative risk reduction, 19 percent; p=2. (Modified from FRISC II Investigators: Lancet 354:701, 1999, with permission.)

recurrent cardiac events in high-risk patients with elevated levels of cardiac troponin T (Lindahl et al., 1997; FRISC II Investigators, 1999a). In addition, among patients with UA (normal CK-MB) in the TIMI 11B trial, elevated levels of troponin I identified patients who derived particular benefit from treatment with enoxaparin (Morrow et al., 2000).

Role of LMWH in Contemporary Management of Unstable Coronary Artery Disease

With predictable pharmacokinetics and high bioavailability, the LMWHs are able to achieve a stable, durable anticoagulant effect without the need for continuous intravenous administration and frequent blood testing. Further, the safety and efficacy

of the LMWHs for the acute management of unstable ischemic heart disease have been demonstrated across multiple randomized clinical trials. In addition, prolonged therapy with some LMWHs may be useful in reducing the risk of recurrent coronary events among selected high-risk populations or in patients awaiting delayed invasive evaluation.

LMWHs in Patients Undergoing Coronary Intervention

Despite these advantages, some clinicians have been reluctant to switch from UFH to LMWHs because of uncertainty regarding the use of LMWHs in patients undergoing invasive evaluation or treatment with glycoprotein IIb/IIIa (GpIIb/IIIa) antagonists. However, emerging evidence regarding use of LMWHs in these settings has been encouraging.

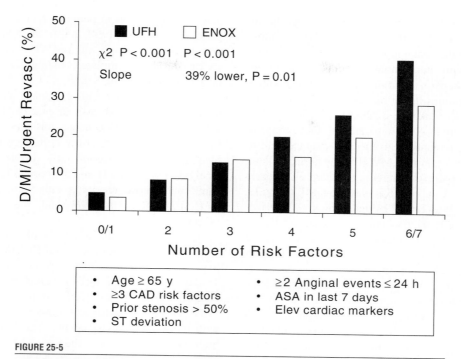

- Age $\geq$ 65 y
- $\geq$3 CAD risk factors
- Prior stenosis > 50%
- ST deviation
- $\geq$2 Anginal events $\leq$ 24 h
- ASA in last 7 days
- Elev cardiac markers

FIGURE 25-5

TIMI Risk Score for Unstable Angina/Non-ST Elevation MI reveals an increasing benefit of enoxaparin (ENOX) compared with unfractionated heparin (UFH) for the reduction of death (D), new myocardial infarction (MI), or urgent revascularization (revasc) among patients enrolled in the TIMI 11B Trial. (Adapted from EM Antman et al: JAMA 284:835, 2000, with permission.)

Data from several clinical trials have demonstrated favorable clinical outcomes among patients undergoing initial medical treatment with LMWHs followed by transition to UFH for percutaneous coronary intervention (PCI) when needed (Fox et al., 2000; FRISC II Investigators, 1999b). In addition, such observations have been extended by experience with LMWHs as the procedural anticoagulant.

For example, reviparin given intravenously was associated with less frequent early thrombotic complications (3.9 vs. 8.2%, $p = .027$) during complicated PCI when compared to UFH for elective catheterization procedures in the REDUCE trial (Karsh et al., 1996). Pilot data also support the safety and efficacy of enoxaparin during coronary intervention performed either electively or in the course of treatment for UA and/or non-ST elevation MI. In a randomized trial of 60 patients undergoing elective PCI, enoxaparin administered as a 1 mg/kg intravenous bolus was associated with similar procedural outcomes to UFH (Rabah et al., 1999). Bleeding complications were infrequent in both groups (1 in 30 patients). The subsequent National Investigators Collaborating on Enoxaparin (NICE) 1 study of 828 patients undergoing PCI confirmed low rates of major bleeding with the same dosing regimen in a larger group of patients (Young et al., 2000). For example, the 1.1% rate of major bleeding in NICE 1 contrasts favorably with the 2.2% rate observed among patients randomized to UFH in the EPISTENT trial. When used in combination with abciximab in the NICE 4 study, an intravenous dose of 0.75 mg/kg was associated with rates of major hemorrhage (0.6%), transfusion (1.8%), and thrombocytopenia (2.3%) that were similar to those reported in other contemporary interventional studies. Data with intravenous administration of 60 IU/kg of dalteparin in combination with abciximab also appear promising for procedural anticoagulation during PCI (Kereiakes et al., 2001).

Several studies have examined the safety of transitioning patients from medical management to PCI while maintaining LMWH as the anticoagulant. Among 293 patients receiving standard enoxaparin dosing for UA or non-ST elevation MI (1 mg/kg subcutaneously every 12 h) undergoing catheterization within 8 h of the morning dose, 97.6% of patients were found to have anti-Xa activity above the lower boundary (0.5 IU/mL) established for efficacy in trials of venous thromboembolism (Collet et al., 2001). One patient undergoing PCI (0.8%), experienced a major bleeding event. In the NICE 3 study, patients being treated with enoxaparin for UA or non-ST elevation MI were also treated with either abciximab, eptifibatide or tirofiban through the time of catheterization and PCI, when indicated (Ferguson, 2001). No additional heparin was administered if the procedure was performed within 8 h of the last subcutaneous dose of enoxaparin, and 0.3 mg/kg was given intravenously if the time of the procedure was >8 h after the most recent dose of LMWH (Ferguson, 2001). Preliminary report of the results showed bleeding rates that were similar to those from prior studies of GPIIb/IIIa inhibitors alone (Ferguson, 2000)

Use of LMWH in Combination with GPIIb/IIIa Antagonists

An additional area of clinical interest is the safety and efficacy of combining LMWHs with GPIIb/IIIa antagonists for the medical management of acute coronary syndromes. Studied in the Antithrombotic Combination Using Tirofiban and Enoxaparin (ACUTE) I and II trials, the administration of enoxaparin with tirofiban vs. UFH with tirofiban was associated with comparable, low rates of major bleeding (0.6% with enoxaparin vs. 0.5% with UFH) as well as with more consistent inhibition of platelet aggregation in patients treated with enoxaparin (Cohen et al., 1999, 2000). Such data indicate a possible advantage of LMWHs in combined antithrombin and antiplatelet therapy. More recently in the GUSTO IV-ACS trial, 974 of 7800 patients enrolled were treated with dalteparin as an adjunct to therapy with abciximab or placebo for patients with non-ST elevation acute coronary syndromes. Rates of non-coronary artery bypass grafting major bleeding were not significantly different in those receiving both LMWH and abciximab (1.3%) compared with those receiving either abciximab and UFH (0.8%) or LMWH and placebo (0.7%) (Simoons, 2001).

Ongoing randomized studies of enoxaparin vs. UFH in combination with GPIIb/IIIa inhibition [e.g., the Aggrastat to Zocor (A to Z) and Synergy Trials] will provide further valuable information regarding the safety and clinical efficacy of LMWHs in the setting of contemporary therapy with potent antiplatelet agents. These data will be important to clinicians as the use of LMWHs for the management of patients with acute coronary syndromes continues to increase.

REFERENCES

Antman EM: The search for replacements for unfractionated heparin. Circulation 103:2310, 2001

Antman EM et al: Enoxaparin prevents death and cardiac ischemic events in unstable angina/non-Q-wave myocardial infarction. Results of the thrombolysis in myocardial infarction (TIMI) 11B trial. Circulation 100:1593, 1999a

Antman EM et al: Assessment of the treatment effect of enoxaparin for unstable angina/non-Q-wave myocardial infarction. TIMI 11B-ESSENCE meta-analysis. Circulation 100:1602, 1999b

Antman EM et al: The TIMI risk score for unstable angina/non-ST elevation MI: A method for prognostication and therapeutic decision making. JAMA 284:835, 2000

Braunwald E et al: ACC/AHA guidelines for the management of patients with unstable angina and non-ST-segment elevation myocardial infarction: A report of the American College of Cardiology/American Heart Association Task Force on Practice Guidelines (Committee on the Management of Patients with Unstable Angina). J Am Coll Cardiol 36:970, 2000

Cohen M et al: A comparison of low-molecular-weight heparin with unfractionated heparin for unstable coronary artery disease. Efficacy and Safety of Subcutaneous Enoxaparin in Non-Q-Wave Coronary Events Study Group. New Engl J Med 337:447, 1997

Cohen M et al: Combination therapy with tirofiban and enoxaparin in acute coronary syndromes. Int J Cardiol 71:273, 1999

Cohen M et al: Anti-thrombotic combination using tirofiban and enoxaparin: The ACUTE II study (abstr). Circulation 102:II-826, 2000

Collet JP et al: Percutaneous coronary intervention after subcutaneous enoxaparin pretreatment in patients with unstable angina pectoris. Circulation 103:658, 2001

Dahlback B: Blood coagulation. Lancet 355:1627, 2000

Ferguson JJ: Combining low-molecular-weight heparin and glycoprotein IIb/IIIa antagonists for the treatment of acute coronary syndromes: The NICE 3 story. National Investigators Collaborating on Enoxaparin. J Invasive Cardiol 12 (Suppl E):E10, 2000

Ferguson JJ 3rd: NICE-3 preliminary results. Presented at the 22nd Congress of the European Society of Cardiology; 2000; Amsterdam

Fox KAA et al: Are treatment effects of enoxaparin (low-molecular weight heparin) more marked in those undergoing percutaneous intervention: Results of the ESSENCE/TIMI 11B? (abstr). Eur Heart J 21:3267A, 2000

FRISC II Investigators: Long-term low-molecular-mass heparin in unstable coronary artery disease: FRISC II prospective randomised multicentre study. Lancet 354:701, 1999a

FRISC II Investigators: Invasive compared with non-invasive treatment in unstable coronary-artery disease: FRISC II prospective randomised multicentre study. Lancet 354:708, 1999b

FRISC Study Group: Low-molecular-weight heparin during instability in coronary artery disease, Fragmin during Instability in Coronary Artery Disease (FRISC). Lancet 347:561, 1996

Gurfinkel EP et al: Low molecular weight heparin versus regular heparin or aspirin in the treatment of unstable angina and silent ischemia. J Am Coll Cardiol 26:313, 1995

Karsch KR et al: Low molecular weight heparin (reviparin) in percutaneous transluminal coronary angioplasty. Results of a randomized, double-blind, unfractionated heparin and placebo-controlled, multicenter trial (REDUCE trial). Reduction of Restenosis After PTCA, Early Administration of Reviparin in a Double-Blind Unfractionated Heparin and Placebo-Controlled Evaluation. J Am Coll Cardiol 28:1437, 1996

Kereiakes DJ et al: Dalteparin in combination with abciximab during percutaneous coronary intervention. Am Heart J 141:348, 2001

Klein W et al: Comparison of low-molecular-weight heparin with unfractionated heparin acutely and with placebo for 6 weeks in the management of unstable coronary artery disease. Fragmin in unstable coronary artery disease study (FRIC). Circulation 96:61, 1997

Lee RT, Libby P: The unstable atheroma. Arterioscler Thromb Vasc Biol 17:1859, 1997

Lindahl B et al: Troponin T identifies patients with unstable coronary artery disease who benefit from long-term antithrombotic protection. Fragmin in Unstable Coronary Artery Disease (FRISC) Study Group. J Am Coll Cardiol 29:43, 1997

Morrow DA et al: Cardiac troponin I for stratification of early outcomes and the efficacy of enoxaparin in unstable angina: A TIMI 11B substudy. J Am Coll Cardiol 36:1812, 2000

Oler A et al: Adding heparin to aspirin reduces the incidence of myocardial infarction and death in patients with unstable angina. JAMA 276:811, 1996

Rabah MM et al: Usefulness of intravenous enoxaparin for percutaneous coronary intervention in stable angina pectoris. Am J Cardiol 84:1391, 1999

Simoons ML: Effect of glycoprotein IIb/IIIa receptor blocker abciximab on outcome in patients with acute coronary syndromes without early coronary revascularisation: The GUSTO IV-ACS randomised trial. Lancet 357:1915, 2001

The FRAXIS Study Group: Comparison of two treatment durations of a low molecular weight heparin in the initial managment of unstable angina of non-Q wave myocardial infarction: FRAX.I.S. Eur Heart J 20:1553, 1999

Weitz JI: Low-molecular-weight heparins. N Engl J Med 337:688, 1997

Young JJ et al: Low-molecular-weight heparin therapy in percutaneous coronary intervention: The NICE 1 and NICE 4 trials. National Investigators Collaborating on Enoxaparin Investigators. J Invasive Cardiol 12 (Suppl E):E14, 2000

THIRD-GENERATION FIBRINOLYTICS

Robert E. Fowles

Value of Fibrinolytic Drugs in Acute Myocardial Infarction

In acute myocardial infarction (AMI), restoration of patency and blood flow in the thrombus-occluded coronary artery is vital to preservation of heart muscle and enhanced survival. Infarct-related coronary arterial flow is gauged angiographically on a scale developed by the Thrombolysis in Myocardial Infarction (TIMI) investigative team: TIMI 3 patency, or "normal" flow (angiographic appearance of contrast similar to nonculprit arterial segments), is associated with the best outcomes and is one of the criteria against which reperfusion therapy is measured. More than 20 years of extensive patient trials and widespread clinical usage have established the crucial role of reperfusion techniques in the treatment of AMI. Fibrinolytic drugs, a foundation of reperfusion therapy, have developed out of increased understanding of the intricacies of the atherothrombotic process and out of improved pharmacologic technology.

The first generation of fibrinolytic drugs included streptokinase, anistreplase (anisoylated plasminogen streptokinase activator complex, or APSAC), and two-chain urokinase-type plasminogen activator (tcu-PA). These agents bring about a "lytic state" by generating systemic plasmin, which in turn degrades fibrinogen, von Willebrand factor, and coagulation factors V, VIII, and XII, and depletes circulating $\alpha2$-antiplasmin. This comprehensive effect upon several elements of the blood clotting system causes the first-generation lytics to be classified *"fibrin-nonspecific."* The most commonly used first-generation fibrinolytic, streptokinase, is limited by antigenicity, risk of hypotension, and a relatively low vessel patency rate.

The second generation of fibrinolytic drugs is essentially represented by alteplase, termed recombinant t-PA, or rt-PA, because it was fashioned after intrinsic tissue-type plasminogen activator (t-PA) using sophisticated gene technology. Alteplase is more fibrin-specific because it activates plasmin by cleaving plasminogen preferentially at the fibrin surface, where high-affinity binding occurs in a ternary complex between fibrin, t-PA, and plasminogen.

Limitations of First- and Second-generation Fibrinolytics

Despite the fact that intravenous first- and second-generation fibrinolytic therapy does not require angiographic or surgical capability and can be given relatively easily and promptly at most emergency facilities, its use is accompanied by several drawbacks, as shown in Table 26-1. AMI mortality at 30 days still hovers around 6.5 to 7.5% in well-controlled trials of fibrinolytic therapy and is higher in "real-world" clinical practice. Only approximately 50% of patients gain TIMI 3 vessel patency 90 min after treatment with fibrinolytics, and they risk reocclusion at a rate of at least 10% or reinfarction in at least 4% of cases. Bleeding remains a significant concern, the most devastating being

TABLE 26-1

LIMITATIONS OF FIBRINOLYTIC DRUGS

First generation (streptokinase)

  Fibrin nonspecific, inducing systemic coagulation
    changes

  Only 32% TIMI 3 90-min coronary patency

  Antigenicity

  Risk of hypotension

Second generation (alteplase)

  Complex infusion scheme (not bolus-delivered)

  Risk of intracranial hemorrhage 0.9%

  Only ~50% TIMI 3 patency at 90 min

  Reocclusion and reinfarction

  30-day mortality still ~7%

  Not all patients are eligible

ABBREVIATION: TIMI, Thrombolysis in Myocardial Infarction Study.

intracranial hemorrhage at a rate of 0.7 to 0.9% of cases, but more frequently in the elderly. Not all AMI patients are eligible for thrombolytic treatment because of such hazards, and not all eligible patients receive treatment. Fibrinolytic regimens can be difficult and error-prone due to complex infusion schemes and weight-based dosing requirements.

Development of New Drugs

Aiming at safer and more effective therapy, development of a third generation of fibrinolytics has moved along several lines. Some new agents are modifications of t-PA; others are hybrids of alteplase and additional plasminogen activators such as prourokinase. A further area of research is the conjugation of plasminogen activators with monoclonal antibodies against fibrin, platelets, or thrombomodulin. New molecules under development include agents originating from bacteria (staphylokinase from staphylococcus) or animals (DS-PA from vampire bat, fibrolase from copperhead snake). Some of the pharmacologic and clinical features of various new fibrinolytics are displayed in Table 26-2.

Reteplase (r-PA)

The first modification of t-PA to be developed was reteplase (r-PA), specifically bioengineered for a more desirable pharmacologic profile: to retain plasminogenolytic activity and fibrin specificity but a longer half-life to permit bolus administration. By deletion of t-PA's finger, epidermal growth factor (EGF), and kringle-1 domains, r-PA has a longer half-life (15 min vs. 4 min for rt-PA), allowing easier administration. In vitro studies showing more extensive clot penetration for r-PA compared with rt-PA suggested that its lower fibrin affinity might be advantageous in accomplishing rapid recanalization. In animal models, including a canine coronary thrombosis preparation, r-PA exhibited faster and more extensive clot lysis than any first- or second-generation fibrinolytic. Its lack of weight-based dosing requirements allows reteplase to be administered

TABLE 26-2

COMPARISONS BETWEEN FIBRINOLYTIC AGENTS[a]

	Plasma half-life	Dose	Fibrin specificity	TIMI 3 coronary patency[b]	ICH
Streptokinase SK	23 min	1.5 MU/60 min	0	32% at 90 min	0.5%
Alteplase t-PA or rt-PA	4 min	15-mg bolus or 0.75 mg/kg per 30 min 0.5 mg/kg per 60 min	++	45–54% at 90 min	0.9%
Reteplase r-PA	15 min	10 U + 10 U 30 min apart	+	60–63% at 90 min	0.9%
Tenecteplase TNK-tPA	20 min	~0.5-mg/kg bolus	+++	64% at 90 min	0.9%
Lanoteplase n-PA	37 min	120-kU/kg bolus or 20-mg bolus	+	57% at 90 min	1.13%
Saruplase r-scu-PA	9 min	60 mg/1 h	+	72% at 90 min	0.9%
Staphylokinase STAR SakSTAR	9 min	15–45 mg/30 min or 5-mg bolus PEG-SakSTAR	++++	58–74% at 90 min	–
DS-PA	2.8 h	0.5-mg/kg bolus	+++	–	–
Monteplase	23 min	0.22-mg/kg bolus	++	53–69% at 60 min	–
Pamiteplase	40 min	0.1–0.3-mg/kg bolus	++	50–54% at 60 min	–

[a]See text for description of drugs.
[b]TIMI (Thrombolysis in Myocardial Infarction) 3 patency (explained in text) is derived from human clinical trials.
Abbreviations: ICH, intracranial hemorrhage; PEG-SakSTAR, polyethylene glycolated Staphylokinase; DS-PA; *Desmodus* salivary plasminogen activator.

as two fixed-dose boluses 30 min apart. Such a regimen was demonstrated in clinical trials to be safe and effective.

RAPID-II, an angiographic AMI trial, found statistically significant better TIMI 3 patency for r-PA at 60 min and 90 min compared with rt-PA (60 min, 51% vs. 37%; 90 min, 60% vs. 45%). The INJECT trial, with 6010 patients in the first fibrinolytic mortality equivalence–designed study, showed a slight numerical advantage of r-PA over streptokinase (9% vs. 9.5%

35-day mortality), statistically concluding that r-PA was at least as effective as streptokinase. (Bode et al, 1996)

The superior early vessel patency found with r-PA in RAPID II was, however, not associated with any demonstrable mortality advantage in the 15,059-patient GUSTO III trial (7.47% 30-day mortality for reteplase vs. 7.24% for alteplase) (GUSTO III Investigators, 1997). Intracranial hemorrhage rates were similar at 0.9% overall. The conclusion was that the main clinically demonstrated advantage of reteplase was the ease of administering the fixed-dose double bolus as opposed to the front-loaded accelerated method for alteplase.

Tenecteplase (TNK-tPA)

Tenecteplase (TNK-tPA) is structurally identical to natural t-PA except for three point mutations, exchanging out the incumbent amino acids threonine (T), asparagine (N), and lysine-histidine-arginine-arginine (KHRR). The T and N substitutions in the kringle-1 domain lengthen the molecule's half-life to approximately 20 min, and the N and KHRR substitutions increase fibrin binding, specificity, and resistance to plasminogen activator inhibitor 1 (PAI-1). As was the case with r-PA, TNK-tPA exhibited better clot lysis than t-PA in animal models. However, in TIMI-10B, a clinical AMI angiographic trial (Cannon et al., 1998), TIMI 3 patency rates were not statistically significantly different from t-PA (30 mg TNK-tPA, 54%; 40 mg TNK-tPA, 63%; 50 mg TNK-tPA, 66%; vs. t-PA, 63%). An intracranial hemorrhage rate of 3.8% in the first 78 patients given 50 mg of TNK-tPA prompted a protocol change, eliminating the 50 mg dose of TNK-tPA and reducing the heparin dose; the subsequent intracranial hemorrhage rate then dropped to 1.9%, the same as the t-PA arm of the TIMI-10B study. Coronary patency appeared to be dose dependent for TNK-tPA, requiring 0.5 to 0.6 mg/kg for maximum TIMI 3 flow rates, the lower dose of 30 mg TNK-tPA showing statistically significantly lower patency than t-PA.

In ASSENT-1, an uncontrolled safety trial testing fixed doses of TNK-tPA, the intracranial hemorrhage rate was no greater than 0.9% but, as in

TIMI-10B, the serious bleeding rate was related to (dose)/(patient weight). The higher bleeding rates seen in fixed-dose regimens that failed to adjust for patient weight prompted a decision to weight-adjust TNK-tPA.

ASSENT-2, a 16,649-patient AMI comparative mortality trial (ASSENT-2 Investigators, 1999), showed equivalence of rt-PA and TNK-tPA with 30-day mortality for both of 6.2% and a similar intracranial hemorrhage rate of 0.9%. Statistically, significantly fewer noncerebral bleeding complications were seen with TNK-tPA (26%) than with rt-PA (29%). In ASSENT-2 the ideal weight-based target dose of TNK-tPA was 0.53 mg/kg, a rather precise figure, from which five dosing tiers were derived in patient weight brackets of 10 kg. The conclusions are that although rt-PA and TNK-tPA are equivalent with respect to mortality outcome and overall intracranial hemorrhage risk, weight-adjusted TNK-tPA has the advantages of slightly lower noncerebral bleeding risk and single-bolus administration. TNK-tPA's features of higher fibrin affinity/specificity and PAI-1 resistance are conceptually appealing, though not yet demonstrated to be of direct clinical superiority with respect to vessel patency, mortality outcome, or intracranial hemorrhage risk.

Lanoteplase (n-PA)

Lanoteplase (n-PA) was structured with deletion of the finger and EGF domains and modification of the kringle-1 glycosylation points of t-PA, resulting in a longer half-life of 37 min. The 602-patient InTIME-1 study showed a numerically higher TIMI 3 patency rate for n-PA of 57% compared to rt-PA at 46% (not statistically significant) and no difference in overall major bleeding. InTIME-2 (Antman et al., 1999), a much larger trial involving more than 15,000 patients, found similar 30-day mortality results for n-PA (6.8%) and rt-PA (6.6%) but a statistically significantly higher intracranial hemorrhage rate (n-PA, 1.13%; rt-PA, 0.62%). Due to this considerable handicap, perhaps caused by a higher than optimal dose, further trials with n-PA have been stopped at this point.

Saruplase (r-scu-PA)

Saruplase (r-scu-PA) is a recombinant human single-chain prourokinase polypeptide that is converted by plasmin into a two-chain urokinase-type plasminogen activator (tcu-PA) or urokinase. Although scu-PA has no fibrin affinity, fibrin-specific clot lysis occurs when the pro-drug is converted to tcu-PA at the fibrin surface; at higher doses systemic effects emerge, rendering scu-PA partially fibrin-specific. The PRIMI study found scu-PA to be superior to streptokinase in patency and speed of reperfusion, with less degradation of systemic fibrinogen. In the SESAM trial, saruplase exhibited patency rates similar to 3-h (not front-loaded) rt-PA. In the 3089-patient COMPASS saruplase-streptokinase equivalence trial (Tebbe et al., 1998), the 30-day mortality rate was numerically but not statistically significantly lower at 5.7% than that of streptokinase at 6.7%. The rate of hemorrhagic stroke of 0.9% for saruplase was similar to that of other plasminogen activators, though higher than the streptokinase risk of 0.3%, and bleeding rates were similar at approximately 10%. Modifications of saruplase currently underway include chimeric conjugation with t-PA and with antiplatelet antibodies.

Staphylokinase

Staphylokinase was produced by recombinant technology initially as STAR (recombinant staphylokinase), which combines with plasminogen and then is activated to a plasmin-staphylokinase complex at the clot surface for effective fibrinolysis. However, unlike streptokinase, staphylokinase is highly fibrin-specific, being inactive in the absence of fibrin, so no systemic fibrinogen degradation occurs. Pilot studies in AMI showed high patency rates without major side effects, and in a 100-patient patency study, STAR was found to be at least as effective as front-loaded rt-PA, more fibrin-specific, and associated with fewer bleeding complications. However, most STAR-treated patients developed antibodies within 2 weeks. Staphylokinase immunogenicity has now been modified by site-directed recombinant amino acid substitutions and by derivatization with polyeth-

ylene glycol (PEG) to produce PEGylated Sak-STAR, with a plasma half-life long enough to allow single-bolus administration (Collen et al., 2000). In early AMI application, this compound shows 78% 90-min TIMI 3 flow, no systemic fibrinogen degradation or systemic plasminogen activation, and no hemodynamic problems or immediate allergic reactions (there may an undetermined degree of reduced, late antigenicity). PEGylated SakSTAR, with its highly promising reperfusion potency and lack of systemic coagulation effects, has been selected for expanded clinical testing.

Desmodus Salivary Plasminogen Activator (DS-PA)

The vampire bat *Desmodus rotundus* secretes several salivary plasminogen activators, four of which have been chemically and genetically isolated. One of these, DS-PAα1, closely resembles human t-PA except for the absence of the kringle-2 domain. DS-PAα1 is more fibrin-specific than either t-PA or TNK-PA, and in initial animal model testing it exhibits faster and more extensive clot fibrinolysis than t-PA. Reocclusion rates are also lower, probably a result of the long half-life (2.8 h) of DS-PAα1. Its lack of activation by β-amyloid may render DS-PAα1 less likely to cause cerebral bleeding, since β-amyloid stimulation is thought to be linked to the hemorrhagic stroke found with t-PA and other plasminogen activator analogues. Although human phase 1 studies have failed to demonstrate antibodies up to 3 months after administration of subtherapeutic doses of DS-PAα1, its potential immunogenicity is still considerable. Early clinical AMI trials with this drug are now underway.

Other Novel Agents

Several new drugs in addition to those already mentioned are under development. Yet another variation of t-PA is *monteplase,* with an amino acid substitution in the EGF domain of t-PA, yielding a longer half-life of 23 min. This bolus-administrable drug in preliminary AMI use has shown a 90-min TIMI 3 patency rate of 69%, superior to tisokinase (a form of t-PA used in Japan), even though monteplase's fibrin specificity was less.

Pamiteplase is a mutant of t-PA, with kringle-1 deletion and a point mutation at the protease cleavage site of t-PA, rendering the drug resistant to degradation by plasmin. Its half-life of 30 to 47 min allows bolus dosing, and early dose-finding trials have suggested better early patency rates compared to t-PA.

Amideplase (K2tu-PA) is an example of hybridized molecules; it is created from the fibrin-binding kringle-2 (K2) domain of t-PA and the plasminogen-converting protease catalytic site of scu-PA. Preliminary work indicates that amideplase can be single-bolus administered, is fibrin-specific, has greater fibrinolytic activity than rt-PA, and has no significant antigenicity.

Fibrolase is not a plasminogen activator but a direct-acting fibrinolytic enzyme derived from copperhead snake venom. In an animal model of arterial thrombosis, fibrolase was rapidly lytic without excessive bleeding or hypotension and was superior to APSAC. Still another area of potential fibrinolytic improvement is the conjugation of plasminogen activators with antifibrin antibodies, attempting to provide greater fibrin affinity and specificity; such drugs are still in preclinical development.

Importance of the Atherothrombotic Milieu

The efficacy of fibrinolytic agents depends on many factors other than drug structure and pharmacology. Certainly the new third-generation drugs offer several advantages, including longer plasma half-life, which allows safer and more convenient administration. Greater fibrinolytic potency as manifested by faster, more complete patency confers a trend toward reductions in 30-day mortality. Pharmacologic properties such as fibrin specificity theoretically should reduce the risk of bleeding, so far only modestly better with the third-generation lytics. These results may be due to the complexity of the milieu in which

fibrinolytics act. The constitution of thrombi is variable; some are more fibrin-rich, some higher in platelet content. Thrombus aging and fibrinolytic resistance can be greatly influenced by intrinsic coagulation system components with genotypic predispositions such as factors VII (Girelli et al., 2000) and XIII (Robinson et al., 2000). Elevated plasma levels of factor VII, von Willebrand factor, fibrinogen, and plasminogen-activator inhibitor are important risk factors for myocardial infarction and will influence the effects of endogenous or therapeutic fibrinolytics (Kohler and Grant, 2000). Platelet function before, during, and after thrombolytic therapy is also highly dynamic, and platelet activation varies with the fibrinolytic agent given (Moser et al., 1999). The intricate pathophysiologic environment of myocardial infarction will continue to be elucidated as fibrinolytic therapy and its combined application with other drugs such as antiplatelet and antithrombotic agents move forward.

REFERENCES

Antman EM et al: Long-term comparison of lanoteplase and alteplase in ST elevation myocardial infarction: 6 month follow-up in InTIME-II Trial. Circulation 100:I-498, 1999

ASSENT-2 Investigators: Single-bolus tenecteplase compared with front-loaded alteplase in acute myocardial infarction: The ASSENT-2 double-blind randomized trial. Lancet 354:716, 1999

Bode C et al: Randomized comparison of coronary thrombolysis achieved with double-bolus reteplase and front-loaded, accelerated alteplase in patients with acute myocardial infarction. Circulation 94:891, 1996

Cannon CP et al: TNK-tissue plasminogen activator compared with front-loaded alteplase in acute myocardial infarction. Circulation 98:2805, 1998

Collen D et al: Polyethylene glycol-derivatized cysteine-substitution variants of recombinant staphylokinase for single-bolus treatment of acute myocardial infarction. Circulation 102:1766, 2000

Girelli D et al: Polymorphisms in the factor VII gene and the risk of myocardial infarction in patients with coronary heart disease. N Engl J Med 343:774, 2000

GUSTO-III Investigators: A comparison of reteplase with alteplase for acute myocardial infarction. N Engl J Med 337:1118, 1997

Kohler HP, Grant PJ: Plasminogen-activator inhibitor type 1 and coronary artery disease. N Engl J Med 342:1792, 2000

Moser M et al: Platelet function during and after thrombolytic therapy for acute myocardial infarction with reteplase, alteplase, or streptokinase. Circulation 100:1858, 1999

Robinson BR et al: Catalytic life of activated factor XIII in thrombi: Implications for fibrinolytic resistance and thrombus aging. Circulation 102:1151, 2000

Tebbe U et al: Randomized, double-blind study comparing saruplase with streptokinase therapy in acute myocardial infarction: The COMPASS equivalence trial. J Am Coll Cardiol 31:487, 1998

THROMBOLYSIS IN ELDERLY PATIENTS WITH ACUTE MYOCARDIAL INFARCTION

Alan K. Berger & Harlan M. Krumholz

The efficacy of thrombolytic therapy in the setting of an acute myocardial infarction (AMI) has been well established for patients younger than 75 years by randomized clinical trials. As a result, the American College of Cardiology/American Heart Association (ACC/AHA) guidelines for the management of AMI strongly endorse thrombolytic therapy for patients aged <75 years who present to a hospital within 6 to 12 h of the onset of symptoms of an AMI, with electrocardiographic evidence of either ST elevation or left bundle branch block, and without contraindications (Ryan et al., 1999). However, among patients aged ≥75 years, the evidence is not as strong, and as a result, the ACC/AHA guidelines recommend thrombolytic therapy with less enthusiasm. Almost 15 years after the publication of the first large randomized trial of thrombolytic therapy, controversy remains regarding its effectiveness in the elderly.

Randomized Clinical Trial Evidence

The evidence that thrombolytic therapy is beneficial in the elderly is not as strong as for younger patients. The trials enrolled relatively few older patients and, among those studied, the relative impact on mortality appears less than in younger patients. Over 60% of the randomized clinical trials excluded patients aged ≥75 years. In the studies that enrolled older patients, the distribution of age was skewed toward younger patients. In actual practice, 30% of the patients with AMI are at least 75 years old (GUSTO Investigators, 1993), compared with only 10% of the patients enrolled in the trials (Fibrinolytic Therapy Trialists' Collaborative Group, 1994).

The trials have principally shown that the relative reduction in the risk of death associated with thrombolytic therapy decreases with increasing age. This finding is relatively consistent across the studies and was illustrated best in the Fibrinolytic Therapy Trialists' (FTT) collaborative meta-analysis of all randomized clinical trials of more than 1000 patients (Fibrinolytic Therapy Trialists' Collaborative Group, 1994). The 58,600 patients from the trials included 17,000 aged 65 to 74 years and 5754 aged ≥75 years. The authors showed that the relative reduction in mortality associated with thrombolytic therapy decreased from 22% for those aged <55 years; to 19% for those aged 55 to 64 years; to 16% for those aged 65 to 74 years; to 4% for those aged ≥75 years. The reason for the decrement in relative effectiveness with increasing age is not known. While the risk of hemorrhage associated with thrombolytic therapy increases with age, this early risk does not completely explain the decreased relative benefit.

The 4% relative reduction in risk among patients aged ≥75 years in the FTT analysis translated to a 1% absolute reduction in risk, or the need to treat 100 patients to save 1 life. Although this difference was not statistically significant, the magnitude of difference has been deemed to be clinically important, most notably in the Global Use of Streptokinase and t-PA to Open Occluded Coronary Arteries (GUSTO) trial. Because the absolute risk of AMI increases with age, smaller relative reductions in risk can produce a similar magnitude of absolute benefit. For example, a 33% relative reduction in risk for a patient group with a 6% risk of dying will decrease the risk to 4% and save 2 lives per 100 treated. A 10% relative reduction in risk for a patient group with a 30% chance of dying will reduce the risk to 27% and save 3 lives per 100. The smaller relative reduction can produce a more important effect when applied to a group with a higher risk.

This relationship was illustrated in a cost-effectiveness analysis of thrombolytic therapy in the elderly (Krumholz et al., 1994). The authors demonstrated that despite the lower relative reduction in risk and the shorter life expectancy of older patients, thrombolytic therapy was extremely cost-effective compared with many other medical interventions.

Use of Thrombolytic Therapy in the Elderly

Observational studies have provided information about the use of thrombolytic therapy in the elderly. First, the proportion of patients eligible for thrombolytic therapy decreases with age. An analysis of the Multicenter Chest Pain Study demonstrated that the proportion of patients who arrived within 6 h of the onset of pain and ST-segment elevation or new

Q waves decreased significantly with increasing age, from 34% in patients aged <65 years to 18% for those aged ≥75 years (Krumholz et al., 1994). In addition, comorbidities that would have contraindicated thrombolytic therapy were present in an additional 12% of AMI patients who were aged >65 years. A recent analysis of Medicare beneficiaries with an AMI revealed that 76% were not eligible for thrombolysis due to clinical contraindications and absence of electrocardiographic inclusion criteria (Krumholz et al., 1997). Among those who were eligible for thrombolytic therapy, only 44% were treated. Significant characteristics associated with underutilization included advanced age, left bundle branch block, delay in presentation, history of bypass surgery, absence of chest pain, Q-waves, sum ST elevation <6 mm in all leads, ST elevation limited to two leads, and mental status changes.

Observational Studies of Effectiveness

Although the pooled studies have raised questions about the value of thrombolytic therapy in the elderly, no further trials have been conducted. The one trial that focused specifically on the elderly was discontinued because of low enrollment. Investigators have made use of observational study designs to draw inferences about the effectiveness of thrombolytic therapy in actual practice.

Thiemann and colleagues studied the care and outcomes of Medicare beneficiaries who were eligible for thrombolytic therapy at hospitals without the capacity for primary angioplasty (Thiemann et al., 2000). They found that among patients aged 65 to 75 years, thrombolysis was associated with an insignificant reduction in 30-day mortality [hazard ratio (HR) = 0.88; 95% confidence interval (CI): 0.69 to 1.12]; among patients aged >75 years, there was a significant hazard associated with thrombolysis (HR = 1.38; 95% CI: 1.12 to 1.71). In another analysis of Medicare beneficiaries, Berger and co-workers found that thrombolysis was not significantly associated with a lower 30-day mortality among patients aged >65 years (HR = 1.01; 95% CI: 0.94 to 1.09).

Unlike Thiemann and colleagues, Berger et al also examined mortality at 1 year and did observe an association with lower mortality (HR = 0.84; 95% CI: 0.79 to 0.89) (Berger et al: 2000). A recent analysis of the combined Myocardial Infarction Registry (MIR) and the Maximal Individual Therapy in Acute Myocardial Infarction (MITRA) registries demonstrated similar findings among 6815 AMI patients aged ≥75 years (Gitt et al., 2001). While thrombolytic therapy had no impact on in-hospital mortality [odds ratio (OR) = 0.95; 95% CI: 0.81 to 1.12], its use was associated with a reduction in 18-month mortality (OR = 0.58; 95% CI: 0.39 to 0.88). Similar results were obtained in a retrospective review of 5428 Swedish AMI patients aged 75 and older; there was a 12% relative risk reduction in 1-year mortality [(RR) = 0.88; 95% CI: 0.79 to 0.97] (Stenestrand et al., 2001).

Unfortunately, these studies have not provided clear guidance about the use of thrombolytic therapy in older patients. From a historic standpoint, randomized clinical trials have been considered a stronger source of evidence for the development of clinical guidelines. The observational studies question the efficacy of thrombolytic agents in the elderly and raise the possibility of an increased risk of mortality.

increasing risk of stroke with advancing age (0.8% in patients aged <65 years, 2.1% in patients aged 65 to 74 years, 3.4% in patients aged 75 to 84 years, and 2.9% in the small sample of patients aged ≥85 years) was demonstrated (White et al., 1996). Increasing age was the most powerful predictor of hemorrhagic stroke in GUSTO-1, and 60% of patients who developed intracranial hemorrhage subsequently died (Gore et al., 1995).

Observational studies have reported higher rates of stroke than those observed in the clinical trials. In the National Registry for Myocardial Infarction-2 (NRMI-2), the incidence of intracranial hemorrhage increased with age (0.4% in patients aged <65 years; 1.24% in patients aged 65 to 74 years; 2.13% in patients aged ≥75 years) (Gurwitz et al., 1998). In the multivariate analysis, age was the most powerful predictor of intracranial hemorrhage [OR = 1.00 in patients aged <65 years; OR = 2.71 (95% CI: 2.18 to 3.37) in patients aged 65 to 74 years; OR = 4.34 (95% CI: 3.45 to 5.45) in patients aged ≥75 years]. Brass and colleagues examined the risk of hemorrhagic stroke among Medicare beneficiaries with AMI who were treated with thrombolytic therapy (Brass et al., 2000). They identified a 1.5% rate of intracranial hemorrhage and determined that some older patients with high-risk characteristics had a risk as high as 4%.

Risks of Thrombolysis in the Elderly

Thrombolytic therapy poses an increased risk of bleeding, including gastrointestinal hemorrhage and vascular injury at the site of arterial punctures, and is associated with a higher rate of blood transfusion. It is the risk of stroke in the elderly, particularly intracranial bleeding, that raises the greatest concern. Early clinical trials—GUSTO-1 and Myocardial Infarction Triage and Intervention (MITI)—documented stroke in 0.6 to 2.0% of patients and intracranial bleeding in 0.3% of patients (Gore et al., 1995; Gebel et al., 1998; Longstreth et al., 1993). In the FTT pooled analysis, thrombolytic therapy in patients aged ≥75 years was associated with an increased risk of stroke compared with younger patients (2.0% vs. 1.2%). In another study, an

Selection of Thrombolytic Agent

While several trials have compared the efficacy and safety profile of the thrombolytic agents, no study to date has focused on the elderly (GUSTO Investigators, 1993; Gruppo Italiano, 1990; ISIS-2 Collaborative Group, 1988). In a subgroup analysis of GUSTO-1, patients aged >75 years treated with tissue plasminogen activator (+-PA) had an insignificantly lower mortality (19.3% vs. 20.6%, p = NS) compared with those treated with streptokinase. The absolute magnitude of the difference was similar to the overall trial result.

The randomized clinical trials have raised concern about the increased risk of intracranial hemorrhage among patients treated with t-PA. Due to differences in trial design, particularly the use of the anticoagulant heparin, it has been difficult to combine the results of the clinical trials. GUSTO-1, in an analysis of patients aged >75 years, found that patients treated with t-PA had an increased risk of all strokes (3.9% vs. 3.1%, 95% CI: 0.90 to 1.87) and hemorrhagic stroke (2.1% vs. 1.2%; 95% CI: 1.01 to 2.88) compared with patients treated with streptokinase. When death and nondisabling stroke were combined, t-PA provided an insignificant benefit over streptokinase in the elderly (20.2% vs. 21.5%, p = NS).

Newer thrombolytic agents, including reteplase and TNK-tPA, have received U.S. Food and Drug Administration approval on the basis of comparative trials with existing thrombolytic agents (streptokinase, t-PA) (The GUSTO 3 Investigators, 1997; The ASSENT-2 Investigators, 1999). Other agents—lanoteplase, staphylokinase, and saruplase—are undergoing evaluation in clinical trials. Relatively little information is available about the therapeutic effectiveness of these agents in the elderly.

Primary Coronary Intervention in the Elderly

Any review of thrombolytic therapy in the elderly should also consider primary percutaneous intervention, the alternative reperfusion therapy. Subgroup analyses of both the Primary Angioplasty in Myocardial Infarction (PAMI) and GUSTO-2B trials demonstrated a strong trend for the benefit of primary percutaneous transluminal coronary angioplasty (PTCA) compared with thrombolysis for patients aged >70 years (Grines et al., 1993; GUSTO-2B Investigators, 1997). The lack of statistical significance may be related to the small proportion of elderly patients enrolled in both of these trials. While the MITI registry failed to show a benefit of coronary intervention among the elderly, analyses of the NRMI registry, the Cooperative Cardiovascular Project (CCP) database, and MIR and MITRA registries also found a strong trend favoring primary PTCA over thrombolysis (Gitt et al., 2001; Every et al., 1996; Tie Fenbrunn et al., 1998; Berger et al., 1999). In spite of the documented benefit of primary PTCA in the

elderly, recent data suggest that elderly patients are far less likely to be offered coronary intervention than younger patients (Regueiro et al., 2001). These studies emphasize the need for a randomized clinical trial of primary PTCA/stenting versus thrombolytic therapy in the elderly.

Conclusions

The decision to utilize thrombolytic agents in the elderly remains a controversial issue. In spite of the finding of a lower relative reduction of risk in the elderly compared with younger patients in the clinical trials, thrombolytic therapy is associated with a greater or equal absolute reduction in risk. Given the incidence of AMI in the elderly, the absolute reduction in risk translates into the potential to save thousands of lives per year. However, the observational studies have provided some cautionary data. As a result, after decades of study, the current literature does not provide clear guidance on the use of thrombolytic therapy in older patients.

REFERENCES

Berger AK et al: A comparison of primary coronary angioplasty with thrombolysis for the management of acute myocardial infarction in the elderly: An analysis of the Cooperative Cardiovascular Project. JAMA 282:341, 1999

Berger AK et al: Thrombolytic therapy in older patients. J Am Coll Cardiol 36:366, 2000

Brass LM et al: Intracranial hemorrhage associated with thrombolytic therapy for elderly patients with acute myocardial infarction: Results from the Cooperative Cardiovascular Project. Stroke 31:1802, 2000

Every NR et al: A comparison of thrombolytic therapy with primary coronary angioplasty for acute myocardial infarction. N Engl J Med 335:1253, 1996

Fibrinolytic Therapy Trialists' Collaborative Group: Indications for fibrinolytic therapy in suspected acute myocardial infarction: Collaborative overview of early mortality and major morbidity results from all randomised trials of more than 1000 patients. Lancet 343:311, 1994

Gebel JM et al: Thrombolysis-related intracranial hemorrhage. A radiographic analysis of 244 cases from the GUSTO-1 trial with clinical correlation. Stroke 29:563, 1998

Gitt A et al: Thrombolysis for acute myocardial infarction in patients older than 75 years: Lack of benefit for hospital mortality but improvement of long-term mortality: Results of the MITRA- and MIR- registries. J Am Coll Cardiol 37 (Suppl A):323A, 2001

Gore JM et al: Stroke after thrombolysis. Mortality and functional outcomes in the GUSTO-1 trial. Circulation 92:2811, 1995

Grines C et al: A comparison of immediate angioplasty with thrombolytic therapy for acute myocardial infarction. The Primary Angioplasty in Myocardial Infarction Study Group. N Engl J Med 328:673, 1993

Gruppo Italiano per lo Studio della Sopravvivenza Nell'-Infarto Miocardico: GISSI-2: A factorial randomized trial of alteplase versus streptokinase and heparin versus no heparin among 12,490 patients with acute myocardial infarction. Lancet 336:65, 1990

Gurwitz JH et al: Risk for intracranial hemorrhage after tissue plasminogen activator treatment for acute myocardial infarction. Participants in the National Registry of Myocardial Infarction 2. Ann Intern Med 129:597, 1998

GUSTO Investigators: An international randomized trial comparing four thrombolytic strategies for acute myocardial infarction. N Engl J Med 329:673, 1993

GUSTO-2B Investigators: A clinical trial comparing primary coronary angioplasty with tissue plasminogen activator for acute myocardial infarction. N Engl J Med 335:1621, 1997

ISIS-2 Collaborative Group: Randomised trial of intravenous streptokinase, oral aspirin, both, or neither among 17,187 cases of suspected acute myocardial infarction: ISIS-2. Lancet II:349, 1988

Krumholz HM et al: Cost effectiveness of thrombolytic therapy with streptokinase in elderly patients with suspected acute myocardial infarction. N Engl J Med 327:7, 1992

Krumholz HM et al: Relationship of age with eligibility for thrombolytic therapy and mortality among patients with suspected acute myocardial infarction. J Am Geriatr Soc 42:127, 1994

Krumholz HM et al: Thrombolytic therapy for eligible elderly patients with acute myocardial infarction. JAMA 277:1683, 1997

Longstreth WT et al: Myocardial infarction, thrombolytic therapy, and stroke. A community-based study. The MITI Project Group. Stroke 24:587, 1993

Regueiro C et al: Primary angioplasty in acute myocardial infarction: Does age matter? J Am Coll Cardiol 37 (Suppl A):360A, 2001

Ryan TJ et al: 1999 update: ACC/AHA guidelines for the management of patients with acute myocardial infarction. A report of the American College of Cardiology/American Heart Association Task Force on Practice Guidelines (Committee on Management of Acute Myocardial Infarction). J Am Coll Cardiol 34:890, 1999

Stenestrand U et al: Thrombolysis is beneficial in elderly acute myocardial infarction patients. J Am Coll Cardiol 37 (Suppl A):323A, 2001

The ASSENT-2 Investigators: Single-bolus tenecteplase compared with front-loaded alteplase in acute myocardial infarction: The ASSENT-2 double-blinded randomised trial. Lancet 354:716, 1999

The GUSTO-3 Investigators: A comparison of reteplase with alteplase for acute myocardial infarction. N Engl J Med 337:1118, 1997

Thiemann DR et al: Lack of benefit of intravenous thrombolysis in patients with myocardial infarction who are older than 75. Circulation 101:2239, 2000

Tiefenbrunn AJ et al: Clinical experience with primary percutaneous transluminal coronary angioplasty compared with alteplase (recombinant tissue-type plasminogen activator) in patients with acute myocardial infarction: A report from the second National Registry of Myocardial Infarction (NRMI-2). J Am Coll Cardiol 31:1240, 1998

White HD et al: Age and outcomes with contemporary thrombolytic therapy. Results from the GUSTO-1 trial. Circulation 94:1826, 1996

THE PACT TRIAL: IMPLICATIONS FOR A FACILITATED APPROACH TO PRIMARY PTCA IN ACUTE MYOCARDIAL INFARCTION

Allan M. Ross

Patients with acute myocardial infarction (MI) selected to undergo percutaneous transluminal coronary angioplasty (PTCA) to recanalize the infarct-related artery (IRA) have an excellent outcome—provided that there are no substantial delays from triage to intervention. However, due to complex logistics, delays in excess of the AHA/ACC guidelines (90 min) are commonplace. Facilitated angioplasty refers to a two-stage treatment approach beginning with immediate administration of a pharmacologic regimen designed to encourage reperfusion in advance of the start of intervention but followed by angiography/PTCA and often stenting, performed as quickly as possible. In addition to ameliorating what would have been a prolonged period of profound ischemia, evidence now suggests that this approach may result in a higher procedural success rate as well as an improved clinical outcome, compared with traditional standalone primary PTCA (Table 28-1) (Brodie et al., 2000).

Such a strategy was initially evaluated using full doses of systemic streptokinase just before and even during infarct angioplasty (not among patients experiencing considerable delay to PTCA, however) in the SAMI trial (O'Neill et al., 1992). Increased adverse events were encountered, not offset by clinical advantages, and the combination of fibrinolytics with PTCA was discouraged. Tangential endorsement of a lack of synergy or even incompatibility between lysis and intervention appeared in a series of trials performed in the late 1980s in which PTCA was tested as an adjunct to fibrinolysis, performed hours to days after the drug treatment (The TIMI Study Group, 1989). Unsatisfactory outcomes, particularly in the European Cooperative Study, served to reduce further interest in combined approaches (Simoons et al., 1988). Interest in the concept was renewed with the confluence of multiple developments including increasing success with rescue PTCA (i.e., PTCA in patients who have failed thrombolysis), more effective and safer procedures

TABLE 28-1

BETTER PTCA OUTCOME IN MI PATIENTS IN THE PRESENCE OF ANTEGRADE FLOW[a]

	n = 1348	
	IRA Closed, %	Open, %
PTCA success	93	97
Convalescent LVEF	55	59
Mortality	9.3	5.0

[a]All comparisons between PTCA starting with an open vessel (antegrade IRA flow TIMI grade 2 or 3) versus a closed one; $p < .05$.

ABBREVIATIONS: PTCA, percutaneous transluminal coronary angioplasty; MI, myocardial infarction; LVEF, left ventricular ejection fraction; IRA, infarct related artery.

SOURCE: Modified from ER Brodie et al., Am J Cardiol 85:13, 2000, with permission.

in the catheterization laboratories, safer anticoagulation regimens, and the recognition that reduced-dose fibrinolytic treatment is of potential benefit to patients bound for the catheterization laboratory.

PACT Protocol

The PACT trial (Plasminogen Activator Angioplasty Compatibility Trial) evaluated pretreatment with half-dose tissue plasminogen activator (t-PA) prior to arrival at the catheterization laboratory vs. placebo bolus followed by primary PTCA (Ross et al., 1999). In all, 606 patients with ST-elevation acute MI were randomly assigned to one of the two strategies. The t-PA dose was 50 mg given as an intravenous bolus over 3 min. Both groups received aspirin (324 mg) and weight-adjusted heparin. The mean time from symptom onset to hospital arrival was 1.4 h; from arrival to study drug, 49 min; and from drug to the first angiogram of the IRA, an additional 49 min. The protocol recommended PTCA for all patients with absent or sluggish IRA flow. In the presence of brisk flow, if PTCA was not undertaken, a second bolus of study drug was encouraged.

The prespecified end-points were IRA patency on arrival in the catheterization laboratory, procedural success rate, adverse events, acute and convalescent left ventricular (LV) function, and reocclusion of the IRA (the latter two determined at a repeat angiographic study 5 to 7 days following treatment).

Results

Total patency at initial angiography (TIMI grades 2 and 3) was 61% in the t-PA group and 34% following aspirin, heparin, and placebo ($p < .001$). The frequency of brisk normal flow (TIMI grade 3), however, was modest following half-dose t-PA: 33%. It was 15% in the placebo group ($p < .001$). When PTCA was required to restore flow, it was technically successful with equivalent rates (93 and 95%) in both strategies. The adverse events experienced by patients in both groups (Table 28-2) were infrequent and equivalent. Reocclusion of the IRA was observed in 5.9 and 3.7% of cases, cerebral hemorrhage in one patient in each group, and major

TABLE 28-2

ADVERSE EVENTS IN THE PACT TRIAL

	t-PA, % (n = 302)	Placebo, % (n = 304)
Reinfarction	3.0	2.6
Angiographic reocclusion	5.9	3.7
Emergency revascularization	7.9	8.3
Major (non-CABG) bleeding	8.5	8.2
Intracranial bleeding	0.3	0.3
In-hospital mortality	3.6	3.0
30-day mortality	3.6	3.3

ABBREVIATION: PACT, Plasminogen Activator Angioplasty Compatibility Trial; t-PA, tissue plasminogen activator; CABG, coronary artery bypass grafting.

TABLE 28-3

ACUTE AND CONVALESCENT LEFT VENTRICULAR EJECTION FRACTION (LVEF) BY TREATMENT ASSIGNMENT AND BY METHOD/TIMING OF RESTORED TIMI GRADE 3 FLOW

LVEF	t-PA, %	Placebo, %	TIMI 3 on cath lab arrival, %	TIMI 3 achieved by PTCA, %
Acute ($p < .001$)	59.4	57.7	60.5	58.7
Convalescent ($p < .004$)	58.2	58.4	62.4	57.9

ABBREVIATIONS: TIMI, Thrombosis in Myocardial Infarction Study; t-PA, tissue plasminogen activator; PTCA, percutaneous transluminal coronary angioplasty.

noncerebral bleeding (excluding coronary artery bypass grafting patients) in 8.5 and 8.3% of cases. Mortality at 30 days was 3.6 and 3.3%.

Global and regional convalescent LV function was remarkably well preserved in both treatments, and the modest TIMI 3 patency advantage following t-PA treatment did not translate into an advantage for the entire group (Table 28-3). However, considerable benefit for early restoration of normal flow on LV function was observed. Ejection fraction at 1 week in patients arriving in the catheterization laboratory with normal flow (two-thirds had received active lytic drug; one-third had received placebo) was 62.4% compared with 57.9% in those whose restoration of normal flow was delayed until PTCA was carried out ($p < .001$).

Limitations

Caution—particularly related to potential bleeding risk—dictated that the PACT trial, which reopened the issue of combining fibrinolysis and PTCA, utilize a modest t-PA dose. Furthermore, the use of antiplatelet agents other than aspirin [specifically, the platelet glycoprotein IIb/IIIa (GpIIb/IIIa) receptor antagonists] was strongly discouraged (similarly out of concern for bleeding). Incorporation of the newer potent regimens capable of acting faster and producing higher rates of patency would presumably enhance the benefits of this type of strategy.

A second major limitation was the population studied. Facilitated PTCA would be applied most appropriately to the considerable number of patients who experience delays >2 h in getting to a catheterization laboratory. While not planned, most patients in the PACT trial reached the laboratory after a rather short delay. The result may have been that the fibrinolytic had little time to promote patency prior to angiography. Additionally, the control (placebo) group in this trial did not endure the long ischemic time that appears to lessen the myocardial salvage in many primary PTCA candidates.

Relevant Recent Reports

Enhancement of fibrinolytic success rates has recently been demonstrated by combining reduced doses of plasminogen activators administered in combination with intravenous platelet GpIIb/IIIa receptor antagonists (Antman et al., 1999). These combinations have been used on top of aspirin and heparin, suggesting that platelets are important targets for improved infarct therapy. The fact that better TIMI 3 patency rates are achieved despite a reduction in the fibrinolytic dose holds the promise of reduced bleeding, specifically intracerebral hemorrhage, compared with the use of full-dose plasminogen activators. The trials available thus far were sized only to evaluate angiographic patency, and so the proof of a favorable safety profile must await the completion of large studies (which are ongoing). If the safety expectations were met, such pharmacologic regimens would be ideally suited for use in a facilitated PTCA strategy. An additional advantage would derive from the benefits broadly reported when such platelet antagonists are employed in percutaneous interventions in general.

A preliminary experience with facilitated infarct angioplasty following administration of such combinations has been reported from the SPEED trial (Herrmann et al., 2000), the pilot study for GUSTO V, a large clinical end-point trial (see below). The results were favorable for patients who underwent intervention following drug therapy—specifically for those whose treatment included both a fibrinolytic (r-PA) and a GpIIb/IIIa antagonist (abciximab). Of such patients, 47% arrived at the catheterization laboratory with normal IRA flow; the intervention was successful in 88% of patients, and the combined end-point of death, reinfarction, and subsequent need for urgent repeat intervention was 5.9%—lower than in patients who received only the platelet inhibitor or only the fibrinolytic.

Unfortunately, the recent publication of the full, 16,588-patient GUSTO V clinical end-point trial (The Gusto V Investigators, 2001) has significantly dampened enthusiasm for combining full dose abciximab with half-dose r-PA. The primary objectives of the study had been to identify a combination of therapies with greater efficacy (lower mortality) and greater safety (less bleeding, fewer strokes) than achieved in ST-elevation MI patients treated with standard (full-dose) fibrinolytic therapy and no glycoprotein receptor antagonist. Neither goal was accomplished, and the important measures of bleeding were clinically and statistically significantly more frequent with the combined therapy. It is not yet established whether these disappointing results portend a similar outcome when ongoing studies of combinations using other fibrinolytics and other GpIIb/IIIa antagonists are completed.

There is also an interest in exploring the use of full-dose glycoprotein receptor blocker treatment in advance of infarct intervention, employing these agents as the pharmacologic component of a facilitated approach. In the randomized placebo controlled ADMIRAL trial, abciximab was given to patients prior to performing angioplasty, and usually stenting, of the infarct artery (Montalescot et al., 2001). In one-fourth of the patients the drug was administered in the prehospital setting. The abciximab-treated group had an increased patency (TIMI grade 3) rate before (17% vs. 5%; $p = .01$) as well as after the intervention, which correlated to a superior angiographic and clinical outcome compared with the placebo group. While GpIIb/IIIa agents may encourage infarct artery patency by suppressing neothrombosis, the angiographic observations in this trial would indicate that the therapy produces arterial patency more often than the rate of true spontaneous recanalization (that of placebo patients) but less often than reduced-dose fibrinolytic therapy.

It was mentioned in the discussion of limitations in the PACT trial that a very modest dose of t-PA had been used (out of concern for bleeding complications). In an experience acquired in France, Loubeyre and colleagues gave full-dose t-PA to 131 MI patients and at a median time of 95 min later treated the infarct-related artery by angioplasty and stenting (Loubeyre et al., 2001). They reported that 49% had normal flow restored prior to the intervention (92% after PCI), with impressively low mortality (4.6%) and major bleeding in only 2.3%. Thus it would appear that intervention after even full-dose fibrinolysis may be more successful and associated with fewer adverse events in the current era of improved procedures, anticoagulation, and puncture site management than was the case a decade ago.

A less salutary experience in a small number of patients ($n = 100$) was observed in the PRAGUE study (Widimsky et al., 2000). These patients received a full dose of streptokinase at a community hospital and were then transferred to undergo PTCA. They were compared with transfer for primary PTCA without fibrinolytic therapy or with fibrinolytic therapy and no intervention. There were more complications associated with the combination approach (streptokinase plus PTCA) and no offsetting clinical benefits. When comparing this trial with the aforementioned SAMI study, (O'Neill et al., 1992) it might be postulated that the use of fibrinolytics with prolonged systemic effects (plasminemia) and/or given in full doses is not as favorable a regimen for facilitated intervention as is the administration of a reduced dose of a more fibrin-selective agent.

New Initiatives

It is fully recognized that due to a relatively low frequency of adverse events and the considerable variability of patient factors (age, time to treatment, history of prior infarction, etc.) favorable results in small angiographic trials are not adequate to provoke a significant change in the way in which infarct patients are managed. However, there is an increasing amount of evidence to generate enthusiasm for facilitated infarct intervention utilizing second- and third-generation fibrinolytics combined with effective antiplatelet therapy. What has been lacking are sufficiently large trials to measure more accurately the frequency of adverse events and clinical results (i.e., mortality and morbidity) in patients referred for infarct artery intervention in whom a considerable delay to the start of the procedure has occurred. At least two such studies have now been designed, and their results will determine the utility of this interesting strategy.

REFERENCES

Antman EM et al: Abciximab facilitates the rate and extent of thrombolysis. The Thrombosis in Myocardial Infarction (TIMI)-14 Investigators. Circulation 99:2720, 1999

Brodie BR et al: Benefit of coronary reperfusion before intervention on outcomes after primary angioplasty for acute myocardial infarction. Am J Cardiol 85:13, 2000

Herrmann HC et al: Facilitation of early percutaneous coronary intervention after reteplase with or without abciximab in acute myocardial infarction. J Am Coll Cardiol 36:1489, 2000

Loubeyre C et al: Outcome after combined reperfusion therapy for acute myocardial infarction, combining pre-hospital thrombolysis with immediate percutaneous coronary intervention and stent. Eur Heart J 22:1128, 2001

Montalescot G et al: Platelet glycoprotein IIb/IIIa inhibition with coronary stenting for acute myocardial infarction. N Engl J Med 344:1895, 2001

O'Neill WW et al: A prospective placebo controlled randomized trial of intravenous streptokinase and angioplasty versus lone angioplasty therapy of acute myocardial infarction. Circulation 86:1710, 1992

Ross AM et al: A randomized trial comparing primary angioplasty with a strategy of short-acting thrombolysis and immediate planned rescue angioplasty in acute myocardial infarction: The PACT trial. J Am Coll Cardiol 99:1954, 1999

Simoons ML et al: Thrombolysis with tissue plasminogen activator in acute myocardial infarction: No additional benefit from immediate coronary angioplasty. Lancet 1:197, 1988

The GUSTO V Investigators: Reperfusion therapy for acute myocardial infarction with fibrinolytic therapy or combination reduced fibrinolytic therapy and platelet glycoprotein IIb/IIIa inhibition: The GUSTO V randomised trial. Lancet 357:16, 2001

The TIMI study group: Comparison of invasive and conservative strategies after treatment with intravenous tissue plasminogen activator in acute myocardial infarction: Results of the Thrombolysis in Myocardial Infarction (TIMI) phase II trial. N Engl J Med 320:618, 1989

Widimsky P et al: Multicentre randomized trial comparing transport to primary angioplasty vs immediate thrombolysis vs combined strategy for patients with acute myocardial infarction presenting to a community hospital without a catheterization laboratory. The PRAGUE study. Eur Heart J 21:823, 2000

29

EMERGENCY REVASCULARIZATION IN ACUTE MYOCARDIAL INFARCTION COMPLICATED BY CARDIOGENIC SHOCK— RESULTS OF THE SHOCK TRIAL

Harvey White / Judith S. Hochman

Cardiogenic shock occurs in 7 to 10% of patients suffering an acute myocardial infarction (MI), and the incidence has not changed in 25 years (Goldberg et al., 1999). It is the leading cause of death in patients hospitalized with acute infarction, with a hospital mortality rate of 70 to 85% (Goldberg et al., 1999). Nonrandomized studies of selected lower-risk patients have reported reduced mortality rates with percutaneous coronary intervention (44%) (Hibbard et al., 1992; Hochman et al., 1995; Hochman and Gersh, 1998; Lee et al., 1988) or coronary artery bypass surgery (36%) (Hochman et al., 1995; Hochman and Gersh, 1998; Kirklin et al., 1985). However, prior to the Should We Emergently Revascularize Occluded Coronaries For Cardiogenic Shock (SHOCK) trial, there had been no completed randomized trials comparing revascu-

larization with medical management of patients with cardiogenic shock (Hochman et al., 1999).

Design of the SHOCK Trial

From April 1993 to November 1998, 302 patients from 30 international centers were randomized into the SHOCK trial, which was supported by a grant from the National Heart, Lung, and Blood Institute. Patients were required to have cardiogenic shock due to left ventricular dysfunction following MI associated with ST-segment elevation, Q-wave infarction, new left bundle branch block, or posterior infarction with ST-segment depression on the electrocardiogram. The clinical criteria for the diagnosis of shock were (1) a systolic blood pressure of

<90 mmHg for 30 min or the need for vasopressors to maintain the blood pressure above 90 mmHg, and (2) end-organ hypoperfusion manifested by cool extremities or a urine output of <30 mL/h. The hemodynamic criteria for the diagnosis of shock were a cardiac index ≤2 L/min per m² and a pulmonary wedge pressure ≥15 mmHg. Patients had to be randomized within 12 h of the onset of shock, and shock had to have occurred within 36 h of the onset of infarction.

Patients randomized into the emergency revascularization group underwent percutaneous coronary intervention or bypass surgery as soon as possible within 6 h after randomization. Patients randomized into the initial medical stabilization group were recommended to receive fibrinolytic therapy, and delayed revascularization was permitted at a minimum of 54 h after randomization if clinically indicated. Intraaortic balloon counterpulsation was recommended for both groups.

The primary end-point was mortality at 30 days, with secondary end-points at 6 months and 1 year. The study was designed to detect a 20% difference in mortality at 30 days.

Results

More than 75% of eligible patients were randomized. The only difference between the two groups was that more patients in the initial medical stabilization group had had previous bypass surgery. The mean age was 66 ± 10 years, and 32% of patients were women. Cardiogenic shock developed at a median time of 5.6 h after the onset of MI.

Treatment

In the emergency revascularization group, 87% of patients underwent a revascularization procedure. Of these, 64% had a percutaneous coronary intervention as their first revascularization procedure at a median time of 54 min after randomization into the trial. Surgery was performed in 36% at a median time of 2.7 h after randomization. Nine patients had

both procedures. In all, 77% of percutaneous interventions were successful (defined as 50% stenosis, stenosis improvement of 20%, and partial or normal coronary flow). Delayed revascularization procedures were performed in 21.3% of patients in the initial medical stabilization group, and 4% had their procedures within 54 h.

Survival

A total of 44% of the initial medical stabilization group and 53.3% of the emergency revascularization group survived the first 30 days ($p = .11$). At 6 months and 1 year, the survival rate was significantly higher in the emergency revascularization group (6 months: 49.7 vs. 36.9%; $p = .03$); 1 year: 46.7 vs. 33.6% $p < .03$ (Hochman et al., 2001). Emergency revascularization significantly improved survival in patients age <75 years (58.6 vs. 43.2% at 30 days, interaction p value .012; and 51.6 vs. 33.3% at 1 year, interaction p value .03), but not in those ≥75 years (25.0 vs. 46.9% at 30 days and 20.8 vs. 34.4% at 1 year). The survival benefit with emergency revascularization in all other subgroups reflected the overall trial results.

Adverse Events

Acute renal failure was less common in the emergency revascularization group (13 vs. 24%, $p = .03$). Five patients in the emergency revascularization group and three in the initial medical stabilization group had strokes.

Relevance to Clinical Practice

The SHOCK trial is the only completed randomized trial comparing an emergency revascularization strategy with medical management of patients with cardiogenic shock. The only previous randomized trial—the Swiss Multicenter Evaluation of Angioplasty for Shock (SMASH) trial—was terminated early after randomizing only 55 patients, and reported 30-day survival rates of 31% with percutaneous intervention and 25% with medical management (p = NS) (Urban et al., 1999). Medical management in the SHOCK trial included fibrinolytic therapy, intraaortic balloon counterpulsation, and revascularization if clinically indicated after 54 h. The 30-day mortality rate in the initial medical stabilization group (56%) was relatively low and may be related to the high rate of adjunctive therapy use. Although the primary endpoint of 30-day mortality was not significantly reduced by emergency revascularization, there was a significant (20%) reduction in mortality at 1 year, equivalent to 131 lives saved for every 1000 patients randomized. Patients < 75 years of age appeared to benefit the most, with 183 lives saved at 1 year for every 1000 patients randomized. Patients over the age of 75 years did not appear to benefit from emergency revascularization, but then only 56 patients in this age group were randomized, so the optimal management of elderly patients remains unclear.

The associated SHOCK Registry shows that the patients randomized into the SHOCK trial were representative of the broad population of patients with cardiogenic shock. The success rate of percutaneous intervention was high, and the results can therefore be extrapolated to other experienced centers. It is worth noting that elderly patients in the SHOCK Registry who were clinically selected to undergo percutaneous coronary intervention or bypass surgery had a risk reduction with emergency revascularization similar to that of younger registry patients. It is therefore important that treatment be individualized in elderly patients.

Limitations

Only a small number of patients were randomized very early after the onset of shock, and it is possible that the benefits of emergency revascularization would have been greater had more patients been randomized earlier. Although the rates of coronary artery stenting and platelet glycoprotein IIb/IIIa receptor antagonist use were reasonably high given the period during which the trial was conducted, it is also likely that the benefits of emergency revascularization would have been even greater had these treatments been used more frequently.

In view of the 6-month and 1-year results of this trial, emergency revascularization with intraaortic balloon counterpulsation should be strongly considered for patients with acute MI complicated by cardiogenic shock.

REFERENCES

Goldberg RJ et al: Temporal trends in cardiogenic shock complicating acute myocardial infarction. N Engl J Med 340:1162, 1999

Hibbard MD et al: Percutaneous transluminal coronary angioplasty in patients with cardiogenic shock. J Am Coll Cardiol 19:639, 1992

Hochman JS, Gersh BJ: Acute myocardial infarction: Complications, in *Textbook of Cardiovascular Medicine*, EJ Topol (ed). Philadelphia, Lippincott-Raven, 1998, pp 437–480

Hochman JS et al: Current spectrum of cardiogenic shock and effect of early revascularization on mortality: Results of an international registry. Circulation 91:873, 1995

Hochman JS et al: Early revascularization in acute myocardial infarction complicated by cardiogenic shock. N Engl J Med 341:625, 1999

Hochman JS et al: One year survival following early revascularization for cardiogenic shock. JAMA 285: 190, 2001

Kirklin JK et al: Intermediate-term results of coronary artery bypass grafting for acute myocardial infarction. Circulation 72:II175, 1985

Lee L et al: Percutaneous transluminal coronary angioplasty improves survival in acute myocardial infarction complicated by cardiogenic shock. Circulation 78:1345, 1988

Urban P et al: A randomized evaluation of early revascularization to treat shock complicating acute myocardial infarction: The (Swiss) Multicenter Trial of Angioplasty for Shock—(S)MASH. Eur Heart J 20:1030, 1999

WHEN SHOULD STATIN THERAPY BEGIN FOLLOWING AN ACUTE CORONARY SYNDROME?

Scott Kinlay

Patients who survive an acute coronary syndrome face a much higher short-term risk of a recurrent coronary event than patients with stable coronary syndromes. For example, medically managed patients with unstable angina or myocardial infarction in the TACTICS-TIMI 18 trial (Treat Angina with Aggrastat and Determine Cost of Therapy with an Invasive or Conservative Strategy–Thrombolysis in Myocardial Infarction 18) had a 20% risk of a recurrent event over the following 6 months (Cannon et al., 2001). In contrast, patients with stable angina have a much lower short-term risk of an event, and risk factor modification is justified for reducing risk over the long term. In the acute coronary setting, the high absolute risk of adverse outcomes means that any successful intervention is likely to have an important clinical impact.

Basic Mechanisms of Lipid Lowering

To understand why early statin therapy should have an effect on outcomes, it is first important to understand the mechanisms that underlie most acute coronary syndromes. The majority of acute coronary syndromes arise from the disruption of vulnerable atherosclerotic plaques in the coronary arteries (Libby, 2001). The characteristics of these plaques have been well described in a number of pathologic studies. These plaques typically have a thin fibrous cap, which is the result of decreased synthesis and increased degradation of collagen mediated by activated inflammatory cells that accumulate, particularly at the shoulder regions of plaques. When the thin fibrous cap ruptures, it exposes the blood to a thrombogenic lipid core that contains abundant tissue factor produced by macrophages. Thrombus formation occludes or subtotally occludes the vessel lumen to impair coronary blood flow and precipitate the acute coronary syndrome. Coronary blood flow can also be affected by vasomotor dysfunction that promotes vasoconstriction and further impedes blood flow to the distal myocardium. Vasomotor dysfunction is more apparent in the culprit lesions of patients with unstable compared to stable coronary syndromes, with vasoconstriction being the predominant finding in the former.

The activated inflammatory cells within plaques, vasomotor dysfunction, and a prothrombotic milieu are consequences of several cellular changes in the vessel wall, including a reduction in endothelium-dependent nitric oxide. The bioavailability of nitric oxide in the vessel wall is decreased by risk factors, in particular by increased low-density lipoprotein (LDL) cholesterol and the subsequent oxidation of LDL cholesterol in the vessel wall.

Lowering LDL cholesterol by dietary and pharmacologic methods is a potent method to reverse this cellular aberration; it also improves endothelial function and promotes plaque stability (Libby, 2001). For example, studies have shown that intensive lowering of LDL cholesterol can rapidly improve endothelial vasomotor function within hours. LDL lowering also decreases the density and activity of inflammatory cells in plaque by reducing recruitment into the vessel wall and increasing apoptosis. It also reduces a number of prothrombotic pathways, including plasminogen activator inhibitor (Kinlay et al., 2001). In addition to these effects mediated by a decrease in LDL cholesterol, HMG-CoA reductase inhibitors (statins) also have a number of nonlipid effects that have been demonstrated in experimental studies and could potentially provide further benefits in clinical treatment (Kinlay et al., 2001; Libby, 2001). These studies demonstrate the basic mechanisms that explain why lipid-lowering therapy stabilizes atherosclerosis and improves clinical outcomes after acute coronary syndromes. Drugs from the statin class are particularly likely to translate these mechanisms into clinical benefits, primarily because of their potent and rapid action on lipid levels but also because of their relative safety.

Clinical Evidence Supporting Early Statin Therapy

Observational studies of patients after acute coronary syndromes have recently documented an impressive reduction in the risk of recurrent events in patients who are discharged from hospital on statin therapy. In one large registry study of patients admitted to hospital with myocardial infarction, those discharged on statin therapy had a 25% reduction in the risk of death over the subsequent year (Stenestrand et al., 2001).

More recently, several randomized trials have demonstrated that statin therapy started during hospitalization for an acute coronary event can produce a decrease in recurrent events over as little as 4 months. In the L-CAD study, 135 patients with an acute coronary syndrome and very high LDL cholesterol [5.2 to 10.4 mmol/L (200 to 400 mg/dL)] were randomized to pravastatin with niacin or placebo in an open design during admission for myocardial infarction. Over the subsequent 2 years there was a decrease in recurrent coronary events, driven primarily by a reduction in the need for revascularization (Arntz et al., 2000). More impressively, intensive LDL reduction with high-dose (80 mg/d) atorvastatin led to a reduction in cardiovascular events over 4 months in the MIRACL study (Schwartz et al., 2001). In this double-blind, randomized placebo-controlled trial of 3086 patients with unstable angina or non-Q wave myocardial infarction, statin therapy significantly reduced by 16% over 4 months the combined coronary end-point of death, myocardial infarction, resuscitated cardiac arrest, or readmission to hospital with unstable angina and objective evidence of ischemia (Table 30-1). This end-point was primarily driven by a reduction in hospitalization for new ischemic events, but there was also a reduction in a secondary end-point of stroke over this short time period. Results from the smaller FLORIDA study in 540 patients, which was presented at the American College of Cardiology meeting in 2000 and has yet to be published, are also consistent with a reduction in ischemic events with lipid-lowering commenced during hospitalization for an acute ischemic event. In the FLORIDA study, a less intensive lipid-lowering regimen of fluvastatin was associated with an approximately 20% reduction in ischemic events over 1 year, with a trend to significant difference from placebo ($p = .08$). Although this study had less power than the MIRACL study, the results were consistent with a clinical benefit from early lipid-lowering with statins.

TABLE 30-1

PRINCIPAL RESULTS FROM THE MIRACL STUDY OF INTENSIVE LIPID LOWERING WITH ATORVASTATIN IN PATIENTS WITH AN ACUTE CORONARY SYNDROME AND THE RISK OF CLINICAL EVENTS OVER 4 MONTHS.

End-point	Placebo ($n = 1548$), % events	Atorvastatin ($n = 1538$), % events	Relative risk reduction,%
Primary end-point			
Death, myocardial infarction, cardiac arrest, hospitalization for unstable angina	17.4	14.8	16[a]
Secondary end-points			
Hospitalization for unstable angina	8.4	6.2	26[a]
Death	4.4	4.2	6
Nonfatal myocardial infarction	7.3	6.6	10
Fatal and nonfatal stroke	1.6	0.8	50[a]

[a] $p < .05$
SOURCE: From GG Schwartz et al: JAMA 285:1711, 2001.

Early Therapy for Long-term Goals

The recent studies suggest that the high short-term risk of recurrent events in patients with acute coronary syndromes can be reduced with intensive lipid-lowering therapy started during hospitalization for the index event. Another justification for commencing statin therapy during the initial hospitalization would be to improve compliance with long-term goals of secondary prevention. Numerous large clinical trials of statins in the secondary prevention setting have documented a reduction in coronary events, stroke, and all-cause death with long-term statin therapy over several years. However, community surveys of patients with coronary artery disease continue to show that many of these patients are not taking lipid-lowering drugs. The reasons for this discrepancy are likely to be many. However, poor communication between medical staff in hospitals and the community practitioners, a perceived lack of importance of lipids by doctors and patients among those who are not discharged on statins, or the cost of therapy will potentially contribute to this poor preventive effort.

The recent short-term studies described above have not only demonstrated a reduction in short-term risk but have also removed any doubts of adverse effects from starting statin therapy soon after an acute coronary event. Patients who are discharged on statin therapy are not subject to doubts about which medical practitioner (the hospital doctor, cardiologist, internist, or endocrinologist) has jurisdiction over the initiation of lipid-lowering therapy—a dilemma that could prevent many patients from being started on these drugs. Furthermore, patients may be more receptive to the importance of risk factor modification and lipid lowering during a hospitalization for an acute coronary event and less likely to discontinue this treatment if it was considered important enough to be started during their index admission.

Regardless of the reasons that support hospital initiation of therapy, it is clear that patients who are discharged from hospital taking statins are more likely to be taking them over the subsequent years. In the CHAMP study, a coordinated attempt at risk factor modification in patients during their initial hospitalization led to higher rates of statin use at discharge and at 1-year follow-up (Fonarow et al., 2001). Similarly, in another study, patients discharged on statins were twice as likely to be taking statins 3 years later than those not discharged on statin therapy (Muhlestein et al. 2001). Thus, a strategy that implements statin therapy in hospital for patients with acute coronary syndromes is likely to lead to improved secondary prevention in the long as well as short term.

Acute Changes in Lipids

Another potential barrier to considering lipid-lowering therapy in patients with acute coronary syndromes is the concern that lipid levels are in a state of flux shortly after an acute coronary event. Total cholesterol, LDL cholesterol, and high-density lipoprotein (HDL) cholesterol fall approximately 24 h after a myocardial infarction and return to baseline levels over 2 to 3 months. This effect is related to the acute-phase response to injury; however, the decrease in total cholesterol is only about 10% on average. Thus, a lipid level taken within 24 h of an acute coronary event is likely to represent the baseline levels before the event, and after this time the small decline in lipids is unlikely to affect the identification of patients with hyperlipidemia. Perhaps more intriguing is an implication of the MIRACL study where statin therapy had a benefit in a population with LDL cholesterol levels previously considered to be "normal." The average LDL cholesterol level on entry into the study was approximately 3.2 mmol/L (125 mg/dL), which suggests that our concept of high LDL cholesterol may be inappropriate in the acute coronary setting. International comparisons suggest that LDL levels in countries with low rates of heart disease are closer to an average of 1.6 mmol/L (60 mg/dL). In the acute coronary setting, where the risk of recurrent events is very high, lower LDL thresholds may be justified when determining the need for statin therapy. Furthermore, the nonlipid effects that are seen with high doses of all statins in experimental studies may contribute to the clinical benefit beyond that of lipid lowering seen in the acute coronary setting.

Incremental Benefit Beyond Invasive Strategies

Several studies have shown that invasive strategies of revascularization offer greater benefits in acute coronary syndromes than more conservative strategies (Cannon et al., 2001). However, percutaneous coronary interventions offer a targeted intervention to the focal region of the coronary artery with the culprit lesion. Risk factor modification is likely to offer incremental benefits because it is a systemic intervention that affects the whole vascular system. This concept is currently being tested in several randomized controlled trials, but the potential short-term and known long-term benefits of statins suggest that lipid lowering should be initiated in patients with acute coronary syndromes treated invasively.

Conclusions

Lipid lowering, in particular with the statin class of drugs, helps to reduce the high risk of recurrent ischemic events when started during the hospital admission for an acute coronary syndrome. The basic mechanisms underlying this clinical benefit likely lie in an improvement in vasomotor function, a decrease in plaque inflammation, and a reduction in prothrombotic factors. These changes in vascular biology affect not only the culprit lesion but plaques elsewhere in the coronary arteries. Initiation of this therapy during the hospital admission is also likely to improve long-term compliance with these drugs and decrease the long-term risks of recurrent cardiovascular events and death.

REFERENCES

Arntz HR et al: Beneficial effects of pravastatin (+/− colestyramine/niacin) initiated immediately after a coronary event (the randomized Lipid-Coronary Artery Disease [L-CAD] Study). Am J Cardiol 86: 1293, 2000

Cannon CP et al: Comparison of early invasive and conservative strategies in patients with unstable coronary syndromes treated with the glycoprotein IIb/IIIa inhibitor tirofiban. N Engl J Med 344: 1879, 2001

Fonarow GC et al: Improved treatment of coronary heart disease by implementation of a Cardiac Hospitalization Atherosclerosis Management Program (CHAMP). Am J Cardiol 87: 819, 2001

Kinlay S et al: Endothelial function and coronary artery disease. Curr Opin Lipidol 12: 383, 2001

Libby P: Current concepts of the pathogenesis of the acute coronary syndromes. Circulation 104: 365, 2001

Muhlestein JB et al: Usefulness of in-hospital prescription of statin agents after angiographic diagnosis of coronary artery disease in improving continued compliance and reduced mortality. Am J Cardiol 87: 257, 2001

Schwartz GG et al: Effects of atorvastatin on early recurrent ischemic events in acute coronary syndromes: The MIRACL study: A randomized controlled trial. JAMA 285: 1711, 2001

Stenestrand U et al: Early statin treatment following acute myocardial infarction and 1-year survival. JAMA 285: 430, 2001

THE ECHOCARDIOGRAPHIC TECHNIQUE OF CHOICE IN THE ASSESSMENT OF CORONARY ARTERY DISEASE

Theodore J. Kolias & William F. Armstrong

Coronary artery disease (CAD) is one of the most common problems faced by the clinician. The need to identify and evaluate CAD frequently prompts diagnostic testing. Over the past 20 years, stress testing with concurrent imaging of the heart has become a standard method of evaluation. One such technique is stress echocardiography, which is the merger of two-dimensional echocardiography with stress electrocardiography (ECG). The addition of two-dimensional echocardiographic imaging to stress testing allows the identification of regional wall-motion abnormalities induced by exercise or other forms of cardiac stress. These new wall-motion abnormalities occur in response to the development of myocardial ischemia from a supply-demand mismatch. They

occur before the onset of chest pain or ECG abnormalities, and they serve as accurate markers for the presence and location of CAD.

Methodology

Exercise Echocardiography

Exercise echocardiography is typically performed using either treadmill testing or bicycle ergometry. Treadmill echocardiography is performed in the same fashion as treadmill ECG, using one of the standard exercise protocols such as the Bruce or Cornell protocol. Echocardiographic images are obtained prior to and immediately after exercise. As with exercise ECG, the adequacy of cardiac stress during exercise echocardiography is determined by the percent of maximal predicted heart rate attained or the pressure-rate product. Bicycle stress echocardiography differs from treadmill exercise echocardiography in that the echocardiographic images are obtained at each stage, including during peak exercise, rather than immediately postexercise. This is feasible because the patient remains more stationary during bicycle stress echocardiography, allowing clear echocardiographic images to be obtained. With bicycle ergometry, 2-min stages are typically used, with incremental workload increases of 25 to 50 W, up to a maximum of 200 W.

Nonexercise Stress Echocardiography

Because many patients are unable to exercise, other forms of stress echocardiography have also been developed. The most common is dobutamine stress echocardiography, which is performed using a graded intravenous infusion of dobutamine, typically starting at 10μg/kg per min and increasing every 3 min by increments of 10μg/kg per min to a maximum of 40 or 50μg/kg per min. In cases where dobutamine alone is unable to achieve the desired heart rate response, atropine can also be administered intravenously in doses of 0.25 mg every 1 to 2 min, to a maximum of 1 to 2 mg, to achieve the desired heart rate. Other modalities of pharmacologic stress echocardiography include dipyridamole and adenosine echocardiography. More recently, an alternative nonpharmacologic method of stress echocardiography has been developed using transesophageal pacing. Finally, transesophageal echocardiography has also been used in combination with dobutamine to evaluate myocardial ischemia in obese patients for whom transthoracic imaging is nondiagnostic.

Imaging Protocol and Interpretation

With each modality, baseline and stress images are obtained in four standard views, as outlined by the American Society of Echocardiography. The resultant images are displayed in a side-by-side manner so as to allow direct comparison of baseline and stress images. A normal response is characterized by normal wall motion at baseline, with subsequent hyperdynamic motion with stress. In contrast, an abnormal response occurs when a segment has normal or hypokinetic wall motion at baseline and develops a new or worse wall-motion abnormality with stress; this abnormal response is consistent with inducible ischemia. Alternatively, when a segment is abnormal at rest and remains unchanged with stress, the response is consistent with a prior myocardial infarction. Using the 16-segment model of the left ventricle, the segments corresponding to each major coronary perfusion territory can be identified, allowing for determination of which coronary artery is likely to be responsible for the observed wall-motion abnormality.

Two recent technical advances in imaging have improved the feasibility and accuracy of stress echocardiography. The first is tissue harmonic imaging, in which second harmonic frequencies are received back from the ultrasound reflector instead of the transmitted frequencies, allowing for reduction of noise in the reflected signal. This technique allows for improved endocardial border detection and better visualization of wall motion. The second advance is the development of intravenous microbubble contrast agents, which also allow for improved delineation of the endocardial border in patients with suboptimal images, thus allowing better assessment of wall motion during stress echocardiography. The ongoing technological advances in the field of echocardiography will likely continue to improve the feasibility and accuracy of stress echocardiography in the future.

Stress Echocardiography to Detect Coronary Artery Disease

The feasibility of using exercise echocardiography to detect CAD was demonstrated in the 1980s by several investigators. In one of the original studies,

rong and colleagues demonstrated that exer-
hocardiography identified patients with CAD
sensitivity of 87% and a specificity of 86%,
coronary angiography as a "gold standard"
rong et al., 1987). Subsequently, Sawada and
kers demonstrated that dobutamine stress
rdiography could also be used to accurately
CAD, with a sensitivity (89%) and speci-
5%) similar to that for exercise echocardiog-
Sawada et al., 1991). Ryan and colleagues
to demonstrate the feasibility as well as the
nsitivity (91%) and specificity (78%) of
exercise echocardiography (Ryan et al.,
Many investigators have subsequently gone
onfirm the accuracy of stress echocardiog-
unselected patients (Figs. 31-1, 31-2 and
well as in selected subgroups, such as
with dilated cardiomyopathy, end-stage

renal disease, or diabetes. Furthermore, studies
evaluating only women demonstrated that both
exercise and dobutamine echocardiography had a
reasonably high sensitivity and specificity for the
detection of CAD. Dobutamine echocardiography
was also shown to be accurate in patients with
hypertension or left ventricular hypertrophy, as well
as in patients who were pacemaker-dependent and
chronotropically insufficient.

Stress echocardiography is particularly useful
for the identification of CAD in patients with multivessel disease. Several studies have documented the
increased sensitivity of the stress echocardiogram in
these patients compared to those with single-vessel
disease, a not surprising finding since multivessel
disease is associated with a greater number of
stress-induced regional wall-motion abnormalities.
Armstrong's team documented a sensitivity of 81%

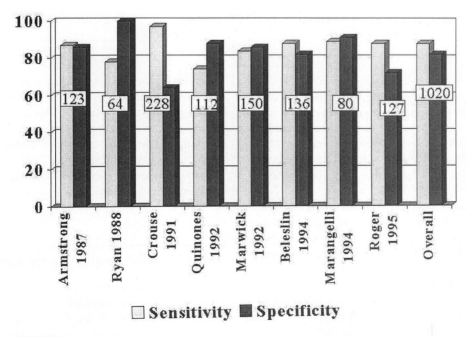

FIGURE 31-1

Selected studies demonstrating the sensitivity (%) and specificity (%) of treadmill stress echocardiography. The numbers in the boxes represent the number of patients in each study.

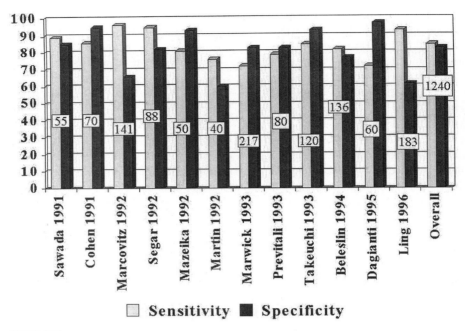

FIGURE 31-2

Selected studies demonstrating the sensitivity (%) and specificity (%) of dobutamine stress echocardiography. The numbers in the boxes represent the number of patients in each study.

for patients with single-vessel disease and 93% for patients with multivessel disease (Armstrong et al., 1987), while Quinones and co-workers reported a sensitivity of 58% for single-vessel disease and 94% for triple-vessel disease (Quinones et al., 1992). These studies confirm the utility of stress echocardiography in identifying this high-risk subset of patients.

The accuracy of stress echocardiography and radionuclide perfusion imaging for the detection of CAD has been compared in several studies. One study demonstrated that the sensitivities and specificities of exercise echocardiography and exercise thallium scintigraphy were similar (sensitivity 74% vs. 76%, specificity 88% vs. 81%) (Quinones et al., 1992). Other investigators have also found comparable sensitivities and specificities between the two techniques, with dobutamine echocardiography having a slightly higher specificity in female patients and in patients with hypertension.

Stress echocardiography has also been used evaluate patients prior to and after percutaneo coronary intervention. Testing prior to the procedu can be used to identify the location of ischem allowing for targeted intervention. After the proc dure, stress echocardiography can be used diagnose the occurrence of restenosis in patie with recurrent symptoms.

Stress Echocardiography and Prognosis

Several investigators have documented the progno tic value of the exercise echocardiogram. One gro studied 463 patients undergoing exercise echoc diography who were followed for a mean of 44 11 months (Marwick et al., 1997). They found th spontaneous cardiac events (cardiac death, myoca dial infarction, and unstable angina) during the fo

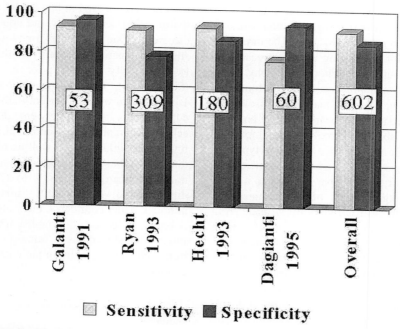

FIGURE 31-3

Selected studies demonstrating the sensitivity (%) and specificity (%) of bicycle stress echocardiography. The numbers in the boxes represent the number of patients in each study.

low-up period were predicted by ischemia on the exercise echocardiogram (relative risk 8.2). Other studies have confirmed the increased risk conferred by the presence of inducible ischemia seen during exercise echocardiography. In addition, several investigators have demonstrated the prognostic value of the dobutamine echocardiogram. Poldermans and co-workers followed 1659 patients who underwent dobutamine stress echocardiography for an average of 36 months (Poldermans et al., 1999). They found that stress-induced ischemia was associated with an increased risk of cardiac death or myocardial infarction (hazard ratio 3.3), and a normal dobutamine echocardiogram was associated with an annual event rate of only 1.3% over a 5-year period. The prognostic value of pharmacologic stress echocardiography has also been demonstrated in subsets of women, hypertensive patients, and patients with single-vessel disease. Finally, both exercise and dobutamine stress echocardiography have been shown to provide prognostic information in patients immediately after a myocardial infarction, with both the presence of inducible ischemia and the presence of viability in the infarct zone affecting prognosis.

Stress Echocardiography and Myocardial Viability

Viable myocardium is defined as myocardium that is dysfunctional at rest but has the potential to recover normal function if adequate blood flow is restored. It may consist of various combinations of infarcted myocardium and myocardium that is either stunned or chronically ischemic ("hibernating"). The identification of myocardial viability is clinically important because patients with left ventricular dysfunction and viable myocardium that is not revascularized have a poor prognosis compared to those who undergo revascularization. The three primary modalities for identifying viable myocardium are low-dose dobutamine echocardiography, thallium scintigraphy, and position emission tomography (PET) scanning. Viability may be assessed from the standard dobutamine echocardiography protocol or a specialized viability protocol may be employed. For the latter, the dobutamine infusion typically starts at 5 μg/kg per min and proceeds in incremental stages of 2.5 or 5 μg/kg per min, up to a maximum of 20 μg/kg per min of dobutamine. The interpretation of myocardial viability is made from the assessment of wall motion at rest and during dobutamine infusion. Augmentation of contractility of a segment during dobutamine infusion implies viability of that segment. A biphasic response consisting of initial augmentation of a segment followed by deterioration at a higher dose of dobutamine is more specific for myocardial viability with a residual obstructive lesion of the coronary artery perfusing the segment and is considered the most accurate measure for subsequent recovery of function.

A number of investigators have compared the various imaging techniques used to assess myocardial viability. Bax and colleagues conducted a meta-analysis of 37 studies from 1980 to 1997, comparing low-dose dobutamine echocardiography, thallium scintigraphy, technetium-MIBI, and F-18 FDG PET scanning for the assessment of myocardial viability (Bax et al., 1997). This meta-analysis revealed that all the techniques had comparable sensitivities ranging from 83 to 90%, although low-dose dobutamine echocardiography had a higher specificity of 81% (range of the other techniques was 47 to 73%).

mon modalities used in this regard are dipyridamole thallium-201 scintigraphy and dobutamine echocardiography. One group performed a meta-analysis of studies comparing the ability of the two techniques to risk-stratify patients prior to vascular surgery (Shaw et al., 1996). This meta-analysis included 1994 patients who underwent thallium imaging and 445 patients who underwent dobutamine stress echocardiography. The odds ratios for death or myocardial infarction as well as for secondary cardiac end-points were greater for a positive dobutamine echocardiogram (14- to 27-fold) than for dipyridamole thallium-201 imaging (fourfold), although wider confidence intervals were noted with dobutamine echocardiography. This meta-analysis illustrates the prognostic value provided by dobutamine echocardiography in patients undergoing noncardiac surgery.

SUMMARY

Stress echocardiography is useful for the identification of CAD, the assessment of its severity, the determination of viability, the prediction of future cardiac events, and risk stratification prior to noncardiac surgery. The sensitivity and specificity of stress echocardiography are comparable to competing nuclear techniques. In addition, the ease of applicability and relatively low cost of stress echocardiography make it an attractive option for noninvasive cardiac testing. As such, stress echocardiography remains the echocardiographic technique of choice in the assessment of coronary artery disease.

Stress Echocardiography and Preoperative Risk Assessment Before Noncardiac Surgery

The evaluation of perioperative cardiac risk prior to noncardiac surgery is a common indication for stress testing with imaging. Two of the most com-

REFERENCES

Armstrong WJ et al: Effect of prior myocardial infarction and extent and location of coronary disease on accuracy of exercise echocardiography. J Am Coll Cardiol 10:531, 1987

Bax JJ et al: Accuracy of currently available techniques for prediction of functional recovery after revascularization in patients with left ventricular dysfunction due to chronic coronary artery disease: Comparison of pooled data. J Am Coll Cardiol 30:1451, 1997

Marwick TH et al: Use of exercise echocardiography for prognostic evaluation of patients with known or suspected coronary artery disease. J Am Coll Cardiol 30:83, 1997

Poldermans D et al: Long-term prognostic value of dobutamine-atropine stress echocardiography in 1737 patients with known or suspected coronary artery disease: A single-center experience. Circulation 99:757, 1999

Quinones MA et al: Exercise echocardiography versus 201T1 single-photon emission computed tomography in evaluation of coronary artery disease. Analysis of 292 patients [see comments]. Circulation 85:1026, 1992

Ryan T et al: Detection of coronary artery disease with upright bicycle exercise echocardiography. J Am Soc Echocardiogr 6:186, 1993

Sawada SG et al: Echocardiographic detection of coronary artery disease during dobutamine infusion. Circulation 83:1605, 1991

Shaw LJK et al: Meta-analysis of intravenous dipyridamole-thallium-201 imaging (1985 to 1994) and dobutamine echocardiography (1991 to 1994) for risk stratification before vascular surgery [see comments]. J Am Coll Cardiol 27:787, 1996

CORONARY HEART DISEASE AND DIABETES MELLITUS

Steven P. Marso / Stephen G. Ellis

The incidence of diabetes mellitus continues to increase worldwide. Currently, 100 million persons have a history of diabetes mellitus, and this number is projected to double in the next decade (Wingard and Barret-Connor, 1995). Since 1960, there has been a tenfold increase in the prevalence of diabetes (Kenny, 1995), and the number continues to rise among children, adults, and the elderly. In the United States, 15.7 million people have diabetes, and approximately one-third remain unrecognized. Although diabetes is present in only 8% of the world population, approximately 15 to 20% of patients presenting with acute coronary syndromes or for percutaneous coronary revascularization procedures have a reported history of diabetes.

Diabetes mellitus, whether type 1 or type 2, is a potent risk factor for the development of atherosclerosis. In fact, atherosclerotic vascular complications account for nearly 80% of all deaths, significant morbidity, and premature mortality among diabetic patients. In the past 15 years there have been numerous advances in the field of cardiovascular medicine such that there has been a marked decline in the age-adjusted mortality rate among patients with cardiovascular disease. Unfortunately, these improvements have not been realized among patients with diabetes mellitus.

According to the National Center for Health Statistics, there has been an increase in the age-adjusted death rate since 1985 for patients with diabetes (McKinlay and Marceau, 2000). Similarly, data from the National Health and Nutrition Examination Survey (NHANES) epidemiologic surveys suggest that the age-adjusted mortality rate for men with diabetes has remained relatively constant in recent years, while there has been a 15.2% increase in the all-cause age-adjusted mortality rate among women with diabetes (Gu et al., 1999).

There is no doubt that patients with a history of diabetes and coronary artery disease remain at a heightened risk. A Finnish-based population study demonstrated an 18.5% annual vascular event rate including death, stroke, or nonfatal myocardial infarction (MI), compared with a 6.8% event rate among diabetic and nondiabetic patients with a history of prior MI (Haffner et al., 1998). These data highlight the high-risk nature of diabetes and the importance of adopting an aggressive secondary prevention strategy. A broad-based strategy including preventive measures, risk factor modification, an aggressive pharmacologic strategy, and appropriate use of coronary revascularization procedures will be required in order to improve the outcomes among diabetic patients.

Insulin Resistance

Over 90% of patients with diabetes mellitus have type 2 diabetes, which, unlike type 1, is a direct result of insulin resistance at the peripheral tissue level. Insulin resistance precedes the onset of overt diabetes by many years, has been linked with the development of atherosclerosis, and is readily identified and modifiable. The clinical hallmarks of insulin resistance are central adiposity, hypertension, elevated triglycerides, and increased levels of circulating free fatty acids (FFA). The beta cells of the pancreas secrete increased amounts of insulin in order to maintain euglycemia. Eventually the beta cells fail, insulin levels plateau (then decline), and hyperglycemia ensues while tissues remain relatively insulin resistant.

The causes of insulin resistance are varied and mostly unexplained. The insulin receptor gene is located on chromosome 19, and there have been no fewer than 50 mutations in this gene described, which, taken in total, cause only rare forms of insulin resistance. However, insulin resistance does appear, in part, to be genetically pre-determined. Young, nonobese, and glucose-tolerant relatives of patients with type 2 diabetes have been shown to be insulin resistant (Warram et al., 1990; Martin et al., 1992). Approximately 50% of first-degree relatives are insulin resistant many decades prior to the onset of diabetes (Kahn, 1994). The genetic drivers of insulin resistance do not appear to be absolute, as environmental factors are clearly contributory in the development of diabetes.

While the molecular underpinnings of insulin resistance are not yet defined, numerous agents have been implicated. Insulin resistance among obese individuals is accounted for partly by increased levels of FFAs and perhaps tumor necrosis factor α (TNF-α). FFAs result in insulin resistance likely via inhibition of muscle glucose metabolism and inducing hyperinsulinemia. TNF-α down regulates GLUT 4 (a membrane-bound receptor glucose transporter) and impairs the tyrosine kinase activity of the insulin receptor (Hofmann et al., 1994). This "prediabetic" insulin-resistant state undoubtedly contributes to the development of atherosclerosis.

Insulin resistance appears to be modifiable by changing life-style and by treatment with newer antidiabetic agents. Identification and treatment of insulin resistance will likely be a key component for the prevention of type 2 diabetes. Thus, numerous methods have been developed for the detection of insulin resistance, including identification of clinical characteristics, calculation of insulin sensitivity index (using euglycemic clamp), fasting insulin homeostasis model assessment (HOMA), insulin-to-glucose ratio, and the Bennett index. These previously described methods are quite involved and are not well suited for implementation into large-scale trials or for use in clinical practice. However, there have been recent reports using a simplified approach utilizing insulin levels alone coupled with triglyceride levels (McAuley et al., 2001; Raynaud et al., 1999). A simplified and validated schema for the identification of insulin resistance will be an important step forward in the understanding of type 2 diabetes and will offer a new technique for disease modification and treatment.

Fortunately, there are numerous clinical markers of insulin resistance. When three or more of these clinical markers are present, there is a high likelihood of that patient being insulin resistant. In fact, the recently updated guidelines from the National Cholesterol Education Program recognize insulin resistance as an important and modifiable cardiovascular risk factor (NCEP III, 2001). The recognized clinical markers of insulin resistance include a fasting glucose of >6.1 mmol/L (>110 mg/dL); triglycerides >1.7 mmol/L (>150 mg/dL); central adiposity [abdominal girth >102 cm (>40 in.) in men and > 89 cm (> 35 in.) in women], hypertension (>130/85), and depressed levels of high-density lipoprotein (HDL) [<1.03 mmol/L (<40 mg/dL) in men and <1.29 mmol/L (<50 mg/dL) in women].

Insulin-resistance syndrome has been implicated in the development of atherosclerosis and is likely a modest predictor of adverse cardiovascular outcomes, with a relative risk of approximately 1.18 (1.08 to 1.29) for the development of coronary heart disease (Ruige et al., 1998). Insulin resistance has also been linked with target vessel revascularization following percutaneous coronary intervention (PCI)

(Nishimoto et al., 1998; Marso et al., 1999). Until recently, insulin and the sulfonylurea agents have been the agents of choice for managing hyperglycemia among patients with type 2 diabetes. Although these agents remain the cornerstone of therapy, newer agents, including metformin and the thiazolidinediones (TZDs), have evolved as important antidiabetic agents; they improve glycemic control through improved insulin sensitivity at the peripheral tissue level. Although the TZDs were initially developed for their antioxidant properties, it became apparent early in development that they had a beneficial effect on serum glucose levels in insulin-resistant animals (Fujita et al., 1983; Fujiwara et al., 1991, 1995; Yoshioka et al., 1989).

Although there are numerous thiazolidinedione (TZD) agents in development, there are only two agents currently approved for use in the United States: rosiglitazone (Avandia) and pioglitazone (Actos). Troglitazone (Rezulin) was voluntarily withdrawn from the market in March of 2000 due to unexpected, severe hepatotoxicity. The molecular target of the TZD agents is their ability to bind to a family of nuclear receptors named *peroxisome proliferator-activated receptors* (PPARs). These receptors are members of the steroid/thyroid hormone receptor superfamily of transcription factors and appear to be important in adipocyte differentiation (Issemann and Green, 1990; Chawla et al., 1994).

The PPAR family consists of three distinct receptors: PPAR-α, PPAR-γ, and PPAR-δ. Once activated, PPAR forms a heterodimer with the retinoic acid receptor, binds to DNA regulatory regions of target genes, and results in differential gene expression and protein synthesis. Each PPAR subtype appears to bind specific ligands. The TZDs' binding affinity for PPAR-γ appears to correlate with their glucose-lowering ability. PPAR-γ receptors are abundantly populated upon adipocytes, intestinal cells, and macrophages. The molecular cascade linking PPAR-γ to adipocyte differentiation and insulin resistance is as yet undefined. However, there is mounting evidence that adipocyte-derived hormones play a key role in the development of obesity and insulin resistance.

Adipose tissue is more than a passive storage tank; it is a complex endocrine organ that releases hormones that play an active role in metabolic homeostasis. As these adipocyte-derived hormones have a similar structure to cytokines, they are collectively referred to as *adipokines* (Saltiel, 2001). These identified proteins include TNF-α, leptin, adipsin, resistin, and adiponectin. In particular, resistin has been linked to the development of insulin resistance in *ob/ob* and *db/db* (inherited obesity and diabetes traits) mouse models (Steppan et al., 2001), while adiponectin has been linked with insulin sensitivity in similar diabetic (as well as nondiabetic) mouse models. (Berg et al., 2001; Yamauchi et al., 2001). Both of these adipokines appear to be regulated by the administration of PPAR-γ agonists. If the results of these preliminary observations are replicated and the molecular pathways further delineated, modulation of the "adipokine" axis may prove to offer a new therapeutic strategy for the treatment of obesity, insulin resistance, and type 2 diabetes mellitus.

The glucose-lowering effects of the TZDs have been extensively studied in humans. It appears that, as a class, they improve glycemic control somewhat less than the sulfonylurea agents or metformin. On average, the fasting plasma glucose level is decreased by approximately 2.5 mmol/L (45 mg/dL) and the HbA1c by about 1.0% (Patel et al., 1999; Matthaei et al., 2000). The glucose-lowering effects of these agents appear to plateau at doses greater than 8 mg for rosiglitazone and 45 mg for pioglitazone. There appears to be no dose dependency for pioglitazone from 15–30 mg/day, but the 45 mg/day dose appears to significantly lower glucose. Both of these agents also have similar efficacy in their glucose-lowering properties.

In addition to the insulin-sensitizing affects, there are numerous other beneficial cardiovascular affects of these agents. They have a favorable impact upon lipoprotein metabolism, endothelial function, anti-inflammatory properties, and have recently been demonstrated to reduce neointimal proliferation among patients undergoing intracoronary stenting (Takagi et al., 2000). Patients with type 2 diabetes have a characteristic lipid profile of elevated triglycerides and low HDL and have modestly elevated low-density lipoprotein (LDL) levels. However, the LDL pool among patients with diabetes has greater amounts of small, dense, oxidized particles, which are thought to be quite atherogenic. As a general rule, the TZD agents decrease triglyceride levels (if markedly elevated), elevate HDL, and decrease the oxidized LDL pool.

Given the perceived and potentially broad-spectrum cardiovascular benefits of these agents, there are currently six large-scale clinical trials evaluating the cardiovascular effects of rosiglitazone. DREAM is projected to enroll 4000 nondiabetic patients with impaired glucose tolerance to ramipril or placebo and rosiglitazone or placebo. The primary end-point is all-cause mortality. ACCORD is a National Institutes of Health multicenter trial projected to enroll 10,000 patients to evaluate the efficacy of intensive (versus conventional) control of serum glucose, lipids, and blood pressure among patients with type 2 diabetes. The VA-COOP is a multicenter, randomized, open-label trial evaluating the effects of intensive versus standard glycemic control in reducing cardiovascular events. Within the BARI 2D trial, there will be an insulin-providing versus an insulin-sensitizing arm. The insulin-providing arm will utilize sulfonylurea agents and insulin while the insulin-sensitizing arm will include glucophage and rosiglitazone. The RECORD trial and the ADOPT trial are also evaluating the effects of rosiglitazone in the setting of combination therapy or with the addition of a newly diagnosed type 2 diabetic patients respectively. The TZDs will certainly evolve to be a mainstay of therapy among patients with diabetes. However, there remain several important clinical limitations with the use of these agents. They are contraindicated in the presence of congestive heart failure as they are often associated with significant weight gain and fluid retention, often resulting in discontinuation.

Diabetes Mellitus and Coronary Revascularization

No subgroup of patients has generated more controversy in recent years than diabetic patients requiring coronary revascularization. Interest was piqued when the National Heart, Lung, and Blood Institute (NHLBI) issued a clinical alert to physicians stating that coronary artery bypass grafting (CABG) should be considered the preferred revascularization procedure in medically treated diabetic patients with multivessel disease requiring an initial coronary revascularization procedure (NHLBI, 1995). These comments were predicated upon the BARI trial, which demonstrated an improved 5-year survival for treated diabetic patients with multivessel disease undergoing bypass surgery compared with balloon angioplasty (80.6% vs. 65.5%, $p = .003$) (BARI Investigators, 1996, 2000). This trial was published against the background of multiple observational studies demonstrating that diabetic patients had prohibitive rates of late MI, mortality, and restenosis following percutaneous balloon angioplasty. Subsequent studies have reported restenosis rates ranging from 40 to 70%, with an overall odds ratio of restenosis among diabetics compared to nondiabetic patients estimated to be 1.3.

Data from Stein and colleagues demonstrated a marked increase in the 5-year mortality rate (12% vs. 7%, $p < .001$) and nonfatal MI rate (19% vs. 11%, $p < .001$) for diabetics compared with nondiabetics following percutaneous transluminal coronary angioplasty (PTCA) (Stein et al., 1995). Kip and colleagues, utilizing long-term follow-up NHLBI registry data, also confirmed these data. (Stein et al., 1995). Although the mechanism of increasing mortality following percutaneous intervention is unknown, significant disease progression likely contributes to the increased late mortality seen among diabetic patients. In addition the late vessel occlusion rate, following conventional balloon angioplasty, approaches 15% among patients with diabetes (compared with 3 to 4% among patients without diabetes) (Van Belle et al., 1999) and is associated with a decrement in left ventricular function and a resultant increase in both all cause and cardiovascular mortality (Van Belle et al., 2001). Multivariate analysis in this study demonstrated that late coronary occlusion was an independent correlate of long-term all-cause mortality (hazard ratio, 2.16; 95% CI, 1.43 to 3.26; $p = .0003$). These compelling data suggest that the relatively uncommon occurrence of late vessel occlusion among nondiabetic patients is frequent among diabetic patients, results in abnormal left ventricular function and remodeling, and is associated with poor survival. These phenomena may explain the propensity for adverse events among diabetic patients following conventional balloon angioplasty.

Balloon Angioplasty or Bypass Surgery for Diabetic Patients

The benefit of CABG in diabetic patients in the BARI trial appeared to be confined to diabetic patients with more than three significant lesions, insulin treatment, and those receiving an internal mammary artery at the time of surgery. Of interest, the 5-year survival rate was similar for nondiabetics and diet-controlled diabetics following either CABG or PTCA (91.4% vs. 91.1%). In contrast to the BARI trial, the BARI registry did not clearly demonstrate a survival advantage for treated diabetics undergoing CABG compared with conventional balloon angioplasty (Detre et al., 1999). The 5-year all-cause mortality for diabetic patients undergoing PTCA was 14.4% and was 14.9% for those undergoing surgical revascularization ($p = .86$). Even following multivariable risk adjustment, PTCA was not associated with a statistically significant increased risk of mortality in the registry. The difference in outcomes for the registry and the randomized trial are very likely due to the differing patient populations and physician choice. The registry patients were more often Caucasian, better educated, less likely to smoke, more physically active, and had a higher reported quality-of-life score and less congestive heart failure compared with the patients in the randomized trial. Furthermore, the patients within the registry who underwent CABG were quite different than those who underwent PTCA. The PTCA group had a lower prevalence of triple-vessel disease, less incidence of more than four lesions, a lower frequency of significant proximal left anterior descending coronary artery stenosis, and fewer ostial coronary lesions.

Based on the BARI randomized and registry data, the long-term outcome of diabetic patients appears to be optimized when physicians and patients decide on which of the two revascularization strategies are more appropriate for the individual patient. Although the BARI experience is becoming obsolete in the current era of percutaneous and surgical revascularization strategies, this trial has generated a great deal of discussion and has been a catalyst for important research in the area of diabetes mellitus and coronary revascularization. The BARI 2D trial is currently underway and evaluating a "stand alone" aggressive medical treatment strategy with early coronary revascularization and aggressive medical therapy. A second randomization scheme compares treatment with an insulin-sensitizing drug (e.g., metformin or a thiazolidinedione) or an insulin-providing drug (e.g., sulfonylurea).

Diabetes in the Stent Era

Restenosis following balloon angioplasty is a result of early elastic recoil, maladaptive arterial remodeling, and neointimal proliferation. As stenting effectively prevents both recoil and late remodeling, restenosis following stenting is a direct function of neointimal formation. This is true for both diabetic and nondiabetic patients. It appears that stenting among diabetic patients results in improved arterial patency compared with conventional balloon angioplasty (Van Belle et al., 1997). While it is unclear whether stenting will improve the long-term clinical outcome of diabetic patients, emerging data suggest that stenting confers added benefit among this cohort of patients. The ARTS trial randomized 1205 patients to either multivessel stenting or CABG (Serruys et al., 2001). The 2-year event-free survival rate (event = death, MI, or cerebrovascular accident (CVA) was similar among the diabetic patients undergoing CABG or multivessel stenting, 85.4% vs. 83.9%, respectively. Although the composite event-rate was similar, there was a trend for an increased 2-year mortality rate among the diabetic cohort in the multivessel stenting group and an increased rate of perioperative stroke rate among diabetic patients undergoing CABG. The freedom from 2-year mortality rate was 92.9% for the stent diabetic cohort. Surgery was associated with an increased rate of stroke. The 2-year freedom from CVA rates were 93.7% and 97.3% for the CABG and stent groups, respectively. However, there remains an increased need for repeat revascularization procedures among the diabetic stent group. The 2-year composite of freedom from death, MI, CVA, or repeat revascularization procedures was 82.3% among the CABG cohort and 56.3% among the stent group, $p < .001$. The long-term follow-up of this cohort will be essential as the mortality benefit of coronary surgery is often not evident for many years following the index revascularization procedure.

Perhaps the most compelling data that stenting improves the outcome for diabetic patients comes form the EPISTENT trial (EPISTENT Investigators, 1998). Patients were randomly assigned to receive either conventional angioplasty with abciximab, stent-placebo, or stent-abciximab. Of the 2399 subjects there were 491 diabetic patients within EPISTENT, and diabetes was a prespecified subset within this trial. The composite event rate of 6-month death, MI, or target vessel revascularization (TVR) occurred in 25.2% of stent-placebo, 23.4% of balloon-abciximab, and 13.0% of stent-abciximab patients ($p = .005$). Abciximab, irrespective of balloon angioplasty or stenting, resulted in a significant reduction in the 6-month death or MI rate (12.7% for stent-placebo, 7.8% for balloon-abciximab, and 6.2% for the stent-abciximab group, $p = .029$). Importantly, stenting with adjunctive abciximab therapy resulted in a significant reduction in the 6-month TVR rate compared with the other two revascularization strategies. Furthermore, the benefit of abciximab among the diabetic cohort persisted through 1-year follow-up (Figure 32-1). The angiographic substudy of the EPISTENT trial provides further corroborating data that abciximab likely reduces restenosis rates in diabetic patients undergoing intracoronary stenting.

Furthermore, there was a trend for an improved mortality in the stent-abciximab diabetic cohort. The 1-year mortality was 4.1% for the stent-placebo group compared with 1.2% for the stent-abciximab group ($p = .11$). The PTCA-abciximab group had an intermediate mortality of 2.6%. These preliminary findings from EPISTENT have been extended with an analysis of all the "EPI" trials, including EPIC, EPILOG, and EPISTENT. In total, there were 1462 patients with diabetes in

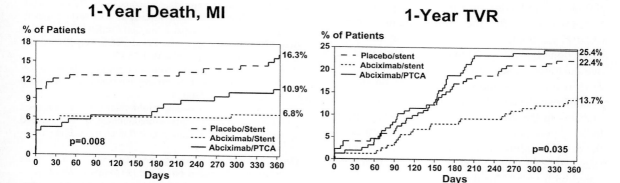

FIGURE 32-1

This figure depicts the Kaplan-Meier 1-year event rates including death, myocardial infarction, and target vessel revascularization (TVR) for patients with diabetes enrolled in EPISTENT (Evaluation of platelet IIb/IIIa inhibitor for stenting).

these three trials. The 1-year mortality rate among the abciximab-treated diabetic patients was 4.5% compared with 2.5% for the placebo-treated diabetic patients, $p = .031$ (Bhatt et al., 2000). High-risk diabetic patients in this analysis derived significant reduction in mortality with abciximab administration. These subgroups included insulin treatment, insulin-resistance syndrome, and multivessel revascularization.

As previously stated, restenosis (arterial renarrowing following PCI) remains a significant problem following PCI among patients with diabetes. Although stenting has resulted in a significant reduction in restenosis rates compared with balloon angioplasty, diabetes remains a potent clinical predictor of restenosis following PCI in the modern stentera. Numerous pharmacologic agents have failed to demonstrate a reduction in the restenosis rates following PCI. However, the administration of intracoronary radiation (brachytherapy) has been shown to significantly reduce the in-stent restenosis rates. Randomized trials have evaluated the efficacy of both intracoronary gamma- and beta-emitting ionizing radiation following percutaneous mechanical recanalization. It appears that brachytherapy is quite effective in reducing restenosis among diabetic patients.

The Gamma 1 trial evaluated the efficacy of iridium 192 administration among patients with significant in-stent restenosis and demonstrated a significant reduction in the subsequent binary restenosis rates for the iridium-treated patients (32.4% vs. 55.3%, $p = .01$) (Leon et al., 2001). Work done by Moses, Moussa and colleagues have demonstrated that gamma radiation reduces the restenosis rates among diabetic patients to near nondiabetic levels. There were 79 patients with diabetes in the Gamma 1 trial, and there appeared to be a potentiated response to irradiation among the diabetic cohort. The 9-month in-stent restenosis rate was 25% for the iridium 192 cohort, compared with 65.5% for the placebo treated cohort, $p = .002$. Of interest, the in-stent restenosis rates were 20.3% for the nondiabetic iridium 192 group, compared with 43.1% for the nondiabetic placebo group, $p = .004$. Although wide spread implementation of intracoronary radiation is problematic and remains limited to patients with instent restenosis, it appears to be quite effective among patients with diabetes.

SUMMARY

The prevalence of diabetes throughout the world continues to increase, and cardiovascular complications remain the leading cause of death among patients with diabetes. Although there have been enormous advances in the medical and surgical treatment of patients with cardiovascular disease, with a resultant decrease in the age-adjusted mortality, this has not translated into improved long-term outcome for patients with diabetes. In order to substantially impact the natural history of diabetes and coronary heart disease, there will need to be a vigorous commitment for continuing diabetes and vascular research and an aggressive clinical implementation of the current therapeutic modalities.

REFERENCES

BARI Investigators: Comparison of coronary bypass surgery with angioplasty in patients with multivessel disease. The Bypass Angioplasty Revascularization Investigation. N Engl J Med 335:217, 1996

BARI Investigators: Seven-year outcome in the Bypass Angioplasty Revascularization Investigation (BARI) by treatment and diabetic status. J Am Coll Cardiol 35:1122, 2000

Berg AH et al: The adipocyte-secreted protein Acrp30 enhances hepatic insulin action. Nat Med 7:947, 2001

Bhatt DL et al: Abciximab reduces mortality in diabetics following percutaneous coronary intervention. J Am Coll Cardiol 35;922, 2000

Chawla A et al: Peroxisome proliferator-activated receptor (PPAR) gamma: Adipose-predominant expression and induction early in adipocyte differentiation. Endocrinology 135:798, 1994

Detre KM et al: Coronary revascularization in diabetic patients: A comparison of the randomized and observational components of the Bypass Angioplasty Revascularization Investigation (BARI). Circulation 99:633, 1999

EPISTENT Investigators: Randomized placebo-controlled and balloon-angioplasty-controlled trial to assess safety of coronary stenting with use of platelet glycoprtein IIb/IIIa blockade. Evaluation of Platelet IIb/IIIa Inhibitor for Stenting. Lancet 352:87, 1998

Executive Summary of The Third Report of The National Cholesterol Education Program (NCEP) Expert Panel on Detection, Evaluation, And Treatment of High Blood Cholesterol In Adults (Adult Treatment Panel III). JAMA. 2001; 285:2486

Ferguson JJ BARI clinical alert on diabetics treated with angioplasty. Circulation 92:3371, 1995

Fujita T et al: Reduction of insulin-resistance in obese and/or diabetic animals by 5- [4-(1-methylcyclohexylmethoxy) benzyl]-thiazolidine-2,4-dione (ADD-3878, U-63,287, ciglitazone), a new antidiabetic agent. Diabetes 32:804, 1983

Fujiwara T et al: Characterization of CS-045, a new oral antidiabetic agent, II. Effects on glycemic control and pancreatic islet structure at a late stage of the diabetic syndrome in C57BL/KsJ-*db/db* mice. Metabolism 40:1213, 1991

Fujiwara T et al: Suppression of hepatic gluconeogenesis in long-term Troglitazone-treated diabetic KK and C57BL/KsJ-db/db mice. Metabolism 44:486, 1995

Gu K et al: Diabetes and decline in heart disease mortality in US adults. JAMA 281:1291, 1999

Haffner SM et al: Mortality from coronary heart disease in subjects with type 2 diabetes and in nondiabetic subjects with and without prior myocardial infarction. N Engl J Med 339:229, 1998

Hofmann C et al: Altered gene expression for tumor necrosis factor-alpha and its receptors during drug and dietary modulation of insulin-resistance. Endocrinology 134:264, 1994

Issemann I, Green S: Activation of a member of the steroid hormone receptor superfamily by peroxisome proliferators. Nature 347:645, 1990

Kahn CR: Banting Lecture: Insulin action, diabetogenes, and the cause of Type II diabetes. Diabetes 43:1066, 1994

Kenny SJ et al: *Diabetes in America.* Bethesda, MD, National Institutes of Health, NIH 95-1468:47, 1995

Leon MB et al: Localized intracoronary gamma-radiation therapy to inhibit the recurrence of restenosis after stenting. N Engl J Med 344:250, 2001

Marso SP et al: Optimizing the percutaneous interventional outcomes for patients with diabetes mellitus: Results of the EPISTENT (Evaluation of Platelet IIb/IIIa Inhibitor for Stenting Trial) diabetic substudy. Circulation 100:2477, 1999

Martin BC et al: Role of glucose and insulin-resistance in development of type 2 diabetes mellitus: Results of a 25-year follow-up study. Lancet 340:925, 1992

Matthaei S et al: Pathophysiology and pharmacological treatment of insulin-resistance. Endocr Rev 21:585, 2000

McAuley KA et al: Diagnosing insulin-resistance in the general population. Diabetes Care 24:460, 2001

McKinlay J, Marceau L: US public health and the 21st century: Diabetes mellitus. Lancet 356:757, 2000

Nishimoto Y et al: Enhanced secretion of insulin plays a role in the development of atherosclerosis and restenosis of coronary arteries: Elective percutaneous transluminal coronary angioplasty in patients with effort angina. J Am Coll Cardiol 32:1624, 1998

Patel J et al: Rosiglitazone monotherapy improves glycemic control in patients with type 2 diabetes: A twelve-week, randomized, placebo-controlled study. Diabetes Obes Metab 1:165, 1999

Raynaud E et al: Revised concept for the estimation of insulin sensitivity from a single sample. Diabetes Care 22:1003, 1999

Ruige JB et al: Insulin and risk of cardiovascular disease: A meta-analysis. Circulation 97:996, 1998

Saltiel AR: You are what you secrete. Nat. Mod; 7:887, 2001.

Serruys PW et al: Comparison of coronary-artery bypass surgery and stenting for the treatment of multivessel disease. N Engl J Med 344:1117, 2001

Stein B et al: Influence of diabetes mellitus on early and late outcome after percutaneous transluminal coronary angioplasty. Circulation 91:979, 1995

Steppan CM et al: The hormone resistin links obesity to diabetes. Nature 409:307, 2001

Takagi T et al: Troglitazone reduces neointimal tissue proliferation after coronary stent implantation in patients with non-insulin dependent diabetes mellitus: A serial intravascular ultrasound study. J Am Coll Cardiol 36:1529, 2000

Van Belle E et al: Restenosis rates in diabetic patients: A comparison of coronary stenting and balloon angioplasty in native coronary vessels. Circulation 96:1454, 1997

Van Belle E et al: Restenosis, late vessel occlusion and left ventricular function six months after balloon angioplasty in diabetic patients. J Am Coll Cardiol 34:476, 1999

Van Belle E et al: Patency of percutaneous transluminal coronary angioplasty sites at 6-month angiographic follow-up: A key determinant of survival in diabetics after coronary balloon angioplasty. Circulation 103:1218, 2001

Yamauchi T et al: The fat-derived hormone adiponectin reverses insulin resistance associated with both lipoatrophy and obesity. Nat Med 7:941, 2001

Warram JH et al: Slow glucose removal rate and hyperinsulinemia precede the development of type II diabetes and the offspring of diabetic parents. Ann Intern Med 113:909, 1990

Wingard DL, Barret-Connor E: *Disease and Diabetes. Diabetes in America.* Washington, DC: US Department of Health and Human Services, NIH 95–68:429, 1995

Yoshioka T et al: Studies on hindered phenols and analogues: Hypolipidemic and hypoglycemic agents with ability to inhibit lipid peroxidation. J Med Chem 32:421, 1989

CARDIOVASCULAR DISEASE AND ERECTILE DYSFUNCTION

Robert A. Kloner

Physiology of Erection

Erection of the penis is a vascular event; therefore, cardiovascular disease and the risk factors for cardiovascular disease can contribute to erectile dysfunction. In the flaccid or nonerect state, the smooth muscle surrounding the arteries and sinusoids of the penis are contracted, limiting blood flow into the penis. During sexual stimulation, nerves and endothelial cells within the penis release nitric oxide (NO), which activates the enzyme gluanylate cyclase that causes an increase in cyclic guanosine monophosphase (GMP) levels. Cyclic GMP relaxes the smooth-muscle cells in the arteries, arterioles, and sinusoids of the two corpus cavernosa (erectile bodies) of the penis. The sinusoidal tissue becomes engorged with blood (like a sponge); it expands within the tough tunica albuginea, compressing veins and thus trapping blood within the corpus cavernosum. Following orgasm and ejaculation, cyclic GMP is broken down by phosphodiesterase 5 (PDE5), a phosphodiesterase that is concentrated in the genitalia. Inhibitory efferent nerves also fire, contributing to contraction of smooth-muscle cells within the arterial walls and sinusoids, reducing blood flow into the corpus cavernosum. The veins reopen and drain the sinusoidal spaces, causing detumescence.

Prevalence and Causes of Erectile Dysfunction

Erectile dysfunction is defined as the consistent inability to achieve and/or maintain an erection sufficient for satisfactory sexual activity. It is estimated that 10 to 30 million men in the United States suffer from erectile dysfunction (ED). While ED often was thought to be primarily psychogenic, it is now clear that organic disease, including vascular disease, is a major contributor. A National Institutes of Health Consensus Conference (NIH Consensus Development Panel on Impotence, 1993) pointed out that "most of the medical disorders associated with erectile dysfunction affect the arterial system." Among the causes linked to cardiovascular disease are diabetes, smoking, hypertension, hypercholesterolemia, low levels of high-density lipoprotein (HDL), atherosclerotic vascular disease, vascular surgery, and certain antihypertensive and other cardiac drugs.

Link between Cardiovascular Risk Factors and Erectile Dysfunction

One of the first studies suggesting a link between cardiovascular risk factors and erectile dysfunction was a study by Virag and colleagues (1985). They showed that smoking, diabetes, and hyperlipidemia were more common among 440 impotent men (average age, 48 years) than among the overall population. Diabetes alone and combinations of other risk factors (smoking, abnormal fasting glucose test, hyperlipidemia, and hypertension) were associated with reduced penile blood pressure index, which is the ratio of blood pressure in the penis compared to the brachial artery. The effect of two or more arterial risk factors appeared to further worsen this index of blood flow into the penis.

The Massachusetts Male Aging study was a community-based multidisciplinary survey of 1290 normal men age 40 to 70 years (Feldman et al., 1994). The prevalence of ED was reported to be 52% for the entire cohort; this included men with complete ED (10%), moderate ED (25%), and mild ED (17%). ED increased with age, from 39% among 40-year olds to 67% among 70-year-olds. Complete ED increased from 5% among 40-year-olds to 15% among 70-year-olds. Cardiovascular risk factors that correlated with the development of ED included low HDL, diabetes, hypertension, and heart disease. Smoking also played a significant role. The probability of complete ED in men with heart disease was 56% for smokers and 21% for nonsmokers. Cardiac drugs also significantly increased the risk of ED.

Other studies have supported the concept that lipid abnormalities contribute to ED. Wei and colleagues found that men with total cholesterol levels >6.2 mmol/L (>240 mg/dL) were more likely to have ED than men with total cholesterol levels <4.7 mmol/L (<180 mg/dL) (Wei et al., 1994). Furthermore, HDL appeared to confer protection. Men with HLD > 1.6 mmol/L (>60 mg/dL) were less likely to have ED than men with HDL levels <0.8 mmol/L (<30 mg/dL). An experimental study showed that rabbits fed a high-cholesterol diet did not maintain high intracavernosal pressures following penile injections of vasodilators, whereas animals fed control diets had no trouble maintaining erections (Azadzoi et al., 1996). Of note, ED associated with a high-cholesterol diet was observed in some animals before anatomic vascular stenoses could be visualized by angiography. This study suggests that the high cholesterol levels induced endothelial dysfunction or other vascular abnormalities that impeded normal vasodilation of the penile vasculature, even before atherosclerotic lesions had developed.

The prevalence of ED in diabetic men is as high as 75% by age of 60. Of course, diabetes accelerates vascular disease, but the diabetic neuropathy that occurs also appears to be important in causing ED. On physical examination of diabetic men, loss of vibratory sensation correlates most closely with development of ED.

Numerous antihypertensive drugs have been associated with ED. Diuretics, specifically the thiazide diuretics, may cause ED. Other antihypertensives have been implicated, including spironolactone, clonidine, guanethidine, methyldopa, reserpine, and beta blockers. A recent study (Fogari et al., 2001) suggested that the antihypertensive valsartan (an angiotensin receptor blocker) actually improved ED. The cardiac drugs clofibrate, gemfibrozil, and digoxin have also been associated with ED.

A recent follow-up study, published by the Massachusetts Male aging study (Feldman HA et al., 2000), strengthened and extended the concept that erectile dysfunction is associated with cardiovascular risk factors. They interviewed men between the ages of 40 and 70 in 1987 to 1989 and then reinterviewed them in 1995 to 1997. These 513 men had no ED at baseline and no history of heart disease, related medicines for heart disease, or diabetes at baseline. Cigarette smoking at baseline nearly doubled the likelihood of the men developing moderate or complete ED by the time of follow-up (24% vs. 14%). Passive smoking and cigar smoking were also predictors of the development of ED. Being overweight (body-mass index ≥ 28 kg/m^2) contributed, as did a composite coronary risk score based on the Framingham study, which took into account age, systolic blood pressure, serum cholesterol, and cigarette smoking. The authors concluded that ED and coronary heart disease share behaviorally modifiable determinants. A likely explanation is that these vascular risk factors contribute to endothelial dysfunction, which then impedes blood flow to the corpus cavernosum (hence ED = endothelial dysfunction = erectile dysfunction).

In another recent study, authors from the Massachusetts Male Aging Study (Derby CA et al., 2000) sought to determine whether life-style changes could modify the risk of ED in men ages 40 to 70. They examined changes in smoking, heavy alcohol use, sedentary life-style, and obesity. Baseline obesity was associated with a higher risk of ED regardless of subsequent weight loss. Men who remained physically active or initiated physical activity were less likely to develop ED. Surprisingly, changes in smoking and alcohol use did not alter the incidence of ED. The authors concluded that changes in midlife may be too late to reverse the deleterious effects of smoking, obesity, and alcohol consumption, while physical activity may decrease the risk of ED, even when begun in midlife. Adoption of healthy life-styles must occur early in life to limit the development of ED.

More men are now seeking treatment for ED as oral medicines become available. This is a good opportunity for the health-care professional to evaluate these patients for cardiovascular risk factors (Kloner and Jarow, 1999). If the patient with ED is evaluated and is found to have cardiovascular risk factors such as smoking, lipid abnormalities, hypertension, and/or diabetes, these risk factors can be controlled and the patient may benefit by reducing his risk of cardiovascular disease. Therefore, it is important to ask patients with ED about their cardiovascular risk factors and their cardiovascular health. Conversely, it is important to ask patients with cardiovascular disease about their sexual health (Levine and Kloner, 2000). Often, patients are not asked about this issue or are embarrassed to discuss it. As more therapies that work become available, it is likely that more and more patients will seek help.

Therapy and Implications for Patients with Cardiac Disease

When a cardiovascular specialist sees a patient with ED, he or she should take a careful history of cardiovascular risk factors, realizing that patients with ED are more likely to have risk factors for cardiovascular disease. Signs and symptoms of vascular disease should be sought on the physical examination. It is important to palpate the lower extremity pulses and auscultate bruits. Details on other aspects of the history and physical examination as well as laboratory workup of ED can be found in standard textbooks.

The available therapies of ED include oral phosphodiesterase 5 inhibitors such as sildenafil (Viagra) and others under study, phentolamine, and apomorphine (also under study); constriction bands; vacuum tumescence devices; intracavernosal injections of vasoactive medicines (such as prostaglandin E_1); intraurethral suppositories of alprostadil; vascular surgery; penile implants; and counseling and sex therapy. Both oral and injected vasodilators have the potential for interaction with systemic vasculature and may therefore affect the cardiac patient.

Sildenafil was the first oral agent approved for ED by the U.S. Food and Drug Administration. It was found to be effective in 63 to 82% of patients at the 25- to 100-mg dose and worked in patients with vascular, neurogenic, and psychogenic ED. Sildenafil is an inhibitor of PDE5 and therefore causes an increase in the crucial cyclic GMP messenger. Its hemodynamic profile resembles that of a weak nitrate; in normal human volunteers it causes drops in systolic/diastolic blood pressure by 8/5.5 mmHg. In patients already on antihypertensive medicines, it induces about the same degree of drop in blood pressure (additive but not synergistic). However, when sildenafil is combined with NO donors (such as organic nitrates, including nitroglycerin, isosorbide dinitrate or mononitrate, and others), a large drop in blood pressure can occur, causing symptomatic hypotension. Therefore, organic nitrates are an absolute contraindication to sildenafil (Jarow et al., 1998). Patients who come into an emergency room with chest pain should be questioned about the use of sildenafil; in those who have taken this drug within 24 h, non-nitrate antianginals should be used.

While there have been some cardiac deaths in men using sildenafil, this does not come as a surprise. There is a small but increased risk for myocardial infarction with sexual activity, and sexual activity is associated with a physiologic cost: an increase in heart rate to about 120 to 130 beats per minute, an increase in systolic blood pressure to about 150 to 180 mmHg, and expenditure of 4 to 6 METS (metabolic equivalents). It is likely that sildenafil enabled men who had been sexually inactive to become active and experience what is essentially moderate physical exertion in the setting of coronary artery disease. Some deaths were related to concomitant use of sildeanfil plus nitrates. In addition, death may have been coincidental. For example, in a population of 1 million men followed for 1 month,

TABLE 33-1

MANAGEMENT RECOMMENDATIONS BASED ON GRADED CARDIOVASCULAR (CV) RISK ASSESSMENT

Grade of risk	Categories of CVD	Management recommendations
Low risk	Asymptomatic, <3 major risk factors for CAD Controlled hypertension Mild, stable angina Post-successful coronary revascularization Uncomplicated post MI (>6–8 wk) Mild valvular disease LVD/CHF (NYHA class I)	Primary-care management Consider all first-line therapies Reassess at regular intervals (6–12 mo)
Intermediate risk	≥3 major risk factors for CAD, excluding gender Moderate, stable angina Recent MI (>2, <6 wk) LVD/CHF (NYHA class II) Noncardiac sequellae of atherosclerotic disease (e.g., CVA, peripheral vascular disease)	Specialized CV testing (e.g., ETT, Echo) Restratification into high risk or low risk based on the results of CV assessment
High risk	Unstable or refractory angina Uncontrolled hypertension LVD/CHF (NYHA class III/IV) Recent MI (<2 wk), CVA High-risk arrhythmias Hypertrophic obstructive and other cardiomyopathies Moderate/severe valvular disease	Priority referral for specialized CV management Treatment for sexual dysfunction to be deferred until cardiac condition stabilized and dependent on specialist recommendations

ABBREVIATIONS: CAD, coronary artery disease; CHF, congestive heart failure; CVA, stroke; CVD, cardiovascular disease; Echo, echocardiogram; ETT, exercise tolerance test; LVD, left ventricular dysfunction; MI, myocardial infarction; NYHA, New York Heart Association.

SOURCE: From R DeBusk et al: Am J Cardiol 86:175, 2000, with permission.

there will be several hundred deaths from heart disease and even more in a population of men in the age range seen with ED. Death rates on sildenafil were well within the expected death rates of men in the appropriate age range. Studies from phase II/III trials did not observe increased rates of myocardial infarction in men receiving sildenafil, compared to placebo (Morales et., 1998). Nevertheless, the American Heart Association and American College of Cardiology released a consensus statement (Cheitlin et al., 1999) suggesting that physicians "exercise caution" in prescribing the drug to patients with active coronary ischemia, heart failure, borderline hypotension, and hypovolemia; patients on multiple antihypertensive drugs; and patients taking drugs that can prolong the half-life of sildenafil (erythromycin, cimetidine, and certain antifungal agents).

For patients who inadvertently receive nitrates plus sildenafil, the consensus statement suggests placing them in Trendelenburg's position, using intravenous fluids, consideration of adrenergic agents, and intraaortic balloon counterpulsation. Other cardiovascular effects may occur with other vasodilators. For example, symptomatic hypotension was reported in 3% of patients who received transurethral alprostadil, and vasodilator side effects also may occur with oral forms of phentolamine.

A recent analysis by Shakir and colleagues of prescription event monitoring for sildenafil in England revealed outcomes in about 5600 users (Shakir et al., 2001). The average age of the patients was 57 years. There was no evidence of a higher rate of fatal myocardial infarction or coronary events among men taking sildenafil. Another group reported the effects of sildenafil on coronary dynamics in 14 men with

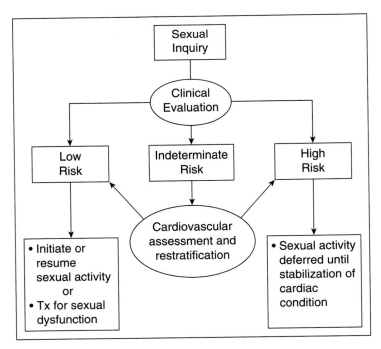

FIGURE 33-1

Sexual activity and cardiac risk: A simplified algorithm. Tx, therapy. (From R DeBusk et al: Am J Cardiol 86:175, 2000, with permission.)

angiographically documented coronary artery disease (Hermann et al., 2000). Sildenafil did not change coronary artery flow, flow velocity, coronary diameter, or coronary vascular resistance. Sildenafil increased coronary flow reserve (hyperemia induced with intracoronary adenosine) by about 13% in both stenosed and nonstenosed coronary arteries. Kloner and colleagues showed that sildenafil improved ED in 70% of hypertensive men taking antihypertensive medicines (Kloner et al., 2001). There was no increase in adverse events from sildenafil in men taking antihypertensives (even multiple antihypertensives) versus those not taking antihypertensives. There were no myocardial infarctions or cardiac deaths among men who had hypertension, were on antihypertensive medicines, and who took sildenafil.

The recent Princeton Consensus Panel (DeBusk et al., 2000) has offered new guidelines for the approach to management of sexual dysfunction in patients with cardiovascular disease (Table 33-1, Fig. 33-1).

REFERENCES

Azadzoi KM et al: Study of etiologic relationship of arterial atherosclerosis to corporal veno-occlusive dysfunction in the rabbit. J Urol 155:1795, 1996

Cheitlin MD et al: Use of sildenafil (Viagra) in patients with cardiovascular disease. J Am Coll Cardiol 33:273, 1999

DeBusk R et al: Management of sexual dysfunction in patients with cardiovascular disease: Recommendations of the Princeton Consensus Panel. Am J Cardiol 86:175, 2000

Derby CA et al: Modifiable risk factors and erectile dysfunction: Can lifestyle changes modify risk? Urology 56:302, 2000

Feldman HA et al: Impotence and its medical and psychosocial correlates: Results of the Massachusetts Male Aging Study. J Urol 151:54, 1994

Feldman HA et al: Erectile dysfunction and coronary risk factors: Prospective results from the Massachusetts Male Aging Study. Prev Med 30:328, 2000

Fogari R et al: Sexual activity in hypertensive men treated with valsartan or carvedilol: A crossover study. Am J Hypertens 14:27, 2001

Hermann HC et al: Hemodynamic effects of sildenafil in men with severe coronary artery disease. N Engl J Med 342:1622, 2000

Jarow JE et al: *Viagra*. New York, M Evans, 1998

Kloner RA, Jarow JD: Erectile dysfunction and sildenafil citrate and cardiologists. Am J Cardiol 83:576, 1999

Kloner RA et al: Effect of sildenafil in patients with erectile dysfunction taking antihypertensive therapy. Am J Hypertens 14:70, 2001

Levine LA, Kloner RA: Importance of asking questions about erectile dysfunction. Am J Cardiol 86:1210, 2000

Morales A et al: Clinical safety of oral sildenafil citrate (Viagra) in the treatment of erectile dysfunction. Int J Impot Res 10:69, 1998

NIH Consensus Development Panel on Impotence: NIH Consensus Conference. Impotence. JAMA 270:83, 1993

Shakir SA et al: Cardiovascular events in users of sildenafil: Results from first phase of prescription event monitoring in England. BMJ 322:651, 2001

Virag R et al: Is impotence an arterial disorder? A study of arterial risk factors in 440 impotent men. Lancet 1(8422):181, 1985

Wei M et al: Total cholesterol and high density lipoprotein cholesterol as important predicators of erectile dysfunction. Am J Epidemiol 140:930, 1994

34

SINGLE-PHOTON EMISSION COMPUTED TOMOGRAPHY MYOCARDIAL IMAGING FOR THE DETECTION OF HIBERNATING MYOCARDIUM

Vasken Dilsizian

Paradigms concerning the relationship between myocardial perfusion and left ventricular (LV) function have changed considerably over the past two decades with the introduction of the concept of stunned and hibernating myocardium. These pathophysiologic states have challenged the conventional wisdom that impaired LV function at rest in ischemic heart disease is an irreversible process.

It is now well established that impaired LV function is reversible in patients with stunned or hibernating myocardium and irreversible in patients with scarred or necrotic myocardium. Because improvement in LV function after revascularization is associated with improved survival, diagnostic procedures that identify reversible LV dysfunction prospectively may provide significant prognostic information. Thus, accurate distinction between viable (hibernating or stunned) and scarred (necrotic) myocardium has important clinical implications. Ideally, such information would be used to guide therapeutic decisions for revascularization and risk stratification.

Although a number of strategies have emerged in the literature for differentiating viable from nonviable myocardium, the finding of reduced regional blood flow but preserved cell membrane integrity and/or metabolism (using nuclear techniques) in dysfunctional myocardial regions provides the most direct evidence of myocardial hibernation.

Myocardial Hibernation

The relationship between myocardial perfusion and LV function differs between patients with stunned and hibernating myocardium. *Hibernating myocardium* refers to chronic LV dysfunction arising from prolonged myocardial hypoperfusion, in which myocytes remain viable but contraction is depressed (Rahimtoola, 1985). Although the mechanism responsible for the depressed contractile function has not been established, hibernation is thought to represent an adaptive response of the myocardium (reduced oxygen demand in the setting of reduced oxygen availability) in the absence of clinically evident ischemia. Interventions that favorably alter the supply/demand relationship of the hibernating myocardium—either by improving blood flow or reducing demand—would improve LV function.

Unlike hibernation, *stunning* refers to an injurious rather than an adaptive response of the myocardium, where transient ischemia followed by reperfusion results in LV dysfunction (Braunwald et al., 1982). Thus, in the case of stunning, myocardial perfusion is normal at rest. Intervention aimed at reducing the number, severity, or duration of ischemic episodes (repetitive stunning) should improve LV function. Because the relationship between myocardial perfusion and LV function differs among patients with stunned and hibernating myocardium, this may have significant implications regarding the technique used to assess myocardial viability.

Myocardial Perfusion Imaging

In patients with chronic coronary artery disease and LV dysfunction, myocardial perfusion imaging with single-photon emission computed tomography (SPECT) can identify patients with potentially reversible LV dysfunction. Although the operative risk of coronary artery bypass surgery is increased in this patient population, it is these same individuals who benefit most from revascularization. Short- and long-term surgical survival benefits are greatest in patients with the most severe LV dysfunction (Alderman et al., 1983). Patients with advanced symptomatic coronary artery disease that is not amenable to standard mechanical revascularization strategies present special challenges. Innovative approaches to address ischemia include compounds that promote the growth of new myocardial blood vessels and novel delivery vectors. Recently, recombinant fibroblast growth factor 2 (rFGF-2) was shown to have a favorable therapeutic effect by stimulating angiogenesis in patients with advanced symptomatic coronary artery disease (Udelson et al., 2000).

Assessment of Myocardial Cell Membrane Integrity

Potassium

Uptake of potassium by myocardial cells is dependent on both regional perfusion and cell membrane integrity. Because potassium is the major intracellular cation in muscle and is virtually absent in scar tissue, it is a particularly well-suited radionuclide for differentiating normal and ischemic but viable myocardium from fibrotic or scarred myocardium.

Earlier studies with potassium showed an association between abnormalities in regional potassium metabolism and acute myocardial injury. In animals studied under conditions of normal flow, ischemia, and infarction, a linear relationship was demonstrated between the distribution of potassium 43 and microspheres. These animal studies led to the use of potassium 43 to detect coronary artery disease and myocardial injury. In clinical studies, the combination of exercise treadmill testing with potassium 43 imaging was able to identify patients with angina pectoris and myocardial territories supplied by significantly narrowed coronary arteries (Zaret et al., 1973). However, the relatively high-energy gamma spectrum of potassium 43 (373 to 619 keV) limits image quality and has impeded routine clinical application for detection of coronary artery disease.

Thallium

Thallium 201 has biological properties similar to potassium 43 but with lower photon energy (80 keV mercury x-ray emission) and shorter physical half-life (74 h). Thallium is a monovalent cation that is transported across the myocyte sarcolemmal membrane both by Na^+, K^+-ATPase transport and by facilitative diffusion. The cellular extraction of thallium across the cell membrane is unaffected by hypoxia unless irreversible injury is present. Similarly, pathophysiologic conditions of chronic hypoperfusion (hibernating myocardium) and postischemic dysfunction (stunned myocardium) do not adversely alter extraction of thallium.

While the initial distribution of thallium is primarily a function of blood flow (either during stress or at rest), the later distribution of thallium, termed the *redistribution phase,* is a function of regional blood volume and is unrelated to flow (Pohost et al., 1977). The distribution of viable myocytes and the extent of scarred myocardium are reflected by regional thallium activity on redistribution images, acquired either 2 to 4 h or 8 to 72 h after stress or rest. During the redistribution phase, there is a continuous exchange of thallium between the myocardium and the extracardiac compartments, driven by the concentration gradient of the tracer and myocyte viability. Thus, the extent of defect resolution, from the initial to delayed redistribution images over time, termed *reversible defect,* reflects one index of myocardial viability.

The impact of a rest-redistribution thallium study for identifying viability in an asynergic, underperfused region at rest (hibernation) is outlined in Color Plate 4 (Fig. 34-1) (*upper panel*). When only scarred myocardium is present, the degree of the initial thallium defect persists over time without redistribution; this is termed an *irreversible defect.* When both viable and scarred myocardium are present, thallium redistribution is incomplete, giving the appearance of partial reversibility on delayed images. As a result of its favorable physical and biological properties, thallium has occupied a rather unique place in cardiac diagnostic imaging for both detecting reductions in flow caused by coronary artery narrowing and distinguishing viable from scarred myocardium.

Technetium 99m–Labeled Perfusion Tracers

Despite the excellent myocardial extraction and flow kinetic properties of thallium for evaluating myocardial blood flow and viability, the energy spectrum of thallium is suboptimal, especially in patients with large body habitus. The higher energy spectrum of technetium 99m (140 keV) results in less scatter and soft tissue attenuation with improved spatial resolution when compared to thallium.

Several classes of technetium 99m–labeled complexes have been developed since 1981 for myocardial perfusion imaging. Sestamibi, teboroxime, and tetrofosmin have all received U.S. Food and Drug Administration approval for detection of coronary artery disease. Sestamibi and tetrofosmin have similar myocardial uptake and blood clearance kinetics, but unlike thallium, they do not redistribute significantly over time. Two injections of the tracers are required to image the heart at peak exercise and at rest. There is limited clinical experience using teboroxime and tetrofosmin for the detection of hibernating myocardium. Whether technetium 99m–labeled perfusion tracers also provide similar information to thallium with regards to myocardial perfusion defect size, defect reversibility, and viability in patients with chronic coronary artery disease remains controversial.

Sestamibi

Sestamibi is a lipophilic cationic complex that is taken up across sarcolemmal and mitochondrial membranes of myocytes by passive distribution, but at equilibrium it is retained within the mitochondria due to a large negative transmembrane potential. Despite the recognized metabolic or transmembrane trapping of sestamibi, the relationship between myocardial tracer uptake and blood flow is not significantly altered except during acute myocardial ischemia, conditions of extremely low pH, or hyperemic flow.

Because accumulation and retention of sestamibi are related to energy-dependent processes that maintain mitochondrial membrane polarization, myocardial uptake of sestamibi may also be a marker of cellular viability. However, a growing number of studies suggest that sestamibi underestimates defect reversibility and myocardial viability in patients with chronic coronary artery disease. The potential underestimation of viability may be particularly evident in regions with severe dysfunction or regions supplied by severely stenosed coronary arteries. In view of the limitations of rest-injected sestamibi for assessing myocardial viability, dual-isotope imaging that combines rest-redistribution thallium with stress sestamibi has been proposed (Berman et al., 1993). Others have proposed injection of sestamibi during nitrate infusion, quantitation of regional radiotracer uptake, and/or acquisition of delayed images (Dilsizian et al., 1994).

Metabolic Imaging With SPECT

The principle of using a metabolic tracer is based on the concept that viable myocytes in hypoperfused and dysfunctional regions are metabolically active, while scarred or fibrotic tissue is metabolically inactive. Because fatty acids are the primary source of myocardial energy production in the *fasting state,* early studies focused on the characterization of myocardial kinetics of ^{11}C-palmitate using positron emission tomography (PET). Fatty acid imaging with radioiodine-labeled fatty acid analogues, such as iodophenylpentadecanoic acid (IPPA) and β-methyliodopentadecanoic acid (BMIPP) using SPECT is the subject of ongoing investigations. In the *fed state,* insulin levels increase and result in profound alterations in myocardial metabolism. Glucose metabolism is stimulated, and tissue lipolysis is inhibited, resulting in reduced fatty acid delivery to the myocardium. The combined effects of insulin on these processes and the increased arterial glucose concentration associated with the fed state result in an increase in myocardial glucose uptake.

Breakdown of fatty acids via beta-oxidation in the mitochondria is exquisitely oxygen dependent. Therefore, in the setting of reduced oxygen supply, the myocytes compensate for the loss of oxidative potential by shifting toward greater glucose utilization to generate high-energy phosphates. Although the amount of energy produced by glycolysis may be adequate to maintain myocyte viability and preserve the electrochemical gradient across the cell membrane, it may not be sufficient to sustain contractile function.

^{18}F-Fluorodeoxyglucose

^{18}F-2-fluoro-2-deoxyglucose (FDG) is a glucose analogue that competes with glucose for hexokinase. Once phosphorylated, FDG-6-phosphate does not enter glycolysis, fructose-pentose shunt, or glycogen synthesis. Since the dephosphorylation rate of glucose is slow, FDG becomes essentially trapped in the myocardium, reflecting regional glucose utilization. In the setting of reduced regional blood flow at rest, myocardial glucose utilization may be increased in hibernating but viable myocardium. Thus, increased FDG uptake in asynergic myocardial regions with reduced blood flow at rest has become a scintigraphic marker of hibernation (See Color Plate 4, Fig. 34-1 *lower panel*).

In clinical practice, the pattern of perfusion-metabolism mismatch (reduced blood flow with preserved or enhanced FDG uptake) in an asynergic region is predictive of functional recovery after revascularization. The overall accuracy of FDG mismatch pattern (using PET) for predicting recovery of function after revascularization is in the 80 to 90% (Tillish et al., 1986). The prognostic significance of perfusion-metabolism mismatch pattern has been demonstrated in several nonrandomized, retrospective studies with PET. Patients with perfusion-metabolism mismatch pattern who were treated medically had higher ischemic events and deaths when compared to those treated with revascularization (DiCarli et al., 1994). Patients with matched defects (concordant reduction in regional perfusion and metabolism), indicating scarred myocardium, displayed no such difference in outcomes between medical and surgical management.

In recent years, advances in SPECT technology have made acquisition of high-energy positron emitting tracers such as FDG possible. It is now possible to image FDG with SPECT systems using either high-energy collimators or with coincidence detection capability (Dilsizian et al., 2001).

Clinical Studies in Chronic Ischemic Heart Disease: Hibernation

Among patients with known chronic coronary artery disease and LV dysfunction, if the clinical question is one of myocardial viability, then a rest-redistribution thallium protocol along with quantitative analysis of the severity of the thallium defect may suffice (Ragosta et al., 1993). In most cases, however, the documentation of the presence and extent of myocardial ischemia is much more important clinically in terms of patient management and risk stratification than knowledge of myocardial viability. Regional

LV dysfunction arising from a transient period of myocardial ischemia (repetitive stunning) and/or a prolonged period of myocardial hypoperfusion at rest (hibernation) may be reversible after revascularization, while regional dysfunction arising from transmural myocardial infarction or mixed scarred and viable myocardium may be irreversible after revascularization. The distinction between reversible and irreversible asynergic regions may be accomplished by demonstrating stress-induced ischemia (reversible defect) in regions that are asynergic on the basis of repetitive stunning and/or hibernation, and scar or lack of ischemia (irreversible thallium defect) in regions that are asynergic as a result of transmural infarction or mixed scarred and viable myocardium (Kitsiou et al., 1998). Such a distinction, prospectively, can be accomplished with a stress-redistribution-reinjection thallium protocol (Dilsizian et al., 1990), which provides information regarding myocardial perfusion during stress, regional myocardial blood volume and potassium space, and myocardial perfusion at rest.

Reinjection of thallium at rest after stress-redistribution imaging improves the detection of ischemic but viable myocardium in up to 49% of the apparently irreversible defects on 3- to 4-h redistribution images. When taking into consideration regions with reversible defects (ischemia) and success of revascularization (reexamining regional perfusion or vessel patency after revascularization) stress-redistribution-reinjection thallium imaging yields excellent positive and negative predictive accuracy (80 to 90% range) for recovery of function after revascularization. Patterns of normal, reversible, and irreversible thallium uptake after reinjection correlate well with the magnitude of collagen replacement (See Color Plate 5 (Fig. 34-2), segmental wall thickness, and severity of coronary artery narrowing in patients with chronic ischemic heart disease undergoing heart transplantation (Shirani et al., 2001). The concordance of stress-redistribution-reinjection thallium and FDG metabolic imaging is excellent (up to 88%) when quantitative image analysis is employed (Bonow et al., 1991). However, in regions judged scarred by thallium (severe irreversible defects), metabolic imaging with FDG may provide incremental information regarding myocardial viability, especially in patients with severely impaired LV function in whom the effects of thallium attenuation would be particularly problematic (Srinivasan et al., 1998).

In the future, parallel advances in technology and radiochemistry may permit even more elegant studies of tissue biochemistry in vivo and thereby elucidate further the relationship between myocardial perfusion, function, and metabolism. Such biochemically based studies would enhance our understanding of hibernation, stunning, and other disease processes.

REFERENCES

Alderman EL et al: Results of coronary artery surgery in patients with poor left ventricular function (CASS). Circulation 68:785, 1983

Berman DS et al: Separate acquisition rest thallium-201/stress technetium-99m sestamibi dual-isotope myocardial perfusion single-photon emission computed tomography: A clinical validation study. J Am Coll Cardiol 22:1455, 1993

Bonow RO et al: Identification of viable myocardium in patients with chronic coronary artery disease and left ventricular dysfunction. Comparison of thallium scintigraphy with reinjection and PET imaging with F-18 fluorodeoxyglucose. Circulation 83:26, 1991

Braunwald E, Kloner RA: The stunned myocardium: Prolonged, postischemic ventricular dysfunction. Circulation 66:1146, 1982

DiCarli MF et al: Value of metabolic imaging with positron emission tomography for evaluation prognosis in patients with coronary artery disease and left ventricular dysfunction. Am J Cardiol 73:527, 1994

Dilsizian V et al: Enhanced detection of ischemic but viable myocardium by the reinjection of thallium after stress-redistribution imaging. N Engl J Med 323:141, 1990

Dilsizian V et al: Myocardial viability in patients with chronic coronary artery disease: Comparison of ^{99m}Tc-sestamibi with thallium reinjection and ^{18}F-fluorodeoxyglucose. Circulation 89:578, 1994

Dilsizian V: Perspectives on the study of human myocardium: Viability, *Myocardial Viability: A Clinical and Scientific Treatise*, In V Dilsizian (ed). Armonk, NY, Futura Publishing, 2000

Dilsizian V et al: Fluorine-18-deoxyglucose SPECT and coincidence imaging for myocardial viability: Clinical and technological issues. J Nucl Card 8:75, 2001

Kitsiou AN et al: Stress-induced reversible and mild-to-moderate irreversible thallium defects: Are they equally accurate for predicting recovery of regional left ventricular function after revascularization? Circulation 98:501, 1998

Pohost GM et al: Differentiation of transiently ischemic from infarcted myocardium by serial imaging after a single dose of thallium-201. Circulation 55:294, 1977

Ragosta M et al: Quantitative planar rest-redistribution ^{201}Tl imaging in detection of myocardial viability and prediction of improvement in left ventricular function after coronary artery bypass surgery in patients with severely depressed left ventricular function. Circulation 87: 1630, 1993

Rahimtoola SH: A perspective on the three large multicenter randomized clinical trials of coronary bypass surgery for chronic stable angina. Circulation 72(Suppl V):V-123, 1985

Shirani J et al: Relation of thallium uptake to morphologic features of chronic ischemic heart disease: Evidence for myocardial remodeling in non-infarct myocardium. J Am Coll Cardiol 38:84, 2001

Srinivasan G et al: ^{18}F-fluorodeoxyglucose single photon emission computed tomography: Can it replace PET and thallium SPECT for the assessment of myocardial viability? Circulation 97:843, 1998

Tillish J et al: Reversibility of cardiac wall-motion abnormalities predicted by positron tomography. N Engl J Med 314:884, 1986

Udelson JE et al: Therapeutic angiogenesis with recombinant fibroblast growth factor-2 improves stress and rest myocardial perfusion abnormalities in patients with severe symptomatic chronic coronary artery disease. Circulation 102:1605, 2000

Zaret BL et al: Noninvasive regional myocardial perfusion with radioactive potassium: Study of patients at rest with exercise and during angina pectoris. N Engl J Med 288: 809, 1973

DETECTION OF VULNERABLE CORONARY ARTERY PLAQUE USING MAGNETIC RESONANCE IMAGING

Zahi A. Fayad & Valentin Fuster

Atherosclerotic Plaques

Atherosclerosis is a systemic disease of the vessel wall that occurs in the aorta and in the carotid, coronary, and peripheral arteries (Fuster et al., 1999). The study of atherosclerosis during its natural history and after therapeutic intervention will enhance our understanding of disease progression and regression and aid in the selection of appropriate treatments.

The main components of the atherosclerotic plaques are (1) connective tissue extracellular matrix, including collagen, proteoglycans, and fibronectin elastic fibers; (2) crystalline cholesterol, cholesteryl esters, and phospholipids; and (3) cells such as monocyte-derived macrophages, T lymphocytes, and smooth-muscle cells. Varying proportions of these components occur in different plaques, thus giving rise to a spectrum of lesions. For example, rupture-prone plaques, the so-called vulnerable plaques in the coronary arteries, tend to have a thin fibrous cap with a large lipid core; often acute ischemic coronary syndromes result from the rupture of a modestly stenotic coronary artery vulnerable plaque.

Among the imaging techniques employed to assess atherosclerotic plaques in humans, high-resolution magnetic resonance (MR) has emerged as the leading in vivo modality (Pohost et al., 1998).

Imaging Techniques

Several invasive imaging techniques such as x-ray angiography, intravascular ultrasound, angioscopy, and optical coherence tomography can be applied to evaluate atherosclerotic vessels; as can noninvasive techniques such as surface B-mode ultrasound and ultrafast computed tomography. Most of these techniques identify luminal diameter, stenosis, wall thickness, and plaque volume; however, none can characterize plaque composition and therefore identify the high-risk or vulnerable plaques (Fayad et al., 2000a, 2001a and b).

Magnetic Resonance Imaging

Introduction

MR differentiates plaque components on the basis of biophysical and biochemical parameters such as chemical composition and concentration, water content, physical state, molecular motion, or diffusion. MR provides imaging without ionizing radiation and thus can be repeated sequentially over time.

Most MR studies are of the hydrogen nuclei (protons) in water as hydrogen is the simplest and most abundant element in the human body. During the examination, the patient is subjected to a high local magnetic field, usually 1.5 tesla, which aligns the protons in the body. These protons (or spins) are excited by a radiofrequency pulse and subsequently detected by receiver coils. Detected signals are influenced by such factors as the relaxation times (T1 and T2); proton density, motion, and flow; molecular diffusion; magnetization transfer; changes in susceptibility. Three additional magnetic fields (gradient fields) are applied during MR imaging: one selects the slice and two encode spatial information. The timing of the excitation pulses and the successive magnetic field gradients determine the image contrast. The ability to obtain images of the atherosclerotic vessels is dependent on the amount of available signal, contrast, and the lack of noise.

The MR images can be "weighted" to the T1, T2, or proton density values through manipulation of the MR parameters (i.e., repetition time and echo time). In a T1-weighted (T1W) image, tissues with low T1 values are displayed as hyperintense picture elements, or pixels (high signal intensity), and conversely, high T1 values are displayed as hypointense pixels (low signal intensity). In a T2W image, tissues with high T2 values are perceived as hyperintense pixels and those with low T2 values as hypointense pixels. Thus, a T1W and a T2W image of the same anatomy can appear quite different since an MR image is not a photograph but a computed map of radio signals emitted by the body. Finally, a proton density–weighted (PDW) image is an image where the differences in contrast are proportional to the density of water and fat protons within the tissue. It is also referred to as an intermediate-weighted image because the contrast in the image is a combination of mild T1 and T2 contrast.

Multicontrast MR Plaque Imaging

The advancements of MR imaging realized the possibilities of high resolution and contrast imaging and fostered the study of different plaque components using multicontrast MR generated by T1W, T2W, and PDW (Fayad et al., 2000a, 2001a

TABLE 35-1

PLAQUE CHARACTERIZATION WITH MAGNETIC RESONANCE

	Relative MR signal intensity[a]		
	T1W	**PDW**	**T2W**
Calcium	Hypointense	Very hypointense	Very hypointense
Lipid	Very hyperintense	Hyperintense	Hypointense
Fibrous	Isointense to slightly hyperintense	Isointense to slightly hyperintense	Isointense to slightly hyperintense
Thrombus[b]	Variable	Variable	Variable

[a]Relative to that of immediately adjacent muscle tissue.
[b]In some cases surface irregularities; the variable signal intensity may be due to the thrombus age.
ABBREVIATIONS: T1W and T2W, T1 and T2 weighted; PDW, proton density weighted.

and b). Atherosclerotic plaque characterization by MR is based on the signal intensities (Table 35-1) and morphologic appearance of the plaque on T1W, PDW, and T2W images as previously validated (Shinnar et al., 1999; Fayad et al., 2000c; Rogers et al., 2000; Worthley et al., 2000a; Fayad et al., 2001a and b).

Coronary Artery Plaque Studies

Previous studies have revealed that in vivo MR imaging can characterize the atherosclerotic plaque in the carotid arteries (Toussaint et al., 1996; Yuan et al., 1998; Hatsukami et al., 2000) (Fig. 35-1) and aorta (Fayad et al., 2000c) (Fig. 35-2). However, the ultimate goal is the imaging of plaque in vivo in the coronary arteries. Preliminary studies in a pig model proclaimed that the difficulties of coronary wall imaging are due to the combination of cardiac and respiratory motion artifacts, as well as the nonlinear course, small size, and location of the coronary arteries (Worthley et al., 2000a and b).

The black-blood MR methods used in the human carotid artery and aorta were extended for imaging of the coronary arterial lumen and wall (Fayad et al., 2000b). This method was validated in swine coronary

lesions induced by balloon angioplasty (Worthley et al., 2000a and b). The intra- and interobserver variability assessment by intraclass correlation for both MR imaging and histopathology showed good reproducibility, with the intraclass correlation coefficients ranging from 0.96 to 0.99. MR imaging was also able to visualize intralesion hematoma (sensitivity 82%, specificity 84%).

High-resolution black-blood MR of both normal and atherosclerotic human coronary arteries was performed. The difference in maximum wall thickness between the normal subjects and patients (40% stenosis) was statistically significant. Fig. 35-3 shows an in vivo MR image of a patient with a plaque in the left anterior descending coronary artery. The coronary MR plaque imaging study was performed during breath-holding to minimize respiratory motion (Fayad et al., 2000b). To alleviate the need for breath-holding, another group combined the black-blood fast spin echo method and a real-time navigator for respiratory gating and real-time slice-position correction (Botnar et al., 2000). Further studies are necessary to identify the different plaque components and to assess the lesions of asymptomatic patients and their outcomes.

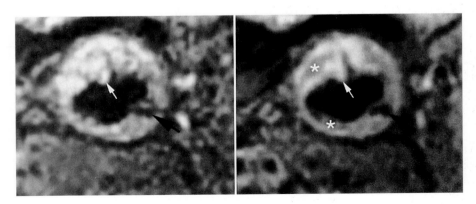

FIGURE 35-1

A 67-year-old male with atherosclerotic disease in the common carotid artery imaged with in vivo high-resolution MR. Multicontrast (T1W, PDW, and T2W) MR images are obtained to characterize all the plaque components. *(A)* T1W image; *(B)* T2W image. A complex lesion is detected with a fissure (at 12 o'clock), calcium (black arrows), lipid deposits (*), and thrombus (white arrows).

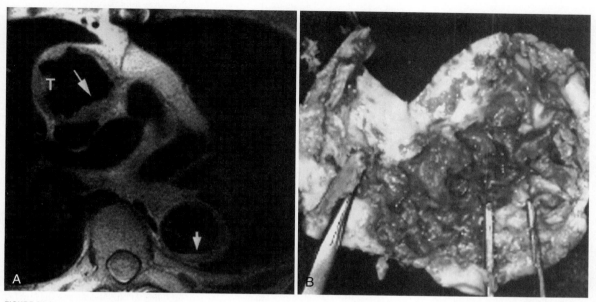

FIGURE 35-2

(A) T2-weighted magnetic resonance (MR) images from a patient with disease in both the ascending and descending thoracic aorta. Plaque characterization was based on the information obtained from T1-, proton density–, and T2-weighted MR images. This shows a severely thrombotic plaque with a very irregular surface and increased wall thickness in the ascending aorta. A thrombus (T) in the arterial lumen is also shown. In the descending aorta a fibrous-rich plaque, with increased wall thickness (arrow) is present. *(B)* The gross pathology of the ascending aorta collected post surgery confirms the presence of thrombus.

In vivo Monitoring of Therapy with MR Imaging

As shown in experimental studies (Skinner et al., 1995; Fayad et al., 1998, McConnell et al., 1999; Worthley et al., 2000c), MR is a powerful tool used to investigate serially and noninvasively the progression and regression of atherosclerotic lesions in vivo. It has been shown recently that MR can be employed to measure the effect of lipid-lowering therapy (statins) in asymptomatic untreated hypercholesterolemic patients with carotid and aortic atherosclerosis (Corti et al., 2001). Atherosclerotic plaques were assessed with MR at different time points after initiation of lipid-lowering therapy. Significant regression of atherosclerotic lesions was observed. Despite the early and expected hypolipidemic effect of the statins, a minimum of 12 months was needed to observe changes in the vessel wall; no changes were detected at 6 months. In agreement with previous experimental studies, there was a decrease in the vessel wall area and no change in the lumen area at 12 months (McConnell et al., 1999; Worthley et al., 2000c).

MR imaging of the popliteal artery and its response to balloon angioplasty has been reported (Coulden et al., 2000). The extent of plaque could be defined in all patients; even in segments of vessel that were angiographically normal, atherosclerotic lesions with cross-sectional areas ranging from 4 to 76% of potential lumen area were identified. Following angioplasty, plaque fissuring and local dissection were easily detected as were serial changes in lumen diameter, blood flow, and lesion size. This study illustrated that MR imaging can define the extent of atherosclerotic plaque in the peripheral vasculature

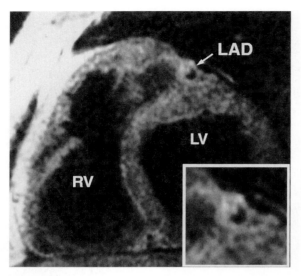

FIGURE 35-3

In vivo MR image of a patient with a plaque (arrow) in the left anterior descending artery (LAD). The insert represents a magnified view of the large eccentric LAD plaque with heterogeneous signal intensity. The MR images are acquired using a long-echo train fast-spin echo sequence with velocity-selective flow suppression during suspended respiration (<16 s). The in-plane spatial resolution was 450 μm and slice thickness was 3 mm. RV, right ventricle; LV, left ventricle. (Adapted from Fayad et al. 2000.)

and demonstrate the remodeling and restenosis following angioplasty.

Conclusions

Assessment of atherosclerotic plaques by imaging techniques is essential for in vivo identification of vulnerable plaques. Several invasive and noninvasive imaging techniques are available. Most techniques identify luminal diameter or stenosis, wall thickness, and plaque volume and are ineffective in identifying the high-risk plaques that are vulnerable to rupture and thrombosis. In vivo, high-resolution, multicontrast, MR imaging holds the best promise of noninvasively imaging high-risk plaques. MR allows serial assessment of progression and regression of atherosclerosis. Application of MR imaging opens new areas for diagnosis, prevention, and treatment (e.g., lipid-lowering drug regimens) of atherosclerosis in all arterial locations.

REFERENCES

Botnar RM et al: Noninvasive coronary vessel wall and plaque imaging with magnetic resonance imaging. Circulation 102:2582, 2000

Corti R et al: Effects of lipid-lowering by simvastatin on human atherosclerotic lesions: A longitudinal study by high-resolution, noninvasive magnetic resonance imaging. Circulation 104:249, 2001

Coulden RA et al: High resolution magnetic resonance imaging of atherosclerosis and the response to balloon angioplasty. Heart 83:188, 2000

Fayad ZA et al: Noninvasive in vivo high-resolution magnetic resonance imaging of atherosclerotic lesions in genetically engineered mice. Circulation 98:1541, 1998

Fayad ZA et al: Characterization of atherosclerotic plaques by magnetic resonance imaging. Ann N Y Acad Sci 902:173, 2000a

Fayad ZA et al: Noninvasive in vivo human coronary artery lumen and wall imaging using black-blood magnetic resonance imaging. Circulation 102:506, 2000b

Fayad ZA et al: In vivo MR evaluation of atherosclerotic plaques in the human thoracic aorta: A comparison with TEE. Circulation 101:2503, 2000c

Fayad ZA et al: Clinical imaging of the high-risk or vulnerable atherosclerotic plaque. Circ Res 2001; 89:305-316

Fayad ZA et al: The human high-risk plaque and its detection by magnetic resonance imaging. Am J Cardiol 88(2 Suppl 1):42, 2001b

Fuster V et al: Acute coronary syndromes: Biology. Lancet 353 (Suppl 2):SII5–9, 1999

Hatsukami TS et al: Visualization of fibrous cap thickness and rupture in human atherosclerotic carotid plaque in vivo with high-resolution magnetic resonance imaging. Circulation 102:959, 2000

McConnell MV et al: MRI of rabbit atherosclerosis in response to dietary cholesterol lowering. Arterioscler Thromb Vasc Biol 19:1956, 1999

Pohost GM et al: From the microscope to the clinic: MR assessment of atherosclerotic plaque. Circulation 98:1477, 1998

Rogers WJ et al: Characterization of signal properties in atherosclerotic plaque components by intravascular MRI. Arterioscler Thromb Vasc Biol 20:1824, 2000

Shinnar M et al: The diagnostic accuracy of ex vivo magnetic resonance imaging for human atherosclerotic plaque characterization. Arterioscler Thromb Vasc Biol 19:2756, 1999

Skinner MP et al: Serial magnetic resonance imaging of experimental atherosclerosis detects lesion fine structure, progression and complications in vivo. Nat Med 1:69, 1995

Toussaint JF et al: Magnetic resonance images lipid, fibrous, calcified, hemorrhagic, and thrombotic components of human atherosclerosis in vivo. Circulation 94:932, 1996

Worthley SG et al: High resolution ex vivo magnetic resonance imaging of in situ coronary and aortic atherosclerotic plaque in a porcine model. Atherosclerosis 150:321, 2000a

Worthley SG et al: Noninvasive in vivo magnetic resonance imaging of experimental coronary artery lesions in a porcine model. Circulation 101:2956, 2000b

Worthley SG et al: Serial evaluation of atherosclerosis with in vivo MRI: Study of atorvastatin and avasimibe in WHHL rabbits. Circulation 102:II-809, 2000c

Yuan C et al: Measurement of atherosclerotic carotid plaque size in vivo using high resolution magnetic resonance imaging. Circulation 98:2666, 1998

ELECTRON BEAM TOMOGRAPHY FOR EARLY DETECTION OF CORONARY HEART DISEASE

Tracy Q. Callister & Paolo Raggi

Rationale

In the asymptomatic population, event rates from coronary heart disease (CHD) remain unacceptably high even though the concept of "risk factor" has been entrenched in the minds of both the population at large and the medical community. Data from the literature suggest that approximately 40% of all hard cardiac events (myocardial infarction and death) occur in the top 20% of the population at risk and that almost no events occur in the 10% of the population with no known risk factors. Consequently, the remaining 70% of the population, at low to intermediate risk, suffers nearly 60% of the hard events. This middle group requires careful risk stratification strategies beyond the scope offered by current techniques. To this end, investigators' attention has recently focused on new technologies for the early detection of CHD.

Over the past two decades, computed tomography (CT) and magnetic resonance have emerged as the premier imaging modalities for the human body. The application of these tools to cardiac imaging has been severely limited by motion artifacts. At a heart rate of 60 beats per minute, the heart completes an entire cycle of contraction, torsion, and relaxation in 1 s. The coronary arteries are presented as small moving targets that cannot be visualized without subsecond scanning times. Electron beam tomography (EBT) has the capability of acquiring CT images in one-tenth of a second (100 ms). At this speed, the coronary arteries are clearly seen and arterial calcification, a marker of atherosclerosis, is easily visualized and its extent quantified (Fig. 36-1). Modern multihead, helical CTs now also approach scan times of 250 to 750 ms, producing clear images of the coronary arteries.

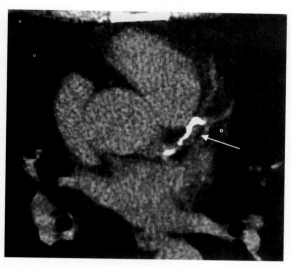

FIGURE 36-1

Electron beam tomography image of the heart obtained in the axial view showing a calcified plaque in the left anterior descending coronary artery (arrow).

Technical Considerations

EBT (formerly ultrafast CT) utilizes a fourth-generation computerized imaging process that does not require a moving x-ray source (Fig. 36-2). A beam of electrons emitted from a stationary source is swept by electromagnets across a 210° arc of tungsten placed below the patient. This creates a fan of x-rays that passes through the body to an opposing 210° ring of detectors located directly above the patient. The acquisition of each image slice is triggered by the electrocardiogram, and imaging occurs during mid-diastole when the heart motion is at a minimum. One image is acquired per heartbeat. To limit chest motion, patients are asked to hold their breath for the 30 to 40 s required to complete the entire examination.

In western countries, changes in the arterial walls begin very early in life. The Pathobiological Determinants of Atherosclerosis in Youth Study examined necropsy data from 2876 subjects between the ages

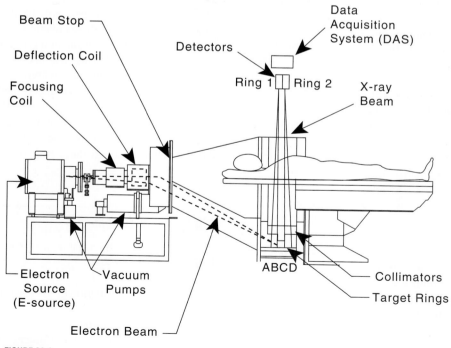

FIGURE 36-2

Diagram of the configuration and function of an electron beam tomography scanner.

of 14 and 34 (Strong et al., 1999). Almost all males between 30 and 34 years of age had fatty deposits, 50% were found to have fibrous plaque, and 3% had calcified lesions. Questions exist about the differing advantages of imaging each of these deposit materials. Cardiac EBT can image only the calcified portions of the complex plaque matrix and this is a potential limitation, as noncalcified and lipid-rich lesions prone to rupture are not visualized. However, any test with "abnormal" results in 50 to 100% of a very young population would clearly be too nonspecific to be useful.

While it appears true that the calcified regions are often stable regions, calcific deposits in the coronary artery walls are invariably associated with the presence of advanced stages of atherosclerosis. Calcium is not an aging phenomenon as it is found even in children with severe familial hyperlipidemias. Rather, it reflects a healing response to the hemorrhage and inflammation caused by the continuing process of plaque rupture and repair (Stary, 2000). The process of coronary calcification is currently believed to be an active process of mineral deposition resembling bone formation, which occurs in response to oxidization injury of the vascular intimal layer (Wexler, 1996).

EBT not only identifies the presence of calcium but also can accurately quantify the extent of calcification, which correlates closely with the total plaque burden (Sangiorgi et al., 1998). To be able to follow the current literature as well as interpret individual patient results requires a basic understanding of at least three quantification techniques: calcium scores, age-sex percentiles, and calcium volumes.

The calcium score is the most common of the three and has been widely used in research and clinical trials (Agatston et al., 1990). It is a unitless number derived by multiplying the summed area of calcification by an arbitrarily chosen density coefficient rated 1 to 4. Repeated comparisons with autopsy data suggest that this score may be interpreted as representing the extent of advanced atherosclerosis present. A score of 0 suggests absence of advanced plaque, while 1 to 99 is considered evidence for the presence of mild, 100 to 400 moderate, and >400 extensive, atherosclerotic disease.

The calcium score distribution is nonuniform and varies widely with both age and gender. The presence of calcium and the mean total calcium score in women is essentially half of that in men until age 60 when the difference rapidly diminishes; by age 65, it becomes virtually identical. By utilizing large databases of patients screened with EBT, it is possible to construct tables of age-sex percentiles. These results rank individuals against matched populations, suggesting an "anatomic age" for their coronary arteries. While a calcium score of 50 would be very common in a 65-year-old male, it would be very rare in a 45-year-old female, placing her at >99th percentile. Table 36-1, an age-sex nomogram of calcium score percentiles, can be used to classify patients based on the extent of their atherosclerotic advancement compared to the expected norm. A >75th age-sex percentile suggests rapid plaque growth and has been associated with an increased risk of a hard cardiac event.

The traditional calcium score has inherent weaknesses. Stable plaques will not change in area but will increase in density as they age. On the other hand, new and expanding plaques will have an increased area of calcification while maintaining a relatively low density. As the traditional calcium score combines the plaque area and the density data into a single abstract number, it becomes difficult to follow changes over time in these divergent measurements. For this reason, direct measurements of the volume of a calcified plaque have been shown to be more reliable (Callister et al., 1998). Calcium volumes are given in hundredths of mm^3 and may range from 0 to >4000.

Clinical Applications

Currently cardiac EBT is being used for the following indications:

1. Detection of subclinical disease in asymptomatic individuals
2. Chest pain evaluation
3. Tracking the progression of the coronary atherosclerotic process

TABLE 36-1

CALCIUM SCORE NOMOGRAM FOR 9728 CONSECUTIVE SUBJECTS

Percentile	Age						
	35–39	40–44	45–49	50–54	55–59	60–64	65–70
Men							
(5433)	(479)	(859)	(1066)	(1085)	(853)	(613)	(478)
25	0	0	0	0	3	14	28
50	0	0	3	16	41	118	151
75	2	11	44	101	187	434	569
90	21	64	176	320	502	804	1178
Women							
(4295)	(288)	(589)	(822)	(903)	(693)	(515)	(485)
25	0	0	0	0	0	0	0
50	0	0	0	0	0	4	24
75	0	0	0	10	33	87	123
90	4	9	23	66	140	310	362

(number of subjects)

Despite the growing interest on the part of the medical and popular communities for new diagnostic tools, many question if there is adequate evidence to support these applications.

Pathologic and EBT findings closely agree on the prevalence of arterial calcifications; coronary calcification seen on the cardiac images of 1242 hearts correlated well (r = 0.97) with the prevalence of atherosclerosis in pathologic specimens of patients of the same age and sex. Serial sectioning of the coronary arteries in autopsied hearts demonstrated that the correlation of calcium with the extent of plaque burden is very high (r > 0.9). These findings were expanded by researchers who demonstrated that the extent of coronary artery calcium, estimated by means of calcium scores, correlates closely with the severity of coronary artery disease detected at angiography. Indeed, recent studies have shown that EBT findings are more predictive of angiographic luminal stenosis than known risk factors for CHD.

Beyond identification of coronary atherosclerosis, EBT may be useful for stratifying asymptomatic as well as symptomatic patients for the risk of developing cardiac events. In a recent publication, the severity of calcification was predictive of the presence of silent myocardial ischemia as detected by stress perfusion tomography (He et al., 2000). In this study, He and colleagues reported the results of 411 asymptomatic patients who were submitted to sequential EBT and single-photon emission CT imaging. Of the patients with calcium scores >400, 46% demonstrated significant inducible perfusion defects (Table 36-2). Arad and colleagues conducted an

TABLE 36-2

CALCIUM SCORES VS. SPECT[A] FINDINGS OF SILENT MYOCARDIAL ISCHEMIA IN 411 ASYMPTOMATIC PATIENTS

Calcium Score	Abnormal SPECT, %
0–10	0
11–100	2.6
101–400	11.3
>400	46

[a]SPECT, single-photon emission computed tomography.
SOURCE: From Zx He et al: Circulation 101:244, 2000.

outcome analysis of 1173 asymptomatic patients (mean age, 53 ± 11 years) followed for a mean of 19 months from the time of EBT screening (Arad et al., 1996). Eighteen patients experienced a total of 26 events. The presence of coronary artery calcification was the strongest predictor of any adverse event. The sensitivity, specificity, negative predictive value, and odds of an event with a calcium score >160 were 89, 82, 99, and 35.4%, respectively. The same investigators continued to follow their patients and reported on the outcome of 1172 subjects followed for an average of 3.6 years (Arad et al., 2000). Again, an absolute calcium score >160 at screening was associated with high likelihood of suffering a soft (odds ratio: 15.8) or a hard event (odds ratio: 20.2). While these studies were challenged for combining both hard and soft (revascularization) events, the authors concluded that coronary artery calcium was a significantly better predictor of subsequent events than the traditional risk factors listed in the National Cholesterol Education Program II guidelines.

A more recent cohort study further examined the ability of EBT screening to identify asymptomatic patients at increased risk of myocardial infarction and cardiac death (Raggi et al., 2000). Primary care physicians selected 632 patients (mean age, 53 ± 8 years) as being at moderate risk and referred them for EBT screening. After a mean follow-up of 3 years the investigators recorded 27 hard events. In this analysis, coronary calcification was more preva-

lent in patients with hard events than in those without (96% of 8 fatal and 19 nonfatal infarctions vs. 50% in patients without events) and therefore predictive. While patients with high calcium scores carried increased risk, not all events occurred at high scores. In fact, nearly two-thirds of events occurred among patients with mild or moderate scores. However, after using a nomogram to convert the individual calcium scores to age- and sex-specific centiles (Table 36-1), it became evident that patients with high percentiles were at higher risk of events irrespective of the total calcium score. The authors concluded that a high age-sex percentile (>75th percentile) conferred a significant risk and might indicate the presence of an accelerated atherosclerotic process.

Several investigators have submitted patients with atypical chest pain symptoms and no evidence of acute ischemia to EBT screening upon arrival in the emergency department. Georgiou and colleagues conducted a prospective study of 192 such patients followed for an average of 50 ± 10 months from the time of EBT imaging (Georgiou et al., 2001). The presence of coronary calcium and increasing score values were strongly related to the occurrence of hard events ($p < .001$) and all cardiovascular events ($p < .001$). The patients with the highest scores had a relative risk of 13.1 for new cardiovascular events as compared to patients with calcium scores in the lowers quartile ranks ($p < .001$). The annualized cardiovascular event rate was 0.6% for subjects with a score of 0, compared with 13.9% per year for the patients with a calcium score >400 ($p < .001$).

Tracking CHD Progression

An attractive application of EBT imaging for both research and patient care is the noninvasive tracking of CHD progression. Serial angiographic studies have demonstrated that among patients in whom drug therapy resulted in lesion stabilization, cardiovascular event rates were significantly reduced. Calcium volume scores, which provide more stability on repeat analyses (overcoming the poor reproducibility of traditional calcium scores), were used in a study of

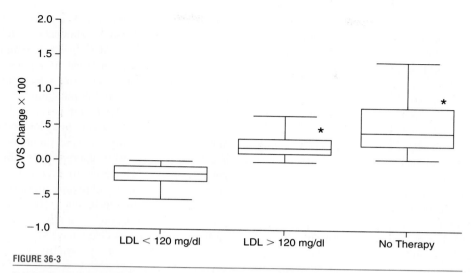

FIGURE 36-3

Relative change in calcium volume score (CVS) in one year in patients treated aggressively with lipid-lowering therapy (mean LDL, <120 mg/dL), patients treated less aggressively (mean LDL, >120 mg/dL) and untreated patients (LDL = low density lipoprotein cholesterol, * = p < 0.05 compared to LDL < 120 mg/dl).

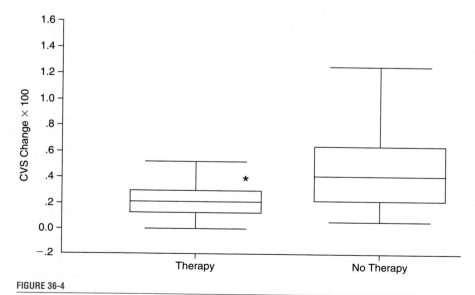

FIGURE 36-4

Relative change in calcium volume score (CVS) in one year in patients treated with lipid-lowering therapy but with inadequate lowering of low density lipoprotein cholesterol (mean LDL = 140 mg/dL) and untreated patients with similar average LDL level.* p = <0.05, compared to no therapy.

149 patients referred by primary physicians for CHD screening (Callister et al., 1998). All patients were asymptomatic and had coronary artery calcification on the baseline EBT study. Initiation of HmG-CoA reductase inhibitors was left to the discretion of the referring physician, and EBT scanning was repeated after 12 months. Figure 36-3 summarizes the outcome in patients treated aggressively with lipid-lowering therapy [low-density lipoprotein (LDL) <3.1 mmol/L (<120 mg/dL)], patients treated more moderately [LDL >3.1 mmol/L (>120 mg/dL)], and untreated patients [mean LDL, 3.6 mmol/L (140 mg/dL)]. The change over time in the calcium volume score was proportional to the degree of aggressiveness with which medical therapy was applied (mean −7 ± 22, 25 ± 22, and 52 ± 36%, respectively). In a comparison of score progression between treated and untreated patients matched for the same LDL levels during the follow-up period [3.6 mmol/L (140 mg/dL)], calcium progression was significantly greater in the untreated group, indicating that slowing of CHD can be obtained even when insufficient therapy is applied (Fig. 36-4). Similarly, another group noted slowing of disease progression in a group of patients treated with HmG-CoA reductase inhibitors compared to untreated patients (15 ± 8% treated vs. 39 ± 12% untreated; $p < .001$) (Budott et al., 2000). These observations may bear important prognostic information if continued accumulation of coronary calcium can be shown to be a harbinger of adverse cardiac events. In two recent abstracts, the incidence of coronary events has been shown to be much greater in patients with continued growth of coronary calcification on sequential EBT scans than in patients where halting of the disease could be demonstrated (Raggi et al., 1999; Shah et al., 2000) See Color Plate 6, Fig. 36-5. Events occurred even in the presence of adequate therapy when vascular calcification continued to progress at rapid rates.

Until recently, only the pathologist knew the state of an individual patient's arteries. As cardiac CT (both EBT and multihead helical scanners) become increasingly available, clinicians will have access to similar knowledge. Although still controversial, the data strongly suggest that the presence of coronary calcium has both diagnostic and prognostic signifi-

cance, predicting future events and the probability of silent ischemia. Measured amounts of calcium correspond to the presence and extent of plaque burden, while a negative test represents a very low risk state. It is alarming that death from CHD presents frequently in an undetected population. Morbidity and mortality due to CHD might be reduced by 30 to 50% if smoking cessation, lipid-lowering therapy, angiotensin-converting enzyme inhibitors, aspirin, and beta blockers were appropriately offered to all patients at risk. However, to accomplish this in a cost-effective manner will require improved detection and risk-stratification techniques. The field of atherosclerotic plaque imaging is rapidly evolving, and the early identification of CHD in asymptomatic individuals may provide an opportunity to reduce both events and cost.

REFERENCES

Agatston AS et al: Quantification of coronary artery calcium using ultrafast computed tomography. J Am Coll Cardiol 15:827, 1990

Arad Y et al: Predictive value of electron beam computed tomography of the coronary arteries: 19-month follow-up of 1173 asymptomatic subjects. Circulation 93:1951, 1996

Arad Y et al: Prediction of coronary events with electron beam computed tomography. J Am Coll Cardiol 36:1253, 2000

Budoff MJ et al: Rates of progression of coronary calcium by electron beam tomography. Am J Cardiol 86:8, 2000

Callister TQ et al: Effect of HMG-CoA reductase inhibitors on coronary artery disease as assessed by electron-beam computed tomography. N Engl J Med 339:1972, 1998

Georgiou D et al: Screening patients with chest pain in the emergency department using electron beam tomography: A follow-up study. J Am Coll Cardiol 38:105, 2001

Guerci A et al: Comparison of electron beam computed tomography and conventional risk factors assessment for the prediction of angiographic coronary artery disease. J Am Coll Cardiol 32:673, 1998

He ZX et al: Severity of coronary artery calcification by electron beam computed tomography predicts silent myocardial ischemia. Circulation 101:244, 2000

Raggi P et al: Cardiac events in patients with progression of coronary calcification on electron beam computed tomography (abstr.). Radiology 213: 351, 1999

Raggi P et al: Identification of patients at increased risk of first unheralded acute myocardial infarction by electron beam computed tomography. Circulation 101:850, 2000

Sangiorgi G et al: Arterial calcification and not lumen stenosis is highly correlated with atherosclerotic plaque burden in humans: A histologic study of 723 coronary artery segments using non-decalcifying methodology. J Am Coll Cardiol 31:126, 1998

Shah A et al: Cardiac events and progression of coronary calcium score using electron beam tomography (abstr.). Circulation 102:II-604, 2000

Stary HC: Natural history of calcium deposits in atherosclerosis progression and regression. Z Kardiol 89:28, 2000

Strong J et al: Prevalence and extent of atherosclerosis in adolescent and young adults. Implications for prevention from the Pathobiological Determinants of Atherosclerosis in Youth Study. JAMA 281:727, 1999

Wexler L et al: Coronary artery calcification: Pathophysiology, epidemiology, imaging methods, and clinical implications. A statement for health professionals from the American Heart Association. Circulation 94:1175, 1996

THE HEART OUTCOMES PREVENTION EVALUATION (HOPE) STUDY, TESTING RAMIPRIL AND/OR VITAMIN E IN SUBJECTS AT HIGH RISK OF CARDIOVASCULAR EVENTS

Peter Sleight

Introduction

The HOPE study tested two plausible preventive measures, vitamin E (400 IU/d) and/or the angiotensin-converting enzyme (ACE) inhibitor ramipril (titrated up to 10 mg/d) or matching placebos in high-risk subjects. The high risk was determined by (1) age >55 years; (2) known vascular disease; or (3) diabetes plus one other risk factor: blood pressure >140/90 mmHg, serum cholesterol >5.2 mmol (>200 mg/dL); microalbuminuria, or cigarette smoking. Exclusion criteria were: uncontrolled hypertension, impaired left ventricular function or heart failure, or existing treatment with an ACE inhibitor or vitamin E.

After observational studies on the use of vitamin E in health professionals there was much interest in the possibility that an antioxidant might reduce risk (Stampfer et al., 1993; Steinberg, 1992). Similarly,

there has been growing interest in the possibility that ACE inhibitors might be protective by some actions unrelated to blood pressure lowering. These include improvement in endothelial function or plaque stabilization as a result of reductions in tissue, as opposed to serum, angiotensin II levels (Davies, 1998; Mancini et al., 1996).

Retrospective analysis of previous studies of ACE inhibition in heart failure such as SOLVD (SOLVD Investigators, 1991, 1992) and SAVE (Pfeffer et al., 1992) had shown an unexpected reduction in myocardial infarction in patients with left ventricular dysfunction (Garg and Yusuf, 1995).

The initial three papers from the HOPE investigators were published recently (The Heart Outcomes Prevention Evaluation Study Investigators, 2000a,b,c). Two articles describe the main results of the vitamin E and ACE inhibitor (ramipril) arms of the study, while the third describes the results of these interventions in the large diabetic subgroup. A series of more detailed analyses has now been published.

The first, SECURE (Study to Evaluate Carotid Ultrasound changes in patients treated with Ramipril and vitamin E), was a substudy of HOPE that followed the progression of carotid atheroma and intima-media thickening in about 750 patients who were randomized to placebo or a high (10 mg) or low (2.5 mg) dose of ramipril in a factorial 3×2 design with vitamin E or placebo, as in the main HOPE study. Progression was significantly reduced only by the 10-mg dose of ramipril (Lonn et al., 2000), despite the fact that the lower and higher doses caused identical falls in blood pressure. This extra benefit, which appeared unrelated to blood pressure change, led to examination of the extent to which the small fall in blood pressure seen in the HOPE study with ramipril (3.3/1.4 mmHg) could account for the large benefits. It was concluded that the blood pressure reduction accounts for no more than about one-third of the benefit.

This chapter synthesizes these results and suggests that the indications for ACE inhibition should now be considerably expanded beyond their current use in hypertension, left ventricular dysfunction, and diabetics with microalbuminuria. These new studies indicate that ramipril substantially reduces the risk of death, stroke, and myocardial infarction in a wide range of patients with normal blood pressure and normal left ventricular function.

Patients currently receiving aspirin for secondary prevention could also benefit from ACE inhibition; the benefits or ramipril in the HOPE study were additive to, and independent of, those seen with proven drugs such as aspirin, lipid-lowering agents, and drugs for the treatment of hypertension (diuretics, beta blockers, and/or calcium channel blockers).

Methods

Eligible patients were recruited in 129 centers in 19 countries from North and South America and Europe. The study was designed and coordinated from the office of the Canadian Cardiovascular Collaboration, McMaster University. In all, 10,576 initially eligible patients first entered a run-in period on 2.5 mg of active ramipril for 7 to 10 days. This was to test compliance and also to eliminate those who had adverse effects on blood pressure, serum creatinine, or potassium. Around 1000 patients were excluded at this stage, but of these only about 150 were because of side effects (hypotension, dizziness, cough) or from abnormal electrolytes or creatinine. The vast majority were due to noncompliance or were patients who had second thoughts about continuing in a 5-year study. The study excluded patients with known left ventricular dysfunction or with uncontrolled blood pressure (except the diabetic cohort, where hypertension was one of the eligibility risk factors). The remaining 9641 subjects were then allocated to ramipril or placebo, beginning with a titration phase of 2.5 mg/d for 1 week, 5 mg/d for 3 weeks, and 10 mg/d thereafter.

The SECURE substudy randomized around 750 patients to vitamin E/placebo as above, but additionally to a high (10 mg) and low (2.5 mg) dose of ramipril or placebo in a 3×2 factorial design. Carefully standardized carotid ultrasound measurements (12 measures each time) were repeated every 6 months to measure intima-media thickness and plaque progression. SECURE also measured left ventricular volume and thickness by ultrasound.

Analysis of Changes in Blood Pressure

The relation between baseline blood pressure, change in blood pressure, and risk were analyzed using Cox multiple regression analysis in HOPE, MicroHOPE, and SECURE. In a further unpublished analysis, the benefits in HOPE were related to the "usual" quartiles of systolic and diastolic blood pressures (i.e., allowing for regression to the mean from the baseline measures). Systolic pressure was measured in duplicate (with a 5-mm gap) by arm cuff sphygmomanometry in a standard way, after sitting for 10 min, as in many previous epidemiologic studies or clinical trials of hypertension treatment. To avoid digit preference the baseline blood pressure was divided into quartiles. The "usual" blood pressures in these quartiles was obtained by calculating the mean blood pressure for all measurements in these quartiles in the placebo group over the whole trial period. The regression dilution factor (RDF) was calculated for the placebo group as the ratio of the spread of the average blood pressure between the top to bottom quartiles at baseline, and that in the same subjects at 2 years. The slope of the baseline blood pressure/risk relation over these quartiles was then multiplied by 1.9 (the RDF) to obtain the steeper relation between risk and "usual" blood pressure in the quartiles of systolic blood pressure and diastolic blood pressure.

Results

The main HOPE results have been published (The HOPE Investigators, 2000a,b,c). The patient population randomized in the HOPE study had a mean age of 66 years and a mean entry blood pressure of 139/79 mmHg; approximately 25% were female. About 80% had prior coronary disease, with 50% having had a prior myocardial infarction (usually >1 year prior to entry); almost 50% had a history of hypertension, 11% a prior cerebrovascular event or transient ischemic attack, and 40% had evidence of peripheral vascular disease or abnormal arm/ankle blood pressure ratio (percent not mutually exclusive). Almost 40% of subjects were diabetic because of overrecruitment.

Concomitant nontrial treatment at baseline consisted of aspirin in around 76%, calcium channel blockers in 47%, beta blockers in 40%, diuretics in 15%, and lipid-lowering therapy in 30%. These changed respectively to 75, 40, 45, 25, and 40% by the study end. Compliance with allocated treatment was good; 70% were taking the full 10 mg dose of ramipril at study end.

There were highly statistically significant relative risk reductions in the ramipril-allocated patients compared to placebo in the primary composite outcome of cardiovascular death, nonfatal stroke, and nonfatal myocardial infarction and in each of these three individually (22, 25, 32, and 20% respectively). In contrast, there were no significant effects with vitamin E, but no harm.

The Kaplan-Meier estimates for each of the four outcomes for ramipril diverged rather early (within 3 to 9 months) and continued diverging throughout the 4.5 years of follow-up, until the study was terminated prematurely on the advice of the data monitoring committee.

These benefits were independent of all other patient characteristics examined — diabetic or not; history of hypertension or not; male or female; over or under 65 years; or whether treated or not by aspirin, lipid-lowering drugs, or any or all of diuretics, beta blockers, or calcium channel blockers. The proportional benefit was not statistically different in any of these categories (except for a slightly less, but still significant, benefit if the patient was on aspirin); in other words, the benefit of ramipril was additive to that of other well-proven treatments.

Reassuringly, noncardiovascular mortality was not significantly different between ramipril and placebo, so that even total mortality was significantly reduced by ramipril, by 16% ($p = .005$) — remarkable in an older population like this. There were also significant relative risk reductions in many prespecified secondary end-points, such as revascularization procedures (-16%), heart failure (-23%), and diabetic complications (-16%). The effects were remarkably consistent over many prespecified subgroups. Rather surprisingly, there was no reduction in unstable angina.

Importantly, the results were the same in those patients (4772) who had had an ejection fraction measured as part of their clinical workup; the mean ejection fraction in these patients was normal (at 61%). Ramipril was well tolerated, with an excess of only 2% discontinuing for any cause, compared with placebo, with 5% excess discontinuation for cough, an expected side effect of ACE inhibition.

The SECURE substudy (Lonn et al., 2000) showed a significant reduction in the rate of progression of carotid arteriosclerosis only with the 10-mg ramipril dose. The 2.5-mg dose showed a nonsignificant trend for less progression, intermediate between placebo and the 10-mg dose. Interestingly, the blood pressure reduction was identical with each dose of ramipril, so that the effect in reducing arteriosclerosis was dissociated from the blood pressure reduction. Vitamin E was identical to placebo on the carotid measurements, consistent with the similar lack of effects on the end-points in the main HOPE trial. In a further analysis from the SECURE group that measured left ventricular dimensions, there were similar graded findings, with preservation of left ventricular volumes only on the 10-mg dose of ramipril.

Left Ventricular Hypertrophy

The prognostic impact of baseline left ventricular hypertrophy and of subsequent regression/prevention were examined (Mathew et al., 2001). It was found that development/persistence of left ventricular hypertrophy was highly significantly related to all primary outcomes and to new heart failure (left ventricular dysfunction was a baseline exclusion criterion). Persistence/development of left ventricular hypertrophy was significantly reduced by ramipril.

Micro-HOPE: Outcomes in Diabetics

The Micro-HOPE study (in 3577 diabetic subjects in HOPE) showed similar or slightly greater relative risk reductions in the primary end-point or its constituents of cardiovascular death, stroke, or myocardial infarction, by 25, 37, 33, and 22%, respectively (The HOPE Investigators, 2000c). Overt nephropathy was significantly reduced (by 24%), as was microalbuminuria ($p = .02$). Unexpectedly, over the 4.5 years of the study, there was a 33% reduction in the onset of new diabetes in those not diabetic at baseline. In both the Micro-HOPE and SECURE studies the benefit of ramipril was independent of change in blood pressure (The HOPE Investigators, 2000c; Lonn et al., 2000).

Impact On Renal Insufficiency

Clinicians have been concerned about the risks of ACE inhibitor treatment, particularly in older patients who might have covert renal artery stenosis. For this reason, our group undertook an analysis that related future risk and benefit from ramipril to baseline mea-

sures of renal insufficiency. (Mann et al., 2001). 980 patients had baseline serum creatinine over the pre-specified level of 124 μmol/L (1.4 mg/dL). Their risk of experiencing a subsequent primary outcome was 22%, compared with a risk of 15% for the 8307 patients with normal renal function ($p = < .001$). Ramipril reduced the relative risk by the same amount (20%) in each group. The increased risk from renal insufficiency was independent of other known risk factors. Dipstick-positive proteinuria was an exclusion criterion in HOPE, so the renal insufficiency was likely to be due mainly to nephrosclerosis. The benefits (and also adverse events) were seen in both hypertensive and normotensive patients. Ramipril was as well tolerated in patients with mild renal insufficiency as in those with normal renal function. The authors concluded that the practice of withholding ACE inhibition in those patients with mild renal insufficiency was unwarranted.

Blood Pressure Reduction Does Not Account for Most of the Benefit From Ramipril

Overall in the main HOPE study the reduction in blood pressure was modest (3.3/1.4 mmHg). An analysis of the previous epidemiology and trial data in hypertension studies showed that a 10- to 15-mmHg reduction in "usual" systolic blood pressure was associated with a roughly 40% reduction in stroke and 15% reduction in myocardial infarction (Guidelines Subcommittee, 1999). From this one would expect that a 3.3-mmHg systolic blood pressure reduction would result in a much smaller reduction in stroke and myocardial infarction than was observed.

Because the HOPE study was not a hypertension trial, and because the population in HOPE differed markedly from that in the hypertension trials, an analysis was made of the usual blood pressure/risk relation in the placebo arm of HOPE, over the 4.5 years of follow-up. Unpublished data show that the blood pressure/risk relation in the HOPE placebo population was not remarkably steep; it was if anything rather flatter than the calculations of the World Health Organization/International Society of Hypertension, so that it is unlikely that the HOPE results are due to an unusually large effect of the small reduction in blood pressure in a rather different population, at higher risk than those in the previous hypertension trials.

It was also found that if the HOPE population was divided into two halves, above and below the median baseline blood pressure of 138/80 mmHg, there was a significant 17% reduction in the primary outcome in the lower half with quite normal entry blood pressure of 126 to 129 mmHg.

Discussion

The blood pressure reduction in HOPE was rather modest and less than might have been expected from a full dose of an ACE inhibitor. However, it should be noted that HOPE was not a hypertension trial and the baseline blood pressure was normal. Additionally, many patients were already on a substantial amount of blood pressure–lowering treatment, which would reduce the impact of a second or third agent. Another concern has been the method for measurement of blood pressure, but this was very similar to that used in many of the trials and epidemiologic studies on which the blood pressure/risk estimates are based. This, together with the Cox regression analyses and the SECURE ultrasound results (which showed different effects of 2.5-mg and 10-mg doses of ramipril despite similar blood pressure change) suggest that the ACE inhibitor benefits were largely independent of the fall in blood pressure, useful as this may be (Lonn et al., 2000).

More recently the PROGRESS trial (presented at the June 2001 meeting of the European Society of Hypertension, He and MacGregor 2001) showed similar modest reduction of blood pressure in the ACE inhibitor arm (perindopril). The reductions in stroke or in major cardiovascular events were also rather modest, and nonsignificant, when compared with HOPE and with the dual-therapy arm of PROGRESS (perindopril plus indapamide, a diuretic). It is not clear whether the less impressive result with perindopril is due to a difference in the drug or to the population studied (post-stroke vs. post-coronary disease in HOPE) or to the play of chance.

Opponents of a non-blood pressure effect of ramipril quote the new overview of hypertension trials (Blood Pressure Lowering Treatment Trialists' Collaboration, 2000), which shows no clear advantage from any particular class of antihypertensive drug. But, as the authors point out, this latest overview has low power to examine particular subgroups such as those with baseline coronary disease (as in HOPE). It seems inherently implausible that all drugs that lower blood pressure have identical benefits in different populations.

A submitted analysis of the HOPE stroke data (Bosch et al., 2001) also finds that the 32% reduction in stroke by ramipril could not be explained by the reduction in blood pressure and was found at all entry levels of blood pressure.

The results of the HOPE study have been compared with landmark trials in cardiovascular protection, such as 4S, SAVE, SOLVD, AIRE, CARE, and LIPID trials, and found to be equally powerful and of similar or greater statistical significance.

Implications for Cardiovascular Prevention

These results considerably extend the range of patients for whom ACE inhibition is indicated. ACE inhibitors are clearly useful for patients with reduced left ventricular function or acute myocardial infarction and for patients with hypertension. The HOPE results suggest that in the type of patients studied, namely older patients, mostly with known coronary disease but with preserved left ventricular function, ACE inhibition should be used as widely as is aspirin to prevent future events, unless there are clear contraindications. The treatment was well tolerated and safe, but it is important to note that it should be carefully titrated, with measurement of electrolytes and creatinine. With these provisos the danger of problems with patients with renal artery stenosis appear minimal. It is important to emphasize this, as ACE inhibition may be underused (especially in elderly subjects with known atherosclerotic disease or with mild to moderate renal insufficiency) due to an overestimated fear of potential problems.

Implications for Future Research

The impressive results of the HOPE studies throw no clear light on the mechanisms for this remarkably large benefit (considering the large amount of effective treatment that the patients were already receiving).

The early divergence of the Kaplan-Meier curves suggests an effect on endothelium, plaque stability, coagulation factors, or all three, as opposed to an effect on the development of new atheromatous lesions. There is good experimental evidence for the presence of angiotensin and associated enzymes in plaques. Angiotensin is known to stimulate the production of cytokines from macrophages, and these in turn stimulate metalloproteinases, which dissolve the collagen cap (Davies, 1998). However, this is speculation, and future studies will be needed to determine what mechanisms are involved, particularly in the unexpected finding of prevention of the onset of new diabetes (The HOPE Investigators, 2000c). The study of Mathew et al. (2001) shows that regression/prevention of left ventricular hypertrophy — a known risk factor — may also play a part.

Future studies will determine whether (as seems likely from the SOLVD and SAVE data) this is a class effect or whether it is specific to ramipril. A large study (DREAM) in patients at high risk for diabetes will reexamine the effect of ramipril in the prevention of new diabetes — an unexpected finding in HOPE. Other planned studies (e.g., ONTARGET) will compare ramipril with the angiotensin receptor blocker, telimisartan, to determine whether this has similar benefits, without the side effect of cough, and will also compare in a third arm the combination of telmisartan with ramipril.

Conclusion

The HOPE studies have demonstrated unequivocally that in high-risk subjects ACE inhibition in a full dose with ramipril has a powerful preventive action on a range of important cardiovascular outcomes, which is only partly related to the modest reduction in blood pressure. It is additive to, and as powerful as, other proven treatments such as aspirin, statins, and treatments for hypertension. Prophylactic ACE inhibition is applicable to the type of patient who is currently eligible for aspirin prophylaxis.

REFERENCES

Blood Pressure Lowering Treatment Trialists' Collaboration: Effects of ACE inhibitors, calcium antagonists, and other blood-pressure-lowering drugs: Results of prospectively designed overviews of randomised trials. Lancet 355:1955, 2000

Bosch J et al: Use of Ramipril in preventing stroke: double blind randomised trial. BMJ 324:699, 2002

Davies MJ: Reactive oxygen species, metalloproteinases, and plaque stability. Circulation 97:2382, 1998

Garg R, Yusuf S: Overview of randomized trials of angiotensin-converting enzyme inhibitors on mortality and morbidity in patients with heart failure. JAMA 273:1450, 1995

Guidelines Subcommittee: 1999 World Health Organization–International Society of Hypertension Guidelines for the Management of Hypertension. Hypertension 17:151, 1999

He FJ, MacGregor GA. Blood pressure and stroke, the PROGRESS trial. J Renin Angiotensin Aldosterone Syst 2:153, 2001

Lonn E et al: Effects of ramipril and of vitamin E on atherosclerosis: Results of the prospective, randomized Study to Evaluate Carotid Ultrasound changes in patients treated with Ramipril and vitamin E (SECURE). Circulation 103:919, 2001

Mancini GBJ et al: Angiotensin-converting enzyme inhibition with quinapril improves endothelial vasomotor dysfunction in patients with coronary artery disease. The TREND (Trial on Reversing Endothelial Dysfunction) study. Circulation 94:258, 1996

Mann JFE et al: Renal insufficiency as a predictor of cardiovascular outcomes and the impact of ramipril: The HOPE randomized trial. Ann Intern Med 134:629, 2001

Mathew J et al: Reduction of cardiovascular risk by regression of electrocardiographic markers of left ventricular hypertrophy by the angiotensin converting enzyme inhibitor, ramipril. Circulation 104:1615, 2001

Otterstad JE & Sleight P: The HOPE study: Comparison with other trials of secondary prevention. Eur Heart J 22:1307, 2001

Pfeffer MA et al: Effect of captopril on mortality and morbidity in patients with left ventricular dysfunction after myocardial infarction. Results of the Survival and Ventricular Enlargement Trial (SAVE). N Engl J Med 327:669, 1992

Stampfer MJ et al: Vitamin E consumption and the risk of coronary disease in women. N Engl J Med 328:1444, 1993

Steinberg D: Antioxidants in the prevention of human atherosclerosis. Summary of the proceedings of a National Heart, Lung and Blood Institute workshop: September 5–6, 1991, Bethesda, Maryland. Circulation 85:2338, 1992

The Heart Outcomes Prevention Evaluation Study Investigators: Effects of an angiotensin-converting enzyme inhibitor, ramipril, on death from cardiovascular causes, myocardial infarction, and stroke in high-risk patients. N Engl J Med 342:145, 2000a

The Heart Outcomes Prevention Evaluation Study Investigators: Vitamin E supplementation and cardiovascular events in high risk patients. N Engl J Med 342:154, 2000b

The Heart Outcomes Prevention Evaluation (HOPE) Study Investigators: Effects of ramipril on cardiovascular and microvascular outcomes in people with diabetes mellitus: Results of the HOPE study and MICRO-HOPE substudy. Lancet 355:253, 2000c

The SOLVD Investigators: Effect of enalapril on survival in patients with reduced left ventricular ejection fractions and congestive heart failure. N Engl J Med 325:293, 1991

The SOLVD Investigators: Effect of enalapril on mortality and the development of heart failure in asymptomatic patients with reduced left ventricular ejection fractions. N Engl J Med 327:685, 1992

ADVANCES IN CLINICAL THERAPEUTIC MYOCARDIAL ANGIOGENESIS

Shmuel Fuchs, Eugenio Stabile,
Richard Baffour, Stephen E. Epstein

Recent progress achieved in understanding the complex mechanisms inherent in the development of new blood vessels, in conjunction with major biotechnology advances, has facilitated the initiation of a new treatment strategy—therapeutic angiogenesis. The emergence of this novel approach reflects the current dearth of effective treatment strategies for the increased number of patients with advanced symptomatic coronary artery disease not amenable to conventional revascularization approaches. It is estimated that 5 to 10% of patients referred to tertiary centers for coronary interventions may be candidates for therapeutic angiogenesis. This chapter summarizes the initial clinical experience with this new approach.

Mechanisms of Collateral Formation

Three different processes contribute to new blood vessels formation: vasculogenesis, angiogenesis, and arteriogenesis.

Vasculogenesis

This earliest stage of blood vessel development occurs in the developing embryo and is associated with the differentiation of primitive hemangioblasts into angioblasts. Under the influence of multiple factors that include vascular endothelial growth factor (VEGF), fibroblast growth factor (FGF), the angiopoietins, and multiple other factors both known and unknown, these cells undergo differentiation into an endothelial cell network forming a primitive blood vessel plexus.

Angiogenesis

This is the main postembryogenesis mechanism responsible for new capillary formation. The process occurs in various physiologic conditions, such as menstruation, and in pathologic conditions, such as diabetic proliferative retinopathy, rheumatoid arthritis, and tumor growth. Angiogenesis encompasses sprouting of preexisting capillaries to form a new capillary network, a process tightly regulated by a large number of proangiogenic factors, including VEGF, FGF, and placental growth factor, which act in concert in a time-dependent manner. The changes induced by these growth factors and cytokines include an initial process of degradation of the basement membrane, remodeling of the perivascular matrix, endothelial cell migration and proliferation, and endothelial cell tube formation, resulting ultimately in a new capillary network.

Arteriogenesis

This postembryogenesis mechanism of resistance and conductance blood vessel growth involves remodeling of preexisting small arterioles into larger vessels. This phenomenon is triggered in part by an increase in shear stress, which occurs in the small, high-resistance, low-flow arterioles that are in parallel with the main arterial channel. Following narrowing or occlusion of the main artery, the pressure gradient across the in-parallel arterioles increases, establishing flow and thereby increasing shear stress. Endothelial shear-stress-responsive elements mediate increased expression of many genes, including macrophage chemoattractant protein 1 (MCP-1), granulocyte-macrophage colony stimulating-factor (GM-CSF), and intercellular cell adehesion molecule (ICAM-1), which act in concert to recruit monocytes into the subintimal space of the vessel wall, where they differentiate into macrophages. The macrophages produce abundant angiogenic growth factors that lead to endothelial and smooth-muscle cell proliferation, migration, vessel remodeling, and synthesis of extracellular matrix. This time- and concentration-dependent coordinated process results in a functioning collateral network establishing connections between feeding and receiving vessels.

Clinical Trials

The results of several clinical trials have now been reported and are summarized in Table 38-1. The studies vary in their underlying strategies, reflecting the uncertainties surrounding the field. For example,

some of the many questions still to be answered are which angiogenic factor(s) will turn out to produce an optimal effect, will the protein or gene be a superior means of delivering the factor, does optimization of response require a multiple-factor strategy, and what is the optimal delivery strategy (e.g., intracoronary, intramyocardial, or transepicardial)? It is therefore not surprising that the current strategies involve administration of proteins (both VEGF and FGF), plasmid DNA-encoding VEGF, and adenoviral vectors containing either VEGF or one of the FGF transgenes and that they utilize a variety of delivery approaches.

Surgical Approach

The initial experience was in patients undergoing coronary artery bypass grafting (Schumacher et al., 1998). Patients had to have a proximal left anterior descending artery stenosis and a narrowing at its distal third and/or at the origin of one of its branches. FGF-1 protein (0.01 mg/kg) was injected intramyocardially distal to the anastomotic site of the left internal mammary artery with the left anterior descending artery of 20 patients at the time of the surgery, with denatured FGF-1 injected as a control ($n = 20$). At 12 weeks' follow-up, coronary angiography was interpreted as showing increased myocardial blush deriving from new vessels sprouting from the coronary artery at the site of injection and filling the distal vessel. Such changes were observed in the intervention group only.

The safety and feasibility of direct intramyocardial injection of replication-deficient adenovirus-mediated $VEGF_{121}$ genetransfer as an adjunct to coronary artery bypass grafting ($n = 15$) or as a sole therapy (minithoracotomy, $n = 6$) was subsequently reported (Rosengart et al., 1999). The injections were targeted to myocardial zones with reversible ischemia that were not amenable to bypass grafting. Five dose-groups were evaluated, and all groups showed similar safety. The six patients who underwent $VEGF_{121}$ injection as sole therapy showed improved anginal status and a trend for improved angiographic collateral scoring. However, ^{99mb}Tc-sestamibi images showed no improvement in the segments subjected to gene administration.

TABLE 38-1

CLINICAL TRIALS OF GENE THERAPY FOR MYOCARDIAL ANGIOGENESIS

Author	Reference	n	Angiogenic factor	Route of administration	Randomized	Results
FGF Studies						
Schumacher et al.	Circulation, 1998	20	aFGF protein	IM; thoracotomy	Yes	"Improved"
Sellke et al.	Ann Thorac Surg, 1998	8	bFBF protein	Hep-al pellets; thoracotomy	No	"Improved"
Laham et al.	Circulation, 1999	24	bFBF protein	Hep-al pellets; thoracotomy	Yes	"Improved"
Unger et al.	Am J Cardiol, 2000	25	bFGF protein	Intracoronary	Yes	Safe
Laham et al.	Presented: ACC, 1999	52	bFGF protein	Intracoronary	No	"Improved"
FIRST Trial	Presented: ACC, 2000	337	bFGF protein	Intracoronary	Yes	1° end-pt: neg
AGENT Trial	Circulation, 2002	79	FGF-4 gene-adeno	Intracoronary	Yes	1° end-pt: neg
VEGF Studies						
Rosengart et al.	Circulation, 1999	21	VEGF$_{121}$ gene-adeno	IM; thoracotomy	No	"Improved"
Losordo et al.	Circulation, 1998	5	VEGF$_{165}$ gene-plasmid	IM; thoracotomy	No	"Improved"
Gibson et al.	Presented: ACC, 1999	28	VEGF$_{165}$ protein	Intravenous	No	"Improved"
Henry et al.	Presented: ACC, 1998	15	VEGF$_{165}$ protein	Intracoronary	No	"Improved"
Henry et al.	Presented: ACC, 1999	178	VEGF$_{165}$ protein	Intracoronary plus IV	Yes	No effect
Vale et al.	Circulation, 2001	6	VEGF-2 plasmid	Transendocardial, catheter based	No	"Improved"

ABBREVIATIONS: FGF, fibroblast growth factor; IM, intramuscular; hep-al, heparin alginate; ACC, American College of Cardiology Annual Meeting; adeno, adenovirus; 1°, primary; IV, intravenous; VEGF, Vascular endothelial growth factor.

In order to achieve prolonged exposure to angiogenic growth factor without the need to administer a viral vector, one team implanted sustained-release heparin-alginate microcapsules containing bFGF protein around ungraftable vessels that were supplying viable myocardial segments (Laham et al., 1999). Twenty-four patients were randomized to either low bFGF dose (10 μg/pellet), high dose (100 μg/pellet), or placebo. Placement of the microspheres (10 pellets per patient) had no significant short-term hemodynamic effects, and blood analysis revealed no increase in baseline bFGF. At 3 months, most patients remained free of angina, and stress nuclear perfusion imaging showed a decrease in the ischemic area, compared to baseline, only in patients receiving the high bFGF dose.

It should be emphasized that all these surgically based interventional studies consist of few patients, and all treated patients were undergoing concomitant coronary bypass surgery (except for six patients in one trial), making it impossible to determine efficacy of the angiogenesis therapy. More recently, however, less invasive approaches were employed that allowed assessment of angiogenesis intervention as sole therapy. Direct myocardial injection of plasmid DNA-encoding $VEGF_{165}$ via minithoracotomy was performed in 20 patients with class III-IV angina. These patients had reversible ischemia on stress nuclear imaging and were considered as "no-option" patients in terms of conventional revascularization procedures (Symes et al., 1999). All patients underwent uneventful procedures and were followed for 90 days. The results of this study were interpreted as showing symptomatic relief, a reduction in stress perfusion score, and angiographic improvement in collateral filling of at least one occluded vessel. A major limitation to this study is the lack of a control group, a defect making it impossible to draw any definitive conclusions about efficacy.

Systemic and Intracoronary Administration

The design of only two of the studies reported to date rise to a phase II status, as they had most of the elements that would permit at least tentative efficacy conclusions to be drawn—the study initiated by Genentec (VIVA) (Henry et al., 1999), and that of Chiron (FIRST) (Simons et al., 2000). Although these studies in their nonrandomized phase I iterations were reported as showing very encouraging positive results, phase II of each of these studies demonstrated *no treatment effect* on the primary end-point (treadmill exercise performance). Although exercise performance improved, it improved in the untreated patients as much as it did in the treated patients.

In the VIVA trial, a single bolus intracoronary (ic) injection of $VEGF_{165}$ protein was administered [17 or 50 (ng/kg)/min] followed by 4 h intravenous infusions of $VEGF_{165}$ [17 or 50 (ng/kg)/min] delivered at day 3, 6, and 9. In the Chiron study a single bolus ic injection of bFGF protein was administered. These negative results underscore the lack of efficiency of the specific therapeutic strategies tested when evaluated in several animal studies; thus, although there are divergent results from different laboratories, the results of at least one laboratory predicted from the results of animal studies that single-bolus ic injections of either FGF or VEGF proteins and the intravenous administration of angiogenesis factors, would *not* result in a myocardial angiogenesis effect. The reason for the lack of efficacy was probably due to the likelihood that enhanced collateral development requires longer duration of exposure to the angiogenesis agent than that provided by bolus injections.

This led to the concept that delivery of a *gene* encoding an angiogenesis factor might be more efficacious, as the encoding protein would be expressed over days or weeks (see Chap. 40, this volume). This concept was recently tested by the study initiated by Berlex Pharmaceuticals (AGENT). It was the first phase I/II, dose-escalating, double-blind randomized trial of myocardial angiogenesis and involved the intracoronary injection of adenovirus carrying as a transgene FGF-4 (Grines et al., 2002). The study demonstrated safety and feasibility, and although it was not powered to detect differences in efficacy, a subgroup analysis of patients with baseline exercise duration of <10 min suggested a treatment-related significant improvement in exercise duration. A definitive test of efficacy is planned to be tested in a phase II/III trial that will be adequately powered specifically for this purpose.

Percutaneous Transendocardial Injections

The clinical experience with percutaneous trans-endocardial approaches for delivery of angiogenesis factors, the least invasive direct intramyocardial injection technique, is limited. The initial experience with a very few patients demonstrated the feasibility of this potentially attractive approach. Most recently, Vale and colleagues summarized their initial experience in six patients who underwent catheter-based transendocardial injection of VEGF-2 plasmid (six injections, 200-μg total dose) directed into the ischemic territory (Vale et al., 2001). At 3-month follow-up, there was statistically significant improvement in multiple end-points including angina score, need for nitroglycerin, exercise stress test parameters, and perfusion (assessed by nuclear imaging) and electromechnaical mapping parameters. It is obviously impossible, however, to draw any conclusions from a group of only six patients.

Summary of the Clinical Trials of Myocardial Angiogenesis

To summarize the clinical studies that have been performed to date on myocardial angiogenesis, in virtually every one the investigators concluded the studies demonstrated efficacy or, more modestly, showed extremely encouraging results. However, these studies accomplished only what phase I studies are designed to accomplish—they demonstrated safety and feasibility. Conclusions regarding efficacy are not possible.

Potential Deleterious Effects

The biologic activity of most of the angiogenic agents currently being tested clinically is very potent, and it is likely that the same activities that lead to a therapeutic effect could also cause unwanted side effects. If this concept is true, then the critical question to be addressed in large clinical trials is whether the incidence of these risks is sufficiently low so that the risks will be outweighed by the therapeutic benefits (Epstein et al., 2001).

Among the side effects that might occur as a result of the biologic effects of these agents are the following:

1. Development of new blood vessels in nontargeted tissues, a complication that would be particularly devastating if it were to occur, for example, in the retinae. This probably applies only to patients with some other vascular disease involving the retinae, such as those with diabetic retinopathy. In this condition the vascular cells are "primed," insofar as it has been demonstrated that there are increased levels of one of the receptors for VEGF.
2. Increased vascular permeability, which by itself may be a necessary component of the angiogenic process but may also cause serious consequences. In this regard, the multiple-organ edema and high mortality observed in adult mice in which VEGF overexpression was achieved by injecting an adenovirus carrying the VEGF transgene raises some concern.
3. Expansion and destabilization of an atherogenic plaque, which may result in atherosclerotic progression and plaque rupture.
4. Facilitated growth of microvessels into dormant and/or unrecognized tumors through angiogenesis processes, a critical process for tumor growth.
5. Growth of in situ vascular tumors (hemangiomatous-like), which were observed in several experimental studies at the sites of direct intra-tissue injection.
6. Hypotension through, at least in part, a nitric oxide–mediated pathway. This effect has resulted in (a) the death of pigs that had chronic myocardial ischemia and were treated with the intracoronary injection of $VEGF_{165}$ protein, and (b) a prolonged hypotensive episode of a patient entered into a phase I study testing the safety of intracoronary administration of bFGF protein.

Future Directions

The molecular mechanisms responsible for angiogenesis are extraordinarily complex: multiple genes must coordinately express their products in appropriate amounts and in an appropriate time-dependent manner. The complexity of the natural process of collateral formation raises the question of what "multiple factor" strategies can be employed. One approach might be to utilize genes that express products that activate or lead to the expression of multiple factors involved in angiogenesis, such as hypoxia inducible factors (HIF-1β, -1α, and -2α). Another multifactor approach is to attract or deliver to ischemic tissue cells that nature has imbued with the capacity to express multiple angiogenic factors in appropriate sequence and concentration. Ito and colleagues have demonstrated the importance of the monocyte in promoting arteriogenesis (Ito et al., 1997). The monocyte, upon phenotypic differentiation to a tissue macrophage, expresses such potentially angiogenic factors as VEGF, nitric oxide, MCP-1, and various cytokines. Yet another multifactor cellular approach is based on the hypothesis that bone marrow cells have angiogenic properties that will enhance collateral flow in ischemic tissue. In testing this concept, it was found that in culture these cells do in fact secrete angiogenic factors, including VEGF and MCP-1, and that when the conditioned medium derived from these cells is applied to endothelial cells, the endothelial cells proliferate, migrate, and form tubes. Most important, it was found that when autologous bone marrow is injected transendocardially into ischemic porcine myocardium, collateral flow and myocardial function improve significantly (Fuchs et al., 2001). Based on these data, a phase I clinical trial assessing the feasibility and safety of this approach was recently initiated.

Conclusions

Therapeutic angiogenesis for myocardial ischemia is a novel treatment strategy aimed at enhancing myocardial blood flow in patients who are not candidates for conventional revascularization. Early excitement, derived from anecdotal case reports or phase I studies, has been somewhat tempered by subsequent negative phase II trials, which were blinded and randomized. The ability to optimize therapeutic angiogenesis is based on concepts that are still in the process of being explored experimentally. Therefore, considerably more experimental work needs to be undertaken in the animal laboratory; at the same time, carefully controlled randomized and blinded large clinical trials must be completed to ascertain efficacy definitively and to determine whether the incidence of serious complications is sufficiently low such that the attendant risks of therapy are outweighed by the benefits attained.

REFERENCES

Epstein SE et al: Angiogenesis therapy: Amidst the hype, the neglected potential for serious side effects. Circulation 104:115, 2001

Fuchs S et al: Transendocardial delivery of autologous bone marrow enhances collateral perfusion and regional function in pigs with chronic experimental myocardial ischemia. J Am Coll Cardiol 37:1726, 2001

Grines CL et al: Angiogenic Gene Therapy (AGENT) trial in patients with stable angina pectoris Circulation 105:1291, 2002

Henry TD et al: Results of intracoronary recombinant human vascular endothelial growth factor (rhVEGF) administration trial. J Am Coll Cardiol 31:65A, 1998

Ito WD et al: Monocyte chemotactic protein-1 increases collateral and peripheral conductance after femoral artery occlusion. Circ Res 80:829, 1997

Laham RJ et al: Local perivascular delivery of basic fibroblast growth factor in patients undergoing coronary bypass surgery: Results of a phase I randomized, double-blind, placebo-controlled trial. Circulation 100:1865, 1999

Rosengart TK et al: Angiogenesis gene therapy: Phase I assessment of direct intramyocardial administration of an adenovirus vector expressing VEGF121 cDNA to individuals with clinically significant severe coronary artery disease. Circulation 100:468, 1999

Schumacher B et al: Induction of neoangiogenesis in ischemic myocardium by human growth factors: First clinical results of a new treatment of coronary heart disease. Circulation 97:645, 1998

Simons M et al: Angiogenesis therapy with recombinant bFGF (personal communication). Presented at the Late Breaking Clinical Trials Session at the 49th

Annual meeting of the American College of Cardiology, March, 2000

Symes JF et al: Gene therapy with vascular endothelial growth factor for inoperable coronary artery disease. Ann Thorac Surg 68:830, 1999

Vale P et al: Randomized, single blind, placebo-controlled pilot study of catheter-based myocardial gene transfer for therapeutic angiogenesis using left ventricular electromechanical mapping in patients with chronic myocardial ischemia. Circulation 103:2138, 2001

BASIC FIBROBLAST GROWTH FACTOR TRIALS FOR PATIENTS WITH ADVANCED CORONARY DISEASE

Michael Simons / Mark J. Post /
Roger J. Laham / Frank W. Sellke

Biology of Basic Fibroblast Growth Factor

Basic fibroblast growth factor (FGFB, or FGF2) is a 16.5-kDa 146-amino-acid protein that belongs to the fibroblast growth factor family, which now comprises more than 22 structurally related polypeptides (Ornitz and Itoh, 2001). As do all members of the FGF family, FGF2 binds with high affinity to cellular heparan sulfates and with even higher affinity ($10^{-11}\ M$) to its specific tyrosine kinase receptor, FGF receptor 1. Heparan sulfate–binding properties of FGF2 serve both to prolong effective tissue half-life of the FGF2 protein (Rosenberg et al., 1997) and to facilitate its binding to its high-affinity receptors. The growth factor is present in the normal myocardium, and its expression is stimulated by hypoxia (Padua et al., 1995) and hemodynamic stress.

Basic FGF is a potent mitogen for cells of mesenchymal, neural, and epithelial origin. In addition to this mitogenic activity, FGF2 possesses a plethora of other biologic effects including antiapoptotic activity and the ability to (1) stimulate nitric oxide (NO) release by both endothelial and inducible NO synthase-dependent pathways; (2) stimulate endothelial production of various proteases, including plasminogen activator and matrix metalloproteinases; and (3) induce chemotaxis. Because of these properties, FGF2 is a powerful angiogenic agent, both in vitro and in vivo. Despite these multiple biologic activities, homozygous deletion of the FGF2 gene is not associated with any significant phenotype except for decreased vascular smooth-muscle contractility, low blood pressure, and thrombocytosis (Zhou et al., 1998).

Despite FGF2's presence in normal tissues, the growth factor does not appear to be biologically active, as suggested by the absence of ongoing angiogenesis. While the precise explanation for this lack of activity of the endogenous growth factor is uncertain, contributing factors probably include very low levels of expression of FGF receptor 1 as well another transmembrane protein involved in FGF2-dependent signaling, syndecan-4. In addition, endogenous FGF2 may be sequestered in the extracellular matrix by binding to the heparan sulfate–carrying proteoglycan perlecan and thus be unavailable to bind to its signaling receptors.

Preclinical Evaluation

The ability of FGF2 to induce angiogenesis in mature tissues was suggested by studies in the canine and porcine infarction models. Early studies documented significantly higher vessel counts following intracoronary injections of FGF2 in the setting of acute coronary thrombosis in dogs and pigs (Battler et al., 1993, Unger et al., 1994). These initial studies were followed by more detailed functional evaluation of therapeutic efficacy of FGF2 in chronic myocardial ischemia that employed the ameroid constrictor model. The placement of ameroid constrictor leads to gradual narrowing of the instrumented artery, which occludes completely over about 3 weeks. This gradual occlusion together with the formation of native collateral vessels results in development of chronic myocardial ischemia accompanied by myocardial hibernation in the affected coronary territory with only limited subendocardial infarction (Post et al., 2001).

Continuous administration of FGF2 in these settings either directly into the occluded coronary artery or into the left atrium resulted in augmentation of coronary flow in the growth factor–treated dogs (Lazarous et al., 1996). Similar studies in pigs showed that sustained-release perivascular administration or intrapericardial delivery of FGF2 not only improved myocardial blood flow in the ischemic myocardium but also improved regional left ventricular function in the ischemic zone (Lopez et al., 1997). Despite the relatively systemic nature of these deliveries, the angiogenic effect of FGF2 was limited to the ischemic myocardium, with no increase in the vessel number or changes in coronary blood flow noted in nonischemic areas of the heart.

Detailed morphology documented an increase in vessel density predominantly in larger vessels, and coronary angiography clearly demonstrated the occurrence of new visible collaterals. Thus, increased coronary perfusion following FGF2 treatment is probably predominantly mediated by formation of epicardial collaterals (neoarteriogenesis) and not by a large increase in myocardial capillaries (true angiogenesis) as suggested by the lack of increase in capillary density.

Delivery Strategies

Despite these promising results, translation of FGF2 therapy, so successful in animal studies, requires delivery strategy that can be implemented in patients. This requirement essentially eliminates all forms of prolonged or frequent repetitive intracoronary infusions. Local perivascular delivery is more easily adaptable to clinical trials but requires open-chest surgery. The feasibility of this form of FGF2 delivery was evaluated in a porcine model using heparin-alginate microcapsules. Heparin alginate provides prolonged (4 to 5 weeks) release of the growth factor with first-order kinetics of growth factor from the polymer (Edelman et al., 1993). The polymer is easily implantable, and its use is not associated with inflammatory reaction (Lopez et al., 1997). Furthermore, perivascular growth factor delivery has the potential advantage of bypassing the endothelial barrier and avoiding rapid washout of growth factor due to rapid arterial blood flow. When delivered using this approach in ameroid-instrumented pigs, FGF2 induced dose-dependent increase in myocardial perfusion of the ischemic myocardium that, at higher dosages, led to improved myocardial function (Lopez et al., 1997). An alternative approach to perivascular administration of FGF2 involves intrapericardial instillation of the growth factor. Osmotic pump delivery into the pericardium led to enhanced growth of new epicardial small vessels in a rabbit model of angiotensin II-induced left ventricular hypertrophy (Landau et al., 1995), and intrapericardial injection resulted in increased vascularity in the setting of acute myocardial infarction. More significantly, transthoracic intrapericardial delivery of FGF2 (30 μg up to 2 mg) in a porcine LCX ameroid occlusion model resulted in significant increases in the number of left-to-left angiographic collaterals and improvement in blood flow to the ischemic myocardium, which was accompanied by improvements in myocardial perfusion as measured by magnetic resonance imaging (MRI), improved microvascular function, and histologic evidence of increased myocardial vascularity (Laham et al., 2000b). However, clinical application of intrapericardial delivery, while technically feasible with the development of several new catheter-based approaches (Waxman et al., 2000), is limited to a small number of patients currently being enrolled in coronary angiogenesis trials because of high prevalence (80 to 90%) of prior coronary artery bypass grafting (CABG) in this group of patients.

The remaining possibilities include short-duration intracoronary or intravenous infusions and endomyocardial injections. Intravenous infusions are appealing because of their practicality, low cost, and applicability to broad groups of patients. Furthermore, treatment can be easily repeated and may not require any special facilities. A disadvantage includes systemic exposure to a growth factor and potential for side effects such as NO-mediated hypotension (Yu and Edelman, 1999). Intracoronary infusions are easily carried out in any cardiac catheterization laboratory and are also applicable in most patients with coronary disease. However, the need for left heart catheterization limits this approach to a single session or, at most, infrequent repetitions. While somewhat more "local" than intravenous infusions, intracoronary infusions are also likely to result in systemic exposure to the growth factor and may precipitate systemic hypotension. A variation on the same theme is transvascular intracoronary administration with a local delivery catheter. This approach, while potentially feasible, remains experimental at this time.

Detailed evaluation of tracer-labeled growth factor uptake and retention in the myocardium and its systemic distribution following intracoronary and intravenous infusions demonstrated that both forms of delivery are associated with relatively low uptake in the target (ischemic) area of the heart. Thus, 1 h after injection, 0.9% of the injected FGF2 was found in the ischemic myocardium following intracoronary and 0.26% following intravenous administration. Perhaps more important, 24 h later, very small amounts of the growth factor remained in the myocardium (0.05% for intracoronary and 0.04% for intravenous) (Laham et al., 1999a). Nevertheless, efficacy studies in the pig ameroid model suggested that single-bolus intracoronary but not intravenous administration results in improved myocardial blood flow and function in the ischemic areas of the heart (Sato et al., 2000).

Intramyocardial delivery of growth factors (Fig. 39-1) is the least evaluated form of therapy at this time. A variety of delivery devices are being investigated (Bao et al., 2001). The appeal of this mode of delivery includes the possibility of targeting the desired areas of the heart, likely higher efficiency of delivery, and prolonged tissue retention (Kornowski et al., 2000). The drawbacks are its invasive nature and the requirement for highly specialized equipment and high skill level of the operator. Furthermore, to date no conclusive data regarding the physiologic efficacy of this mode of administration are available.

Side Effects and Toxicity

Animal studies as well as early clinical trials suggested several characteristic toxicities associated with

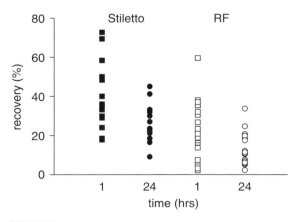

FIGURE 39-1

Scattergram of ^{125}I FGF2 recovery from the myocardium following injection with either Stiletto or RF-PMR delivery catheters.

exposure to FGF2. In particular, renal insufficiency, due to membranous nephropathy accompanied by proteinuria, may be the most significant long-term side effect of FGF2 administration. While the mechanism of this side effect is not known, it likely related to FGF2 deposition in heparan sulfate–rich glomerular membrane. Another well-documented side effect is severe hypotension due to FGF2-induced NO release and arteriolar vasodilation. However, it should be pointed out that this safety profile has been obtained almost exclusively in studies of normal animals and thus may not be fully applicable to patients with advanced atherosclerotic disease. In fact, the pleiotrophic nature of FGF2 activity raises concerns regarding the cytokine's effect on vascular smooth muscle, in particular in patients who have recently undergone coronary angioplasty and bypass surgery. FGF2 administration in normal dogs in the setting of arterial injury resulted in decreased neointimal proliferation compared to that in untreated animals, presumably due to faster reendotheliazation of the denuded arterial segment (Lazarous et al., 1996). Studies in cholesterol-fed pigs demonstrated reasonable safety of intrarterial FGF2 administration at time of arterial injury in terms of accelerated neointimal formation and restenosis.

Another theoretical concern associated with FGF2 or, indeed, the administration of any angiogenic growth factor is the development of plaque angiogenesis (O'Brien et al., 1994) that may precipitate plaque growth or destabilization due to broad-spectrum mitogenicity and chemotactic activity, especially towards macrophages (Libby et al., 1995, Celletti et al., 2001). The latter possibility may be particularly relevant given the ability of FGFs to induce angiogenesis in vasa vasorum and the association between plaque angiogenesis and its growth as well as stability.

Other areas of concern include proliferative retinopathy and occult malignancies. Proliferative retinopathy has been associated with the appearance of angiogenic growth factors (predominantly vascular endothelial growth factor) in the orbital fluid (Aiello et al., 1994). The role of angiogenesis in tumor growth and metastasis is well documented (Folkman, 1997), and facilitation of this process may theoretically lead to tumor growth or metastatic spread. However, clinical experience with various growth factors so far has not substantiated these fears (Henry et al., 1999).

Clinical Evaluation

Given efficacy data in animal models and delivery considerations discussed above, the initial clinical study of FGF2 in patients with coronary disease employed heparin-alginate delivery in patients undergoing CABG (Sellke et al., 1998). Growth factor–containing bead implantation added on average 2.8 ± 1.1 min to operative time and was well tolerated. In particular, there were no hemodynamically significant changes and no significant increase in the serum FGF2 levels. To assess the efficacy of this approach, patients requiring CABG were selected who had an area of ischemic but viable myocardium subtended by a major coronary artery that was not likely to be bypassed at the time of surgery for technical reasons. The 24 patients meeting these criteria were randomized at the time of surgery in a double-blind fashion to implantation of 10 heparin-alginate microspheres containing 10 or 100 μg of FGF2 or placebo controls. Nuclear and MRI perfusion scans were performed prior to hospital discharge and then again at 90 days (Laham et al., 1999b). Two patients in the trial died at the time of CABG (one in the control and one in the 100-μg FGF2 group). At the time of the 90-day evaluation, all seven remaining patients in the 100-μg FGF2 group were symptom free, while three of the seven patients in the control group continued to experience angina and two required additional revascularization procedures. Nuclear perfusion imaging demonstrated a significant reduction in the size of the target zone in the 100-μg FGF2 group but not in the 10-μg FGF2 or control groups. Thus, this small study demonstrated the safety and feasibility of this mode of FGF2 therapy (Fig. 39-2). A larger randomized phase II study is currently ongoing.

The safety and feasibility of intracoronary and intravenous FGF2 delivery were tested in two

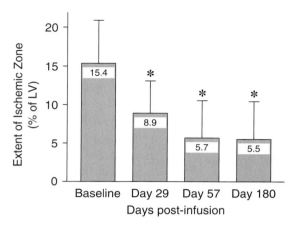

FIGURE 39-2

Magnetic resonance perfusion imaging allowed the determination of the extent of the myocardial area with delayed contrast arrival, which was significantly reduced at days 29, 57, and 180, as compared to baseline. Data presented as mean ±SEM. *denotes statistical significance with p < 0.001. Laham et al. JACC 2000; 36:2132

TABLE 39-1

CHANGES IN NUCLEAR PERFUSION DEFECT AT 90 DAYS COMPARED TO BASELINE

	Placebo	bFGF 10 µg	bFGF 100 µg
Follow-up scans	6/7	8/8	6/7
Worse	3	2	0
Unchanged	3	2	1
Better	0	4	5

Laham et al. Circulation 1999; 100:1865

open-label dose-escalation phase I studies. In one study, 25 patients with known but not critical coronary artery disease were randomized (2:1) to increasing doses of FGF2 (3 to 100 µg/kg) or placebo infused into the left main coronary artery (Unger et al., 2000). In the other trial, 52 patients with severe coronary disease who were suboptimal candidates for conventional therapeutic approaches were given intracoronary FGF2 in dose from 0.33 µg/kg to 48 µg/kg divided between two major arterial conduits (Laham et al., 2000a, Udelson, et al., 2000). In both trials basic FGF infusions were well tolerated over a 2 log range of doses, with systemic hypotension becoming the dose-limiting toxicity at 48 µg/kg. Clinical follow-up over 6 months documented mortality in four patients (two sudden deaths in patients with ejection fractions of 22 and 30%, one death following cardiac transplant for progressive failure symptoms, and one from non-Hodgkin's lymphoma diagnosed 8 days after FGF2 infusion). There was no significant toxicity such as irreversible proteinuria, renal failure, or deteriorating proliferative retinopathy (Laham et al., 2000a). Efficacy evalua-

tion was assessed using exercise testing, nuclear and MRI perfusion imaging, and the Seattle Angina Questionnaire (SAQ) at 60 days and 6 months. Symptom assessment demonstrated significant improvement in patients receiving intracoronary infusions. In particular, angina frequency score increased (denoting improvement) from 39.8 ± 27.0 at baseline to 69 ± 27.9 and 64.3 ± 30.2 at 57 and 180 days, respectively ($p < .001$), and exertional capacity score increased from 49.3 ± 19.8 at baseline to 65.0 ± 21.8 at 57 days and 73.5 ± 24.6 at 6 months ($p < .001$). None of the scores demonstrated significant deterioration from day 57 to day 180. Exercise testing documented mean exercise time improvement by 39 s at day 29 ($p = .046$), 135 s by day 57 ($p < .001$), and 140 s by day 180 ($p < .001$). MRI perfusion imaging demonstrated a significant reduction in the size of the ischemic territory (Table 39-1, Fig. 39-3) and improved left ventricular wall thickening in this territory. Taken together, these results suggest that intracoronary infusions of FGF2 are reasonably safe and may produce functionally significant benefits (Laham et al., 2000a).

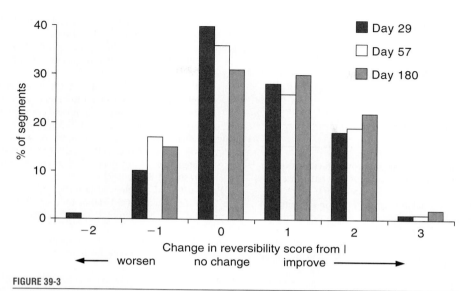

FIGURE 39-3

Distribution of segments according to the change from baseline in the segmental reversibility score, a measure of the magnitude of inducible ischemia. At all time points during the serial follow-up myocardial perfusion studies, the majority of segments which were ischemic at baseline improved. Udelson et al. Circulation 2000; 102:1605

These claims were evaluated in a 337-patient double-blind phase II trial that examined three different intracoronary dosages of FGF2 (0.3, 3.0, and 30 μg/kg) vs. placebo controls. Exercise tolerance was increased at 90 days in all four groups and was not significantly different between placebo and FGF-treated groups. At the same time, FGF2 significantly reduced angina symptoms as measured by the angina frequency score (AFS) of the SAQ (overall, $p = .035$), Canadian Cardiovascular Society (CCS) class score in the mid-dose group (pair-wise, $p = .012$ in the 3.0 μg/kg group), and the Physical Component Summary Scale of the SF-36 (pair-wise, $p = .033$), all FGF groups vs. placebo. These differences were more pronounced in highly symptomatic patients (baseline AFS ≤ 40 and/or CCS score of 3 or 4). No differences were significant at 180 days due to continued improvement in the placebo group (M. Simons and N. Chronos, American College of Cardiology 2001 presentation). Adverse events were similar across all groups, except for hypotension that

occurred with higher frequency in the 30-μg/kg FGF2 group. In summary, single intracoronary FGF2 infusion appears to result in short-term symptomatic improvement most pronounced in the more symptomatic patient subgroups. Given the favorable safety profile, additional trials of intracoronary FGF2 among highly symptomatic patients are needed to further assess this mode of angiogenic growth factor therapy.

Summary and Conclusions

The development of angiogenic growth factor therapy over the past few years promises to revolutionize the approach to treatment of chronic myocardial ischemia. Nevertheless, while initial results are clearly exciting, we have much to learn about this form of therapy (Simons et al., 2000). In particular, delivery issues are likely to play an important role as these therapies continue to evolve. Furthermore, careful documentation of side effects and toxicities over an extended period of time will be important to the ultimate acceptance of these therapies.

REFERENCES

Aiello LP et al: Vascular endothelial growth factor in ocular fluid of patients with diabetic retinopathy and other retinal disorders. N Engl J Med 331:1480, 1994

Bao J et al: Intramyocardial delivery of FGF2 in combination with radio frequency transmyocardial revascularization. Cathet Cardiovasc Interv 53:429, 2001

Battler A et al: Intracoronary injection of basic fibroblast growth factor enhances angiogenesis in infarcted swine myocardium. J Am Coll Cardiol 22:2001, 1993

Celletti FL et al: Vascular endothelial growth factor enhances atherosclerotic plaque progression. Nat Med 7:425, 2001

Edelman ER et al: Perivascular and intravenous administration of basic fibroblast growth factor: Vascular and solid organ deposition. Proc Natl Acad Sci USA 90:1513, 1993

Folkman J: Angiogenesis and angiogenesis inhibition: An overview, EXS 79:1, 1997

Henry T et al: Double blind placebo controlled trial of recombinant human vascular endothelial growth factor—the VIVA trial. J Am Coll Cardiol 33:384A, 1999

Kornowski R et al: Delivery strategies to achieve therapeutic myocardial angiogenesis. Circulation 101:454, 2000

Laham RJ et al: Intracoronary and intravenous administration of basic fibroblast growth factor: Myocardial and tissue distribution. Drug Metab Dispos 27:821, 1999a

Laham RJ et al: Local perivascular delivery of basic fibroblast growth factor in patients undergoing coronary bypass surgery: Results of a phase I randomized, double-blind, placebo-controlled trial. Circulation 100:1865, 1999b

Laham RJ et al: Intracoronary basic fibroblast growth factor (FGF-2) in patients with severe ichemic heart disease: Results of a Phase I open-label dose escalation study. J Am Coll Cardiol 36:2132, 2000a

Laham RJ et al: Intrapericardial delivery of fibroblast growth factor-2 induces neovascularization in a porcine model of chronic myocardial ischemia. J Pharmacol Exp Ther 292:795, 2000b

Landau C et al: Intrapericardial basic fibroblast growth factor induces myocardial angiogenesis in a rabbit model of chronic ischemia. Am Heart J 129:924, 1995

Lazarous DF et al: Comparative effects of basic fibroblast growth factor and vascular endothelial growth factor on

coronary collateral development and the arterial response to injury. Circulation 94:1074, 1996

Libby P et al: Cytokines regulate vascular functions related to stability of the atherosclerotic plaque. J Cardiovasc Pharmacol 25:S9, 1995

Lopez JJ et al: Basic fibroblast growth factor in a porcine model of chronic myocardial ischemia: A comparison of angiographic, echocardiographic and coronary flow parameters. J Pharmacol Exp Ther 282:385, 1997

Nugent MA, Edelman ER: Kinetics of basic fibroblast growth factor binding to its receptor and heparan sulfate proteoglycan: A mechanism for cooperactivity. Biochemistry 31:8876, 1992

O'Brien ER et al: Angiogenesis in human coronary atherosclerotic plaques. Am J Pathol 145:883, 1994

Ornitz DM, Itoh N: Fibroblast growth factors. Genome Biol 2:Reviews 3005, 2001

Padua RR et al: Basic fibroblast growth factor is cardioprotective in ischemia-reperfusion injury. Mol Cell Biochem 143:129, 1995

Post MJ et al: Therapeutic angiogenesis in cardiology using protein formulations. Cardiovasc Res 49:522, 2001

Rosenberg RD et al: Heparan sulfate proteoglycans of the cardiovascular system. J Clin Invest 99:2062, 1997

Sato K et al: Efficacy of intracoronary versus intravenous FGF-2 in a pig model of chronic myocardial ischemia. Ann Thorac Surg 70:2113, 2000

Sellke FW et al: Therapeutic angiogenesis with basic fibroblast growth factor: Technique and early results. Ann Thorac Surg 65:1540, 1998

Simons M et al: Clinical trials in coronary angiogenesis: Issues, problems, consensus: An expert panel summary. Circulation 102:E73, 2000

Udelson, JE et al: Therapeutic angiogenesis with recombinant fibroblast growth factor-2 improves stress and rest myocardial perfusion abnormalities in patients with severe symptomatic chronic coronary artery disease. Circulation 102:1605, 2000.

Unger EF et al: Basic fibroblast growth factor enhances myocardial collateral flow in a canine model. Am J Physiol 266:H1588, 1994

Unger EF et al: Effects of a single intracoronary injection of basic fibroblast growth factor in stable angina pectoris. Am J Cardiol. 85:1414, 2000

Waxman S et al: Preclinical safety testing of percutaneous transatrial access to the normal pericardial space for local cardiac drug delivery and diagnostic sampling. Cathet Cardiovasc Interv 49:472, 2000

Yu C, Edelman ER: Growth factor delivery strategies, in JA Ware, M Simons (eds): *Angiogenesis and Cardiovascular Disease.* New York, Oxford Univ Press, 1999

Zhou M et al: Fibroblast growth factor 2 control of vascular tone. Nat Med 4:201, 1998

40

VEGF GENE THERAPY IN PATIENTS WITH SEVERE CORONARY DISEASE

Douglas W. Losordo, Peter R. Vale,
James F. Symes & Jeffrey M. Isner

For patients in whom antianginal medications fail to provide sufficient symptomatic relief, a percutaneous transluminal coronary intervention or coronary artery bypass graft (CABG) surgery may be required. However, considerable numbers of patients, estimated to number over 200,000 each year in the United States alone, may not be candidates for either intervention due to diffusely obstructed native vessels and/or bypass grafts.

Folkman and colleagues established that endothelial cells may migrate, proliferate, and remodel in response to certain growth factors, and in doing so form new sprouts from parent vessels, i.e., angiogenesis (Folkman, 1971). It is now clear that bone marrow–derived endothelial progenitor cells also contribute to such neovascular networks (Isner and Asahara, 1999). Vascular endothelial growth factor (VEGF), identified by Ferrara and others (Ferrara, 1991; Keck, 1989; Plouet, 1989) as an endothelial cell–specific mitogen, has been shown to play a critical role in regulating endogenous neovascularization in response to tissue ischemia (Couffinhal et al., 1998; Carmeliet, 1999, see also Chap. 38, this volume).

Gene Transfer

Gene transfer (GT) is introduction of genetic material into somatic cells of an organism. The clinical goals include achieving high levels of sustained gene expression without provoking adverse host reactions. For several reasons, ischemic muscle represents a promising target for GT. First, both cardiac and striated muscles have been shown to absorb and express naked plasmid DNA (as well as transgenes incorporated into viral vectors). Second, previous studies have shown that the transfection efficiency of intramuscular GT is augmented more than fivefold when injected into ischemic muscle (Takeshita, 1996; Tsurumi et al., 1996). Viral vectors enhance transfection efficiency and yield higher levels of gene expression. However, in vitro (Takeshita, 1994) and in vivo (Losordo et al., 1994) models have demonstrated that low-efficiency (<1% of cells), but site-specific, transfection with a naked plasmid DNA encoding for a *secreted* protein (e.g., VEGF) may overcome the handicap of inefficient transfection by paracrine and autocrine effects. Thus GT of a secreted protein may achieve therapeutic effects not realized by transfection with genes encoding for proteins that remain intracellular (e.g., basic fibroblast growth factor, or FGF2). Furthermore, unlike certain viral vectors, plasmid DNA does not induce inflammation.

The preclinical and phase 1 clinical studies that employed GT with naked plasmid DNA encoding for VEGF are reviewed below.

Preclinical Studies with VEGF

Direct myocardial gene transfer of plasmid human VEGF$_{165}$ (Vale, 1999a; Tio, 1999) or VEGF-2 (Vale, 1999b) via a minimally invasive chest wall incision in a swine model of chronic myocardial ischemia resulted in enhanced collateral vessel filling and improved perfusion to ischemic myocardium assessed by colored microspheres. Intramyocardial injection of adenovirus encoding VEGF$_{121}$ (Mack et al., 1998; Lee, 2000) via thoracotomy in a pig ameroid model also improved collateral perfusion and function. Intracoronary adenoviral VEGF gene delivery produced much lower gene and VEGF levels in the myocardium with poor localization (Lee, 2000), while intracoronary adenoviral delivery of FGF5 was shown to improve blood flow and contractile function in the swine chronic ischemia model (Giordano et al., 1996). Pericardial delivery of adenovirus encoding VEGF$_{165}$ in a dog model did not increase collateral flow.

Preliminary preclinical studies in swine, utilizing a navigation system and catheter mapping technology (NOGA) integrated with an injection catheter (Biosense-Webster, Warren, NJ) to deliver plasmid DNA encoding a reporter gene to the myocardium (Vale, et al., 1999a), established that *percutaneous* myocardial GT could be successfully achieved in normal and ischemic myocardium in a relatively site-specific fashion without significant morbidity or mortality. Similar findings were demonstrated by a study utilizing adenoviral-assisted GT of a reporter gene (Kornowski et al., 2000). Safe and effective GT was also demonstrated in studies utilizing catheter-based

delivery of naked plasmid DNA encoding for VEGF-1 and VEGF-2 (Vale, 1999b), as evidenced by reduced ischemia on NOGA mapping.

Clinical Trials of Direct Myocardial VEGF Gene Transfer

Published studies of VEGF GT for therapeutic angiogenesis in human subjects have thus far been limited to phase I dose-escalating, nonrandomized trials involving naked plasmid DNA and adenoviral vectors. Patients in these trials generally have severe angina refractory to medical therapy, demonstrate ongoing myocardial ischemia, and are unsuitable for conventional revascularization. Other angiogenic cytokines have been administered via a wide variety of routes that include intravenous (Henry, 1999), intracoronary (Henry, 2000), or transepicardial at time of bypass surgery (Rosengart, 1999a); or via thoracotomy (Rosengart, 1999b), intrapericardial (March, 1996), or periadventitial at time of bypass surgery; and most recently transendocardial by catheter (Vale, 2001a).

The first trial of phVEGF$_{165}$ myocardial GT as sole therapy (i.e., without percutaneous transluminal coronary angiography or CABG surgery) was a phase 1, dose-escalating, open label clinical study in 30 "no-option" patients (Losordo, 1998; Symes, 1999). VEGF was administered by direct injection via a limited anterior thoracotomy. Injections were performed under continuous guiance of transesophageal echocardiographic monitoring. The patients in this phase 1 study demonstrated symptomatic improvement, increased exercise time, and objective evidence of reduced ischemia on single-photon emission computed tomography (SPECT) sestamibi myocardial perfusion scanning. Importantly, an improvement in resting perfusion defects was seen post-GT, suggesting improvement in areas of severly ischemic or hibernating viable myocardium (Shen, 1995; Wijns, 1998; Dilsizian and Bonow, 1993) as a result of therapeutic neovascularization. This observation was supported by the findings of electromechanical mapping (Vale et al., 2000), which demonstrated that resting perfusion defects on the SPECT images corresponded to foci of ischemia (reduced wall motion with preserved viability) on the endocardial maps; these maps showed significant improvement in wall motion abnormalities post-GT.

An open-label, dose-escalating, multicenter clinical trial of VEGF-2 plasmid DNA gene transfer was completed in 30 patients with refractory class III or IV angina. Significant symptomatic improvement occurred in 25/29 (86%) patients who improved by two or more angina classes and increased their mean duration of exercise by more than 2 min at 12 months post-GT (J. Isner, unpublished data).

The only other reported study of direct myocardial VEGF GT employed an adenoviral vector expressing VEGF$_{121}$, which was injected into patients undergoing bypass graft surgery ($n = 15$) and as sole therapy via minithoracotomy ($n = 6$). Symptoms and exercise duration improved in both bypass surgery and sole therapy groups, but stress-induced nuclear perfusion images remained unchanged. (Rosengart et al., 1999)

A single-blind pilot study of percutaneous, catheter-based VEGF-2 DNA gene transfer vs. a control/sham procedure, guided by the NOGA mapping system, was performed in six patients with medically refractory myocardial ischemia who were not candidates for conventional revascularization procedures (Vale et al., 2001b). VEGF-2-transfected patients reported a significant reduction in weekly anginal episodes and nitrate tablet consumption at 12 months post-GT. In contrast, while the blinded patients randomized to the control group reported an *initial* reduction in these parameters, this changed clinical profile was not sustained past 30 days, suggesting that the continued reduction in angina in the VEGF-2-treated group was not a placebo effect. The symptomatic improvement seen in the active treatment group was again accompanied by objective evidence of improved myocardial perfusion by both SPECT-sestamibi perfusion scanning and electromechanical mapping See Fig. 40-1 Color Plate 13 (Vale et al., 2001). While the clinical findings of this pilot trial concerning efficacy are similarly encouraging, the number of patients and the single-blinded design preclude firm conclusions in this regard. Consequently, a

multicenter randomized, double-blind, placebo-controlled trial of catheter-based VEGF-2 GT is underway that has thus far enrolled 19 patients. There have been no complications associated with a total of 150 injections among the 25 patients given either VEGF-2 or placebo in these two studies.

This preliminary experience thus suggests that it is feasible to replace currently employed operative approaches with minimally invasive techniques for applications of cardiovascular gene therapy designed to target myocardial function and perfusion. Such an approach may have at least three advantages compared to an operative approach. First, it potentially allows more selective delivery of the transgene to targeted ischemic zones, including sites that could not be accessed by an operative approach. Second, the catheter-based approach facilitates placebo-controlled, double-blind testing of myocardial GT. Third, the intervention could be performed as an outpatient procedure.

Potential Safety Concerns

Many angiogenic factors are known to be involved in tumor growth secondary to enhancing angiogenesis. Hence, in theory, angiogenic growth factors may lead to development of tumors, and they may be too small to be recognized. Even so, there are neither in vitro nor in vivo data to suggest that VEGF increases the risk of neoplastic growth and/or metastases, although longer term follow-up will be required to address this issue in clinical trials. Nevertheless, one must be vigilant about the possibility of cancer in patients treated with these angiogenic growth factors.

It is theoretically possible that VEGF may exacerbate proliferative and/or hemorrhagic retinopathy in patients with diabetes in view of the high VEGF levels demonstrated in the ocular fluid of patients with active proliferative retinopathy, leading to loss of vision (Aiello, 1994). With up to a 4-year follow-up, this adverse effect of therapeutic angiogenesis has not been observed in more than 100 patients (one-third with diabetes and/or remote retinopathy) treated with local delivery of naked plasmid VEGF-1 or VEGF-2 DNA at one institution; there was no effect on the visual acuity or fundoscopic findings as evidenced by serial funduscopic examinations pre- and post-GT by an independent group of retinal specialists (Vale, 1998a).

Experiments in transgenic mice engineered to overexpress VEGF ± angiopoietin have demonstrated lethal permeability-enhancing effects of VEGF (Thurston, 1999). However, even though VEGF has been reported to cause local edema, which manifests as pedal edema in patients treated with VEGF for critical limb ischemia, it responds well to treatment with diuretics (Baumgartner et al., 2000).

Another concern stems from the recent demonstration that inhibitors of angiogenesis tested in an apolipoprotein E–deficient mouse model of atherosclerosis inhibited plaque growth and intimal neovascularization (Moulton et al., 1999), and that VEGF administration accelerated aortic plaque formation in the same model (Celletti et al., 2001). However, data available from four separate animal studies and two clinical studies of human subjects (Vale 1998b; Laitinen et al., 2000) fail to support the notion that accelerated atherosclerosis is a likely consequence of administering angiogenic cytokines; the outcome, in fact, is quite the opposite, in that administration of VEGF led to a statistically significant reduction in intimal thickening due to accelerated reendothelialization, thereby refuting the notion that acceleration of atherosclerosis will be a consequence of VEGF-induced stimulation of angiogenesis (Losordo, 2001).

this early stage of clinical trials into myocardial gene therapy, it has been shown that direct myocardial GT utilizing different doses of naked plasmid DNA encoding for $VEGF_{165}$ and VEGF-2 can be performed safely, and this approach has shown objective evidence of improving myocardial perfusion. On-going clinical studies will determine the potential for neovascularization GT to be performed by nonsurgical, catheter-based delivery and will provide the opportunity to evaluate clinical efficacy in double-blind, placebo controlled trials.

The current clinical strategies employed for critical limb and chronic myocardial ischemia constitute an extrapolation from initial applications of GT to animal models with limb ischemia utilizing the 165-amino acid isoform of the VEGF-1 gene. These results, however, likely have generic implications for strategies of therapeutic neovascularization using alternative candidate genes, vectors, and delivery strategies; all of these are being actively studied in on-going clinical trials. Furthermore, the relative merits of GT versus recombinant protein administration remain to be clarified.

For the most part, clinical studies of therapeutic angiogenesis have been restricted to patients with myocardial or limb ischemia who have no other options. Although this is the group to target in the near future, it is not difficult to foresee a time when the sizeable population of patients who undergo bypass surgery but are not optimal candidates for that procedure may be eligible for therapeutic angiogenesis, which might be performed at an earlier stage of disease and thus provide a greater possibility of a successful outcome.

Conclusions

It is clear that site-specific VEGF GT can be employed in an attempt to achieve physiologically meaningful *therapeutic* modulation of vascular disorders. Intramuscular injection of naked plasmid DNA achieves constitutive overexpression of VEGF that may be sufficient to induce therapeutic angiogenesis in selected patients with critical limb ischemia (Vale et al., 1998; Tsurumi et al., 1996). Furthermore, at

ACKNOWLEDGEMENTS

This work was supported in part by NIH grants HL-63414, AG-16332, and HL-63695 (Dr. Losordo); HL-53354, HL-57516, and HL-60911 (Dr Isner); and a grant from the E.L.Weigand Foundation, Reno, NV, and the Peter Lewis Educational Foundation. Dr. Vale is the recipient of a fellowship from Bracco Diagnostics Inc./Society for Cardiac Angiography and Interventions.

REFERENCES

Baumgartner I et al: Lower-extremity edema associated with gene transfer of naked DNA vascular endothelial growth factor. Ann Intern Med 132: 880, 2000

Celletti FL et al: Vascular endothelial growth factor enhances atherosclerotic plaque progression. Nat Med 7: 425, 2001

Couffinhal T et al: A mouse model of angiogenesis. Am J Pathol 152: 1667, 1998

Dilsizian V, Bonow RO: Current diagnostic techniques of assessing myocardial viability in patients with hibernating and stunned myocardium. Circulation 87: 1, 1993

Giordano FJ et al: Intracoronary gene transfer of fibroblast growth factor-5 increases blood flow and contractile function in an ischemic region of the heart. Nat Med 2: 534, 1996

Isner JM, Asahara T: Angiogenesis and vasculogenesis as therapeutic strategies for postnatal neovascularization (perspective). J Clin Invest 103: 1231, 1999

Kornowski R et al: Electromagnetic guidance for catheter-based transendocardial injection: A platform for intramyocardial angiogenesis therapy. J Am Coll Cardiol 35: 1031, 2000

Laitinen M et al: Catheter-mediated vascular endothelial growth factor gene transfer to human coronary arteries after angioplasty. Hum Gene Ther 11: 263, 2000

Losordo DW et al: Use of the rabbit ear artery to serially assess foreign protein secretion after site specific arterial gene transfer in vivo: Evidence that anatomic identification of successful gene transfer may underestimate the potential magnitude of transgene expression. Circulation 89: 785, 1994

Mack CA et al: Biologic bypass with the use of adenovirus-mediated gene transfer of the complementary deoxyribonucleic acid for vascular endothelial growth factor 121 improves myocardial perfusion and function in the ischemic porcine heart. J Thorac Cardiovasc Surg 115: 168, 1998

Moulton KS et al: Angiogenesis inhibitors endostatin and TNP-470 reduce intimal neovascularization and plaque growth in apolipoprotein E-deficient mice. Circulation 99: 1726, 1999

Rosengart TK et al: Angiogenesis gene therapy: phase I assessment of direct intramyocardial administration of an adenovirus vector expressing VEGF121 cDNA to individuals with clinically significant severe coronary artery disease. Circulation 100:468, 1999

Tsurumi Y et al: Direct intramuscular gene transfer of naked DNA encoding vascular endothelial growth factor augments collateral development and tissue perfusion. Circulation 94: 3281, 1996

Vale PR et al: Arterial gene therapy for inhibiting restenosis in patients with claudication undergoing superficial femoral artery angioplasty (abstr.). Circulation 98: I-66, 1998

Vale PR et al: Catheter-based myocardial gene transfer utilizing nonfluoroscopic electromechanical left ventricular mapping. J Am Coll Cardiol 34: 246, 1999a

Vale PR et al: Percutaneous electromechanical mapping demonstrates efficacy of pVGI.1 (VEGF2) in an animal model of chronic myocardial ischemia (abstr.). Circulation 100: I-22, 1999b

Vale PR et al: Left ventricular electromechanical mapping to assess efficacy of phVEGF$_{165}$ gene transfer for therapeutic angiogenesis in chronic myocardial ischemia. Circulation 102: 965, 2000

Vale PR et al: Randomized, single-blind, placebo-controlled pilot study of catheter-based myocardial gene transfer for therapeutic angiogenesis using left ventricular electromechanical mapping in patients with chronic myocardial ischemia. Circulation 103: 2138, 2001a

CATHETER-BASED RADIATION THERAPY TO PREVENT RESTENOSIS FOLLOWING PERCUTANEOUS CORONARY INTERVENTIONS

Paul S. Teirstein

The need for repeat procedures because of restenosis continues to be the Achilles' heel of coronary angioplasty. An enormous body of investigative work has been directed at potential restenosis therapies. Scores of pharmaceutical agents have been tested in clinical trials. Despite initial promising results in the animal laboratory, most clinical trials to date have been disappointing. Coronary stents are currently the only intervention proven to decrease restenosis. In the STRESS and BENESTENT trials, implantation of a single Palmaz-Schatz coronary stent was associated with a 30% reduction in restenosis rates.

Radiotherapy is one of the latest in a long line of potential antiproliferative therapies to be enthusiastically tested as an adjunct to angioplasty. In more than 100 years of clinical experience, radiotherapy has proved highly effective in inhibiting cellular proliferation, both in malignant and benign disease. Examples of benign hyperplastic entities effectively treated with radiotherapy include the exuberant fibroblastic activity of keloid scar formation, heterotopic ossification, desmoid/aggressive fibromatosis, Peyronie's disease, and pterygium. In these benign proliferative disorders, doses of 700 to 1000 cGy in one treatment or fractionated treatments after the stimuli have proved effective in inhibiting fibroblastic activity without significantly interfering with the normal healing process.

Clinical Trials

Clinical data derived from trials of intravascular radiation therapy are rapidly accumulating. In one very early study, Bottcher and colleagues used ^{192}Ir to treat 13 patients with angioplasty plus stent implantation for femoral artery restenosis (Bottcher et al., 1994; Liermann et al., 1994). All 13 patients also received 12-Gy radiation immediately after the procedure. Clinical follow-up indicated no recurrent restenosis over 3 to 27 months. Steidle also used ^{192}Ir to treat 24 patients following stent implantation for femoral artery stenosis (Steidle, 1994). Percutaneous radiation therapy with 2.5 Gy per day for 5 days for a total of 12.5 Gy was administered to 11 of 24 patients. Over a 7-month follow-up period, reocclusion occurred in 2 of 11 patients in the radiation group and in 5 of 13 patients in the no-radiation group.

Condado and coworkers treated 21 patients undergoing coronary angioplasty with [192]Ir (Condado et al., 1997). While there was no control group, 1-year follow-up results were very encouraging, with a reported late loss index of 0.19 and restenosis rate of 27.3%. These results have remained essentially stable at 5-year angiographic follow-up.

In the Scripps Coronary Radiation to Inhibit Proliferation Post-Stenting (SCRIPPS) trial, patients with previous restenosis and stent implantation were randomized to receive a 0.03-in. ribbon containing either ^{192}Ir sealed sources at its tip or a ribbon containing placebo, inactive sources (Best Industries, Springfield, VA). [192]Ir dosimetry was calculated using intravascular ultrasound (IVUS) measurements. The radiation oncologist and physicist used information from the IVUS image to determine a dwell time that provided 800 cGy to the internal elastic membrane furthest from the radiation source, provided that no more than 3000 cGy was delivered to the internal elastic membrane closest to the radiation source. All angiographic and IVUS measurements were performed at an independent core ultrasound laboratory by investigators blinded to procedural information and patient assignment (Teirstein et al., 1997).

Between March and December 1995, 55 patients were randomized; 26 were assigned to ^{192}Ir and 29 to placebo. Angiographic indices of restenosis at 6 months were markedly different in treated vs. placebo patients. Late luminal loss was significantly lower in the ^{192}Ir group (0.38 ± 1.06 mm vs. 1.03 ± 0.97 mm; $p = .009$). Notably, the late lumen loss index (a sensitive measure of a therapy's ability to preserve the postprocedural luminal diameter) was significantly lower in the ^{192}Ir group (0.12 ± 0.63 vs. 0.60 ± 0.43; $p = .002$). Using a dichotomous definition, angiographic restenosis ($\geq 50\%$ diameter stenosis at follow-up) either within the stent or at the stent border (outside the stent but still covered by the study ribbon) was only 16.7% in the ^{192}Ir group compared to 53.6% for placebo patients ($p = .025$). Restenosis limited to the stented segment occurred in only 8.3% of the ^{192}Ir group compared to 35.7% of placebo patients ($p = .024$). The difference in angiographic restenosis rates was supported by a reduction in target lesion revascularization in the ^{192}Ir group (11.5% vs. 44.8%; $p = .008$). Composite clinical events (death, myocardial infarction, stent thrombosis, or target lesion revascularization) were also significantly less frequent in ^{192}Ir patients (15.4% vs. 48.3%; $p = .011$).

The angiographic results were supported by the independent IVUS analysis, which showed that there was no significant change in stent area or stent volume between the immediate postprocedure and follow-up period. The decrease in mean lumen area at follow-up was smaller in the ^{192}Ir group (0.7 ± 1.0 mm^2 vs. 2.2 ± 1.8 mm^2; $p = .003$), as was the increase in area of tissue growth within the stent struts (0.7 ± 0.9 mm^2 vs. 2.2 ± 1.8 mm^2; $p = .003$). The decrease in lumen volume was also smaller in the ^{192}Ir group (16.4 ± 24.0 mm^3 vs. 44.3 ± 34.6 mm^3; $p = .008$), as was the increase in volume of tissue growth within stent struts (15.5 ± 22.7 mm^3 vs. 45.1 ± 39.4 mm^3; $p < .01$).

Clinical and angiographic follow-up were obtained at the 3-year time point (Teirstein et al., 2000; Williams and Sharaf, 2000). At 3 years there was some late angiographic "catch up" in the irradiated group. The reduction in restenosis fell from 69% to 48%. However, at 3 years there was still a significant difference in restenosis rates (33% vs. 64%). Importantly, at 3 years the clinical benefits were durable (Fig. 41-1). Target lesion revascularization was 15.4% in treated compared to 4.3% in placebo patients ($p < .01$).

The Washington Radiation for In-Stent Restenosis Trial (WRIST) randomized 130 patients with in-stent restenosis to ^{192}Ir or placebo. At 6 months, the clinical and angiographic results were nearly identical to the SCRIPPS trial, with a 67% reduction in angiographic restenosis ($p < .001$) and a 78% reduction in the need for target lesion revascularization. The GAMMA I trial randomized

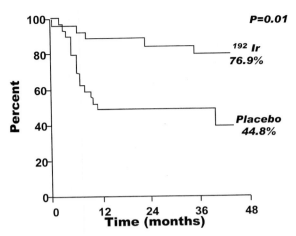

FIGURE 41-1

Kaplan-Meier curves for event-free survival in ¹⁹²Ir and placebo groups of the SCRIPPS trial. Event-free survival was defined as survival without myocardial infarction or repeated revascularization of the target lesion. The curves diverge at 3 months, differences increase over the next 7 months, after which clinical events are infrequent.

252 patients with native coronary in-stent restenosis up to 45 mm in length to ¹⁹²Ir, a gamma emitter, versus placebo. (Leon et al., 2001). The results were consistent with the previous single-center

gamma radiation trials. Restenosis was reduced from 55.3% in placebo patients to 32.4% in treated patients ($p = .01$) (Fig. 41-2). Target lesion revascularization was reduced from 42.1 to 24.4% ($p < .011$). There was remarkable consistency between the results of the above three gamma vascular brachytherapy trials. Thus, gamma radiation using ¹⁹²Ir is the very first therapeutic agent of more than 50 clinically tested to demonstrate an impact on neointima formation after angioplasty (Handley, 1995).

Beta emitters differ from the gamma energy used in the above trials in that they are less penetrating and easily shielded, making them somewhat easier to handle in the catheterization laboratory environment. However, questions have been raised concerning the ability of a beta emitter to provide therapeutic radiation doses to the required depth. Nonetheless, the results to date have been very encouraging (Teirstein, 1997). One group initially treated 15 patients undergoing coronary angioplasty with ⁹⁰Y, a beta emitter (Verin et al., 1997). The results were disappointing due to a loss index of 50% and restenosis rate of 40% at 6 months. However, this led to the more encouraging European dose-finding study. This trial randomized 181 patients with de novo disease, 28 of whom

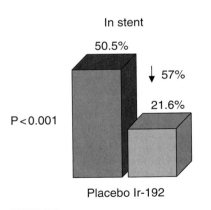

FIGURE 41-2

Restenosis rate in ¹⁹²Ir versus placebo patients at 6-month angiography in the GAMMA I trial. When the angiographic analysis is confined to the stented, treatment with ¹⁹²Ir reduced restenosis by 57%. When the angiographic analysis was extended to include the radioactive source margins outside of the stents (the edge effect) the restenosis rate was reduced by 41.4%.

received stents, to four doses of ^{90}Y (9, 12, 15, and 18 Gy at 2 mm from the source). A pronounced dose-response effect was observed, with 6-month restenosis rates falling from 27.5% in the lowest dose group to only 8.3% in the highest dose group, (Erbel et al., 1999). Another group used ^{90}Sr/Y, also a beta emitter, to treat 21 patients undergoing coronary angioplasty in the BERT I trial (King et al., 1998). Although there was no control group, the reported 6-month restenosis rate of 17% and loss index of 0.05% were very encouraging. In the expanded BERT II trial, 82 patients were treated with the same radiation delivery system. At 6-month follow-up, the restenosis rate was 17% and the late loss index was only 9% (Joyal et al., 2000). The BERT trial similarly reported encouraging results and documented a pattern of favorable remodeling after beta radiation in nonstented patients (Sabaté et al., 1999). These favorable results inspired a 476-patient randomized trial (the START trial, Popma JJ et al., in press, Circulation) to test ^{90}Sr/Y in patients with in-stent restenosis. Compared to placebo, patients with in-stent restenosis receiving radiation sustained a 36% reduction in subsequent restenosis, from 45 to 29% ($p = .001$). Clinical results were also impressive, with the need for target vessel revascularization falling from 24% in placebo to 16% in treated patients ($p = .026$).

The PREVENT trial used a balloon-centered beta-emitting source to treat patients undergoing balloon angioplasty or stent placement (Raizner et al., 2000). Patients were randomized to either placebo or three different doses of ^{32}P. At 6-months angiography, patients treated with ^{32}P had a significant reduction in restenosis (44 vs. 25%). However, these results were somewhat mitigated by the presence of new disease of the treatment margins (the "edge effect"). Thus, the need for target vessel revascularization was similar in both the placebo and treated groups. A larger, multicenter trial (The INHIBIT trial, Waksman R. et al., 2002) randomized 332 patients with in-stent restenosis up to 40 mm in length to the same ^{32}P emitter versus placebo. At 9 months, the need for target vessel revascularization was reduced from 31% in placebo patients to 20% in treated patients ($p = .033$).

Another potentially effective beta emitter is a radioactive, beta-emitting coronary stent. Beta-emitting radioactive stents hold the promise of a simple, easy-to-use, efficient radiotherapy delivery system. Metal stents have been made radioactive by implanting ^{31}P ions beneath the metal surface and then exposing them to neutron irradiation to convert ^{31}P into ^{32}P (Laird et al., 1996), or by activating stainless steel stents in a cyclotron (Hehrlein et al., 1995). The beta-emitting radioactive stent is applied directly to the vessel wall, which may provide more favorable dosimetry.

The IRIS feasibility trial (ISOSTENT, San Carlos, CA) tested escalating doses of a ^{32}P radioactive stent for patients with de novo native coronary stenoses (Moses et al., 1998; Serruys and Kay, 2000). While doses <0.22 MBq ($<6\ \mu$Ci) were ineffective, at higher doses the hyperplastic response was nearly abolished within the stent body. Unfortunately, at the stent margins this device elicited an intense hyperplastic response, resulting in clinically significant "edge restenosis" in approximately 50% of patients. A variety of creative remedies for this edge, or "candy-wrapper," effect have been tested including very high doses, low-pressure delivery inflations, and nonradioactive stent margins ("cold ends"); none, to date, have been successful.

Challenges to Radiotherapy

Despite the encouraging data emanating from the numerous clinical vascular radiation trials, challenges remain. The most significant remaining issues are late thrombosis and the so-called edge effect. Late vessel thrombosis was not appreciated until larger studies were undertaken. Most vascular radiation trials have documented a 5 to 10% rate of late vessel thrombosis occurring more than 30 days after the initial procedure (Costa et al., 1999; Waksman, 1999). This is an important clinical problem because most patients with late thrombosis present with acute myocardial infarction. Late thrombosis has occurred almost exclusively in patients who receive new stents at the time of the index radiation procedure. Presumably, radiation is so effective in preventing smooth-muscle proliferation that, in some cases, these stent struts remain bare or poorly endothelialized. Nearly all patients who sustain late stent thrombosis have discontinued antiplatelet therapy There are several potential solutions to this problem. Clearly, in the setting of radiation therapy, placement of new stents should, if possible, be avoided. Furthermore, antiplatelet therapy with aspirin and clopidogrel (or ticlopidine) should be continued for 3 to 6 months in the absence of new stents and, when new stents are placed, an even longer treatment period may be necessary. Finally, newer treatment modalities such as heparin-coated stents or antiplatelet stent coatings may be beneficial.

The problem of edge effect has been reported at varying rates depending on the device used and procedural technique. At one end of the spectrum, the beta-emitting ^{32}P stent has been particularly susceptible to this problem (Albiero et al., 2000). Nearly 50% of patients treated with this stent sustained very significant restenosis at one or both of the stent edges. One cause of edge effect may be failure to cover the entire injured vessel segment with the radioactive device. This phenomena, termed *geographical miss* by the radiation oncology community, is undoubtedly responsible for some of the edge restenoses observed in clinical trials. However, in most trials, geographical miss does not explain all of the edge effect observed. Other mechanisms, such as stimulation of neointimal proliferation by low doses of radiation at the source margins, may need to be invoked. Ultimately, edge effect will be limited in part by careful documentation of vessel injury during the preradiation angioplasty procedure and meticulous coverage of the entire injured segment plus an adequate margin by the radiation device. However, despite perfect procedural technique, edge effect may still be a persistent limitation of vascular radiation therapy.

Long-Term Consequences of Vascular Radiotherapy

While early safety and efficacy has been demonstrated in numerous animal studies and several human trials, the long-term efficacy and, most important, safety of this technique have been questioned. The possibility of late untoward consequences such as aneurysm formation, perforation, or accelerated vascular disease are significant concerns (Wiedermann et al., 1995; Waksman et al., 1995). In addition, it is not known if the beneficial effects of radiation therapy will be durable or if radiation will only delay and not permanently reduce restenosis. With the prospect of an increasing number of patients being exposed to intravascular radiation, it is essential to obtain long-term clinical follow-up.

Presently, long-term follow-up of patients enrolled in clinical trials using vascular radiotherapy is very limited. Five-year angiographic follow-up after intracoronary gamma radiation has been reported (Condado et al., 2000). The restenosis rate was low at 28%, but this study lacked a control group for comparison. Several coronary aneurysms and one definite pseudoaneurysm reported in the Condado series developed possibly because the vessels were potentially exposed to very high radiation doses (up to 92 Gy at 2 mm from the source) compared to the lower 12 to 20 Gy at 2 mm from the source used in most other clinical experiences. In other reports, long-term follow-up has documented high patency rates in femoropopliteal arteries undergoing angioplasty plus intravascular gamma radiation (Bottcher et al., 1994; Liermann et al., 1994). The SCRIPPS trial obtained angiographic follow-up in 19 patients treated with gamma radiation at 3 years. There were no perforations, aneurysms, pseudoaneurysms, or other special safety concerns (Teirstein et al., 2000).

Conclusions

Vascular radiotherapy is the first proven, clinically effective, antirestenosis therapy. Despite its established efficacy, there is much room for improvement. The optimum dose and isotope have not yet been established for any of the radiotherapy devices in clinical use. Dose-finding studies and randomized comparisons between devices will be required to optimize safety and effectiveness. While the role of antiplatelet therapy in minimizing late thrombotic events has been established, the optimum duration of therapy must be clearly defined. Continued long-term follow-up is required to define the long-term consequences of this new therapy accurately.

While vascular radiotherapy is rapidly evolving, other competitive antiproliferative technologies have emerged. Very possibly, radiotherapy has ushered in a new era in percutaneous revascularization where effective mechanical devices are coupled with equally effective antiproliferative and antithrombotic agents to dramatically improve long-term outcomes for patients with coronary artery disease.

REFERENCES

Albiero R et al: Edge restenosis after implantation of high activity ^{32}P radioactive β-emitting stents. Circulation 101:2454, 2000

Bottcher HD et al: Endovascular irradiation—a new method to avoid recurrent stenosis after stent implantation in peripheral arteries: Technique and preliminary results. Int J Radiat Oncol Biol Phys 29:183, 1994

Condado JA et al: Long-term angiographic and clinical outcome after percutaneous transluminal coronary angioplasty and intracoronary radiation therapy in humans. Circulation 96:727, 1997

Condado JA et al: Five year clinical and angiographic follow-up after intracoronary 192-Iridium radiation therapy (abstr.). Circulation 102 (Suppl II):II-750, 2000

Costa MA et al: Late coronary occlusion after intracoronary brachytherapy. Circulation 100:789, 1999

Erbel R et al: Intracoronary beta-irradiation to reduce restenosis after balloon angioplasty: Results of a multicenter European dose-finding study (abstr.). Circulation 100 (Suppl I):1, 1999

Handley DA: Experimental therapeutics and clinical studies in (re)stenosis. Micron 26:51, 1995

Hehrlein C et al: Low-dose radioactive endovascular stents prevent smooth muscle cell proliferation and neointimal hyperplasia in rabbits. Circulation 92:1570, 1995

Joyal M et al: Two year follow-up after post-PTCA β-radiation: A QCA analysis (abstr.). J Am Coll Cardiol 35(Suppl A):1A, 2000

King SB, III et al: Endovascular β-radiation to reduce restenosis after coronary balloon angioplasty. Results of the Beta Energy Restenosis Trial (BERT). Circulation 97:2025, 1998

Laird JR et al: Inhibition of neointimal proliferation with low-dose irradiation from a β-particle-emitting stent. Circulation 93:529, 1996

Leon MB et al: Localized intracoronary gamma-radiation therapy to inhibit the recurrence of restenosis after stenting. N Engl J Med 334:250, 2001

Liermann DD et al: Prophylactic endovascular radiotherapy to prevent intimal hyperplasia after stent implantation in femoro-popliteal arteries. Cardiovasc Intervent Radiol 17:12, 1994

Moses JW et al: Short-term (1 month) results of the dose response IRIS feasibility study of a beta-particle emitting radioisotope stent (abstr.). J Am Coll Cardiol 31 (Suppl):3 350A, 1998

Popma JJ et al: A randomized trial of ^{90}strontium/^{90}yttrium beta radiation versus placebo control for treatment of in-stent restenosis. Circulation, in press

Raizner AE et al: Inhibition of restenosis with β-emitting radiotherapy: Report of the proliferation reduction with vascular energy trial (PREVENT). Circulation 102:951, 2000

Sabaté M et al: Geometric vascular remodeling after balloon angioplasty and β-radiation therapy. A three-dimensional intravascular ultrasound study. Circulation 100:1182, 1999

Serruys PW, Kay IP: I like the candy, I hate the wrapper. The ^{32}P radioactive stent. Circulation 101:3, 2000

Steidle B: Preventive percutaneous radiotherapy for avoiding hyperplasia of the intima following angioplasty together with stent implantation [in German]. Strahlenther Onkol 170:151, 1994

Teirstein P: β-radiation to reduce restenosis. Too little, too late. Circulation 95:1095, 1997

Teirstein PS et al: Catheter-based radiotherapy to inhibit restenosis after coronary stenting. N Engl J Med 336:1697, 1997

Teirstein PS et al: Three-year clinical and angiographic follow-up after intracoronary radiation. Results of a randomized clinical trial. Circulation 101:360, 2000

Verin V et al: Feasibility of intracoronary β-irradiation to reduce restenosis after balloon angioplasty. A clinical pilot study. Circulation 95:1138, 1997

Waksman R: Late thrombosis after radiation: Sitting on a time bomb. Circulation 100:780, 1999

Waksman R et al: Endovascular low-dose irradiation inhibits neointima formation after coronary artery balloon injury in swine. A possible role for radiation therapy in restenosis prevention. Circulation 91:1533, 1995

Waksman R et al: Use of localized intracoronary beta radiation in treatment of in-stent restenosis: the inhibit randomized controlled trial. Lancet 359:543, 2002

Wiedermann JG et al: Intracoronary irradiation markedly reduces neointimal proliferation after balloon angioplasty in swine: Persistent benefit at 6-month follow-up. J Am Coll Cardiol 25:1451, 1995

Williams DO, Sharaf BL: Intracoronary radiation. It keeps on glowing. Circulation 101:350, 2000

COMPARISON OF ANGIOPLASTY AND CORONARY BYPASS SURGERY IN DIABETICS: SEVEN-YEAR OUTCOME OF THE BARI TRIAL

Katherine M. Detre, Robert C. Brooks, & Maria Mori Brooks

Coronary artery bypass graft surgery (CABG) was developed in the late 1960s and established as the primary invasive treatment for patients with symptomatic multivessel coronary artery disease (CAD). In 1977, percutaneous transluminal coronary angioplasty (PTCA) was introduced as a less invasive method of revascularization, principally to treat patients with single-vessel disease. By 1986, the second National Heart, Lung, and Blood Institute (NHLBI) PTCA registry found that the coronary anatomy of PTCA patients was becoming increasingly similar to that of patients undergoing CABG (Detre et al., 1989). Several randomized trials were initiated between 1986 and 1991 comparing PTCA and CABG for patients eligible for the two revascularization approaches (The RITA Investigators, 1993; King et al., 1994; CABRI Trial Participants, 1995). The largest of these studies, the NHLBI-sponsored Bypass Angioplasty Revascularization Investigation (BARI), was designed to compare long-term survival among patients with multivessel disease and severe angina or ischemia randomly assigned to an initial revascularization strategy of balloon angioplasty versus CABG. The most provocative result from the BARI trial was the revascularization treatment comparison in the subgroup of patients treated for diabetes (The BARI Investigators, 1996; The BARI Investigators, 2000).

Methods

Patients were eligible for the BARI randomized trial if they had angiographically documented multivessel CAD, clinically severe angina or objective evidence of ischemia, required nonemergent revascularization, and were judged to be anatomically suitable both for PTCA and for CABG as an initial revascularization procedure. Patients with prior PTCA or CABG were excluded from the trial, as were patients with single-vessel disease or left main artery disease.

Patients were enrolled between August 1988 and August 1991 at 18 North American clinical centers. New interventional devices and drugs, such as stents and glycoprotein IIb/IIIa receptor antagonists, were not available during initial revascularization.

The primary end-point of BARI was all-cause mortality. Each patient was contacted to determine vital status as of September 15, 1997; as a result, the average patient follow-up time was 7.8 years. Secondary end-points included Q-wave myocardial infarction (Q-MI), subsequent revascularizations, angina, and cause-specific mortality determined by an independent committee. Treated diabetes was defined as having a history of diabetes and receiving insulin or oral hypoglycemic drugs at study entry.

Treatment comparisons were made by the intention-to-treat principle. Kaplan-Meier estimates and log-rank tests were used to compare cumulative rates of survival, survival free of Q-MI, and repeat revascularization. Angina rates were compared cross-sectionally at each follow-up for surviving patients who completed that follow-up using chi-square statistics. Angina was classified as stable or unstable, and stable angina was further classified according to the criteria of the Canadian Cardiovascular Society, (CCS).

Results

Enrollment

Among 12,530 multivessel CAD patients who were clinically eligible for BARI, only one-third ($n = 4107$) were considered angiographically suitable for both procedures. Of these 4107 eligible patients, 1829 patients were enrolled in the BARI randomized trial. At the time of randomization, 353 patients had been treated for diabetes with insulin or oral hypoglycemic drugs; 180 were randomized to CABG and 173 to PTCA. The 94 patients with a history of diabetes who did not require medication at baseline were included in the analysis as nondiabetic subjects.

Baseline Profiles

Compared to nondiabetic patients in BARI, treated diabetic patients had significantly higher risk profiles (The BARI Investigators, 1997). A larger proportion of diabetic patients were women (43 vs. 23%) and minorities (18 vs. 8%), had less than a high school education (80 vs. 70%), had clinical histories of congestive heart failure (19 vs. 6%), peripheral vascular disease (23 vs. 15%), hypertension (65 vs. 45%), and renal dysfunction (6 vs. 2%), and had triple-vessel disease (46 vs. 40%). At the time of randomization, 163 (46%) of the treated diabetics were receiving insulin and 190 (54%) were receiving oral hypoglycemic drugs only. No significant differences were seen between diabetic patients randomized to CABG and PTCA.

In-Hospital Outcomes

Diabetic and nondiabetic patients had similar in-hospital outcomes in BARI (The BARI Investigators, 1997). Moreover, the occurrence of in-hospital death was similar for the two treatment groups within the subgroup of diabetic patients (1.2% with CABG vs. 0.6% with PTCA) and within the subgroup of nondiabetic patients (1.4% with CABG vs. 1.2% with PTCA).

Primary and Secondary Outcomes

In the BARI randomized trial, there was a steady divergence between the survival curves for the 914 patients assigned to CABG and the 915 patients assigned to PTCA (7-year survival: 84.4% CABG vs. 80.9% PTCA, $p = .043$) (The BARI Investigators, 2000). This difference could be attributed to a substantial and statistically significant treatment difference in the subgroup of the 353 patients with treated diabetes mellitus ($p = .0011$; Fig. 42-1). Estimates of 7-year survival were 76.4% for diabetic patients assigned to CABG and 55.7% for those assigned to PTCA. Among patients without treated diabetes, cumulative survival was virtually identical (7-year survival: 86.4% CABG vs. 86.8% PTCA group).

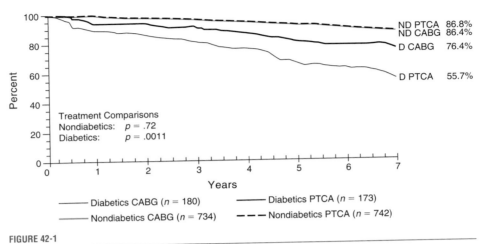

FIGURE 42-1

Survival by assigned treatment and diabetic status. Kaplan-Meier estimates of survival comparing the BARI randomized treatment groups, CABG vs. PTCA, stratified by diabetes status. D, diabetes; ND, no diabetes; CABG, coronary artery bypass graft; PTCA, percutaneous transluminal coronary angioplasty.

For diabetic patients randomized to CABG, those who received at least one internal mammary artery (IMA) graft had better 7-year survival (83.2%, $n = 140$) compared to those who received only saphenous vein grafts (SVGs) (54.5%, $n = 33$) (The BARI Investigators, 2000). The survival rate in the diabetic SVG group was almost identical to that for diabetic patients who received PTCA (55.5%, $n = 170$). Among the nondiabetic patients who received their assigned treatment, these three groups had nearly identical survival rates (86.5% IMA vs. 85.2% SVG only vs. 86.8% PTCA).

When the diabetic subgroup was stratified according to diabetes treatment (i.e., insulin versus oral agents only), the effects of both diabetes treatment and revascularization on long-term survival were evident (Fig. 42-2). Patients receiving insulin were at higher risk than those receiving oral agents alone regardless of method of revascularization, and patients assigned to CABG had better survival than those assigned to PTCA within the oral and insulin groups. Diabetic CABG patients receiving oral agents only had the best 7-year survival (84.1%), while PTCA patients receiving insulin had the worst

(49.4%); survival for the other two groups, CABG patients receiving insulin and PTCA patients receiving oral agents only, was similar (67.8 and 60.6%, respectively).

Long-term survival free of Q-MI was also worse for diabetic patients compared to nondiabetic patients. Among patients treated for diabetes, there was a statistically significant treatment difference regarding survival free of Q-MI favoring CABG (65.2% CABG vs. 50.0% PTCA, $p = .049$), while among nondiabetic patients these curves were similar (77.8% CABG vs. 78.9% PTCA, $p = .57$).

As expected, subsequent procedures, both PTCA and CABG, were much more common among patients receiving PTCA as their initial revascularization (Table 42-1) (The BARI Investigators, 2000). For patients initially assigned to CABG, repeat revascularization rates were similar for those with and without treated diabetes (11.1 vs. 13.5%, $p = .45$). In contrast, for patients initially assigned to PTCA, repeat revascularization rates were higher for those with treated diabetes than for nondiabetic patients (69.9 vs. 57.8%, $p = .0078$), and in particular, the rate of subsequent CABG was higher for diabetic

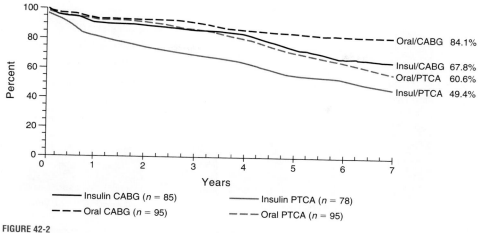

FIGURE 42-2

Survival by assigned treatment and diabetic treatment at baseline. Kaplan-Meier estimates of survival comparing the BARI randomized treatment groups, CABG vs. PTCA, in patients with treated diabetes stratified by diabetic treatment (insulin vs. oral agents only). Solid lines indicate patients receiving insulin and dashed lines indicate patients receiving oral agents only. Grey dashed lines indicate patients randomized to coronary artery bypass graft (CABG) and Grey solid lines indicate patients randomized to percutaneous transluminal coronary angioplasty (PTCA).

TABLE 42-1

ESTIMATED SUBSEQUENT REVASCULARIZATION PROCEDURES RATES AT SEVEN YEARS FROM THE BARI RANDOMIZED TRIAL

Subsequent procedure	Diabetic patients		Nondiabetic patients	
	CABG ($n = 180$)	PTCA ($n = 173$)	CABG ($n = 734$)	PTCA ($n = 742$)
None	88.9	30.1	86.5	42.2
PTCA only	9.3	21.9	11.8	24.5
1 PTCA	6.7	12.8	7.7	16.3
≥2 PTCAs	2.6	9.1	4.1	8.2
CABG only	1.7	27.0	0.8	21.8
Both CABG and PTCA	0.0	21.0	0.9	11.5

ABBREVIATIONS: CABG, coronary artery bypass graft; PTCA, percutaneous tranluminal coronary angioplasty.

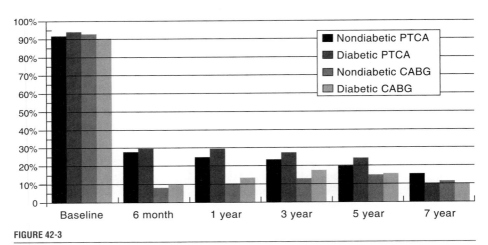

FIGURE 42-3

Angina rates among surviving patients. The percentage of patients with angina at baseline, 6 months, 1 year, 3 years, 5 years, and 7 years after study entry in BARI patients randomized to percutaneous transluminal coronary angioplasty (PTCA) and coronary artery bypass graft (CABG) and stratified by diabetes status at baseline.

PTCA patients compared to nondiabetic PTCA patients (48.0 vs. 33.3%, $p = .014$). Much of this difference can be attributed to the fifth and sixth years of follow-up, when a sharp rise in the number of CABG procedures for diabetics occurred.

Patients assigned to CABG were significantly less likely to have angina during the first 5 years; however, the difference between the treatment groups narrowed over time (Fig. 42-3) (The BARI Investigators, 2000). Among survivors who completed their 7-year follow-up ($n = 1072$), the 7-year treatment difference in angina was not statistically significant overall (15.1% PTCA vs. 11.4% CABG, $p = .075$) or within the subgroup of surviving diabetic patients (11.0 vs. 9.5%, $p > .10$). The large majority of angina reported throughout follow-up was stable CCS class I or II.

Discussion

Seven-year follow-up in BARI showed an overall mortality benefit among patients with multivessel coronary disease randomized to initial revascularization with CABG compared to those randomized to initial PTCA. The survival benefit, however, was entirely limited to the subset of patients with treated diabetes.

Among diabetic patients, an impressive survival benefit was seen with initial CABG therapy compared to PTCA, with an absolute mortality reduction of 20.7% at 7 years. This survival benefit was entirely attributable to a decrease in cardiac mortality and was limited to patients who received an IMA graft. The mortality benefit was consistently observed across other subgroups of diabetic patients, including those with or without proximal left anterior descending coronary artery disease, with normal or abnormal left ventricular function, and with varying degrees of baseline angina severity.

Hypoglycemic treatment regimen (insulin vs. oral agents) at the time of randomization appeared to be an important prognostic variable for diabetic patients undergoing revascularization in the BARI trial. Patients using oral agents only had improved survival compared to insulin-treated patients within each revascularization treatment arm. The survival advantage with initial CABG therapy was seen for both diabetic treatment subgroups but was apparent much earlier among patients treated with insulin. Insulin treatment thus appeared to be a marker of increased overall mortality and of increased benefit from initial CABG therapy. Information on the degree of baseline hyperglycemia and the overall glycemic control was unfortunately not available from this study.

Long-term MI rates were higher in diabetic patients than in nondiabetic patients (20.9 vs. 14.0% at 5.4 years of follow-up, $p = .004$) (Chaitman et al., 1997). However, MI rates were similar for patients randomized to PTCA vs. CABG within either the diabetic or nondiabetic groups. MIs occurred during the initial hospitalization more frequently with CABG patients and more frequently during the follow-up period for the PTCA group. Among diabetic patients, CABG therapy improved long-term survival free of Q-MI compared to PTCA therapy because of the survival benefit, rather than because of improved MI incidence.

The other smaller, randomized studies of CABG vs. PTCA in patients with multivessel coronary disease have shown results consistent with, but less striking than, BARI. The Emory Angioplasty versus Surgery Trial (EAST), a single-center trial with 392 patients, showed no difference in overall mortality between revascularization strategies. Among 59 diabetic subjects, however, the survival curves diverged after 5 years, with a trend toward improved overall survival with CABG (75.5% survival with CABG vs. 60.1% with PTCA at 8 years, $p = .23$) (King et al., 2000). A similar trend toward higher mortality with PTCA was seen among diabetic patients after 2 years of follow-up in the Coronary Angioplasty versus Bypass Revascularization Investigation (CABRI) (Bertrand, 1995). In contrast, data from the Randomised Intervention Treatment of Angina (RITA-1) trial suggest that the benefit from CABG may not extend to patients with single-vessel disease (Henderson et al., 1998).

SUMMARY

The BARI results demonstrate that diabetic patients with multivessel disease and unstable or severe symptoms should receive CABG using an IMA graft rather than balloon PTCA. However, the results leave many unanswered issues regarding revascularization choices in diabetic patients, including the optimal treatment of diabetic patients for whom revascularization is an option but whose symptoms do not yet require immediate intervention. The appropriate impact of newer percutaneous devices such as coronary stents, minimally invasive surgical techniques, and adjunctive antiplatelet therapies on revascularization decisions also needs to be defined. The increasing incidence of diabetes in the overall population and the high risk for cardiovascular morbidity and mortality among diabetic patients make further research on CAD treatment in patients with diabetes imperative.

REFERENCES

Bertrand M: Long-term follow-up of European revascularization trials. Presented at the 68th Scientific Sessions, Plenary Session XII, of the American Heart Association, Anaheim, Calif, November 16, 1995

CABRI Trial Participants: First-year results of CABRI (Coronary Angioplasty versus Bypass Revascularization Investigation). Lancet 346:1179, 1995

Chaitman BR et al: Myocardial infarction and cardiac mortality in the Bypass Angioplasty Revascularization Investigation (BARI) randomized trial. Circulation 96:2162, 1997

Detre KM et al: One-year follow-up results of the National Heart, Lung, and Blood Institute's Percutaneous Transluminal Coronary Angioplasty Registry. Circulation 80:421, 1989

Henderson RA et al: Long-term results of RITA-1 trial: Clinical and cost comparison of coronary angioplasty and coronary-artery bypass grafting. Lancet 352:1419, 1998

King SB et al: A randomized trial comparing coronary angioplasty with coronary bypass surgery. N Engl J Med 331:1044, 1994

King SB et al: Eight-year mortality in the Emory Angioplsty Surgery Trial (EAST). J Am Coll Cardiol 35:1116, 2000

The BARI Investigators: Comparison of coronary bypass surgery with angioplasty in patients with multivessel disease. N Engl J Med 335:217, 1996

The BARI Investigators: Influence of diabetes on 5-year mortality and morbidity in a randomized trial comparing PTCA and CABG in patients with multivessel disease. The Bypass Angioplasty Revascularization Investigation (BARI). Circulation 96:1761, 1997

The BARI Investigators: Seven-year outcome in the Bypass Angioplasty Revascularization Investigation (BARI) by treatment and diabetic status. J Am Coll Cardiol 35:1122, 2000

The RITA Investigators: Coronary angioplasty versus coronary artery bypass surgery: The Randomised Intervention Treatment of Angina (RITA) trial. Lancet 341:573, 1993

CORONARY ANGIOPLASTY VOLUMES AND OUTCOMES*

Charles Maynard, Nathan R. Every, & James L. Ritchie

Since its introduction in 1977, the use of percutaneous transluminal coronary angioplasty (PTCA) has expanded rapidly, with 539,000 procedures performed in the United States in 1998. In addition, 376,000 procedures using coronary artery stents were performed in that year. Given the large number of procedures performed, and the associated risk of both mortality and morbidity, many studies have addressed possible risk factors for adverse events. Hirshfeld and colleagues, representing the Technology and Practice Executive Committee of the American College of Cardiology, have conducted an extensive review of these studies and have made specific recommendations for the assessment and maintenance of proficiency in coronary interventional procedures (Hirshfeld et al., 1998).

One of the key findings from the review was support of the volume-outcome hypothesis for PTCA; that is, institutions performing a higher volume of PTCAs generally have a lower incidence of complications, most notably death and the need for emergent coronary artery bypass graft (CABG) surgery. The committee also concluded that on average there is an inverse relationship between individual operator caseload and the likelihood of complications, although this association is not as distinct as the one for institutional volumes and outcomes (Hirshfeld et al., 1998). The first purpose of this chapter is to summarize the results of key studies that have evaluated the volume-outcome hypothesis for hospitals and individual operators. Attention will be given to studies that have been published since the committee report was published in 1998.

A second purpose is to examine whether coronary artery stents have altered the volume-outcome hypothesis. Two studies reported that stents were associated with a reduced need for same-admission bypass surgery in the Medicare population from 1994 to 1996 and in California hospitals from 1993 to 1996 (Ritchie et al., 1999b; Maynard et al., 1999). How this result impacts the volume outcome-association will be assessed.

* This work was sponsored in part by the Department of Veterans Affairs Quality Enhancement Research Initiative Ischemic Heart Disease Center. The views expressed in this article are those of the authors and do not necessarily represent the views of the Department of Veterans Affairs.

Methodology: Administrative Databases and Definitions of Outcomes and Volumes

Throughout this chapter, outcomes or complications are defined as hospital mortality or the need for CABG surgery during the same hospital admission. These particular events have been selected because they are often all that is available in so-called administrative databases, which contain limited information on the hospitalization for PTCA. Typically, the occurrence of same-admission bypass surgery is obtained from International Classification of Diseases (ICD)-9 procedure codes.

Many of the studies investigating the volume-outcome hypothesis have used administrative databases from different settings, including the state of California, the Nationwide Inpatient Sample of varying numbers of states from the Healthcare Cost and Utilization Project, and Medicare. Information on operator volumes and survival beyond hospital discharge is usually not included in these data sets, although Medicare files with highly restricted access contain this information. The principal value of these databases is that they are comprehensive, i.e., they report on all procedures in a large population, such as Medicare. Special data registries, such as the one established in New York State, typically contain operator volumes and long-term survival status, as well as more detailed information on patient characteristics, which allows for risk adjustment.

The definition of institutional or operator volumes varies from study to study. In most studies cited in this chapter, low institutional volume refers to annual caseloads of ≤200, the minimum standard established by the American College of Cardiology/ American Heart Association (ACC/AHA) guidelines (Smith et al., 2001). Medium volumes are usually defined as 201 to 400 cases per year, and high volume as >400 cases per year. In Medicare, these criteria are often reduced by about half, since only patients 65 years and older are included. In New York State, where relatively few centers perform PTCA, different standards of low (<600), medium (600 to 999), and high (≥1000) have been used. Operator volumes of at least 75 cases per year have been established as the standard for acceptable practice by the ACC/AHA guidelines. In New York, operator volumes were categorized as low (<75), medium (75 to 174), or high (≥175). In Medicare, accounting for lower overall volumes, low operator volumes were defined as <25 per year, medium as 25 to 50, and high as >50.

Institutional Volumes and Outcomes

Ritchie and colleagues, using hospital discharge abstract data from the state of California for 1989, were the first to show that institutions with higher PTCA volumes had lower rates of same-admission bypass surgery (Ritchie et al., 1993). Although there was a trend toward reduced hospital mortality in high-volume centers, this difference was not statistically significant. Similar findings for California hospitals in 1993 and 1996 were also evident, as seen in Table 43-1.

Two groups, one using data from the state of New York and the other using Medicare data, concluded that PTCA outcomes were better in high-volume institutions (Hannan et al., 1997; Jollis et al., 1997). A third group, using a 20% random sample of U.S. hospitals from the Healthcare Cost and Utilization Project for 1993–1994, reported that rates of hospital mortality and same-admission bypass surgery were lower in high-volume centers (Table 43-1) (Ritchie et al., 1999a). This study of 163,527 procedures is among the largest and most representative reported, since it was not restricted with respect to patient age, geographic location, or type of medical center. On a national basis, the authors estimated that if all procedures performed in low- and medium-volume facilities had been done in high-volume facilities, the number of deaths for the 2 years would have decreased by 1.9% from 14,238 to 13,965, and the number of same-admission surgeries would have declined by 7.3% from 30,116 to 27,929. These estimates do not take into account the shifting of low-volume operators from low-volume to high-volume centers. These findings for 1993–1994 have been updated with results from the

TABLE 43-1

THE ASSOCIATION BETWEEN INSTITUTIONAL VOLUMES AND OUTCOMES FOR CORONARY ANGIOPLASTY

Study	AMI			No AMI		
	Death	CABG	n	Death	CABG	n
California 1989 (Ritchie, 1993)						
Low	4.5%	8.9%	1744	0.8%	5.8%	5201
Medium	4.3%	6.7%	1751	0.7%	4.2%	6549
High	3.6%	5.2%	1297	0.8%	3.9%	8314
			4792			20,064
p	.42	<.0001		.94	<.0001	
California 1993 (unpublished)						
Low	3.8%	5.6%	1490	1.2%	4.2%	3168
Medium	4.1%	6.8%	4030	0.9%	4.3%	10,367
High	3.6%	5.2%	3650	0.9%	3.1%	12,645
			9170		<.0001	26,180
p	.39	.19		.26		
California 1996 (Maynard, 1999)						
Low	3.5%	5.3%	1086	0.7%	3.5%	2171
Medium	4.0%	6.0%	4099	0.9%	3.3%	8993
High	3.4%	4.8%	6470	0.8%	3.2%	20,221
			11,655			31,385
p	.27	.05		.45	<.0001	
US 1993–1994 (Ritchie, 1999a)						
Low	4.6%	4.6%	2875	1.0%	4.0%	5791
Medium	3.7%	5.3%	10,484	0.9%	3.5%	23,914
High	3.8%	4.3%	30,911	0.8%	2.8%	89,552
			44,270			119,257
p	.0005	<.0001		.01	<.0001	
US 1996 (Maynard, 2001)						
Low	4.0%	3.2%	1607	1.0%	2.8%	2422
Medium	4.2%	5.9%	4111	1.0%	3.1%	7062
High	3.5%	3.5%	24,427	0.8%	2.0%	60,688
			30,145			70,172
p	.036	<.0001		.039	<.0001	
Rural Medicare, 1996 (Maynard, 2000)						
Low	8.2%	3.3%	330	1.6%	3.3%	509
Medium	10.1%	4.3%	822	1.8%	2.9%	1573
High	6.7%	3.9%	1217	1.2%	1.7%	3201
			2369			5283
p	.08	.91		.15	.002	

ABBREVIATIONS: AMI, acute myocardial infarction; CABG, coronary artery bypass graft surgery during the same admission.

1996 Nationwide Inpatient Sample from the Health-care Cost and Utilization Project (Maynard et al., 2001), as seen in Table 43-1.

A relevant question is whether low-volume centers should continue to exist, given the fact that high-volume centers achieve better results. It is important to recognize that not all low-volume centers have poor outcomes; this may be particularly true for low-volume centers that have high-volume operators. It is also possible that patients are treated in low-volume centers because they live in isolated areas in which there is only a single medical center. Maynard and colleagues reported that among all U.S. hospitals in 1996 there were 51 rural centers that performed PTCA in individuals 65 years and older; there were 13 high-, 18 medium-, and 20 low-volume hospitals (Maynard et al., 2000). In general, hospital mortality and same-admission surgery rates were lower in high-volume centers in rural areas, as seen in Table 43-1.

Concerning low-volume centers, Maynard and colleagues reported that in California from 1989 to 1996, the percent of hospitals performing >200 cases per year increased from 42 to 72% (Maynard et al., 1999). In 1996, 34 (28%) of 122 California hospitals performing PTCA were low-volume, and only 8% of patients were treated in centers performing ≤200 cases per year. Although low-volume centers continued to exist, >90% of patients were treated in higher volume centers. In comparison, in the state of New York, only 31 centers performed PTCA in 1994, and 13 of them performed ≥600 or more cases per year (Hannan et al., 1997). Ho, who examined the California experience with PTCA, concluded that the disparity in outcomes between low- and high-volume centers lessened from 1984 to 1996 (Ho, 2000).

Two studies have examined the volume-outcome association for primary PTCA or angioplasty performed in the setting of acute myocardial infarction (AMI). Every and colleagues, using data from the Cooperative Cardiovascular Project that included 6124 individuals 65 years and older undergoing primary PTCA, found that 82% of U.S. hospitals performed fewer than three primary procedures per month (Every et al., 2000). There was an association

between admission to higher volume hospitals and lower short- and long-term mortality; this association was independent of total PTCA volumes. Using the National Registry of Myocardial Infarction that included 36,535 primary PTCAs, Canto and colleagues concluded that in comparison to the lowest volume hospitals, mortality was 28% lower in the highest volume centers (Canto et al., 2000).

Operator Volumes and Outcomes

Several studies have demonstrated an inverse association between operator volumes and complication rates, although the association is not as clear-cut as the one for hospital volumes. In the state of New York, operator volumes of <75 patients per year were associated with higher rates of hospital death and same-admission bypass surgery (Hannan et al., 1997). In Medicare, higher rates of bypass surgery were associated with lower operator volumes of ≤50 total cases per year, although hospital mortality was not associated with Medicare operator volume (Jollis et al., 1997). These results for New York and Medicare are presented in Fig. 43-1. Ellis and colleagues, using data from five high-volume centers, reported that risk-adjusted death and a composite measure of outcome were inversely related to annual operator volume but not to years of operator experience (Ellis et al., 1997).

The association between operator volume and outcome is potentially modified by institutional volume, as seen in Fig. 43-2, which displays hospital mortality and same-admission surgery rates for operators performing <75 cases per year in New York State. Complication rates for low-volume operators in centers with >1000 cases per year were lower than for low-volume operators in centers performing <600 cases per year. In addition, other factors may influence the operator volume-outcome association. Little is known about the relation between operator volume and case selection, long-term outcome, periprocedural myocardial infarction, or measures of cost effectiveness (Hirshfeld et al., 1998). Consequently, the volume-outcome hypothesis for operators must be considered in light of these limitations.

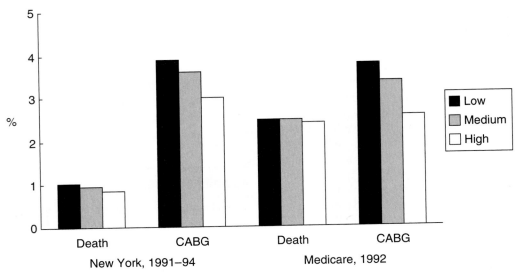

FIGURE 43-1

Operator volumes and outcomes for coronary angioplasty in New York and Medicare. In New York State, there was an inverse association between higher operator volumes and both lower mortality and same-admission surgery rates. In Medicare, this finding applied only to same-admission surgery. Rates for New York are risk-adjusted. Medicare rates are not risk-adjusted. CABG, coronary artery bypass graft surgery during the same admission. (From Hannan et al: JAMA 279:892, 1997, for New York data; and Jollis et al: Circulation 95:2485, 1997, for Medicare data.)

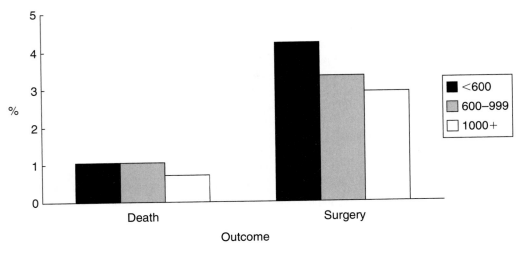

FIGURE 43-2

Outcomes in low-volume operators by categories of hospital volume. Outcomes for low-volume operators were better in high-volume hospitals. Low volume is defined as <75 cases per year. Rates are risk-adjusted. (From Hannan et al: JAMA 279:892, 1997.)

The Impact of Coronary Artery Stenting

Stents were first approved by the U.S. Food and Drug Administration in late 1994 to limit restenosis, although prior to that time a "bail out" device was approved for patients who had complete occlusion and required emergency surgery. In just a few short years, there has been dramatic growth in the use of stenting, such that it is now the major method of nonsurgical revascularization. The introduction of the ICD-9 procedure code for stents (36.06) in October 1995 permitted the identification of these procedures in Medicare and hospital discharge abstract databases.

Stents were associated with decreases in same-admission surgery rates but not in hospital mortality, in both Medicare (Ritchie et al., 1999b) and the state of California (Maynard et al., 1999). In Medicare from 1994 to 1996, same-admission bypass surgery rates decreased from 4.7 to 4.0% in the group with AMI and from 2.8 to 2.1% in the group without infarction. In California from 1993 to 1996, surgery rates decreased from 6.0 to 5.2% in the group with AMI and from 3.7 to 2.6% in the group without infarction. In 1996 in both Medicare and California, hospital mortality and same-admission surgery rates were lower in the stent group in comparison to the one undergoing PTCA without stenting. Adjustment for differences between those who did and did not undergo stenting was not optimal. In the Nationwide Inpatient Sample from the Healthcare Cost and Utilization Project for 1996, stenting was associated with decreases in both mortality and same-admission surgery rates in both the AMI and no-AMI groups (Maynard et al., 2001).

An important question is whether stenting, by its ability to "bail out" threatened closure, altered the hospital volume-outcome hypothesis. As can be seen for Medicare patients in Fig. 43-3, in the

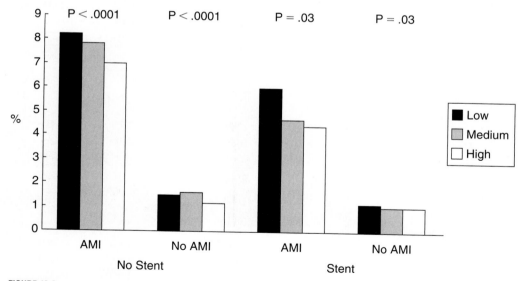

FIGURE 43-3

Institutional volumes and hospital mortality in patients with and without stents in Medicare, 1996. Hospital mortality was lower in high-volume centers for patients with AMI. The association is not as clear in the stent, no-AMI group where mortality was low. *p* value is by chi-square for trend statistic. AMI, acute myocardial infarction. (From Ritchie et al: Am Heart J 138:437, 1999b.)

no-stent group, hospital mortality was lower in high-volume centers in groups both with and without a principal diagnosis of AMI. The same result was true for Medicare patients in the stent group for patients with and without myocardial infarction, although the numbers of patients receiving stents was lower. Similar results were obtained for same-admission CABG surgery, as seen in Table 43-2. In California in 1996, hospital mortality was similar across categories of stent volumes for both AMI and no-AMI groups, although same-admission surgery rates were inversely associated with stent volumes in the no-AMI group (Table 43-2). In the 1996 Healthcare Cost and Utilization Project, the association between outcomes and stent volume was not evident, although there was a trend toward lower mortality and CABG rates in high-volume centers. Smaller numbers of procedures may have limited the ability to detect statistically significant differences. Given results from Table 43-2, it does not appear that stents have altered the volume-outcome association, although more numbers are needed to support this contention. McGrath and colleagues, using 1997 Medicare claims data,

TABLE 43-2

THE ASSOCIATION BETWEEN INSTITUTIONAL VOLUMES AND OUTCOMES FOR CORONARY ARTERY STENTING

Study	AMI			No AMI		
	Death	CABG	*n*	Death	CABG	*n*
Medicare 1996 (Ritchie, 1999)						
Low	6.0%	1.8%	1057	1.2%	1.3%	2931
Medium	4.7%	1.9%	3128	1.1%	1.4%	10,092
High	4.4%	1.4%	12,349	1.1%	1.1%	45,279
			16,534			58,302
p	.03	.08		.47	.07	
California 1996 (Maynard 1999)						
Low	1.0%	2.4%	287	0.6%	2.2%	1337
Medium	2.7%	3.3%	1488	0.7%	2.3%	5014
High	2.6%	2.4%	2565	0.8%	1.4%	10,699
			4340			17,050
p	.33	.21		.35	<.0001	
US 1996 (Maynard, 2001)						
Low	2.6%	0.4%	462	0.8%	1.8%	969
Medium	3.1%	2.3%	1408	0.8%	1.8%	3149
High	2.6%	1.6%	9751	0.7%	1.4%	28,227
			11,621			32,345
p	.46	.94		.65	.08	

ABBREVIATIONS: AMI, acute myocardial infarction; CABG, coronary artery bypass graft surgery during the same admission.

concluded that in the era of the coronary stent, patients treated by high-volume physicians and at high-volume centers had better outcomes (McGrath et al., 2000).

Conclusion

The preponderance of evidence supports the conclusion that complications of PTCA are reduced in high-volume centers. However, not all low-volume centers have poor outcomes. Because of geographic isolation, some low-volume centers are necessary. In addition, the performance of low-volume centers may be improved by the presence of high-volume operators who perform PTCA at more than one center. The inverse relationship between complication rates and operator volume is confused by several factors, including hospital volume. The fact that low-volume operators do better at high-volume centers must be considered when evaluating the hypothesis for operators. Whether or not this applies to primary PTCA, in which volumes are lower, has not been determined. Finally, while stents have reduced the need for same-admission bypass surgery and mortality in some cases, they have not altered the basic relationship between higher hospital and operator volumes and better outcomes.

REFERENCES

Canto JG et al: The volume of primary angioplasty procedures and survival after acute myocardial infarction. N Engl J Med 342:1573, 2000

Ellis SG et al: Relation of operator volume and experience to procedural outcome of percutaneous coronary revascularization at hospitals with high interventional volumes. Circulation 96:2479, 1997

Every NR et al: The association between institutional primary angioplasty procedure volume and outcome in elderly Americans. J Invasive Cardiol 12:303, 2000

Hannan EL et al: Coronary angioplasty volume-outcome relationships for hospitals and cardiologists. JAMA 279:892, 1997

Hirshfeld JW et al: Recommendations for the assessment and maintenance of proficiency in coronary interventional procedures. Statement of the American College of Cardiology. J Am Coll Cardiol 31:722, 1998

Ho VT: Evolution of the volume-outcome relation for hospitals performing coronary angioplasty. Circulation 101:1806, 2000

Jollis JG et al: Relationship between physician and hospital coronary angioplasty volume and outcome in elderly patients. Circulation 95:2485, 1997

Maynard C et al: Institutional volumes and coronary angioplasty outcomes in California: Results before and after the introduction of stenting. Eff Clin Pract 2:108, 1999

Maynard C et al: Coronary angioplasty outcomes in rural hospitals: Results from the Medicare Provider Analysis and Review Files. Am J Med 108:710, 2000

Maynard C et al: Improved outcomes associated with stenting in the Healthcare Cost and Utilization Project. J Interv Cardiol 14:159, 2001

McGrath PD et al: Relation between operator and hospital volume and outcomes following percutaneous coronary interventions in the era of the coronary stent. JAMA 284:3139, 2000

Ritchie JL et al: Coronary angioplasty statewide experience in California. Circulation 88:2735, 1993

Ritchie JL et al: Association between percutaneous transluminal coronary angioplasty volumes and outcomes in the Healthcare Cost and Utilization Project, 1993–1994. Am J Cardiol 83:493, 1999a

Ritchie JL et al: Coronary artery stent outcomes in a Medicare population: Less emergency bypass surgery and lower mortality in stent patients. Am Heart J 138:437, 1999b

Smith SC Jr et al: ACC/AHA guidelines for percutaneous coronary interventions (revision of the 1993 PTCA guidelines)—executive summary. J Am Coll Cardiol 37:2115, 2001

MINIMALLY INVASIVE CORONARY SURGERY

Valavanur A. Subramanian, Nilesh U. Patel

Introduction

Coronary artery bypass grafting (CABG) surgery is the most exhaustively studied operation in the history of surgery, and it has achieved widespread use because its benefits have been so thoroughly documented. The paradox is that the more elderly and debilitated patients who benefit the most from cardiac surgery, compared with medical therapy, are the ones who sustain greater risk of morbidity and mortality after cardiac surgery. Challenges brought on by an aging population, an increase in the number of patients with comorbidities requiring primary and repeat CABG surgery, the emphasis on clinical outcomes, the competitive status of coronary stenting, and cost containment in cardiac surgery have driven considerable changes and refinements in the surgical treatment of coronary artery disease. Though complete revascularization is associated with improved quality of life, fewer ischemic events, and increased overall survival in patients, the trauma of access often exceeds the trauma of surgical treatment while achieving complete revascularization. Other trade-offs are often increases in morbidity, mortality, cost, and post-operative stay. Outcomes after incomplete revascularization are also highly satisfactory if the patient is offered appropriate, optimum, targeted revascularization.

The most recent changes aim towards less invasiveness and the avoidance of the trauma- and inflammation-producing aspects of conventional CABG surgery while maintaining the safety and efficacy of proven surgical procedures.

The invasive aspects of conventional CABG are:

- Full midline sternotomy
- Aortic cannulation and manipulation
- Use of cardiopulmonary bypass.

In good-risk patients, the deleterious effects of these invasive manipulations are minimized due to the physiologic ability of these patients to cope with this surgical insult. As preoperative comorbid conditions increase, the risk of a surgical procedure significantly increases by the degree of surgical invasiveness. A full midline sternotomy usually heals without any adverse consequences in the majority of patients (<2% infection rate), but becomes an increasing problem particularly in cancer patients with irradiated chest walls; in patients with diabetes mellitus, renal failure, chronic obstructive pulmonary disease (COPD) or immunocompromising diseases; in older patients with decalcified, brittle sternums; and in patients undergoing reoperations. Cardiopulmonary bypass with its well-documented systemic inflammatory response also becomes a significant risk factor for those patients with renal, pulmonary, hepatic, hematologic, and neurologic dysfunction. Cannulation, cross-clamping, and aortic manipulation are also significant risk factors in most patients.

Atheroma of the ascending aorta and aortic arch is the most important risk factor for perioperative stroke in elderly patients undergoing CABG with cardiopulmonary bypass. This incidence may be as high as 6% for gross neurologic injury or 57% for mild cognitive changes (Roach et al., 1996). The cause of postoperative neurologic dysfunction is not fully understood but is believed to be a result of both embolic phenomena and hypoperfusion during cardiopulmonary bypass (Stump et al., 1996). Those with severely calcified ascending aorta, ascending luminal aortic atheroma, prior history of neurologic disease, or peripheral vascular disease are at a particularly increased risk for permanent neurologic injury (Roach et al., 1996). Between 1978 and 1988, teams led by Benetti and Buffolo popularized beating heart coronary surgery with full sternotomy (Benetti et al., 1991; Buffolo et al., 1985). The first multicenter report of minimally invasive direct coronary artery bypass (MIDCAB) grafting with mini-thoracotomy by Subramanian and co-workers brought minimally invasive cardiac surgery to the attention of cardiologists and cardiac surgeons (Subramanian et al., 1995). Minimally invasive coronary surgery currently falls into two basic categories:

1. Port-access coronary artery bypass surgery
2. Beating heart surgery
   a. MIDCAB, with minimal access incisions
   b. OPCAB—off-pump coronary artery bypass surgery with full sternotomy.

Approximately 7% of all CABG operations performed today (540,000 per year, worldwide) are done through a minimally invasive approach. Of these procedures, 85% are performed on a beating heart without cardiopulmonary bypass support.

Port-Access Coronary Artery Bypass Surgery

In this technique the patient is placed on total cardiopulmonary bypass with direct femoral artery and vein cannulation, and the heart is stopped with cardioplegic arrest and occlusion of the ascending aorta with an endoluminal balloon catheter placed with fluoroscopic and transesophageal echocardiographic assistance. The coronary artery target sites are approached through a fourth left intercostal space [5.0- to 7.5-cm (2- to 3-in.)] incision, and single or multiple coronary anastomoses are performed under a bloodless and motionless field with arterial and venous grafts, similar to the conventional method. Advantages of this technique are avoidance of sternotomy, feasibility of multivessel bypasses, and technical accuracy of anastomoses. The disadvantages are the requirements of cardiopulmonary bypass, femoral artery cannulation, and aortic manipulation with their known complications of aortic dissection, atherosclerotic emboli, postoperative bleeding, stroke, infection, and pulmonary and renal insufficiency. Data from a port-access international registry from 92 centers on 1036 patients have shown a stroke rate of 2.1 to 2.6 % and reoperation for bleeding in 2.3 to 5.5 % of patients requiring one to three bypass grafts, respectively (Shemin et al., 1999). These disadvantages have precluded its liberal application in high-risk patients with peripheral vascular disease, aortic atherosclerosis, renal failure, COPD, and coronary reoperations and in patients with hepatic, hematologic, and neurologic dysfunction. A steeper operator learning curve and substantial increased expense for the necessary equipment are required.

Beating Heart Surgery
MIDCAB Approach

In the MIDCAB approach, coronary bypass is performed through strategically placed thoracic and extrathoracic minimal-access incisions without cardiopulmonary bypass and aortic manipulation. The type of incision depends on the target vessel being revascularized (See Figs. 44-1 and 44-2, Color Plates 7 and 8). The advantage of MIDCAB is the avoidance of all the invasive aspects of conventional CABG surgery; the disadvantage is limited access to multivessel revascularization. Before April 1996, the so-called prestabilizer era, liberal use of beta blockers and calcium channel blockers and intermittent transient cardiac standstill, accomplished by means of bolus infusion of adenosine, helped to facilitate the coronary anastomoses. But pharmacologic stabilizers did not completely eliminate vertical and transverse movements of the target site, thus predisposing to the formation of multiple intimal tears and thrombi with unpredictably low patency rates (Subramanian et al., 1997). Hemodynamic instability was another major problem. The most important innovation in the MIDCAB technique was the introduction of regional cardiac wall and coronary artery target vessel stabilization with specially designed devices to hold the coronary artery site motionless while the heart continued to beat. Stabilizers not only improved anastomotic patency rates to become comparable to those of conventional bypass surgery but

also made this approach widely acceptable and helped to advance the learning curve more quickly for beginners. In addition, use of a rib cage retractor system along with a stabilizer allowed for easier harvesting of the mammary artery up to its origin.

Anterior MIDCAB is the most standardized of all MIDCAB procedures at present Fig. 44-3. It is performed through a minithoracotomy incision [5 to 7.5 cm (2 to 3 in.)] in the fourth intercostal space underneath the nipple See Fig. 44-4 Color Plate 9. The procedural success rate of this operation is >98% in most centers. Appropriate use of mechanical stabilizers has improved the early patency rate of left internal mammary to left anterior descending artery (LIMA-LAD) graft to well over 96% by many surgeons. (Shemin et al., 1999; Subramanian et al., 1997). In addition, an event-free interval rate of >95% has been reported by several investigators (Subramanian, 1998; Calafiore et al., 1998). In one recent series of 420 patients using the MIDCAB approach plus the use of mechanical stabilizers for LIMA-LAD graft, the event-free survival was 95.6% at follow-up of 1 to 60 months, with acute target lesion reintervention (TLR) of 1.2% and late TLR of 3.1%.

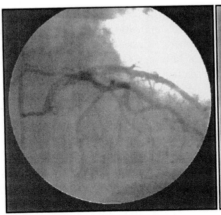

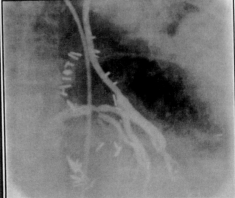

Preop   **Postop**

FIGURE 44-3

Anterior MIDCAB. *(Left)* Postoperative angiogram. *(Right)* Angiogram of the same patient's left mammary artery to left anterior descending coronary artery graft.

Indications for MIDCAB have been widening and they are:

1. Proximal lesions unsuitable for angioplasty or failed catheter-based intervention
2. Prior CABG with occluded vein grafts and patent mammary artery
3. Multivessel disease in patients for whom cardiopulmonary bypass is considered high risk because of associated risk factors (COPD, chronic renal failure, aortic atheroma, diffuse cerebral and peripheral vasculopathy)
4. Ischemic cardiomyopathy with documented ischemia of the anterior wall
5. "Hybrid therapy" for multivessel disease i.e., MIDCAB and concomitant percutaneous transluminal coronary angioplasty (PTCA)
6. As an adjunct to major noncardiac procedure such as ascending aortic aneurysm repair.

Although there are no absolute contraindications for MIDCAB, relative contraindications are an intramyocardial course of the vessel and small diffusely diseased vessel.

Early results with the grafting of the inferior wall with the right internal mammary artery or right gastroepiploic artery by either a subxiphoid incision or by a ministernotomy on the right side have been encouraging with an early graft patency of 92%. A newly developed high mid-lateral MIDCAB incision in the third or fourth space above the nipple in the lateral position to approach both the circumflex marginal and the left anterior descending coronary artery has been especially gratifying for the treatment of left main stenosis with the use of LIMA to LAD with composite radial artery graft to the circumflex marginal artery. In a limited number of patients, bilateral mammary artery graft harvest has been done through this incision for treatment of left main coronary artery stenosis. In the same fashion, the lateral MIDCAB incision for reoperative CAGB surgery with the radial artery graft from the descending thoracic aorta to the marginal branches has been good, with an early patency rate of nearly 100% Fig. 44-5 Color Plate 10. During the past 2 years, an extrathoracic transabdominal [small 5.0- to 7.5-cm (2- to 3-in.) incision in the upper abdomen] approach to MIDCAB Fig. 44-6,

Color Plate 11 has been fully developed at the authors' institution and successfully applied in 90 patients for double or triple CABG for primary and reoperative patients, with good clinical results (Fig. 44-7 Color Plate 12) (Subramanian and Patel, 2000). The authors believe that this will lead to true outpatient MIDCAB procedures similar to laparoscopic herniorrhaphy, appendectomy, and cholecystectomy.

Off-Pump Coronary Artery Bypass

OPCAB has significant advantages in patients for whom cardiopulmonary bypass and aortic manipulation present an increased risk (renal, pulmonary, hepatic and neurologic injury and/or insufficiency; aortic atheroma/calcification) and multivessel revascularization is required (Puskas et al., 1998). The disadvantages of this approach are the technical difficulty of bypassing the posterior and lateral wall vessels and the need for a full midline sternotomy. Some of the maneuvers used to facilitate anastomoses on the posterior and lateral wall include single-lung anesthesia, extreme Trendlenberg position with rotation of the table to the right, pericardial sutures (R. Lima stitch), traction sponges and slings (Calafiore, Spooner), wide division of the pleura and pericardium on the right side, and detachment of costal attachments of the diaphragm. Experimental work is now being conducted on a right heart assist device, to allow lifting and dislocation of the heart without reduction in preload or hemodynamic compromise. Also, introduction of the cardiac dislocating device, EXPOSE, has given a lot of freedom to expose various surfaces of the heart without significant hemodynamic changes. It is basically a suction device that lifts up the heart from the apex so that it can be maneuvered in various directions.

Endoscopic Vein and Artery Harvesting

Saphenous Vein

Sometimes morbidity of vein harvesting is much more than sternotomy and is mostly seen in diabetic or obese patients and those with peripheral vascular disease. Endoscopic saphenous vein harvesting involves harvesting the vein through a 2.5-cm (1-in.) wide incision made just above the knee with endoscopic and other specially developed equipment. Up to 65 cm (26 in.) of greater quality saphenous vein can be removed. A significant reduction in postoperative leg wound infection, decreased patient discomfort, earlier ambulation, and increased patient satisfaction have been demonstrated when compared to the standard open method (Connolly, 1997).

Endoscopic Radial Artery Harvesting

Endoscopic harvesting of the radial artery has been developed at the authors' institute and features a 2-cm (0.75-in.) incision at the wrist crease. The radial artery in this method is harvested using endoscope, harmonic scalpel, and hemoclips. Preliminary clinical experience with this technique has shown feasibility of harvesting the radial artery endoscopically, with early good clinical results and also better vascular intimal preservation in older patients.

Robotic MIDCAB

The initial notion of robotics in surgery involved operating at a site remote from the surgeon. The ability to transpose surgical and technical proficiency from one site to a distant site was thought to expand surgical application. Currently there is no clear path to practical application because of expense, transmission delay, and medical and legal issues. Application of telepresence surgery in the foreseeable future will probably be limited to telementoring rather than to remote manipulation. Telementoring will allow the surgeon to teach or proctor the performance of an advanced or new technique at a remote site using real-time teleobservation and monitoring.

Current applications of robotics include surgical assistance, dexterity enhancement, systems networking, and image-guided therapy. Dexterity is enhanced by placing a microprocessor between the surgeon's hand and the tip of the surgical instrument. Doing so allows performance of precise micromovement inside a patient's chest without putting a hand inside the chest. "Motion scaling," in which gross hand movements can be reduced and made more precise, and also unintentional movements can be eliminated by filter. For now, robotic coronary surgery requires cardiopulmonary bypass and an arrested heart, but soon, with the development of an endoscopic stabilization system, totally endoscopic closed-chest robotic coronary surgery on a beating heart may be a reality.

SUMMARY

Minimally invasive CABG surgery techniques are still under intense clinical investigation. Some studies have shown cost savings, especially with the MID-CAB technique, due to decreased length of hospital stay (2 days), decreased need for heart-lung machines and the personnel to run them, elimination of the need for ventilators in post-recovery; and fewer blood tests and blood transfusions. Stroke rate with these procedures is essentially zero, and the risk of heart attack is halved without a heart-lung machine. Chance of infection is cut down to about one-fourth of what it is using cardiopulmonary bypass. Although these benefits of minimally invasive coronary surgery are becoming apparent, more studies are needed to validate the claims that it is at least as safe and effective as open-heart procedures.

Currently there is rapid development in enabling technology, i.e., robotic assistance and facilitating coronary anastomotic devices (staples, surgical glue.) This will lead further towards truly noninvasive coronary surgery with ports. Hybrid MIDCAB in combination with PTCA and stent has become increasingly frequent. A new paradigm for CABG may consist of LIMA-LAD MIDCAB and/or of the circumflex or right coronary artery, combined with risk-factor prevention.

REFERENCES

Benetti FJ et al: Direct myocardial revascularization without extracorporeal circulation. Chest 100:312, 1991

Buffolo E et al: Direct myocardial revascularization without cardiopulmonary bypass. Thorac Cardiovasc Surg 26:33, 1985

Calafiore AM et al: The LAST operation: Techniques and results before and after the stabilization era. Ann Thorac Surg 66:998, 1998

Connolly MW: Endoscopic subcutaneous saphenous vein harvest: Lessons learned from 350 cases. Presented at the Third Annual New York Symposium on Vascular and Endovascular Techniques, New York, NY, September 1997

Puskas JD et al: Off pump multivessel coronary bypass via sternotomy is safe and effective. Ann Thorac Surg 66:1068, 1998

Roach GW et al: Adverse cerebral outcomes after coronary bypass surgery. N Engl J Med 335:1587, 1996

Shemin RJ et al: World's largest registry of minimally invasive CABG with endo CBP demonstrates excellent results with minimal morbidity and mortality (Abstr.). J Am Coll Cardiol 33:2, 567A, Feb 1999

Stump D et al: Cerebral emboli and cognitive outcome after cardiac surgery. J Cardiothorac Vasc Anesth 10:113, 1996

Subramanian VA: Minimally invasive coronary artery bypass grafting on the beating heart: the American experience, in MC Oz, DJ Goldstein (eds). *Contemporary Cardiology: Minimally Invasive Cardiac Surgery,* Totowa, NJ, Humana Press, 1998, pp 89–103

Subramanian VA et al: Minimally invasive coronary artery bypass surgery: A multi-center report of preliminary clinical experience. Circulation 92(Suppl):1645, 1995

Subramanian VA et al: Minimally invasive direct coronary artery bypass grafting: Two year clinical experience. Ann Thorac Surg. 64:1648, 1997

Subramanian VA, Patel NU: Transabdominal minimally invasive direct coronary artery bypass grafting (MIDCAB). Eur J Cardiothorac Surg 17: 485, 2000

INTRAVASCULAR ULTRASOUND INSIGHTS INTO TRANSPLANT VASCULOPATHY

Samir R. Kapadia, E. Murat Tuzcu

Cardiac transplantation is an important therapeutic alternative for patients with severe irreversible congestive heart failure. Transplant vasculopathy continues to be a troublesome long-term complication of heart transplantation, being the major cause of death in patients surviving 1 year after transplantation.

Coronary angiography, despite its well-recognized limitations, has served as an important tool to investigate coronary anatomy in normal and diseased states (Ziada et al., 1999). Rapid progress in technology has led to emergence of intravascular ultrasound (IVUS) as a widely utilized tool to study a number of morphologic and developmental questions regarding transplant coronary artery disease (CAD). The major advantage of IVUS imaging is its ability to visualize the vessel wall in vivo, whereas angiography can only discern the effects of the disease process on the vessel lumen (Ziada et al., 1999).

Basic Principles of IVUS
Image Interpretation

Ultrasound images are generated by reflections of waves from interfaces between tissues having different acoustic properties. The strength and signal quality of the ultrasound beam returning to the transducer (backscatter) determine whether the ultrasound scanner visualizes a particular structure. The acoustic impedance of tissue determines the amplitude of the backscatter and the intensity of image. Acoustic properties of the tissues are determined by specific gravity, compressibility, and viscosity. In a normal coronary artery, the discrete echodense layer at the lumen-wall interface separates lumen from echolucent media, which is referred to as *intima*. The tunica media is visualized as a distinct subintimal sonolucent layer, which is limited by an outer echodense media-adventitia interface. The outer, or trailing, edge of the adventitia is indistinct, as it merges into the surrounding perivascular connective tissue. The echodense intima and adventitia with the sonolucent medial layer in between give the arterial wall a trilaminar appearance. In young populations, the internal elastic membrane is not dense enough to reflect an ultrasound signal, giving a monolayer appearance. Subtle, finely textured echoes moving in a characteristic swirling pattern characterize the blood within the vessel lumen.

Lesion Morphology

There are no standard definitions to describe the morphology of the lesions in transplant CAD. The longitudinal extent (focal vs. diffuse) of disease can be described using the classification of coronary artery segments as defined in the Coronary Artery Surgery Study (CASS). A lesion can be defined as focal if there is at least one normal site in the same CASS segment. A lesion is diffuse when it involves the entire segment (Kapadia et al., 1998). A lesion is circumferential if it involves the entire circumference of a vessel and noncircumferential if any arc of the vessel wall is free of disease.

Quantitative IVUS Analysis

Intimal thickness is defined as the distance from the intimal leading edge to the external elastic membrane (adventitial leading edge) (Fig. 45-1) The measurement of intima therefore includes media. Lumen cross-sectional area (L_{csa}), external elastic membrane cross-sectional area (EEM_{csa}) or vessel area, maximal intimal thickness (IT_{max}), and minimal intimal thickness (IT_{min}) are commonly measured at the sites of interest. Intimal (or plaque) cross-sectional area (IT_{csa}) is calculated from the difference between EEM_{csa} and L_{csa}. IT_{max} is a commonly used measure to describe the severity of

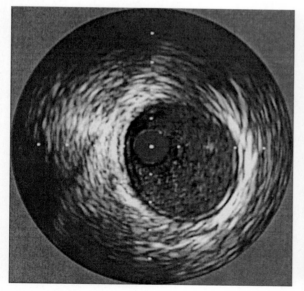 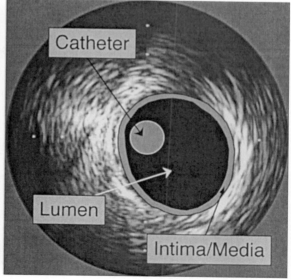

FIGURE 45-1

Intravascular ultrasound (IVUS) image of a normal coronary artery. On the right panel the IVUS catheter, the lumen, and the intima/media are illustrated. The intima/media appears as a thin rim of tissue between the lumen and the adventitia.

lesions. A standardized classification for extent of transplant vasculopathy has been proposed using the severity of intimal thickening and the degree of circumferential involvement (Botas et al., 1995).

Although IVUS examination of a single coronary artery yields thousands of cross-sectional images, some cross-sectional images have to be selected for measurement in order to express this information quantitatively. Various approaches for sampling the sites have been proposed. One approach is to select multiple sites, at least 1 cm apart, from the proximal coronary segments to represent the entire coronary tree. The sample is neither derived according to predefined criteria; nor is it randomly selected and therefore is subject to selection bias. An alternative method is to select sites according to predefined criteria; two sites, one with the least intimal thickness and another with the greatest intimal thickness are selected from each segment of a coronary artery. The third approach, morphometry, allows three-dimensional information to be obtained from data collected in two dimensions. The pullback sequence of a coronary artery of interest is divided in approximately equal time intervals, and a site is randomly selected closest to the time of interest. Using mathematical modeling, volumes are calculated; they can be calculated precisely by performing automated pullback with a known pullback speed. For this, lumen and intimal areas are measured at sites that are 1 to 2 mm apart. The volumes are calculated using Simpson's formula. All these approaches have been employed in cross-sectional and serial study designs.

Safety of IVUS Examination

The safety of intracoronary ultrasound imaging has been well documented with rare complications. The most frequently encountered complication is a focal coronary spasm (2 to 5% of cases), which usually responds rapidly to intracoronary nitroglycerin. Data from multiple European centers performing IVUS examinations reported a 1.1% complication (spasm, vessel dissection, or guidewire entrapment) rate in a total of 718 examinations. All complica-

tions occurred in patients with atherosclerotic coronary disease undergoing percutaneous intervention (Batkoff and Linker, 1996). In another multicenter report from 28 centers in 2207 IVUS studies, where 505 (23%) studies were performed in heart transplant recipients and 1702 (77%) in nontransplant patients, spasm was reported in 63 (2.9%) patients. None of the transplant patients had any other complication in this series (Hausmann et al., 1995). Moreover, the long-term safety of this procedure has also been studied in transplant patients. It has been shown that instrumentation of the coronary arteries does not lead to development or progression of transplant vasculopathy (Son et al., 1999).

Rationale for using IVUS for Studying Transplant CAD

Transmitted lesions of donor atherosclerosis and newly developed lesions of vasculopathy contribute to transplant CAD. These lesions are difficult to study with angiography because they are small, eccentric lesions that frequently do not encroach upon the lumen due to arterial remodeling. Further, these early lesions do not produce ischemia on stress testing. By the time vasculopathy manifests as ischemia on functional studies, the disease process is usually well advanced. IVUS imaging, due to its ability to visualize arterial wall structure in vivo, provides a sensitive tool to study early transplant vasculopathy lesions. Whether noninvasive functional studies to assess endothelial function can accurately predict morphologic changes remains unknown (Allen-Auerbach et al., 1999).

Insights into Transplant Vasculopathy

The lesions of transplant vasculopathy have different characteristics compared to the lesions of donor atherosclerosis (Table 45-1) (Billingham, 1992). However, due to vast heterogeneity in the morphology of both these lesions types, it is impossible to ascertain the origin of each lesion by the morphology alone

TABLE 45-1

COMPARISON OF TRANSPLANT VASCULOPATHY WITH CONVENTIONAL ATHEROSCLEROSIS

Characteristics	Transplant Vasculopathy	Donor Atherosclerosis
Intimal proliferation	Circumferential	Non-circumferential
Internal elastic lamina	Intact	Disrupted
Calcium deposition	Absent	Frequently present
Intramyocardial vessels	Involved	Spared
Rate of development	Months	Years

(Kapadia et al.,1998). IVUS examination performed soon after transplantation allows accurate identification of donor atherosclerosis. Serial IVUS examinations performed thereafter can spot newly developing lesions of transplant vasculopathy. Accurate information on the extent and severity of these lesions can be obtained by including proximal and distal segment imaging of all three epicardial vessels (Kapadia et al., 2000).

Donor Disease

Lesions seen on IVUS examination performed within the first 2 months after transplantation are thought to represent donor atherosclerosis because the prevalence and severity of these lesions are dependent on donor age, gender, and donor atherosclerosis risk factors and *not* on recipient characteristics.

Typically, a lesion is defined as a site in the coronary artery with $IT_{max} > 0.3$ to 0.5 mm. This somewhat arbitrary threshold has been derived from necropsy studies performed on war casualties. Despite the young donor age, atherosclerosis is detected in >50% of transplanted patients (Tuzcu et al., 2001). Age and male gender of donor are the most important predictors of atherosclerosis. Not surprisingly, most of these lesions are angiographically silent (Tuzcu et al., 1995). Donor atherosclerosis lesions are frequently focal, noncircumferential, and involve proximal coronary artery segments with predilection for bifurcation (Kapadia et al., 1998).

The long-term natural history of donor atherosclerosis lesions after transplantation remains largely unknown. In a serial study, donor disease progression, defined as ≥ 0.3-mm increase in IT_{max}, was seen in 42% of patients during the first year after transplantation (Kapadia et al., 1998). The progression of the donor lesions was insignificant between the first and second year after transplantation (Kapadia et al., 1999). This "progression" may represent transplant vasculopathy lesions developing over atherosclerosis or actual progression of atherosclerosis. Rarely, regression of donor atherosclerosis has also been documented.

Factors determining the progression of donor lesions have not been adequately studied. A small study of 36 patients with donor lesions investigated the role of conventional atherosclerosis risk factors on the progression of these lesions. In the multivariate analysis, recipient pretransplant body mass index and posttransplant serum triglyceride level were significant predictors for the progression of donor atherosclerosis. Older recipient age showed a trend in predicting progression; however, donor age did not affect disease progression (Kapadia et al., 2001).

Scarcity of organs has led to more frequent acceptance of older donors, which in turn has increased the prevalence of donor atherosclerosis in transplanted hearts. Fortunately, careful selection of older donors does not affect graft survival adversely (Drinkwater et al., 1996). Even the incidence of angiographically detectable transplant CAD on 5 years' follow-up is similar in recipients of older hearts compared to younger donors (Drinkwater et al., 1996). This finding is in accordance with the observation that evidence of atherosclerosis on IVUS examination is not associated with more frequent or severe transplant vasculopathy.

Transplant Vasculopathy

The incidence of angiographically detected transplant vasculopathy ranges from 10 to 20% at 1 year and up to 50% by 5 years. This is an underestimation of the true disease prevalence as vasculopathy lesions are detected in almost 50% of the patients after 1 year of transplantation with multivessel IVUS imaging (Kapadia et al., 1998).

Vasculopathy lesions are defined as lesions appearing at previously normal sites, underscoring the value of baseline examination soon after transplantation (Fig. 45-2). Without a baseline study, accurate identification of vasculopathy lesions is not feasible because they cannot be confidently differentiated from early atherosclerosis by morphology alone. The early lesions of vasculopathy are frequently located in the proximal segments and commonly involve vessel bifurcation. These lesions are

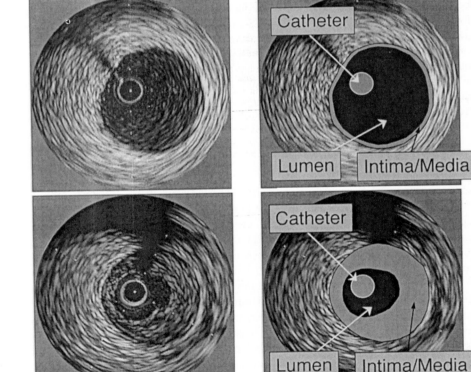

FIGURE 45-2

Development of severe transplant vasculopathy. The upper panels show IVUS images at baseline (less than 6 weeks after transplantation). The lower panels show the same site at 1-year follow-up. The vessel site is normal at baseline, but at follow-up substantial proliferation has developed occupying the entire circumference of the vessel.

more frequently diffuse and circumferential compared to the donor lesions (Kapadia et al., 1998).

The natural history of transplant vasculopathy has been investigated in cross-sectional studies where only one IVUS examination is performed after variable time interval from transplantation. In such studies, it has been shown that the intimal thickness and intimal area increase progressively with time. In a serial study of a relatively small number of patients, it appeared that lesion severity did not increase rapidly after the first year of transplantation, but new lesions continued to develop at previously normal sites (Kapadia et al., 1999). This finding underscores the importance for continued surveillance for transplant vasculopathy.

IVUS imaging has been used to evaluate factors affecting the development of vasculopathy lesions. In a study by Mehra and colleagues, significant independent predictors of severe intimal hyperplasia included donor age >35 years, first-year mean biopsy score >1, and hypertriglyceridemia. Additionally, subjects with severe intimal thickening had a fourfold higher cardiac event rate than those without severe intimal proliferation on IVUS (Mehra et al., 1995a). In another study, in patients with evidence of rejection, the rate of progression of transplant vasculopathy correlated with the severity of rejection (Jimenez et al., 2001). One group reported total cholesterol, low-density lipoprotein (LDL) cholesterol, triglyceride levels, obesity indexes, donor age, and years following cardiac transplantation to be independent predictors of the severity of cardiac allograft vasculopathy (Escobar et al., 1994). Similarly, another study demonstrated significant correlation between fasting plasma triglyceride level and weight with severity of intimal thickening (Rickenbacher et al., 1996). Further, male recipients of female allografts have worse vasculopathy compared with either male or female recipients of male allografts at 1 year after heart transplantation (Mehra et al., 1994).

IVUS imaging has also provided insight into the effectiveness of various therapies influencing transplant vasculopathy. A subgroup analysis from a randomized trial showed that the decrease in cholesterol levels and improvement in survival with pravastatin therapy was associated with a decrease in the rate of progression of vasculopathy lesions (Kobashigawa et al., 1995). Another small study reported reduction in the intimal thickness with treatment utilizing diltiazem, angiotensin-converting enzyme inhibitors, or both (Mehra et al., 1995b). In a retrospective study, conventional atherosclerosis risk factors did not predict development of allograft vasculopathy, but greater increase in serum LDL cholesterol level during the first year after transplant was associated with more severe vasculopathy. This may suggest that maintenance of LDL cholesterol as close to pretransplant values as possible may help to limit the rate of progression of acquired allograft vasculopathy (Kapadia et al., 2001).

The findings of IVUS imaging are shown to predict long-term clinical outcome. In a study of 74 patients, patients with severe intimal thickening (>0.5 mm) had more events (death, myocardial infarction, and retransplantation) at approximately 4-years' follow-up (Mehra et al., 1995c). Another study reported that patients with intimal thickness >1 mm had the worst survival (Wiedermann et al., 1994). On the other hand, others have reported an increased cardiac event rate in patients with mean intimal thickening of >0.3 mm in 145 heart transplant recipients at 48 months' follow-up (Rickenbacher et al., 1995). The experience at Cleveland Clinic Foundation with 100 patients at approximately 4-years' follow-up also demonstrated a higher event rate, with rapidly progressive intimal thickening in the first year of transplantation (Kapadia et al., 1999).

Remodeling in Transplant CAD

Glagov and colleagues originally described coronary artery remodeling in a necropsy study of left main coronary arteries as a compensatory enlargement of vessel to prevent lumen loss in early stages of atherosclerosis. In recent years, histopathologic and IVUS studies have demonstrated that at some lesion sites the vessel may shrink in size and contribute to, instead of compensate for, the degree of luminal stenosis, a phenomenon described as negative remodeling, or arterial shrinkage. Both these phenomena have been studied in transplant population using serial and cross-sectional study designs.

In a cross-sectional study design, remodeling can be studied using comparison of lesion sites with reference sites. Serial measurements of lumen, plaque, and vessel area at the lesion site can provide the most rigorous evidence for remodeling, but the logistics of this type of study, variability of measurement, and the practical difficulties in identifying the same exact site on follow-up examination limit the usefulness of this methodology (Kapadia et al., 1999). Positive and negative remodeling have both been demonstrated in cross-sectional and serial studies in transplant patients (Lim et al., 1997). The rate of remodeling has shown to be dependent on the time interval from transplantation. Ziada and colleagues have reported the rate of remodeling of donor lesions to be different from that of vasculopathy lesions in a 3-year serial follow-up (Ziada et al., 1999). Further, vessel remodeling appears to be more pronounced in eccentric lesions than in concentric lesions (Schwartzacher et al., 2000). Negative remodeling may be important in large coronary segments because it appears to be a major contributor of lumen loss in the first year after transplantation in one study (Wong et al., 2001). However, in a study with 5-year follow-up, a biphasic response, consisting of early expansion and late constriction, was seen (Tsutsui et al., 2001).

SUMMARY

IVUS imaging is a safe, feasible, and sensitive method to investigate transplant CAD. It can be used to identify patients with rapidly progressive vasculopathy in whom aggressive timely measures may help to prolong graft survival. Further, serial IVUS information can be used to judge response to therapy. In future trials with newer immunosuppressive therapies and other measures to halt transplant vasculopathy, IVUS examination may provide useful surrogate end-points for long-term survival of transplant recipients. With the development of newer catheters with easier automated pullback systems, it will be possible to encourage more widespread use of IVUS imaging.

REFERENCES

Allen-Auerbach M et al: Relationship between coronary function by positron emission tomography and temporal changes in morphology by intravascular ultrasound (IVUS) in transplant recipients. J Heart Lung Transplant 18:211, 1999

Batkoff BW, Linker DT: Safety of intracoronary ultrasound: Data from a Multicenter European Registry. Cathet Cardiovasc Diagn 38:238, 1996

Billingham ME: Histopathology of graft coronary disease. J Heart Lung Transplant 11 (3 Pt 2):S38, 1992

Botas J et al: Influence of preexistent donor coronary artery disease on the progression of transplant vasculopathy. An intravascular ultrasound study. Circulation 92:1126, 1995

Drinkwater DC et al: Outcomes of patients undergoing transplantation with older donor hearts. J Heart Lung Transplant 15:684, 1996

Escobar A et al: Cardiac allograft vasculopathy assessed by intravascular ultrasonography and nonimmunologic risk factors. Am J Cardiol 74:1042, 1994

Hausmann D et al: The safety of intracoronary ultrasound. A multicenter survey of 2207 examinations. Circulation 91: 623, 1995

Jimenez J et al: Cellular rejection and rate of progression of transplant vasculopathy: A 3-year serial intravascular ultrasound study. J Heart Lung Transplant 20:393, 2001

Kapadia SR et al: Development of transplantation vasculopathy and progression of donor-transmitted atherosclerosis: Comparison by serial intravascular ultrasound imaging. Circulation 98:2672, 1998

Kapadia SR et al: Impact of intravascular ultrasound in understanding transplant coronary artery disease. Curr Opin Cardiol 14:140, 1999

Kapadia SR et al: Intravascular ultrasound imaging after cardiac transplantation: Advantage of multi-vessel imaging. J Heart Lung Transplant 19:167, 2000

Kapadia SR et al: Impact of lipid abnormalities in development and progression of transplant coronary disease: A serial intravascular ultrasound study. J Am Coll Cardiol 38:206, 2001

Kobashigawa JA et al: Effect of pravastatin on outcomes after cardiac transplantation [see comments]. N Engl J Med 333:621, 1995

Lim TT et al: Role of compensatory enlargement and shrinkage in transplant coronary artery disease. Serial intravascular ultrasound study. Circulation 95:855, 1997

Mehra MR et al: Influence of donor and recipient gender on cardiac allograft vasculopathy. An intravascular ultrasound study. Circulation 90(5 Pt 2):II78, 1994

Mehra MR et al: Predictive model to assess risk for cardiac allograft vasculopathy: An intravascular ultrasound study. J Am Coll Cardiol 26:1537, 1995a

Mehra MR et al: An intravascular ultrasound study of the influence of angiotensin-converting enzyme inhibitors and calcium entry blockers on the development of cardiac allograft vasculopathy. Am J Cardiol 75:853, 1995b

Mehra MR et al: Presence of severe intimal thickening by intravascular ultrasonography predicts cardiac events in cardiac allograft vasculopathy. J Heart Lung Transplant 14:632, 1995c

Rickenbacher PR et al: Prognostic importance of intimal thickness as measured by intracoronary ultrasound after cardiac transplantation. Circulation 92:3445, 1995

Rickenbacher PR et al: Coronary artery intimal thickening in the transplanted heart. An in vivo intracoronary untrasound study of immunologic and metabolic risk factors. Transplantation 61:46, 1996

Schwarzacher SP et al: Determinants of coronary remodeling in transplant coronary disease: A simultaneous intravascular ultrasound and Doppler flow study. Circulation 101:1384, 2000

Son R et al: Does use of intravascular ultrasound accelerate arteriopathy in heart transplant recipients? Am Heart J 138(2 Pt 1):358, 1999

Tsutsui H et al: Lumen loss in transplant coronary artery disease is a biphasic process involving early intimal thickening and late constrictive remodeling: Results from a 5-year serial intravascular ultrasound study. Circulation 104:653, 2001

Tuzcu EM et al: Occult and frequent transmission of atherosclerotic coronary disease with cardiac transplantation: Insights from intravascular ultrasound. Circulation 91:1706, 1995

Tuzcu EM et al: High prevalence of coronary atherosclerosis in asymptomatic teenagers and young adults: Evidence from intravascular ultrasound. Circulation 103:2705, 2001

Wiedermann JG et al: Severe intimal thickening by intravascular ultrasonography predicts early death in cardiac transplant recipients. Circulation 90:193, 1994

Wong C et al: Role of vascular remodeling in the pathogenesis of early transplant coronary artery disease: A multicenter prospective intravascular ultrasound study. J Heart Lung Transplant 20:385, 2001

Ziada KM et al: The current status of intravascular ultrasound imaging. Curr Probl Cardiol 24:541,1999

46

PRINZMETAL'S VARIANT ANGINA: A CONTEMPORARY PERSPECTIVE

John Beltrame

Prinzmetal and coworkers made a major contribution to the clinical understanding of coronary artery disease when they reviewed 32 cases of angina occurring at rest (Prinzmetal et al., 1959); they described how these differed from classic angina of effort, as characterized by Heberden. In particular, they noted ST-segment elevation (rather than depression) during pain and a preserved effort tolerance. To emphasize these differences, they coined the term *variant angina* and suggested that an altered coronary vascular tone might be responsible. Today, variant angina is considered a chronic disorder of coronary vasomotor reactivity attributable to epicardial artery spasm, which manifests as recurrent episodes of rest angina typically associated with ST-segment elevation.

Pathophysiology

With the advent of coronary angiography, the presence of coronary spasm during a spontaneous episode of rest pain in a patient with variant angina was confirmed (Oliva et al., 1973). However, subsequent progress in defining the underlying mechanism responsible for the coronary spasm has been slow. Initial investigations focused on disturbances in the autonomic nervous system and/or humoral factors, but more recent studies have evaluated the role of the endothelium and cellular mechanisms.

The Autonomic Nervous System

Sympathetic and possibly parasympathetic efferent fibers innervate the coronary vessels. Surgical cardiac denervation has been reported as an effective therapy for refractory coronary spasm (Bertrand et al., 1980), suggesting a role for the autonomic nervous system. However, spasm has also been reported in a denervated transplant heart (Buda et al., 1981). Other data implicating the autonomic nervous system include heart rate variability studies, which described altered autonomic activity preceding spontaneous episodes of coronary spasm. Also, acetylcholine has been shown to provoke coronary spasm, and atropine to suppress this response (Yasue, 1983). Other vasospastic stimuli, such as ergonovine and cold pressor stimulation, have sympathomimetic properties, although the response to α-adrenergic blockers (e.g., prazosin and phentolamine) has been variable.

Humoral Mechanisms

Histamine, serotonin, and prostanoids have been implicated in the pathogenesis of coronary artery spasm. Histamine has been of interest since (1) mast cells have been identified at vasospastic sites (Forman et al., 1985), (2) endogenous levels are increased in variant angina patients, and (3) histamine is a provocative stimulus for coronary artery spasm (Ginsburg et al., 1981). However, enthusiasm for its pathogenetic role in variant angina declined when it was found to be a less sensitive provocative stimulus than ergonovine or acetylcholine.

Platelet aggregation has been demonstrated in the coronary circulation during episodes of spontaneous coronary spasm (Miyamoto et al., 2000). Whether this is cause or effect is unclear, but it has bought attention to the vasoactive platelet products serotonin and thromboxane. Ergonovine has serotonergic properties, and serotonin per se may provoke coronary spasm in variant angina patients. However, serotonin antagonists are ineffective in preventing ergonovine-induced spasm. Similarly, inhibition of the thromboxane pathway with aspirin does not prevent coronary spasm.

The studies described above were conducted with the aim of identifying a specific receptor-mediated mechanism responsible for coronary spasm. Another study used multiple sequential provocative stimuli in 28 variant angina patients and found that spasm could be induced with two or more stimuli in the same patient in 82% of the study patients (Kaski et al., 1986). They therefore concluded that coronary spasm was due to a local nonspecific supersensitivity to provocative stimuli rather than to a specific mechanism.

Racial Differences in Coronary Vasomotor Reactivity

Extensive pathophysiologic studies of variant angina patients have been undertaken by Japanese investigators. These have demonstrated (1) diffuse vasospasm of the spastic vessel, (2) hyperreactivity of nonspastic vessels, and (3) increased basal vasomotor tone in spastic and nonspastic vessels. In contrast, compa-rable studies in Caucasian patients have shown focal coronary spasm with normal vasomotor reactivity and basal tone in nonspastic vessels (Beltrame et al., 1999). These and other differences raise the possibility of a "Japanese variant" and highlight the potential pitfall of generalizing study findings.

Endothelial Function

The endothelium releases local vasodilators (e.g., nitric oxide) and vasoconstrictors (e.g., endothelin) that regulate vascular smooth-muscle function. Although increased endothelin levels have been demonstrated in variant angina patients, most investigations have focused on the role of nitric oxide in this disorder.

One group of Japanese investigators has proposed coronary endothelial dysfunction resulting in impaired nitric oxide production as an important mechanism for coronary spasm. They have demonstrated impaired coronary flow–mediated dilation at vasospastic sites (Kugiyama et al., 1997) and a blunted constrictor response to a nitric oxide synthase inhibitor, suggesting deficient nitric oxide production by endothelial nitric oxide synthase (eNOS). Furthermore, they have identified three linked mutations in the 5′ flanking region of the eNOS gene in variant angina patients (Nakayama et al., 1999). More recently, this group has demonstrated improved endothelial function (Kugiyama et al., 1998) and suppression of coronary spasm (Motoyama et al., 1998) in some variant angina patients, using vitamins C and E, respectively. These antioxidants protect nitric oxide from degradation by oxidative stress; thus, the low vitamin E levels reported in variant angina patients may contribute to endothelial dysfunction.

Despite these comprehensive studies suggesting that endothelial dysfunction has an important role in the pathogenesis of coronary spasm, other Japanese investigators have demonstrated intact endothelial function in these patients (Egashira et al., 1996). These disparate findings may reflect methodologic differences but once more underscore the complexity of the underlying pathophysiology of variant angina and why it still remains elusive.

Cellular Mechanisms

A chronic porcine model of coronary artery spasm has been developed and provides valuable insights into the pathophysiology and cell biology of coronary spasm. The original model (the atherosclerotic model) involved a high-cholesterol diet following localized balloon-induced coronary endothelial injury. In a later model (the inflammatory model), the proximal left coronary artery is wrapped with a cotton mesh containing recombinant human interleukin-1β (Ito et al., 1995). In both models, coronary artery spasm can be consistently provoked with intracoronary histamine or serotonin at treated but not control sites. These models demonstrate the potential importance of atherosclerosis and inflammation in the pathogenesis of coronary artery spasm.

Extensive studies utilizing these models have provided the following insights into the cellular mechanisms of coronary artery spasm (Fig. 46-1):

1. Endothelial-dependent vasodilatory responses are intact at the spastic site in the inflammatory model (Miyata et al., 1999), adding to the controversy of the role of the endothelium in coronary spasm. Furthermore, endothelin-1 does not provoke epicardial artery spasm in this model nor does it play a role in serotonin-induced spasm.

2. The enhanced reactivity of the vasospastic site is due to an altered signal transduction between receptor and contractile proteins, since isolated smooth-muscle cell preparations from these sites show similar responses with increasing calcium concentrations as do controls, suggesting that the contractile proteins are unaltered per se.

3. The intracellular calcium concentration is fundamental to vasomotor signal transduction and can be derived extracellularly or from intracellular sarcoplasmic reticulum stores. In this model, coronary spasm is primarily mediated via calcium influx through L-type calcium channels,

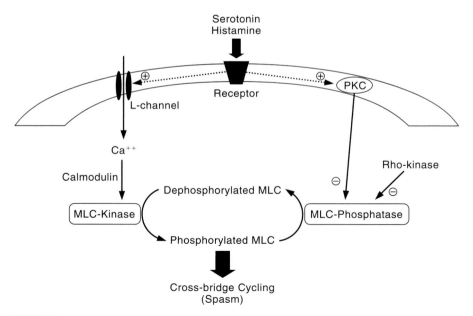

FIGURE 46-1

Cellular mechanisms in coronary spasm. Proposed signal transduction pathway for provoked spasm (smooth-muscle contraction) based upon findings from a chronic porcine model of coronary artery spasm (see text) PKC = Protein kinase C; MLC = myosin light chain kinase.

and the intracellular calcium stores appear to play little role. Furthermore, there is increased *L*-channel expression at the vasospastic sites (Kuga et al., 2000).

4. Myosin light chain (MLC) phosphorylation is critical to smooth-muscle cross-bridge cycling and is regulated by myosin light chain kinase (MLC-K), which phosphorylates, and myosin light chain phosphatase (MLC-P), which dephosphorylates the contractile protein (Fig. 46-1). At the vasospastic site there is increased MLC monophosphorylation and unique MLC diphosphorylation compared with control sites (Katsumata et al., 1997). The generation of diphosphorylated MLC may be central to the pathogenesis of spasm in this model and has been shown to occur with the inhibition of MLC-P. In turn, inhibition of this enzyme may occur via a protein kinase C or Rho-kinase, which is upregulated at the spastic site.

The insights derived from these models not only provide a better understanding into the mechanism of coronary spasm but may also lead to other potential therapies.

Clinical Features

History

Patients with variant angina usually present with recurrent episodes of angina at rest that respond promptly to sublingual nitrates. Patients may be woken up by their angina due to the circadian pattern of coronary vasomotor reactivity, since peak spastic activity occurs between midnight and 6 A.M. Palpitations, presyncope, or syncope occurring with the chest pain may reflect associated bradyarrhythmias or malignant tachyarrhythmias, which may result in sudden cardiac death. Unlike effort angina there is no predictable relationship with the level of exertion, although the pain may occur occasionally during activity. Potential triggers for an anginal episode may include hyperventilation, exposure to cold, alcohol ingestion, or acute psychological stress.

Of the traditional atherosclerotic risk factors, only cigarette smoking has been shown to predispose to coronary spasm. As discussed above, racial origin may also be a predisposing factor. Whereas patients with exertional angina experience a gradual deterioration with pain occurring at progressively lower workloads, variant angina is characterized by periods of waxing and waning over weeks or months. During the "hot phase," there is heightened coronary vasomotor reactivity resulting in frequent anginal episodes that may be precipitated by stimuli that are inconsequential during the quiescent or "cold phase."

The Electrocardiogram

Patients with variant angina classically exhibit ST-segment elevation during spontaneous or provoked episodes of angina. This reflects abrupt occlusion of a large epicardial artery resulting in transmural myocardial ischemia. In contrast, classic exertional angina is characterized by ST-segment depression reflecting subendocardial ischemia from the increased myocardial metabolic demand. While these electrocardiographic patterns have traditionally been considered as distinguishing features of the two syndromes, the distinction is not decisive since ST-segment depression may occur with spasm of smaller epicardial vessels.

The evolution of the electrocardiogram (ECG) changes during spontaneous episodes of variant angina has been carefully documented (Chierchia et al., 1980). The initial ECG finding is a peaking of T waves followed by progressive ST-segment elevation, with T-wave inversion occurring after resolution of the episode. Over the following days, the inverted T waves become progressively less deep until they are isoelectric and finally return to their normal morphology. Should a further anginal episode occur while the T wave is inverted, then the T wave will rapidly become upright and recommence the sequence with peaking of the T wave. During this transition, an isolated ECG may appear "normal" although the evolving pattern is ischemic, a phenomenon referred to as *pseudonormalization*. Other ECG phenomena that have been occasionally reported during episodes of variant angina include (1) transient Q waves, (2) increasing R wave voltage, and (3) ST-segment alternans.

Continuous ECG monitoring of ST segments for 24 to 48 h is useful in the diagnosis of variant angina, particularly when there are frequent episodes of pain. Ambulatory ECG studies in patients with variant angina have demonstrated the following differences from exertional angina: (1) an absence of a precipitating tachycardia prior to the ischemic changes; and (2) a circadian pattern of disease activity with most ischemic episodes occurring in the early morning, even though they may be asymptomatic (silent ischemia).

Since effort tolerance is generally preserved in variant angina, it would be expected that exercise stress testing would usually be negative. However, various studies have reported ischemic changes during or shortly after testing in 30 to 60% of patients (Kaski and Maseri, 1990). This may occur because of coexistent atherosclerotic coronary artery disease or an increased sensitivity to catecholamines during the "hot phase" of the disorder. Repeating the stress test under nitrate cover should abolish the ischemic changes in variant angina patients.

Noninvasive Imaging Techniques

Myocardial scintigraphic techniques have been used to support or complement ECG findings in establishing the presence of spasm-induced ischemia. New radioactive tracers that allow delayed scanning may extend the availability of this modality. Dobutamine stress echocardiography has a very limited role in the diagnosis of variant angina since only 14% of affected patients show asynergy with dobutamine provocation (Kawano et al., 2000). The role of magnetic resonance imaging in the diagnosis of variant angina remains to be defined.

Coronary Angiography

Many clinicians consider the diagnosis of variant angina only when angiography demonstrates normal coronary morphology. However, Prinzmetal's original description included patients with atherosclerotic disease. The absence of atherosclerosis was only described later when it was referred to as a "variant of variant angina" (Cheng et al., 1973). Hence angiogra-

phy in variant angina patients may reveal significant atherosclerosis, although the presence of a severe, fixed, flow-limiting lesion may provide an alternative explanation for the patient's angina. If lesions are demonstrated, intracoronary nitrates should be administered to determine if they are "fixed" or "dynamic" in nature.

As described above, coronary spasm can be demonstrated directly by coronary angiography during a spontaneous or provoked episode. Catheter-induced spasm must be distinguished, as its clinical implications are unclear. The term *vasospastic angina* is often used to describe patients with rest angina and inducible coronary spasm (independent of the presence of ST-segment elevation). Coronary spasm should be diagnosed only when there is a total or subtotal occlusion of an epicardial artery, since less severe reductions in luminal diameter would not be expected to impair resting coronary blood flow and are therefore unlikely to produce angina at rest. It is important to delineate this pathologic state from mild coronary vasoconstriction (e.g., <30% reduction in the vessel lumen), which may be a "physiologic" response under certain circumstances.

Diagnosis

Variant angina should be suspected in patients presenting with recurrent episodes of rest angina, particularly if these episodes occur in the early morning. To make a diagnosis of variant angina, coronary artery spasm must be either directly demonstrated by coronary angiography or inferred by documenting ECG (reversible ST-segment elevation) or scintigraphic evidence of ischemia in the absence of a critical fixed stenosis. To document coronary spasm objectively during a spontaneous episode of rest angina would be fortuitous; diagnosis often requires provocative spasm testing, as outlined below.

Differential Diagnosis

Before undertaking provocative spasm testing, the differential diagnosis should be considered. *Evolving myocardial infarction* presents with rest pain and

ST-segment elevation but differs from variant angina since the ST-segment elevation is persistent and unresponsive to nitrates. Furthermore, variant angina patients may have a history of recurrent episodes. However, differentiation may be difficult as variant angina patients also experience myocardial infarction (MI). In contemporary clinical practice, variant angina patients may often be misdiagnosed as having an evolving MI and promptly treated with thrombolytics.

Mixed pattern angina represents a continuum of the spectrum between variant angina and stable exertional angina (Maseri, 1995). It is characterized by episodes of both rest and exertional pain, often with a variable exercise tolerance reflecting the dynamic vasomotor nature of the coronary artery stenosis. Distinguishing these patients from those with variant angina may be difficult and requires careful detailing of the history, particularly in relation to nocturnal/early morning episodes.

Microvascular spasm is characterized by rest angina with ST-segment elevation despite the absence of epicardial artery spasm. Such patients often exhibit a slow passage of contrast during angiography, referred to as the *coronary slow-flow phenomenon* (Beltrame and Horowitz, 1999). Further investigation of this disorder is required to understand its microvascular pathophysiology and clinical features.

A number of *other cardiac disorders* (e.g., syndrome X, pericarditis) may present with rest pain but are readily differentiated from variant angina by their clinical features and/or provocative test findings. Similarly, *noncardiac disorders* such as gastroesophageal reflux and esophageal spasm need to be considered.

Provocative Testing

Provocative spasm testing requires (1) an agent/maneuver that provokes coronary spasm, and (2) a method for assessing the response (see Table 46-1). Of the large variety of spasmogens available, ergonovine, acetylcholine, and hyperventilation are the most commonly used and have similar sensitivities (93%, 90%, and 83%, respectively) in identifying variant angina patients (Heupler et al., 1978; Okumura et al., 1988; Previtali et al., 1989).

The traditional provocation study involves incremental intravenous administration of ergonovine (25 to 400 μg) and ECG monitoring for ST-segment elevation. Similarly, the hyperventilation test involves ECG monitoring during this maneuver. Intracoronary acetylcholine (25 to 100 μg) administered during coronary angiography has been extensively used in Japan and allows angiographic demonstration of spasm as well as ECG monitoring.

Bedside ergonovine provocative testing is hazardous, and associated deaths have been reported. In more recent years, provocative testing has been largely confined to the cardiac catheterization laboratory with the following inherent safety advantages over bedside testing:

TABLE 46-1

TECHNIQUES FOR PROVOCATIVE CORONARY SPASM TESTING

Provocative Agent/Maneuver

Intravenous Agents	Ergonovine, methylergonovine, histamine, phenylephrine, epinephrine/norepinephrine + β blocker, dopamine
Intracoronary Agents	Acetylcholine, methylcholine, ergonovine serotonin, histamine
Maneuvers	Hyperventilation ± TRIS buffer infusion, cold pressor stimulus, isometric handgrip, exercise stress testing.

Response Assessment

Clinical	Chest pain
Ischemic Markers	ECG (12 lead)
	Myocardial scintigraphy
Angiography	Coronary spasm

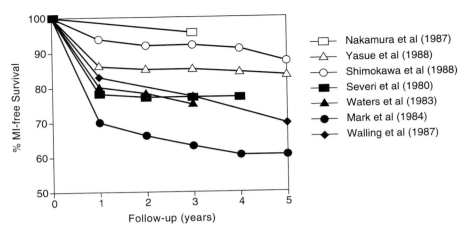

FIGURE 46-2

Survival without myocardial infarction in patients with variant angina. Major prognostic studies examining 5-year infarct-free survival amongst Japanese (open shapes) and Caucasian (filled shapes) patients with variant angina. Details of the studies cited in the figure are to be found in the References. (Adapted from J Beltrame et al: Am Coll Cardiol 33:1442, 1999, with permission.)

1. Documentation of coincident atherosclerotic coronary disease
2. Ability to assess each coronary artery selectively
3. Prompt detection of coronary spasm, thereby allowing rapid termination of testing rather than awaiting ECG evidence of ischemia
4. Rapid delivery of intracoronary nitrates/calcium antagonists to alleviate spasm

Prognosis and Natural History

Large studies following up patients with variant angina reveal a guarded prognosis. Five-year infarct-free survival has been reported to be as low as 60% (Fig. 46-2). The use of calcium antagonists, the extent/severity of atherosclerotic coronary disease, and the presence of multivessel spasm (i.e., simultaneous inferior and anterior ST-segment elevation) have been shown to be independent predictors of infarct-free survival (Yasue et al., 1988). Furthermore, as shown in Fig. 46-2, infarct-free survival is better among Japanese patients than among their Caucasian counterparts (Beltrame et al., 1999).

The natural history of variant angina exhibits a waxing and waning pattern over a period of weeks to months. Complications such as MI, arrhythmias, or sudden cardiac death typically occur during the "hot phase" and usually within the first 3 months. While bouts of angina may recur, spontaneous remission may occur in some patients and thus medical therapy withdrawn. Spontaneous remission is more likely to occur in patients who cease smoking and who do not have significant underlying atherosclerotic coronary artery disease.

Therapeutic Measures
Conventional Therapy

As mentioned above, calcium antagonists have a major impact on the morbidity/mortality of variant angina and are therefore used as the primary therapy for this disorder. The dosage should be titrated to symptoms and may require substantially higher doses than for stable/mixed pattern angina (e.g., daily dosages of up to 480 mg for verapamil or diltiazem, and 80 mg for nifedipine).

Nitrates have long been used in the management of variant angina although they are less potent than the calcium antagonists. Sublingual nitrates are the first-line therapy during an acute episode of variant angina. Should the episode persist, then intravenous nitrates or calcium antagonists may be required.

Refractory Variant Angina

Potential therapies for variant angina patients refractory to high-dose nitrates/calcium channel blockers include the use of additional antianginals, percutaneous coronary interventions, or cardiac denervation. Perhexilene, guanethidine, clonidine, and high-dose amiodarone have been described as being beneficial in case reports. Coronary angioplasty and stent deployment have been utilized on spasm-associated stenoses with reputedly good effect (Leisch et al., 1986; Gaspardone et al., 1999). However, angioplasty of vasoreactive lesions is associated with a higher frequency of restenosis (Leisch et al., 1986), and spasm has been shown to recur at sites adjacent to the deployed stent. As mentioned above, cardiac denervation has been reported to be beneficial in the management of variant angina (Clark et al., 1977). However, the procedure has been associated with a significant mortality.

REFERENCES

Beltrame JF, Horowitz JD: ST elevation secondary to microvascular dysfunction. J Am Coll Cardiol 34:312, 1999

Beltrame JF et al: Racial heterogeneity in coronary artery vasomotor reactivity: Differences between Japanese and Caucasian patients. J Am Coll Cardiol 33:1442, 1999

Bertrand M et al: Surgical treatment of variant angina: Use of plexectomy with aortocoronary bypass. Circulation 61:877, 1980

Buda A et al: Coronary artery spasm in the denervated transplanted human heart. Am J Med 70:1144, 1981

Cheng T et al: Variant angina of Prinzmetal with normal coronary arteriograms. A variant of the variant. Circulation 47:476, 1973

Chierchia S et al: Sequence of events in angina at rest: Primary reduction in coronary flow. Circulation 61:759, 1980

Clark D et al: Coronary artery spasm: Medical manangement, surgical denervation and autotransplantation. J Thorac Cardiovasc Surg 73:332, 1977

Egashira K et al: Basal release of endothelium-derived nitric oxide at site of spasm in patients with variant angina. J Am Coll Cardiol 27:1444, 1996

Forman M et al: Increased advential mast cells in a patient with coronary spasm. N Engl J Med 313:1138, 1985

Gaspardone A et al: Coronary artery stent placement in patients with variant angina refractory to medical treatment. Am J Cardiol 84:96, A8, 1999

Ginsburg R et al: Histamine provocation of clinical coronary artery spasm: Implications concerning the pathogenesis of variant angina pectoris. Am Heart J 102:819, 1981

Heupler F et al: Ergonovine maleate provocative test for coronary arterial spasm. Am J Cardiol 41:631, 1978

Ito A et al: Tyrosine kinase inhibitor suppresses coronary arteriosclerotic changes and vasospastic responses induced by chronic treatment with interleukin-1 beta in pigs in vivo. J Clin Invest 96:1288, 1995

Kaski J, Maseri A: Coronary artery spasm: European view. J Coronary Artery Dis 1:660, 1990

Kaski JC et al: Local coronary supersensitivity to diverse vasoconstrictive stimuli in patients with variant angina. Circulation 74:1255, 1986

Katsumata N et al: Enhanced myosin light chain phosphorylations as a central mechanism for coronary artery spasm in a swine model with interleukin-1beta. Circulation 96:4357, 1997

Kawano H et al: Myocardial ischemia due to coronary artery spasm during dobutamine stress echocardiography. Am J Cardiol 85:26, 2000

Kuga T et al: Increased expression of L-type calcium channels in vascular smooth muscle cells at spastic site in a porcine model of coronary artery spasm. J Cardiovasc Pharmacol 35:822, 2000

Kugiyama K et al: Nitric oxide-mediated flow-dependent dilation is impaired in coronary arteries in patients with coronary spastic angina. J Am Coll Cardiol 30:920, 1997

Kugiyama K et al: Vitamin C attenuates abnormal vasomotor reactivity in spasm in coronary arteries in patients with coronary spastic angina. J Am Coll Cardiol 32:103, 1998

Leisch F et al: Influence of a variant angina on the results of percutaneous transluminal coronary angioplasty. Br Heart J 56:341, 1986

Mark D et al: Clinical characteristics and long-term survival of patients with variant angina. Circulation 69: 880, 1984

Maseri A: Transient myocardial ischemia and angina pectoris: Classification and diagnostic assessment, in *Ischemic Heart Disease. A Rational Basis for Clinical Practice and Clinical Research,* New York, Churchill Livingstone, 1995, pp 451–76

Miyamoto S et al: Formation of platelet aggregates after attacks of coronary spastic angina pectoris. Am J Cardiol 85:494, A10, 2000

Miyata K et al: Endothelial vasodilator function is preserved at the spastic/inflammatory coronary lesions in pigs. Circulation 100:1432, 1999

Motoyama T et al: Vitamin E administration improves impairment of endothelium-dependent vasodilation in patients with coronary spastic angina. J Am Coll Cardiol 32:1672, 1998

Nakamura M et al: Clinical characteristics associated with myocardial infarction, arrhythmias, and sudden death in patients with vasospastic angina. Circulation 75:1110, 1987

Nakayama M et al: T-786→C mutation in the 5'-flanking region of the endothelial nitric oxide synthase gene is associated with coronary spasm. Circulation 99:2864, 1999

Okumura K et al: Sensitivity and specificity of intracoronary injection of acetylcholine for the induction of coronary artery spasm. J Am Coll Cardiol 12:883, 1988

Oliva P et al: Coronary arterial spasm in Prinzmetal angina: Documentation by coronary arteriography. N Engl J Med 288:745, 1973

Previtali M et al: Hyperventilation and ergonovine tests in Prinzmetal's variant angina pectoris in men. Am J Cardiol 63:17, 1989

Prinzmetal M et al: A variant form of angina pectoris: Preliminary report. Am J Med 27:375, 1959

Severi S et al: Long-term prognosis of "variant" angina with medical treatment. Am J Cardiol 46:226, 1980

Shimokawa H et al: Clinical characteristics and long-term prognosis of patients with variant angina. A comparative study between western and Japanese populations. Int J Cardiol 18:331, 1988

Walling A et al: Long-term prognosis of patients with variant angina. Circulation 76:990, 1987

Waters D et al: Factors influencing the long-term prognosis of treated patients with variant angina. Circulation 68:258, 1983

Yasue H: Role of autonomic nervous system in the pathogenesis of angina pectoris. Arch Mal Coeur Vaiss 76:3, 1983

Yasue H et al: Long-term prognosis for patients with variant angina and influential factors. Circulation 78:1, 1988

CHAPTER

47

MANAGEMENT OF ATRIAL SEPTAL DEFECT

Abraham Rothman

Atrial septal defects (ASDs) are communications between the right and left atria. In children, ASDs constitute 5 to 10% of congenital heart disease. In adults, ASDs comprise 30% of congenital cardiac lesions, second in prevalence only to bicommissural aortic valves.

Anatomy

Secundum defects, located centrally in the region of the fossa ovalis (Fig. 47-1), represent 70 to 80% of all ASDs. Primum defects, located in the lower portion of the atrial septum near the crux of the heart, constitute 10 to 15% of ASDs. Primum defects are frequently associated with a cleft in the mitral valve and a superior QRS axis. Sinus venosus defects, located posteriorly near the orifice of either the superior or inferior vena cava, constitute 10 to 15% of ASDs. The superior type of sinus venosus defect is more common than the inferior type and is frequently associated with partial anomalous venous return of one or more right pulmonary veins.

Physiology

In an uncomplicated ASD, flow between the atria is predominantly or exclusively left to right. Such a shunt results in a volume load to the right side of the heart, the pulmonary circulation, and the left atrium. In childhood, this atrial shunt is tolerated well. Over many years, however, the potential adverse effects of the shunt include right-sided cardiac failure, atrial arrhythmias, and pulmonary vascular disease with reversal of the atrial shunt. In addition, mitral valve abnormalities may develop if ASDs are not repaired early, with a prevalence of 15% in adults compared with 0.4% in children.

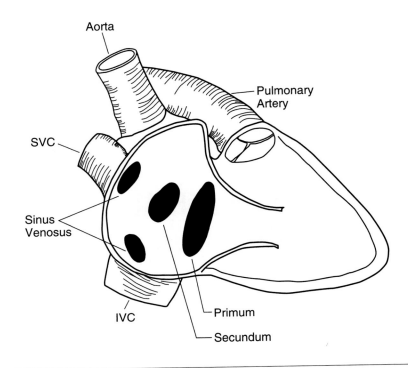

FIGURE 47-1

Anatomic location of atrial septal defects. Primum defects are located adjacent to the tricuspid and mitral valves; secundum defects are found centrally in the fossa ovalis; and sinus venosus defects are located posteriorly, adjacent to one of the vena cavae, in the area derived from the embryologic sinus venosus. IVC, inferior vena cava; SVC, superior vena cava.

Presentation

Children with ASDs rarely have symptoms. Their lesions are frequently discovered because of a murmur or a chest roentgenogram performed for another reason. In contrast, more than 95% of adults older than 40 years with ASDs have symptoms, including fatigue, dyspnea, frequent respiratory illnesses, and supraventricular arrhythmias. On physical examination, there is fixed splitting of the second heart sound, an ejection murmur at the left upper sternal border (secondary to increased flow across the pulmonary outflow), and sometimes a middiastolic tricuspid valve flow rumble. There may be a mitral regurgitation murmur. If pulmonary vascular disease has developed, ASDs may be associated with a loud second heart sound (P_2) and cyanosis.

Diagnosis

In children, conventional transthoracic echocardiography is generally diagnostic for the number, size, location, and flow pattern of ASDs. For adults in whom transthoracic imaging is less commonly diagnostic, agitated-saline contrast echocardiography or transesophageal echocardiography may be necessary to confirm the diagnosis. Recently, three-dimensional echocardiography has been applied to imaging of ASDs with promising results. Cardiac catheterization is performed only if the echocardiogram is not diagnostic, to evaluate pulmonary vascular resistance, or for transcatheter intervention. At the time of ASD diagnosis in adults, one-third of patients have pulmonary vascular disease, 50% of patients age 50 to 60 years have significant atrial arrhythmias, 15% have mitral valve abnormalities, and a few patients (often familial cases) have complete heart block.

Natural History

Between 20 and 30% of secundum ASDs close spontaneously in the first few years of life. Primum ASDs and sinus venosus ASDs have no chance for spontaneous closure. Elective closure of ASDs, either surgically or by catheter device, is generally recommended before children reach school age.

A commonly cited observational study of the natural history of unrepaired ASDs reported a survival of less than 50% beyond age 40 years, and only 10% by the age of 60 years (Campbell, 1970). The morbidity and mortality associated with untreated ASDs was attributed to arrhythmias, pulmonary vascular disease, and diminished left ventricular function.

Therapy

Intervention is recommended for patients with ASDs who have a $\dot{Q}_p/\dot{Q}_s$ (pulmonary to systemic flow ratio) of at least 1.5/1.0 and no significant elevation of pulmonary vascular resistance.

Surgical Treatment

In children, closure of ASDs is clearly beneficial. The 30-year survival of patients with ASDs repaired in childhood is the same as that of the general population (97%). At follow-up, exercise tolerance is good, pulmonary hypertension is rare, residual ASD flow is uncommon (5 to 10%), and atrial arrhythmias, while common (39%), are serious (requiring antiarrhythmic medications or pacemakers) in only 5 to 7% of patients.

In adults, results of ASD closure are less compelling. Early surgical mortality, which approaches 0% in children, is about 1% in the fifth decade of life, and 5 to 10% in patients >60 years. One group

performed a retrospective comparison of the results of surgery and medical therapy in 179 patients older than 40 years with ASDs (Konstantinides et al., 1995). The 10-year survival among the 84 patients who underwent surgery was 95%, compared with 84% for the 95 patients who were followed medically. As compared with medical therapy, surgery also prevented functional deterioration. There was no difference in atrial arrhythmias or cerebrovascular insults between the two groups. The conclusion of the authors, supported by an accompanying editorial (Perloff, 1995), was that surgical repair was superior to medical therapy.

Another group reported 27-year survival after ASD surgery in two adult age groups (Murphy et al., 1990). If the ASD was repaired surgically between ages 25 and 40, survival rate was 84%, compared with 91% for normal controls. For patients who underwent surgical ASD repair after 41 years of age, survival was 40%, compared with 59% for normal controls. Repair performed in older patients was associated with a higher risk for late cardiac failure, stroke, and atrial fibrillation.

Other studies that support surgical intervention in adults with ASDs include a report describing surgical repair in 166 patients (mean age 44 years) with 2 operative deaths (1.2%), and perioperative complications in 13%. At a mean follow-up of 90 months, there were eight late deaths (5%) and 12% morbidity (mostly arrhythmias). Survival was 98% at 5 years and 94% at 10 years (Horvath et al., 1992). Another group repaired ASDs in 49 patients over the age of 50, without operative deaths but with 2 neurologic events. At a mean follow-up of 9.7 years, most patients had improved functional class, three patients (6%) had late strokes, and three patients (6%) had significant arrhythmias (Shibata et al., 1996). A third team described ASD repair results in 39 patients (mean age, 35 years) with no operative deaths, one pulmonary embolism, and symptomatic improvement in 82% of the patients (Gatzoulis et al., 1996).

Two studies addressed the change in exercise capacity after ASD closure in adults. One found improvement in exercise capacity in patients who had large left-to-right atrial shunts preoperatively (Kobayashi et al., 1997). In the other, 31 patients with an average $\dot{Q}_p/\dot{Q}_s$ ratio of 2.8/1.0 who underwent ASD repair at a mean age of 40 years were studied (Helber et al., 1997). Ten years after surgery, mean ventilatory function improved from 80% of normal to normal, and mean exercise capacity increased from 50 to 60% of normal to normal.

In contrast to several studies supporting ASD repair in adults, one group proposed that surgical closure of ASDs in adults is not indicated (Shah et al., 1994). The authors tracked the course at one institution of all 105 patients with ASDs diagnosed since 1955. The patients were >25 years old at diagnosis and had reached >45 years at follow-up. Data were available for 83 patients, 34 treated medically and 49 surgically. At a mean follow-up of 25 years, the mean age was 63 years for the medical patients and 62 years for the surgical patients. There was no difference between the two groups in terms of survival, stroke, or cardiac failure. There were no operative deaths, but there were three late cardiac deaths (one medical, two surgical). No patient developed progressive pulmonary vascular disease. Lost to follow-up were 7 medical and 15 surgical patients. At follow-up, there was no significant difference between the two groups in terms of symptoms (medical, 41%; surgical, 44%), prevalence of atrial fibrillation (medical, 35%; surgical, 33%), or supraventricular tachycardia (medical, 26%; surgical, 21%). The only significant difference was the prevalence of tricuspid regurgitation (medical, 43%; surgical, 17%). The authors concluded that ASD surgery in patients age >25 years was not justified.

Pulmonary Vascular Disease

Pulmonary vascular disease, which rarely develops in adult patients with ASDs, can complicate the decision to intervene surgically. The outcome of 40 patients with ASDs and a total pulmonary vascular resistance >7 Wood units has been described (Steele et al., 1987). Surgery was performed in 26 patients, and 14 patients were followed medically. Median follow-up was 12 years. Among the surgical patients, 19 of 22 survived if the preoperative pul-

monary resistance was <15 Wood units, compared with 0 of 4 patients surviving with a preoperative pulmonary resistance >15 Wood units. Among the medically followed patients, only one of five patients survived despite a pulmonary resistance at the time of diagnosis <15 Wood units, compared with three of nine patients who survived with a pulmonary resistance at the time of diagnosis of >15 Wood units. Based on these findings, the authors recommended surgical ASD repair if the total pulmonary vascular resistance was <15 Wood units.

Postoperative Complications

Common complications after ASD surgical repair in adults are arrhythmias and pericardial effusions. Following secundum ASD repair, transient postoperative arrhythmias are frequent. The incidence of arrhythmias increases with length of follow-up. In patients with preoperative arrhythmias, ASD surgery rarely results in a conversion to sinus rhythm. In patients with preoperative atrial fibrillation, the arrhythmia generally persists postoperatively unless a concomitant Maze procedure is performed. One team performed simultaneous ASD surgery and Maze procedures in 26 patients (mean age, 58 years) with atrial fibrillation (Kobayashi et al., 1998). There were no deaths. At a mean follow-up of 2.7 years, sinus rhythm was present in 22 of the 26 patients. Another team performed ASD repair and Maze procedures in 21 patients (mean age 42 years) (Sandoval et al., 1996). At a mean follow-up of 8 months, there was one death, but 90% of the patients were in sinus rhythm. Following repair of primum ASDs, complete heart block occurs in 5 to 10% of patients. Due to the defect's proximity to the sinus node, surgical repair of sinus venosus ASDs may be complicated by sinus node injury.

The incidence and severity of pericardial effusions after ASD repair in 339 patients have been examined (Yip et al., 1997). Pericardial effusions were present in 54 patients (16%), with cardiac tamponade in 5 (1.5%). The majority of pericardial effusions occurred 4 to 12 days after ASD repair, with a peak occurrence at 10 days.

Noncardiac Surgery in the Adult with an Unrepaired ASD

An unrepaired ASD in the adult patient may increase the risk of several complications following noncardiac surgery. These complications include paradoxical embolus, atrial arrhythmias, increased left-to-right atrial shunting (if there is significant blood loss), difficulties with lung compliance (when there is abundant pulmonary blood flow), increases in pulmonary vascular resistance (resulting in an acute pressure load to the right ventricle), and bacterial endocarditis (in patients with primum defects and associated clefts in the mitral valve).

ASD and Pregnancy

Pregnancy is generally well tolerated in women with ASDs, despite an increase in stroke volume and cardiac output of 40 to 50%. However, particularly in women >40 years, there is an increased risk of elevated pulmonary vascular resistance, arrhythmias, right ventricular failure, and thrombosis. Peripartum hemorrhage may cause a significant increase in left- to-right shunting across the ASD.

The outcome of pregnancies in 80 women (mean age, 20 years) before and after ASD surgery have been reviewed (Actis Dato et al., 1998). Sixty women who had undergone ASD repair had 115 postoperative pregnancies, and 20 women who had not undergone ASD repair had 48 pregnancies. The women who had unrepaired ASDs had a higher incidence of miscarriage, preterm delivery, and cardiac symptoms during pregnancy compared with the women who had previously undergone surgical ASD repair. There was no difference between the two groups in terms of stillbirths, offspring malformations, or long-term maternal cardiac complications.

Recurrence Risk

Approximate recurrence risks for congenital heart disease are about 2.5% if one sibling was previously born with an ASD and 8% if two prior siblings were affected. In the offspring of parents with an ASD, the risk of congenital heart disease approaches 4 to 5% if the mother is affected, compared with 1.5% if the father is affected.

Newer Therapeutic Techniques

Limited-Access Surgery

Recently, surgeons have devised smaller skin and osteal incisions for ASD repair (Fig. 47-2). Even though the term *minimally invasive surgery* has been used for these modifications, perhaps a more accurate term would be *limited-access surgery*. These new techniques, frequently performed with femoral cardiopulmonary bypass, include the following: right parasternal incision with excision of several costal cartilages, right anterior thoracotomy with thoracoscopic video assistance, right anterolateral submammary thoracotomy, bilateral submammary incision, limited ministernotomies (upper, middle, or lower), transxiphoid approach without sternotomy, and combinations of the above. These newer ASD closure techniques, compared with conventional midline sternotomies, have provided improved aesthetic results with similar success and complication rates.

Transcatheter Devices

Although the first successful percutaneous closure of an ASD was described in 1974, only in the past decade has there been a resurgence in interest and design of a variety of devices to close ASDs by transcatheter techniques. The five major devices tested in patients have included (in alphabetical order) the Amplatzer device, the Angel-Wings device, the ASDOS device, the Buttoned device, and the CardioSeal device (Fig. 47-3). Each device consists of one or two occlusive structures and a supportive frame, all of which can be collapsed and introduced through an 8F to 11F delivery sheath. These devices are best suited for secundum atrial septal defects which are <20 mm in diameter and surrounded by circumferential rims of at least 4 to 5 mm. The current devices are not designed for closure of primum

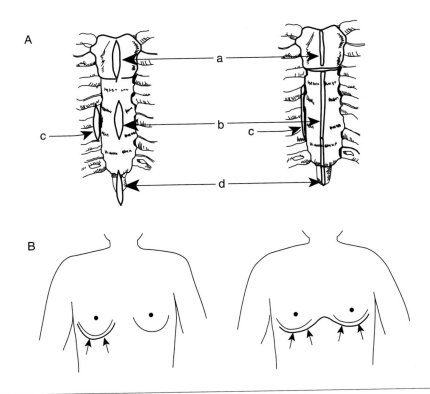

FIGURE 47-2

Diagrammatic representation of limited-access surgical sites. A. Limited skin (left) and osteal (right) access sites for cardiac surgery: a, upper skin incision with manubrial osteal access; b, middle skin incision with sternal access; c, right parasternal incision with access through costal cartilages; d, lower skin incision with transxyphoid osteal access. B. Left: right anterolateral submammary thoracotomy (arrows). Right: bilateral submammary incision (arrows).

or sinus venosus defects, which lack circumferential rims, are too close to valve structures, or have associated surgical lesions (partial anomalous pulmonary venous return or atrioventricular valve abnormalities).

All of these devices have been used in adults in preliminary studies. The current success rate for implantation is 90 to 95%, with a complication rate, including device embolization, of <5%. While residual leaks immediately after implantation are common, the rate of residual flow across the devices decreases with length of follow-up (5 to 15%, 5 years after implantation). Advantages of the devices over surgery include less incisional discomfort, faster ambulation and return to routine activities, and potentially lower hospital costs (shorter stay in the intensive care unit and hospital).

Future

Despite nearly half a century since the first open-heart surgical closure of an ASD, there remains controversy about the role of surgical closure of ASDs in adults. There is little doubt that surgeons will increase the use of limited access techniques and

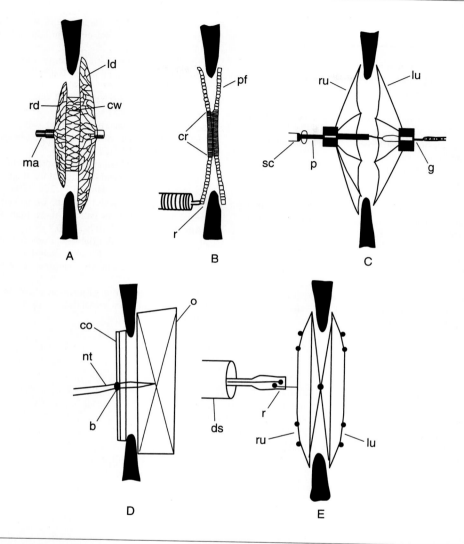

FIGURE 47-3

Devices used for transcatheter closure of atrial septal defects. A. Amplatzer Septal Occluder (cw, connecting waist; ld, left atrial disc; ma, microscrew adapter; rd, right atrial disc). B. AngelWings device (cr, central conjoint ring; pf, polyester fabric; r, release mechanism). C. ASDOS device (g, guidewire; lu, left atrial umbrella; p, pusher; ru, right atrial umbrella; sc, screwdriver catheter). D. Buttoned device (b, button; co, counter-occluder; nt, nylon thread; o, occluder). E. CardioSeal device (ds, delivery sheath; lu, left atrial umbrella; r, release mechanism; ru, right atrial umbrella).

that interventional cardiologists will continue to improve the percutaneous technique. For now, though, the question that remains unanswered is whether intervention is indicated and, if so, by which method. Lest there be another half-century without an answer, large prospective randomized studies are necessary to compare medical management with newer surgical techniques and transcatheter devices to ascertain the optimal management of the adult with an ASD.

REFERENCES

Actis Dato GM et al: Atrial septal defect and pregnancy: A retrospective analysis of obstetrical outcome before and after surgical correction. Minerva Cardioangiol 46:63, 1998

Campbell M: Natural history of atrial septal defect. Br Heart J 32:820, 1970

Gatzoulis MA et al: Should atrial septal defects in adults be closed? Ann Thorac Surg 61:657, 1996

Helber U et al: Atrial septal defect in adults: Cardiopulmonary exercise capacity before and 4 months and 10 years after defect closure. J Am Coll Cardiol 29:1345, 1997

Horvath KA et al: Surgical treatment of adult atrial septal defect: Early and long-term results. J Am Coll Cardiol 20:1156, 1992

Kobayashi J et al: Maze procedure for atrial fibrillation associated with atrial septal defect. Circulation 98(Suppl 19):II399, 1998

Kobayashi Y et al: Pre- and postoperative exercise capacity associated with hemodynamics in adult patients with atrial septal defect: A retrospective study. Euro J Cardio-thorac Surg 11:1062, 1997

Konstantinides S et al: A comparison of surgical and medical therapy for atrial septal defect in adults. N Engl J Med 333:469, 1995

Murphy JG et al: Long-term outcome after surgical repair of isolated atrial septal defect-follow-up at 27–32 years. N Engl J Med 323:1645, 1990

Perloff JK: Surgical closure of atrial septal defect in adults. N Engl J Med 333:513, 1995

Sandoval N et al: Concomitant mitral valve or atrial septal defect surgery and the modified Cox-Maze procedure. Am J Cardiol 77:591, 1996

Shah D et al: Natural history of secundum atrial septal defect in adults after medical or surgical treatment: A historical prospective study. Br Heart J 71:224, 1994

Shibata Y et al: Surgical treatment of isolated secundum atrial septal defect in patients more than 50 years old. Ann Thorac Surg 62:1096, 1996

Steele PM et al: Isolated atrial septal defect with pulmonary vascular obstructive disease—long-term follow-up and prediction of outcome after surgical correction. Circulation 76:1037, 1987

Yip ASB et al: Pericardial effusion in adults undergoing surgical repair of atrial septal defect. Am J Cardiol 79:1706, 1997

COARCTATION OF THE AORTA IN THE ADULT

Gordon Mack, Grant H. Burch, & David J. Sahn

Coarctation of the aorta in the adult is a narrowing of the thoracic descending aorta with thickening of the media layer commonly located just beyond the remnant of the ductus arteriosus (95%). This postductal restriction stimulates collateral vessel development from subclavian branches of intercostal, internal mammary, internal thoracic, and spinal arteries to supply the lower extremities. Often, a longer narrowed portion of the transverse aorta and isthmus occurs (tubular hypoplasia), affecting the method of repair. Infantile coarctation (preductal) is often a more diffuse narrowing proximal to the patent ductus arteriosus. Juxtaductal coarctation is an infolding of the posterior lateral wall opposite the area of insertion of the ligamentum or ductus arteriosus. The much less common abdominal coarctation is associated with severe hypertension and may involve the origin of the renal arteries (Morriss and McNamara, 1998).

An associated bicuspid aortic valve occurs in 50 to 85% of patients with coarctation; the association of anomalies of the mitral valve is also unexpectedly high, with clinically significant mitral stenosis or regurgitation in 5 to 10 percent. The mitral valve anomalies are abnormal size, restriction of the free margins of anterior leaflet, abnormal apposition of papillary muscle, or a true parachute mitral valve.

Clinical Findings

Patients can present with a heart murmur or hypertension, but the majority are asymptomatic. Symptoms may include headache, cold feet, leg cramps, paresthesia, pain, muscle weakness, epistaxis, and rarely claudication. The suspicion of coarctation arises if systolic pressure in the arm is >10 mmHg greater than in the leg when measured with the appropriate sized cuffs. The severity of hypertension depends on the degree of coarctation and the collaterals developed. Collaterals may be visualized and palpated over the thorax. The upper extremities and torso can be more developed than the lower extremities. A brachial-femoral delay and differential pulses can be palpated, depending on the relation between the coarctation and the origin of the left subclavian artery. A high-frequency midsystolic ejection murmur is audible over the chest and upper back and along the spine. It becomes longer as the obstruction increases and is continuous if sufficiently narrow. Collaterals or valvular stenosis can contribute to the systolic murmurs.

A chest roentgengram may reveal a dilated ascending aorta and a pre- to poststenotic dilation of the descending aorta, typified as the "A3" sign. Rib notching appears with dilated collateral vessels.

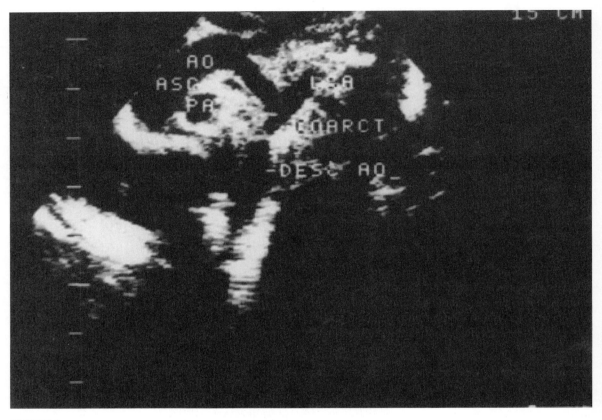

FIGURE 48-1

Echocardiogram view from the suprasternal notch of a discrete coarctation. (Asc Ao, ascending aorta; PA, pulmonary artery; LSA, left subclavian artery; Coarct, coarctation; Desc Ao, descending aorta.)

The electrocardiogram may be normal or show left ventricular hypertrophy with strain.

Two-dimensional and Doppler echocardiography are usually sufficient for a gross anatomical diagnosis of the coarctation (Fig. 48-1) and possible isthmus hypoplasia. The pressure gradient across the coarctation can be estimated by the Bernoulli formula using continuous-wave Doppler recordings. Associated anomalies and the size and function of the left ventricle can be measured. If further anatomical definition is required, magnetic resonance imaging (Fig. 48-2) and/or cardiac catheterization can be performed. Cardiac catheterization allows direct angiographic visualization of the lesion, defines associated valvular or coronary disease, directly determines the gradient across the coarctation, delineates the collateral circulation, and can offer an opportunity for transcatheter intervention with balloon dilation, which will be discussed further.

Natural History

Aneurysms develop after long-standing hypertension at intercostal or subclavian arteries, proximal and distal thoracic aorta, and in the circle of Willis

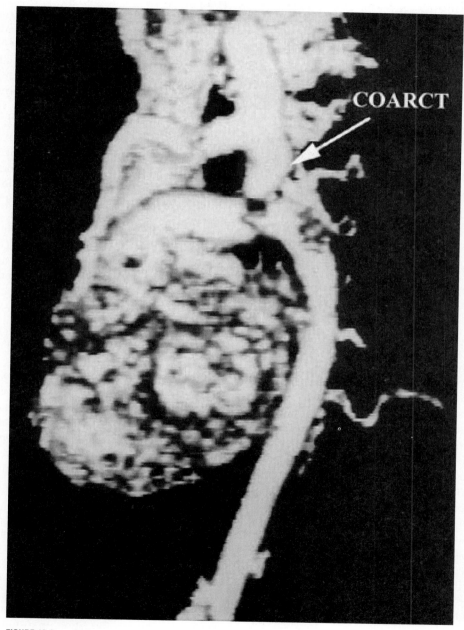

FIGURE 48-2

Three-dimensional display from magnetic resonance imaging: reconstructed image obtained from scan with gadolinium time-of-flight contrast enhancement. (Coarct, coarctation of the aorta.)

(berry aneurysms, 10%). Aneurysmal dilation of the ascending aorta can occur. Cystic medial necrosis, as seen in ascending aorta specimens from patients with the Marfan syndrome, is also seen in resected coarctation specimens.

Unoperated coarctation of the aorta has a 90% mortality by age 50, and the average age of death is 35 years. Principal causes are aortic rupture or dissection, endocarditis or endarteritis, congestive heart failure, and intracranial hemorrhage (Campbell, 1970). Further morbidity occurs with calcific aortic stenosis and premature coronary disease. *Coarctation in the adult should be anatomically relieved and the residual hypertension should be treated pharmacologically.*

Treatment

Surgery

Surgery for coarctation of the aorta in the adult can be quite challenging, because the aorta is more sclerotic, inelastic, and friable than normal and may require a Dacron tube replacement or prosthetic bypass graft. Resection and end-to-end anastomosis or a subclavian flap angioplasty are commonly performed. Patch aortoplasty using Dacron or polytetrafluoroethylene (Teflon) appears to be more likely associated with late aneurysm formation. The problem may be due to compliance mismatch and disintegration of the elastic lamina at the level of the aneurysm due to stretching of the scar tissue interposed between the patch and aortic tissue. Prosthetic bypass grafts are used for recurrent coarctation, for long hypoplastic segments, or if endarteritis requires a long segment resection. Aneurysms and false aneurysms can form at suture lines.

Intra- and postoperative complications are infrequent but include recurrent laryngeal nerve palsy, phrenic nerve palsy, bleeding from collateral vessels, paradoxical (postductal) hypertension, chylothorax, mesenteric arteritis, and paraplegia. Repair in the adult with poor collateral flow with prolonged crossclamp time may require femoral-femoral bypass to ensure spinal artery perfusion (Morriss and McNamara, 1998).

Residual or late hypertension can develop in one-third of patients with surgical repair. The lowest rate of residual hypertension (6%) occurred with surgical repair performed in children between 1 and 5 years of age. If the repairs were performed at 6 to 18 years, 19 to 40 years, or >40 years of age, the residual hypertension rates were 30, 47, and 50%, respectively. Higher morbidity and mortality rates were noted with operations performed at >40 years of age (Liberthson et al., 1979). Abnormal aortic stiffening and pulse wave propagation in the upper segment can contribute to hypertension and residual gradients, even without significant anatomical recoarctation. The wall stress inherent in the aortic wall fragility or weakness can be exacerbated by external forces, such as hypertension, and lead to aneurysm formation, dissection, or rupture of the aorta.

Balloon Angioplasty

Balloon angioplasty as treatment for coarctation of the aorta was initially limited to postoperative restenosis. It was believed that postoperative scarring and fibrosis of the aorta and surrounding tissues would prevent rupture of the aorta. Long-term follow-up (10 years) of balloon angioplasty for postoperative recoarctation by Siblini and colleagues showed 2 of 33 restenosis patients with a narrowed isthmus, none with aneurysm formation, and one with aortic perforation due to dilation with an oversized balloon (Siblini et al., 1998). Mortality after balloon angioplasty for recoarctation ranges from 0 to 2.5%, compared to mortality in surgery of 3 to 41%.

Dilation of native coarctation once appeared to require disruption and dissection of the intima and media (Fig. 48-3). Initially, there was a 43% incidence of aneurysm formation. In a study by Fawzy and colleagues with adolescent and adult native coarctation patients, a small aneurysm developed in 2 of 22 patients with no change in gradient and size at a mean follow-up of 25 months (Fawzy et al., 1992). Two-thirds of resected aneurysms have cystic medial necrosis on pathologic examination,

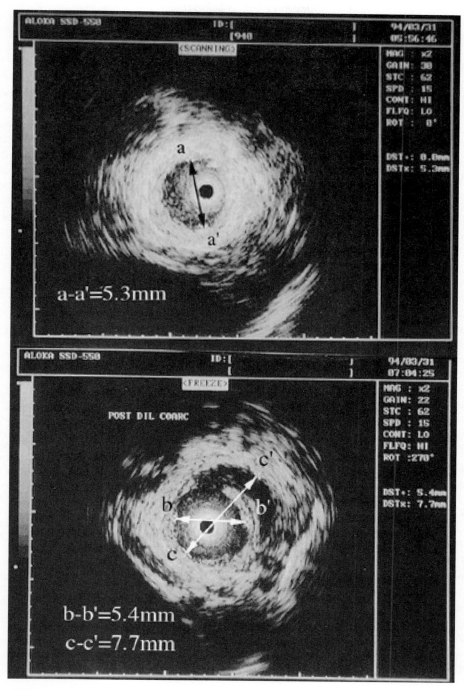

FIGURE 48-3

Intravascular ultrasound (IVUS), pre- and postdilation, with increased luminal diameter resulting from disruption of intima and a dissection space.

which may be the underlying cause of aneurysm formation regardless of the type of repair (Ebeid et al., 1997).

Restenosis occurs in 9 to 25% of native coarctation balloon aortoplasty patients. In two studies, factors identified for recoarctation were age <1 year, absolute size of the isthmus and relative size to the descending aorta (>0.65), absolute size of the coarctation, and size of the coarctation after balloon angiography (Rao et al., 1989; Shaddy et al., 1993). In addition, if the postcatheterization gradient exceeded 12 mmHg, restenosis was anticipated. There was no effect due to the presence of a ductus arteriosus, the type of coarctation, whether the lesion was discrete or diffuse, the preangiography gradient (even if >50 mmHg), or the systolic pressure after balloon dilation. The complication rates were similar between surgical or balloon angioplasty repair; however, the latter was not associated with nerve injury or spinal ischemia. No progression of the aneurysm was seen with intermediate-term follow-up. Pooled data since 1980 showed comparable or lower rates of initial and late mortality, recoarctation, and aneurysm formation with balloon angioplasty (Shaddy et al., 1993).

For coarctation of the aorta not amenable to ballon dilation alone, balloon-expandable stents have been used with some success by Suarez de Lezo and colleagues (1999) and Ebeid and colleagues (1997). Distorted, angulated, and hypoplastic distal transverse segments are remodeled, and a damaged aortic wall may be lent support. Flow to the major branches of the aortic arch crossed by the stent are maintained without obstruction, even at 3-year follow-up. Reexpansion of the stent is possible but limited to the size of the largest stent able to be placed. The stents are not associated with thrombus formation and are rapidly covered by a neointimal layer. Recent experience shows excellent stenting results in young adults and children, with a 27% incidence of some intimal thickening inside the stent on follow-up intravascular ultrasound and 10% of patients with mild restenosis and 7% with late small aneurysm formation (Suarez de Lezo et al., 1999).

Pre- and postoperative hypertension were independent risk factors of mortality. The most common causes of late death in patients with repaired coarctation were coronary artery disease, sudden death, heart failure, cerebrovascular accident, or ruptured aortic aneurysm. Considering the risk of late hypertension, aneurysm formation, and increased risk of associated cardiac disease, all patients require long-term monitoring after surgical or transcatheter treatment of coarctation of the aorta. A review of the literature and the authors' experience suggest that coarctation of the aorta should be managed initially by the transcatheter approach.

REFERENCES

Campbell M: Natural history of coarctation of the aorta. Br Heart J 32:633, 1970

Ebeid MR et al: Use of balloon-expandable stents for coarctation of the aorta: Initial results and intermediate follow-up. J Am Coll Cardiol 30(7):1847, 1997

Fawzy ME et al: Balloon coarctation angioplasty in adolescents and adults: Early and intermediate results. Am Heart J 124(1):167, 1992

Liberthson RR et al: Coarctation of the aorta: Review of 234 patients and clarification of management problems. Am J Cardiol 43:835, 1979

Morriss MJH, McNamara DG: Coarctation of the aorta and interrupted aortic arch, in *The Science and Practice of Pediatric Cardiology,* 2d ed, A Garson et al (eds). New York, Williams & Wilkins, 1998, pp 1317–1346

Rao PS et al: Causes of recoarctation after balloon angioplasty of unoperated aortic coarctation. J Am Coll Cardiol 13(1):109, 1989

Shaddy RE et al: Comparison of angioplasty and surgery for unoperated coarctation of the aorta. Circulation 87(3):793, 1993

Siblini G et al: Long-term follow-up results of balloon angioplasty of postoperative aortic recoarctation. Am J Cardiol 81:61, 1998

Suarez de Lezo J et al: Immediate and follow-up findings after stent treatment for severe coarctation of aorta. Am J Cardiol 83:400, 1999

THE CHANGING SPECTRUM OF VALVULAR HEART DISEASE PATHOLOGY

William D. Edwards

For industrialized countries, valve repair and valve replacement are now so commonplace that their use is generally taken for granted. Nevertheless, it is sobering to consider that within five millennia of recorded human history, only during the past five decades have successful treatments become available that have substantially improved the quality of life and increased the longevity of people with symptomatic valvular heart disease. Although the *basic causes* of valvular disease have not changed appreciably (except for the addition of iatrogenic disorders), their *relative frequencies* have changed dramatically; this fact has important implications for the practice of medicine in the 21st century. However, before gazing into the future, it would behoove us to glance into the past to glean any temporal trends.

The following comments are based on data compiled from several published studies of left-sided cardiac valves surgically excised at Mayo Clinic Rochester between 1965 and 1990 and on previously unpublished data from 1995 and 2000. Three factors may distort how accurately the data reflect valvular heart disease in North America as a whole. First, our surgical referrals may be some-

what biased toward elderly patients, thus favoring age-related diseases. Second, valves that are repaired without the removal of tissue will not be recorded in the data. And third, the causes of medically treated valve disease may have a different relative distribution than surgically treated disease. Nonetheless, the above three potential sources of bias are probably of minor importance, such that the following information is considered to be adequately representative of valvular heart disease in North America.

The Past: Temporal Trends from 1965 to 2000

Functional States

For aortic valves excised in 1965, pure stenosis, combined stenosis and insufficiency, and pure regurgitation each accounted for about one-third of the cases. Since then, pure aortic stenosis has progressively increased in prevalence, representing over one-half of the cases in the 1970s and nearly two-thirds during the 1980s and 1990s (Dare et al., 1993b; Passik et al., 1987). In 2000, pure aortic stenosis accounted for 71% of all of our surgically excised aortic valves (Fig. 49-1A).

In contrast, for mitral valves excised in 1965, about three-fifths had combined stenosis and insuffi-

ciency and about one-fifth each had pure stenosis or pure regurgitation. During the 1970s, each functional category accounted for about one-third of the cases. Since then, however, pure regurgitation has increased steadily (Dare et al., 1993; Olson et al., 1987) and represented 78% of our cases in 2000 (Fig. 49-1B).

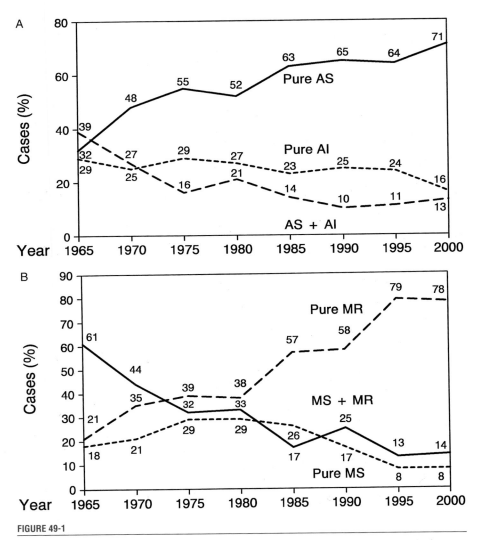

FIGURE 49-1

Temporal changes in the relative frequencies of the three functional disease states, for left-sided valves surgically excised at Mayo Clinic Rochester during 5-year intervals from 1965 to 2000. (A) Aortic valves (1978 cases). (B) Mitral valves (1238 cases). AI, aortic insufficiency; AS, aortic stenosis; MR, mitral regurgitation; MS, mitral stenosis.

Thus, over the past 35 years, the relative frequencies of the various functional states have changed remarkably. In 2000, surgeons at Mayo Clinic Rochester removed 442 aortic valves and 261 mitral valves, among which 312 (44%) had pure aortic stenosis and 205 (29%) had pure mitral regurgitation. Currently, these two disorders account for nearly three-fourths of all surgically excised left-sided cardiac valves.

Rheumatic Valvular Disease

When successful prosthetic valves first became available in the early 1960s, the most common etiology of valvular dysfunction in North America (and worldwide) was chronic rheumatic disease. However, since that time, the most prevalent causes have shifted from rheumatic to nonrheumatic disorders for all left-sided dysfunctional states except pure mitral stenosis and combined mitral stenosis and regurgitation (Dare et al., 1993a, b). The reasons for this change are numerous and include a decreased prevalence of acute rheumatic fever in North America, a concomitant increase in the frequencies of age-related and iatrogenic valvular disorders, and an increased willingness for surgeons to operate on the elderly and on patients with active infective endocarditis.

By 1945, the revised Jones criteria were established for the diagnosis of acute rheumatic fever and penicillin had become readily available for the prevention of its recurrences. Knowing that severe chronic rheumatic valvular heart disease generally takes about 30 to 40 years to develop and lead to surgical intervention in North America, one would predict that a significant decrease in the relative frequency of rheumatic disease should have occurred between 1975 and 1985. Indeed, this was observed in the surgical population at Mayo Clinic Rochester for all forms of aortic valve dysfunction and for pure mitral regurgitation (Fig. 49-2).

This trend has continued, such that by 2000 the frequency of postinflammatory (rheumatic) disease was only 7% for pure aortic stenosis, 16% for combined aortic stenosis and insufficiency, 14% for pure aortic incompetence, and 9% for pure mitral regurgitation. In contrast, chronic rheumatic disease has remained quite prevalent among patients with pure mitral stenosis and with combined mitral stenosis and insufficiency, accounting for 90% and 81%, respectively, in 2000 (compared to 100% for each in 1965).

Despite the continued prominence of postinflammatory (rheumatic) disease as the leading cause of mitral stenosis, the absolute number of patients with mitral stenosis has been declining steadily in our surgical population. Thus, although mitral stenosis (with or without mitral regurgitation) represented 79% of all surgically excised mitral valves in 1965, it accounted for only 18% in 2000. As a result, when all surgically excised mitral valves are considered together, the percentage with rheumatic disease has decreased from 89 in 1965 to only 25 in 2000.

Nonrheumatic Valvular Disease

As postinflammatory (rheumatic) disease has progressively decreased since 1965, the relative frequency of nonrheumatic disorders has increased proportionately. For pure aortic stenosis, the prevalence of degenerative disease increased from 0% in 1965 to 61% in 2000; for pure mitral regurgitation, myxomatous disease increased from 17% to 71% during the same time interval (Fig. 49-2).

Among 703 left-sided valves that were excised at Mayo Clinic Rochester in 2000, the primary *mechanisms* of valvular dysfunction were calcification (59%), structural weakening (27%), and fibrosis (14%). The major *causes* of left-sided valve disease were age-related processes, accounting for 49% of the valves (Table 49-1). These included degenerative aortic valvular calcification (211 cases), myxomatous mitral valvular disease (145 cases), and aortic root dilation (14 cases).

For the 442 aortic valves excised in 2000, age-related degenerative calcification was the most commonly encountered cause of pure stenosis (61%) and combined stenosis and insufficiency (38%); age-related dilation of the ascending aorta was the most frequent cause of pure regurgitation (19%). Resected ascending aortic tissue usually showed cystic medial

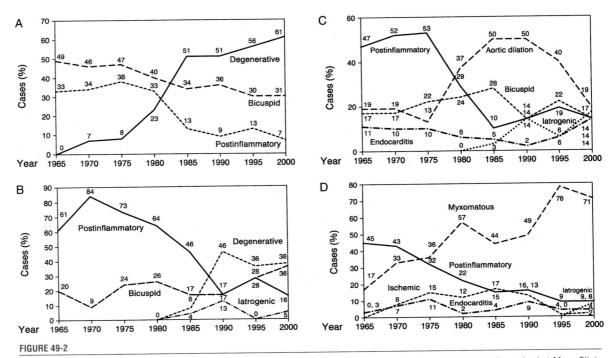

FIGURE 49-2

Temporal changes in the relative frequencies of the most common causes of disease, for left-sided valves surgically excised at Mayo Clinic Rochester during 5-year intervals from 1965 to 2000. (*A*) Pure aortic stenosis (1159 cases). (*B*) Combined aortic stenosis and regurgitation (346 cases). (*C*) Pure aortic regurgitation (473 cases). (*D*) Pure mitral regurgitation (694 cases). Data for the 544 cases of mitral stenosis, with or without mitral regurgitation, are not shown because postinflammatory (rheumatic) disease accounted for ≥80% during each year. (For each year, the sum of the percentages may be less than 100% because only data for the most common causes are included.)

degeneration or, less often, giant cell aortitis. Congenitally bicuspid aortic valves were a frequent cause of combined stenosis and insufficiency (36%), pure stenosis (31%), and pure regurgitation (14%) (Table 49-2). For patients with aortic valvular disease, the mean age at operation has increased from 49 years in 1965 to 67 years in 2000.

Of the 205 purely regurgitant mitral valves excised in 2000, the most frequently observed cause was myxomatous disease (71%). Among patients with myxomatous valves, 82% were older than 50 years and most had a clinical history of mitral valve prolapse. In about 25% of the cases, cordal rupture had contributed to valvular insufficiency. Thus, valve weakness and age-related factors set the stage for pure mitral regurgitation in most cases.

TABLE 49-1

CAUSES OF DYSFUNCTION IN 703 LEFT-SIDED CARDIAC VALVES SURGICALLY EXCISED IN 2000 AT MAYO CLINIC ROCHESTER

Cause	No.	%
Age-related valvular disease	341	49
Congenitally bicuspid aortic valve	132	19
Postinflammatory (rheumatic) disease	108	15
Iatrogenic valvular disease	39	6
Infective endocarditis	18	3
Other valvular disease	65	9
Total	703	100

TABLE 49-2

MOST COMMON CAUSES OF VALVULAR DYSFUNCTION IN 703 LEFT-SIDED CARDIAC VALVES SURGICALLY EXCISED IN 2000 AT MAYO CLINIC ROCHESTER

Functional state	Most common causes	%
Pure AS	Degenerative and bicuspid	92
AS + AI	Degenerative and bicuspid	74
Pure AI	Aortic dilation, iatrogenic, bicuspid	50
Pure MS	Postinflammatory (rheumatic)	90
MS + MR	Postinflammatory (rheumatic)	81
Pure MR	Myxomatous (floppy, prolapse)	71

ABBREVIATIONS: AI, aortic insufficiency; AS, aortic stenosis; MR, mitral regurgitation; MS, mitral stenosis.

Of the 39 valves excised in 2000 for iatrogenic disease, 64% were purely regurgitant. The most common etiology was previous surgical valve repair (72%); other causes included drugs, irradiation, and previous balloon valvuloplasty. Iatrogenic disease accounted for 17% of all purely regurgitant aortic valves and 8% of all purely regurgitant mitral valves.

The Future: Predictions for the Twenty-First Century

Cautionary Note

The future is unknown. Any number of unexpected and unpredictable factors may develop and appreciably alter the occurrence and treatment of valvular heart disease during the twenty-first century. Nonetheless, the trends identified in the preceding paragraphs allow one to make reasonable predictions concerning the probable course of valvular heart disease.

Age-Related Valvular Disease

The population of elderly persons in the United States is increasing exponentially; this will have an important impact on health care costs (Schneider and Guralnik, 1990). Undoubtedly, there will be a substantial increase in the number of citizens with age-related valvular disease—particularly aortic stenosis, aortic insufficiency, and mitral regurgitation.

Calcification is the chief cause of degenerative aortic stenosis and those cases of mitral regurgitation due to mineralization of its annulus. Recent studies have demonstrated that calcification is not a passive process but rather entails the upregulation of enzyme systems commonly associated with bone formation (Srivatsa et al., 1997). Perhaps interference with this process could appreciably slow the progression of age-related calcification and thereby contribute to the prevention of degenerative aortic stenosis and mitral annular calcification.

Currently, little is known concerning the aging factors that weaken the ascending aorta, thereby causing its progressive dilation and leading to aortic valvular incompetence. Cystic medial degeneration and giant cell aortitis represent the most frequently observed microscopic counterparts of aortic root dilation, although their pathogenesis is also poorly understood. Perhaps the discovery of effective means to detect and retard these degenerative and inflammatory processes in the ascending aorta may allow a significant reduction in the frequency of aortic insufficiency in the elderly.

Myxomatous mitral valve disease is another disorder in which aging appears to weaken the valve and lead to progressive regurgitation. The aortic valve may also become involved. Genetic and metabolic factors may play pathogenetic roles. To the extent that the causes of myxomatous degeneration can be identified in the future, preventative measures may become available to control this increasingly prevalent form of valve disease in the elderly.

Congenitally Bicuspid Aortic Valves

Bicuspid aortic valves affect 1 to 2% of the general population and most commonly occur as isolated anomalies. Their usually normal function at birth belies the fact that virtually all will become dysfunctional as the ravages of mechanical stress, degenerative calcification, and infection take their toll. Eventually, about 85% will become stenotic (with or without coexistent insufficiency) due to progressive calcification. Most of the remaining 15% will become purely regurgitant due to cusp prolapse, annular dilation, or infection, although a few will become associated with an acute aortic dissection (Sabet et al., 1999). Clearly, however, the most common fate of a congenitally bicuspid aortic valve is calcific stenosis.

There is no reason to believe that the frequency of bicuspid aortic valves in the population will change appreciably during this century. Consequently, if no strategy is devised to control the development of valvular calcification, one would predict that most patients with bicuspid valves will eventually need aortic valve replacement. Currently, about 4 million U.S. citizens have congenitally bicuspid aortic valves, and this number is expected to increase as our population continues to grow.

Rheumatic Valvular Disease

In North America (and in most industrialized countries), the incidence of acute rheumatic fever has decreased dramatically over the past 50 years. With it, a substantial decrease in the number of persons with symptomatic chronic rheumatic heart disease has also occurred—or is beginning to do so. Thus, barring any unexpected outbreak of rheumatic fever, the relative percentage of valve dysfunction due to postinflammatory (rheumatic) disease should continue to decrease.

For underdeveloped countries, however, the predictions are considerably different. Worldwide, it is estimated that 15 to 20 million new cases of acute rheumatic fever occur annually. In nonindustrialized nations, chronic rheumatic valve disease generally progresses more rapidly than in North America and will probably continue to be a major cause of morbidity and mortality for many years to come. Where available, antibiotics will be used prophylactically for acute rheumatic fever, and balloon valvuloplasty and surgical interventions will be used to treat chronic rheumatic valvular disease. Only over the course of decades will its prevalence begin to diminish, region by region.

Other Valvular Disease

Valve diseases due to drugs, irradiation, infection, and ischemic heart disease occur less commonly than the disorders discussed above, but they have increased in relative frequency in recent years (Fig. 49-2). They tend to produce valvular regurgitation more often than stenosis.

Iatrogenic Valvular Disease

Most iatrogenic valve disease develops unpredictably. This is particularly true for drug-related injury, such as that associated with various migraine medications (ergotamine or methysergide) and certain appetite suppressants (fenfluramine, with or without phentermine). With mediastinal irradiation for various malignancies, it was hoped that newer methods and lower dosages would lessen the likelihood of cardiac injury, but cases with extensive fibrosis of the valves and other regions of the heart continue to be reported (Veinot and Edwards, 1996).

For the above exposures, some individuals seem to be more predisposed to develop valvular injury than others. Currently, the detection of hyperresponders is limited, but perhaps future identification of genetic markers may allow the selective use of specific therapies only in individuals who are unlikely to develop complications. It is to be expected, however, that new drugs will be developed and marketed that will cause unpredictable and adverse valvular reactions.

Infective Endocarditis

Valves that have been chronically deformed by congenital or acquired disorders, such as bicuspid aortic valves and myxomatous mitral valves, will continue to be at risk for infective endocarditis, as will valves exposed to highly virulent organisms such as *Staphylococcus aureus*. Immunosuppression, intravenous drug abuse, chronic alcoholism, and male gender will also remain important risk factors.

Newly discovered organisms may also be identified as important causes of active infective endocarditis or of chronic valvulitis.

Ischemic Heart Disease

Mitral regurgitation due to ischemic heart disease may develop either acutely, due to rupture of an infarcted papillary muscle, or chronically, as a result of papillary muscle fibrosis, subjacent regional wall motion abnormalities, or left ventricular dilation.

Chronic ischemic mitral regurgitation appears to occur considerably more often in the medical population than in the surgical population. Any future decrease in the incidence of ischemic mitral insufficiency will likely depend on the overall effectiveness of preventing coronary atherosclerosis, myocardial infarction, and left ventricular remodeling.

Conclusions

In North America (and most industrialized nations), as the number of elderly citizens continues to increase, the number of patients with age-related forms of valvular disease will also increase. This trend will plateau or decrease only as we learn to control the processes that lead to valvular calcfication and to valvular and aortic weakening. New insights into the causes of age-related changes may be discovered, including genetic, metabolic, infectious, and atherosclerotic factors. Bicuspid aortic valves will also contribute substantially to health care costs unless valvular calcification can be controlled. Rheumatic valvular disease will progressively decrease in industrialized nations but will most likely remain prevalent in underdeveloped countries. Iatrogenic, infectious, and ischemic forms of valvular disease will probably continue to account for a small percentage of surgical cases. Clearly, the new century holds both exciting opportunities and difficult challenges for the treatment, control, and prevention of valvular heart disease. Documentation of the temporal changes in prevalences will be important for monitoring any successful preventative measures.

REFERENCES

Dare AJ et al: Evaluation of surgically excised mitral valves: Revised recommendations based on changing operative procedures in the 1990s. Hum Pathol 24:1286, 1993a

Dare AJ et al: New observations on the etiology of aortic valve disease: A surgical pathologic study of 236 cases from 1990. Hum Pathol 24:1330, 1993b

Olson LJ et al: Surgical pathology of the mitral valve: A study of 712 cases spanning 21 years. Mayo Clin Proc 62:22, 1987

Passik CS et al: Temporal changes in the causes of aortic stenosis: A surgical pathologic study of 646 cases. Mayo Clin Proc 62:119, 1987

Sabet HY et al: Congenitally bicuspid aortic valves: A surgical pathology study of 542 cases (1991 through 1996) and a literature review of 2,715 additional cases. Mayo Clin Proc 74:14, 1999

Schneider EL, Guralnik JM: The aging of America. Impact on health care costs. JAMA 263:2335, 1990

Srivatsa SS et al: Increased cellular expression of matrix proteins that regulate mineralization is associated with calcification of native human and porcine xenograft bioprosthetic heart valves. J Clin Invest 99:996, 1997

Veinot JP, Edwards WD: Pathology of radiation-induced heart disease: A surgical and autopsy study of 27 cases. Hum Pathol 27:766, 1996

ECHOCARDIOGRAPHY AND THE SELECTION OF PATIENTS FOR MITRAL BALLOON VALVULOPLASTY

Charles J. Bruce, Charanjit S. Rihal

Noninvasive imaging using two-dimensional and Doppler echocardiography, both transthoracic and transesophageal, has revolutionized the assessment of patients with mitral stenosis (MS) and is considered the diagnostic tool of choice in this clinical setting (Table 50-1) (Bonow et al., 1998). Echocardiography not only confirms the presence of MS but also provides an objective assessment of the severity of obstruction and guides selection of further therapies (Bruce and Nishimura, 1998a, 1998b).

For symptomatic patients with severe MS, the major treatment options include surgery (open or closed commissurotomy or mitral valve replacement) or percutaneous balloon mitral valvuloplasty (PMBV). In recent years, PMBV has increasingly been performed instead of surgical commissurotomy because it is less invasive and has excellent short- and intermediate-term results in carefully selected patients. Results compare favorably to surgical mitral commissurotomy. However, not all patients with severe MS are suitable for this procedure. It is now recognized that PMBV relieves mitral valve

obstruction by commissurotomy, which is the splitting of the fused mitral commissures (as opposed to a plastic remolding of the stenotic valve). Patients with unfavorable mitral apparatus morphology or dense commissural calcification are less likely to achieve a good anatomic result. Careful preprocedural patient selection using echocardiography is thus crucial to evaluate the morphology of the mitral valve apparatus and the extent of commissural calcification and to detect the presence and severity of concomitant conditions such as mitral regurgitation and pulmonary hypertension. Echocardiographic examinations also provide ancillary anatomic information important in planning the technical approach, such as left atrial size, presence or absence of left atrial or left atrial appendage thrombus and thickness, and morphology of the atrial septum and fossa ovalis membrane.

Finally, echocardiography is ideally suited for follow-up of patients with MS, either to determine the optimal timing of intervention or to document the hemodynamic response after intervention and to detect complications.

TABLE 50-1

ACC/AHA RECOMMENDATIONS FOR ECHOCARDIOGRAPHY IN MITRAL STENOSIS (MS)

Indication	Class
Transthoracic	
Diagnosis of MS, assessment of hemodynamic severity (mean gradient, mitral valve area, pulmonary artery pressure), and assessment of right ventricular size and function	I
Assessment of valve morphology to determine suitability for percutaneous mitral balloon valvotomy	I
Diagnosis and assessment of concomitant valvular lesions	I
Reevaluation of patients with known MS with changing symptoms or signs	I
Assessment of hemodynamic response of mean gradient and pulmonary artery pressures by exercise Doppler echocardiography in patients when there is a discrepancy between resting hemodynamic and clinical findings	IIa
Reevaluation of asymptomatic patients with moderate to severe MS to assess pulmonary artery pressure	IIb
Routine reevaluation of the asymptomatic patient with mild MS and stable clinical findings	III
Transesophageal	
Assessment for presence or absence of left atrial thrombus in patients being considered for percutaneous mitral balloon valvotomy or cardioversion	IIa
Evaluation of mitral valve morphology and hemodynamics when transthoracic echocardiography provides suboptimal data	IIa
Routine evaluation of mitral valve morphology and hemodynamics when complete transthoracic echocardiographic data are satisfactory	III

Mitral Stenosis: Diagnosis and Severity

The diagnosis of MS is reliably made from two-dimensional echocardiography, which demonstrates restricted opening of the mitral valve leaflets due to diastolic "doming" of the anterior leaflet ("hockey-stick" deformity) and immobility of the posterior leaflet (Fig. 50-1). A "fish mouth" appearance is seen on the parasternal short-axis views. The two major parameters used to assess severity of MS are mitral valve area (MVA) and the diastolic transmitral-filling gradient. Until the development of echocardiography, both parameters required invasive cardiac catheterization for measurement.

While the severity of MS can be directly measured using two-dimensional cross-sectional planimetry, this measurement is technically challenging and prone to error. Severity of MS is better assessed with Doppler velocity signals. Using the noninvasive Doppler technique, the transmitral gradient, MVA, and pulmonary artery pressure (all indicators of the hemodynamic consequence of MS) can be estimated reliably and accurately.

The transmitral gradient is measured by continuous-wave Doppler interrogation of the flow during diastole across the mitral valve (Hatle et al., 1978). Using the modified Bernoulli equation ($\triangle P = 4 \times velocity^2$), the instantaneous gradient between the left atrium and left ventricle is determined (Fig. 50-2).

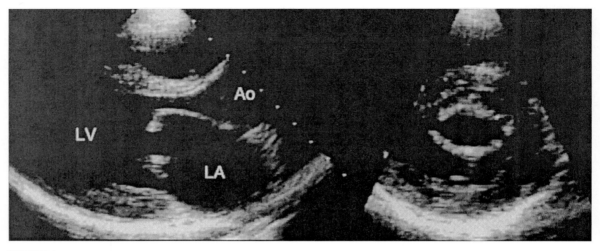

FIGURE 50-1

Two-dimensional echocardiogram of a patient with mitral stenosis shown during diastole. The parasternal long-axis view (left) shows diastolic doming and the typical "hockey stick" deformity of the anterior mitral valve leaflet. The posterior leaflet is immobile and the left atrium is enlarged. The parasternal short-axis view (right) demonstrates the typical "fish mouth" deformity of the mitral valve with narrowing of the mitral orifice. From this view, an estimate of the mitral valve area can be made using planimetry. Ao, aorta; LA, left atrium; LV, left ventricle. (From CJ Bruce, RA Nishimura: Curr Probl Cardiol 23:125, 1998, with permission.)

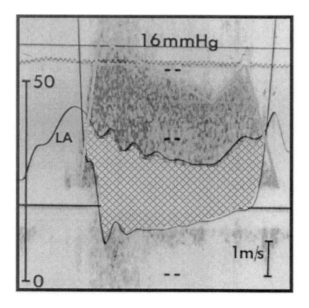

This Doppler measurement is more accurate than conventional cardiac catheterization using the pulmonary artery wedge pressure and compares favorably with transseptal left atrial–left ventricular pressure gradients (Nishimura et al., 1994). Since the transmitral gradient is dependent on R-R interval, it is also important to report the heart rate at which the measurement was obtained.

Less affected by heart rate is the MVA. The most common method of determining valve area by Doppler echocardiography is using the diastolic half-time (Hatle et al., 1979). The half-time is a measurement of the rate of fall of pressure between the left

FIGURE 50-2

Shown are the cardiac catheterization left atrial and left ventricular pressure recordings and simultaneous transmitral Doppler gradient in a patient with mitral stenosis. The gradient between the left atrium and left ventricle, as calculated at catheterization, is depicted by the hatched area. The mean gradient determined by Doppler echocardiography is calculated by planimetering the transmitral velocity curve and applying the modified Bernoulli equation. In this patient, a transmitral gradient of 16 mmHg was present, indicative of severe mitral stenosis.

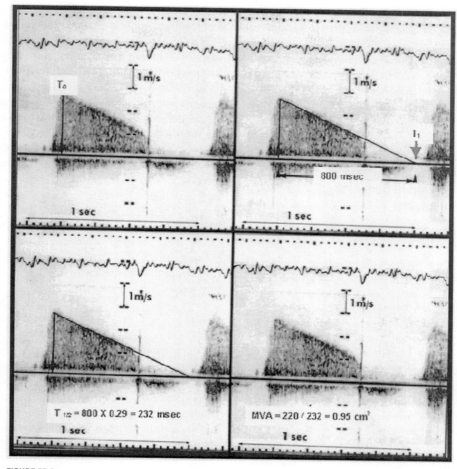

FIGURE 50-3

Echocardiogram illustrating the method by which diastolic half-time and mitral valve area (MVA) are derived from the transmitral Doppler flow velocity curve in a patient with atrial fibrillation. The deceleration time is measured by extrapolating the fall in velocity from the peak initial velocity (T_0) to the baseline (T_1). The deceleration time is the time from the T_0 to the point where this extrapolation meets the baseline (T_1). The diastolic half-time ($T_{1/2}$) is calculated by multiplying the deceleration time by a constant of 0.29. The MVA is calculated by dividing the diastolic half-time into a constant of 220. In this patient, severe mitral stenosis is present with a MVA of 0.95 cm2. (From CJ Bruce, RA Nishimura: Curr Probl Cardiol 23:125, 1998, with permission.)

atrium and left ventricle and can be estimated from the Doppler transmitral flow velocity curve by the "deceleration time" (Fig. 50-3). The diastolic half-time is the product of the deceleration time × 0.29, or the time it takes the peak pressure gradient to drop by 50%. Using an empirically derived constant (220), the MVA can be derived from the Doppler-derived diastolic half-time as MVA = 220/diastolic half-time.

This Doppler-derived valve area correlates closely with the valve area obtained at cardiac catheterization and is now universally applied to determine MVA.

The third echocardiographic method to measure MVA is based on the continuity of flow principle (Nakatani et al., 1988). Simply put, this concept maintains that flow remains constant through all the heart valves in the absence of regurgitation or shunts. This method is dependent on accurate measurement of volumetric flow and thus should be used only by laboratories experienced in the technique of quantitative Doppler measurements.

Exercise with simultaneous Doppler estimation of transmitral and pulmonary pressures can aid in the hemodynamic assessment of MS in borderline cases (Bruce and Nishimura, 1998a, 1998b).

Mitral Valve and Mitral Apparatus Morphology in Patient Selection for Balloon Valvuloplasty

PMBV was first described by Inoue et al in 1984 (Inoue et al., 1984). (See Chap. 51) This is a catheter-based procedure in which an inflatable balloon is introduced into the left atrium via a transseptal puncture and advanced across the stenotic mitral valve. A specially designed balloon catheter (Inoue catheter, Toray Corporation, Japan) is most commonly used for the procedure around the world. Once the catheter is in position across the stenotic mitral valve, the balloon is inflated, resulting in splitting of the fused commissures. This procedure reduces the transmitral gradient, increases the MVA, and typically results in marked clinical improvement in well-selected patients. Double-balloon techniques are rarely used now.

Although many factors have been associated with outcome after valvotomy (age, New York Heart Association class, pulmonary pressure, comorbid conditions), morphology of the mitral apparatus is most important. Patients with a pliable anterior mitral leaflet and little subvalvular disease have the highest likelihood of an optimal result from the procedure. An echocardiographic score is commonly used (Abascal et al., 1988), in which four factors are evaluated and graded on an ordinal scale of 1 to 4. These are summed to provide an overall assessment of degree of rheumatic involvement ranging from 4 (least) to 16 (most). These factors consist of the leaflet thickness, leaflet mobility, leaflet calcification, and the degree of subvalvular fusion. This scoring grade has been shown to predict the acute and intermediate-term outcome of PMBV. Patients with a score ≤8 have good acute results and a low incidence of complications. Patients

with a score ≥10 have a higher likelihood of suboptimal results, complications, and subsequent restenosis.

Despite the overall predictive value of the mitral valve score, there remain a number of patients with a relatively high mitral valve score who benefit from PMBV. Conversely, there are also patients with low scores who do less well. It has been reported that the appearance of the commissures as assessed from the short axis transthoracic view is a very important predictor of outcome (Cannan et al., 1997). Among patients with no calcification in the commissures, there is a >95% chance of a successful procedure with excellent long-term outcome, while those with commissural calcification have a significantly higher complication rate and lower event-free survival. This finding emphasizes that successful balloon valvotomy results from splitting open the fused commissures, a factor not taken into account in standard scoring systems.

For these reasons, patients with anatomically favorable morphology are the ideal candidates for PMBV, have high procedural success rates (>90%) with low complication rates (<2 to 3%), and can expect sustained clinical improvement (80 to 90% event-free survival) over follow-up periods of 3 to 7 years (Bruce and Nishimura, 1998a). As stated earlier, patients with calcified, thickened, poorly mobile leaflets and subvalvular disease and calcified commissures have a high risk of complications and high rates of restenosis. Patients with such unfavorable anatomy, particularly those with heavily calcified commissures, should undergo mitral valve replacement unless they have other coexisting medical problems that place them at higher risk for surgery.

Echocardiographic Assessment of Coexistent Cardiac Disease

Once the decision has been made to proceed with PMBV (based on history, hemodynamics, and valve morphology), transesophageal echocardiography is performed to rule out left atrial thrombus, measure left atrial dimension, further assess any mitral regurgitation, and assess the interatrial septum for suitability for transseptal puncture and passage of the catheter (Bonow et al., 1998). Left atrial thrombus is readily detected by the use of transesophageal echocardiography. If thrombus is detected, PMBV should be deferred. These patients should be anticoagulated with warfarin for 2 to 3 months and thereafter undergo repeat transesophageal echocardiography. If resolution of the thrombus is confirmed, PMBV can be performed safely. Left atrial dimension is important for technical reasons; the larger the left atrium, the more difficulty can be expected manipulating catheters across the stenotic mitral valve. Rarely, a huge left atrium, out of proportion to the degree of mitral stenosis, is the only clue to otherwise unrecognized severe mitral regurgitation. This scenario can occur if the regurgitation jet courses alongside the wall of the left atrium (Coanda effect), making detection by color-flow Doppler difficult. The morphology of the interatrial septum is important in planning the technique of transseptal puncture and anticipating difficulties. Important factors include presence and size of a patent foramen ovale; thickness of the membrane and limbus; and whether the fossa is normal, effaced, or bulging.

The most frequent complication of PMBV is mitral regurgitation, but this is seldom severe enough (<3% in the North America Inoue Balloon Registry) to warrant mitral valve replacement during the same hospitalization. However, as many as one-third of patients can be expected to have a one-grade increase in mitral regurgitation after the procedure. Thus, detection of mitral regurgitation and measurement of its severity is an essential part of the preprocedural evaluation. When present, it can be semi-quantitatively assessed using transthoracic or transesophageal echocardiography by measuring the regurgitant volume, regurgitant fraction, and effective orifice area using volumetric or color flow Doppler [proximal isovelocity surface area (PISA)] methods. If significant mitral regurgitation is present (grade 3+ to 4+), PMBV should not be performed.

Finally, another consideration in the selection of patients for PMBV is the presence or absence of associated valvular and/or coronary artery disease. The transthoracic echocardiogram can (1) provide an assessment of overall left ventricular size and function, (2) detect regional wall motion abnormalities if present, and (3) detect associated nonmitral valvular disease. These factors are important to take into account when considering how best to treat the MS, i.e., whether to proceed with a less invasive percutaneous procedure vs. open-heart surgery and mitral valve replacement.

Echocardiography and Follow-Up

Immediately following PMBV, the hemodynamic response can be measured by determining the transmitral gradient using continuous-wave Doppler and the modified Bernoulli equation; however, these should be interpreted carefully and in conjunction with invasive measurements performed at the time of the procedure (Fig. 50-4). The diastolic half-time method may be inaccurate when there are significant abnormalities of left atrial or left ventricular compliance (as may occur immediately post PMBV). Also, if mitral regurgitation is present (which commonly occurs after PMBV), mitral valve area calculated using the continuity principle is inaccurate.

A baseline postprocedural echocardiogram is usually performed at least 72 h after the procedure to allow equilibration of the acute changes in atrial and ventricular compliance (Bonow et al., 1998). Baseline measurements of postprocedural hemodynamics are recorded, and complications such as mitral regurgitation, atrial septal defect, or ventricular dysfunction are noted.

Serial echocardiography after uncomplicated PMBV is not necessary. However, repeat echocardiography is indicated should symptoms recur.

Conclusion

Echocardiography has an established role in the noninvasive preprocedural evaluation of patients undergoing percutaneous mitral balloon valvuloplasty. The diagnosis and severity of mitral stenosis can be confirmed by echocardiography, as

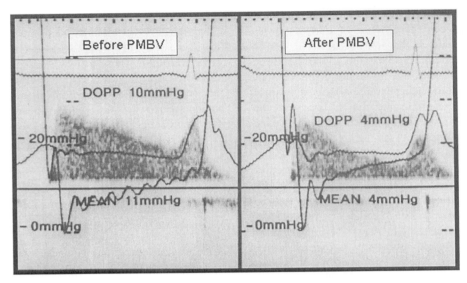

FIGURE 50-4

Simultaneous transmitral Doppler echocardiogram and left atrial and left ventricular pressure recordings in a patient with mitral stenosis before (left) and after PMBV (right). There is a significant decrease in transmitral gradient (10 mmHg to 4 mmHg) after the procedure. (*From CJ Bruce, RA Nishimura: Curr Probl Cardiol 23:125, 1998, with permission.*)

can identification of coexistent cardiac pathology (multivalve involvement, concomitant mitral regurgitation, or presence of left atrial thrombus) and suitability for PMBV. All of these factors, identified by echocardiography, influence the outcome (acute and longer-term) of the procedure. Thus, echocardiography plays a pivotal role in the assessment of the risk, success rate, and outcome of the procedure on an individual basis in the patient with clinically significant MS undergoing PMBV.

REFERENCES

Abascal VM et al: Mitral regurgitation after percutaneous balloon mitral valvuloplasty in adults: Evaluation by pulsed Doppler echocardiography. J Am Coll Cardiol 11:257, 1988

Bonow RO et al: ACC/AHA practice guidelines: Guidelines for the management of patients with valvular heart disease. Circulation 98:1949, 1998

Bruce CJ, Nishimura RA: Clinical assessment and management of mitral stenosis. Cardiology Clin 16:375, 1998a

Bruce CJ, Nishimura RA: Newer advances in the diagnosis and treatment of mitral stenosis. Curr Probl Cardiol 23:125, 1998b

Cannan CR et al: Echocardiographic assessment of commissural calcium: A simple predictor of outcome after percutaneous mitral balloon valvotomy. J Am Coll Cardiol 29:175, 1997

Hatle L et al: Noninvasive assessment of pressure drop in mitral stenosis by Doppler ultrasound. Br Heart J 40:131, 1978

Hatle L et al: Noninvasive assessment of atrioventricular pressure half-time by Doppler ultrasound. Circulation 60:1096, 1979

Inoue K et al: Clinical application of transvenous mitral commissurotomy by a new balloon catheter. J Thorac Cardiovasc Surg 87:394, 1984

Nakatani S et al: Value and limitations of Doppler echocardiography in the quantification of stenotic mitral valve area: Comparison of the pressure half-time and the continuity equation methods. Circulation 77:78, 1988

Nishimura RA et al: Accurate measurement of the transmitral gradient in patients with mitral stenosis: A simultaneous catheterization and Doppler echocardiographic study. J Am Coll Cardiol 24:152, 1994

PERCUTANEOUS MITRAL COMMISSUROTOMY

Zoltan G. Turi

The theoretical benefits of splitting rheumatically fused mitral commissures have been understood since the initial successful surgical valvulotomy by Cutler and Levine in 1923. Closed-heart procedures by Bailey, Harken, and Brock in the late 1940s led to the well-accepted closed commissurotomy technique, still commonly performed in developing countries. Effective and low cost, it is a suitable alternative to open surgical commissurotomy, which was adopted as the definitive surgical technique nearly 30 years ago in the industrialized nations. The pioneering work of Rashkind, who introduced balloon septostomy, led Inoue in 1979 to develop a "pillow" shaped balloon for the same purpose. Realizing its potential for percutaneous mitral commissurotomy, he performed the first such procedure in 1982. Made of nylon but constrained by a fiber mesh, the device inflates sequentially: first distally, followed by its proximal portion, leaving a "dog-bone" shaped appearance as it straddles the valve (Fig. 51-1). Subsequent work in the mid-1980s with cylindrical balloon dilatation by Lock and colleagues, and the introduction of double-balloon commissurotomy by Al Zaibag and colleagues led to the most commonly performed techniques currently available. Retrograde dilatation, which avoids the need for transseptal puncture, has been championed by Stefanidis and co-workers, and most recently Cribier and colleagues introduced a nonballoon technique (Cribier et al., 1999). The latter employs a metal valvulotome, similar to the Tubbs dilator used extensively in the surgical treatment of mitral stenosis in the 1950s and 1960s, mounted on a cable, which has the particular virtue of being extensively resterilizable.

Indications

Recent American College of Cardiology/American Heart Association guidelines define percutaneous mitral commissurotomy as indicated in symptomatic patients with moderate or severe mitral stenosis (defined as mitral valve area ≤ 1.5 cm^2), favorable valve morphology, <moderate mitral regurgitation, and no thrombus (Table 51-1). Patients with severe pulmonary hypertension, even if asymptomatic, and severely symptomatic patients with nonpliable calcified valves who are at high risk for surgery are categorized as class IIa. Relative contraindications are severe subvalvular disease and calcification. More controversial contraindications are eccentric fusion of the commissures and presence of clot in the left atrial appendage. The mechanism of action is primarily commissural splitting, although stretching of the valvular orifice contributes and, where present, fracture of calcification may play a role as well.

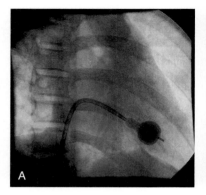 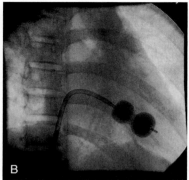 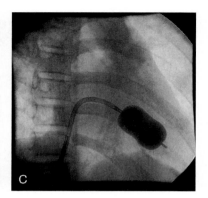

FIGURE 51-1

The Inoue balloon. A. Distal portion inflated in the left ventricle is pulled back against the mitral orifice B. Continued inflation creates the classic "dog bone" appearance which secures balloon position across the mitral orifice. C. Full inflation expands the midportion of the balloon and exerts force along the commissural planes.

Several algorithms for evaluating the suitability of the mitral apparatus to percutaneous dilatation have been developed. The scoring system of Wilkins and colleagues has been most widely adopted (Table 51-2), although it does not take mitral regurgitation, presence of thrombus, or a number of other important anatomic and physiologic factors into account (Wilkins et al., 1988). More recent revisions to this scoring system designed to account for these omissions have not been incorporated widely.

Procedure

Preprocedure transesophageal echocardiography (TEE) should be performed routinely (See Chap. 50); at a minimum those patients with atrial fibrillation, large left atria, severe pulmonary hypertension, or known prior embolic episode should have TEE immediately before the procedure. TEE is significantly more sensitive for clot detection than transtho-

TABLE 51-1

INDICATIONS FOR PERCUTANEOUS BALLOON MITRAL COMMISSUROTOMY

Class	NYHA class	MVA ≤ 1.5 cm²	PHT	Ca²⁺	Surgical risk	Atrial fibrillation
I	II–IV	+		−		
IIa	I	+	+	−		
IIa	III–IV	+		+	+	
IIb	I	+		−		+
IIb	III–IV	+		+	−	
III		−				

NOTE: MVA, mitral valve area; PHT, pulmonary hypertension defined as pulmonary artery systolic pressure >50 mmHg at rest or >60 mmHg with exercise; Ca²⁺, calcified nonpliable mitral valve; surgical risk, patients at high risk of perioperative morbidity or mortality; atrial fibrillation, new onset. SOURCE: Based on recommendations from RO Bonow et al: Circulation 98:1949, 1998.

TABLE 51-2

ECHOCARDIOGRAM-BASED SCORING SYSTEM OF SUITABILITY FOR PERCUTANEOUS COMMISSUROTOMY

Grade	Mobility	Subvalvular disease	Leaflet thickening	Calcification
1	Normal except leaflet tips	Minimal thickening	Near normal	Localized to single area
2	Midleaflet and base normal	Thickening of one-third of chord	Thickening of leaflet margins	Scattered along leaflet margins
3	Mobility mostly at base	Thickening to distal one-third	Thickening throughout leaflet (5–8 mm)	Extending into midleaflets
4	Minimal leaflet movement	Thickening down to papillary muscles	8–10 mm thickening throughout leaflet	Extensive throughout leaflets

SOURCE: Based on an echocardiographic score described by GT Wilkins et al: Br Heart J 60:299, 1988.

racic echo. In the setting of thrombus limited solely to the left atrial appendage, some groups have proceeded to perform balloon commissurotomy without reported complications. Nevertheless, in most cases a minimum of 6 weeks of adequate anticoagulation should be tried first or consideration given to open commissurotomy if the patient needs the procedure urgently.

With the exception of the retrograde arterial technique, performed in a very limited number of centers, procedures are performed via transseptal puncture, almost invariably via the right femoral venous approach (left femoral, internal jugular, subclavian, and transhepatic approaches have also been described). After dilation of the interatrial septum, the dilating device is advanced across the mitral orifice and the commissures are split. Most operators employ a stepwise dilating technique, with progressive increase in balloon size until gradient reduction is optimal or a significant increase in mitral regurgitation is noted. Transesophageal echo performed during the procedure provides sensitive feedback on development of mitral regurgitation, can aid in transseptal puncture, and provides additional catheter position, structural, and hemodynamic information to the operator. If TEE

is not available, transthoracic echo between inflations is a similarly useful, although less sensitive, adjunct.

Results

Regardless of the percutaneous technique used, the results in patients with relatively ideal valve anatomy include approximate doubling of the initial valve area and at least 50% reduction of the initial gradient (Fig. 51-2). Analysis of >8000 patients in 14 studies reveals initial valve areas of 1.0 ± 0.3 cm^2 predilatation increasing to 2.1 ± 0.6 cm^2. In patients with less than ideal valve anatomy, results are less impressive: these subsets include patients with high echo scores and prior commissurotomy (balloon or surgical). Complications are primarily related to two aspects of the procedure: first, transseptal puncture, and second, mitral regurgitation. The procedure involves a steep learning curve, with substantial improvement in results and decrease in complications with increasing experience; tamponade is particularly common early in operators' practices. In experienced

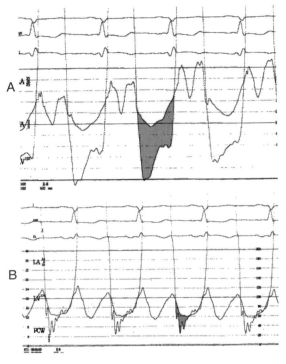

FIGURE 51-2

Gradient between left atrium and left ventricle in a patient with mitral stenosis in sinus rhythm. (*A*) Typical gradient. (*B*) After balloon inflation the gradient has resolved. A small rise in left ventricular end-diastolic pressure is typical because of increased volume loading, even in the absence of secondary mitral regurgitation.

cally apparent cerebral infarcts may occur much more commonly.

Long-term results have been reported through 10 years. In general, predictors of good outcome include ideal valve anatomy (low echo score), good initial results, and absence of atrial fibrillation at initial commissurotomy. Restenosis based on actuarialized analysis and clinical or noninvasive evaluation has been reported to occur in <10% of patients, although preliminary analysis of cardiac catheterization data from the author's database suggests that this may underestimate a true restenosis rate in the 30 to 40% range. Event-free survival at 7 years has been reported to be 65% (survival without mitral valve replacement or repeat commissurotomy), and overall survival as 95%.

Inferior results are seen when balloon valvuloplasty is performed in patients who have undergone prior commissurotomy, although these patients have typically had higher echo scores; when adjusted for underlying valve morphology, the results have generally been similar. Percutaneous commissurotomy has been performed successfully during pregnancy, with minimal x-ray or with purely noninvasive guidance, and represents a suitable nonsurgical alternative to potentially teratogenic medical regimens or valve surgery. Dilatation of bioprosthetic mitral valves has yielded unimpressive hemodynamic results and is associated with considerable theoretical risk of debris embolization. Dilatation of mildly stenotic mitral valves has been reported to result in dramatic improvement in valve area, although there is no evidence to support a hypothesized resultant delay in onset of atrial fibrillation or pulmonary hypertension.

Controversy exists regarding the predictive value of atrial fibrillation on outcome after mitral valvuloplasty. Two recent studies have failed to confirm prior findings that this arrhythmia is an independent predictor of unfavorable outcome; a third study (Langerveld et al., 2001) showed a strong independent correlation with postprocedure adverse events. At a minimum, atrial fibrillation represents a marker for multiple other factors associated with less favorable short- and long-term results.

hands, in-hospital mortality should be in the 1 to 2% range, tamponade in 2%, and severe mitral regurgitation in <5%, depending on technique, operator experience, and patient population. Predictors of mitral regurgitation include eccentric commissural fusion, severe calcification, and severe subvalvular disease; mortality is associated with age, high echo score, and atrial fibrillation. Patients with high echo scores and poor overall valve morphology do show moderate improvement in hemodynamics and symptoms; however, there is concomitantly higher morbidity and mortality. Stroke has been reported in 2 to 4%, although hyperintensive foci demonstrated by magnetic resonance imaging suggest that small, nonclini-

Long-term follow-up is now available on patients who underwent balloon dilatation despite the presence of significant calcification as well as on patients who were deemed inoperable and therefore underwent balloon dilation despite unfavorable anatomy. In general, the procedure is relatively safe in these settings, but the immediate and long-term results are markedly inferior. Thus the procedure appears at best to be palliative in such patients.

Comparison with Surgery

Several randomized trials have compared percutaneous balloon commissurotomy with surgical commissurotomy. In general, these studies have confirmed the equivalence or superiority of balloon to *closed* surgical commissurotomy, including better valve areas, restenosis rates, functional classification, and freedom from reintervention. Less expected was the finding that mitral valve area after ballooning is superior to *open* commissurotomy, including through 3- and 7-year follow-up. This finding has not been explained. It is hypothesized that catheterization laboratory operators have intraprocedural hemodynamic feedback and can increase the extent of dilatation using a stepwise dilating technique until an ideal valve opening is achieved or increasing mitral regurgitation is noted. This continuous information loop is traditionally not available to surgeons performing open or closed commissurotomy.

Other Considerations

Mitral stenosis is endemic in developing countries where medical resources are scarce and basic medical care may not be available. The disease is particularly common among persons from lower socioeconomic strata who may not have access to health care and may not be able to afford basic preventive measures such as penicillin prophylaxis. In this setting, closed surgical commissurotomy may be a suitable alternative given its relatively low cost,

minimal equipment needs, and lack of reliance on disposables. Without reuse of balloon catheters, the cost is approximately one-sixth that of percutaneous balloon valvuloplasty. While balloon catheters are widely reused in developing nations, arguable concerns regarding infection are preventing this practice in an increasing number of countries. Thus, although a double-balloon monorail technique was developed by Bonhoeffer and tested in East Africa in an area with a high prevalence of HIV infection, it is only modestly less expensive than the Inoue device. The recently developed percutaneous metal valvulotome (Fig. 51-3), designed for heat resterilization and reuse 30 to 50 times, may have a significant impact on the availability of treatment for the millions of poor with this disease.

There have been a number of comparison studies between the Inoue and the double-balloon techniques. The techniques have similar hemodynamic improvement and complication profiles. In general, the Inoue technique is simpler and faster at a cost of somewhat lower gradient reduction and a slightly higher incidence of mitral regurgitation (Leon et al., 1999). Some complications, such as perforation of the ventricle and residual atrial septal defect, occur significantly less frequently with the Inoue balloon.

The beneficial effect on the pulmonary circulation of relief of mitral obstruction has been well documented in the surgical literature. The author's data suggest that improvement after valvuloplasty is similar to that seen after surgery but occurs earlier, possibly because the potentially deleterious effects of thoracotomy are avoided. Patients with severe pulmonary hypertension have more severe mitral stenosis but sustained improvement corresponding to the relief of mitral obstruction. Using nitric oxide inhalation, Mahoney and colleagues recently demonstrated significant reduction of pulmonary artery pressure and pulmonary vascular resistance in patients with mitral stenosis (Mahoney et al., 2000). After relief of the obstruction with balloon valvuloplasty, pulmonary artery pressure but not pulmonary resistance decreased. These findings suggest that endothelium-dependent elevation in pulmonary vascular tone is a significant component of pulmonary hypertension in mitral stenosis.

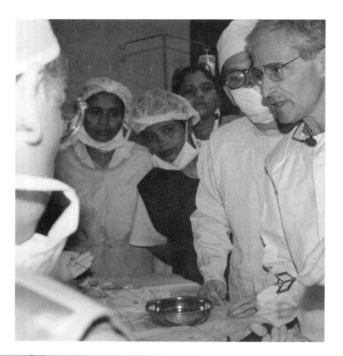

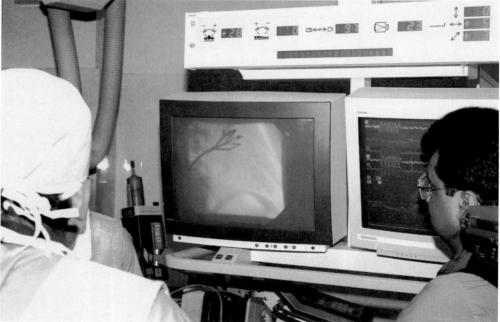

FIGURE 51-3

The percutaneous metal mitral commissurotome. (*A*) Demonstrated by Dr. Cribier. (*B*) Deployed across the mitral valve.

There is limited effort being directed to the development of new technologies for percutaneous treatment of mitral stenosis. Disease prevalence is low in the industrialized nations; thus there is little financial stimulus for medical device developers. New intracardiac ultrasound catheters that can be placed in the right heart during the procedure may allow for pre-procedure interrogation of the left atrium for thrombus and for monitoring transseptal puncture, catheter passage, hemodynamic and anatomic changes, and development of mitral regurgitation between dilatations. The further development of the percutaneous metal valvulotome may have not only cost implications, but if the safety profile and learning curve can be optimized, may represent a suitable alternative to balloon valvuloplasty in the next several years.

REFERENCES

Ben Farhat M et al: Percutaneous balloon versus surgical closed and open mitral commissurotomy. Seven year follow-up of a randomized trial. Circulation 97:245, 1998

Bonow RO et al: Guidelines for the management of patients with valvular heart disease. A report of the American College of Cardiology/American Heart Association Task Force on Practice Guidelines. Circulation 98:1949, 1998

Cribier A et al: Percutaneous mechanical mitral commissurotomy with a newly designed metallic valvulotome. Circulation 99:793, 1999

Glazier JJ et al: Percutaneous balloon mitral valvuloplasty. Prog Cardiovasc Dis 40:5, 1997

Iung B et al: Late results of percutaneous mitral commissurotomy for calcific mitral stenosis. Am J Cardiol 85:1308, 2000

Kang DH et al: Long-term clinical and echocardiographic outcome of percutaneous mitral valvuloplasty: Randomized comparison of Inoue and double-balloon techniques. J Am Coll Cardiol 35:169, 2000

Langerveld J et al: The predictive value of chronic atrial fibrillation for the short- and long-term outcome after percutaneous mitral balloon valvotomy. J Heart Valve Dis 10:530, 2001

Leon MN et al: Comparison of immediate and long-term results of mitral balloon valvotomy with the double-balloon versus Inoue techniques. Am J Cardiol 83:1356, 1999

Mahoney PD et al: Hemodynamic effects of inhaled nitric oxide in women with mitral stenosis and pulmonary hypertension. Am J Cardiol 87:188, 2000

Orrange SE et al: Actuarial outcome after catheter balloon commissurotomy in patients with mitral stenosis. Circulation 95:382, 1997

Reyes VP et al: Percutaneous balloon valvuloplasty compared with open surgical commissurotomy for mitral stenosis. N Engl J Med 331:961, 1994

Sutaria N et al: Long term outcome of percutaneous mitral balloon valvotomy in patients aged 70 and over. Heart 83:433, 2000

Tarka EA et al: Hemodynamic effects and long-term outcome of percutaneous balloon valvuloplasty in patients with mitral stenosis and atrial fibrillation. Clin Cardiol 23:673, 2000

Turi ZG et al: Percutaneous balloon versus surgical closed commissurotomy for mitral stenosis: A prospective, randomized trial. Circulation 83:1179, 1991

Wilkins GT et al: Percutaneous balloon dilatation of the mitral valve: An analysis of echocardiographic variables related to outcome and the mechanism of dilatation. Br Heart J 60:299, 1988

52

PREDICTORS OF OUTCOME IN SEVERE, ASYMPTOMATIC AORTIC STENOSIS

Raphael Rosenhek, Helmut Baumgartner

Symptomatic patients with severe aortic stenosis (AS) have a very poor outcome. Average survival after the onset of symptoms has been reported to be less than 2 to 3 years (Ross and Braunwald, 1968). Valve replacement not only results in dramatic symptomatic improvement but also in enhanced long-term survival (Horstkotte and Loogen, 1980). This holds true even for patients with impaired left ventricular (LV) function, as long as functional impairment is indeed caused by AS (Connolly et al., 1997). Thus, there is general agreement that, in the absence of serious comorbid conditions, surgery is strongly recommended for patients with severe AS who develop symptoms of congestive heart failure (CHF), angina, or syncope. In contrast, the management of asymptomatic patients with severe AS remains a matter of controversy (Bonow et al., 1998). Many are reluctant to send asymptomatic patients for surgery, whereas others are concerned about following these patients conservatively.

Should asymptomatic patients with severe aortic stenosis undergo early elective surgery?

Pros

Risk of Sudden Cardiac Death

When following asymptomatic patients with AS conservatively, sudden death is probably the major concern. Prospective data in this respect are still limited. In three studies where significant numbers of patients with nonsevere stenosis were included, no sudden death was reported. Otto and colleagues followed 123 patients with an average peak aortic jet velocity of 3.6 ± 0.6 m/s for 30 months (Otto et al., 1997). The two other series with 51 and 37 patients (Kelly et al., 1988, and Faggiano et al., 1992, respectively) had follow-up periods of 1.5 and 2.0 years, respectively.

Only two studies reported the outcome of larger cohorts of patients with exclusively severe stenosis as defined by a peak aortic jet velocity ≥4.0 m/s. Pellikka and colleagues (1990) observed two sudden deaths among 113 patients during a mean follow-up of 20 months. Both patients, however, had developed symptoms at least 3 months before death. Rosenhek and co-workers reported one sudden death that was not preceded by any symptoms among 104 patients followed for 27 months on average (Rosenhek et al., 2000). Thus, sudden death may indeed occur even in the absence of preceding symptoms in patients with AS, but this appears to be a very uncommon event, with a rate of probably less than 1% per year. Finally, it has to be considered that sudden death has even been reported after successful valve replacement, and thus this risk cannot be entirely eliminated by surgical treatment (Engelstein and Zipes, 1998).

Risk of Developing Irreversible Myocardial Damage

In contrast to valvular regurgitation, patients with asymptomatic severe AS who have already developed impaired systolic LV function are very frequently encountered. It has been speculated that myocardial fibrosis and severe LV hypertrophy that may not be reversible after delayed surgery could preclude an optimal postoperative outcome. However, there are currently no data to support this hypothesis. Considering the excellent outcome after valve replacement, it is unlikely that the risk of developing irreversible myocardial damage may play a major role.

Risk of Death between Onset of Symptoms and Surgical Treatment

One important concern is the fact that patients do not always promptly report their symptoms but are already at a high risk of abrupt deterioration and sudden death. In addition, it has to be considered that, at least in some countries, patients may wait several months for surgery. In a Scandinavian study, for example, 7 of 99 patients with severe AS who were scheduled for surgery died during an average waiting period of 6 months (Lund et al., 1996).

Rapid Development of Symptoms

Some studies have reported a very rapid development of symptoms, with up to 80% of the patients requiring valve replacement within 2 years (Otto

et al., 1997). Such observations have also questioned whether it is worthwhile to delay surgery in asymptomatic patients. However, other investigators have reported better outcome; individual outcome varies widely. Survival free of death or valve replacement required for the development of symptoms was 56 ± 5% at 2 years in the series reported by Rosenhek and colleagues (2000).

Increased Operative Risk in Severely Symptomatic Patients

Patients with severe symptoms (NYHA classes III and IV) have been found to have a significantly higher operative mortality than those with no or only mild symptoms (NYHA classes I and II). Urgent or emergent valve replacement carries a significantly higher risk than elective surgery (STS National Database, 2000).

Cons
Operative Risk

Although the operative risk has dramatically decreased over the past few decades, it must be considered to be in the range of at least 2 to 3% (Lindblom et al., 1990). In an asymptomatic patient, this risk has to be outweighed by a proven benefit.

Prosthetic Valve-Related Long-Term Morbidity and Mortality

After valve replacement with a mechanical or bioprosthetic valve, significant valve-related complications such as thromboembolism, bleeding, endocarditis, valve thrombosis, paravalvular regurgitation, and valve failure occur at the rate of 2 to 3% per year. Death directly related to the prosthesis has been reported at a rate of approximately 1% per year (Bonow et al., 1998).

Individual Variation of Outcome

The individual course of the disease is highly variable, and some patients have been followed for many years without developing symptoms. Considering that valve replacement is not a cure for this disease, general recommendation of early surgery is inappropriate.

To summarize, the decision for valve replacement in asymptomatic patients with AS remains difficult. Waiting too long can put the patient at an increased risk of sudden death and higher operative mortality, whereas operating on a patient too early puts him or her at an unnecessary operative risk and risk of prosthetic valve–related complications. Thus, predictors of outcome that can help to select patients who are likely to benefit from early elective surgery would be highly desirable.

Predictors of Outcome in Asymptomatic, Severe Aortic Stenosis

Clinical Predictors

Several clinical variables have been evaluated with respect to their value as predictors of outcome. However, age, gender, hypertension, hypercholesterolemia, diabetes mellitus, LV hypertrophy, ventricular ectopic activity, coronary artery disease, cigarette smoking, use of digoxin, use of a diuretic drug, and the cause of AS could not be found to be independent predictors and may not be helpful in the selection of asymptomatic patients for surgery (Otto et al., 1997; Pellikka et al., 1990; Rosenhek et al., 2000).

Echocardiographic Predictors

Among echocardiographic parameters, peak aortic jet velocity and ejection fraction (Pellikka et al., 1990), as well as the rate of hemodynamic progression (Otto et al., 1997), were identified as independent predictors of outcome. However, these findings do not specify any recommendations on how to select high-risk patients who may benefit from early elective surgery.

In a more recent study (Rosenhek et al., 2000), aortic valve calcification proved to be a powerful independent predictor of outcome. Event-free survival at 4 years was $75 \pm 9\%$ in patients with no or only mild calcification vs. $20 \pm 5\%$ in those with moderately or severely calcified valves. The worse outcome of patients with more severe calcification appeared to parallel a more rapid hemodynamic progression. However, even in the presence of calcification, the rate of hemodynamic progression varies widely. In addition to the degree of calcification, the hemodynamic progression documented by serial echocardiographic examination appeared to yield important prognostic information. The combination of a calcified valve with a rapid increase in velocity of 0.3 m/s between visits less than 1 year apart identified a high-risk group of patients. Approximately 80% of them required surgery or died within 2 years.

Exercise Test

Although Otto and colleagues reported in their group of asymptomatic patients with AS that those with an end-point had a smaller exercise increase in valve area, blood pressure, and cardiac output, none of these variables were an independent predictor of outcome by multivariate analysis (Otto et al., 1997). Nevertheless, exercise testing has been shown to be helpful for the evaluation of reportedly asymptomatic patients. Das and colleagues recently reported that 36% of 58 consecutive patients with AS who had denied symptoms experienced significant symptoms during exercise testing (Das et al., 2001). In addition, despite the lack of solid evidence, most physicians believe that an abnormal hemodynamic response to exercise (e.g., hypotension) in a patient with severe AS is sufficient reason to consider surgery (Bonow et al., 1998). It has to be emphasized that exercise testing is only appropriate in asymptomatic patients and is contraindicated in symptomatic patients.

Current Practice Guidelines for the Management of Asymptomatic Patients with Severe Aortic Stenosis and Clinical Impact of Recently Identified Predictors of Outcome

Based on the data showing that it is relatively safe to delay surgery until symptoms develop, current AHA/ACC practice guidelines recommend aortic valve replacement only in asymptomatic patients with severe AS who undergo cardiac surgery for any other reason such as coronary artery bypass surgery, surgery of the aorta, or other heart valves (class I) (Bonow et al., 1998). Although controversial, weight of evidence/opinion is considered in favor of surgery (class IIa) in those asymptomatic patients with severe AS who present with impaired systolic LV function and in patients with an abnormal response to exercise (e.g., hypotension). Ventricular tachycardia, marked or excessive LV hypertrophy (15 mm), and a valve area <0.6 cm^2 are less well established as indications for surgery and, thus, considered a class IIb indication.

More recent findings suggest expansion of the recommendations for managing patients with asymptomatic severe AS by using echocardiography for risk stratification in the following way:

- Patients with no or only mild calcification of a stenosed aortic valve represent a group with low likelihood of developing symptoms and requiring surgery in the near future. They may remain asymptomatic for many years. Annual follow-up visits and the advice to report promptly the development of any exertional chest discomfort, dyspnea, or lightheadedness during exercise appear to be appropriate for these patients.
- Patients with moderately or severely calcified valves represent a group of patients with poor outcome. Rapid progression must be expected, and close follow-up is required.
- Patients with moderately or severely calcified valves in whom serial echocardiographic testing reveals rapid progression with a steep increase in jet velocity ($\geq$0.3 m/s per year) identifies a high-risk group with an 80% rate of symptom development in 2 years. Considering the fact that

patients do not always promptly report the development of symptoms, the risk of death on the waiting list for surgery, and the higher operative risk in severely symptomatic patients, it may be desirable to consider elective valve replacement instead of waiting for symptoms in this high-risk subgroup.

REFERENCES

Bonow RO et al: ACC/AHA guidelines for the management of patients with valvular heart disease. A report of the American College of Cardiology/American Heart Association. Task Force on Practice Guidelines (Committee on Management of Patients with Valvular Heart Disease). J Am Coll Cardiol 32:1486, 1998

Connolly HM et al: Aortic valve replacement for aortic stenosis with severe left ventricular dysfunction. Prognostic indicators. Circulation 95:2395, 1997

Das P et al: The value of treadmill exercise testing in apparently asymptomatic aortic stenosis. J Am Coll Cardiol 37 (Suppl A):489A, 2001

Engelstein ED, Zipes DP: Sudden cardiac death, in *The Heart, Arteries, and Veins,* RW Alexander, RC Schlant, V Fuster (eds). New York, McGraw-Hill, 1998, pp 1081–1112

Faggiano P et al: Rate of progression of valvular aortic stenosis in adults. Am J Cardiol 70:229, 1992

Horstkotte D, Loogen F: The natural history of aortic valve stenosis. Eur Heart J 9 (Suppl E):57, 1988

Kelly TA et al: Comparison of outcome of asymptomatic to symptomatic patients older than 20 years of age with valvular aortic stenosis. Am J Cardiol 61:123, 1988

Lindblom D et al: Long-term relative survival rates after heart valve replacement. J Am Coll Cardiol 15:566, 1990

Lund O et al: Mortality and worsening of prognostic profile during waiting time for valve replacement in aortic stenosis. Thorac Cardiovasc Surg 44:289, 1996

Otto CM et al: Prospective study of asymptomatic valvular aortic stenosis. Clinical, echocardiographic, and exercise predictors of outcome. Circulation 95:2262, 1997

Pellikka PA et al: The natural history of adults with asymptomatic, hemodynamically significant aortic stenosis. J Am Coll Cardiol 15:1012, 1990

Rosenhek R et al: Predictors of outcome in severe, asymptomatic aortic stenosis. N Engl J Med 343:611, 2000

Ross J Jr, Braunwald E: Aortic stenosis. Circulation 38 (Suppl 1):61, 1968

STS National Database: STS U.S. cardiac surgery database: 1997 Aortic valve replacement patients: Preoperative risk variables. Chicago, Society of Thoracic Surgeons, 2000 (See http://www.ctsnet.org/doc/3031)

THE STENTLESS AORTIC PROSTHESIS FOR AORTIC VALVE REPLACEMENT

Donald B. Doty & John R. Doty

The porcine aortic valve was originally proposed for human aortic valve replacement by Binet and associates and was implanted directly into the aortic root (Binet et al., 1965). O'Brien subsequently developed a heterograft valve bank for continued use of both bovine and porcine nonstented valves (O'Brien, 1967). Unsatisfactory results, most likely due to less than optimal tissue preservation techniques, led to the abandonment of direct xenograft valve implantation in favor of such valves mounted on a stent frame. The stented bioprostheses are manufactured to provide a standard device that is easily implanted and provides reproducible results in the aortic position. With long-term follow-up, however, stented xenograft failure due to calcification and cusp rupture is apparent, particularly in younger patients. Stent-mounted porcine valves have less than ideal hemodynamic performance when the aortic root is small.

David and associates revived the concept of direct insertion of a nonstented porcine xenograft into the aortic root (David et al., 1990). This valve was manufactured on a limited trial basis by Hancock Laboratory and subsequently for full-scale clinical trial by St. Jude Medical as the *Toronto SPV* (stentless porcine valve) (Fig. 53-1). This device is derived from the porcine aortic root. The porcine tissue is fixed in glutaraldehyde with the aortic valve in the closed position by applying low pressure to the fixative solution. The aorta is removed from all three sinuses of Valsalva, and the exterior is covered completely with fine polyester fabric. The Medtronic *Freestyle* Bioprosthesis (Fig. 53-2) was designed, tested, and approved for implantation in human trials beginning in 1992. This valve is a stentless valve derived from a porcine aortic root preserved in glutaraldehyde and has a ring of polyester at the inflow and covering the septal myocardium, which provides strength and ease of implantation. The hemodynamic properties of the device have been tested in vitro (Yoganathan et al., 1994) and in vivo.

Operative Technique

Three basic techniques are used for implantation of a stentless porcine bioprosthesis: (1) subcoronary valve replacement, (2) root inclusion, and (3) root replacement.

ST. JUDE TORONTO SPV

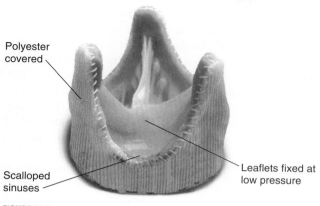

FIGURE 53-1

St. Jude Toronto SPV stentless aortic valve bioprosthesis. Manufacturer's photograph, digitally enhanced.

FREESTYLE BIOPROSTHESIS

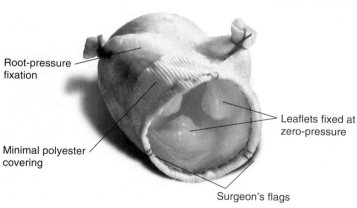

FIGURE 53-2

Medtronic Freestyle aortic root bioprosthesis. Manufacturer's photograph, digitally enhanced.

Subcoronary Valve Replacement

In this technique the bioprosthesis is used only as a valve supported by the sinus aorta of the patient (David et al., 1998; Doty et al., 1998; Krause, 1997; Pepper, 1998; Sintek et al., 1996; Westaby et al., 1995). A transverse aortotomy is made 5 to 10 mm above the sinus rim. Alternatively, the ascending aorta is transected for exposure of the aortic root and coronary arteries. The diseased aortic valve is excised, and calcium depositions are thoroughly debrided from the aortic root.

The Toronto SPV device is pretrimmed and ready for immediate implantation. The Freestyle valve must be tailored by removing the aortic sinus from the right and left coronary sinuses of the bioprosthesis. The bioprosthesis is implanted in its anatomic position without rotation unless the right coronary artery is positioned so low that the prosthesis will not fit under it.

Root Inclusion

The root inclusion technique refers to placement of the Freestyle bioprosthesis as a tube inside the native aorta in an attempt to reduce the distortion of the graft (Huysmans, 1997). The only modification to the graft is openings made in the sinus aorta to accommodate anastomosis of the patient's coronary arteries to the graft. This technique is useful for patients with a dilated aortic root and an ascending aorta that is not aneurysmal.

Root Replacement

In root replacement the entire native aortic root and valve are excised and replaced with the Freestyle bioprosthesis (Kon et al., 1995). Full-root replacement technique is employed for treatment of aortic root pathology that precludes the use of other techniques that require relatively normal patient aorta to support the graft. It is also employed because there is the least chance for aortic valve distortion of any of the implant techniques. Root replacement technique is possible only with the Freestyle device.

Clinical Results

The Toronto SPV bioprosthesis and the Medtronic Freestyle aortic root bioprosthesis have been implanted in large numbers of patients, mostly over the age of 61 years. Follow-up extends to 10 years for the Toronto SPV valve (David et al., 1998) and over 7 years in some patients with the Freeestyle

valve (Doty et al., 1999, 2001). Investigators have compared these two stentless bioprostheses in single institution trials and have found very little difference in hemodynamic or clinical results. One team found no differences in clinical outcome or hemodynamic performances of these two valves, and both devices offer excellent results with normalization of left ventricular function (Del Rizzo and Abdoh, 1998). Another group reported excellent hemodynamic performances, which were equivalent, of both valves, but there was slightly more aortic valve regurgitation with the Toronto SPV valve (Legare et al., 1998). Bach and associates recently presented data suggesting increased aortic valve regurgitation 8 years postoperatively using the Toronto SPV valve, which may be attributed to dilation of the unsupported sinotubular junction (Fig. 53-3) (Bach et al., 2001). At midterm follow-up, however, there seems to be little difference in clinical results for the two valves so that inferences may therefore be assumed to be the same for both valves at this point in time. Hence, for the remainder of this chapter, only the results of the Freestyle bioprosthesis in 1100 patients at 5 years (Doty et al., 1999) or at 7 years after operation in 700 patients (Doty et al., 2001) will be considered.

There was an acceptable risk of operation (5.7% overall), considering that most of the patients were elderly. The aortic valve lesion for which aortic valve replacement was required was pure stenosis in 43% or mixed stenosis and regurgitation in 45% (total stenotic lesions, 88%). There was a remarkable improvement in functional capacity after operation, with 95% of patients in functional class I or II where there had been 73% in class III or IV prior to operation.

The most popular method of implantation was the subcoronary valve replacement. While this method requires knowledge of the spatial relationships of the aortic root, it does not alter the natural tissues of the aortic root substantially. In that sense, it is a somewhat less difficult procedure than aortic root replacement techniques, but in another sense, it may be more difficult to perform reproducibly. There is remarkably high probability (95 to 100%) that the bioprosthetic valve will be competent or have no more than mild regurgitation regardless of the technique chosen for implantation. Risk of hemorrhage may be less

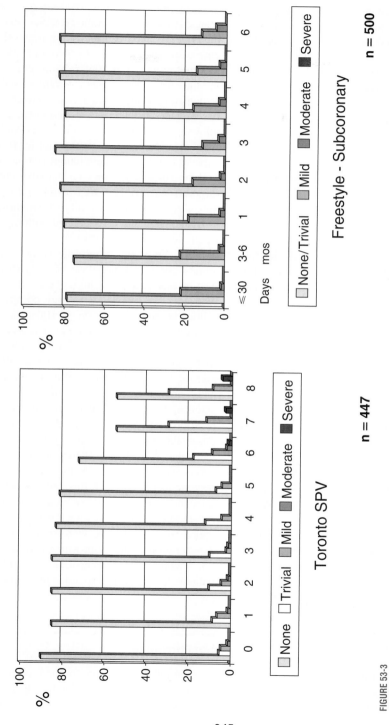

FIGURE 53-3

Aortic valve regurgitation estimated by echocardiography up to 8 years for the Toronto SPV and up to 6 years for the Freestyle bioprostheses. (Adapted from DS Bach et al., and DB Doty et al.)

and more easily controlled with subcoronary valve replacement or root inclusion technique than with full-root replacement technique because the bioprosthesis is completely enclosed within the natural aorta so that the only source of major bleeding is the readily accessible aortotomy. Risk of operation was lowest using subcoronary valve implant techniques (5.0% vs. 9.3% full root), even though the patients were older with two-thirds being over the age of 70 years. The subcoronary technique also required about 20 min less myocardial ischemia time than aortic root techniques. Less xenograft aorta is inserted when the subcoronary valve replacement is used and may account for a somewhat lower frequency of thromboembolism. Xenograft aorta will ultimately calcify even though α-aminooleic acid is added to the fixative, because this substance retards calcification in the aorta less well than in the leaflet tissue. This may also be in favor of using a subcoronary valve implantation technique so that more of the patient's own flexible aorta is preserved. On the other hand, the most perfect early and late implants in terms of valve competence were achieved by full-root replacement technique. No valvular regurgitation was observed in 96% of patients when full-root implant technique was employed.

Aortic root pathology encountered at operation surely affects the choice of operation because the data show that there were more patients with primary aortic valve regurgitation and many more patients requiring ascending aorta repair in the full-root replacement group compared to the other techniques in which the bioprosthesis is enclosed within the aortic root. Aortic root replacement operations, however, took more time to perform, as reflected in about 20 min longer ischemic time. This was especially important when aortic valve replacement was accompanied by aortocoronary bypass. Taken in sum, a longer procedure, more complex aortic root pathology, and more exposed suture lines in complete aortic root replacement procedures may account for the higher early mortality rate after operation than when the other methods were employed. At 7 years, however, actuarial analysis indicated little difference in survival when subcoronary implant technique is compared to full-root technique (62.0 vs. 67.7% freedom from death).

The remarkable functional improvement is likely related to excellent hemodynamic performance of the stentless bioprosthesis. Low transvalvular gradients were sustained to the 4-year mark. Previously reported reduction in transvalvular gradient observed in the first year after operation stabilized and remained constant up to 4 years. Effective valve area has been consistently good even in small-size valves, allowing implantation of 19- or 21-mm prostheses without enlargement of the aortic root with the expectation that excellent hemodynamic performance will be sustained. Low transvalvular gradients and large effective orifice areas even in 19- and 21-mm valves reduces the possibility of patient-to-prosthesis size mismatch and is associated with rapid resolution of left ventricular hypertrophy.

The Freestyle bioprosthesis not only demonstrates good forward flow hemodynamics but can also be inserted with a high degree of diastolic competence. The bioprosthesis was competent or only mildly incompetent in 96 to 100% of the patients, with the highest levels of competence achieved when the device was implanted by the full-root replacement technique. Moderate valve insufficiency was present in only 8% of patients at the 6-year mark, and there were no patients with severe valve incompetence. There were eight valves explanted for technical problems resulting in valvular incompetence or unsatisfactory hemodynamic performance. This low incidence of valve explantation indicates that surgeons can master the techniques of insertion and become confident that this bioprosthesis will have good hemodynamic performance and will not leak. An additional six valves were explanted for infective endocarditis, and none were removed for structural deterioration of the bioprosthesis. Total valve explant rate was 0.5% per patient-year, leaving 92 to 99% of patients free of valve explant at the 7-year mark.

Complications

The thromboembolic rate for the Freestyle bioprosthesis was low, in spite of the fact that patients were not given warfarin unless there was persistent atrial fibrillation or flutter. Early thromboembolism was noted in only 1.9% of patients having subcoronary valve implantation when very rigid criteria were applied. Late thromboembolism occurred at a rate of 1.6 events per patient-year, with permanent neurologic events at an even lower rate of 0.6 per patient-year. Actuarial analysis of thromboembolism rate showed 78 to 87% of patients free of this complication at 7 years after valve implantation.

Endocarditis was an infrequent event. The freedom from endocarditis was >94.5% at 7 years. This indicates that the Freestyle bioprosthesis is quite resistant to infection, and infection on this bioprosthesis can be successfully treated. Endocarditis, however, accounted for nearly one-half of the valves that were explanted (6 of 14).

Structural deterioration during the 5-year follow-up has been rare, with no valves explanted for this cause. These data imply that if the Freestyle bioprosthesis can be implanted with technical accuracy and without bacterial contamination, it can be expected to function very well for at least 7 years. It is too early to know if the long-term durability of the Freestyle bioprosthesis will compare favorably with other bioprostheses. The hope and expectation that zero-net pressure fixation of the porcine aortic valve leaflets and the addition of α-aminooleic acid to the tissues, technology unique to this bioprosthesis, will favorably affect durability requires additional follow-up, and at the 7-year mark the results are very encouraging.

REFERENCES

Bach DS et al: Eight year hemodynamic follow-up after aortic valve replacement with the Toronto SPV stentless aortic valve. Abstract presented at Stentless Bioprostheses, fourth International Symposium, San Diego CA. May 2001

Binet JP et al: Heterologous aortic valve transplantation. Lancet 2:1275, 1965

David TE et al: Aortic valve replacement with stentless porcine aortic bioprosthesis. J Thorac Cardiovasc Surg 99:113, 1990

David TE et al: Aortic valve replacement with stentless porcine aortic valves: A ten-year study. J Heart Valve Dis 7:250, 1998

Del Rizzo DF, Abdoh A: Clinical and hemodynamic comparison of the Medtronic Freestyle and Toronto SPV stentless valves. J Card Surg 13:398, 1998

Doty JR et al: Aortic valve replacement with Medtronic Freestyle bioprosthesis: Operative technique and results. J Card Surg 13:208, 1998

Doty DB et al: Aortic valve replacement with Medtronic Freestyle bioprosthesis: 5-year results. Semin Thorac Cardiovasc Surg 2(Suppl 1):35, 1999

Doty DB et al: Aortic valve replacement with Medtronic Freestyle bioprosthesis: Seven year results. Medtronic Freestyle Valve Symposium, San Diego CA. June 2001

Huysmans H: Implanting the Freestyle bioprosthesis: Root-inclusion technique. *The Freestyle Aortic Root Bioprosthesis Implant Technique Monograph.* Medtronic, Minneapolis, Minn. 1997

Kon ND et al: Comparison of implantation techniques using Freestyle stentless porcine aortic valve. Ann Thorac Surg 59:857, 1995

Krause AH Jr: Technique for complete subcoronary implantation of the Medtronic Freestyle porcine bioprosthesis. Ann Thorac Surg 64:1495, 1997

Legare JF et al: St. Jude SPV versus Medtronic Freestyle: A single institution comparison of two stentless aortic valves. J Card Surg 13:392, 1998

O'Brien MF: Heterograft aortic valves for human use. J Thorac Cardiovasc Surg 53:392, 1967

Pepper JR: The stentless porcine valve. J Card Surg 13:352, 1998

Sintek CF et al: Small aortic root in the elderly: Use of stentless bioprosthesis. J Heart Valve Dis 5(Suppl III):S308, 1996

Westaby S et al: Aortic valve replacement with the Freestyle stentless xenograft. Ann Thorac Surg 60:S422, 1995

Yoganathan AP et al: Hydrodynamic performance of the Medtronic Freestyle aortic root bioprosthesis. J Heart Valve Dis 3:571, 1994

BALLOON VALVULOPLASTY FOR AORTIC STENOSIS

Andrew D. Michaels & Thomas A. Ports

Surgical mechanical dilatation of the stenotic adult aortic valve has been attempted since the 1950s. Various valvotomy approaches have failed to provide durable benefit for calcific aortic stenosis, and aortic valve replacement clearly has emerged as treatment of choice in adults. Because of the high morbidity associated with percutaneous aortic valvuloplasty, which is followed by restenosis in most patients within 6 to 12 months, this therapy is considered an alternative only for those patients who cannot undergo aortic valve replacement. Open surgical valvotomy does remain an option for infants and children with critical congenital aortic stenosis when it is desirable to postpone definitive valve replacement.

Noncalcific Congenital Aortic Stenosis

The fibrotic nature of noncalcific congenital stenotic aortic valves makes them well suited for percutaneous balloon valvuloplasty. Lababidi first performed percutaneous balloon aortic valvuloplasty in children and young adolescents, resulting in a significant decrease in the peak aortic valve gradient (Lababidi, 1984). Excellent short-term and satisfactory long-term clini-

cal results have been reported using balloon valvuloplasty in children and adolescents with congenital aortic stenosis. The procedure has an 80 to 90% success rate, with a mortality rate of 0.7%. Survival at 8 years is 95%. One-quarter of patients require repeat intervention after 4 years, and one-half of patients develop restenosis by 8 years (Moore et al., 1996).

For young adults with severe congenital aortic stenosis without significant calcification of the aortic valve, balloon valvuloplasty may offer some benefit. In a cohort of young adults (age range, 17 to 40; mean, 23 years) with noncalcified congenital aortic stenosis, balloon aortic valvuloplasty significantly reduced the aortic valve gradient and increased the aortic valve area (Rosenfeld et al., 1994). No deaths or embolic cerebrovascular events were reported. After a mean follow-up of 38 months, 50% of patients required no further intervention. The absence of significant valvular calcification is an important predictor of improved short- and long-term results. While aortic valve replacement remains the treatment of choice for young adults with aortic stenosis, an attempt at balloon valvuloplasty may be an alternative if there is no significant valvular calcification.

Calcific Aortic Stenosis

The adult cardiologist typically encounters the elderly patient with acquired calcific aortic stenosis. Since its introduction seventeen years ago, percutaneous balloon aortic valvuloplasty has been shown to be moderately effective in increasing the aortic valve orifice and decreasing the aortic valve gradient in elderly patients with severe aortic stenosis (Cribier et al., 1986). However, the postprocedural valve area typically does not exceed 1.0 cm^2. This procedure is currently restricted to nonsurgical candidates primarily because of the high procedural morbidity and discouraging midterm restenosis rate.

Patient Selection and Practice Guidelines

Symptomatic patients with calcific aortic stenosis should be considered for aortic valve replacement as the treatment of choice. However, there are particular patient groups in which balloon valvuloplasty may have an important palliative role. The most recent American College of Cardiology/American Heart Association (ACC/AHA) guidelines for management of patients with valvular heart disease clearly state that there are no class I indications (defined when there is evidence and/or general agreement that the procedure is useful and effective) for percutaneous aortic valvuloplasty in adults (Bonow et al., 1998). Performing balloon aortic valvuloplasty in hemodynamically unstable patients with refractory cardiogenic shock as a "bridge" to aortic valve replacement is a class IIA recommendation (defined when there is a weight of evidence/opinion in favor of usefulness/efficacy). The indication for palliative valvuloplasty in patients with serious comorbid condition is a class IIB indication (defined when usefulness/efficacy is less well-established by evidence/opinion). Patients who are poor surgical candidates due to comorbid conditions (i.e., malignancy, end-stage liver disease, severe obstructive lung disease), advanced age, or terminal illness may be considered for aortic valvuloplasty.

The technique is also listed as a class IIB indication for patients with critical aortic stenosis who require emergent noncardiac surgery, if it is felt that conservative medical therapy presents excessive perioperative risk.

Contraindications for aortic valvuloplasty include moderate or greater aortic insufficiency, left ventricular thrombus, aortic valve endocarditis, severe peripheral vascular disease, and a contraindication to periprocedural anticoagulation (typically with heparin). The risk of the procedure is increased in patients with severe left ventricular systolic dysfunction or peripheral vascular disease.

Mechanisms of Improved Aortic Valve Area

Intraoperative and postmortem aortic valve dilatations have demonstrated the mechanisms of how balloon aortic valvuloplasty improves the aortic valve orifice. Balloon dilatation increases leaflet mobility, leading to an enlargement of the aortic valve orifice. The mechanism of dilatation predominantly involves fracturing of the calcific aortic valve deposits. In some patients, stretching of the annulus and separation of the calcified or fused commissures may also occur.

Technique

The retrograde transfemoral approach for balloon aortic valvuloplasty is most commonly used. Aortic valvuloplasty has also been performed by an antegrade transatrial septal approach using conventional balloon catheters. Recently, an initial experience utilizing the antegrade transseptal approach with the Inoue mitral valvuloplasty balloon catheter has been reported (Eisenhauer et al., 2000). While this approach avoids a larger femoral arteriotomy, it is a longer, more technically demanding procedure with the added risks of transseptal puncture. A brachial arterial approach is not recommended because of the large arteriotomy required. Placement of a temporary

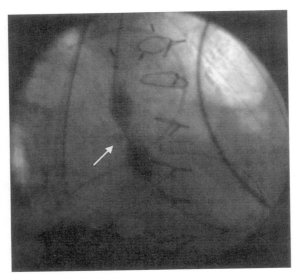

A

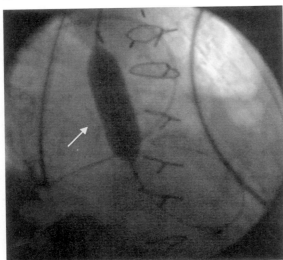

B

FIGURE 54-1

(A) An 82-year-old woman with metastatic vulvar carcinoma is referred for aortic valvuloplasty prior to pelvic and abdominal palliative tumor resection. The patient has developed congestive heart failure refractory to medical therapy. This anteroposterior projection shows passage of the deflated aortic valvuloplasty balloon across a calcified stenotic aortic valve. One inflation with a 20-mm diameter by 5.5-cm length balloon (shown here) resulted in a significant improvement in her aortic valve gradient. Balloon markers are positioned so the balloon is centered across the calcified aortic valve (arrows). A pulmonary artery catheter is seen in the right pulmonary artery. (B) Using the retrograde single-balloon technique, the balloon is fully inflated across the stenotic aortic valve (arrow).

transvenous pacemaker may be considered in patients with right or left bundle branch block. Intraaortic balloon pump insertion may also be considered in patients with severely depressed left ventricular systolic function and in those with decompensated congestive heart failure.

The aortic valve gradient is typically measured from simultaneous pressure recordings from the left ventricle and ascending aorta. The aortic valve area is calculated using the Gorlin formula. The proximal and distal markers of the valvuloplasty balloon are used to position the midballoon at the level of the calcified aortic valve (Fig. 54-1A). An exchange-length guidewire is kept in the left ventricle during balloon positioning and inflation. Once a good position is achieved, the balloon is rapidly filled to its maximum diameter (Fig. 54-1B) with diluted contrast media. The balloon is rapidly deflated and withdrawn into the descending aorta over the exchange-length guidewire. Repeat measurements of the aortic valve gradient (Fig. 54-2) and cardiac output are performed.

The usual hemodynamic goal is to increase the aortic valve area by >100% and to achieve an aortic valve area of at least 1.0 cm². If this goal has not been achieved and no procedural complications have occurred, the procedure may be repeated using a larger balloon catheter. If an inadequate result still is not achieved, a dual-balloon technique may then be attempted. Following the procedure, the arterial sheaths are removed and hemostasis achieved with Perclose arteriotomy sutures (Michaels and Ports, 2001) or external compression. The use of percutaneous suture closure devices for these 10 French arteriotomies has reduced the vascular complications associated with balloon aortic valvuloplasty.

Procedural Results and Complications

In the Mansfield Scientific Aortic Valvuloplasty Registry, data was collected from 27 U.S. and European centers on 492 patients with calcific aortic stenosis undergoing balloon aortic valvuloplasty between 1986 and 1987 (McKay, 1991). Balloon aortic valvuloplasty resulted in a decrease in the mean aortic valve pressure gradient from 60 ± 23 to 30 ± 13 mmHg, and an increase in aortic valve area from 0.50 ± 0.18 to 0.82 ± 0.30 cm². There was also an accompanying increase in cardiac output from 3.86 ± 1.26 to 4.05 ± 1.31 L/min.

In this registry, complications occurred in 20.5% of patients. The procedural death rate was 4.9%. Death occurred within 7 days in an additional 2.6% of patients, emboli in 2.2%, ventricular perforation in 1.8%, massive aortic insufficiency in 1%, and emergency aortic valve replacement in 1.2%. The most common complication was local vascular injury, requiring surgical repair in 5.7% of patients.

The National Heart, Lung, and Blood Institute (NHLBI) Balloon Valvuloplasty Registry enrolled 674 patients at 24 centers from 1987 to 1989 (NHLBI, 1991). Similar acute hemodynamic results were obtained. Balloon aortic valvuloplasty led to a decrease in the mean aortic valve pressure gradient from 55 ± 21 to 29 ± 13 mmHg, an increase in aortic valve area from 0.5 ± 0.2 to 0.8 ± 0.3 cm², and an increase in cardiac output from 3.9 ± 1.2 to 4.1 ± 1.2 L/min. Complications occurred in 25% of patients. Complications included procedural death (3%), cardiac arrest (5%), emergency aortic valve replacement (1%), left ventricular perforation (2%), cerebrovascular accident (3%), and other systemic embolus (2%).

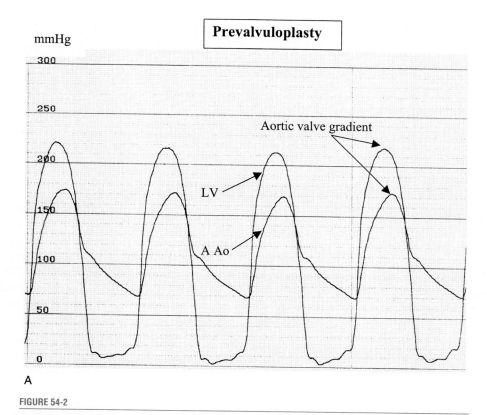

A

FIGURE 54-2

(*A*) The baseline pressure gradient across the patient's calcified aortic valve is shown, measured by simultaneous pressure monitoring from the left ventricle (LV) and ascending aorta (A Ao) with an 8 French double-lumen pigtail catheter. There is a 42-mmHg mean gradient and a 45-mmHg peak-to-peak gradient across the aortic valve (arrows). (*B*) There is a marked reduction in the aortic valve gradient (a 10-mmHg mean gradient and a 15-mmHg peak-to-peak gradient) following balloon aortic valvuloplasty with 20-mm and then 23-mm diameter balloons. The aortic valve area increased from 0.66 cm² at baseline to 1.76 cm² following valvuloplasty.

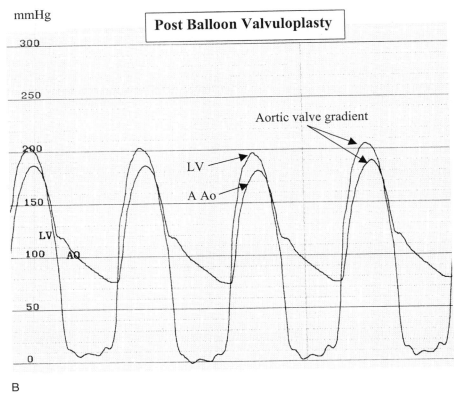

FIGURE 54-2 *(continued)*

Vascular complications again were common, with 23% requiring transfusion and 7% requiring vascular surgery. At 30 days, the overall mortality rate was 14%. Of the survivors at 30 days, 75% experienced at least one functional class improvement in congestive heart failure, and 53% experienced at least one quartile improvement in overall functional status.

The use of newer balloons with lower deflated balloon profiles, improved vascular sheaths, and percutaneous suture closure techniques may decrease the incidence of vascular trauma.

Long-Term Results

In most patients, restenosis with recurrent symptoms occurs in the first 6 to 12 months following balloon valvuloplasty for calcific aortic stenosis, accompanied by clinical deterioration. The 1-year survival rate in the Mansfield registry was 64%, with an event-free survival of 43% (McKay, 1991). In the NHLBI registry, the survival at 1, 2, and 3 years was 55%, 35%, and 23%, respectively (NHLBI, 1991). Therefore, it must be emphasized that, when feasible, definitive aortic valve replacement is the technique of choice for managing the adult patient with severe calcific aortic stenosis.

REFERENCES

Bonow BO et al: ACC/AHA guidelines for the management of patients with valvular heart disease: A report of the American College of Cardiology/American Heart Association Task Force on Practice Guidelines (Committee on Management of Patients with Valvular Heart Disease). J Am Coll Cardiol 32:1486, 1998

Cribier A et al: Percutaneous transluminal valvuloplasty in acquired aortic stenosis in elderly patients: An alternative to valve replacement? Lancet 1:63, 1986

Eisenhauer AC et al: Balloon aortic valvuloplasty revisited: The role of the Inoue balloon and transseptal antegrade approach. Cathet Cardiovasc Intervent 50:484, 2000

Lababidi Z et al: Percutaneous balloon aortic valvulo-plasty: Results in 23 patients. Am J Cardiol 53:194, 1984

McKay RG, for the Mansfield Scientific Aortic Valvuloplasty Registry Investigators: The Mansfield Scientific Aortic Valvuloplasty Registry: Overview of acute hemodynamic results and procedural complications. J Am Coll Cardiol 17:485, 1991

Michaels AD, Ports TA: Use of a percutaneous arterial suture device (Perclose) in patients undergoing percutaneous balloon aortic valvuloplasty. Cathet Cardiovasc Intervent 53:445, 2001

Moore P et al: Midterm results of balloon dilation of congenital aortic stenosis: Predictors of success. J Am Coll Cardiol 27:1257, 1996

NHLBI Balloon Valvuloplasty Registry Participants: Percutaneous balloon aortic valvuloplasty: Acute and 30 day follow-up results in 674 patients from the NHLBI Balloon Valvuloplasty Registry. Circulation 84:2383, 1991

Rosenfeld HM et al: Balloon aortic valvuloplasty in the young patient with congenital aortic stenosis. Am J Cardiol 73:1112, 1994

TIMING OF OPERATION FOR ASYMPTOMATIC SEVERE AORTIC REGURGITATION

Robert O. Bonow

The management of patients with chronic severe aortic regurgitation (AR) represents a series of challenging considerations for the physician. Patients with this condition characteristically remain asymptomatic for many years, even decades, despite the severe left ventricular (LV) volume overload. During this time, the left ventricle adapts to the volume load through recruitment of hypertrophy and chamber dilatation; through these mechanisms, it is able to maintain systolic function in the normal range. In the majority of patients, aortic valve replacement (AVR) can be safely postponed until the onset of symptoms, and in these patients long-term functional and survival results are excellent. However, it is also possible for LV systolic dysfunction to develop in the absence of symptoms; by the time symptoms develop, a subset of patients will have developed irreversible LV systolic dysfunction. Thus, if the development of symptoms is used as the sole indication for AVR, some patients will be at risk of persistent LV dysfunction, heart failure, and death despite a technically successful operation. This has led to a temptation on the part of many physicians to recommend AVR in the early stages of the natural history of severe AR. Such an aggressive approach is not warranted.

Major advances in cardiac valve replacement surgery over the past three decades have resulted in improved outcomes of patients undergoing surgery for chronic severe AR, but AVR continues to entail both the immediate perioperative risks and the long-term risks associated with prosthetic heart valves. These risks clearly are not justified in all patients with chronic severe AR.

Cumulative data from a large number of clinical studies have identified factors that predict survival and LV function after AVR and have identified subgroups of asymptomatic patients who may benefit from AVR (Bonow et al., 1998). These findings have prompted a movement toward early operation in patients with minimal or no cardiac symptoms who manifest extreme LV dilatation and/or evidence of LV systolic dysfunction. Thus, the improved outcome of patients undergoing AVR over the past 30 years reflects improvement in selection of patients for AVR as well as improvements in surgical techniques.

In determining the optimal timing of AVR in asymptomatic patients with AR, the physician must consider two important factors. These are the post-operative survival and LV function of patients undergoing AVR (and the determinants of these survival and LV functional results) and the natural history of asymptomatic patients with severe AR.

Determinants of Outcome after Aortic Valve Replacement

Preoperative LV systolic function and severity of preoperative symptoms have an important impact on postoperative survival and postoperative LV function (Bonow et al., 1998). Several lines of reasoning support the position for operation in asymptomatic patients with evidence of LV systolic dysfunction:

- In *symptomatic* patients undergoing AVR, preoperative measures of LV "pump" function at rest (i.e., resting ejection fraction) are the most sensitive in identifying patients at risk of postoperative LV dysfunction and congestive heart failure (Bonow et al., 1985, 1998; Carabello et al., 1987; Klodas et al., 1996). Patients with normal preoperative ejection fraction have an excellent outcome, whereas those with depressed preoperative ejection fraction represent a group at higher risk after AVR.
- In *asymptomatic* patients, the time course between the development of LV dysfunction at rest and the onset of symptoms is relatively short: two-thirds or more of patients with LV dysfunction develop symptoms requiring operation within 2 to 3 years (Bonow et al., 1998).
- Long-term postoperative prognosis and improvement in LV function are enhanced in asymptomatic patients or mildly symptomatic patients with LV dysfunction, as compared to more severely symptomatic patients (Bonow et al., 1985, 1998).
- Survival and reversibility of LV dysfunction after AVR is also dependent upon the severity and duration of preoperative LV dysfunction (Bonow et al., 1985; Carabello et al., 1987).

These data support the concept that postoperative survival and postoperative LV function will be enhanced favorably if asymptomatic or mildly symptomatic patients with LV dysfunction undergo operation without waiting for the development of more significant symptoms or more severe LV dysfunction (Bonow et al., 1998).

Natural History of Asymptomatic Patients

Although the concern that some asymptomatic patients with AR may develop irreversible LV dysfunction is valid, and although some asymptomatic patients may benefit from early AVR, it must be understood that this concern pertains only to a small minority of asymptomatic patients with this disease. The vast majority of asymptomatic patients who are encountered in clinical practice maintain normal LV contractile function at rest for many years and usually develop symptoms before or coincident with the onset of depressed contractile function. Asymptomatic patients with normal LV ejection fractions have an excellent prognosis, with only a gradual rate of deterioration during conservative, nonoperative management. Several lines of evidence from seven natural history studies support these concepts (Bonow et al., 1998):

- Fewer than 6% per year require AVR because symptoms or LV dysfunction develop at rest.
- Fewer than 3.5% per year develop asymptomatic LV systolic dysfunction.
- Fewer than 0.2% per year die suddenly.

Although the overall outcome of asymptomatic patients with severe AR and normal LV ejection fraction is excellent, there is a higher-risk subgroup that can be identified by noninvasive testing:

- Patients likely to require operation over a 10-year period because of symptoms or LV dysfunction can be identified on the basis of severity of LV dilatation by echocardiography and progressive increases in LV cavity dimensions or decreases in resting ejection fraction during the course of serial follow-up studies (Bonow et al., 1991; Siemienczuk et al., 1989; Tornos et al., 1995).

- Patients at risk of sudden death during the natural history of AR are those with evidence of extreme LV dilatation on echocardiography (Siemienczuk et al., 1989), with LV cavity dimensions ≥80 mm at end diastole (normal, ≤ 55 mm), and/or LV dimensions >55 mm at end systole (normal, ≤35 mm).

- Patients with extreme LV dilatation who undergo AVR have an excellent outcome if surgery is performed while they are asymptomatic with normal LV systolic function; however, postoperative survival is significantly reduced if AVR is performed in such patients after the onset of symptoms and/or LV dysfunction (Klodas et al., 1996).

Indications for Aortic Valve Replacement

AVR is clearly indicated in symptomatic patients with severe AR, even if LV systolic function is normal. In the absence of symptoms, AVR is also warranted in patients who develop LV systolic dysfunction (ejection fraction below normal at rest) or extreme LV dilatation (Table 55-1). AVR is also indicated in patients with severe AR who have other associated cardiovascular conditions requiring surgery on the heart or proximal aorta, such as those who require coronary artery bypass surgery, aortic root repair, or surgical replacement or repair of other heart valves.

If asymptomatic patients are followed carefully and undergo operation only after the development of symptoms, LV systolic dysfunction, and/or extreme LV dilatation, the operative mortality is very low, long-term postoperative survival is excellent, and LV function after operation improves in virtually every patient. Hence, although asymptomatic patients with *depressed* LV contractile function at rest or extreme LV dilatation should undergo AVR before the onset of symptoms, the great majority of asymptomatic patients with *normal* LV contractile function at rest can be followed carefully

TABLE 55-1

INDICATIONS FOR AORTIC VALVE REPLACEMENT IN CHRONIC SEVERE AORTIC REGURGITATION

Patients developing important symptoms (angina, dyspnea, presyncope, or syncope)

Patients developing LV systolic dysfunction (ejection fraction below normal at rest)

Patients developing extreme LV dilatation[a]

Aortic root dilatation (aortic root diameter >50 mm)

Patients undergoing coronary artery bypass surgery or surgery on the aorta or other heart valves

[a]Defined as an end-diastolic dimension of ≥75 mm (normal, ≤55 mm) or an end-systolic dimension of ≥55 mm (normal, ≤35 mm) by echocardiography.

and do not require "prophylactic" valve replacement to preserve LV function. A proposed management strategy, including the timing of serial clinical evaluations and echocardiograms (based on the severity of LV dilatation), can be found in the *American College of Cardiology/American Heart Association Guidelines for the Management of Patients with Valvular Heart Disease* (Bonow et al., 1998). This strategy is outlined in Fig. 55-1.

Medical Therapy

It has been known for nearly two decades that vasodilating agents [nitroprusside, hydralazine, nifedipine, and angiotensin-converting enzyme (ACE) inhibitors] are effective in reducing the regurgitant volume in patients with AR and, in doing so, reducing LV volumes and preserving LV ejection fraction. However, the number of patients reported in vasodilator trials is small, and only one long-term study has been conducted to determine if the hemodynamic effects of vasodilating agents translate into a beneficial effect on the natural history of chronic severe AR. In a randomized

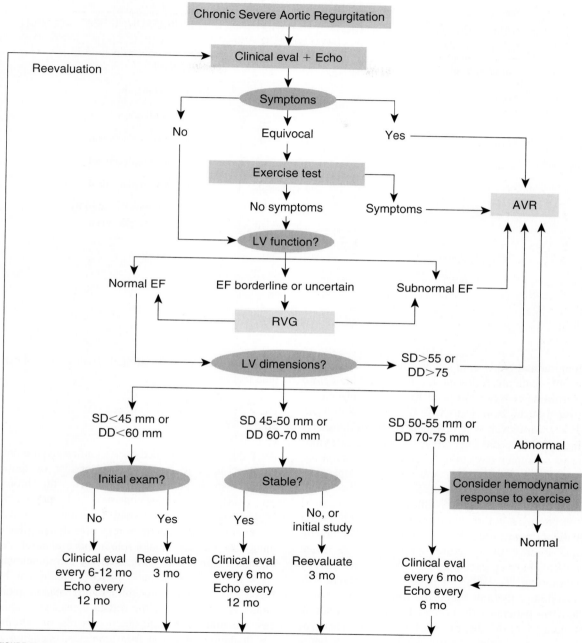

FIGURE 55–1

Management strategy for patients with chronic severe aortic regurgitation. AVR, aortic valve replacement; DD, end-diastolic dimension; EF, ejection fraction; LV, left ventricular; RVG, radionuclide ventriculography; SD, end-diastolic dimension. (From ACC/AHA Guidelines for the Management of Patients with Valvular Heart Disease, RO Bonow et al: J Am Coll Cardiol 32:1486, 1998.)

TABLE 55-2

INDICATIONS FOR MEDICAL THERAPY IN PATIENTS WITH CHRONIC AORTIC RE-GURGITATION

Severity of AR	Symptoms	LV function	Management
Mild-moderate	No	Normal	No medical therapy
Severe	No	Normal	Vasodilator therapy
Severe	No	Depressed	Aortic valve replacement
Severe	Yes	Normal	Aortic valve replacement
Severe	Yes	Depressed	Aortic valve replacement
Severe	Severe	Severely depressed	Medical therapy followed by aortic valve replacement

NOTE: AR, aortic regurgitation.

longitudinal study comparing nifedipine to digoxin in 143 patients followed for 6 years, long-acting nifedipine reduced the need for valve replacement over 6 years from 34 to 15% (Scognamiglio et al., 1994). Moreover, when patients receiving long-acting nifedipine did undergo AVR because of symptoms or impaired systolic function, all survived operation and LV size and function improved considerably in all patients.

Vasodilator therapy with nifedipine or ACE inhibitors is not recommended for asymptomatic patients with mild AR and normal LV function in the absence of systemic hypertension, as these patients have an excellent outcome with no therapy (Bonow et al., 1998). In patients with severe AR, vasodilator therapy should be reserved for asymptomatic patients with normal LV systolic function (Table 55-2). Medical therapy is not an alternative to surgery in symptomatic patients or in patients with LV systolic dysfunction, as such patients should be considered surgical candidates rather than candidates for long-term medical therapy (Bonow et al., 1998), unless AVR is not recom-

mended because of additional cardiac or noncardiac factors.

SUMMARY

AVR should be performed once significant symptoms develop. Lacking important symptoms, operation should also be performed in patients with chronic severe AR who manifest consistent and reproducible evidence of either LV contractile dysfunction at rest or extreme LV dilatation. Noninvasive imaging techniques should play a major role in this evaluation. An important clinical decision, such as recommending AVR in the asymptomatic patient, should not be based on a single echocardiographic measurement alone. However, when these data consistently indicate impaired contractile function at rest or extreme LV dilatation on repeat measurements, operation is indicated in the asymptomatic patient (Bonow et al., 1998). This strategy should reduce the likelihood of irreversible LV dysfunction in these patients and enhance long-term postoperative survival.

REFERENCES

Bonow RO et al: Survival and functional results after valve replacement for aortic regurgitation from 1976 to 1983: Impact of preoperative left ventricular function. Circulation 72:1244, 1985

Bonow RO et al: Serial long-term assessment of the natural history of asymptomatic patients with chronic aortic regurgitation and normal left ventricular systolic function. Circulation 84:1625, 1991

Bonow RO et al: *ACC/AHA Guidelines for the Management of Patients with Valvular Heart Disease.* A report of the American College of Cardiology/American Heart Association Task Force on Practice Guidelines (Committee on Management of Patients with Valvular Heart Disease). J Am Coll Cardiol 32:1486, 1998

Carabello BA et al: Predictors of outcome for aortic valve replacement in patients with aortic regurgitation and left ventricular dysfunction: A change in the measuring stick. J Am Coll Cardiol 10:991, 1987

Klodas E et al: Aortic regurgitation complicated by extreme left ventricular dilation: Long-term outcome after surgical correction. J Am Coll Cardiol 27:670, 1996

Scognamiglio R et al: Nifedipine in asymptomatic patients with severe aortic regurgitation and normal left ventricular function. N Engl J Med 331:689, 1994

Siemienczuk D et al: Chronic aortic insufficiency: Factors associated with progression to aortic valve replacement. Ann Intern Med 110:587, 1989

Tornos MP et al: Clinical outcome of severe asymptomatic chronic aortic regurgitation: A long-term prospective follow-up study. Am Heart J 130:333, 1995

SURGERY FOR TRICUSPID REGURGITATION

Charles J. Mullany

The diagnosis and management of tricuspid valve disease in the adult still remain a challenge for the clinician. The indications for surgery and the appropriate surgical procedure are less well defined and understood than the more common problems of left-sided valvular heart disease. In part, this is related to the unique pathophysiology of the tricuspid valve, which functions in a low-pressure system compared to the aortic and mitral valves (Duran et al., 1980). In addition, tricuspid valve disease in isolation is uncommon and is more frequently associated with the more serious and common pathology of the left-sided valves, which tend to dominate a patient's clinical presentation. Moreover, less than perfect surgical results, particularly for tricuspid regurgitation, are generally well tolerated and may cause minimal symptoms, if any, for the patient.

Etiology

Causes of tricuspid regurgitation can be divided into two main groups—patients with normal leaflets and those with abnormal leaflets (Table 56-1) (Bonow et al., 1998). The most important cause of tricuspid regurgitation in the adult is tricuspid annular dilatation secondary to pulmonary hypertension combined with pathology of the mitral and/or the aortic valve. This is commonly referred to as *functional tricuspid regurgitation*. In such instances, the leaflets are usually normal and most of the annular dilatation involves the annulus to which the anterior and septal leaflets are attached.

Acquired tricuspid regurgitation related to abnormal leaflets is less common and the causes are much more varied (Table 56-1). Carcinoid heart disease produces thickening and retraction of the tricuspid leaflets with subsequent severe tricuspid regurgitation. Histologically the valve leaflets are encased by plaques containing spindle-shaped cells and collagen material within a mucopolysaccharide ground substance (Color Plate 14, Figure 56-1). Similar changes are seen in patients with valvular disease related to ergotamine and anorectic medication. As the incidence of rheumatic heart disease declines in the United States and other western countries, rheumatic disease of the tricuspid valve has become less common.

Indications for Surgery

Tricuspid valve surgery is strongly indicated for patients who have moderate to severe tricuspid regurgitation and who are undergoing surgery for either mitral and/or aortic valve disease. Intraoperative trans-

TABLE 56-1

CAUSES OF TRICUSPID REGURGITATION

Normal leaflets
  Pulmonary hypertension
    Left ventricular failure
    Mitral/aortic valvular disease
    Acute and chronic cor pulmonale (e.g., pulmonary
      thromboembolism)
  Right ventricular infarction
Abnormal leaflets
  Rheumatic heart disease
  Infective endocarditis
  Carcinoid heart disease
  Trauma
  Pacemaker/catheter-induced regurgitation
  Medication (ergotamine, anorectic drugs)
  Myxomatous degeneration
  Congenital abnormalities (e.g., Ebstein's anomaly)

esophageal echocardiography is very useful in determining the need for tricuspid surgery as well as in evaluating the success of the subsequent repair. Annuloplasty, using a ring (Carpentier/Duran/Cosgrove) or a suture technique (Kay/deVega), is almost always sufficient in these patients (Duran et al., 1980; Grondin et al., 1975). Tricuspid valve replacement is rarely warranted for functional tricuspid regurgitation. In patients with mild tricuspid regurgitation, tricuspid surgery is not required since it usually resolves once the mitral and/or aortic valve problem is corrected and there is subsequent resolution of the secondary pulmonary hypertension (Bonow et al., 1998).

Failure to correct moderate to severe tricuspid regurgitation at the same time as other valvular surgery may result in a poor functional result and a need for subsequent surgery, with a high mortality (King et al., 1984; Hornick et al., 1996; Mullany et al., 1987). In patients who develop significant tricuspid regurgitation after previous valvular surgery, careful investigation of the left-sided valves (particularly the mitral) is essential. Prosthetic mitral valve dysfunction or perivalvular leak with resultant pulmonary hypertension is the usual cause for the recurrent tricuspid regurgitation. On the other hand, if the left-sided valves are normal and significant tricuspid regurgitation has recurred, fixed pulmonary hypertension or severe left ventricular dysfunction may exist. These patients often have a poor prognosis (King et al., 1984). At the Mayo Clinic, in a recent review of 34 patients undergoing isolated tricuspid valve surgery for severe tricuspid regurgitation following prior valvular surgery for left-sided valvular disease, hospital mortality was 8.8% and the 5-year survival was only 48.8% (Staab et al., 1999). In this study, pulmonary hypertension was not found to be a risk factor for an adverse outcome. However, in this series there were no patients with a systolic pulmonary artery pressures greater than 67 mmHg.

For patients with severe tricuspid regurgitation, without mitral or aortic pathology, the decision for surgery is less clear cut. In the totally asymptomatic patient, surgery is most probably not indicated, particularly in the absence of pulmonary hypertension (Bonow et al., 1998). In the symptomatic patient, diuretic therapy may be useful initially. However, if symptoms persist, then surgery should be undertaken before irreversible right ventricular failure develops. Tricuspid valve replacement may be preferable to valve repair and annuloplasty in such patients.

Surgery for infective endocarditis of the tricuspid valve is not often required but should be undertaken for uncontrolled sepsis, recurrent pulmonary emboli, and significant tricuspid regurgitation with symptoms. Tricuspid valve replacement is usually required, although repair may be possible. However, for patients whose infective endocarditis is related to intravenous drug use, tricuspid valve excision without replacement can be undertaken, with subsequent valve replacement for hemodynamic symptoms at a later date. Such a decision needs to be individualized depending on whether the patient is also cured of the drug addiction.

Carcinoid heart disease is becoming more common because of the effective management of the carcinoid syndrome with somatostatin and its analogues. Severe tricuspid regurgitation due to thickening and retraction of the leaflets is the usual manifestation, often associated with pulmonary valve stenosis. For patients with severe tricuspid regurgitation and symptoms, tricuspid valve replacement will be required. Additionally, pulmonary valvectomy with patch enlargement of the pulmonary outflow tract is often undertaken. In carcinoid patients who require extensive hepatic surgery or hepatic artery embolization for metastatic disease and who have significant tricuspid regurgitation, tricuspid valve replacement should be undertaken first, in order to prevent the subsequent hemodynamic instability that may occur following the hepatic procedure if severe uncontrolled tricuspid regurgitation is left untreated.

Ebstein's anomaly not uncommonly presents in adult life. In a 25-year experience reported from the Mayo Clinic, 323 patients underwent surgical treatment for this condition (Theodoro et al., 1987). The median age was 17 years, and the oldest patient was 70 years. Whenever possible, valvuloplasty was preferred to valve replacement inasmuch as it avoided the subsequent problems of prosthetic valve dysfunction and anticoagulation. In 43% of patients, tricuspid valve repair was possible, while 55% underwent valve replacement, usually with a bioprosthesis. The 10-year survival of patients undergoing a bioprosthetic valve replacement was 93% (Danielson et al., 1992; Kiziltan et al., 1998).

Choice of Valve

For most patients undergoing tricuspid valve surgery for tricuspid regurgitation, valve repair or annuloplasty is usually sufficient. Valve replacement is usually reserved for those patients with abnormal leaflets (carcinoid syndrome, rheumatic disease, bacterial endocarditis) or for patients who require reoperation for severe tricuspid regurgitation after previous tricuspid surgery. The type of valve inserted in the tricuspid position, mechanical vs. tissue, continues to be a source of controversy

(Ratnatunga et al., 1998; Kawano et al., 2000; Shapira et al., 2000; Ohata et al., 2001; Dalrympl-Hay et al., 1999; Nakano et al., 2001), although more recent data tend to favor the bioprosthetic valves (Dalrympl-Hay et al., 1999). Mechanical valves are more prone to thrombosis in the tricuspid position than when the corresponding valve is placed in the aortic or mitral position. This also applies to the current generation of bileaflet valves (Kawano et al., 2000; Shapira et al., 2000). In addition, tissue valves appear to be less likely to undergo tissue degeneration in the tricuspid position than on the left side of the heart, even in young patients (Kiziltan et al., 1998; Williams et al., 1982).

Figure 56-2 shows freedom from reoperation after tricuspid bioprosthesis replacements for patients ≤18 years of age undergoing surgery for Ebstein's anomaly at the Mayo Clinic, compared with freedom from reoperation from bioprosthesis replacement in all cardiac positions (in the same age group) previously reported from the same institution (Kiziltan et al., 1998; Williams et al., 1982). For patients who require a mechanical valve in the aortic or mitral position or who need chronic anticoagulation for atrial fibrillation, a low-profile bileaflet tilting disk valve (e.g., St. Jude Medical) could be considered for the tricuspid position. However, even in these circumstances a bioprosthesis may be preferable given the relatively high incidence of valve thrombosis that occurs despite adequate anticoagulation (Kawano et al., 2000).

Although there are data to suggest that preserving the subvalvular apparatus (chordae and papillary muscles) in mitral valve surgery is beneficial and helps retain left ventricular geometry and function, corresponding data for tricuspid valve surgery and the right ventricle are lacking. Nevertheless, it would seem reasonable to preserve the subvalvular apparatus during tricuspid valve replacement. On many occasions minimal excision of valvular tissue is required. If the patient already has a permanent right ventricular pacing system in place, then pacing leads can be positioned between the sewing ring of the prosthesis and the annulus. If permanent pacing

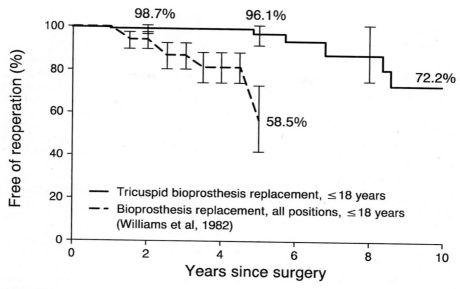

FIGURE 56-2

Freedom from reoperation for tricuspid bioprosthesis replacement for patients ≤18 years in the Mayo Clinic series compared with freedom from reoperation for bioprosthesis replacement in all cardiac positions in patients ≤18 years previously reported from the same institution (Williams et al., 1982). (Reprinted with permission from Kiziltan HT et al: Ann Thorac Surg 66:1539, 1998.)

is anticipated postoperatively, permanent epicardial ventricular pacing leads should be placed. This will avoid subsequent placement of transvenous pacing leads across a tissue prosthesis. Clearly this cannot be done if a mechanical valve is in place.

Results of Surgery

Early mortality and long-term survival after tricuspid valve replacement or annuloplasty depend to a large part upon variables which are independent of the tricuspid valve itself. These include patient age, NYHA class, pulmonary hypertension and degree of pulmonary resistance, right ventricular function, right heart failure, number of valves operated upon, and number of previous operations. For patients who undergo mitral valve replacement or repair together with tricuspid annuloplasty for functional regurgitation, mortality is generally low (5%). However, the operative mortality may be as high as 20 to 25% for patients who undergo repeat tricuspid surgery, particularly in the presence of pulmonary hypertension, or who require surgery for uncorrected tricuspid regurgitation after previous mitral valve replacement (King et al., 1984; Mangoni et al., 2001; Do et al., 2000). The U.K. Heart Valve Registry identified 425 patients who underwent tricuspid valve replacement with a 30-day mortality of 17.3% (Ratnatunga et al., 1998). However, this included patients having single-, double-, or triple-valve surgery, with those having single isolated tricuspid valve replacement having the lowest mortality. A report from the Mayo Clinic cited an 8.8% mortality for patients having isolated tricuspid surgery after previous left-sided valvular surgery (Staab et al., 1999).

Long-term survival is again dependent upon many factors often related to age, number of previous operations, and the patient's left-sided disease. The 10-year survival in the U.K. Heart Valve Registry was 43%, which is significantly less than for patients having aortic valve replacement (63%) or mitral valve replacement (57%) (Ratnatunga et al., 1998). For most patients who survive surgery, functional class is significantly improved. Staab et al., showed that for patients who are alive at a mean follow-up of 71 months, the mean NYHA class was 2.1 compared to 3.4 preoperatively (Staab et al., 1999). In Ebstein's anomaly, at a mean follow-up of 9.4 years, 92% of patients were in class I or II (Theodoro et al., 1997).

SUMMARY

Surgery for tricuspid regurgitation continues to be a surgical challenge. Functional regurgitation, usually related to pulmonary hypertension and left-sided valvular disease, remains the most common problem and, if severe, should be treated by annuloplasty at the same time as mitral and/or aortic valve surgery. For patients requiring valve replacement, the choice of prosthesis is controversial, but the data suggest that a tissue valve is the preferred prosthesis. For patients who present with tricuspid regurgitation after previous aortic or mitral valve surgery, a careful evaluation of left-sided valves needs to be undertaken. Valvular dysfunction of left-sided valves is a common cause of subsequent tricuspid regurgitation. Operative mortality varies and depends upon many factors, often unrelated to the valve. Mortality for tricuspid valve repair associated with mitral valve repair may be as low as 5%. However, mortality for repeat tricuspid surgery, in the presence of pulmonary hypertension, may be as high as 20%. Long-term survival is less than that for isolated aortic or mitral valve replacement.

REFERENCES

Bonow RO et al: ACC/AHA Guidelines for the Management of Patients With Valvular Heart Disease. A report of the American College of Cardiology/American Heart Association Task Force on Practice Guidelines (Committee on Management of Patients with Valvular Heart Disease). J Am Coll Cardiol 32:1486, 1998

Dalrympl-Hay MJ et al: Tricuspid valve replacement: Bioprostheses are preferable. J Heart Valve Dis 8:644, 1999

Danielson GK et al: Operative treatment of Ebstein's anomaly. J Thorac Cardiovasc Surg 104:1195, 1992

Do QB et al: Clinical outcome after isolated tricuspid valve replacement: 20 year experience. Can J Cardiol 16:489, 2000

Duran CMG et al: Is tricuspid valve repair necessary? J Thorac Cardiovasc Surg 80:849, 1980

Grondin P et al: Carpentier's annulus and deVega's anuloplasty. The end of the tricuspid challenge. J Thorac Cardiovasc Surg 70:852, 1975

Hornick P et al: Tricuspid valve replacement subsequent to previous open heart surgery. J Heart Valve Dis 5:20, 1996

Kawano H et al: Tricuspid valve replacement with the St. Jude Medical valve: 19 years of experience. Eur J Cardiothorac Surg 18:565, 2000

King RM et al: Surgery for tricuspid regurgitation late after mitral valve replacement. Circulation 70(Suppl I):I-193, 1984

Kiziltan HT et al: Late results of bioprosthetic tricuspid valve replacement in Ebstein's anomaly. Ann Thorac Surg 66:1539, 1998

Mangoni AA et al: Outcome following isolated tricuspid valve replacement. Eur J Cardiothorac Surg 19:68, 2001

Mullany CJ et al: Repair of tricuspid valve insufficiency in patients undergoing double (aortic and mitral) valve replacement: Perioperative mortality and long-term (1–20 years) follow-up in 109 patients. J Thorac Cardiovasc Surg 94:740, 1987

Nakano K et al: Tricuspid valve replacement with bioprostheses: Long-term results and causes of valve dysfunction. Ann Thorac Surg 71:105, 2001

Ohata T et al: Comparison of durability of bioprostheses in tricuspid and mitral positions. Ann Thorac Surg 71:S240, 2001

Ratnatunga CP et al: Tricuspid valve replacement: UK heart valve registry mid-term results comparing mechanical and biological prostheses. Ann Thorac Surg 66:1934, 1998

Shapira Y et al: Mid-term clinical and echocardiographic follow-up of patients with CarboMedics valves in the tricuspid position. J Heart Valve Dis 9:396, 2000

Staab ME et al: Isolated tricuspid valve surgery for severe tricuspid regurgitation following prior left heart valve surgery: Analysis of outcome in 34 patients. J Heart Valve Dis 8:567, 1999

Theodoro DA et al: Surgical management of Ebstein's anomaly: A 25-year experience. Circulation 96(Suppl l):I-507, 1997

Williams DB et al: Porcine heterograft valve replacement in children. J Thorac Cardiovasc Surg 84:446, 1982

CHAPTER

57

THE GENETICS OF ATRIAL FIBRILLATION

Robert Roberts & Ramon Brugada

Atrial fibrillation (AF) is the most common sustained cardiac dysrhythmia. It is estimated that between 2 and 3 million Americans suffer from atrial fibrillation. The prevalence increases with age from 2.3% between the ages of 40 and 60 years to 5.9% over the age of 65 (National Heart, Lung, and Blood Institute Working Group on Atrial Fibrillation, 1993; Wolf et al., 1987). The common and most dreaded complication of AF is cerebral embolic stroke. Indeed, atrial fibrillation accounts for one-third of all strokes in patients over the age of 65 (Albers, 1994).

There are repeated examples in the history of medicine in which the etiology of a disease has been solved by studying a familial form of the disorder. Elucidation of the molecular defect in familial hypercholesterolemia formed the framework for our understanding and treatment of hypercho-lesterolemia, despite the fact that <3% of coronary artery disease is due to the familial form. It is often easier to understand nature when it wanders off the beaten path than when everything is working normally. While there have been rare reports in the literature about familial AF, it is not felt by cardiologists to be familial, although it was first reported to be familial in 1943. In 1996, the first family with this arrhythmia was identified. Since then, identification and collection of blood samples from over 20 families with AF has taken place; through other physicians, 100 other families with AF have been identified. It appears that patients with AF without known structural or functional heart disease are more likely to have a genetic basis due to either a de novo mutation (sporadic) or passed on from the previous generation (familial). (R. Brugada and Roberts, 1999; Roberts and Brugada, 2000.)

Clinical Features—Phenotype

In addition to the original family identified in Spain, four other related families were identified from this region for a total of 102 individuals. There were 42 individuals in the family affected with AF, and 6 had died from complications that may be attributed to the atrial fibrillation—namely, five died from cerebral vascular accident and one patient had a cardiac arrest at age 35. The disease was chronic in all but one patient, and the heart rate varied from 90 to 150 beats per minute. At the time of diagnosis, the ages of affected patients ranged from 1 to 45 years. Most of the patients were asymptomatic, with only six patients complaining of palpitations. There were no echocardiographic abnormalities, but on follow-up, two patients had developed dilated cardiomyopathy, presumably secondary to poorly controlled heart rate. Electrocardioversion was attempted unsuccessfully in three patients with chronic AF. Two of the patients who subsequently developed dilated cardiomyopathy had ejection fractions of 51 and 54%, with increased internal diameters of the left ventricle and the left atria. The remainder had no abnormalities on echocardiography, and the average ejection fraction was 69%.

Familial Mode of Transmission

The disease in the initial families was transmitted in an autosomal dominant pattern. The same pattern of inheritance has been observed in all of the subsequent families. Thus, the disease affects males and females equally and is transmitted vertically across each successive generation, with about 50% of the offspring inheriting the defective gene (Fig. 57-1). It is characteristic in autosomal dominant disorders that the clinical manifestations (phenotype) are highly variable, including age of onset, severity, and the extent of disease. It is expected, as in most adult autosomal dominant disorders, that the mutation will involve the substitution of a single base in most affected individuals with the remainder being due to deletions or insertions.

Identification of the Gene

Utilizing genetic linkage analysis, it has been possible to map the chromosomal location of the gene responsible for AF in the initial five families (Brugada et al., 1997). This involved genotyping normal and affected patients for 300 chromosomal DNA markers. These markers are of known location on a chromosome and are selected to cover the full length of each of the 23 chromosomes. As these markers are inherited in a pattern identical to that of gene inheritance, i.e., by chance alone, only 50% of affected individuals with the disease will inherit a particular marker. It was found, however, that all of the individuals affected with AF also inherited a set of markers on the long arm of chromosome 10 in band region 2.3. This indicates that the gene responsible for AF is in close physical proximity to these markers and thus must reside in the region of chromosome 10q23. Through analysis of genetic crossovers (recombinations), the region containing the gene has since been narrowed to about 1 cM (1 million bp). Known genes mapped to the region such as the β-adrenergic receptor have been analyzed and shown not to contain a mutation. Thus, it will be necessary to clone and sequence the complete region to identify what is, at this time, an unknown gene responsible for AF in this family. It is anticipated that the gene is likely to encode a channel protein that is involved in conduction of impulses throughout the atria. However, until it is identified, other possibilities also exist. Studies are underway to complete the sequencing of this region. In the meantime, some genetic analyses in other families have been done and have shown that the chromosomal locus 10q23 is not the site responsible for disease in one family; thus, it establishes that other genes are also responsible for AF.

Implications from Genetic Studies

The action potential generated in the human ventricle is associated with multiple ionic currents, including sodium, potassium, chloride, and others.

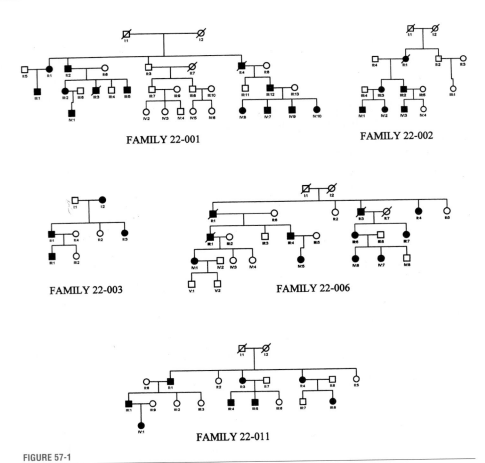

FIGURE 57-1

Shown here are five family trees in which atrial fibrillation was common. The squares refer to males and the circles refer to females. The slashed squares and circles refer to those who have died, and the black squares and circles indicate individuals affected with atrial fibrillation.

The recent avalanche of material from identification of the genes responsible for the long QT syndrome is rapidly elucidating the channels responsible for the inward and outward transport of various ions that generate the ventricular action potential and also those responsible for variations in the action potential associated with a predisposition to ventricular arrhythmias and sudden death. It is anticipated that with further intensity of the study of genetics in AF and other supraventricular arrhythmias, a series of genes will be identified from which pathways for the conduction and generation of the atrial action potential will be determined. While familial etiology is likely to account for only a very small proportion of AF, nevertheless it could lay the groundwork for the treatment of both familial and acquired forms. As mentioned above, the cholesterol theory was proved by the results of initial studies performed in familial disorders that accounted for <3% of all patients with coronary artery disease. This formed the framework and foundation for the now-proven cholesterol hypothesis and the development of drugs specifically targeted to inhibit cholesterol synthesis, which have markedly reduced the incidence of coronary artery disease, myocardial infarction, and mortality.

REFERENCES

Albers GW: Atrial fibrillation and stroke: Three new studies, three remaining questions. Arch Intern Med 154:1443, 1994

Brugada R et al: Identification of a genetic locus for familial atrial fibrillation. N Engl J Med 336:905, 1997

Brugada R, Roberts R. Molecular biology and atrial fibrillation. Curr Opin Cardiol. 14:269, 1999

National Heart, Lung, and Blood Institute Working Group on Atrial Fibrillation: Atrial fibrillation: Current understandings and research imperatives. J Am Coll Cardiol 22: 1830, 1993

Roberts R, Brugada R. Genetic aspects of arrhythmias. Am J Med Genet. 97:310, 2000

Wolf PA et al: Atrial fibrillation: A major contributor to stroke in the elderly: The Framingham Study. Arch Intern Med 147:1561, 1987

THE BRUGADA SYNDROME

Ihor Gussak,
Bernard R. Chaitman

Introduction

In the United States alone, sudden cardiac death (SCD) due to cardiac arrest occurs with an incidence of more than 300,000 per year. Recent interest has focused on unexpected arrhythmogenic death occurring in individuals with minimal or no structural heart disease, estimated to represent 3 to 9% of out-of-hospital cases of ventricular fibrillation (VF) unrelated to myocardial infarction (Viskin et al., 1997). In addition to the ventricular preexcitation syndrome and the long QT syndrome, the *Brugada syndrome* (BRS) represents a new electrocardiographic (ECG) marker of SCD in otherwise healthy individuals (Brugada and Brugada, 1992).

The prevalence of VF associated with the BRS has been estimated as high as 40 to 60% of all cases of idiopathic VF (Chen et al., 1998). Certain electrophysiologic similarities have been found between ECG markers of the BRS, early repolarization syndrome, and hypothermia (Gussak et al., 1999). A strong link has been identified between the BRS and sudden and unexpected death syndrome (SUDS) in Southeast Asian males (Nademanes et al., 1997). Possible overlap with arrhythmogenic right ventricular dysplasia has been suggested (Scheinman, 1997).

Recent genetic data link the BRS to an ion channel gene mutation resulting in heterogeneous loss of the action potential dome in the right ventricular epicardium, a mechanism underlying both idiopathic ST-segment elevation in the right precordial leads and the dispersion of repolarization that predisposes the heart to the development of malignant reentrant ventricular arrhythmias. (Chen et al., 1998).

Patients with the *concealed* and the *asymptomatic* forms of the syndrome, in whom preclinical diagnosis and risk stratification are vital to the prevention of the fatal ventricular arrhythmias, present a great challenge, both in establishing the diagnosis and determining the prognosis.

Clinical Assessment of Patients with Suspected or Documented Brugada Syndrome: Diagnosis and Risk Stratification

Traditionally, diagnosis of *apparent* BRS was based on the presence of *idiopathic* J-point elevation followed by downsloping ST segments in the right-sided chest leads in patients with clinically documented episodes of ventricular tachycardia/ventricular fibrillation (VT/VF) or unexpected syncope of unknown origin (Gussak et al., 1999). However, the initial optimism that a diagnosis of BRS could be made simply on the basis of distinct ECG changes (see below) has been tempered, both by a high incidence of false-positive and false-negative cases related to "waxing" and "waning" ECG signature (Gussak and Chaitman, 1999; Gussak et al., 2001; Brugada et al., 2000a) and by drug- or disease-induced ECG abnormalities resembling those in BRS (Littman et al., 2000; Bolognesi et al., 1997; Tarin et al., 1999). Diagnostic criteria for BRS are summarized in Table 58-1. One major and one minor criterion are associated with increased likelihood of BRS. (Gussak et al., 2001).

The clinical presentation of BRS should be considered when (1) a resting 12-lead ECG has shown changes compatible with BRS, or (2) symptoms or family history suggests increased risk of SCD in the setting of a structurally normal heart.

Resting ECG

The ECG marker of BRS has three components:

1. Elevated terminal portion of the QRS complex (prominent J wave)

TABLE 58-1

DIAGNOSTIC CRITERIA FOR BRUGADA SYNDROME

Major criteria

1. Presence of the ECG marker of Brugada syndrome in patients with structurally normal heart

2. Appearance of the ECG marker of Brugada syndrome after administration of sodium channel blockers

Minor criteria

1. Family history of sudden cardiac death

2. Syncope of unknown origin

3. Documented episodes of ventricular tachycardia/ventricular fibrillation

4. Positive programmed electrocardiostimulation test on ventricular tachycardia/ventricular fibrillation

5. Genetic mutations of ion channels

2. Non-injury-related ("idiopathic") elevated descending ST segment

3. Negative T wave in the same right-sided precordial leads.

Leads V_1 to V_3 show the most prominent changes, with the degree of ST-segment elevation tapering off in adjacent leads. These peculiar ECG abnormalities of ventricular repolarization are often more prominent in the right chest leads placed one intercostal space higher than usual, and often associated with normal QT interval (Gussak et al., 1999; Bjerregaard et al., 1994; Gussak et al., 1995). It is also a characteristic finding that the ST-segment elevation in the right precordial leads is not accompanied by reciprocal ST-segment depression in opposite leads (Fig. 58-1A) and is often associated with varying degrees of conduction block in the right bundle branch.

The role of the conduction defect in the right ventricle is a matter of some controversy. It has been pointed out that in patients with BRS, early repolarization abnormalities, but not right bundle branch block (RBBB), are an integral part of its ECG signature (Bjerregaard et al., 1994; Gussak et al., 1995). There is no correlation between RBBB and SCD, whereas a definite link exists between the magnitude of ST-segment elevation and incidence of the life-threatening arrhythmic events in patients with BRS (Itoh et al., 2001). More prominent ST-segment elevation in the right chest leads has been observed immediately before (Fig. 58-1B) and after episodes of aborted SCD in some patients (Gussak et al., 1999).

J-point elevation followed by downsloping ST segment and negative T wave have also been reported in some patients with arrhythmogenic right ventricular dysplasia (Scheinman, 1997; Fontaine, 1995). In patients with BRS, this would occur without obvious pathologic findings; in patients with arrhythmogenic right ventricular dysplasia, myocardial cells are replaced by fatty tissue.

In many patients with the BRS, the ECG manifestations transiently normalize, leading to underdiagnosis of the syndrome. Strong sodium channel blockade can unmask the ST-segment elevation in leads V_1 to V_3 and conduction disturbances in the right ventricle in many patients (Fig. 58-2). A number of other

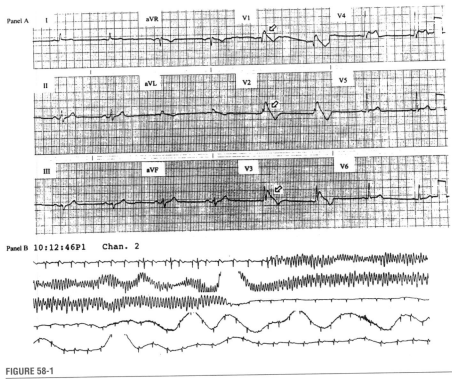

FIGURE 58-1

(*A*) Twelve-lead ECG of a patient with Brugada syndrome. The right precordial leads, V₁-V₃, display J-point elevation and downsloping ST segments. The QRS is normal, but QT dispersion between V₂ and V₆ is larger than normal (120 ms). (*B*) Self-terminating polymorphic ventricular tachycardia (continuous recording) in a patient with the Brugada syndrome. Closely coupled premature ventricular contractions precede the onset of tachyarrhythmia. Note the disappearance of the repolarization abnormalities following the arrhythmia. (Adapted from I Gussak et al: J Am Coll Cardiol 33:5, 1999, with permission.)

agents, including adrenergic and cholinergic neurohormones, are also capable of modulating the degree of ST-segment elevation in BRS. β-Adrenoreceptor stimulation and α-adrenoreceptor blockade reduce the magnitude of ST-segment elevation, whereas β-adrenergic blockade, α-adrenergic stimulation, sodium channel blockade, and muscarinic stimulation augment the ST-segment elevation it (Antzelevitch; 1998; Brugada et al.; 1998; Miyazaki et al., 1996).

The prevalence of the ECG marker for BRS in persons with idiopathic VF and in healthy controls is the subject of ongoing investigation (Viskin et al., 2000; Hermida et al., 2000). Many clinical cases have been reported in countries worldwide, particularly in Japan and Southeast Asia, with a tendency to familial predisposition (Brugada and Brugada, 1992; Chen et al., 1998; Nademanee et al., 1997; Gussak et al., 2001). The incidence of SUDS among Asians living in the United States varies among different ethnic groups from 1:2500 to 1:1087. In the majority of victims of SUDS, apparent or concealed BRS as well as strong family history of unexpected and unexplained death have been well documented, (Nademanee et al., 1997).

Thus, as in the case of long QT syndrome, a diagnosis of BRS can be established with only a degree of certainty and must rely on both clinical presentation and diagnostic findings. The ECG

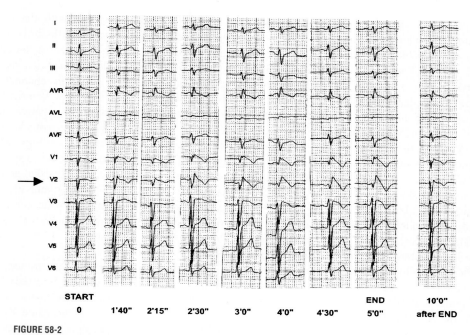

FIGURE 58-2

The effect of the sodium channel blocker Ajmaline in a patient with concealed Brugada syndrome. Note: Transient appearance of the elevated downsloping ST-segment elevation in V$_1$-V$_3$ leads accompanied by conduction deterioration in the right ventricle. (Courtesy of Dr. P. Brugada).

findings described above are the cornerstones for the diagnosis and must occur either spontaneously or following provocative testing with sodium-blocking drugs. Since there are false-positive findings, other possible causes for such ECG changes must be considered.

Signal-Averaged ECG

Positive late potentials on the signal-averaged ECG are a common finding in BRS, particularly in patients in whom an elevated ST segment is accompanied by apparent RBBB, and their role, as noninvasive markers, in risk stratification is of interest (Ikeda et al., 2001).

However, the sensitivity and specificity for late potentials to predict arrhythmogenic events varies, depending on the clinical setting (Borggrefe et al., 1997; Englund et al., 1998), the arrhythmogenic mechanisms that underlie the disease process, and

the presence of the intraventricular conduction defects, which reduce diagnostic accuracy (Gussak et al., 2001). The signal-averaged ECG is a reasonable test in the diagnostic workup of suspected BRS: positive detection of late potentials could strengthen the indication for invasive electrophysiologic testing.

Programmed Electrical Stimulation and Sodium Channel Blockade

Sodium channel blocking drugs have been used to unmask ECG changes in *concealed* forms of BRS (Hermida et al., 2000). Antiarrhythmic drugs such as ajmaline, flecainide, propafenone, and procainamide have been shown to produce or augment ECG changes typical of BRS, and also to evaluate the inducibility of VT/VF during programmed electrical stimulation in both apparent and concealed forms of BRS (Brugada et al., 2000b). Programmed electrical stimulation (positive predictive value: 50%, negative predictive value: 46%) and pharmacologic challenge with sodium channel blockers (positive predictive value: 35%) are of limited value in identifying patients at risk (Priori et al., 2000). However, electrophysiologic testing, including provocative tests of inducibility of VT/VF and drug effects on (1) the magnitude of ST-segment elevation and (2) inducibility of VT/VF, are still the most appropriate tests for confirmation of the diagnosis and for risk stratification for SCD in patients with BRS at the current time (Gussak et al., 1999; Gussak et al., 2001; Brugada et al., 2000a, 2000b).

Since sodium channels blockers do not normally provoke malignant ventricular tachyarrhythmias, electrophysiologic testing is primarily indicated for evaluating the inducibility of VT/VF before or after drug administration. Drug challenge is best applied to cases of concealed BRS. Since ajmaline is not available in the United States, procainamide or flecainide could be the agents of choice in this country (Gussak et al., 2001).

Other diagnostic tools are of limited value; imaging techniques, endocardial biopsy, and cardiac catheterization are useful mainly in ruling out structural cardiac abnormalities. Finally, extension of the testing to family members is also important because of a high incidence of familial occurrence.

Thus, any BRS patient with either spontaneous or inducible ventricular tachyarrhythmias should be considered at high risk for SCD, and a reasonable approach would be to treat with an implantable cardiac defibrillator.

Etiology, Pathogenesis, and Genetics

Possible Ionic and Cellular Mechanisms

Accentuation of ST-segment elevation in patients with BRS following vagal maneuvers or sodium channel blockers, as well as normalization of ST-segment elevation following β-adrenergic agents, are concordant with the findings in isolated myocardial tissue preparations. The appearance of ST-segment elevation only in right precordial leads in patients

with BRS is also consistent with the observation that loss of the action potential dome is much more easily induced in right vs. left ventricular epicardium because of the higher density of I_{to} in right vs. left ventricular epicardium. Sodium channel blockers also facilitate loss of the right ventricular action potential dome as a result of a negative shift in the voltage at which phase 1 begins (Antzelevich, 1998). These similarities in electrophysiology, pharmacology, and ECG have prompted some to speculate that a depressed right ventricular epicardial action potential dome underlies the ST-segment elevation and that phase 2 reentry may provide the trigger for episodes of VF in patients with BRS (Gussak et al., 1999; Gussak and Chaitman, 1999; Antzelevitch, 1998).

The BRS is genetically determined. Approximately 60% of patients with (aborted) SCD with the typical ECG have a family history of SCD or have family members with the same ECG abnormalities. In 25% of families, there appears to be an autosomal dominant mode of transmission with variable expression of the abnormal gene; sporadic cases of the de novo mutation have also been reported (www.brugada.crtia.be/aboutthissite/index2.html). The first gene to be linked to BRS was reported in early 1998 (Chen et al., 1998). Mutations in the cardiac sodium channel gene, *SCN5A*, the same gene responsible for the long QT syndrome, have been identified (Fig. 58-3). Mutations have been identified in the gene that encodes the α subunit of the sodium channel *(SCN5A)* on chromosome 3. This genetic defect causes a reduction in the density of the sodium current and explains the worsening of the above ECG abnormalities when patients are treated with sodium channel blocking antiarrhythmic agents, which further diminish the already reduced sodium current (Naccarelli and Antzelevitch, 2001). *SCN5A* was excluded as the gene causing BRS in at least one family, leading to the speculation that genetic heterogeneity exists in BRS (Chen et al., 1998).

These genetic findings provide further support for a primary electrical disease as the basis for the BRS form of idiopathic VT/VF.

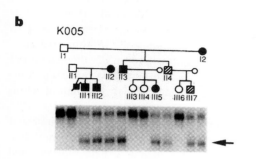

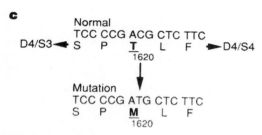

FIGURE 58-3

Cardiac sodium channel gene *SCN5A* missense mutation co-segregating with the Brugada syndrome. (*A*) ECG of an affected individual. Note the elevated ST segment in leads V₁-V₃. (*B*) Pedigree structure and mutation analysis using single-strand conformation polymorphism (SSCP) analysis with primers amplifying exon 28 of the cardiac sodium channel gene, SCN5A. Affected individuals are filled circles (females) and filled squares (males). Unaffected individuals are empty symbols, and individuals without clinical data are shown as hatched. The individual who suffered sudden cardiac death is slashed. (*C*) DNA and amino-acid sequences of the SCN5A missense mutation associated with the Brugada syndrome. DNA sequence analysis revealed a C-to-T substitution, which causes the substitution of a highly conserved threonine by a methionine at codon 1620 (T1620M mutation) in the extracellular loop between DIVS3 and DIVS4. (Adapted from Q Chen et al: Nature 392:293, 1998, with permission.)

Mechanisms of Arrhythmia: Delayed Conduction Versus Early Repolarization Abnormalities.

The finding of a variable degree of intraventricular conduction in patients with BRS delay is not a surprising finding when the well-documented genetic mutations of the sodium ion channels are considered (Chen et al., 1998; Bezzina et al., 1999; Deschenes et al., 2000). While no correlation between RBBB and SCD has yet been established in a population other than that with BRS, the magnitude of ST-segment elevation has been linked to the incidence of life-threatening arrhythmic events, particularly in BRS patients (Gussak and Chaitman, 1999; Bolognesi et al., 1997; Itoh et al., 2001).

The reentry mechanism that underlines the arrhythmogenic potential in BRS has been considered based on the high inducibility and reproducibility of VT/VF during electrophysiologic testing (Brugada and Brugada, 1992; Gussak et al., 1999; Nademanee et al., 1997; Brugada et al., 2000a, 2000b). Whether development and maintenance of reentry are due to a delayed conduction and/or its degree or to dispersion of repolarization, however, is not known. Moreover, it must be emphasized that all mechanisms currently proposed to explain the full scope of arrhythmogenic potential in BRS are speculative (Gussak et al., 2001).

The Brugada Syndrome and Early Repolarization Syndrome

Early repolarization syndrome has been identified predominantly in young, otherwise healthy males and has a predisposition to familial occurrence. Its ECG manifestation may normalize transiently in many individuals, and the syndrome shows a response to drugs and autonomic modulation similar to that of BRS (Gussak et al., 1999; Gussak and Antzelevitch, 2000). In experimental models, the ECG signature of early repolarization syndrome may mimic that of BRS (Gussak and Antzelevitch, 2000).

Clinical interest in early repolarization syndrome has been rekindled recently because of its similarities with the ECG manifestations of the highly arrhythmogenic BRS and the potential for misdiagnosis (Gussak and Antzelevitch, 2000). In some clinical instances, it is difficult to distinguish patients with early repolarization syndrome from those with BRS, based solely on a resting ECG. The former, although characterized by idiopathic ST-segment elevation, is different from BRS in that it is generally not associated with arrhythmias. Electrocardiographically, both syndromes resemble a pattern of reversed Wolff-Parkinson-White syndrome, with a distinct slur or notch on the downstroke of the R wave. Two major features permit differentiation of the ECG signatures of early repolarization syndrome and BRS: *pattern* and *lead specificity*. The elevated ST-segment in early repolarization syndrome is usually localized in leads V_2-$V_{4(5)}$ and has an upward concavity with positive T-wave polarity accompanied by a notched J point (Gussak et al., 1999; Gussak and Antzelevitch, 2000). In contrast, the ECG of BRS patients generally displays a prominent J-point elevation, followed by a downsloping ST segment and negative T wave in the right precordial leads (V_1-V_3) only (Gussak et al., 1999; Gussak and Antzelevitch, 2000).

Electrophysiologically, the early repolarization and Brugada syndromes share some common mechanisms of drug and neuromodulation. As with BRS, isoproterenol is known to reduce or even eliminate the ST-segment elevation in individuals with early repolarization syndrome, whereas propranolol increases the magnitude of ST-segment elevation (Myazaki et al., 1996).

Clinical Course, Prognosis, and Current Concepts of the Treatment Strategy

The mean age of affected individuals is in the mid to late thirties, ranging from newborn to 70 years. All clinical manifestations of BRS are attributed exclusively to the life-threatening ventricular tachyarrhythmias and their complications. Tragically, in some patients, SCD is the first and only clinical event. In the majority of cases, malignant tachyarrhythmias occur at rest and in many cases at night time, especially in Japan and Southeastern Asia (Nademanee et al., 1997; Itoh et al., 2001; Ikeda et al., 2001; Miyazaki et al., 1996). A sudden rise in vagal activity has been reported to occur just before VF episodes in some patients. Among other manifestations of the electrical instability are frequent premature ventricular complexes and paroxysmal atrial fibrillation (Itoh et al., 2001).

The prognosis is poor in BRS with documented arrhythmias, with up to a 10% per year mortality. Antiarrhythmic drugs including beta blockers and amiodarone have not shown benefit in prolonging survival. (Naccarelli and Antzelevitch, 2001). The incidence of arrhythmic events is similar in patients receiving either an implantable cardiac defibrillator, amiodarone, or β-adrenergic blockers. However, only patients with the defibrillator are protected from SCD (Gussak et al., 1999; Brugada et al., 2000a, 2000b).

Thus, at present there are no specific pharmacologic treatments for preventing SCD in patients with BRS. Diagnosis and prevention of life-threatening ventricular tachyarrhythmias and their complications is one of the main objectives of therapy. The only treatment presently known to be effective against SCD in these patients is the implantable cardiac defibrillator (Viskin et al., 1997; Gussak et al., 1999; Brugada et al., 2000a, 2000b).

SUMMARY

The Brugada syndrome is a malignant primary electrical disease of the heart caused by a defect in an ion channel gene, resulting in abnormal electrophysiologic activity in the right ventricle and characterized by (1) a phenotypic ST-segment elevation in the right-sided precordial leads often accompanied by apparent conduction block in the right ventricle, (2) grossly structurally normal heart, and

(3) a propensity for life-threatening ventricular tachyarrhythmias.

Due to clinical and genetic heterogeneity of the syndrome, patients with BRS present a great challenge, both in establishing the diagnosis and determining the prognosis. Patients at risk often show periodic normalization of their ECG, leading to underestimation of incidence of BRS. Sodium channel blockers can be used to unmask the syndrome. The only unequivocally effective treatment to date is an implantable cardiac defibrillator, which should be considered in symptomatic and asymptomatic individuals with positive electrophysiologic testing.

REFERENCES

Antzelevitch C: The Brugada syndrome. J Cardiovasc Electrophysiol 9:513, 1998

Bezzina C et al: A single Na(+) channel mutation causing both long-QT and Brugada syndromes. Circ Res 85:1206, 1999

Bjerregaard P et al: Recurrent syncope in a patient with prominent J wave. Am Heart J 127:1426, 1994

Bolognesi R et al: Abnormal ventricular repolarization mimicking myocardial infarction after heterocyclic antidepressant overdose. Am J Cardiol 79:242, 1997

Borggrefe M et al: Prediction of arrhythmia risk based on signal-averaged ECG in postinfarction patients. Pacing Clin Electrophysiol 20:2566, 1997

Brugada P, Brugada J: Right bundle-branch block, persistent ST segment elevation and sudden cardiac death: A distinct clinical and electrocardiographic syndrome. A multicenter report. J Am Coll Cardiol 20:1391, 1992

Brugada J et al: Right bundle-branch block and ST-segment elevation in leads V_1 through V_3. A marker for sudden death in patients without demonstrable structural heart disease. Circulation 97:457, 1998

Brugada P et al: Sudden death in patients and relatives with the syndrome of right bundle branch block, ST segment elevation in the precordial leads V(1) to V(3) and sudden death. Eur Heart J 21:321, 2000a

Brugada R et al: Sodium channel blockers identify risk for sudden death in patients with ST-segment elevation and right bundle branch block but structurally normal hearts. Circulation 101:510, 2000b

Chen Q et al: Genetic basis and molecular mechanism for idiopathic ventricular fibrillation. Nature 392:293, 1998

Deschenes I et al: Electrophysiological characterization of SCN5A mutations causing long QT (E1784K) and Brugada (R1512W and R1432G) syndromes. Cardiovasc Res 46:55, 2000

Englund A et al: Wavelet decomposition analysis of the signal-averaged electrocardiogram used for risk stratification of patients with hypertrophic cardiomyopathy. Eur Heart J 19:1383, 1998

Fontaine G: Arrhythmogenic right ventricular dysplasia. Curr Opin Cardiol 10:16, 1995

Gussak I, Antzelevitch C: Early repolarization syndrome: Clinical characteristics and possible cellular and ionic mechanisms. J Electrocardiol 33:299, 2000

Gussak I et al: ECG phenomenon called the J wave: History, pathophysiology, and clinical significance. J Electrocardiol 28:49, 1995

Gussak I et al: The Brugada syndrome: Clinical, electrophysiologic and genetic aspects. J Am Coll Cardiol 33:5, 1999

Gussak I et al: Clinical diagnosis and risk stratification in patients with Brugada syndrome. J Am Coll Cardiol 37:1635, 2001

Hermida JS et al: Prevalence of the Brugada syndrome in an apparently healthy population. Am J Cardiol 86:91, 2000

Ikeda T et al: Assessment of noninvasive markers in identifying patients at risk in the Brugada syndrome: Insight into risk stratification. J Am Coll Cardiol 37:1628, 2001

Itoh H et al, for the Hokuriku Brugada Study Group: Arrhythmias in patients with Brugada-type electrocardiographic findings. Jpn Circ J 65:483, 2001

Littmann L et al: Brugada-type electrocardiographic pattern induced by cocaine. Mayo Clin Proc 75: 845, 2000

Miyazaki T et al: Autonomic and antiarrhythmic drug modulation of ST segment elevation in patients with Brugada syndrome. J Am Coll Cardiol 27:1061, 1996

Naccarelli GV, Antzelevitch C: The Brugada syndrome: Clinical, genetic, cellular, and molecular abnormalities. Am J Med 110:573, 2001

Nademanee K et al: Arrhythmogenic marker for the sudden unexplained death syndrome in Thai men. Circulation 96:2595, 1997

Priori SG et al: Clinical and genetic heterogeneity of right bundle branch block and ST-segment elevation syndrome: A prospective evaluation of 52 families. Circulation 102:2509, 2000

Scheinman MM: Is Brugada syndrome a distinct clinical entity? J Cardiovasc Electrophysiol 8:332, 1997

Tarin N et al: Brugada-like electrocardiographic pattern in a patient with a mediastinal tumor. Pacing Clin Electrophysiol 22:1264, 1999

Viskin S et al: Mode of onset of malignant ventricular arrhythmias in idiopathic ventricular fibrillation. J Cardiovasc Electrophysiol 8:1115, 1997

Viskin S et al: Prevalence of the Brugada sign in idiopathic ventricular fibrillation and healthy controls. Heart 84:31, 2000

ARRHYTHMOGENIC RIGHT VENTRICULAR DYSPLASIA/ CARDIOMYOPATHY

Hugh Calkins, Frank Marcus

Arrhythmogenic right ventricular dysplasia or cardiomyopathy (ARVD/C) is an inheritable heart muscle disease characterized by ventricular arrhythmias and structural abnormalities of the right ventricle due to progressive replacement of right ventricular myocardium with fatty and fibrous tissue. The precise prevalence of ARVD/C is unknown as patients with a clinical diagnosis of ARVD/C represent only one spectrum of the disease. However, the prevalence of the disease has been estimated to be 6/10,000 in one region of Italy. Since the initial description of ARVD/C approximately two decades ago, much has been learned about this disease. The purpose of this chapter is to review our current understanding of ARVD/C and also to highlight those questions that remain unanswered.

Clinical Presentation and Natural History

The first large series of patients with ARVD/C was reported by Marcus and colleagues (Marcus et al., 1982). The information about ARVD/C has increased significantly since then as a result of studies by Corrado and others (Corrado et al., 1997, 2000). ARVD/C most commonly comes to clinical attention because of the presence of ventricular arrhythmias, which range from isolated premature beats to sustained ventricular tachycardia or ventricular fibrillation. These ventricular arrhythmias, which are of right ventricular (RV) origin, may be asymptomatic and detected by a routine electrocardiogram (ECG) or they may cause palpitations, syncope, or sudden cardiac death (SCD). Although ARVD/C is a relatively uncommon cause of SCD, it accounted for up to one-fifth of all episodes of SCD that occurred in patients below the age of 35 in the Veneto region of Italy (Thiene et al., 1988). Patients with ARVD/C usually present with ventricular arrhythmias after puberty and before the age of 45 years. There is a predominance of males. Exercise has been identified as a common precipitant of the arrhythmias that occur in patients with ARVD/C. The natural history of patients with ARVD/C is primarily a function of the degree of cardiac electrical instability. The natural history of the disease appears to be highly variable. SCD is the first manifestation of the disease in some patients with ARVD/C. Other patients have mild asymptomatic disease, which may or may not progress over several decades and result in sustained ventricular arrhythmias, while yet other patients develop progressive right and occasionally biventricular heart failure as a late manifestation. At the present time, very little is known about the typical clinical course of ARVD/C in patients with overt disease or in those who are asymptomatic family members of an ARVD/C patient. The factors that determine rate and degree of progression from one stage to another remain undefined.

Diagnosis

Diagnosis of ARVD/C is based on the identification of electrical, anatomical, and functional abnormalities that predominantly affect the right ventricle in a person with ventricular arrhythmias. Standardized major and minor diagnostic criteria have been established (Table 59-1) (McKenna et al., 1994). The diagnosis of ARVD/C is established by the presence of two major criteria or one major plus two minor criteria, or no major and four minor criteria. Specific cardiac tests that are usually recommended in all patients with suspected ARVD/C include an ECG, a signal-averaged ECG, an exercise stress test, an echocardiogram, a Holter monitor, and a chest x-ray. Additional tests performed by many centers include cardiac magnetic resonance imaging, a multiple-gated acquisition blood pool scan, cardiac catheterization with right ventriculography, an endomyocardial biopsy, and/or an electrophysiology study.

The major condition that needs to be differentiated from ARVD/C is ventricular tachycardia arising from the RV outflow tract in the absence of structural heart disease. This type of ventricular tachycardia has many similarities with ARVD/C: (1) it occurs during exercise; (2) it has a left bundle branch block inferior axis morphology consistent with an origin from the RV outflow tract (this is one of the several types of ventricular tachycardia morphologies that may be seen in ARVD/C); and (3) it occurs predominantly in young, otherwise healthy people (Table 59-2). Other entities that need to be considered in the differential diagnosis of ARVD/C are abnormalities that primarily affect the right side of the heart such as an atrial septal defect, anomalous pulmonary venous return, and Ebstein's malformation.

Pathology/Etiology

The most striking morphologic feature of ARVD/C is segmental or diffuse replacement of epicardium and midmyocardium of the free wall of the right ventricle by fatty or fibrofatty tissue. The endocardium and the septum are usually spared. The RV wall thickness is usually normal, but there may be focal thinning of the right ventricle. Histologic evaluation reveals myocardial atrophy with residual myocytes interspersed with fibrofatty tissue. As the disease progresses, the left ventricle may become involved, particularly the epicardium of the left ventricle. Aneurysms that typically affect the inflow, apical, and outflow portions of the right ventricle (referred to as the *triangle of dysplasia*) have been reported in approximately half of autopsy cases. Evidence of patchy and acute inflammation with myocyte death and focal round cell infiltrates, mostly lymphocytes, are present in two-thirds of cases (Thiene et al., 1991). It is not known whether this inflammation represents evidence of viral myocarditis or is the response to the process that causes destruction of the myocardium. The diagnosis of ARVD/C may be overlooked by routine autopsy because the limit between normal and pathologic fatty infiltration is unclear.

Three mechanisms have been proposed for the replacement of RV myocardium with fibrofatty tissue that occurs in patients with ARVD/C. The first mechanism, outlined above, is inflammation of the myocardium. This may be due to myocarditis and may cause fibrous healing. The second mechanism proposed is apoptosis (Mallat et al., 1996). And the third proposed mechanism for ARVD/C is genetically determined myocardial atrophy.

Genetics

A family history of ARVD/C is present in up to 50% of cases (Marcus et al., 2000). Linkage analysis has identified six genetic loci on chromosomes 1, 2, 3, 10, and 14 for the autosomal dominant form. Some families are not linked to these loci, which suggests further genetic heterogeneity. There is

TABLE 59-1

CRITERIA FOR DIAGNOSIS OF ARRHYTHMOGENIC RIGHT VENTRICULAR DYSPLASIA/CARDIOMYOPATHY

I. Global and/or regional dysfunction of the right ventricle.

   A. Major

      1. Severe dilation and reduction of the RV ejection fraction with no (or only mild) LV impairment

      2. Localize RV aneurysms (akinetic or dyskenetic areas with diastolic bulging)

      3. Severe segmental dilation of the right ventricle

   B. Minor

      1. Mild global RV dilation and/or ejection fraction reduction with normal left ventricle

      2. Mild segmental dilation of the right ventricle

      3. Regional RV hypokinesia

II. Tissue characterization of walls

   A. Major

      1. Fibrofatty replacement of myocardium on endomyocardial biopsy

III. Repolarization Abnormalities

   A. Minor

      1. Inverted T waves in the right precordial leads (V_2 and V_3) (age $>$12 years, in absence of RBBB)

IV. Depolarization/Conduction Abnormalities

   A. Major

      1. Epsilon waves or localized prolongation ($>$110 ms) of the QRS complex in the right precordial leads (V_1-V_3)

   B. Minor

      1. Late potentials on signal-averaged ECG

V. Arrhythmias

   A. Minor

      1. Left bundle branch block type ventricular tachycardia (sustained and nonsustained) (ECG, Holter, exercise testing)

      2. Frequent ventricular extrasystoles ($>$1000/24 h) (Holter)

VI. Family History

   A. Major

      1. Familial disease confirmed at necropsy or surgery

   B. Minor

      1. Familial history of premature sudden death ($<$35 years) due to suspected RV dysplasia

      2. Familial history (clinical diagnosis based on present criteria)

ABBREVIATIONS: ECG, electrocardiogram; LV, left ventricular; RBBB, right bundle branch block; RV, right ventricular.
SOURCE: From WJ McKenna et al: Br Heart J 71:215, 1994.

evidence that there may be different phenotypic expressions of the different genes. There are both intra- and interfamilial variation in disease presentation and severity. Thus, screening of first-degree relatives is recommended and should be repeated every 3 to 5 years, as signs and symptoms may have a later onset. A patient with ARVD/C has a 50% risk of passing the disease to a child.

TABLE 59-2

DIFFERENTIATION OF ARVD/C FROM RVOT TACHYCARDIA FROM THE SURFACE ECG

	ARVD/C	RVO-VT	Control
T inversion > V_2	54%[a]	33%	1%
Max. QRS duration ($V_1 - V_3$)	114 ± 19 ms	104 ± 13 ms	98 ± 11 ms
Max QRS > 110 ms ($V_1 - V_3$)	52%[a]	21%	13%
Epsilon potential	23%[a]	3%	0%
Late potential (25 Hz)	41%[a]	12%	3%
QRS dispersion	40 ± 13 ms[a]	34 ± 10 ms	33 ± 9 ms
QT dispersion	54 ± 21 ms	47 ± 16 ms	40 ± 13 ms

[a]$p < .001$ ARVD/C vs. RVOT tachycardia and control
ABBREVIATIONS: ARVD/C, arrhythmogenic right ventricular dysplasia/cardiomyopathy; ECG, electrocardiogram; RVO-VT, right ventricular outflow tract ventricular tachycardia.
SOURCE: Adapted from T Wichter et al: Pacing Clin Electrophysiol 22:A69, 1999.

A mutation in the cardiac ryanodine receptor gene (RYR2) on chromosome 1 has been reported in four Italian families with ARVD/C and effort-induced polymorphic ventricular tachycardia (Tiso et al., 2001). These families appear to be clinically distinct from other patients with ARVD/C in the type of tachycardia (the pathology being limited to the RV apex), the high penetrance rate, and the equal numbers of males and females affected (Bauce et al., 2000). Genetic testing for RYR2 mutations is not available on a clinical basis at this time, and there are no published reports of patients with ARVD and monomorphic ventricular tachycardia being screened for RYR2 mutations. RYR2 is activated by calcium and induces the release of calcium from the sarcoplasmic reticulum into the cytosol (Tiso et al., 2001). The theory is that a mutation in the receptor would lead to calcium leakage. RYR2 is related to the RYR1 receptor found in skeletal muscle and involved in malignant hyperthermia susceptibility.

There is a rare autosomal recessive form of ARVD that is always found in combination with palmoplantar keratoderma and woolly hair, called *Naxos disease* (Coonar et al., 1998). It is an extremely rare condition, with the majority of patients being from Naxos, Greece. The gene for Naxos disease was identified as plakoglobin when a homozygous mutation causing frameshifts was found in 19 patients and unaffected family members were heterozygous for the mutation (McKoy et al., 2000). Subsequently, 8 of 40 heterozygous family members were reported to show minor cardiac abnormalities; 5 of the 8 had woolly hair phenotype but none had palmoplantar keratoderma (Protonotarios et al., 2001). Patients with the autosomal dominant form of ARVD have been tested for mutations in plakoglobin, but none have been found (McKoy et al., 2000). Plakoglobin is involved in cell adhesion and possibly in the formation of desmosomal junctions. Three families in Ecuador with dilated cardiomyopathy, woolly hair, and keratoderma, also inherited in an autosomal recessive form, were found to have a mutation in a related gene called desmoplakin (Norgett et al., 2000).

Management

The management of patients with ARVD/C is typically directed at treating their ventricular arrhythmias. This may involve antiarrhythmic drug therapy, catheter ablation, and/or placement of an implantable defibrillator. To date, there have been no prospective trials to determine the relative safety and efficacy of these approaches. There have also been no prospective trials to determine which of the many antiarrhythmic agents is optimal for treatment of the arrhythmias that occur in patients with ARVD/C. If a patient has a benign form of the disease, no specific treatment may be needed. Placement of an implantable defibrillator is generally recommended for ARVD/C patients who are considered to be at increased risk for SCD. These risk factors include: (1) a prior cardiac arrest; (2) syncope due to ventricular tachycardia; (3) evidence for extensive RV disease (T-wave inversion in V_3 or beyond, markedly abnormal late potentials, RV enlargement and wall motion abnormalities on echocardiography); (4) left ventricular involvement; and (5) presentation with polymorphic ventricular tachycardia and a RV apical aneurysm (which is associated with a genetic locus on chromosome 1q42–43). Turrini and colleagues recently reported that increased QRS dispersion (longest minus shortest QRS duration in 12 leads $\geq$ 40 ms) was the strongest independent predictor of sudden death in ARVD/C patients, followed by a history of syncope (Turrini et al., 2001).

Implantable defibrillators are also often placed in patients with ARVD/C who have had a family member die of SCD. Whether these individuals are at increased risk of sudden death has not been determined. It is not known whether patients with ARVD/C who have experienced sustained ventricular tachycardia in the absence of syncope benefit from placement from an implantable cardioverter defibrillator. Catheter ablation is generally not relied on as primary therapy because of a high incidence of recurrence, which reflects in part the progressive nature of the disease.

It is also not known whether other types of medical therapy, such as angiotensin-converting enzyme inhibitors or beta blockers, may alter the course of ARVD/C. Similarly, it is unknown whether avoidance of exercise may alter the clinical course of the disease. There is, however, at least some evidence that vigorous exercise may exacerbate the disease and for this reason it is generally recommended that patients with ARVD/C avoid competitive athletics.

Unanswered Questions

A large number of questions remain unanswered regarding the diagnosis and treatment of ARVD/C. For example, it remains uncertain how best to diagnose or exclude the diagnosis of ARVD/C in patients with a mild form of the disease and in relatives of affected individuals. The natural history of ARVD/C has also not been well defined. In addition, the optimal approach to treatment of patients with ARVD/C has not been defined. Which patients should have an implantable defibrillator inserted? Should patients with possible ARVD/C cease exercising? The ultimate goal is to localize the genes that cause ARVD. This information would greatly facilitate diagnosis of the disease and would also allow for genotype/phenotype correlations. In addition, the identification of the specific genetic defect may ultimately have specific therapeutic implications for gene therapy. In an effort to address some of these questions, a European registry and a U.S. registry for ARVD/C are now underway (Corrado et al., 2000). In the United States, the ARVD/C registry has been funded by the National Heart, Lung, and Blood Institute and will start enrolling ARVD/C patients in 2002. More information concerning these registries is available at ARVD.org and ARVD.com. Hopefully, this effort and others in the years ahead will provide answers to the many unanswered questions concerning ARVD/C.

REFERENCES

Bauce B et al: Familial effort polymorphic ventricular arrhythmias in arrhythmogenic right ventricular cardiomyopathy map to chromosome 1q42–43. Am J Cardiol 85:573, 2000

Coonar AS et al: Gene for arrhythmogenic right ventricular cardiomyopathy with diffuse nonepidermolytic palmoplantar keratoderma and woolly hair (Naxos disease) maps to 17q21. Circulation 97:2049, 1998

Corrado D et al: Spectrum of clinicopathologic manifestations of arrhythmogenic right ventricular cardiomyopathy/dysplasia: A multicenter study. J Am Coll Cardiol 30:1512, 1997

Corrado D et al: Arrhythmogenic Right Ventricular Dysplasia/Cardiomyopathy: Need for an International Registry. J Cardiovasc Electrophysiol 11:827-832, 2000

Mallat Z et al: Evidence of apoptosis in arrhythmogenic right ventricular dysplasia. N Engl J Med 335:1190, 1996

Marcus FI et al: Right ventricular dysplasia: A report of 24 adult cases. Circulation 65:384, 1982

Marcus FI et al: Arrhythmogenic right ventricular dysplasia/cardiomyopathy, in *Molecular Genetics of Cardiac Electrophysiology,* CI Berul, JA Towbin (eds). Boston Kluwer Academic, pp 239–250, 2000

McKenna WJ et al: Diagnosis of arrhythmogenic right ventricular dysplasia/cardiomyopathy. Br Heart J 71:215, 1994

McKoy G et al: Identification of a deletion in plakoglobin in arrhythmogenic right ventricular cardiomyopathy with palmoplantar keratoderma and woolly hair (Naxos disease). Lancet 355:2119, 2000

Norgett EE et al: Recessive mutation in desmoplakin disrupts desmoplakin-intermediate filament interactions and causes dilated cardiomyopathy, woolly hair and keratoderma Hum Mol Genet 9:2761, 2000

Protonotarios N et al: Genotype-phenotype assessment in autosomal recessive arrhythmogenic right ventricular cardiomyopathy (Naxos disease) caused by a deletion in plakoglobin. J Am Coll Cardiol 38:1477-84, 2001

Thiene G et al: Right ventricular cardiomyopathy and sudden death in young people. N Engl J Med 318:129, 1988

Tiso N et al: Identification of mutations in the cardiac ryanodine receptor gene in families affected with arrhythmogenic right ventricular cardiomyopathy type 2 (ARVD2). Hum Mol Genet 10:189, 2001

Turrini P et al: Dispersion of ventricular depolarization-repolarization: A noninvasive marker for risk stratification in arrhythmogenic right ventricular cardiomyopathy. Circulation 103:3075, 2001

Wichter T et al: Identification of arrhythmogenic right ventricular cardiomyopathy from the surface ECG: Parameters for discrimination from idiopathic right ventricular tachycardia. Pacing Clin Electrophysiol 22:A69, 1999

SUDDEN DEATH IN HYPERTROPHIC CARDIOMYOPATHY

Barry J. Maron

Hypertrophic cardiomyopathy (HCM) is a genetic cardiac disease with particularly heterogeneous presentation and diverse natural history (Maron, 1997). Sudden and unexpected death has been recognized as a prominent and devastating component of the natural history of HCM since the initial description of this disease over 40 years ago (Frank and Braunwald, 1968). Many authors have emphasized that these catastrophic events occur not uncommonly in young asymptomatic patients; as a consequence, there has been intense interest in the stratification of risk and in preventive treatment for sudden cardiac death (SCD).

Historic Context and Occurrence

Since Teare's original pathologic report of this disease in a small number of patients who died suddenly (Teare, 1958), the recognition that some HCM patients are at increased risk for SCD has generated concern and considerable study, as well as controversy (Frank and Braunwald, 1968; McKenna and Deanfield, 1984). Even the frequency with which premature SCD occurs in HCM has

been the subject of debate, due largely to the relatively uncommon occurrence of the disease as well as the impact of highly selective referral patterns in which severely affected and high-risk patients have been disproportionately referred to tertiary HCM centers (Maron, 1997). Consequently, a large portion of the HCM literature offers annual mortality rates as high as 3 to 6% (McKenna and Deanfield, 1984), which are not truly representative of the overall HCM disease spectrum. Indeed, if the HCM mortality rate was truly 5 to 6%, virtually none of the patients in a HCM cohort would ultimately survive past age 50 (Maron et al., 1999). Since it is well established that HCM is compatible with normal longevity, we must assume that the earlier mortality estimates were skewed and represented overestimates.

More recent studies of largely unselected regional and nonreferred (i.e., community-based) populations, which are more representative of the overall disease, have reported much lower mortality rates (due largely to SCD) of only about 1% per year (Maron et al., 1999). These data create a different perspective of HCM, in which the overall risk of the disease does not differ significantly from that in the population as a whole. It should be emphasized, however, that while these concepts pertain to the *overall* HCM disease spectrum, specific high-risk subsets exist within that population that may well have mortality rates of 5% per year or more.

Profile of Sudden Death and Risk Stratification

Based on studies in both tertiary and community-based patient populations, SCD in HCM occurs most commonly in young individuals (≤30 years old), usually during sedentary activities or mild exertion but not infrequently with intense exertion, and most often in the absence of significant symptoms

(Maron et al., 1982; Maron et al., 2000a). Indeed, HCM is the most common cause of SCD in young people, including trained competitive athletes (Fig. 60-1); also, SCD occurs frequently in African Americans and most commonly in basketball and football (Maron, 1997). Withdrawal from intense competitive situations is usually recommended to reduce risk. However, based on data from cohorts free of tertiary referral bias, it has become evident that HCM is characterized by an extended period of risk that is not confined to the young but in fact extends into midlife and beyond (Maron et al., 2000a) (Fig. 60-2).

Defining reliable markers for SCD in HCM and isolating the minority who are at risk from the overall patient population have proved challenging because of limitations implicit in the low prevalence of the disease and the striking heterogeneity of expression, prognosis, and genetics. Indeed, there is no single test (invasive or noninvasive) that can reliably assess with precision the level of risk in HCM patients. Myriad risk factors have been proposed in the literature over several decades of investigation, although few are supported by controlled data in sizeable groups of patients.

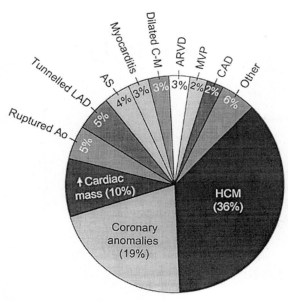

FIGURE 60-1

Causes of sudden cardiac death in young competitive athletes (median age 17), based on systematic tracking of 158 athletes in the United States, primarily from 1985 to 1995. Ao indicates aorta; LAD, left anterior descending coronary artery; AS, aortic stenosis; C-M, cardiomyopathy; ARVD, arrhythmogenic right ventricular dysplasia; MVP, mitral valve prolapse; CAD, coronary artery disease; HCM, hypertrophic cardiomyopathy; ↑, increased. (Adapted from BJ Maron et al: Circulation 94:850, 1996.)

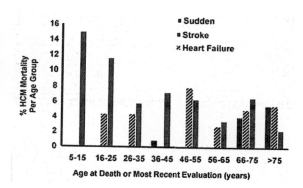

FIGURE 60-2

Distribution of ages at the time of HCM-related death showing that while sudden death occurs most commonly in children and young adults, the risk for sudden death persists throughout mid-life and beyond. Displayed as percent HCM mortality by age group. Percent HCM mortality was calculated by dividing the total number of HCM deaths by the total number of patients at the end of the follow-up (or at death).

Nevertheless, it is possible to regard the high-risk profile for HCM as characterized by one or more of the following clinically identifiable risk factors: (1) prior cardiac arrest or spontaneous sustained ventricular tachycardia (VT); (2) family history of HCM-related death, particularly if sudden, in close relatives or multiple relatives; (3) syncope (particularly if related to exertion, repetitive, and in the young); (4) multiple repetitive or prolonged nonsustained bursts of VT on ambulatory (Holter) electrocardiography (ECG); or (5) extreme left ventricular hypertrophy, particularly in adolescents and young adults (wall thickness ≥30 mm; comprising about 10% of HCM patients) (Figs. 60-3 and 60-4) (Maron et al., 1997; Elliott et al., 2001). Multiple

risk factors convey increasingly greater SCD risk (Elliott et al., 2000)

Proposed risk factors such as hypotensive blood pressure response to exercise (which could potentially trigger reduced coronary flow and ischemia-induced arrhythmias), as well as infrequent runs of nonsustained tachycardia, have been shown to have low positive predictive accuracy (about 15 to 20%), although the absence of either of these findings is associated with high negative predictive accuracy (about 75%). Therefore, while the latter parameters, when positive, may not alone be sufficiently strong markers of SCD to justify a primary prevention intervention, when absent they are useful in identifying a low-risk clinical subset (Maron, 1997).

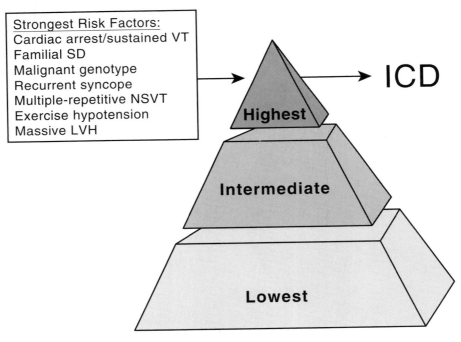

FIGURE 60-3

Assessment of risk for sudden cardiac death in overall HCM population. Treatment for prevention of sudden death is limited to that small subset perceived to be at highest risk compared to all other patients with HCM on the basis of risk factor analysis. Asymptomatic individuals with mild left ventricular hypertrophy, but *without* ventricular tachycardia on ambulatory Holter ECG, hypotensive blood pressure response to exercise, or family history of premature HCM-related death are regarded to be at low risk. ICD, implantable cardioverter-defibrillator; LVH, left ventricular hypertrophy; NSVT, nonsustained ventricular tachycardia; SD, sudden death; VT, ventricular tachycardia. (From BJ Maron et al: Curr Probl Cardiol 23:477, 1998.)

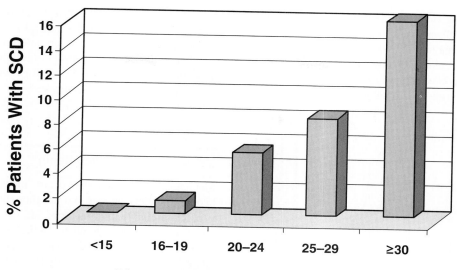

FIGURE 60-4

Relation between maximal left ventricular (LV) wall thickness and the risk of sudden cardiac death (SCD) in 480 patients with HCM. The incidence of sudden death increased progressively and in direct relation to maximal wall thickness ($p = .001$ by the chi-square test for trend). The greatest risk is associated with the most extreme hypertrophy, and the smallest risk linked to the most mild degrees of hypertrophy.

Of note, one report suggests that tunneled (bridged) segments of left anterior descending coronary artery (1 to 3 cm) are independently associated with increased risk for cardiac arrest in children with HCM (mediated by myocardial ischemia).

Furthermore, the presence, absence, or magnitude of outflow obstruction has not proved to be an independent predictor for SCD, nor have other noninvasive indices such as QT interval, QT dispersion, or heart rate variability. Invasive parameters for detecting a substrate for ventricular fibrillation, such as inducible ventricular arrhythmias with programmed electrical stimulation, are not sufficiently specific to be regarded as useful for SCD risk discrimination.

It has been proposed, based on genotype-phenotype correlations, that the individual genetic defects in HCM (in addition to dictating phenotypic expression) could represent the primary determinants of outcome and stratifying markers for SCD risk with specific mutations conveying favorable or adverse prognosis (Maron et al., 1998;

Niimura et al., 1998; Marian and Roberts, 1995; Schwartz et al., 1995; Anan et al., 1994). For example, some β-myosin heavy chain mutations (such as Arg403gin) and troponin-T mutations may be associated with a higher frequency of premature death in comparison to other genetic defects (such as myosin-binding protein C mutations). However, caution is warranted before drawing strong conclusions regarding prognosis based only on the available genetic data, which is skewed toward high-risk families by patient selection. Prognosis attached to adult gene carriers without left ventricular hypertrophy (LVH) or those patients who ultimately develop hypertrophy in adulthood appear to be largely benign. Only a small number of sudden deaths in young people with little or no LVH have been reported, primarily from a few highly selected pedigrees with troponin-T mutations. Assessing risk with genetic markers (ie., mutations in genes encoding sarcomeric proteins) is a promising strategy that nevertheless has not yet proved applicable to clinical practice, given the very limited access to such testing on a routine basis. While more rapid sequencing of gene mutations is not currently available, this technology could eventually alter the landscape of molecular screening for HCM.

Indeed, while emphasis has understandably been placed on high-risk patients, many other HCM patients without risk factors or symptoms and with only mild and localized hypertrophy appear to be at the *lowest* risk for SCD or deterioration. Such patients with favorable prognoses constitute an important proportion of the overall HCM population and generally deserve a measure of reassurance regarding their disease.

Mechanisms of Sudden Death

Mechanisms by which SCD occurs in HCM have not been completely defined but are thought to be complex and probably multifactorial, ultimately involving ventricular tachyarrhythmias. Defining the arrhythmias responsible for sudden and unexpected death in HCM has historically been difficult, given the paucity of ECG recordings during clinical events. However, arrhythmia sequences documented by stored ECG recordings in patients experiencing appropriate defibrillator discharges represent a unique window to understanding SCD events in HCM (Maron et al., 2000b). Ventricular tachycardia or fibrillation have proved to be the rhythms that triggered appropriate device activations in each case, supporting the hypothesis that primary ventricular tachycardia/fibrillation represents the mechanism most commonly responsible for unexpected catastrophes in this disease (Fig. 60-5). It is possible that these arrhythmia sequences may ultimately prove to be more complex, since anecdotal examples of premonitory rhythms

◄ FIGURE 60-5

Primary prevention of sudden cardiac death in HCM. Stored ventricular electrogram from asymptomatic 35-year-old man who received a defibrillator prophylactically due to a family history of HCM-related sudden death and marked ventricular septal thickness (i.e., 31 mm). Electrogram was obtained 4 years and 8 months after the defibrillator implant (at 1:20 A.M. during sleep). Continuous recording at 25 mm/s, shown in four contiguous panels, with the tracing recorded left-to-right in each segment. (A) Begins with 4 beats of sinus rhythm and thereafter ventricular tachycardia begins abruptly (at 200 beats/minute); (B) Device senses ventricular tachycardia and charges; (C) Ventricular tachycardia deteriorates into ventricular fibrillation; (D) Defibrillator discharges appropriately (20-J shock) during ventricular fibrillation and restores sinus rhythm immediately. (From BJ Maron et al: N Engl J Med 342:365, 2000.)

immediately preceding ventricular tachycardia/fibrillation have been reported. (Elliott et al., 1999)

Potentially lethal arrhythmias in HCM probably emanate from (1) an electrophysiologically unstable myocardial substrate in which distorted electrical transmission is created by the disorganized left ventricular architecture, or (2) bursts of myocardial ischemia leading to myocyte necrosis and areas of replacement fibrosis (which is probably ultimately due to "small vessel disease" in the form of abnormal and narrowed intramural arterioles) (Fig. 60-6). In the greatly thickened left ventricle, this unstable substrate may be vulnerable to a variety of triggers, either intrinsic (i.e., related to the HCM disease process, such as an abrupt increase in outflow obstruction) or extrinsic and environmental (e.g., intense physical exertion). It should be emphasized, however, that it is a relatively small subgroup of patients (among all others with HCM) who are truly at high-risk and deserve to be regarded as candidates for preventive treatment.

Sudden Death Prevention

Pharmacologic

Historically, the prophylactic management of high-risk patients has been confined to treatment with drugs, such as beta blockers or verapamil, or antiarrhythmic agents, such as procainamide and quinidine, and, more recently, with amiodarone. However, in HCM, there are very limited data supporting the efficacy of drug treatment as a preventive measure against SCD. For example, since the sole report 15 years ago proposing the protective effects for amiodarone (utilizing retrospective and nonrandomized historic case-control design and short follow-up), there has been virtually no new information regarding the efficacy of this drug in HCM patients (McKenna et al., 1985). Also, the frequent adverse consequences associated with the chronic use of amiodarone severely limit its application to sudden death prevention in young patients with HCM who require coverage over long periods of future risk. Indeed, prevention of SCD in HCM has consistently represented a major management challenge for clinicians.

Implantable Cardioverter-Defibrillator

Since its introduction by Dr. Michel Mirowski 20 years ago, the implantable cardioverter-defibrillator (ICD) has achieved widespread acceptance as a preventive treatment for SCD by indisputably demonstrating efficacy for terminating life-threatening ventricular arrhythmias and prolonging life, principally in high-risk patients with ischemic heart disease. The superiority of the ICD to antiarrhythmic drug treatment has been documented in prospective randomized trials. Of particular importance has been the evolution of the ICD from a thoracotomy-based procedure with epicardial leads to a transvenous endocardial electrode system with pectoral implantation of the pulse generator, greatly facilitating clinical employment particularly with regard to primary prevention of SCD.

Efficacy of the ICD was recently investigated in a group of HCM patients judged to be at high risk for sudden death as part of a multicenter, retrospective study at selected U.S. and Italian centers (Maron et al., 2000b). The study group of 128 HCM patients with ICDs was followed for an average period of just 3 years; appropriate device interventions (either defibrillation shocks or antitachycardia pacing) occurred in almost 25%, with an average discharge rate of 7% per year. About 60% of those patients who received defibrillator therapy experienced multiple appropriate interventions.

Of note, the ICD has proved highly reliable in sensing and interrupting ventricular tachycardia/fibrillation despite the substantially increased heart mass characteristic of HCM (Maron et al., 2000b; Spirito et al., 2000; Elliott et al., 1999). (Fig. 60-5) Also, more than one-half of the study patients were taking amiodarone or other antiarrhythmic drugs at the time of appropriate defibrillator discharge, which underlines the superiority of the ICD.

Annual appropriate ICD intervention rates for HCM are lower than those reported in coronary artery disease. Nevertheless, they are significant since the ICD in HCM must be considered in the context of a much younger patient population, with an average age at implant of only 40 years, and usually free of significant congestive heart failure and systolic dysfunction. These patients are exposed to

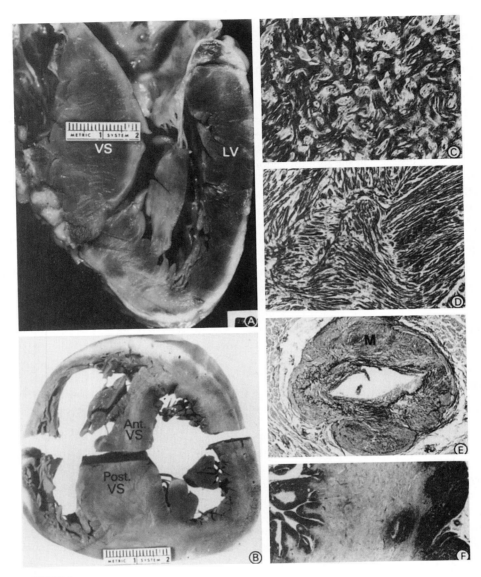

FIGURE 60-6

Morphologic components of the underlying disease process in HCM. *(A)* Gross heart specimen shown in a cross-sectional plane similar to that of the echocardiographic (parasternal) long axis. Pattern of left ventricular hypertrophy is asymmetric, with wall thickening confined primarily to the anterior ventricular septum (VS) which bulges into the left ventricular outflow tract. *(B)* Heart specimen illustrating a different pattern of hypertrophy in which marked left ventricular wall thickening is present in posterior portion of ventricular septum (Post. VS), while the anterior septum (Ant. VS) is only mildly thickened. *(C and D)* These show histologic patterns characteristic of the left ventricle in HCM. In *C,* septal myocardium has markedly disordered architecture with adjacent hypertrophied cardiac muscle cells arranged at perpendicular and oblique angles to each other. In *D,* bundles of hypertrophied cells show a disorganized "interwoven" arrangement. *(E)* Intramural coronary artery with apparently narrowed lumen and thickened wall due primarily to medial (M) hypertrophy. *(F)* Extensive scarring of ventricular septum which is transmural in distribution. LV, left ventricular free wall. (From BJ Maron et al: N Engl J Med 316:780, 844, 1987.)

long periods of potential risk and could survive many decades with normal or near-normal life expectancy, given the protection afforded by an ICD.

Life-saving defibrillator interventions were more frequent in those patients implanted specifically for *secondary prevention* (i.e., following cardiac arrest with documented ventricular fibrillation) and fortuitous resuscitation or with spontaneous, sustained ventricular tachycardia; over 40% of these patients received ICD discharges during the relatively short follow-up period. Such frequent recurrence of potentially lethal ventricular tachyarrhythmias following cardiac arrest is consistent with a previously reported experience in the pre-ICD era with similar HCM patients.

ICDs solely for *primary prevention* showed a substantial appropriate device intervention rate of almost 5% per year (Fig. 60-5). In this context, primary prevention represents purely prophylactic implantation dictated by a perception of high-risk status for SCD based on the patient's clinical profile (i.e., risk factors). However, with regard to primary prevention ICD implants, further studies with much larger numbers of patients will be required to define with greater precision specifically which HCM patients among the broad disease spectrum should be targeted for (and would benefit most from) prophylactic ICD.

Of note, the time interval between implant and first appropriate ICD intervention was quite variable, and some patients experienced particularly long time delays of ≥4 years (and up to 9 years) before for the first life-saving intervention. Therefore, in HCM, the timing of SCD is largely unpredictable, and the ICD may remain dormant for long periods of time before ultimately intervening appropriately. Due to the youth of the patients and the long risk period involved in HCM, the decision to implant an ICD in a high-risk patient with this disease is likely to represent a life-long commitment.

Complete consensus has not been reached regarding when a single risk factor is sufficient to target candidates for preventive treatment with the ICD, and individual clinical judgement may be necessary when considering the appropriateness of a given implant. Also, attitudes toward ICDs (and also the access to such devices) can vary considerably between different countries and cultures, and importantly influence clinical decision-making.

REFERENCES

Anan R et al: Prognostic implications of novel β cardiac myosin heavy chain gene mutations that cause familial hypertrophic cardiomyopathy. J Clin Invest 93:280, 1994

Elliott PM et al: Survival after cardiac arrest in patients with hypertrophic cardiomyopathy. J Am Coll Cardiol 33:1596, 1999

Elliott PM et al: Sudden death in hypertrophic cardiomyopathy: Identification of high risk patients. J Am Coll Cardiol 36:2212, 2000

Elliott PM et al: Relation between severity of left ventricular hypertrophy and prognosis in patients with hypertrophic cardiomyopathy. Lancet 357:420, 2001

Frank S, Braunwald E: Idiopathic hypertrophic subaortic stenosis: Clinical analysis of 126 patients with emphasis on the natural history. Circulation 37:759, 1968

Marian AJ, Roberts R: Recent advances in the molecular genetics of hypertrophic cardiomyopathy. Circulation 92:1336, 1995

Maron BJ: Hypertrophic cardiomyopathy. Lancet 350:127, 1997

Maron BJ et al: Sudden death in hypertrophic cardiomyopathy: Profile of 78 patients. Circulation 65:1388, 1982

Maron BJ et al: Hypertrophic cardiomyopathy as an important cause of sudden cardiac death on the athletic field in African-American athletes (abstr.). J Am Coll Cardiol 29 (Suppl A):462A, 1997

Maron BJ et al: Impact of laboratory molecular diagnosis on contemporary diagnostic criteria for genetically transmitted cardiovascular diseases: Hypertrophic cardiomyopathy, long Q-T syndrome, and Marfan syndrome. Circulation 98:1460, 1998

Maron BJ et al: Clinical consequences of hypertrophic cardiomyopathy in an unselected regional United States cohort. JAMA 281:650, 1999

Maron BJ et al: Epidemiology of hypertrophic cardiomyopathy-related death: Revisited in a large non-referral based patient population. Circulation 102:858, 2000a

Maron BJ et al: Efficacy of implantable cardioverter-defibrillators for the prevention of sudden death in patients with hypertrophic cardiomyopathy. N Engl J Med 342:365, 2000b

McKenna WJ, Deanfield JE: Hypertrophic cardiomyopathy: An important cause of sudden death. Arch Dis Child 59:971, 1984

McKenna WJ et al: Improved survival with amiodarone in patients with hypertrophic cardiomyopathy and ventricular tachycardia. Br Heart J 53:412, 1985

Niimura H et al: Mutations in the gene for human cardiac myosin-binding protein C and late-onset familial hypertrophic cardiomyopathy. N Engl J Med 338:1248, 1998

Schwartz K et al: Molecular basis of familial cardiomyopathies. Circulation 91:532, 1995

Spirito P et al: Magnitude of left ventricular hypertrophy predicts the risk of sudden death in hypertrophic cardiomyopathy. N Engl J Med 342:1778, 2000

Teare D: Asymmetrical hypertrophy of the heart in young patients. Br Heart J 20:1, 1958

61

NEWER APPROACHES TO MANAGEMENT OF THE LONG QT SYNDROME

Peter J. Schwartz & Silvia G. Priori

For several years the therapy for the long QT syndrome (LQTS) has been based primarily on anti-adrenergic interventions, pharmacologic or surgical. This reflected the correct perception that most episodes of life-threatening arrhythmias were triggered by increases in sympathetic activity (Schwartz, 1985). There has also been considerable individual variation in the approach to asymptomatic patients, and the authors had initially taken a conservative approach, recommending initiation of therapy in six specific subgroups (Schwartz et al., 1995a). The availability of new epidemiologic data and the growing understanding of the molecular defects underlying the various genetic subtypes of LQTS (Priori et al., 1999) allows a reappraisal of the therapeutic approach along new lines.

Asymptomatic Patients

The decision to treat or not to treat an asymptomatic patient with LQTS clearly depends on his or her risk of dying during the first event, should the patient ever become symptomatic. For a while this risk seemed to be rather low, and the potential negative psychological effects in children of a nonnecessary and life-long treatment represented a respectable argument against indiscriminate prophylactic treatment.

The authors recently completed the analysis of 570 patients from 197 LQTS families, all followed directly at their center in Pavia. All patients had a prolonged $QT_c > 440$ ms or clinical symptomatology including syncope, cardiac arrest, or sudden cardiac death below age 40. The incidence of sudden death during the first episode was 7% and that of cardiac arrest was 3%, for a total of 10%—certainly higher than expected. Moreover, this analysis was limited to patients >1 year of age because this is the population for which a cardiologist is usually called to make a decision. In the age group <1 year there was an additional 4% of sudden deaths/cardiac arrests, which increased to an unacceptable 12% the risk for sudden death during the first event for an infant diagnosed as affected by LQTS at birth. Conversely, the authors found that 68% of patients who suffered either sudden death or cardiac arrest had previously been asymptomatic. This analysis also showed that almost 50% of the patients are still asymptomatic and that, among these, 60% are already above age 20.

This finding has profoundly affected the authors' policy, and they now initiate treatment, always with

TREATMENT STRATEGY OF LONG QT SYNDROME IN PAVIA

I. Asymptomatic patients and patients with syncope
   A. Start with beta blockers (full dose)
   B. If syncope recurs (15–20% of patients)
      1. Left cardiac sympathetic denervation (LCSD)
      2. Pacemaker (only with evidence of brady-cardia-dependent torsades de pointes)
      3. Mexiletine (only if accompanied by marked QT shortening)

II. Patients presenting with cardiac arrest, with or without therapy
   A. Implant a cardioverter defibrillator
   B. Initiate or continue beta blockers
   C. Perform LCSD

beta blockers, in every asymptomatic individual diagnosed as affected by LQTS (Table 61-1).

Symptomatic Patients

The clinical management of patients who have already had a first syncope or cardiac arrest is different. In the mid-1980s (Schwartz, 1985), the first quantitative evidence was provided to indicate that antiadrenergic treatment, mostly beta blockers, was highly effective in reducing mortality among symptomatic patients when compared to patients untreated or those treated with a variety of non-adrenergic interventions (Fig. 61-1). While the overall efficacy of beta blockers cannot be reasonably disputed (Zareba et al., 1998), the open question concerns the percentage of patients who continue to have recurrences and, most important, the percentage of those who die despite treatment. On this critical point preliminary data exist on several hundred patients enrolled in the International Registry for LQTS. The main limitation of these data lies in the fact that therapy has been administered by physicians with varying degrees of expertise in LQTS, using variable dosages and with variable degrees of

compliance; nonetheless, they are useful to understand the impact of beta blockers when so administered. Recurrences for syncope were observed in one-third of the patients. Most important is the 5-year incidence of cardiac arrest/sudden death (CA/SD). This appears to be strikingly dependent on the type of symptoms prior to the institution of therapy; for patients presenting with syncope the incidence of CA/SD is 3%, but it increases to 13% for those presenting with cardiac arrest. Several among the patients who died had interrupted their therapy and no longer had an active prescription.

These data are especially useful for the identification of a subgroup of patients in whom a high risk for life-threatening recurrences is more likely and for whom a more aggressive therapy is required. Importantly, the recurrence rate for CA/SD is definitely lower in those highly qualified centers that see a large number of patients and where patients return for yearly controls on a routine basis. At the authors' center, with almost 200 families followed very regularly and by the same medical team, the incidence of CA/SD despite therapy during the past 5 years has been below 2%.

A variable percentage of patients, approximately 15 to 20% at the authors' center, has recurrence of syncope despite full-dose beta blockade. What is the next step for them? At the authors' center, left cardiac sympathetic denervation (LCSD) is performed whenever a patient has a recurrence. This procedure with its very strong rationale has been described in detail (Moss and McDonald, 1971; Schwartz et al., 1991), and worldwide data were available in 1994 on 123 patients not fully protected by pharmacologic therapy. The authors perform LCSD on approximately 10 patients/year, mostly referred from other countries. This subgroup is one at particularly high risk because of recurrent syncope or cardiac arrest despite full dose beta blockade. In approximately 40% of these patients there has been one episode of syncope, mostly during the first 6 months, but the 5-year incidence of events has decreased from 21 ± 31 to 1 ± 3. Mortality among these patients has been below 3% during the past 25 years. An ongoing reappraisal, based on almost 150 patients, confirms the high long-term efficacy

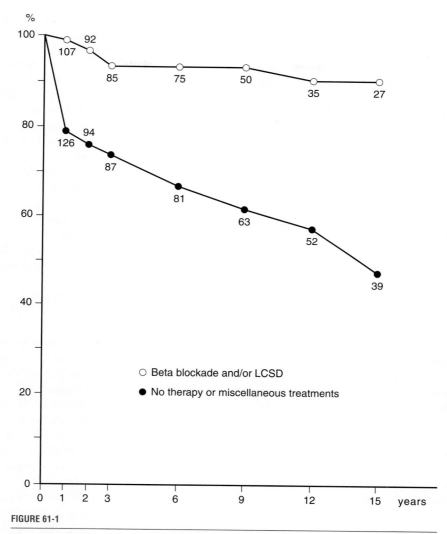

FIGURE 61-1

Effect of therapy on the survival, after the first syncopal episode, of 233 patients affected by congenital long QT syndrome. The protective effect of beta adrenergic blockade and of left cardiac sympathetic denervation (LCSD) is evident. The mortality 3 years after the first syncope is 6% in the group treated with antiadrenergic interventions and 26% in the group treated differently or not treated. Fifteen years after the first syncope, the respective mortality rates are 9% and 53%. (From PJ Schwartz: Am Heart J 109:399, 1985, with permission.) LCSD = left cardiac sympathetic denervation.

of LCSD. A critical point for the outcome lies in the need to remove the first four thoracic ganglia in order to ensure adequate denervation; the authors always leave intact the upper half of the left stellate ganglion to avoid the Horner syndrome. The time to complete this surgery, using the extrapleural approach and without opening the chest, is 35 to 40 min. It is unfortunate that this highly effective treatment is available in only a few centers and that most thoracic surgeons no longer use it, thus depriving LQTS patients from a straightforward approach to permanently reduce their risk.

Cardiac pacing has been used in LQTS patients, mostly for fear of excessive bradycardia resulting from beta blockade. Results have been variable, with most reports suggesting a decrease in the incidence of syncope, but the usual concomitant initiation, or increase in dosage, of beta blockers makes interpretation of the data questionable.

Use of the Internal Cardioverter Defibrillator

The use of the implantable cardioverter defibrillator (ICD) has been debated for years. The main arguments against its widespread use in this population of children and teenagers are the negative psychological impact of such an implant (when not absolutely necessary); the problems related to leads and battery life; and the fact that many patients after an ICD shock suffer from "storms" of arrhythmias (enhanced by sympathetic activation), leading to a series of multiple shocks mostly occurring during episodes of torsade de pointes, which do not produce loss of consciousness. Suicide attempts among teenagers repeatedly shocked are a grim reminder of the impact that medical decisions may have on the quality of life of the very people we try to protect. On the other hand, the life-saving value of the ICD is undeniable. The main question is the identification, with a reasonably positive predictive power, of the patients truly at risk. In this regard, the recent data from the International Registry presented above are quite valuable. The occurrence of a cardiac arrest, prior to or during therapy, mandates the implant of an ICD.

The LQTS Genotype

The identification of several of the LQTS genes (Priori et al., 1999) and the understanding of the electrophysiologic consequences of the various mutations, together with the growing number of genotype-phenotype studies, are opening new perspectives for more tailored therapy. It has to be said, however, that these newer approaches are currently more a promise than a reality. The first issue concerns terminology. The appealing term *gene-specific therapy* is already in vogue but may be a misnomer. It is already evident that, particularly for *SCN5A,* the sodium channel gene, different mutations produce very different effects (some produce LQTS while others produce the Brugada syndrome); some of these mutations produce an excess of Na^+ inward current during the plateau phase and others do not. Obviously, the former may respond to Na^+ channel blockers and the latter probably not. Eventually, this might lead to "mutation-specific" therapy. At this time, *gene-based therapy* may be the appropriate term, deriving from the concept that most mutations on the same gene, particularly on K^+ channel genes, may be expected to produce qualitatively similar losses in repolarizing current.

When dealing with genotyped patients, the new terminology becomes necessary. LQT1 patients are those with mutations on *KvLQT1,* the gene encoding the I_{Ks} current; LQT2 patients have mutations on *HERG,* the gene encoding the I_{Kr} current; LQT3 patients have mutations on *SCN5A,* the gene encoding the cardiac sodium channel gene. In 1995, the authors provided the first evidence on the possibility of shortening the QT interval by the Na^+ channel blocker mexiletine, specifically in the LQT3 patients (Schwartz et al., 1995b). As mexiletine produces some degree of QT shortening in most patients, the specificity lies in the quantity of the effect, which is markedly greater (average shortening 90 ms) for LQT3 patients. There is no evidence yet that this QT shortening, albeit encouraging, provides any protection, and some failures have already occurred. Thus, mexiletine should never be used as sole treatment. The suggestion has been made that the sodium channel blocker flecainide might be more specific than mexiletine for LQT3 patients, particularly those with mutations similar to ΔKPQ (Windle et al., 2001). A troubling finding with flecainide was that in addition to shortening the QT interval it produced the ST-segment elevation typical for the Brugada syndrome in 6 of the 13 LQT3 patients (Priori et al., 2000). More recently, evidence was provided indicating that flecainide potentiates tonic block of I_{Na} in the ΔKPQ mutant, and this was interpreted as supporting proarrhythmic risks (Viswanathan et al., 2001).

The important possibility of correcting the loss in repolarizing current in LQT2 patients by elevating the K^+ plasma level is currently hampered by the difficulty in achieving the target level by chronic oral therapy.

The most practical information for gene-based therapy comes from recent studies on genotype-phenotype correlations (Schwartz et al., 2001). The most relevant data can be summarized as follows:

1. LQT1 patients, as a group, shorten their QT interval less than normal during exercise. Most of their arrhythmic episodes occur during exercise, especially swimming, and the combination of physical and emotional stress accounts for 97% of their cardiac events.
2. LQT3 patients shorten their QT interval during exercise, or with faster heart rates, more than control individuals; they also tend to lengthen their QT markedly at night and when the heart rate is low (Stramba-Badiale et al., 2001).
3. LQT2 patients are at particularly high risk during acoustic stimuli.

Fewer than 15% of the cardiac events of LQT2 and LQT3 patients occur during exercise.

On the basis of these observations, the following recommendations seem appropriate. LQT1 patients, more than LQT2 and LQT3 patients, should be actively discouraged from engaging in any sport and competitive physical activity; adult supervision while swimming is recommended. These patients respond extremely well to beta blockers (Schwartz et al., 2001). LQT2 patients should be closely monitored for K^+ plasma levels. LQT3 patients seem to be at higher risk when their heart rate is low; accordingly, this is the only group in which beta blockers should be administered with caution. The combination of beta blockers and a pacemaker may be useful to allow full dose beta blockade without concerns about ensuing bradycardia. Alternatively, particularly useful in these patients is left cardiac

sympathetic denervation, which prevents the arrhythmogenic neural release of norepinephrine in the ventricles without reducing heart rate because the sympathetic control of heart rate is primarily dependent on right-sided cardiac nerves (Schwartz and Stone, 1979). As cardiac events in LQT3 patients have a high degree of lethality, the consideration of implanting an ICD is also appropriate.

The exciting new perspectives offered by the molecular insights should not modify the positive reality that the more traditional antiadrenergic therapies remain highly effective in protecting >95% of the patients presenting with syncope from life-threatening arrhythmias.

REFERENCES

Moss AJ, McDonald J: Unilateral cervicothoracic sympathetic ganglionectomy for the treatment of long QT interval syndrome. N Engl J Med 285:903, 1971

Priori SG et al: Genetic and molecular basis of cardiac arrhythmias: Impact on clinical management. Circulation 99:518, Parts I and II; 674, Part III, 1999

Priori SG et al: The elusive link between LQT3 and Brugada syndrome. The role of flecainide challenge. Circulation 102:945, 2000

Schwartz PJ, Stone HL: Effects of unilateral stellectomy upon cardiac performance during exercise in dogs. Circ Res 44:637, 1979

Schwartz PJ: Idiopathic long QT syndrome: Progress and questions. Am Heart J 109:399, 1985

Schwartz PJ et al: Left cardiac sympathetic denervation in the therapy of congenital long QT syndrome: A worldwide report. Circulation 84:503, 1991

Schwartz PJ et al: The long QT syndrome, in Cardiac Electrophysiology: From Cell to Bedside, 2nd ed, DP Zipes, J Jalife (eds). Philadelphia, Saunders, 1995a, pp 788–811

Schwartz PJ et al: Long QT syndrome patients with mutations on the SCN5A and HERG genes have differential responses to Na^+ channel blockade and to increases in heart rate. Implications for gene-specific therapy. Circulation 92:3381, 1995b

Schwartz PJ et al: Genotype-phenotype correlation in the long QT syndrome. Gene-specific triggers for life-threatening arrhythmias. Circulation 103:89, 2001

Stramba-Badiale M et al: Gene-specific differences in the circadian variation of ventricular repolarization in the long QT syndrome: A key to sudden death during sleep? Ital Heart J 1:323, 2000

Viswanathan PC et al: Gating-dependent mechanisms for flecainide action in *SCN5A*-linked arrhythmia syndromes.
Circulation 104:1200, 2001

Windle JR et al: Normalization of ventricular repolarization
with flecainide in long QT syndrome patients with
SCN5A:DeltaKPQ mutation. Ann Noninvasive Electrocardiol 6:153, 2001

Zareba W et al, for the International Long-QT Syndrome
Registry Research Group: Influence of the genotype on
the clinical course of the long QT Syndrome. N Engl J
Med 339:960, 1998

IBUTILIDE: A NEW ANTIARRHYTHMIC AGENT

Hakan Oral & Fred Morady

Ibutilide fumarate is a new class III (Vaughan-Williams) antiarrhythmic agent that is used intravenously for conversion of atrial flutter and atrial fibrillation to sinus rhythm by prolonging action potential duration (Fig. 62-1).

Pharmacologic Effects and Pharmacokinetics

Ibutilide increases action potential duration primarily by blocking the rapid component of the cardiac delayed rectifier potassium current (I_{Kr}) without significant reverse-use dependence, i.e., without loss of effect at rapid heart rates (Yang et al., 1995). At nanomolar concentrations, ibutilide also activates a slow, inward-depolarizing sodium current (Lee, 1992).

Ibutilide increases refractoriness of the atrium and the ventricle by prolonging action potential duration; in addition, it decreases conduction velocity. Ibutilide has also been shown to decrease the energy requirement for atrial defibrillation in humans (Oral et al., 1999) and ventricular defibrillation in dogs (Wesley et al., 1993). Although ibutilide may lead to a mild decrease in sinus rate and atrioventricular nodal conduction (Murray, 1998), the drug usu-

ally does not have a clinically significant effect on heart rate, PR interval, or QRS duration in humans. However, ibutilide causes a dose-dependent prolongation of the QT interval, which is a result of the therapeutic effect of the drug, i.e., prolongation of action potential duration and repolarization (Ellenbogen et al., 1996). Excessive QT interval prolongation due to ibutilide may result in a form of polymorphic ventricular tachycardia referred to as *torsade de pointes* (Fig. 62-2).

Ibutilide does not have a clinically significant hemodynamic effect in patients with normal or depressed left ventricular ejection fractions (Stambler et al., 1996; Ellenbogen et al., 1996; Oral et al., 1999).

Ibutilide is available for intravenous use only. The drug has a high systemic plasma clearance that approximates liver blood flow and also has a large volume of distribution with minimal protein binding. Its elimination half-life ranges between 2 and 12 h, with a mean of 6 h. Ibutilide is metabolized in the liver, probably by a cytochrome P450–independent enzyme system, and excreted largely in the urine. There are no apparent drug interactions between ibutilide and digoxin, beta blockers, or calcium channel blockers. In a recent study, there were no adverse arrhythmic events when ibutilide was administered to patients who were already receiving a class I

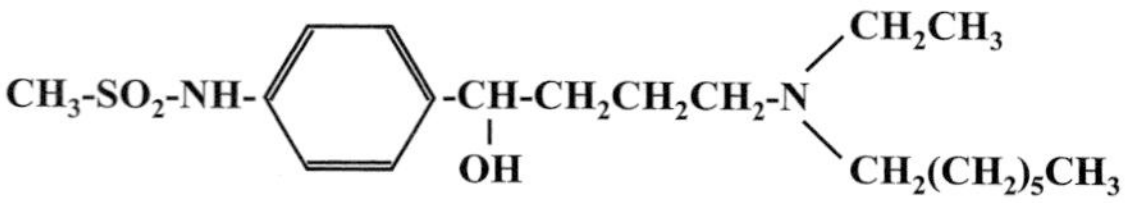

$$CH_3-SO_2-NH-\langle\ \rangle-CH-CH_2CH_2CH_2-N\begin{array}{c} CH_2CH_3 \\ \\ CH_2(CH_2)_5CH_3 \end{array}$$
$$OH$$

FIGURE 62-1

Chemical structure of ibutilide. Ibutilide, *N*-[4-[4-(ethylheptylami-no)-1-hydroxybutyl]phenyl]-methanesulfonamide, has structural similarities to sotalol and dofetilide due to the methanesulfonilide moiety.

antiarrhythmic agent or amiodarone (Oral et al., 1999). In another study, there was only one episode of nonsustained polymorphic ventricular tachycardia after administration of 2 mg ibutilide to 70 patients with atrial fibrillation or flutter who had been treated chronically with amiodarone, despite the presence of a significant prolongation in QT interval (Glatter et al., 2001). There is no need to adjust the dose in the presence of hepatic or renal dysfunction. However, since clearance will be delayed in the presence of hepatic dysfunction, longer periods of electrocardiographic monitoring may be required to detect proarrhythmia. Current recommendations suggest electrocardiographic monitoring for 4 h after ibutilide administration.

In rats, ibutilide is both teratogenic and embryocidal (Murray, 1998). In pregnancy, ibutilide is a category C antiarrhythmic agent and should not be administered to a pregnant woman unless clinical benefit substantially outweighs the risk to the fetus. There are no data regarding the excretion of ibutilide in the breast milk; breastfeeding should be discouraged during and after therapy with ibutilide. The safety and efficacy of ibutilide in pediatric patients have not been established.

Dosage and Administration

Ibutilide is infused intravenously as a 1.0-mg dose over 10 min for chemical cardioversion of atrial flutter or fibrillation in patients who weigh ≥60 kg. If the body weight is <60 kg, the dose is 0.01 mg/kg. The infusion should be stopped as soon as the arrhythmia terminates or if an adverse effect occurs. If the atrial flutter or fibrillation is still present 10 min after completion of the first dose, a second 1.0 mg dose of ibutilide may be administered.

Adverse Effects

The most important adverse effect associated with ibutilide infusion is the development of polymorphic ventricular tachycardia (torsade de pointes), which may be nonsustained or sustained, in association with QT-interval prolongation. The incidence of sustained polymorphic ventricular tachycardia associated with

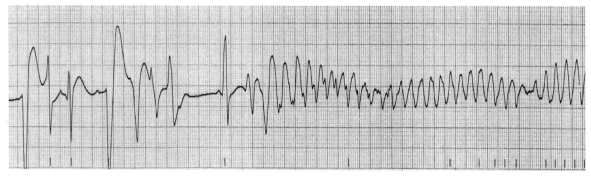

FIGURE 62-2

Torsade de pointes. ECG tracing of a patient who developed polymorphic ventricular tachycardia during sinus rhythm after ibutilide pretreatment. This patient had a left ventricular ejection fraction of 10%.

ibutilide is 2 to 3%, and the incidence of nonsustained polymorphic ventricular tachycardia is 1 to 6%. Almost all of the adverse arrhythmic events occur within the first 40 min after the completion of the infusion. The most significant predictor of ibutilide-associated polymorphic ventricular tachycardia is a decreased left ventricular ejection fraction of <30%. Therefore, ibutilide should be avoided in patients who have a low left ventricular ejection fraction. Ibutilide should also not be used in conditions that predispose to the development of polymorphic ventricular tachycardia, such as occurs in patients with a QT_c interval >480 ms (unless attributable to amiodarone) or hypokalemia.

Clinical Studies

Ibutilide is more effective in cardioversion of atrial flutter than atrial fibrillation. Cardioversion efficacy has been reported to be in the range of 38 to 76% for atrial flutter and 20 to 51% for atrial fibrillation (Stambler et al., 1996; Ellenbogen et al., 1996; Volgman et al., 1998; Oral et al., 1999). The duration of atrial fibrillation appears to be the most significant predictor of successful cardioversion with ibutilide. One study also found a correlation between the left atrial size and the efficacy of cardioversion with ibutilide (Stambler et al., 1996).

The effect of ibutilide on atrial defibrillation energy requirements has been investigated (Oral et al., 1999). In this study, 100 patients with atrial fibrillation for >6 h (mean duration = 117 ± 201 days) were randomized to undergo transthoracic cardioversion with and without pretreatment with 1 mg of ibutilide. Patients with inadequate anticoagulation, a QT_c >480 ms (unless attributable to amiodarone), or who were pregnant were excluded. Since two patients with a left ventricular ejection fraction of ≤20% developed sustained polymorphic ventricular tachycardia early in the study, patients with a left ventricular ejection fraction of <30% were subsequently excluded. Among the 100 patients, 82% had structural heart disease, 23% coronary artery disease, 11% nonischemic cardiomyopathy, 26% valvular heart disease, and 22%

hypertensive heart disease. Forty-seven patients were being treated with amiodarone or sotalol.

In patients who were randomized to undergo cardioversion with ibutilide pretreatment, 1 mg ibutilide was infused over 10 min. If atrial fibrillation was still present after 10 min, transthoracic cardioversion was performed using a step-up protocol of 50, 100, 200, 300, and 360 J. If cardioversion was not successful in patients who were randomized to undergo transthoracic cardioversion without ibutilide pretreatment, 1 mg ibutilide was administered and transthoracic cardioversion was repeated using the same step-up protocol. Anticoagulant therapy was continued for 1 month after cardioversion in patients in whom atrial fibrillation was present for >48 h. Patients were followed for a mean of 218 ± 110 days after the cardioversion.

Transthoracic cardioversion without ibutilide pretreatment was successful in 72% of the patients. In patients who received ibutilide initially, sinus rhythm was restored in 20% by ibutilide alone and in all of the remaining 80% of patients after transthoracic cardioversion. The efficacy of transthoracic cardioversion with ibutilide pretreatment was 100%, whereas the efficacy of transthoracic cardioversion without ibutilide pretreatment was 72% ($p < .001$). In all of the patients in whom transthoracic cardioversion by itself was not successful, sinus rhythm was restored when transthoracic cardioversion was repeated after the administration of 1 mg ibutilide. The mean energy required for atrial defibrillation was 228 ± 93 J without ibutilide pretreatment, and 166 ± 80 J with ibutilide pretreatment ($p < .001$), which corresponded to a decrease of approximately 30% in the transthoracic atrial defibrillation energy requirement with ibutilide. Concomitant antiarrhythmic therapy was not associated with a change in the atrial defibrillation energy requirements.

Recurrence rates of atrial fibrillation were similar in patients who received ibutilide and in those who did not. At 6 months' follow-up, 50% of patients in whom sinus rhythm was restored by transthoracic cardioversion alone, 90% of patients in whom sinus rhythm was restored by ibutilide alone, and 62% of patients in whom sinus rhythm

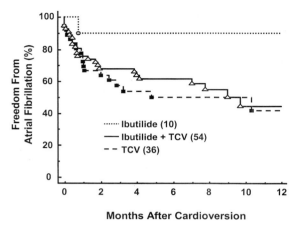

FIGURE 62-3

Freedom from recurrence of atrial fibrillation after cardioversion with and without ibutilide pretreatment. Kaplan-Meier analysis of the percentage of patients remaining free of atrial fibrillation after restoration of sinus rhythm with ibutilide, transthoracic cardioversion (TCV) alone, or transthoracic cardioversion with ibutilide pretreatment. (Reproduced from H Oral et al: N Engl J Med 349:1849, 1999, with permission from the Massachusetts Medical Society.)

was restored by transthoracic cardioversion after ibutilide pretreatment remained in sinus rhythm (Fig. 62-3). Two patients (3%) with a left ventricular ejection fraction of $\leq 20\%$ developed sustained, polymorphic ventricular tachycardia, and another patient had one episode of nonsustained, polymorphic ventricular tachycardia (Fig. 62-2). Concomitant antiarrhythmic therapy with amiodarone or sotalol was not associated with an increase in the incidence of arrhythmic events.

The results of this study demonstrated that the energy requirement for atrial defibrillation is reduced by approximately 30% when 1 mg ibutilide is administered prior to transthoracic cardioversion. Moreover, when conventional transthoracic cardioversion by itself was not effective in restoring sinus rhythm, successful conversion to sinus rhythm could be achieved in a very high percentage of patients when transthoracic cardioversion was repeated after the administration of ibutilide. The recurrence rate of atrial fibrillation is similar in patients who do and do not receive ibutilide.

Therefore, facilitation of transthoracic cardioversion by ibutilide results in a clinically meaningful return to sinus rhythm that is no more or less likely to be long-lived than when sinus rhythm is restored by conventional transthoracic cardioversion alone.

The administration of ibutilide before cardioversion provides a very effective alternative for management of patients with atrial fibrillation who have failed transthoracic cardioversion. In current practice, these patients are either left in permanent atrial fibrillation or referred for internal cardioversion. However, pretreatment with ibutilide is simple, noninvasive, and highly effective in restoring sinus rhythm when compared to internal cardioversion, which requires specialized personnel, hospital facilities, and equipment.

SUMMARY

Ibutilide is a class III antiarrhythmic agent used intravenously for acute conversion of atrial flutter and atrial fibrillation to sinus rhythm. Ibutilide also lowers atrial defibrillation energy requirements and facilitates transthoracic cardioversion of atrial fibrillation. Ibutilide pretreatment usually eliminates the need for internal cardioversion in patients who fail transthoracic cardioversion. Polymorphic ventricular tachycardia associated with ibutilide pretreatment is almost exclusively seen in patients with a low left ventricular ejection fraction and can be avoided if ibutilide is administered only to patients with a left ventricular ejection fraction >30% and a QT_c interval <480 ms.

Because the use of ibutilide is associated with the cost of the drug and continuous electrocardiographic monitoring afterwards to watch for an adverse effect, and because transthoracic cardioversion by itself is effective in restoring sinus rhythm in a majority of patients, pretreatment with ibutilide may be more appropriate and cost-effective in patients who have already failed an attempt at transthoracic cardioversion or in patients with atrial fibrillation of short duration in whom ibutilide by itself is particularly effective in restoring sinus rhythm.

REFERENCES

Ellenbogen KA et al: Efficacy of intravenous ibutilide for acute termination of atrial fibrillation and flutter: A dose response study. J Am Coll Cardiol 28:130, 1996

Glatter K et al: Chemical cardioversion of atrial fibrillation or flutter with ibutilide in patients receiving amiodarone therapy. Circulation 103:253, 2001

Lee KS: Ibutilide, a new compound with potent class III antiarrhythmic activity, activates a slow inward Na^+ current in guinea pig ventricular cells. J Pharmacol Exp Ther 262:99, 1992

Murray KT: Ibutilide. Circulation 97:493, 1998

Oral H et al: Facilitating transthoracic cardioversion of atrial fibrillation with ibutilide pretreatment. N Engl J Med 349:1849, 1999

Stambler BS et al: Efficacy and safety of repeated doses of ibutilide for rapid conversion of atrial flutter of atrial fibrillation. Circulation 94:1613, 1996

Volgman AS et al: Conversion efficacy and safety of intravenous ibutilide compared with intravenous procainamide in patients with atrial flutter or fibrillation. J Am Coll Cardiol 31:1414, 1998

Wesley RC Jr et al: Ibutilide: Enhanced defibrillation via plateau sodium current activation. Am J Physiol 264:H1269, 1993

Yang T et al: Ibutilide, a methanesulfanilide antiarrhythmic, is a potent blocker of the rapidly activating delayed rectifying current (I_{Kr}) in AT-1 cells: Concentration-, time-, voltage-, and use-dependent effects. Circulation 91:1799, 1995

NONPHARMACOLOGIC TREATMENT OF ATRIAL FIBRILLATION

Mark E. Josephson

Atrial fibrillation is the most common sustained arrhythmia in our patient population, affecting 10% of persons over age 75 and even more prevalent in patients with clinical congestive heart failure (up to 25%). Symptoms and sequelae of atrial fibrillation such as palpitations, heart failure, syncope, and stroke impose an immense cost on our health care system. The expected increase in longevity of the population will only add to that burden. In fact, atrial fibrillation may account for at least 25% of strokes in the elderly.

Heretofore, the therapy of atrial fibrillation has been empirical and consists of (1) anticoagulation to decrease the incidence of stroke, (2) atrioventricular (AV) nodal blockade to control the ventricular response, and (3) antiarrhythmic agents to prevent the recurrence of atrial fibrillation. None of these has been totally effective, although anticoagulation does reduce the stroke risk to 1 to 1.5% per year from 5 to 7% per year. Obviously, the most effective way to reduce the incidence of stroke is the prevention of atrial fibrillation. Despite the use of beta blockers, calcium channel blockers, and digoxin, adequate rate control—particularly during exercise—is achievable in only 50% of patients. This is particularly true in patients with cardiomyopathy, heart failure, and pulmonary disease in whom beta blockers are frequently contraindicated and in whom adrenergic agonists are used for therapy.

Prevention of atrial fibrillation by antiarrhythmic agents has had a checkered history with modest efficacy, drug intolerance, and potentially lethal proarrhythmic side effects. Consequently, there has been great interest in the development of nonpharmacologic therapy for both rate control and prevention of atrial fibrillation. These nonpharmacologic approaches may be used alone or in combination with pharmacologic agents. These nonpharmacologic approaches include (1) AV nodal ablation or modification to control the ventricular rate; (2) pacing for prevention of atrial fibrillation; (3) antitachycardia pacing and atrial defibrillation for earlier conversion and prevention of remodeling of the atrium, which potentiates the recurrences of atrial fibrillation; and (4) catheter and surgical ablative procedures to prevent atrial fibrillation.

AV Junctional Ablation and Modification for Ventricular Rate Control

Control of the ventricular response in atrial fibrillation is critical because many of the symptoms associated with atrial fibrillation are related to the rapid ventricular response. Persistently high ventricular rates, often in association with paroxysmal atrial fibrillation, can lead to a tachycardia-mediated cardiomyopathy. Rate control can improve ventricular function dramatically (Rodriguez et al., 1993). Unfortunately, as noted above, in many patients adequate rate control cannot be achieved by pharmacologic agents alone. Moreover, in elderly patients, the combination of agents usually required to control the ventricular response is often poorly tolerated, leading to poor compliance. In the early 1980s, catheter ablation of the AV junction was developed. The precision with which radio frequency (RF) energy can be delivered has led some to consider the use of AV nodal modification to decrease the ventricular response without producing AV block, therefore obviating the need for pacing. There are three problems with this approach. First, it is only applicable in patients in whom no symptoms are associated with the irregularity of ventricular responses. Second, inadvertent complete AV block occurs in 20% of patients. Finally, some data suggest that a regular rhythm is associated with better hemodynamics than an irregular rhythm.

The application of RF energy to produce AV block is rather simple and easily achievable. This procedure is cost effective and improves quality of life (Rokas et al., 2001). Objective benefits include improved exercise tolerance; increased ejection fraction; decreased left ventricular end-systolic, and end-diastolic diameters; and decreased left atrial diameter (Rodriguez et al., 1993). The type of pacemaker required for those patients in whom complete AV block is produced depends on whether chronic atrial fibrillation or paroxysmal atrial fibrillation is present. In the presence of chronic atrial fibrillation, a ventricular demand (VVIR) pacemaker allows for a regular increase in ventricular response on exercise. In cases of paroxysmal atrial fibrillation, particularly those with brady-tachy syndrome, a dual-chamber, rate-responsive pacemaker—preferably with mode switching—is needed. In addition to optimizing AV coordination, atrial pacing may prevent or decrease the episodes of atrial fibrillation.

Currently, AV nodal ablation should be considered when there is failure of multiple AV blocking agents manifested by poor rate control, irregular rhythm that is still symptomatic, drug intolerance, and/or poor compliance preference.

Pacing for Prevention of Atrial Fibrillation

Over the past two decades, it has become generally appreciated that atrial-based pacing for patients with a sick-sinus syndrome, particularly those with brady-tachy syndrome, appears to be associated with low incidence of development of chronic atrial fibrillation. Randomized control studies have demonstrated that atrial-based pacing (atrial demand or dual chambered) in such patients is associated with a lower incidence of chronic atrial fibrillation, strokes, congestive heart failure, and mortality (Anderson et al., 1994). Based on this information, there has been an increased interest in the use of pacemakers to prevent atrial fibrillation in those patients with paroxysmal atrial fibrillation but no bradycardia indications for pacing.

Clinical trials are underway of dual-site right atrial pacing and bicameral (dual atrial) and left atrial (via the coronary sinus) pacing alone to prevent atrial fibrillation in specific patients. (Saksena 1996 & 1998) These are all based on the concept that more synchronized atrial activation will be less arrhythmogenic because electrophysiologic heterogeneity will be reduced. Preliminary data have demonstrated that patients with marked interatrial conduction defects may benefit from simultaneous right and left atrial pacing. One group has shown that pacing from the high right atrium and from the coronary sinus os (dual-site right atrial pacing) decreases recurrences of atrial fibrillation when compared to single-site high right atrial pacing. (Saksena et al., 1996). Other groups suggest that resynchronization of the atria by simultaneously pacing the coronary sinuses and right atrium, particularly during premature atrial complexes, can decrease the incidence of atrial fibrillation in patients with marked interatrial conduction delays (Daubert et al., 1997; D'Allones et al., 2000). These delays can be identified by broad, notched P waves in leads I and II of the electrocardiogram during sinus rhythm. Other investigators have suggested that pacing the interatrial septum, specifically the region of Bachmann's and bundle, may synchronize atrial activation and decrease the incidence of atrial fibrillation. Others suggest that left atrial pacing via the coronary sinus alone might be beneficial. Finally, the role of chronic overdrive pacing and rate smoothing are currently being evaluated as additional pacing modalities to prevent atrial fibrillation. All of these pacing modalities require further evaluation in prospective trials to ascertain their efficacy.

Atrial Defibrillators and Antitachycardia Pacing

It has been recognized for many decades that the longer that atrial fibrillation is present, the harder it is to convert to and maintain sinus rhythm. It has been demonstrated that atrial fibrillation is associated with electrical remodeling, producing a short refractory period, which facilitates the maintenance and/or early recurrence of atrial fibrillation (Wijffels et al., 1995). This led to the concept that "atrial fibrillation begets atrial fibrillation," suggesting that rapid termination of atrial fibrillation can prevent its recurrence.

Two devices have been developed to defibrillate the atrium using rather low energy (106 J). One is a primary atrial defibrillator that employs a right atrial lead and a coronary sinus lead for defibrillation and sensing and a ventricular lead for synchronization. Initial studies using this device suggest that it is safe and effective (Wellens et al., 1998). Despite

the ability to achieve sinus rhythm, a high early recurrence rate was noted, requiring additional antiarrhythmic agents and repeated defibrillation. Nonetheless, the feasibility of defibrillating patients with low-energy shocks has been shown to be safe in normal hearts. Moreover, early data suggest a decrease in recurrent symptomatic episodes of atrial fibrillation. This device has been replaced by one more sophisticated, capable of atrial and ventricular defibrillation, dual-chamber pacing, and antitachycardia pacing (ATP). Theoretically, this device would have a greater capability of preventing atrial fibrillation in view of the atrial pacing capabilities, and it has the advantage of being able to perform ventricular defibrillation. Consequently, this device is applicable to patients with both atrial and ventricular arrhythmias. Recent experience with this device has shown that ATP can effectively terminate rapid atrial tachycardias including flutter and fibrillation (Schoels et al., 2001; Friedman et al., 2001). This device has been shown to decrease the burden of atrial fibrillation, which should consequently decrease the risk of stroke. Although the concept of atrial defibrillation is appealing and early experience is promising, the appropriate patient population still needs to be defined. The combined atrial and ventricular device provides widespread applicability to patients with and without heart disease. Nevertheless, pain, even at low energies, is a concern. Methods to decrease atrial defibrillation thresholds will be necessary to achieve relatively pain-free atrial defibrillation, if this is the primary indication for the device.

Surgery and Catheter Ablation

The ideal therapy for atrial fibrillation is prevention, maintenance of AV synchrony, and restoration of atrial function. By doing this, incidences of palpitations, congestive heart failure, and stroke are decreased. Based on the hypothesis that maintenance of chronic atrial fibrillation is due to multiple reentrant wavelets, a surgical procedure, the *maze operation,* was developed by Cox et al., 1993. The procedure aims to compartmentalize the atrium in order to prevent the critical number of reentrant wavelets required for maintenance of atrial fibrillation. Several iterations of this procedure have evolved, all of them demonstrating the ability to prevent atrial fibrillation in patients with idiopathic atrial fibrillation or fibrillation associated with valvular heart disease. However, the procedures are associated with significant morbidity, including sinus node dysfunction, a complicated postoperative course characterized by fluid retention, and atrial arrhythmias. Nonetheless, the procedure has demonstrated maintenance of sinus rhythm and some, although not normal, atrial function in the majority of patients. The surgical approach has not yet demonstrated adequate atrial mechanical function and freedom from embolic phenomena, a basic goal of the procedure. Long-term follow-up is necessary to demonstrate whether the risk of thromboembolic phenomena is reduced beyond that which anticoagulation can provide. Modifications of the original procedure have evolved to make it simpler to incorporate during mitral valve surgery. Recently the use of RF and other energy sources has been employed to do the modified maze operation. The lesions typically encircle the pulmonary veins and establish a line of block between the pulmonary veins and the mitral annulus.

Electrophysiologists have attempted to mimic the surgical procedure using catheter-based RF energy to deliver linear lesions, either by elongated electrodes or point-by-point sequential RF applications. Currently, this technique is unreliable and may cause significant morbidity, including stroke, cardiac tamponade, and pulmonary hypertension. It is also fraught with the risk of development of other arrhythmias as a consequence of the inability to produce linear lesions without breaks in areas where complete lines of block were intended. While the feasibility of this procedure to "cure" atrial fibrillation has been observed, the success rate is poor. Staged procedures involving first the right atrium and then the left atrium have been proposed, but it appears that one must incorporate lesions in the left atrium in order to be successful in patients with organic heart disease (Haissaguerre, 1996). Currently, these procedures

should be considered highly experimental, in contrast to the surgical procedures which have been demonstrated to be effective.

Detailed mapping data in experimental animals and humans have suggested that there are multiple types of atrial fibrillation. One form of atrial fibrillation is initiated by focal atrial tachycardia, which then results in fibrillatory conduction. Patients with this form of atrial fibrillation have frequent episodes of paroxysmal atrial fibrillation interspersed with sinus rhythm with atrial premature complexes and/or atrial tachycardias, suggesting a common site of initiation of the arrhythmia. The majority of these arise in venous structures, particularly in the pulmonary veins. The high incidence of initiation probably relates to the poorly coupled muscular sheaths surrounding the pulmonary veins and their propagation to the left atrium.

One team demonstrated that RF ablation at mapped sites could not only terminate the atrial tachycardia but prevent atrial fibrillation (Haissaguerre et al., 1998). The exact frequency of patients with atrial fibrillation in whom this approach is applicable is unknown but is probably in the range of 5%. Only patients with paroxysmal episodes of atrial tachycardia are more likely to have successful mapping demonstrating a focal source of origin. The ability to map accurately is limited, many patients have multiple foci, and recurrences are common. This focal procedure is also not free from complications since pulmonary vein thrombosis and pulmonary hypertension have been reported, as well as the usual complications associated with any left-sided approach such as tamponade, cardiac peroration, and stroke. In order to improve the safety and efficacy of pulmonary vein ablation of atrial fibrillation, isolation of the pulmonary vein is currently being undertaken. This may be done by segmental ablation of muscular sheaths around the pulmonary veins, circumferential ablation at the ostia of the pulmonary veins, or encircling the pulmonary veins (Haissaguerre et al., 1998; Chen et al., 1999; Papponne et al., 2000; Haissaguerre, 2000abc; Natale, 2000b). Long-term follow-up will be necessary to assess the efficacy and safety of these procedures. The widespread use of these procedures for atrial fibrillations should be discouraged until safety and efficacy are proven.

Role of Ablation of Flutter in Patients with Atrial Fibrillation

Atrial flutter and fibrillation frequently occur in the same patient. This suggests the possibility that in some patients atrial flutter may initiate and/or perpetuate atrial fibrillation. It is not possible to recognize in which patients flutter plays a role in initiation and/or perpetuation of atrial fibrillation. However, the success and ease with which RF ablation of atrial flutter (Cosio et al., 1996; Lesh et al., 2000) can be accomplished suggests that such an ablation may be useful in patients who have both atrial flutter and fibrillation. Several investigations have shown a decrease in the incidence of atrial fibrillation in such patients undergoing flutter ablation (Movscowitz et al., 1996; Natale et al., 2000a), and the latter group also demonstrated the superiority of RF ablation over pharmacologic therapy for atrial flutter.

Another group of patients in whom a flutter ablation can be particularly helpful are those patients whose fibrillation is converted to flutter by antiarrhythmic drugs. The agents most likely to produce these are class IA and IC and amiodarone. Once the drug is shown to change fibrillation to flutter, a simple flutter lesion is preformed. This combination therapy ("hybrid therapy") has been demonstrated to have an excellent long-term success as long as antiarrhythmic therapy is maintained (Huang et al., 1998).

SUMMARY

In recent years, electrophysiologists have learned that atrial fibrillation is not just one arrhythmia but that it may have multiple mechanisms. Pharmacologic treatment alone has proven inadequate in many patients. Nonpharmacologic therapies are now available as primary therapy, with or without adjunctive pharmacologic therapy. The future of atrial fibrillation management will rely on a better understanding of the type of atrial fibrillation being treated and the appropriate balance of pharmacologic and nonpharmacologic therapy, including the use of hybrid therapy.

REFERENCES

Anderson HR et al: Prospective randomized trial of atrial versus ventricular pacing in sick sinus syndrome. Lancet 344: 1523, 1994

Chen SA et al: Initiation of atrial fibrillation by ectopic beats originating from the pulmonary veins. Electrophysiological characteristics, pharmacological responses and effects of radiofrequency ablation. Circulation 100:1879, 1999

Cosio FG et al: Radiofrequency ablation of atrial flutter. J Cardiovasc Electrophysiol 7:60, 1996

Cox JL et al: Five-year experience with the maze procedure for atrial fibrillation. Ann Thorac Surg 56:814, 1993

D'Allones GR et al: Long-term effects of biatrial synchronous pacing to prevent drug-refractory atrial arrhythmias: A nine year experience. J Cardiovasc Electrophysiol 11:1081, 2000

Daubert C et al: Biatrial synchronous pacing: A new approach to prevent arrhythmias in patients with atrial conduction block, in *Prevention of Tachyarrhythmias with Cardiac Pacing*, JC Daubert et al (eds.) Armonk, NY, Futura Publishing, 1997, pp 99–119

Friedman P et al: Atrial therapies reduce atrial arrhythmia burden in defibrillator patients. Circulation 104:1023, 2001

Haissaguerre M et al: Right and left atrial radiofrequency catheter therapy of paroxysmal atrial fibrillation. J Cardiovasc Electrophysiol 7:1132, 1996

Haissaguerre M et al: Spontaneous initiation of atrial fibrillation by ectopic beats originating in the pulmonary veins. N Engl J Med 339:659, 1998

Haissaguerre M et al: Mapping-guided ablation of pulmonary veins to cure atrial fibrillation. Am J Cardiol 86 (9 Suppl 1):K9, 2000a

Haissaguerre M et al: Electrophysiological end point for catheter ablation of atial fibrillation initiated from multiple pulmonary venous foci. Circulation 101:1409, 2000b

Haissaguerre M et al: Catheter ablation of chronic atrial fibrillation targeting the reinitiating triggers. J Cardiovasc Electrophysiol 11:2, 2000c

Huang DT et al: Hybrid pharmacologic and ablative therapy: A novel and effective approach for the management of atrial fibrillation. J Cardiovasc Electrophysiol 9:462, 1998

Lesh MD: Catheter ablation of atrial flutter and tachycardia, in *Cardiac Electrophysiology: From Cell to Bedside*, DP Zipes, J Jalife (eds). Philadelphia, Saunders, 2000, pp 1009–1027

Movscowitz C et al: The results of atrial flutter ablation in patients with and without a history of atrial fibrillation. Am J Cardiol 78:93, 1996

Natale A et al: Prospective randomized comparison of antiarrhythmic therapy versus first line radiofrequency ablation in patients with atrial flutter. J Am Coll Cardiol 35:1898, 2000a

Natale A et al: First human experience with pulmonary vein isolation using a through-the-balloon circumferential ultrasound ablation system for recurrent atrial fibrillation. Circulation 102:1879, 2000b

Pappone C et al: Circumferential radiofrequency ablation of pulmonary vein ostia: A new anatomic approach for curing atrial fibrillation. Circulation 102:2619, 2000

Rodriguez LM et al: Improvement in left ventricular function by ablation of atrioventricular nodal conduction in selected patients with lone atrial fibrillation. Am J Cardiol 72:1137, 1993

Rokas S et al: Atrioventricular node modification in patients with chronic atrial fibrillation: Role of morphology of RR interval variation. Circulation 103:2942, 2001

Saksena S et al: Prevention of recurrent atrial fibrillation with chronic dual-site right atrial pacing. J Am Coll Cardiol 28:687, 1996

Saksena S et al: Multisite electrode pacing for prevention of atrial fibrillation. J Cardiovac Electrophysiol 9:S155, 1998

Schoels W et al: Worldwide clinical experience with a new dual-chamber implantable cardioverter defibrillator system. J Cardiovasc Electrophysiol 12:521, 2001

Wellens HJJ et al: Atrioverter: An implantable device for the treatment of atrial fibrillation. Circulation 98:1651, 1998

Wijffels MCEF et al: Atrial fibrillation begets atrial fibrillation: A study in awake chronically instrumented goats. Circulation 92:1954, 1995

64

MANAGEMENT OF POSTOPERATIVE ATRIAL FIBRILLATION

David B. Bharucha, Peter R. Kowey

Incidence/Risk Factors

Atrial fibrillation and flutter (AFF) occur frequently after multiple types of cardiac surgery, with an incidence as high as 40% following coronary artery bypass grafting (CABG) (Daudon et al., 1986) and 60% following valvular surgery (Andrews et al., 1991). Patients at the highest risk for developing postoperative AFF have characteristics described in Table 64-1 (Dixon et al., 1986, Leitch et al., 1990). A minimally invasive approach to CABG (vs. via a conventional sternotomy) does not lessen the incidence of postoperative AFF when corrected for disease severity (Tamis et al., 1998).

Risk stratification can be performed using clinical characteristics (Table 64-1) or by laboratory methods. One such test has been based on P wave duration, as calculated directly from the surface electrocardiogram or from signal-averaged data (Oshima et al., 1996).

Prognosis

Postoperative AFF usually arises 1 to 5 days following surgery and often has a self-limited course. Over 90% of patients with AFF following cardiac surgery

who have no prior history of atrial arrhythmias are in sinus rhythm 6 to 8 weeks following their operation (Stebbins et al., 1995).

Mechanism/Pathogenesis

There are multiple perioperative issues that have been implicated in making the atria susceptible to AFF (Table 64-2) but no definitive explanation is available. The pathophysiology of postoperative AFF is likely related to preexisting age-related degenerative changes in many cardiac surgical patients, coupled with perioperative abnormalities in dispersion of atrial refractoriness, atrial conduction velocities, and atrial transmembrane potentials.

Management

Prophylaxis

Given the high incidence of postoperative AFF, it is reasonable to treat prophylactically, especially in the presence of the risk factors described in Table 64-1. Medication with beta blockers, in the presence

TABLE 64-1

CLINICAL CHARACTERISTICS OF PATIENTS AT THE HIGHEST RISK FOR DEVELOPING POSTCARDIAC SURGICAL ATRIAL ARRHYTHMIAS

Advanced age

Left atrial enlargement

Roentgenographic cardiomegaly

Nature of cardioprotection and hypothermia during bypass

Longer bypass times

Previous cardiac surgery

Absence of beta blocker treatment (or withdrawal of previous treatment)

Chronic obstructive pulmonary disease

Chronic renal failure

TABLE 64-2

POTENTIAL PATHOGENESIS/MECHANISMS OF POST CARDIAC SURGICAL ATRIAL ARRHYTHMIAS

Pericarditis

Atrial injury from direct surgical handling or from cannulation

Acute atrial enlargement from pressure or volume overload

Inadequate cardioprotection during bypass

Atrial infarction

Hyperadrenergic postoperative state

Postoperative pulmonary issues

or absence of digitalis, has been demonstrated to decrease AFF from 40% in CABG patients and 60% in valve surgical patients to 20% and 30%, respectively (Andrews et al., 1991). The benefit of beta blockade, alone or with digoxin, has been demonstrated in multiple studies (Kowey et al., 1992). Digitalis given pre- or postoperatively has been shown to be beneficial, although not to the same degree or with the same consistency as beta blockers (Kowey et al., 1992). Postoperative verapamil given to patients in sinus rhythm has been observed to slow the rate of any AFF but not to alter its incidence (Davison et al., 1985).

Other antiarrhythmic agents, such as procainamide (Gold et al., 1996), have been studied in a prophylactic role but have conferred varying benefit in different reports. There are no comprehensive data available regarding propafenone or sotalol, although preliminary data about the latter drug are encouraging.

Oral and parenteral amiodarone have been examined for a potential prophylactic role before and after cardiac surgery. One group showed a possible benefit of outpatient preoperative medication with oral amiodarone in decreasing AFF (Daoud et al., 1997), although their observation of a high incidence of atrial arrhythmias in the control group despite a high rate of use of beta blockers [an approach shown to prevent at least 50% of AFF in almost every trial in which it has been studied (Andrews et al., 1991)] calls their observation into question. Also, distinct disadvantages of preoperative amiodarone treatment exist: the need to identify patients well in advance of their procedure, potential bradyarrhythmic hazards (especially in an outpatient setting and in the elderly), and, although rare, an increased risk of severe perioperative pulmonary toxicity.

Intravenous (IV) amiodarone has been shown to be beneficial in reducing postoperative AFF without significant risk, although the size of the benefit did not result in reduced length of hospital stay in the Amiodarone Reduces Coronary Artery Disease Bypass Grafting Hospitalization (ARCH) trial (Guarnieri et al., 1999); also, the relatively modest benefit of IV amiodarone in this report would have probably been even smaller had a greater number of patients received a beta blocker.

Nonpharmacologic therapy for postoperative AFF has been examined. Although single- and multiple-site atrial pacing has been shown to be helpful in some situations of paroxysmal AFF, this

TABLE 64-3

SUMMARY OF MEASURES FOR PROPHYLAXIS AND TREATMENT OF POSTCARDIAC SURGICAL ATRIAL ARRHYTHMIAS

Prophylaxis
  Definitive: beta blockers
  Possible: digitalis, amiodarone, procainamide
  Unproven: sotalol, propafenone, procainamide, atrial
    pacing
  Ineffective: calcium channel blockers

Treatment
  Rate control with beta blocker, calcium channel
    blocker, digitalis, or amiodarone
  Anticoagulation
  Electrical or pharmacologic conversion, preferably
    after drug-loading

modality has not yet demonstrated a benefit for postoperative AFF (Schweikert et al., 1998).

In summary (Table 64-3), beta blockers have been shown to be the most effective single prophylactic agent (Andrews et al., 1991; Kowey et al., 1992) and carry a lower risk relative to other antiarrhythmic agents.

Treatment for Postoperatively Occurring AFF

Rate Control

Given the self-resolving, natural course of postoperative AFF for the vast majority of patients with no history of atrial arrhythmias (Stebbins et al., 1995), treatment to control the ventricular response rate in postoperative AFF is a useful and relatively safe strategy. Rate control therapy with a beta blocker should be the first-line choice, with the relative benefit partly due to treatment of the hyperadrenergic postoperative state and the well-demonstrated phenomenon of beta blocker withdrawal. Other AV-nodal blocking agents, such as calcium channel blockers and digoxin, have a role in control of ventricular rate in AFF but are not as effective as beta blockers. IV agents with short half-lives (e.g., esmolol) can be particularly useful if

there is the potential for bradyarrhythmias, hypotension, or bronchospasm.

Electrical Conversion

Conversion from well-tolerated postoperative AFF is generally not actively sought, both because of the high recurrence rate and the usual self-resolving course. For patients with symptoms, therapies are similar to those employed in nonpostoperative circumstances, except for the accentuated need for postconversion pharmacologic therapy because of multiple, ongoing triggers for recurrence. If conversion is necessary, defibrillation—or, if atrial flutter or tachycardia is present, pace-termination—can be employed. In a case of atrial fibrillation that is difficult to convert by usual external techniques, consideration should be given to (1) internal defibrillation utilizing transvenous coils, or (2) a "double defibrillator" technique in which two pairs of orthogonally placed external patch electrodes are discharged simultaneously (Saliba et al., 1999). Low-energy atrial defibrillation, via operatively implanted temporary epicardial coils (Liebold et al., 1998), may ultimately be an effective strategy for high-risk patients (Table 64-1) who are preoperatively known to be unable to tolerate otherwise effective pharmacologic prophylaxis.

Pharmacologic Conversion

Consideration of IV pharmacologic measures for the conversion of AFF should be given if the patient's respiratory status would make anesthesia for an electrical conversion potentially difficult. Medications that have been shown to be potentially useful include newer class III agents (such as ibutilide and possibly investigational agents such as tedisamil and trecetilide).

Anticoagulation

Although one might expect a relatively low risk for a thromboembolic event in association with a limited course of postoperative AFF, several studies have shown, with both prospective analyses and case-controlled retrospective analyses, an increased rate of post-CABG stroke in association with postoperative AFF (Reed et al., 1998), even after correction for comorbid risk factors. Thus, given the potentially devastating consequences of a thromboembolic event, anticoagulation with IV heparin and then coumadin is often performed for postoperative AFF. Because of the risk of bleeding in postoperative patients, anticoagulation must be done judiciously. If cardioversion is performed for postoperative AFF, conventional recommendations for anticoagulation (i.e., its need) are applicable.

REFERENCES

Andrews TC et al: Prevention of supraventricular arrhythmias after coronary artery bypass surgery. Circulation 84 (Suppl 5):III236, 1991

Daoud EG et al: Preoperative amiodarone as prophylaxis against atrial fibrillation after heart surgery. N Engl J Med 337:1785, 1997

Daudon P et al: Prevention of atrial fibrillation or flutter by acebutolol after coronary bypass grafting. Am J Cardiol 58:933, 1986

Davison R et al: Prophylaxis of supraventricular tachyarrhythmia after coronary bypass surgery with oral verapamil: A randomized, double-blinded trial. Ann Thorac Surg 39:336, 1985

Dixon FE et al: Factors predisposing to supraventricular tachyarrhythmias after coronary artery bypass grafting. Am J Cardiol 58:476, 1986

Gold MR et al: Efficacy and safety of procainamide in preventing arrhythmias after coronary artery bypass surgery. Am J Cardiol 78:975, 1996

Guarnieri T et al: Intravenous amiodarone for the prevention of atrial fibrillation after open heart surgery: The ARCH (Amiodarone Reduces Coronary Artery Disease Bypass Grafting Hospitalization) trial. J Am Coll Cardiol 34:343, 1999

Kowey PR et al: Meta-analysis of the effectiveness of prophylactic drug therapy in preventing supraventricular arrhythmia early after coronary artery bypass grafting. Am J Cardiol 69:963, 1992

Leitch JW et al: The importance of age as a predictor of atrial fibrillation and flutter after coronary artery bypass grafting. J Thorac Cardiovasc Surg 100:338, 1990

Liebold A et al: Low-energy cardioversion with epicardial wire electrodes: New treatment of atrial fibrillation after open heart surgery. Circulation 98:883, 1998

Oshima H et al: Value of the regional P-wave recorded by signal-averaged ECG on the atrium for predicting atrial fibrillation after cardiac surgery (abstr.). Circulation 94:I-69, 1996

Reed GL et al: Stroke following coronary-artery bypass surgery: A case-control estimate of the risk from carotid bruits. N Engl J Med 319:1246, 1998

Saliba WI et al: High energy synchronized external direct current cardioversion with 720 joules for atrial fibrillation refractory to standard cardioversion (abstr.). J Am Coll Cardiol 33:126A, 1999

Schweikert RA et al: Atrial pacing in the prevention of atrial fibrillation after cardiac surgery: Results of the second postoperative pacing study (POPS-2) (abstr.). J Am Coll Cardiol 31:117A, 1998

Stebbins D et al: Clinical outcome of patients who developed atrial fibrillation after coronary artery bypass surgery (abstr.). Pacing Clin Electrophysiol 18:811, 1995

Tamis JE et al: Atrial fibrillation is common after minimally invasive direct coronary artery bypass surgery (abstr.). J Am Coll Cardiol 31:116A, 1998

65

ATRIAL FIBRILLATION TRIALS

D. George Wyse

Atrial fibrillation (AF) is an extremely common arrhythmia. The prevalence of AF is increasing dramatically in North America, even after adjusting for the aging of the population. Many consider AF to be a benign arrhythmia, but both community (Benjamin et al., 1998) and patient studies (Dries et al., 1998; Wyse et al., 2001) indicate that AF is associated with increased mortality after adjustment for other risk factors. The explanation for such increased mortality is uncertain. It may be partly attributed to stroke. Other potential explanations include underuse of effective therapy, such as warfarin, and adverse effects of treatment (e.g., proarrhythmia). Furthermore, uncontrolled AF can itself lead to worsening ventricular function and heart failure (tachycardia-induced "cardiomyopathy").

It is necessary to have a clinical framework within which to consider AF. A recent Joint Task Force of the American College of Cardiology, American Heart Association, and European Society of Cardiology have completed guidelines on the management of patients with AF (Fuster et al., 2001). The clinical classification scheme used in these guidelines is recommended. The scheme divides AF into four categories: new onset, paroxysmal, persistent, and permanent. *New-onset AF* refers to the first detected episode of AF. It includes the first electrocardiographically documented episode in those who are suspected of having previous episodes. *Paroxysmal AF* starts and stops by itself, usually within 48 h, but can last up to 7 days. *Persistent AF* has been present continuously for more than 7 days but also includes episodes cardioverted in less than 7 days. *Permanent AF* is designated when repeated attempts fail to restore sinus rhythm or no attempt is made to restore sinus rhythm and the patient is left in AF. Note that the term *chronic AF* is not used in this scheme. The reason is that chronic AF had a very specific meaning to arrhythmia specialists, but this term was used differently by others and led to confusion. A particular patient's status within such a scheme can change over time; for example, paroxysmal AF can progress to persistent or permanent AF. However, at any one moment in time an individual patient's status within such a scheme will be a determinant of the treatment strategy. The scheme is also important in interpretation of the literature on the management of AF for application to individual patients.

There are a number of limitations concerning randomized clinical trials of AF management. The main problem is the selection of end-points (Wyse, 2001). There are many from which to choose, including mortality, stroke, bleeding, restoration or maintenance of rhythm, heart rate control, quality of life, and cost. The most useful end-points are those that are clinically important. A consequence of the misconception that AF is a benign arrhythmia has been that many randomized clinical trials have used rhythm control or heart rate control as primary end-points. It should be recognized that these are in fact surrogate end-points in most instances. Indeed, there is no direct evidence that the strategy of rhythm control is uniformly superior to the heart rate control strategy, although this concept is a common bias held by many physicians. Furthermore, it should be emphasized that there is currently no accepted "gold standard" for good heart rate control and good rhythm control (Wyse, 2001). Research on these fundamental issues is badly needed. The trials of anticoagulation therapy were among the first to use clinically important end-points. Only recently have we begun to see trials of rhythm management using such end-points. Restoration of rhythm is an appropriate end-point in studies of cardioversion per se, but such studies frequently have not been placebo-controlled. A lack of an appropriate control group is another serious problem in many studies of AF management. Therefore, although the literature on management of AF is vast, the quality of much of the work is too poor to be the basis for an evidence-based approach to management.

Trials of Antithrombotic Therapy

Stroke is one of the most serious consequences of AF. During the 1990s there were several large randomized trials conducted on the use of warfarin and aspirin for both primary and secondary prevention of thromboembolism in nonvalvular AF. The results of these trials have been condensed into a number of recommendations. At the core of the recommendations is the concept of risk stratification. There are three major schemes for risk stratification for thromboembolism in nonvalvular AF, and these are presented in Table 65-1. Two of these schemes designate high-, intermediate-, and low-risk categories and the third designates only high- and low-risk. The recommendations in each case are for warfarin to be used for the high-risk categories and aspirin or nothing to

TABLE 65-1

RISK STRATIFICATION FOR THROMBOEMBOLISM IN PATIENTS WITH NONVALVULAR ATRIAL FIBRILLATION

Reference	High-risk	Intermediate risk	Low-risk
Atrial Fibrillation Investigators, 1994	Prior stroke, TIA, Age ≥ 65 years History of hypertension Coronary artery disease diabetes	—	Age < 65 years No high-risk features
American College of Chest Physicians: Laupacis et al., 1998	Prior stroke, TIA, Age > 75 years History of hypertension LV dysfunction >1 Intermediate-risk factor	Age 65–75 years Diabetes Coronary artery disease Thyrotoxicosis	Age < 65 years No risk factors
Stroke Prevention in Atrial Fibrillation: The SPAF writing committee, 1988	Prior stroke, TIA, Women >75 years Systolic BP >160 LV Dysfunction	History of hypertension No high-risk factors	No high-risk factors No history of hypertension

ABBREVIATIONS: BP, blood pressure; LV, left ventricular; TIA, transient ischemic attack.

be used in the low-risk categories. For the intermediate-risk categories, the recommendation is to use either warfarin or aspirin. The recommendations of the American College of Chest Physicians are the ones that have most recently been up-dated (Albers et al., 2001). The recommended INR range is 2.0 to 3.0 for warfarin. In the trials, this range of INR reduced the risk of thromboembolism by two-thirds with an acceptable risk of major bleeding. Aspirin is a weakly effective alternative to warfarin but does not appear to be effective in the elderly, who are at greatest risk. There are no substantive trial data for other alternatives to warfarin, such as low-molecular weight heparin, antithrombin agents, or combinations of antiplatelet agents. However, several large trials are in progress or about to start, and effective alternatives to warfarin would be very welcome.

The populations studied in the randomized trials of thromboembolism prophylaxis consisted largely of males in their mid-sixties with persistent or permanent AF. Accordingly, a large number of issues with respect to antithrombotic therapy for AF have not been resolved by well-designed randomized clinical trials. Safety of warfarin with this INR in those over 75 years and particularly in women is uncertain. There is also uncertainty about warfarin therapy for intermittent AF and isolated type 1 atrial flutter. The current consensus is that intermittent AF should be treated the same as persistent or permanent AF, particularly if symptoms are not reliable for determination if AF has recurred. Isolated atrial flutter probably has a lower risk than AF, but the consensus is that atrial flutter should be treated the same as AF, particularly as many patients will have both atrial flutter and AF. Currently, the best approach is to use anticoagulation with warfarin unless there is no doubt the risk is low. Current data suggest that warfarin therapy is underutilized.

The risk for thromboembolism is greatest around the time of cardioversion, whether electric or pharmacologic. There is little information from clinical trials available on this issue. The guidelines in this respect are largely based on consensus of experts. A recently completed trial compared the approach of transesophageal-guided cardioversion followed by anticoagulation to prior anticoagulation for 3 weeks before cardioversion followed by a further period of antico-

agulation (Klein et al., 2001). The study was not as large as originally intended, which has created some uncertainty. The primary end-point was a composite of thromboembolic events. This event rate was low and no different in the two groups. The number of hemorrhagic events was lower in the transesophageal-guided group, but there was a disturbing trend for increased death in this group. Many consider the two approaches equivalent, but equivalence is not established by this single trial.

Trials of Restoration of Sinus Rhythm

Cardioversion has not been studied extensively in clinical trials, with the exception of pharmacologic cardioversion. Subject selection is important in studies of cardioversion, primarily with respect to the duration of AF. The longer the duration of AF, the lower is the likelihood of successful cardioversion. Transthoracic and transvenous electrical cardioversion have been compared in a small, randomized clinical trial. The transvenous technique was more effective. However, it is usually reserved for those situations in which transthoracic electrical cardioversion has failed. This trial was done before the advent of biphasic waveforms in external cardioverter-defibrillators. The need for alternatives to standard transthoracic electrical cardioversion is waning with the wider application of a biphasic waveform for cardioversion.

There has been great interest in pharmacologic cardioversion as an alternative to electrical cardioversion, but they have not been directly compared in a clinical trial. The putative advantages of pharmacologic cardioversion are that it is more acceptable to patients, is more readily available, and does not require a general anesthetic. Some think it is less likely to be associated with stroke, but there is no clear evidence to support this supposition and anticoagulation guidelines for cardioversion are the same for electric and pharmacologic cardioversion. Pharmacologic cardioversion can also be self-administered in selected patients. The disadvantages are that it is less effective and the drugs can potentially cause adverse effects.

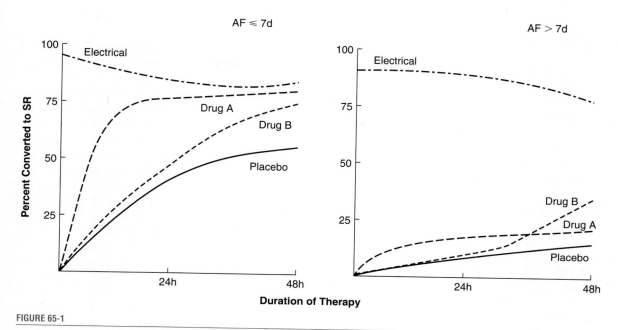

FIGURE 65-1

Hypothetical comparison of the time course of electrical cardioversion and pharmacologic cardioversion, with a rapidly acting drug (Drug A) or a slowly acting drug (Drug B), compared to placebo in recent onset (left panel) and persistent (right panel) atrial fibrillation.

The state of knowledge with respect to pharmacologic cardioversion is summarized in Fig. 65-1 and Table 65-2 (Miller et al., 2000). The hypothetical sketch in Fig. 65-1 illustrates the importance of patient and drug selection. The first point is that the duration of AF is an important determinant of effectiveness. AF of ≤7 days' duration (predominantly paroxysmal AF) is much more likely to respond to drug therapy (left panel). Placebo control is an important aspect of such studies because in recent-onset AF more than half the patients will spontaneously convert to sinus rhythm within 48 h (left panel). Finally, drugs that accelerate the return of sinus rhythm are the most useful (drug A, left panel, e.g., ibutilide, flecainide, propafenone), and more rapid return of sinus rhythm is the expected result. At 48 h there is little difference in the proportion in sinus rhythm in the treated and placebo groups. Drugs that have a slow onset of action (drug B, left panel, e.g., amiodarone, oral dofetilide) are less useful in this setting. As is shown in the right panel, persistent AF is much less likely to convert

spontaneously, and pharmacologic cardioversion is much less effective. Drugs with a slow onset of

TABLE 65-2

STATUS OF ANTIARRHYTHMIC DRUGS TESTED FOR PHARMACOLOGIC CARDIOVERSION

Proven efficacy	Incompletely tested	Proven inefficacy
Amiodarone[a]	Disopyramide	Digoxin[b]
Dofetilide[a]	Procainamide	Sotalol[c]
Flecainide		Verapamil
Ibutilide[a]		
Propafenone		
Quinidine[a]		

[a] Some efficacy for persistent atrial fibrillation.
[b] May be effective combined with diltiazem.
[c] Exception is atrial fibrillation after open-heart surgery.

action (drug B, right panel, e.g., amiodarone, oral dofetilide) are most likely to have an effect, but it may take days or even weeks before cardioversion occurs. Electrical cardioversion is much more effective in persistent AF (right panel) but is plagued by "immediate" and "early" recurrence of AF (IRAF and ERAF) that can occur in minutes or a few days. These phenomena may be the consequence of atrial electrical remodeling that may be altered by prior antiarrhythmic drug treatment (De Simone et al., 1999). More research on this point is needed.

Table 65-2 summarizes the status of individual drugs for pharmacologic cardioversion. Some of these drugs appear to have a differential efficacy for atrial flutter in comparison to AF, although this information is not available for all drugs. Ibutilide, for example, has greater effectiveness for atrial flutter than for AF. On the other hand, flecainide and propafenone have greater effectiveness for AF than for atrial flutter. Although quinidine is effective, it is rarely used anymore and should be considered a rarely used alternative. Flecainide and propafenone are really only useful for recent-onset AF, a point mentioned in discussion of Fig. 65-1. One of the most poorly recognized aspects of pharmacologic cardioversion is the inefficacy of sotalol outside the setting of recent open-heart surgery, even though it is effective for maintenance of sinus rhythm.

Maintenance of Sinus Rhythm

Long-term therapy for maintenance of rhythm is not usually necessary for new-onset AF. Often no treatment or a short period of treatment of the first episode or optimal therapy for underlying problems such as untreated hypertension is all that is needed, and AF may not recur for months or even years. Treatment for maintenance of rhythm becomes an issue only when AF is recurrent. The alleged strengths of this strategy are better relief of symptoms and reduced risk of stroke. However, there are little data to support these putative advantages. The weaknesses of this approach are the inefficacy of the drugs, adverse effects of the drugs—including fatal proarrhythmia—and the lack of a widely applicable

and effective nonpharmacologic therapy. The available data comparing the strategy of rhythm control vs. rate control will be outlined below. The status of the various therapies for maintenance of rhythm as evaluated in randomized clinical trials is outlined in Table 65-3 (Miller et al., 2000). It is important to state that the end-point in the randomized clinical trials that form the basis of Table 65-3 is the surrogate of maintenance of rhythm, not clinical end-points such as death, quality of life, etc.. The actual selection of therapy can be quite complex in an individual patient, and the recent joint guidelines (Fuster et al., 2001) have some algorithms that are helpful. Amiodarone (Roy et al., 2000) and dofetilide (Singh et al., 2001) are probably the most effective drugs and certainly the safest in those with structural heart disease. Dofetilide must be started in hospital. Nonpharmacologic therapies are being aggressively investigated and may soon yield results that will lead to testing in randomized clinical trials. Among the nonpharmacologic therapies, only atrial-based pacing has had limited testing in randomized clinical trials. Atrial-based pacing may help to prevent AF (Connolly et al., 2000), but its role in treatment of patients with AF is less clear.

Trials of Heart Rate Control

Heart rate control has not been as extensively studied in randomized clinical trials as pharmacologic cardioversion and maintenance of rhythm. Until recently, it was not considered a primary alternative to maintenance of rhythm. Its use has largely been confined to patients with permanent AF or those in whom maintenance of rhythm has been deemed a failure. It is also used as a temporary therapy, often while awaiting an appropriate period of anticoagulation before cardioversion. Heart rate-control medications are safer than those used for maintenance of rhythm. There is a highly effective and widely applicable nonpharmacologic therapy. The heart rate control strategy is alleged to be less effective at controlling symptoms and less effective in preventing stroke, but there is no good evidence in support of these suppositions. The available data comparing

TABLE 65-3

STATUS OF ATRIAL FIBRILLATION THERAPIES FOR MAINTENANCE OF RHYTHM BASED ON RANDOMIZED CLINICAL TRIALS

Proven efficacy	Incompletely tested	Not tested
Amiodarone	Atrial-based Pacing	Atrial pacing software
Azimilide	Single site[a]	Prevention
Disopyramide	Dual site[b]	Treatment
Dofetilide		Implantable cardioverter
Flecainide		Radio Frequency ablation
Propafenone		Linear
Quinidine		Focal
Sotalol		Surgery
		Maze
		Others

[a] Prevention of atrial fibrillation (AF) in some subsets but not effective in paroxysmal AF in absence of bradycardia indication.

[b] May be more effective than support pacing or single-site pacing in highly selected subgroup (bradycardia indication + continued aggressive drug therapy: episodes of AF less frequent than weekly).

heart rate vs. rhythm control strategies will be outlined below. One of the deficiencies of the heart rate control strategy is that there is no widely accepted definition to use as a "gold standard." It is clear that there should be criteria for both resting heart rate and heart rate during activity. There are data to suggest that the resting heart rate should be <90 beats per minute. Data on maximum exercise heart rate can be used, but symptom-limited exercise testing is labor-intensive. The strategy of heart rate control is in general labor-intensive for physicians. This may be one of the reasons it is used less often. The status of heart rate control therapies as evaluated in randomized clinical trials is outlined in Table 65-4 (Sharif & Wyse, 1998). It must be emphasized that the end-point for the clinical trials in Table 65-4 is the surrogate of heart rate itself, not clinical end-points such as death, quality of life, etc.. Digoxin is seldom used by itself but is a good adjunctive agent with a beta blocker or calcium channel blocker. Beta-blocker therapy can sometimes lead to chronotropic incompetence, which may require a pacemaker. Amiodarone and sotalol are good agents for heart rate control, although simpler agents should be used if possible. The combination of total atrioventricular node ablation and a permanent pacemaker is a very effective and well-tolerated therapy for heart rate control. It has been found to be more effective than drug therapy in randomized clinical trials using quality of life and left ventricular function as end-points. Atrioventricular node modification has been compared to atrioventricular node ablation and pacemaker and is not as effective.

Rhythm vs. Rate Control

As mentioned above, there is a lot of interest in comparison of these two strategies for the management of AF. Two small studies have recently been completed. The Pharmacological Intervention in Atrial Fibrillation (PIAF) Study (Hohnloser et al., 2000)

TABLE 65-4

STATUS OF AF THERAPIES TESTED FOR HEART RATE CONTROL BASED ON RANDOMIZED CLINICAL TRIALS

Proven efficacy		
Alone	With digoxin	Incompletely tested
Amiodarone	Betaxolol[a]	AVN ablation + pacemaker[b]
Pindolol[a]	Diltiazem	AVN modification ± pacemaker
Sotalol[a]	Nadolol[a]	High-rate VVI(R) pacing
Verapamil	Verapamil	

[a] Probably a beta-blocker class effect. Some beta blockers decrease exercise tolerance.
[b] Randomized clinical trials have shown superiority to drug therapy and AVN modification for quality of life in drug-resistance patients.
ABBREVIATIONS: AVN, Atrioventricular node; VVI, ventricular inhibited.

enrolled 252 patients with persistent AF and randomized them to rhythm control with amiodarone or to rate control with diltiazem. The primary end-point was symptomatic improvement, and there was no difference in this end-point. There was also no difference in quality of life. The amiodarone patients walked further on a 6-min walk test but also had more adverse drug effects and were more frequently hospitalized. The Strategies of Treatment of Atrial Fibrillation (STAF) Study (Carlsson & Tebbe, 2001) has only been presented in abstract form. It was intended to be a pilot study. Two hundred patients were enrolled, and the trial was terminated for futility concerning the primary end-point—a composite of death, stroke/transient ischemic attack, cardiopulmonary resuscitation, or thromboembolism—as there was no difference in this end-point and no likelihood a difference would be shown if the main study was completed. The patients enrolled had persistent AF. In the rhythm control arm, cardioversion, amiodarone, and class 1 drugs were allowed, depending on the patient's clinical status. Digitalis, beta blockers, calcium channel blockers, and atrioventricular node ablation with pacemaker were permitted in the heart rate control arm. In the rhythm control arm, anticoagulation was discontinued after 3 weeks of maintenance of rhythm, but it was continued permanently in the heart rate

control arm. If AF recurred in the rhythm control arm, anticoagulation was restarted prior to cardioversion. After 3 years of follow-up, <25% of the rhythm control patients remained in sinus rhythm, and eight of the nine events in this group occurred while the patients were in AF. The authors concluded that although sinus rhythm might be better, it was not possible to maintain it well enough to make a difference. The Atrial Fibrillation Follow-up Investigation of Rhythm Management (AFFIRM) Trial is the largest trial addressing this issue (Wyse, 2000). The primary end-point of AFFIRM is total mortality. It has enrolled 4060 patients with a mixture of paroxysmal and persistent AF. All the therapies outlined in this chapter are permitted in the trial. The average follow-up is 3.5 years, and the main results will be available in 2002. At least two other smaller studies are also in progress. A large study focused on AF patients with heart failure has just begun.

Until definitive evidence is available concerning the relative merits of these two approaches to rhythm management in AF, physicians need to make a judgment about the best approach in each patient. In general, the rhythm control approach should be the initial approach in highly symptomatic patients, particularly those with paroxysmal AF and relatively normal hearts. In less symptomatic patients, particularly those with persistent AF, the physician may choose to start with the heart rate control approach. This controversy is particularly acute for the patients with heart failure because they are at much greater risk of proarrhythmia from antiarrhythmic drugs.

SUMMARY

North America is currently experiencing an epidemic of AF. Only recently has clinical trial science been applied to this problem in an extensive manner. There is much that remains to be learned. However, better application of the current knowledge would improve the management of this extremely common heart rhythm problem. The information outlined in this chapter should form a good foundation for management using our current knowledge base.

REFERENCES

Albers GW et al: Antithrombotic therapy in atrial fibrillation. Chest 119(Suppl 1): 194S, 2001

Atrial Fibrillation Investigators: Risk factors for stroke and efficacy of antithrombotic therapy in atrial fibrillation. Analysis of pooled data from five randomized controlled trials [published erratum appears in Arch Intern Med 154:2254, 1994]. Arch Intern Med 154:1449, 1994

Benjamin EJ et al: Impact of atrial fibrillation on the risk of death: The Framingham Heart Study. Circulation 98:946, 1998

Carlsson J, Tebbe U: Rhythm control versus rate control in atrial fibrillation: Results from the STAF pilot study (Strategies of Treatment of Atrial Fibrillation) (Abstr.). Pacing Clin Electrophysiol 24(Part II):561, 2001

Connolly SJ et al: Effects of physiologic pacing versus ventricular pacing on the risk of stroke and death due to cardiovascular causes. Canadian Trial of Physiologic Pacing Investigators. N Engl J Med 342:1385, 2000

De Simone A et al: Pretreatment with verapamil in patients with persistent or chronic atrial fibrillation who underwent electrical cardioversion. J Am Coll Cardiol 34:810,1999

Dries DL et al: Atrial fibrillation is associated with an increased risk for mortality and heart failure progression in patients with asymptomatic and symptomatic left ventricular systolic dysfunction: A retrospective analysis of the SOLVD trials. Studies of Left Ventricular Dysfunction. J Am Coll Cardiol 32:695, 1998

Fuster V et al: ACC/AHA/ESC Guidelines for the Management of Patients with Atrial Fibrillation: A report of the American College of Cardiology/American Heart Association Task Force on Practice Guidelines and the European Society of Cardiology (Committee to Develop Guidelines for the Management of Patients with Atrial Fibrillation). J Am Coll Cardiol 38:1231, 2001

Hohnloser SH et al, for the PIAF Investigators: Rhythm or rate control in atrial fibrillation—Pharmacological Intervention in Atrial Fibrillation (PIAF): A randomized trial. Lancet 356:1789, 2000

Klein AL et al, for the Assessment of Cardioversion Using Transesophageal Echocardiography Investigators: Use of transesophageal echocardiography to guide cardioversion in patients with atrial fibrillation. N Engl J Med 344:1411, 2001

Laupacis A et al: Antithrombotic therapy in atrial fibrillation. Chest 114:579S, 1998

Miller MR et al: Efficacy of agents for pharmacologic conversion of atrial fibrillation and subsequent maintenance of sinus rhythm: A meta-analysis of clinical trials. J Fam Pract 49:1033, 2000

Roy D et al: Amiodarone to prevent recurrence of atrial fibrillation. Canadian Trial of Atrial Fibrillation Investigators. N Engl J Med 342:913, 2000

Sharif MN, Wyse DG: Atrial fibrillation: Overview of therapeutic trials. Can J Cardiol 14:1241, 1998

Singh S et al, for the Dofetilide Atrial Fibrillation Investigators: Efficacy and safety of oral dofetilide in converting to and maintaining sinus rhythm in patients with chronic atrial fibrillation or flutter. The Symptomatic Atrial Fibrillation Investigative Research on Dofetilide (SAFIRE-D) Study. Circulation 102:2385, 2000

The SPAF III Writing Committee for the Stroke Prevention in Atrial Fibrillation Investigators: Patients with nonvalvular atrial fibrillation at low risk of stroke during treatment with aspirin: Stroke Prevention in Atrial Fibrillation III Study. JAMA 279:1273, 1998

Wyse DG: The AFFIRM Trial: Main trial and sub studies— what can we expect? J Interv Card Electrophysiol 4 (Suppl 1): 171, 2000

Wyse DG: Selection of endpoints in atrial fibrillation studies. J Cardiovasc Electrophysiol 13:(Suppl) S47, 2001

Wyse DG et al, for the AVID Investigators: Atrial Fibrillation: A risk factor for increased mortality—an AVID Registry analysis. J Interv Card Electrophysiol 5:267, 2001

RECENT CLINICAL TRIALS WITH AMIODARONE

William G. Stevenson

Nonsustained ventricular tachycardia (VT) and depressed left ventricular function are markers for mortality and sudden death in survivors of myocardial infarction (MI) and in patients with heart failure. However, therapy with class I antiarrhythmic agents or D-sotalol can increase mortality even if ventricular ectopy is suppressed. Thus, the risk/benefit ratio favors avoiding antiarrhythmic therapy. Implantable cardioverter defibrillators are the first option for very high risk patients, such as those resuscitated from cardiac arrest or who have sustained VT, but the majority of patients at risk do not fit this profile. There remains a need for effective, safe antiarrhythmic drug therapy both for prevention of sudden death and to alleviate arrhythmia symptoms. Several trials have suggested that amiodarone may have a role in this regard, but they have not been definitive. The well-recognized toxicities of amiodarone mandate a cautious approach to its use. Recently two larger trials, the European Myocardial Infarct Amiodarone Trial (EMIAT) and the Canadian Amiodarone Myocardial Infarction Arrhythmia Trial (CAMIAT), have further clarified the benefit and limitations of amiodarone therapy in high-risk survivors of MI (Julian et al., 1997; Cairns et al., 1997). These studies are particularly relevant because patients were recruited between 1990 and 1995, and their treatment with therapies recently appreciated to reduce mortality (Table 66-1) was closer to current practice than in older trials.

Post-Myocardial Infarction Trials

EMIAT enrolled 1486 patients early after acute MI who had a left ventricular ejection fraction of ≤ 0.4 (Table 66-1) (Julian et al., 1997). Ambient ventricular ectopy was not required. Amiodarone was administered orally in the dose of 800 mg/d for 2 weeks, then 400 mg/d for 14 weeks, then 200 mg/d. The prespecified primary end-point was all-cause mortality, and the primary analysis was by intention to treat. With a median follow-up of 21 months there was no difference in total mortality, which was 14% in both groups. There was a borderline significant reduction in deaths due to arrhythmia of 4.4% versus 6.7% (risk ratio, 0.65; 95% CI, 0.42 to 1.0). Adjusting the analysis for history of prior MI, which was more common in the amiodarone-treated group, and performing an efficacy analysis, which censured patients who withdrew from therapy, yielded similar results.

TABLE 66-1

PATIENT POPULATIONS IN EMIAT AND CAMIAT: AMIODARONE AFTER MYOCARDIAL INFARCTION

	EMIAT, n = 1486	CAMIAT, n = 1202
Entry Criteria.		
Time after MI	5–21 days	6–45 days
Ventricular ectopy	Not required	<10 PVCs/h or NSVT
LV ejection fraction	<0.40	Not required
Prior MI (AM/PI)	32%/26%	33%/35%
Exclusions		
Bradyarrhythmias	+	+
Thyroid dysfunction	+	+
Liver dysfunction	+	+
Need for antiarrhythmic Rx	+	+
Population Characteristics		
Age (mean, years)	60	64
Male/female	84%/16%	82%/18%
LV ejection fraction	0.30	NA
VPB >10/h or NSVT	40%	100%
NSVT	27%	38%
Heart rate (mean)	75/min	>70/min in 43.5% of pts.
Concomitant Therapy (AM/PI)		
Thrombolytics	NA	47%/50%
Aspirin	NA	83%/82%
Beta blockers	45%/44%	60%/59%
ACE inhibitors	58%/59%	32%/31%

ABBREVIATIONS: ACE, angiotensin-converting enzyme; AM, amiodarone group; LV, left ventricular; MI, myocardial infarction; NA, not available; NSVT, nonsustained ventricular tachycardia; PI, placebo group; PVC, premature ventricular complex; Rx, medication; VPB, ventricular premature beats

SOURCE: Amiodarone Trials Meta-Analysis Investigators: Lancet 350:1417 1997; JA Cairns et al: Lancet 349:675, 1997; DG Julian et al: Lancet 349:667, 1997.

CAMIAT enrolled 1202 patients who had frequent ($\geq$10/h) premature ventricular depolarizations or nonsustained VT 6 to 45 days after MI (Table 66-1) (Cairns et al., 1997). Depressed ventricular function was not required but was likely present due to the association with ventricular arrhythmias. Amiodarone was administered orally as 10 mg/kg per day for 2 weeks, followed by 400 mg or 300 mg daily. The primary end-point was resuscitated ventricular fibrillation or arrhythmic death, rather than total mortality. During a median follow-up of 21 months, total mortality was similar in the amiodarone (8%) and placebo (11%) groups (p = .129). However, the primary end-point of arrhythmic deaths or resuscitation from ventricular fibrillation was reduced from 6.5% to 4% (relative risk reduction, 38%; CI, 2.1 to 62.6; p = .029). The findings of the efficacy analysis were similar.

Thus, in both EMIAT and CAMIAT, arrhythmic deaths were reduced by amiodarone, but total mortality was not improved. Amiodarone did not increase mortality and was therefore not harmful, but neither was it clearly beneficial.

Heart Failure Trials

These studies raise questions of whether a small benefit exists that would be demonstrable in a patient population at greater risk, such as patients with heart failure, and/or whether nonarrhythmic causes of death are increased by amiodarone and offset any benefit. The Survival Trial of Antiarrhythmic Therapy in Congestive Heart Failure (CHF-STAT) randomized 674 patients, with symptomatic heart failure, depressed ventricular function and, $\geq$10 premature ventricular contractions per hour to placebo or amiodarone administered orally as 800 mg/d for 14 days, 400 mg/d for 50 weeks, and then 300 mg/d (Table 66-2) (Massie et al., 1996). Although severity of heart failure was mild to moderate, as indicated by symptoms and an average resting heart rate of 80 beats/min, 39% of patients died during a median follow-up of 45 months; 51% of deaths were sudden. Amiodarone had no impact, either beneficial or adverse, on survival (69% vs. 71% at 2 years) or

sudden death (15% vs. 19%; p = .43). There was a trend toward benefit in the subgroup of 193 patients without ischemic heart disease, but no such trend in patients with ischemic heart disease. Left ventricular ejection fraction improved an average of 8 percentage points in the amiodarone-treated patients, associated with a decrease in heart rate (Massie et al., 1996).

The Grupo de Estudio de la Sobrevida en la Insuficiencia Cardiaca en Argentina (GESICA) trial randomized 516 patients with advanced heart failure, average resting heart rate of 90 beats/min (Table 66-2). Amiodarone was administered orally as 600 mg daily for 14 days, then 300 mg daily for 2 years. Treatment was not blinded. The average follow-up was 13 months. Amiodarone therapy reduced total mortality from 41.4% to 33.5% (risk reduction, 28%; 95% CI, 4 to 45%; p = .024). Sudden death accounted for 37% of deaths and was 15.2% vs. 12.3% in the control and amiodarone groups, respectively (p = .16). In contrast to the studies discussed above, only 39% of patients had a history of prior MI; the majority likely had nonischemic causes of cardiomyopathy, including hypertension and Chagas' disease. Consistent with the improvement in ventricular function observed in CHF-STAT, amiodarone reduced the combined end-point of death or hospitalization for heart failure and was associated with an improvement in functional class. A mortality benefit was observed only in the subgroup of patients with a resting heart rate $\geq$90 min. In heart failure, tachycardia has a negative inotropic effect. It is possible that the improvement in ventricular function produced by amiodarone is mediated by heart rate slowing (Nul et al., 1997). These studies suggest that patients with advanced heart failure and elevated resting heart rates and those with nonischemic rather than ischemic cardiomyopathy are more likely to benefit from therapy with amiodarone.

Amiodarone Trials Meta-Analysis

To further address the possibility that a small benefit may have gone undetected in many trials, the Amiodarone Trials Meta-Analysis Investigators analyzed

TABLE 66-2

PATIENT POPULATIONS IN CHF-STAT AND GESICA: AMIODARONE IN PATIENTS WITH HEART FAILURE

Population characteristics	CHF-STAT, n = 674	GESICA, n = 516
Placebo-controlled	Yes	No
Entry criteria	CHF	CHF
Arrhythmia	>10 PVCs/h	Not required
LV ejection fraction	≤0.40	≤0.35
LVEF (mean)	0.25	0.19
Age (mean, years)	65	60–59
Male/female	99%/1%	81%/19%
Prior MI	63%	37%
NYHA class III or IV	41%	79%
Nonsustained VT	77%	33%
Medications		
Digitalis	70%	76%
ACE-inhibitors	78%	90%
Systolic BP, mmHG (mean)	127	115–117
Heart rate, beats/min	80	91–89

ABBREVIATIONS: ACE, angiotensin-converting enzyme; BP, blood pressure; VT, ventricular tachycardia; LV, left ventricular.
SOURCE: HC Doval et al: Lancet 344:493; 1994; SN Singh et al: N Engl J Med 333:77, 1995.

13 randomized controlled trials of amiodarone in 6500 patients with recent MI (78% of reported patients) or heart failure (22% of reported patients). The results of this analysis indicated a 13% reduction in total mortality (odds ratio 0.87; 95% CI, 0.78 to 0.99) and a 29% reduction in sudden death (odds ratio 0.71; 95% CI, 0.59–0.85). There was no evidence for an increase in nonarrhythmic death.

Thus, it appears likely that amiodarone has a small beneficial effect on mortality in "high-risk" patients who have survived an MI and in some subgroups of patients who have heart failure. Should amiodarone therapy be routinely employed in these patients? The enthusiasm for this approach is blunted by amiodarone's side effects. Although many of these are mild and easily managed, their detection requires constant surveillance. The cost, inconvenience, and impact on quality of life of medical surveillance for and treatment of side effects is difficult to quantify (Table 66-3). In placebo-controlled trials, perceived side effects led to drug discontinuation in 41% of patients (Amiodarone Trials Meta-Analysis

TABLE 66-3

AMIODARONE SIDE EFFECTS

Hypothyroidism	7%
Hyperthyroidism	1.4%
Pulmonary infiltrates	1.6%
Peripheral neuropathy	0.5%
Hepatitis	1%
Bradycardia	2.4%
Visual disturbances	1%
Sleep disturbances	1.7%
Gastrointestinal	1–2%
Skin	1–2%

SOURCE: Modified from Amiodarone Trials Meta-Analysis Investigators: Lancet 350:1417, 1997; JA Cairns et al: Lancet 349:675, 1997; HC Doval et al: Lancet 344:493, 1994; DG Julian et al: Lancet 349:667, 1997; SN Singh et al: N Engl J Med 333:77, 1995.

Investigators, 1997). However, 27% of patients receiving placebo also withdrew from treatment, suggesting that actual toxicity occurs much less frequently. Many patients will not tolerate even mild side effects for a theoretical benefit if they do not feel better. In the GESICA trial, drug withdrawal occurred in only 4.6% of patients; the lower maintenance dose, nonblinded therapy, and severity of heart failure may have motivated patients and physicians to continue therapy.

Assuming a 13% 2-year mortality for high-risk MI survivors and a 13% reduction in mortality by amiodarone therapy, 59 patients would need to be treated to save 1 life. Probably eight of these patients would experience a significant side effect; the drug would likely be withdrawn for real or perceived side effects in twice that many patients. Although one death may be prevented, more patients will experience adverse effects. Furthermore, amiodarone side effects will continue to emerge over

time, while mortality and sudden death have their greatest incidence in the first year after acute infarction and then decline. Treating physicians will have to weigh the risks and benefits carefully for the individual patient. The increasing use of thrombolytic therapy, β-adrenergic blockers, angiotensin-converting enzyme inhibitors, and aspirin may further reduce the benefit of amiodarone. It is interesting to note, however, that amiodarone tended to show greater benefit in patients who were receiving β-adrenergic blockers compared to patients not receiving beta blockers (Cairns et al., 1997; Julian et al., 1997).

For patients with chronic heart failure, the risk-benefit ratio may be more favorable. Assuming a 2-year mortality of 30% and a 13% reduction in mortality by amiodarone therapy, 26 patients would need to be treated to save 1 life. Probably four of these would have a significant side effect, and the drug would likely be withdrawn in twice as many patients. It is possible that greater benefit may be seen in the subgroup of patients who have relatively rapid heart rates and in those with nonischemic cardiomyopathy (Nul et al., 1997).

SUMMARY

In summary, routine administration of amiodarone to all high-risk MI survivors and patients with heart failure is not warranted. Rather, each patient should be considered individually (Table 66-4).

All patients should receive those therapies known to improve survival. For MI survivors this includes β-adrenergic blockers, angiotensin-converting enzyme inhibitors, aspirin, and HMG-CoA reductase inhibitors. Amiodarone therapy can be safely used to suppress symptomatic ventricular ectopy and to treat atrial fibrillation, although it is not specifically approved for the latter. In MI survivors with left ventricular ejection fraction ≤0.35 and nonsustained VT, an electrophysiologic study can be considered followed by implantation of a defibrillator if sustained VT is inducible. For patients with nonischemic dilated cardiomyopathy and for all patients with moderate to

TABLE 66-4

SUGGESTED GUIDELINES FOR AMIODARONE THERAPY

Myocardial infarction survivors with mild or no heart failure:

Symptomatic ventricular ectopy despite beta blockers

Atrial fibrillation requiring antiarrhythmic drug therapy

Frequent nonsustained VT and ICD not an option

Moderate or severe heart failure or nonischemic dilated cardiomyopathy:

Resting heart rate ≥90/min after optimization of therapy

Atrial fibrillation requiring antiarrhythmic drug therapy

Frequent nonsustained VT

Symptomatic ventricular ectopy/nonsustained VT

Endstage heart failure with sustained arrhythmias, but ICD not a reasonable option

ABBREVIATIONS: ICD, implantable cardioverter defibrillator; VT, ventricular tachycardia

severe heart failure, amiodarone should be considered if the heart rate remains elevated >90 beats/min after optimization of heart failure therapy. Amiodarone has a role as part of an individualized treatment program for selected patients.

REFERENCES

Amiodarone Trials Meta-Analysis Investigators: Effect of prophylactic amiodarone on mortality after acute myocardial infarction and in congestive heart failure: Meta-analysis of individual data from 6500 patients in randomized trials. Lancet 350:1417, 1997

Cairns JA et al: Randomized trial of outcome after myocardial infarction in patients with frequent or repetitive ventricular premature depolarisations: CAMIAT. The Canadian Amiodarone Myocardial Infarction Arrhythmia Trial Investigators. Lancet 349:675, 1997

Doval HC et al: Randomized trial for low-dose amiodarone in severe congestive heart failure. Grupo de Estudio de la Sobrevida en la Insuficiencia Cardiaca en Argentina (GESICA). Lancet 344:493, 1994

Doval HC et al: Nonsustained ventricular tachycardia in severe heart failure. Independent markers of increased mortality due to sudden death. The GESICA-GEMA Investigators. Circulation 94:3198, 1996

Julian DG et al: Randomized trial of effect of amiodarone on mortality in patients with left ventricular dysfunction after recent myocardial infarction: EMIAT: The European Myocardial Infarct Amiodarone Trial Investigators. Lancet 349:667, 1997

Massie BM et al: Effect of amiodarone on clinical status and left ventricular function in patients with congestive heart failure. The CHF-STAT Investigators. Circulation 93:2128, 1996

Nul DR et al: Heart rate is a marker of amiodarone mortality reduction in severe heart failure. The GESICA-GEMA Investigators. J Am Coll Cardiol 29:1199, 1997

Singh SN et al: Amiodarone in patients with congestive heart failure and asymptomatic ventricular arrhythmias. The Survival Trial of Antiarrhythmic Therapy in Congestive Heart Failure. N Engl J Med 333:77, 1995

TRANSESOPHAGEAL ECHO-GUIDED CARDIOVERSION OF ATRIAL FIBRILLATION

Warren J. Manning

Atrial fibrillation (AF) is the most common sustained arrhythmia and is characterized by a loss of organized electrical and mechanical activity in the atria. The associated loss of the atrial systolic contribution to left ventricular filling leads to depressed cardiac output and symptoms of dyspnea and fatigue, while the resulting atrial stasis predisposes to the formation of atrial thrombi with subsequent migration and clinical thromboembolism.

For patients with sustained AF, cardioversion to sinus rhythm is often recommended to relieve symptoms, improve cardiac output, and (although unproven), decrease the long-term risk of clinical thromboembolism. Unfortunately, both electrical and pharmacologic cardioversion may be associated with clinical thromboembolism, most often occurring during the first 10 days following conversion (Berger and Schweitzer, 1998). Patients with sustained AF for at least 2 days are subjected to a 5 to 7% risk of cardioversion-related clinical thromboembolism if cardioversion is not preceded by several weeks of therapeutic warfarin (INR > 2.0). The use of 3 to 4 weeks of therapeutic warfarin prior to cardioversion results in an 80% relative reduction in clinical thromboembolic risk, to approximately 1.2% (Silverman and Manning, 1998).

Conventional Approach to Cardioversion of Atrial Fibrillation

Although no prospective, randomized studies have been performed to determine the optimal INR or duration of prophylactic warfarin, historic data have led to the widespread use of 1 month of prophylactic warfarin (INR > 2.0) prior to elective cardioversion. The use of this "conservative" strategy comes at the "cost" of a delay in cardioversion for the vast majority of patients who could otherwise undergo early and safe cardioversion. This 1-month delay exposes the patient to prolonged precardioversion warfarin therapy (with associated risk of hemorrhagic complications) and prolongs the period of AF. It has been estimated that up to 25% of patients receiving warfarin in preparation for cardioversion do not undergo cardioversion as planned due to hemorrhagic complications and/or transient subtherapeutic INR levels (Klein et al., 1997). For patients with hemorrhagic complications, the clinician is faced with the difficult choice of reducing the intensity of anticoagulation, often to a subtherapeutic range (with the patient remaining in AF). For the patient with a transient subtherapeutic INR, the dose of warfarin is increased, and the "1-month clock" must be restarted. Finally, the use of 1 month of precardioversion warfarin serves to prolong the duration of AF prior to cardioversion and thus may adversely impact recovery of atrial mechanical function and long-term maintenance of sinus rhythm. The impact on atrial function and long-term maintenance of sinus rhythm appears to be most relevant for those presenting with AF of only several weeks' duration (Manning et al., 1994).

Transesophageal Echocardiography-Facilitated Early Cardioversion

An alternative strategy that uses transesophageal echocardiography (TEE) to guide early cardioversion for those in whom no atrial thrombi can be seen is now used at many centers. This strategy has favorable results and is gaining widespread acceptance (Klein et al., 1997, 2001; Manning et al., 1993; Stoddard et al 1995; Weigner et al., 2001). Among patients with AF, the vast majority of thrombi are located within the left atrial appendage (Fig. 67-1), an area not well seen by transthoracic (surface) echocardiography but easily visualized by multiplane TEE. Thus, TEE offers the opportunity to exclude atrial thrombi and therefore facilitate

early and safe cardioversion. The recommended strategy (Fig. 67-2) is for the patient to be therapeutically anticoagulated with heparin (PTT, $2.0 \times$ control) or warfarin (INR$>$2.0) at the time of TEE and extending to 1 month after cardioversion. The use of systemic anticoagulation in this manner is intended to minimize the formation of microthrombi and to prevent thrombi from forming during the postcardioversion period. It has been demonstrated that conversion to sinus rhythm is associated with relatively depressed atrial and atrial appendage mechanical function—therefore increased risk for new thrombus formation (Stoddard et al., 1995).

At least four independent, prospective studies have now examined the safety of a TEE-guided approach to early cardioversion of atrial fibrillation of 2 days' duration (Klein et al., 1997, 2001; Stoddard et al., 1995; Weigner et al., 2001). These studies demonstrate that 12% of these patients will have TEE evidence of atrial thrombi. This apparent discrepancy between the 12% prevalence of atrial thrombus on TEE and the 6% historic rate of clinical thromboembolism for

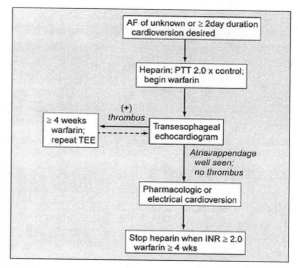

FIGURE 67-2

Management of patients presenting with AF of unknown or $\geq$2 day duration. Patients with a thrombus on the initial TEE should receive 1 month of warfarin followed by a TEE to document complete thrombus resolution prior to elective cardioversion.

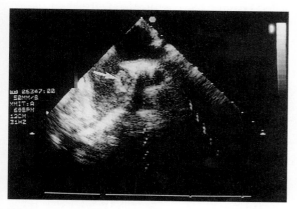

FIGURE 67-1

TEE in a patient with AF demonstrating a 14-mm long thrombus (arrow) within the left atrial appendage.

nonanticoagulated patients is likely explained by (1) the imperfect specificity of TEE, (2) the likelihood that not all thrombi migrate after cardioversion, and (3) the fact that not all thrombus migration is associated with clinical thromboembolism. TEE evidence for atrial thrombus is associated with prior thromboembolism and left ventricular systolic dysfunction (Manning et al., 1993).

Using the anticoagulation strategy described in Fig. 67-2, and based on almost 2000 prospectively studied patients, clinical thromboembolism has been reported in < 0.5% of patients following a "negative" TEE for atrial thrombus. A 1222-patient, prospective, multicenter randomized study comparing the conservative approach of 1 month of warfarin and the TEE-facilitated approach was recently completed and confirmed the "equivalence" of the expedited TEE and the conventional approaches (Klein et al., 2001). Optimal patients for TEE-expedited cardioversion include those with a relatively brief (<1 month) duration of AF or those with an increased risk of hemorrhagic complications. Assuming expeditious performance of TEE and cardioversion, thereby not prolonging the initial hospitalization, the TEE approach has been shown to be cost effective for inpatients (Silverman and Manning, 1998) and for enhancing long-term maintenance of sinus rhythm (Weigner et al., 2001). At some centers, TEE-facilitated cardioversion is offered to nearly all inpatients but to only selected outpatients, primarily those in whom hemorrhagic risk of warfarin is increased. Other centers offer the TEE strategy equally to inpatients and outpatients.

Management of Patients with TEE Evidence of Thrombus

The optimal treatment for patients who have TEE evidence of atrial thrombi remains undefined. Despite warfarin and avoidance of cardioversion, these patients remain at increased risk for adverse events (Silverman and Manning, 1998). As illustrated in Fig. 67-2, it seems most prudent to perform a follow-up TEE (after 4 weeks of warfarin) to document com-plete thrombus resolution prior to elective cardioversion. If residual thrombus is present, cardioversion should not be performed.

TEE-Facilitated Cardioversion Without Anticoagulation

In the absence of the anticoagulation strategy outlined in Fig. 67-2, several centers have reported clinical thromboembolism following a "negative TEE" for atrial thrombus (Black et al., 1994). The mechanism of these adverse events is unknown and may be related to thrombi not visualized by TEE or to thrombi that form during the pericardioversion period (Stoddard et al 1995). Because of these reports, the use of systemic anticoagulation at the time of TEE and extending to 1 month after cardioversion is strongly encouraged.

Patients with nonvalvular AF in whom warfarin is contraindicated can be offered the option of full-dose heparin anticoagulation at the time of TEE and extending to 24 h after cardioversion. Though unproven, this approach is likely to be preferred to "blind" cardioversion.

REFERENCES

Berger M, Schweitzer P: Timing of thromboembolic events after electrical cardioversion of atrial fibrillation or flutter: A retrospective analysis. Am J Cardiol 82:1545, 1998

Black IW et al: Exclusion of atrial thrombus by transesophageal echocardiography does not preclude embolism after cardioversion of atrial fibrillation: A multicenter study. Circulation 89:2509, 1994

Klein AL et al, for the ACUTE Investigators: Cardioversion guided by transesophageal echocardiography: The ACUTE pilot study. A randomized, controlled trial. Ann Intern Med 126:200, 1997

Klein AL et al, for the ACUTE Investigators: Use of transesophageal echocardiography to guide cardioversion in patients with atrial fibrillation. N Engl J Med 344:1411, 2001

Manning WJ et al: Cardioversion from atrial fibrillation without prolonged anticoagulation with use of transesophageal echocardiography to exclude the presence of atrial thrombi. N Engl J Med 328:750, 1993

Manning WJ et al: Impaired left atrial mechanical function after cardioversion: Relationship to the duration of atrial fibrillation. J Am Coll Cardiol 23:1535, 1994

Silverman DI, Manning WJ: Current perspective: Role of echocardiography in patients undergoing elective cardioversion of atrial fibrillation. Circulation 98:479, 1998

Stoddard MF et al: Transesophageal echocardiographic guidance of cardioversion in patients with atrial fibrillation. Am Heart J 129:1204, 1995

Weigner MJ et al: Early cardioversion of atrial fibrillation facilitated by tranesophageal echocardiography: Short-term safety and impact on maintenance of sinus rhythm at 1 year. Am J Cardiol 110:694, 2001

CARDIAC ARREST: NEWER THERAPEUTIC CONCEPTS

Karl B. Kern

Cardiac arrest remains a major cause of morbidity and mortality in the industrialized nations. Significant understanding of cardiac arrest and the physiology of cardiopulmonary resuscitation (CPR) has been steadily advancing since the advent of closed-chest CPR. Recently, several new concepts for treating cardiac arrest have achieved the uncommon position of having not only the interest of the medical community but also some actual clinical data.

Improving Basic Life Support

The importance of early CPR in the treatment of sudden cardiac arrest is well recognized and has led to the development of "Basic Life Support" (BLS) programs adapted for any first responder to such an emergency, including a lay person, or "bystander." It is clear that bystander-performed CPR is an important step in the chain of survival needed for successful community treatment of cardiac arrest. The current paradox is that in spite of evidence that bystander BLS significantly increases neurologically intact survival from cardiac arrest, the incidence of bystander CPR is declining. Previous reports of 40 to 60% incidence of bystander CPR have declined to more recent reports of only 20 to 30% incidence of bystander BLS in communities such as Tucson, AZ,

and suburban Pittsburgh, PA (Valenzuela et al., 1992; Mossesso et al., 1998). This reluctance to perform bystander CPR seems based chiefly on fear of contagious disease through mouth-to-mouth contact, though the complexity of the task is also a definite hindrance. Numerous surveys have demonstrated that many, including American Heart Association BLS instructors, physicians and nurses, as well as lay persons, are anxious about the risks of mouth-to-mouth contact for rescue breathing (Ornato et al., 1990; Brenner and Kauffman, 1993; Locke et al., 1995). In reality, these risks are extremely low (Mejicano GC and Maki DG, 1998). Nonetheless, the perception of risk limits many individuals' willingness to perform mouth-to-mouth breathing as part of an initial response and BLS effort. Not uncommonly today, a potential bystander rescuer will phone 911 and then do nothing but wait for professional help to arrive.

The need to simplify BLS CPR has led to several innovative ideas. First, few BLS first responders, particularly lay persons, can reliably discern the presence or absence of a pulse (Eberle et al., 1996). Valuable time is lost in efforts to feel for and confirm the absence of a pulse before assuming cardiac arrest has occurred and beginning BLS. Doing away with this "feel for a pulse" requirement or suggestion in assessing the collapsed victim is one step towards a more achievable and simplified BLS system (American Heart Association et al., 2000). Second, correct hand positioning for chest compressions can be taught effectively in a more simplified fashion than previously. Instructions given a group of lay persons to "place the hands in the center of the chest, one on top of the other, and push down to compress the chest" resulted in an "effective" hand position more than 75% of the time (Assar et al., 2000). This was not dissimilar from what was achieved by the more complex current BLS teaching instructions.

The most dramatic, and controversial, suggestion for simplifying BLS CPR is to do away with mouth-to-mouth breathing. There is an ever increasing and now convincing body of scientific evidence suggesting that it may not be essential to provide such ventilation during the first few minutes of ventricular fibrillation (VF) cardiac arrest. Adequate oxygen exists in the blood and the lungs to keep reasonable, if not normal, levels of arterial saturation for delivery of oxygen to the tissues. The limiting factor is delivery, i.e., circulation. Hence, most important is to enhance the circulation during the first minutes of cardiac arrest. The fewer interruptions to chest compressions, the greater the opportunity for ample circulation during CPR. Recently Assar and colleagues showed this very principle. In their study comparing lay persons taught standard BLS ($n = 269$) and those taught a simplified BLS ("bronze" CPR—no mouth-to-mouth ventilation) ($n = 236$), they found that the number of chest compressions delivered was doubled when interruptions for mouth-to-mouth ventilation were eliminated (Table 68-1) (Assar et al., 2000).

Six experimental studies of VF cardiac arrest (total $n = 169$) have shown no outcome differences following 6 to 12 min of VF treated by BLS with or without ventilation. Figure 68-1 illustrates the similar return of spontaneous circulation and 24 to 48-h survival between those animals receiving standard BLS (including ventilation) and those receiving just chest compressions-only BLS.

Clinical data continue to mount supporting chest compression-only BLS CPR as well. Van Hoeyweghen and co-workers, in an out-of-hospital resuscitation study, found that if upon arrival of the professional rescue team good quality bystander CPR in some form or another was being performed, enhanced survival rates were seen (Van Hoey-

TABLE 68-1

COMPARISON OF BLS PERFORMANCE AFTER STANDARD AND SIMPLIFIED TRAINING

	Standard BLS	Chest Compression-Only BLS	p
Number of subjects	269	236	NS
"Effective" hand position	77%	79%	NS
Shout for help	44%	70%	.001
Check for breathing	76%	94%	.001
Phone for ambulance	21%	32%	.001
Time to begin CPR	63 ± 25 s	34 ± 11 s	.001
Duration of CC pauses	16 s	9 s	.001
Chest compression/min	39/min	84/min	.001

NOTE: BLS, basic life support; CC, chest compression; NS, not significant.
SOURCE: Adapted from D Assar et al: Resuscitation 45:7, 2000.

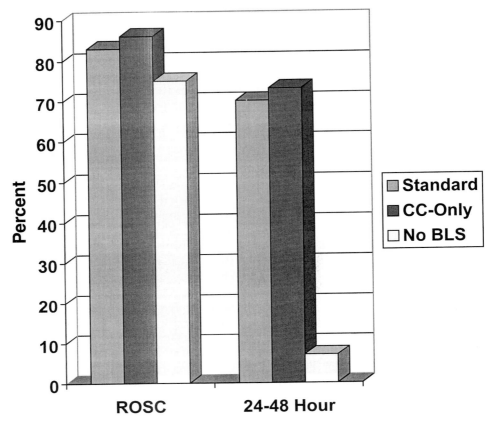

FIGURE 68-1

Outcome in an experimental model of ventricular fibrillation cardiac arrest initially treated with standard BLS CPR versus chest compression-only BLS CPR versus no BLS CPR until arrival of the ACLS-capable professional rescuers. ROSC, return of spontaneous circulation; 24 to 48-h survival. (From Circulation 88:1993, 1993; Ann Emerg Med 26:342, 1995; Chest 108:821, 1995; Circulation 95:1635, 1997; Circulation 96:4364, 1997; Resuscitation 39:179, 1998.)

weghen et al., 1993). Surprisingly, it did not matter if BLS was chest compressions with ventilation or just chest compressions alone. Survival rates for both groups were equal (16% vs. 15%), but if no bystander CPR was being performed, survival decreased (6%; $p <.001$ vs. either).

Using their well-established telephone dispatcher–assisted CPR program in Seattle, Hallstrom and colleagues reported their results with chest compression-only CPR (Halstrom et al., 2000).

Over a period of nearly 10 years they randomized such requests for dispatcher assistance in CPR phone instructions either to standard BLS including mouth-to-mouth breathing or to chest compression only BLS, without any mouth-to-mouth breathing. After approximately 500 such calls, the survival-to-discharge rates were nearly 50% greater with chest compression-only CPR. Although not significantly different (10% vs. 15%, $p = .09$), they showed "no outcome harm" by eliminating mouth-to-mouth breathing by lay rescuers until professional help arrived.

Use of Automatic External Defibrillators

Simplification of BLS CPR will continue to be an area of intense interest in the field of resuscitation. Another area of interest that spans both BLS and advanced cardiac life support (ACLS) resuscitation efforts is achieving early defibrillation. Public-access defibrillation (PAD) is beginning to gain momentum and be more and more acceptable to the medical professional and lay person alike. Data now exist showing feasibility and improved survival from cardiac arrest with the use of automatic external defibrillators (AEDs). Successful PAD programs

involving police as first responders equipped with AEDs exist in Rochester, MN, and suburban Pittsburgh PA (White et al., 1998; Mossesso et al., 1998). Many commercial airlines have equipped their planes with AEDs, and a number of "saves" have already been reported (O'Rourke et al, 1997; Page et al., 2000). Exciting data highlighting the importance of time to defibrillation, even with AEDs, have come from a PAD program in the gaming establishments of Las Vegas (Valenzuela et al., 2000). Valenzuela and co-workers found a 59% survival-to-hospital discharge rate for victims of witnessed VF cardiac arrest in those casinos where security guards were both trained and equipped with AEDs. In their study, they documented a mean time of 4.4 min from collapse to shock. In a subgroup analysis, they showed that unusually short time

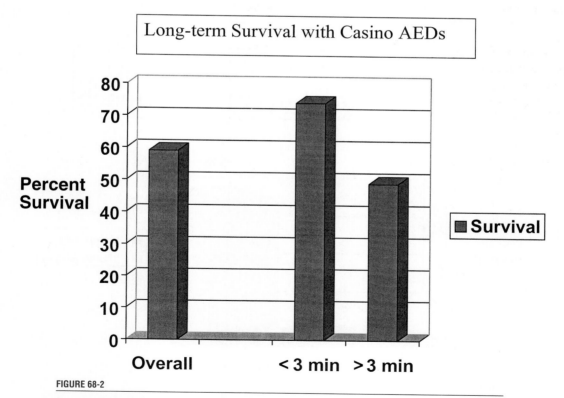

FIGURE 68-2

Survival with automatic external defibrillators (AEDs) in casinos. (From TD Valenzuela et al: N Engl J Med 343:1206, 2000.)

periods to defibrillation resulted in even better long-term survival. Figure 68-2 shows that in those defibrillated before 3 min, the mean survival rate was 74%, while in those defibrillated after 3 min, the mean survival rate dropped to 49% ($p < .01$).

The most recent experience with the use of AEDs in the public sector comes from the major airports in the city of Chicago. With insight and courage, the Chicago Airport Authority decided to provide AEDs in the terminals for any trained individual to access and use. Using an unlocked but alarmed storage system, 51 AEDs have been deployed. These devices were purposefully spaced to allow acquisition from anywhere in the terminal within a 1-min brisk walk. Over 2500 airport personnel have been trained, but the instruction on the storage box is that anyone with training may utilize them. Within the first 10 months of this program, 14 cardiac arrest victims were treated, 12 of

the 14 were in VF upon attachment of the AED, and 9 of the 12 VF cardiac arrest victims were successfully defibrillated and survived long term, neurologically intact (Willoughby and Caffrey; 2000). This 75% successful hospital discharge rate is the highest percentage of long-term survivors from VF cardiac arrest ever reported for a PAD program (Fig. 68-3.)

The key to success in PAD is time to defibrillation. Follow-up care can be important, but if initial defibrillation is delayed, minimum success can be expected. Figure 68-4 shows the same relationship between time to defibrillation and successful outcome with AED use as has been estimated from the use of manual defibrillators. Now actual data support our previous hope: if defibrillation can be rapidly accomplished in the community, excellent long-term results, including central nervous system function, can be achieved.

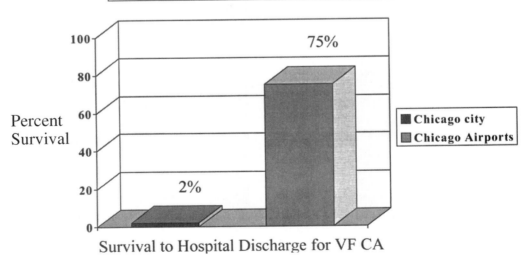

FIGURE 68-3

Difference in long-term survival for victims of ventricular fibrillation cardiac arrest (CA) in Chicago: community and airport locations. (From PJ Willoughby et al: Circulation 102 (Suppl II): II-828, 2000.)

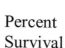
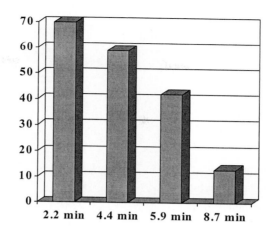

Percent Survival

2.2 min   4.4 min   5.9 min   8.7 min

Time to Defib with an AED

FIGURE 68-4

Effect on survival of time (minutes) to defibrillation (Defib) with an automatic external defibrillator (AED). (From VN Mossesso et al: Ann Emerg Med 32:200, 1998; TD Valenzuela et al: N Engl J Med 343:1206, 2000; RD White et al: Resuscitation 39:145, 1998)

Advanced Cardiac Life Support

ACLS includes a few new concepts as well. Newer resuscitation medications and circulatory adjuncts are appearing, often with significant clinical data obtained by worldwide collaboration and effort. Such drugs include amiodarone for refractory VF; vasopressin as an alternative to epinephrine for improving CPR-generated perfusion and, ultimately, successful outcome; and possibly the use of bolus thrombolytics for the treatment of refractory out-of-hospital cardiac arrest.

The ARREST trial was the first prospective, randomized, placebo-controlled trial of any anti-arrhythmic agent administered during CPR to improve outcome (Kudenchuk et al., 1999). Significantly more patients survived to hospital admission after receiving amiodarone than those receiving placebo. (Of note, the majority of patients received epinephrine and lidocaine before randomization). Table 68-2 shows the major results from this important cardiac arrest trial. The lack of significant

difference in hospital discharge rates between patients receiving amiodarone and those not has been interpreted differently. Some believe this indicates that amiodarone given for refractory VF does not make any significant real difference and hence should be avoided. Others believe it simply indicates the complexity of treating cardiac arrest victims and highlights the need for better and more innovative care of those initially resuscitated but who expire prior to hospital discharge. This is not an inconsequential group, comprising about 60 to 75% of those initially resuscitated. Most resuscitation researchers feel that as the first prospective, randomized evidence showing an improvement over standard drug therapy during ACLS, amiodarone should be given careful consideration for the treatment of cardiac arrest due to refractory VF, even though no longer-term survival benefit was seen in the ARREST trial.

Additional data concerning amiodarone during cardiac arrest were recently reported from the ALIVE trial (Dorian et al., 2001). In this randomized,

TABLE 68-2

SUMMARY OF THE ARREST TRIAL

	Amiodarone	Placebo	p
No. of subjects	246	258	NS
Male	76%	79%	NS
Witnessed	70%	77%	NS
Bystander CPR	68%	59%	NS
EMT arrival (min)	4.3 ± 2.0	4.4 ± 2.3	NS
No. of defibrillator shocks	5 ± 2	5 ± 2	NS
Other antiarrythmic drugs	22%	21%	NS
Time to study drug (min)	21 ± 8	21 ± 7	NS
Admission to hospital	44%	35%	.03
Time to ROSC post Rx (min)	9 ± 9	7 ± 5	NS
Total CPR time (min)	28 ± 14	29 ± 16	NS
Hemodynamic support post ROSC			
Rx for bradycardia	41%	25%	.004
Pressor support	59%	48%	.04
Admission to hospital in pts with transient ROSC before Rx	64%	41%	.03

NOTE: ARREST, Amiodarone in Out-of-Hospital Resuscitation of Refractory Sustained Ventricular Tachyarrhythmia; EMT, emergency medical technician; NS, not significant; ROSC, return of spontaneous circulation.
SOURCE: Adapted from PJ Kudenchuk et al: N Engl J Med 341:871, 1999.

prospective clinical trial, amiodarone was compared to lidocaine for the treatment of refractory VF. Using a similar protocol to the ARREST trial, including a primary end-point of admission to the hospital, this study found amiodarone significantly better than lidocaine for achieving short-term survival in cardiac arrest victims with refractory VF. Together these two trials strongly suggest that amiodarone is the best choice among antiarrhythmic therapies during cardiac arrest.

Alternative vasoconstrictors to replace epinephrine have been sought for three decades. Following encouraging results from numerous experimental studies, Lindner and colleagues have studied two small series of patients treated with vasopressin after failure of epinephrine. The first was a series of refractory cardiac arrest patients who failed to resuscitate after epinephrine but who responded to vasopressin. Next this group performed a pilot prospective, randomized trial ($n = 40$) of vasopressin vs. epinephrine during cardiac arrest. They found significantly greater 24-h survival with vasopressin (Lindner et al., 1997). An ongoing larger randomized trial (anticipated enrollment of 1500 patients) is now underway in Europe, with results expected later in 2002.

An interesting series of patients with refractory out-of-hospital cardiac arrest treated with bolus thrombolytic therapy was reported (Boettiger et al., 2001). In a nonrandomized, unblinded study of 40 patients receiving thrombolytics for refractory cardiac arrest, this group found no increase in bleeding complications and an increase in early resuscitation outcome, including return of spontaneous circulation, and hospital admission rates compared to historic controls.

Continued interest in improving upon standard CPR has produced clinical outcome data for several alternative circulatory adjuncts. Promising therapies in this regard include interposed abdominal compression (IAC) CPR and active compression-decompression (ACD) CPR. IAC CPR, where the abdomen is compressed during the chest relaxation phase of BLS, has shown improved survival, including 24-h survival, and improved survival-to-hospital discharge when applied to in-hospital cardiac arrest patients. (Sack et al., 1992a, 1992b). Out-of-hospital studies have been less convincing. ACD CPR, where the chest wall is actively pulled upward during the relaxation phase of BLS, has produced variable results in different studies, and though some have not shown improved outcome, others have, including a study from Paris where an increase in 1-year survival was found with ACD CPR (Plaisance et al., 1999).

Exciting advances are happening in the field of resuscitation and acute care of cardiac arrest. Continued improvements are anticipated and expected.

REFERENCES

American Heart Association in collaboration with International Liason Committee on Resuscitation: Guidelines 2000 for Cardiopulmonary Resuscitation and Emergency Cardiovascular Care: International Consensus on Science, Part 3: Adult Basic Life Support. Circulation 102(Suppl I):I-39, 2000

Assar D et al: Randomized controlled trials of staged teaching for basic life support: 1. Skill acquisition at bronze stage. Resuscitation 45:7, 2000

Bottiger BW et al: Efficacy and safety of thrombolytic therapy after initially unsuccessful cardiopulmonary resuscitation: A prospective clinical trial. Lancet 357:1583, 2001

Brenner BE, Kauffman J: Reluctance of internists and medical nurses to perform mouth-to-mouth resuscitation. Arch Intern Med 153:1763, 1993

Dorian P et al: ALIVE: A randomized, blinded trial of intravenous amiodarone versus lidocaine in shock resistant ventricular fibrillation (abstr.). Circulation 104(Suppl II):II-765, 2001

Eberle B et al: Checking the carotid pulse: Diagnostic accuracy of first responders in patients with and without a pulse. Resuscitation 33:107, 1996

Hallstrom AP et al: Cardiopulmonary resuscitation by chest compression alone or with mouth-to-mouth ventilation. N Engl J Med 342:1546, 2000

Kudenchuk PJ et al: Amiodarone for resuscitation after out-of-hospital cardiac arrest due to ventricular fibrillation. N Engl J Med 341:871, 1999

Lindner KH et al: Randomized comparison of epinephrine and vasopressin in patients with out-of-hospital ventricular fibrillation. Lancet 349:535, 1997

Locke CJ et al: Bystander cardiopulmonary resuscitation: Concerns about mouth-to-mouth contact. Arch Intern Med 155:938, 1995

Mejicano GC, Maki DG: Infections acquired during cardiopulmonary resuscitation: Estimating the risk and defining strategies for prevention. Ann Intern Med 129:813, 1998

Mossesso VN Jr et al: Use of automated external defibrillators by police officers for treatment of out-of-hospital cardiac arrest. Ann Emerg Med 32:200, 1998

Ornato JP et al: Attitudes of BCLS instructors about mouth-to-mouth resuscitation during the AIDS epidemic. Ann Emerg Med 19:151, 1990

O'Rourke MF et al: An airline cardiac arrest program. Circulation 96:2849, 1997

Page RL et al: Use of automated external defibrillators by a US airline. N Engl J Med 343:1210, 2000

Plaisance P et al: Comparison of standard cardiopulmonary resuscitation and active compression-decompression for out-of-hospital cardiac arrest. N Engl J Med 341:569, 1999

Sack JB et al: Interposed abdominal compression-cardiopulmonary resuscitation and resuscitation outcome during asystole and electromechanical dissociation. Circulation 86:1692, 1992a

Sack JB et al: Survival from in-hospital cardiac arrest with interposed abdominal counterpulsation during cardiopulmonary resuscitation. JAMA 267:379, 1992b

Valenzuela TD et al: Case and survival definitions in out-of-hospital cardiac arrest: Effect on survival rate calculations. JAMA 267:272, 1992

Valenzuela TD et al: Outcomes of rapid defibrillation by security officers after cardiac arrest in casinos. N Engl J Med 343:1206, 2000

Van Hoeyweghen RJ et al, for the Belgian Cerebral Resuscitation Study Group: Quality and efficiency of bystander CPR. Resuscitation 26:47, 1993

White RD et al: Seven years experience with early defibrillation by police and paramedics in an emergency medical services system. Resuscitation 39:145, 1998

Willoughby PJ, Caffrey S: Improved survival with an airport-based PAD program (abstr.). Circulation 102 (Suppl II): II-828, 2000

69

INDICATIONS FOR THE IMPLANTED CARDIOVERTER/ DEFIBRILLATOR—AN UPDATE

Alfred E. Buxton

Mirowski's implantable defibrillator, introduced to clinical medicine in 1980, revolutionized the care of patients with life-threatening cardiac arrhythmias. The use of the implantable cardioverter/defibrillator (ICD) has grown steadily, due to progressive technical refinements and a plethora of clinical trials evaluating its utility (See also Chap. 79). There can be no doubt that the ICD effectively terminates most episodes of ventricular fibrillation (VF) by shock and ventricular tachycardia (VT) by pacing or shock. The current challenge lies in refining indications for the devices in order to understand more completely which patients will benefit from them. Practitioners should be aware that a major change in the approach to treatment of patients with life-threatening ventricular arrhythmias has occurred over the past several years, due in large part to the outcome of large-scale multicenter trials. The result of this sea change is that, in many cases, the ICD has supplanted drugs as first-line antiarrhythmic therapy. No longer is it thought that ICDs should be used only after a test or clinical event suggests drug failure. The indications for ICDs are evolving continuously. This chapter outlines current indications and the data that form the basis for them. They are based in large part on guidelines established by the Committee on Pace-maker Implantation of the joint American College of Cardiology/American Heart Association Task Force on Practice Guidelines (Gregoratos et al., 1998).

There are two major indications for use of the ICD: primary and secondary prevention of sudden cardiac death. Use of the ICD for prophylaxis against sudden death (primary prevention) is far more recent than its indication for secondary prevention in survivors of cardiac arrest. Currently, the major indication for use of the ICD remains cardiac arrest due to VF or VT, that does not result from a transient or reversible cause. The 1998 revision of the guidelines (Gregoratos et al., 1998) no longer requires that cardiac arrest survivors be drug refractory or intolerant, nor is tachycardia required to be inducible by electrophysiologic (EP) testing or hemodynamically unstable before a patient receives an ICD.

Large-Scale Trials of ICDs vs. Drugs

The results of several large-scale randomized trials comparing outcome of cardiac arrest survivors treated with ICDs vs. drugs form the basis for the first-line therapy recommendations. The largest of these trials, the Antiarrhythmics Versus Implantable Defibrillators (The AVID Investigators, 1997), enrolled 1016 patients who survived cardiac arrest, sustained VT with syncope, or sustained VT in the presence of left ventricular ejection fraction (LVEF) <0.40 and symptoms suggesting severe hemodynamic compromise. Patients were randomized to receive therapy with either an ICD or an antiarrhythmic drug. The drug therapy choices were amiodarone (administered empirically, without testing to predict efficacy), or sotalol (administered with either EP testing or ambulatory electrocardiographic monitoring to predict efficacy). However, only 13 patients were discharged taking sotalol, while 483 of the 509 patients randomized to receive drug therapy were treated with amiodarone. Survival throughout the trial was superior for patients randomized to ICD therapy. After a mean follow-up of 18.2 months, 15.8% of patients treated with ICDs had died, compared to 24% of patients randomized to drug therapy.

Two other large-scale randomized trials comparing mortality of cardiac arrest survivors treated with ICDs vs. drugs have now been published. The Cardiac Arrest Study Hamburg (CASH) randomized 346 survivors of cardiac arrest equally among four treatment arms: ICD, amiodarone, metoprolol, or propafenone (Kuck et al., 2000). The propafenone arm was terminated prematurely because of excessive mortality (2.6 times that of the ICD arm). After a mean follow-up of 57 months, total mortality was similar for patients randomized to metoprolol and amiodarone (45.4% and 43.5%, respectively), but 23% lower (not significantly—$p = .081$) in patients randomized to ICD therapy (36.4%).

The Canadian Implantable Defibrillator Study (CIDS) (Connolly et al., 2000b) randomized 659 survivors of cardiac arrest or patients with hemodynamically unstable VT to therapy with amiodarone or ICD. After a mean follow-up of 3 years, a nonsignificant reduction in mortality of 20% was observed in patients treated with ICDs (8.3% per year) compared to that of patients randomized to amiodarone (10.2% per year; $p = .142$).

Meta-Analysis

Although the survival benefit of ICD therapy in the CASH and CIDS trials did not achieve statistical significance, the results of all three studies (including the AVID trial) are consistent. A formal meta-analysis of these three trials (Connolly et al., 2000a) did indeed suggest remarkable similarity across the studies with regard to patient characteristics and outcome. Taken together, therapy with ICDs in the study populations resulted in a 27% reduction in total mortality, and a 51% reduction in arrhythmic mortality. Thus, the ability of implantable defibrillators to treat ventricular tachyarrhythmias effectively not only translates into the expected reduction in arrhythmic deaths but also carries through to reducing total mortality. Of note, analyses of treatment effects in the AVID and CIDS trials, and in the meta-analysis, suggest that the sickest patients—those with most marked left ventricular dysfunction (as reflected by LVEF and advanced heart failure)—are likely to benefit the most from ICD treatment (with regard to survival).

Reversible Causes of Cardiac Arrest

A number of practical questions relating to patient management remain unanswered. For example, whether correcting apparent transient or reversible causes of cardiac arrest constitutes adequate therapy without the use of a defibrillator is not exactly clear. A post hoc analysis from the AVID study suggests that patients experiencing cardiac arrest presumed due to transient metabolic perturbations such as hypokalemia or ischemia are at high mortality risk (this was a substudy of the AVID registry, and detailed information on treatments and causes of death is not currently available) (Wyse et al., 2001). However, numerous studies have shown that primary ventricular fibrillation in the setting of acute myocardial infarction, although associated with increased in-hospital mortality, is not associated with long-term risk of recurrent VF.

It is not necessary to treat all patients with sustained ventricular tachyarrhythmias with implantable defibrillators. Some arrhythmias lend themselves to cure in the electrophysiology laboratory. Tachycardia due to bundle branch reentry may cause syncope or cardiac arrest and is readily cured by radiofrequency catheter ablation. Some cases of monomorphic VT complicating remote myocardial infarction may be cured by radiofrequency catheter ablation or surgical endocardial resection. In addition, as noted above, subgroups of cardiac arrest survivors do not derive equal survival advantages from ICDs over antiarrhythmic drug therapy. For example, patients with LVEF >35% demonstrated significantly less survival advantage when treated with ICDs compared to patients with LVEF <35%. In part this may result from the fact that arrhythmias in patients with higher ejection fractions seem to occur with lower frequency. Therefore, over the relatively short follow-up periods entailed in the clinical trials, it will be harder to demonstrate significant benefit in patient subgroups with lower event rates.

Ventricular Tachycardia

There are several other groups of patients, besides cardiac arrest survivors, in whom use of the ICD is now accepted as first-line therapy. Certain patients with spontaneous sustained VT may be at high risk for sudden death. This group includes some patients with VT associated with syncope or severely symptomatic VT associated with a LVEF <0.40. The AVID trial included 561 patients with VT, and these patients demonstrated a survival benefit similar to patients with VF with ICD treatment. However, not all patients with sustained VT may require an ICD to improve survival. The survival benefit of ICD therapy in patients with prior myocardial infarction and hemodynamically stable sustained monomorphic VT is not clear. These patients may be treated with antiarrhythmic drugs, or surgical or radiofrequency catheter ablation, with relatively low risk of sudden death (on the order of 2 to 3% yearly) (Sarter et al., 1996). Such patients may be identified by their presentation and findings on EP testing. However, the ICD may be useful as adjunctive therapy in such patients by using antitachycardia pacing to terminate tachycardia episodes. Other patients with sustained monomorphic

VT at low risk for sudden death are those with certain types of idiopathic VT in the setting of normal ventricular function. This includes patients with idiopathic VT arising from the right or left ventricular outflow tracts and "fascicular" left ventricular VT. Such patients, when symptomatic, are best treated by radiofrequency catheter ablation, rather than the ICD.

A third group of patients in whom the ICD is accepted as first-line therapy includes patients presenting with syncope of unknown origin who have hemodynamically significant sustained VT or VF induced at EP study. If such patients cannot be treated with pharmacologic antiarrhythmic therapy, an ICD is indicated. This indication is not supported by evidence from multiple prospective clinical trials but rather by observational data documenting high (approximately 20% yearly) cardiovascular mortality in such patients, largely due to sudden death. In addition, observations of patients experiencing syncope of unclear etiology with nonischemic dilated cardiomyopathy who receive ICDs have a 40 to 50% incidence of receiving "appropriate" ICD therapies over 2 years (Knight et al., 1999; Fonarow et al., 2000). This rate of therapy delivery is comparable to that of patients with similar underlying disease who received ICDs as treatment for cardiac arrest (Knight et al., 1999). A related indication includes patients with recurrent syncope of uncertain etiology in the presence of severe ventricular dysfunction, who have no inducible ventricular tachyarrhythmias at EP study if other causes of syncope are excluded. This group of patients also has a high mortality risk, which also seems to be frequently related to sudden death.

Primary Prevention

There are now data from two prospective randomized trials that support a role for the ICD in the primary prevention of sudden death in patients with coronary heart disease. (Moss et al., 1996; Buxton et al., 1999; Table 69-1). These studies evaluated patients with coronary artery disease, left ventricular dysfunction, and asymptomatic nonsustained VT. The first of these,

TABLE 69-1

PRIMARY PREVENTION TRIALS IN PATIENTS WITH CORONARY HEART DISEASE

Trial	Ejection fraction (median)	Total mortality in control group[a] at 2 years	Hazard ratio[b]	p value[c]
MADIT	.26	32%	0.46	.009
MUSTT	.29	28%	0.80/0.73	.06/.043

[a] The control group for the MADIT study was composed of 101 patients randomized to "conventional" antiarrhythmic therapy. The control group for the MUSTT trial was composed of 351 patients randomized to no antiarrhythmic therapy.

[b] The hazard ratio is a representation of the ratio of risk of death over time. The hazard ratio for the MADIT study represents the total mortality risk for patients randomized to ICD therapy vs. those randomized to "conventional" antiarrhythmic therapy over 2 years' follow-up. The hazard ratio for the MUSTT trial represents the 5-year ratio for total mortality/arrhythmic events for patients randomized to EP-guided therapy (including both antiarrhythmic drugs and ICDs) vs. patients randomized to no antiarrhythmic therapy. Thus the MADIT study found a 54% reduction in total mortality for patients given ICDs compared to those treated with conventional therapy. Conversely, the MUSTT trial found a 20% reduction in total mortality, and a 27% reduction in arrhythmic events over 5 years for patients randomized to EP-guided therapy. An observational (nonrandomized) comparison of survival with ICD therapy versus non-ICD therapy in the MUSTT trial showed a >50% reduction in both total mortality and arrhythmic events.

[c] The p value for the MADIT study represents the degree of significance for the hazard ratio for total mortality. The p values for the MUSTT trial represent the degree of significance for the hazard ratios for total mortality/arrhythmic events, respectively.

the Multicenter Automatic Defibrillator Implantation Trial ("MADIT"; Moss et al., 1996) performed EP studies in patients with the characteristics noted above. Patients with inducible sustained VT were given intravenous procainamide. If inducible sustained VT persisted, they were then randomized to receive either an ICD or "conventional" antiarrhythmic therapy. The latter treatment was uncontrolled and left to individual investigators' discretion. Empirical amiodarone was the choice in 74% of cases randomized to this arm. There was no untreated control group in this study of the 196 patients who were enrolled in the trial. After an average follow-up of 27 months, the investigators noted a 54% reduction in total mortality for the patients randomized to the ICD treatment group. The actual mortality in the "conventional" treatment group was 32% at 2 years.

The second prospective trial supporting the use of ICDs for primary prevention of sudden death was the Multicenter Unsustained Tachycardia Trial ("MUSTT"; Buxton et al., 1999). The major purpose of this randomized, controlled trial was to assess the ability of antiarrhythmic therapy (including both ICDs and drugs) guided by EP studies to reduce the risk of sudden death in patients with coronary artery disease and the other characteristics noted above. This trial randomized 704 patients who had inducible sustained VT at a baseline EP study (performed in the absence of antiarrhythmic medications). Patients were randomized equally into two groups: one to receive therapy with β-adrenergic blocking agents and angiotensin-converting enzyme (ACE) inhibitors alone, versus a second group treated with these agents plus antiarrhythmic therapy guided by EP studies. Antiarrhythmic drugs were tested first, and patients who failed to respond to drugs (judged by EP study) then received an ICD. Over a 5-year follow-up the patients randomized to EP-guided therapy experienced a 27% lower risk of arrhythmic death or cardiac arrest (the primary end-point for the trial).

Total mortality was reduced by 20%. This trial was not designed to compare the efficacy of antiarrhythmic drugs versus the ICD for reduction of mortality. However, at the trial's completion, evaluation of treatments given to patients randomized to therapy guided by EP study revealed that the number of patients treated with ICDs was approximately the same as those treated with antiarrhythmic drugs. Further analysis demonstrated that the improved survival of the EP-guided group was due entirely to therapy with ICDs. Patients discharged without ICDs had event rates very similar to those of the untreated control patients, but the ICD reduced the risk of arrhythmic death or cardiac arrest by approximately 74%, while total mortality was reduced by 50%.

The results of these two trials demonstrate, for the first time, the ability of the ICD to reduce mortality of patients at high risk for sudden death who have never experienced a symptomatic arrhythmia. The MUSTT trial also establishes the risk for arrhythmic death or cardiac arrest of patients with coronary disease, left ventricular dysfunction, or asymptomatic nonsustained VT who have inducible sustained VT. The control group in this trial, treated with beta-blocking agents and ACE inhibitors alone, experienced a Kaplan-Meier 5-year arrhythmic event rate of 32% and total mortality of 48%. It should be noted that in both trials ICDs were implanted only in patients who failed to respond to antiarrhythmic drugs, as tested in the EP laboratory. Thus, neither trial proved efficacy in patients who respond to drugs at EP testing. However, given the rather poor outcome of patients treated with antiarrhythmic drugs guided by EP testing in the MUSTT trial, it does not seem reasonable to require drug failure prior to ICD use in appropriate patients.

Other Conditions in Which ICD is Indicated

A number of other less common conditions are also recognized now as appropriate indications for ICDs. These indications are the result of observational data and expert opinion, rather than multiple controlled prospective trials, but are nonetheless accepted at this time (Table 69-2).

TABLE 69-2

INDICATIONS FOR ICD USE NOT SUPPORTED BY DATA FROM RANDOMIZED CONTROLLED TRIALS

Cardiac arrest presumed due to VF in the presence of inability to perform EPS

Severely symptomatic sustained VT in patients awaiting cardiac transplantation

Familial conditions associated with high risk for sudden death, including long QT syndrome

ABBREVIATIONS: EPS, electrophysiologic study; VF, ventricular fibrillation; VT, ventricular tachycardia.

It should be recognized that there are a number of clinical situations in which new indications for ICDs are being investigated. The high risk of sudden death in patients with congestive heart failure and left ventricular dysfunction, even in patients with no symptomatic arrhythmias, has prompted evaluation of the potential utility of the ICD to improve survival in this setting. The Sudden Cardiac Death in Heart Failure Trial ("SCD-HeFT") is an ongoing study comparing the efficacy of amiodarone and ICDs versus placebo to improve survival in patients with severe stable heart failure of any etiology. This trial will complete follow-up in approximately 2.5 years. A second ongoing study in this area is the "MADIT-II" trial, which is comparing survival with ICD treatment to no ICD treatment in patients who have experienced a myocardial infarction at least 1 month previously, have an ejection fraction ≤30%, and no symptomatic arrhythmia. Patients with severe, advanced heart failure symptoms (NYHA class IV) are excluded from both trials (Klein et al., 1999).

Conditions in Which ICD is not Indicated

A number of conditions exist for which it is recognized that the ICD is not indicated at present. These include ventricular tachyarrhythmias for which primary cures exist, such as those associated with rapid atrial tachycardias in patients with Wolff-Parkinson-White Syndrome, VTs due to transient or reversible disorders, and the idiopathic VTs curable by radiofrequency catheter ablation (noted previously). A second group of conditions for which ICDs are not indicated are those in which the ICD would not improve patient survival or overall quality of life. These include incessant VT or VF, significant psychiatric illnesses that could be aggravated by ICD discharges or that preclude adequate ICD follow-up care, terminal illnesses, and class IV refractory congestive heart failure patients who are not candidates for cardiac transplantation.

Finally, one group of potential ICD candidates has been shown by a recent randomized, controlled trial to *not* have a survival benefit from ICDs. These are patients undergoing coronary artery bypass surgery who have left ventricular dysfunction and abnormal signal-averaged ECGs but no symptomatic ventricular arrhythmias. This trial ("CABG-Patch") randomized 900 patients to receive an ICD or no ICD at the time of coronary artery bypass surgery (Bigger, 1997). Over an average follow-up of 32 months, the actuarial total mortality rates in the control and ICD therapy groups were 24% and 27%, respectively ($p = .64$).

Conclusions

In conclusion, multiple well-designed clinical trials have now demonstrated clearly the ability of the ICD to reduce the risk of arrhythmic death and overall mortality in selected patient populations. It is likely that there will be significant growth in the utilization of ICDs for primary prevention of sudden death in the future. In fact, future growth for this indication may well outpace growth in the number of devices implanted for secondary prevention. The challenge for cardiologists and electrophysiologists at this time is to define better the patients who are likely to derive the most benefit from this therapy.

Addendum: Since this chapter was prepared the results of the MADIT II trial were reported. (MADIT II, 2002). See addendum to Chap. 79, p. 507.

REFERENCES

Bigger JT Jr, for the Coronary Artery Bypass Graft (CABG) Patch Trial Investigators: Prophylactic use of implanted cardiac defibrillators in patients at high risk for ventricular arrhythmias after coronary artery bypass graft surgery. N Engl J Med 337:1569, 1997

Buxton AE et al: A randomized study of the prevention of sudden death in patients with coronary artery disease. N Engl J Med 341:1882, 1999

Connolly SJ et al: Meta-analysis of the implantable cardioverter defibrillator secondary prevention trials. Eur Heart J 21:2071, 2000a

Connolly SJ et al: Canadian Implantable Defibrillator Study (CIDS): A randomized trial of the implantable cardioverter defibrillator against amiodarone. Circulation 101:1297, 2000b

Fonarow GC et al: Improved survival in patients with nonischemic advanced heart failure and syncope treated with an implantable cardioverter-defibrillator. Am J Cardiol 85:981, 2000

Gregoratos G et al: ACC/AHA guidelines for implantation of cardiac pacemakers and antiarrhythmia devices: A report of the American College of Cardiology/ American Heart Association Task Force on Practice Guidelines (Committee on Pacemaker Implantation). J Am Coll Cardiol 31:1175, 1998

Klein H et al: New primary prevention trials of sudden cardiac death in patients with left ventricular dysfunction: SCD-HEFT and MADIT-II. Am J Cardiol 83:91D, 1999

Knight BP et al: Outcome of patients with nonischemic dilated cardiomyopathy and unexplained syncope treated with an implantable defibrillator. J Am Coll Cardiol 33:1964, 1999

Kuck K-H et al: Randomized Comparison of Antiarrhythmic Drug Therapy With Implantable Defibrillators in Patients Resuscitated From Cardiac Arrest: The Cardiac Arrest Study Hamburg (CASH). Circulation. 102:748-754, 2000

Moss AJ et al: Improved survival with an implanted defibrillator in patients with coronary disease at high risk for ventricular arrhythmia. N Engl J Med 335:1933, 1996

Sarter BH et al: What is the risk of sudden cardiac death in patients presenting with hemodynamically stable sustained ventricular tachycardia after myocardial infarction? J Am Coll Cardiol 28:122, 1996

The Antiarrhythmics Versus Implantable Defibrillators (AVID) Investigators: A comparison of antiarrhythmic-drug therapy with implantable defibrillators in patients resuscitated from near-fatal ventricular arrhythmias. N Engl J Med 337:1576, 1997

Wyse DG et al: Life-threatening ventricular arrhythmias due to transient or correctable causes: high risk for death in follow-up. Journal of the American College of Cardiology. 38:1718-24, 2001

CHAPTER

70

MYOCYTE APOPTOSIS IN THE DEVELOPMENT OF HEART FAILURE

Piero Anversa

Characteristics of Myocyte Death

Understanding the structural basis of heart failure has proved to be a difficult clinical problem. Cardiac hypertrophy and chamber dilation are usually apparent, but routine histology may show normal myocardium with little damage represented by foci of reparative and interstitial fibrosis. Even in ischemic cardiomyopathy, in which the accumulation of collagen can constitute more than 25% of the ventricle, the volume of intact myocardium often exceeds the muscle mass of control hearts (Anversa et al., 1998). Alterations exist in vascular supply, composition of the myocyte cytoplasm, and muscle contractility, but these modifications develop early experimentally, suggesting that other factors at the cellular level may be implicated in the chronic deterioration of ventricular performance. Morphologic evidence of acute scattered myocyte death has been elusive. Criteria for the recognition of irreversible cellular damage attributed to ongoing necrotic myocyte death have been described, but their application has been limited (Guerra et al., 1999; Frustaci et al., 2000; Kajstura et al., 2001). Apoptosis, i.e., programmed cell suicide, has now been identified in end-stage cardiac failure, raising the possibility that it may contribute to the progression of the pathologic process (Anversa et al., 1998; Haunstetter et al., 1998).

The detection of myocyte death is complicated by the complexity of distinguishing apoptosis, necrosis, and apoptosis-necrosis. With apoptosis, DNA degradation is specific to the spacer region, leaving the DNA associated with the nucleosomes intact. DNA fragments of a size equivalent to that of the mononucleosomes, combined with their multiplicity, are frequently considered the hallmark of apoptosis. Detection of apoptosis requires the application of histochemical methods that are not commonly used in the histology laboratory. Similarly, the recognition of necrosis of single myocytes is difficult in the human heart. Cell necrosis is characterized by loss of plasmamembrane integrity, which remains essentially intact in apoptotic cells. Loss of asymmetry of the sarcolemmal lining occurs with apoptosis, but this does not involve discontinuity of the plasmamembrane. In animals, necrotic myocytes have been identified by in vivo injection of myosin antibody and its subsequent localization to dying cells (Anversa et al., 1998). Obviously, this approach cannot be used in patients.

Double-stranded DNA surrounds by two full turns the histone cores forming the nucleosomes, which are arranged in an organized manner in the chromatin strands (See Color Plate 16, Fig 70-1). During interphase, in the absence of mitosis, chromatin is distributed in this fashion within the nucleus; in mitosis, chromosomes are formed. A region of linker DNA of variable length separates each nucleosome bead from the next. Histones in the nucleosomes protect the DNA from digestion by endonucleases, but these enzymes can degrade the linker DNA. Thus, in the helical twist of DNA, the two strands of the linker region are accessible to endonucleases, which induce staggered ends and blunt ends (for reviews, see Anversa et al., 1998; Buja et al., 1998). Staggered ends consist of double-strand breaks in the internucleosomal DNA, with single-base $3'$ overhangs Color Plate 16 top (A) or longer overhangs involving up to four bases Color Plate 16 center (B). Endonucleases and exonucleases produce cleavage of internucleosomal and nucleosomal DNA, which results in blunt ends of the digested fragments Color Plate 16 bottom (C). The first two aspects of double-strand breaks correspond to the activation of apoptosis by Ca^{2+}-dependent DNase I and pH-dependent DNase II, respectively. The third form reflects cell necrosis mediated by activation of endonucleases and exonucleases.

On this basis, the distinction between apoptosis and necrosis and the recognition of cells affected by both types of cell death can be obtained and applied to the analysis of cell death in tissue sections of the normal and pathologic human heart. Importantly, the relative contribution of myocyte necrosis, apoptosis, and apoptosis-necrosis to the failing human heart was recently measured (Guerra et al., 1999). Although staggered ends in double-strand DNA breaks are produced by DNase I and DNase II, other DNases have been identified (Green et al., 1998; Haunstetter et al., 1998). However, whether they lead to single-base or longer $3'$ overhangs or to a different form of DNA cleavage is currently unknown.

Key events in apoptosis include a class of aspartate-specific proteases termed *caspases,* in which the death effector domain may be activated via the release of cytochrome c from mitochondria (Green et al., 1998; Haunstetter et al., 1998, 2000). Target proteins in the nucleus and cytoskeleton are degraded, triggering the execution of the death signal. Multiple stimuli capable of activating the endogenous cell death pathway converge in the mitochondria where several proapoptotic and antiapoptotic gene products of the Bcl-2 family of proteins are located. Additionally, the mitochondria play an important role in precipitating the apoptotic process through changes in electron transport, abnormalities in transmembrane potential, and defective oxidation-reduction state. The activation of endonucleases and the formation of double-strand DNA cleavage represent the distal determinant of genomic DNA damage.

The activation of mitochondrial permeability pore transition results in the leakage of molecules to the cytosol (Atlante et al., 2000). Translocation of cytochrome c to the extramitochondrial space may be paralleled by an increased expression of the antiapoptotic protease-activating factor (Apaf-1). In the presence of adenosine diphosphate (ADP) and cytochrome c, Apaf-1 participates in a multistage reaction (Cain et al., 1999; Zou et al., 1999; Moroni et al., 2001). Following hydrolysis of adenosine triphosphate (ATP) to ADP, cytochrome c binds to Apaf-1, promoting its multimerization from a monomeric form to a large complex. The functional multimeric complex recruits and cleaves pro-caspase-9; when caspase-9 is activated, cytochrome c and ADP are no longer required (Hu et al., 1999). The decrease in pro-caspase-9 level is accompanied by an increase in the active subunits p35 and p10 (Krajewski et al., 1999). Moreover, activated caspase-9 results in the cleavage of downstream effectors, caspase-3 and DNA fragmentation factor (DFF45) (Zhou et al., 2001) and, thereby, caspase-activated DNase (CAD). CAD is the only endonuclease induced by the caspase cascade (Wolf et al., 1999). These steps in the initiation of myocyte apoptosis have been shown to be operative in experimental dilated cardiomyopathy (Cesselli et al., 2001).

Poly(ADP-ribose)polymerase (PARP) increases shortly after the initiation of apoptosis and is activated by binding to DNA strand breaks (Herceg and Wang, 2001). PARP catalyzes the poly(ADP-ribos)ylation of nuclear peptides and facilitates the recruitment of repair proteins at the site of DNA damage. The positive effect of PARP on DNA integrity is lost in late apoptosis: capase-3 induces proteolysis of the 112-kDa full-length PARP to the inactive subunits, p89 and p24. Similarly, DNA-dependent protein kinase (DNA-PK), an essential component of the repair of double-strand DNA breaks, is enhanced initially during apoptosis (Douglas et al., 2001). With the progression of the cell death process, DNA-PK is cleaved, most likely by caspase-3, losing its ability to repair DNA. The structure of the nuclear envelope is preserved until the late stages of cell death, when the degradation of the two isoforms of lamin, A and B, is orchestrated by caspase-3 (Slee et al., 2001). This chain of biochemical events has been documented in vivo in a model of heart failure (Cesselli et al., 2001).

Myocyte Death and Heart Failure

The decompensated heart is characterized functionally by an increased myocardial load and structurally by myocyte death and reactive growth processes in the viable cells. These cellular events condition acute and chronic ventricular remodeling. Apoptosis is a rapid phenomenon that induces sudden pathologic changes in the anatomy of the heart in response to abrupt alterations in loading (Anversa et al., 1998). This occurs shortly after infarction, in which the increase in diastolic stress is coupled with the acti-

vation of apoptosis, side-to-side slippage of myocytes, mural thinning, and chamber dilation. Whether a similar mechanism is operative chronically, participating in the continuous expansion in cavitary volume of the failing heart, has not been proven; the marked increase in myocyte apoptosis (see Color Plate 17, Figure 70-2) in patients undergoing cardiac transplantation is consistent with this possibility (Olivetti et al., 1997, Guerra et al., 1999). Similarly, heart failure mediated by diabetes alone or in combination with hypertension (Frustaci et al., 2000) is characterized by ongoing myocyte, endothelial cell, and fibroblast death of apoptotic and necrotic origin (See Color Plates 18, 19, and 20, Figures 70-3, 70-4, & 7-5). These conditions are characterized by oxidative stress and the formation of nitrotyrosine.

It is important to recognize that myocyte necrosis occurs over a longer period of time than apoptosis and may not be implicated in the precipitous restructuring of the wall in response to acute changes in ventricular pressure. Myocyte necrosis results in the stimulation of an inflammatory reaction, activation of fibroblasts, and collagen accumulation, chronically altering the volume composition of the myocardium (See Color Plate 21, Figure 70-6). The time-dependent evolution of these processes affects cardiac anatomy. Sustained death stimuli, such as prolonged ischemia, may induce necrotic myocyte cell death and myocardial scarring, which is invariably found in end-stage cardiac failure. With the exception of the infarcted region of the ventricular wall, in which apoptosis and necrosis occur simultaneously in a large number of myocytes, scattered myocyte death is either apoptotic or necrotic; their combination in the same cell is a very rare event (Guerra et al., 1999). However, apoptotic cell death is significantly higher in men than in women affected by terminal failure (Guerra et al., 1999). This difference between genders may be explained, at least in part, by the more pronounced activation of the survival factor serine/threonine protein kinase, Akt, in female than in male myocardium (Camper-Kirby et al., 2001). Although the time required for the completion of apoptosis and necrosis in myocytes is unknown, necrotic myocyte death is seven-fold higher than apoptosis in men and women with cardiac failure (Guerra et al., 1999).

Myocytes possess the various components of the renin-angiotensin system. Stretching of sarcomeres, simulating diastolic overload in vivo, is coupled with the cellular release of angiotensin II (Ang II) in adult cardiac muscle cells (Leri et al., 1998). Ang II triggers myocyte apoptosis in vitro, and angiotensin-converting enzyme (ACE) inhibition prevents this form of cell death in vivo (Li Z et al., 1997). This points to the possibility that the beneficial influence of ACE inhibitors and/or Ang II receptor blocking agents on the failing heart is mediated, at least in part, by attenuation of myocyte death and cardiac restructuring (Barlucchi et al., 2001). In this regard, insulin-like growth factor (IGF) 1, which improves cardiac anatomy and function in idiopathic dilated cardiomyopathy, interferes with the formation and secretion of Ang II from myocytes (Leri et al., 1999a, 1999b), preventing myocyte death in the postinfarcted heart (Li Q et al., 1997). Moreover, this growth factor limits ventricular dilation, reactive hypertrophy, and myocardial loading. However, acromegaly is coupled with an increase in myocyte apoptosis (Frustaci et al., 1999).

In the failing heart, apoptosis affects 0.2% of myocytes (Olivetti et al., 1997; Guerra et al., 1999), a value that may suggest a modest impact of this form of cell death on ventricular hemodynamics; an example of myocyte apoptosis is shown in Color Plate 17, Figure 70-2. As discussed above, myocyte necrosis may be equally relevant and may exceed apoptosis, and together they may reduce severely the number of viable cells in the myocardium, contributing to the continuous decline in function of the diseased heart. Attenuation of myocyte apoptosis and necrosis experimentally interferes with cardiac failure of ischemic or nonischemic origin (Li Q et al., 1997; Li B et al., 1999; Kajstura et al., 2001). Ongoing myocyte necrosis has been assessed quantitatively in the decompensated human heart (Guerra et al., 1999), and its reduction may similarly protect from the progression of cardiac dysfunction. Moreover, the lack of information concerning the duration of distinct forms of myocyte death does not allow the computation of the rates of apoptosis and necrosis with time. In several cell types, apoptosis is completed in between 20 min

and 3 h, but whether myocytes behave in a similar manner remains to be determined. Myocyte necrosis may be more extensive than apoptosis, but its execution may require as much as 24 h. The proportion of cells that die by apoptosis or necrosis is one of the several questions that have to be answered to understand the functional implication of myocyte death in the failing heart. Additionally, we have no knowledge of the susceptibility of cells to die by apoptosis and/or necrosis nor of their capacity to oppose death signals and maintain normal mechanical behavior. These issues constitute a major challenge for future research in this area and for the recognition of the pathophysiologic role of myocyte death in heart failure.

REFERENCES

Anversa P et al: Myocyte death and growth in the failing heart. Lab Invest 78:767, 1998

Atlante A et al: Cytochrome c is released from mitochondria in a ROS dependent fashion and can operate as a ROS scavenger and as a respiratory substrate in cerebellar neurons undergoing excitotoxic death. J Biol Chem 275:37159, 2000

Barlucchi L et al: Canine ventricular myocytes possess a renin-angiotensin system that is upregulated with heart failure. Circ Res 88:298, 2001

Buja LM et al: Modes of myocardial cell injury and cell death in ischemic heart disease. Circulation 98:1355, 1998

Cain K et al: Caspase activation involves the formation of the aposome, a large (~700 kDa) caspase-activating complex. J Biol Chem 274:11549, 1999

Camper-Kirby D et al: Myocardial Akt activation and gender: Increased nuclear activity in females versus males. Circ Res 88:1020, 2001

Cesselli D et al: Oxidative stress-mediated cardiac cell death is a major determinant of ventricular dysfunction and failure in dog dilated cardiomyopathy. Circ Res 89:279, 2001

Douglas P et al: Protein phosphatases regulate DNA-dependent protein kinase activity. J Biol Chem 276:18992, 2001

Frustaci A et al: Cell death in acromegalic cardiomyopathy. Circulation 99:1426, 1999

Frustaci A et al: Myocardial cell death in human diabetes. Circ Res 87:1123, 2000

Green D et al: Mitochondria and apoptosis. Science 281:1309, 1998

Guerra S et al: Myocyte death in the failing heart is gender dependent. Circ Res 85:856, 1999

Haunstetter A et al: Apoptosis: Basic mechanisms and implications for cardiovascular disease. Circ Res 82:1111, 1998

Haunstetter A et al: Toward antiapoptosis as a new treatment modality. Circ Res 86:371, 2000

Herceg Z, Wang Z: Functions of poly(ADP-ribose) polymerase (PARP) in DNA repair, genomic integrity and cell death. Mutat Res 477:97, 2001

Hu Y et al: Role of cytochrome c and dATP/ATP hydrolysis in Apaf-1-mediated caspase-9 activation and apoptosis. EMBO J 18:3586, 1999

Kajstura J et al: IGF-1 overexpression inhibits the development of diabetic cardiomyopathy and Ang II-mediated oxidative stress. Diabetes 50:1414, 2001

Krajewski S et al: Release of caspase-9 from mitochondria during neuronal apoptosis and cerebral ischemia. Proc Natl Acad Sci USA 96:5752, 1999

Leri A et al: Stretch-mediated release of angiotensin II induces myocyte apoptosis by activating p53 that enhances the local renin-angiotensin system and decreases the Bcl-2-to-Bax protein ratio in the cell. J Clin Invest 101:1326, 1998

Leri A et al: Insulin-like growth factor-1 induces Mdm2 and downregulates p53, attenuating the myocyte renin-angiotensin system and stretch-mediated apoptosis. Am J Pathol 154:567, 1999a

Leri A et al: overexpression of insulin-like growth factor-1 attenuates the myocyte renin-angiotensin system in transgenic mice. Circ Res 84:752, 1999b

Li B et al: Insulin-like growth factor-1 attenuates the detrimental impact of non-occlusive coronary artery constriction on the heart. Circ Res 84:1007, 1999

Li Q et al: Overexpression of insulin-like growth factor-1 in mice protects from myocyte death after infarction, attenuating ventricular dilation, wall stress, and cardiac hypertrophy. J Clin Invest 100:1991, 1997

Li Z et al: Increased cardiomyocyte apoptosis during the transition to heart failure in the spontaneously hypertensive rat. Am J Physiol 272:H2313, 1997

Moroni MC et al: Apaf-1 is a transcriptional target for E2F and p53. Nat Cell Biol 3:552, 2001

Olivetti G et al: Apoptosis in the failing human heart. N Engl J Med 336:1131, 1997

Slee EA et al: Executioner caspase-3, -6, and -7 perform distinct, non-redundant roles during the demolition phase of apoptosis. Mol Cell Biol 18:6719, 2001

Wolf BB et al: Caspase-3 is the primary activator of apoptotic DNA fragmentation via DNA fragmentation factor-45/inhibitor of caspase-activated DNase inactivation. J Biol Chem 274:30651, 1999

Zhou P et al: Solution structure of DFF40 and DFF45 N-terminal domain complex and mutual chaperone activity of DFF40 and DFF45. Proc Natl Acad Sci USA 98:6051, 2001

Zou H et al: An Apaf-1-cytochrome c multimeric complex is a functional apoptosome that activates pro-caspase-9. J Biol Chem 274:11549, 1999

TUMOR NECROSIS FACTOR IN HEART FAILURE

Douglas L. Mann

Although clinicians have recognized the potential importance of inflammatory mediators in the pathogenesis of heart disease for well over 200 years, it has taken nearly as many years for clinicians and scientists to focus on the basic biologic mechanisms by which inflammatory mediators contribute to the pathogenesis of cardiac disease states. Nonetheless, despite the relatively delayed onset in interest in the mechanistic role that inflammatory mediators play in heart disease, there has been considerable interest over the past decade in the role that inflammatory mediators play in regulating cardiac structure and function. Accordingly, this chapter summarizes the recent growth of knowledge that has taken place in this field, with a particular emphasis on the potential role that tumor necrosis factor (TNF), a proinflammatory cytokine, plays as a mediator of disease progression in the failing human heart.

TNF in Heart Failure

The current interest in understanding the role of proinflammatory cytokines in heart failure arises from the simple observation that many aspects of the syndrome of heart failure can be explained by the *known* biologic effects of these molecules (Table 71-1). Simply

stated, when expressed at sufficiently high concentrations, such as those that are observed in heart failure, cytokines are sufficient to mimic some aspects of the so-called heart failure phenotype, including (but not limited to) progressive left ventricular (LV) dysfunction, pulmonary edema, LV remodeling, fetal gene expression, and cardiomyopathy. Thus, the "cytokine hypothesis" for heart failure holds that heart failure progresses, at least in part, as a result of the direct toxic effects that cytokines exert on the heart and circulation (Seta et al., 1996). It bears emphasis that the cytokine hypothesis does not imply that cytokines *cause* "heart failure" per se; rather, the overexpression of cytokines contributes to the progression of heart failure once LV dysfunction ensues. Thus, the elaboration of cytokines, much like the elaboration of neurohormones, may represent a biologic mechanism that is responsible for disease progression in patients with heart failure. Indeed, pathophysiologically relevant concentrations of TNF are sufficient to provoke many aspects of the heart failure phenotype, including LV remodeling and LV dilation (Bozkurt et al., 1998). Moreover, recent studies in transgenic mice that overexpress TNF in the cardiac compartment have shown that these animals will develop progressive LV dilation and LV dysfunction (Sivasubramanian et al., 2001).

TABLE 71-1

THE POTENTIAL UNTOWARD EFFECTS OF TNF IN THE HEART

Left ventricular dysfunction in humans
Pulmonary edema in humans
Cardiomyopathy in humans
Reduced leg blood flow in humans
Left ventricular remodeling experimentally
Abnormalities in myocardial metabolism experimentally
Anorexia and cachexia experimentally
β-Receptor uncoupling from adenylate cyclase
  experimentally
Abnormalities of mitochondrial energetics
Activation of the fetal gene program experimentally

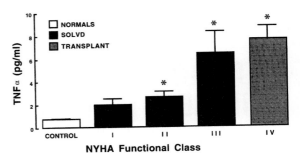

FIGURE 71-1

Tumor necrosis factor (TNF) levels in patients with class I–IV heart failure. In comparison to age-matched control subjects (open bar), there was a progressive increase in serum TNF levels in direct relation to decreasing functional heart failure classification. The solid bars denote values for patients enrolled in SOLVD (Torre-Amione et al., 1996a); the shaded bar denotes values for NYHA class IV patients who were undergoing cardiac transplantation (Torre-Amione et al., 1996b). (Reproduced from Y Seta et al: J Card Fail 2:243, 1996, with permission.)

Elevated levels of TNF have consistently been identified in patients with advanced heart failure. Moreover, several studies suggest that there is increasing cytokine elaboration in direct relation to the severity of the disease process (Torre-Amione et al., 1996a). As shown in Fig. 71-1, there is a progressive increase in TNF levels in direct relation to deteriorating NYHA functional class. Moreover, in an analysis of cytokine levels in the SOLVD data base (Torre-Amione et al., 1996a), there was a trend towards increasing mortality with increasing levels of TNF. Thus, much like elevated levels of neurohormones, TNF levels may be predictive of NYHA class and clinical outcome.

Site and Source of Cytokines in Heart Failure

Following the original description of elevated cytokine levels in heart failure (Levine et al., 1990), there was speculation that activation of the immune system was responsible for this elevation, although the mechanism(s) for immune activation was less than certain. However, this logical thought has been challenged recently by the observation that the heart is capable of elaborating TNF in response to a variety of forms of environmental injury. Thus, an alternative hypothesis for the source of proinflammatory cytokine production is that the failing heart itself may be the source of TNF production in heart failure. In

support of this point of view, several laboratories have reported that TNF mRNA and protein are present in failing human hearts, whereas neither TNF mRNA nor protein are detectable in nonfailing human hearts (Torre-Amione et al., 1996b) See Color Plate (See Color Plate 15, Figure 71-2). These findings suggest that the myocardium may represent an important source for TNF production in heart failure, and that the presence of TNF in the peripheral circulation represents "spillover" of cytokines produced locally within the myocardium. Indeed, a recent report has shown that there is increased TNF production by the heart in patients with mild to moderate heart failure (Tsutamoto et al., 2001).

A third hypothesis for the elaboration of TNF in heart failure is that a decreased cardiac output leads to the elaboration of TNF by underperfused metabolic tissues. However, this premise has not been supported by a clinical study in which there was no evidence for increased peripheral arteriovenous spillover of TNF. (Tsutamoto et al., 1998). A fourth possible source for cytokine production in heart failure is that increased bowel permeability, as a result of mesenteric venous congestion in heart failure, leads to bacterial translocation and endo-toxin release (a potent stimulus for TNF production) (Niebauer et al., 1999). However, while this may remain an important mechanism for TNF production in end-stage heart failure, it is unlikely to explain the increased levels of TNF that are observed in patients with NYHA class II and III heart failure (Torre-Amione et al., 1996a). Given that TNF is produced by virtually all cell types within the body, it would be surprising if there were not multiple sites and sources of cytokine production in patients with heart failure (Mann, 1999).

Cytokines as Potential Therapeutic Targets in Heart Failure

The concept that antagonizing cytokines may be ben-eficial in patients with heart failure is supported by several previous clinical studies. In the first study, patients with dilated cardiomyopathy were random-ized to receive prednisone or placebo. Although there were no significant overall changes in ejection frac-tion after 3 months of therapy, there was >5% increase in ejection fraction in 53% of the patients who received prednisone, whereas only 27% of the control subjects had a similar increase in ejection frac-tion, suggesting that antiinflammatory strategies may benefit certain subsets of patients with dilated car-diomyopathy. More recently, Sliwa and colleagues studied the effects of pentoxifylline (which blocks the transcriptional activation of TNF) in patients with dilated cardiomyopathy and NYHA class II–III heart failure (Sliwa et al., 1998). After 6 months of ther-apy, they observed that four patients in the placebo group died as a result of progressive pump dysfunc-tion, whereas no patient in the pentoxifylline group experienced functional deterioration. They also observed that there was a significant increase in the ejection fraction (from 22.3 ± 9.0 to 38.7 ± 15.0) in the pentoxifylline group, whereas there was no signif-icant change in the placebo group. Importantly TNF levels decreased significantly from 6.5 ± 3.0 pg/mL to 2.1 ± 1.0 pg/mL in the pentoxifylline group, whereas there was no significant change in the TNF levels in the placebo group. Thus, it appears that

modulation of TNF levels via agents that alter intra-cellular cyclic AMP levels, and therefore block the transcriptional activation of TNF, may be a useful strategy for altering cytokine levels in heart failure.

An alternative strategy to suppressing cytokine production is to attempt to neutralize the biologic effects of TNF using soluble TNF receptors as "decoys," to prevent TNF from binding to its cognate receptors on cell surface membranes. The strategy that has been used thus far is to use a soluble TNF antag-onist consisting of the extracellular domains of the type 2 TNF receptor fused in duplicate to the Fc por-tion of the IgG_1 molecule. Although the soluble TNF antagonist (etanercept, ENBREL) was shown to be effective in two small phase I clinical studies (Deswal et al., 1999; Bozkurt et al., 2001), two large-scale clinical trials of etanercept in patients with NYHA class II–IV heart failure were stopped because of lack of efficacy. Thus, although the results of large clinical trials with soluble TNF antagonists have been disap-pointing, agents that block the transcriptional activa-tion of TNF appear to be the most useful strategy for altering cytokine levels in heart failure.

How Should We View the Role of Cytokines in Heart Failure?

The cytokine hypothesis holds that heart failure pro-gresses, at least in part, because cytokine cascades that are activated following myocardial injury exert deleterious effects on the heart and circulation (Seta et al., 1996). It bears emphasis that the cytokine hypothesis does not imply that cytokines cause heart failure per se, but rather that the overexpression of cytokines contributes to the progression of heart fail-ure once LV dysfunction ensues. Based on the avail-able evidence, the excessive elaboration of cytokines appears to be sufficient to produce many of the patho-physiologic hallmarks of heart failure, including LV dysfunction and LV dilatation (see Table 71-1). There is also evidence that proinflammatory cytokine levels can be manipulated in the setting of heart failure. While it is perhaps premature to speculate whether modulating cytokine levels may translate into clinical improvements in morbidity and mortality for patients with heart failure, there is a growing body of evidence that suggests that modulating cytokine levels may represent a new therapeutic paradigm for treating patients with heart failure.

ACKNOWLEDGEMENTS

The author acknowledges the secretarial assistance of Ms Mary Helen Soliz and would also like to acknowledge Dr. Andrew I. Schafer for his past and present support. This work was supported, in part, by research funds from the N.I.H. (P50 HL-O6H and RO1 HL58081–01, RO1 HL61543–01, HL-42250–10/10).

REFERENCES

Bozkurt B et al: Pathophysiologically relevant concentrations of tumor necrosis factor-α promote progressive left ventricular dysfunction and remodeling in rats. Circulation 97:1382, 1998

Bozkurt B et al: Results of targeted anti-tumor necrosis factor therapy with etanercept (ENBREL) in patients with advanced heart failure. Circulation 103:1044, 2001

Deswal A et al: A phase I trial of tumor necrosis factor receptor (p75) fusion protein (TNFR:Fc) in patients with advanced heart failure. Circulation 99:3224, 1999

Levine B et al: Elevated circulating levels of tumor necrosis factor in severe chronic heart failure. N Engl J Med 223:236, 1990

Mann DL: Inflammatory mediators in heart failure: Homogeneity through heterogeneity. Lancet 353:1812, 1999

Niebauer J et al: Endotoxin and immune activation in chronic heart failure: A prospective cohort study. Lancet 353:1838, 1999

Seta Y et al: Basic mechanisms in heart failure: The cytokine hypothesis. J Card Fail 2:243, 1996

Sivasubramanian N et al: Left ventricular remodeling in transgenic mice with cardiac restricted overexpression of tumor necrosis factor. Circulation 2001:826, 2001

Sliwa K et al: Randomized investigation of effects of pentoxifylline on left ventricular performance in idiopathic dilated cardiomyopathy. Lancet 351:1091, 1998

Torre-Amione G et al: Proinflammatory cytokine levels in patients with depressed left ventricular ejection fraction: A report from the studies of left ventricular dysfunction (SOLVD). J Am Coll Cardiol 27:1201, 1996a

Torre-Amione G et al: Tumor necrosis factor-α and tumor necrosis factor receptors in the failing human heart. Circulation 93:704, 1996b

Tsutamoto T et al: Interleukin-6 spillover in the peripheral circulation increases with the severity of heart failure, and the high plasma level of interleukin-6 is an important prognostic predictor in patients with congestive heart failure. J Am Coll Cardiol 31:391, 1998

Tsutamoto T et al: Relationship between tumor necrosis factor-alpha production and oxidative stress in the failing hearts of patients with dilated cardiomyopathy. J Am Coll Cardiol 37:2086, 2001

LAMIN A/C MUTATIONS IN FAMILIAL DILATED CARDIOMYOPATHY

Matthew R. G. Taylor & Luisa Mestroni

Introduction

Dilated cardiomyopathy (DCM) is a disease of the cardiac muscle that results in progressive ventricular dilation and systolic dysfunction leading to congestive heart failure (CHF). The relatively high disease prevalence of 1:2500 individuals and the substantial associated morbidity and mortality make DCM a serious public health concern. In spite of advances in heart failure treatment, DCM remains a leading cause of cardiac transplant and death from progressive heart failure.

Historically, genetic factors contributing to DCM were believed to be rare and of little clinical relevance. More recently, the role of genetics in the pathogenesis of DCM has gained increased prominence. Current evidence suggests that 20 to 50% of DCM may be explained by mutations in genes important for cardiac muscle function. These cases of DCM, formerly referred to as idiopathic DCM, are now being termed *familial DCM* (FDC).

FDC is genetically heterogeneous, and all basic Mendelian inheritance patterns of transmission have been reported (Mestroni et al., 1999). The autosomal dominant pattern of inheritance is most common and accounts for the majority of FDC pedigrees. To date, 10 genes and 19 loci have been associated with FDC (Table 72-1). A common thread connecting several of these genes is their various roles in the makeup of the cellular cytoskeleton. The cytoskeleton is composed of a number of proteins responsible for interacting in a meshlike network that provides structural support for cardiac muscle cells and plays a role in allowing for the transmission of contractile forces across cells and to neighboring cells.

The exact details of how mutations in cytoskeletal genes generate a DCM phenotype remain elusive. However, these findings have led to a *force-transmission* model for FDC that shows that perturbations to the integrity of this network, presumably affecting the transmission of contractile force within and between cells, are sufficient to result in a DCM phenotype. This model stands in contrast to a *force-generation* model that was first described as the cause for hypertrophic cardiomyopathy (HCM), where mutations in genes coding for contractile-related proteins are more relevant. It is now evident that there are genes forming the sarcomere (cardiac

TABLE 72-1

PHENOTYPES, KNOWN LOCI, AND DISEASE GENES FOR FAMILIAL DILATED CARDIOMYOPATHY

Phenotype	Frequency, %	Chromosomal location	LOCUS	OMIM[a]	Known gene
Autosomal dominant FDC	56	1q32	CMD1D	191045	Cardiac troponin T
		2q31	CMD1G	604145	Titin
		2q35	CMD1I	125660	Desmin
		6q12–q16		605582	
		9q13	CMD1B	600884	
(with mitral prolapse)		10q21–q23	CMD1C	601493	
		14q12		160760	β-Myosin heavy chain
		15q14		102540	Cardiac actin
		15q22.1		191010	α-Tropomyosin
Autosomal recessive FDC	16	Unknown		212110	
X-linked DC	10	Xp21		302345	Dystrophin
Autosomal dominant FDC with skeletal muscle disease	7.7	1q11–q23	LGMD1B	159001	Lamin A/C
		5q33–34	LGMD2F	601411	δ-sarcoglycan
		6q23	CMD1F	602067	
Autosomal dominant FDC with conduction defects	2.6	1q1–q1	CMD1A	115200	Lamin A/C
		2q14–q22	CMD1H	604288	
		3p22–p25	CMD1E	601154	
Other:	7.7				
Autosomal dominant left ventricular noncompaction		Xq28		300069	G4.5 (tafazzin)
		18q12.1–q12.2		601239	α-dystrobrevin
Autosomal recessive with retinitis pigmentosa and deafness		6q23–q24	CMD1J	605362	
Autosomal recessive with wooly hair and keratoderma		6p24		605676	Desmoplakin
X-linked congenital DCM		Xq28			G4.5 (tafazzin)
Mitochondrial DCM		mtDNA		510000	

NOTE: [a]OMIM, Online Mendelian Inheritance in Man

actin, cardiac β-myosin heavy chain, troponin T, and α-tropomyosin) that can be implicated in both FDC and familial HCM. This suggests that different mutations in the same protein can change the functional properties of the protein, leading to a hypertrophic or a dilated phenotype. Other mechanisms that can cause DCM include defects in energy production due to mutations in genes that encode transport proteins or enzymes involved in cardiac fatty acid β-oxidation. Finally, the function of the G4.5 gene, causing congenital X-linked dilated cardiomyopathy, remains unknown.

Pathogenesis of *LMNA*-Associated Dilated Cardiomyopathy

Cardiomyopathies have been found to be associated with several forms of muscular dystrophy, including Duchenne, Becker, limb-girdle, and Emery-Dreifuss muscular dystrophy (EDMD). Mutations in the lamin A/C gene, which maps to chromosome 1, were shown to cause the autosomal dominant form of EDMD. Based on phenotype similarities and linkage data suggesting a locus for FDC on chromosome 1, *LMNA*

was selected as a suitable candidate gene for FDC (OMIM#*150330) and mutations were found in affected family members (Brodsky et al., 2000; Fatkin et al., 1999). The carriers of the gene mutations were characterized by DCM, frequently by conduction system disease, and by absent to variable involvement of the skeletal muscle (OMIM#*150330).

As shown in Fig. 72-1, *LMNA* encodes two isoforms (lamin A and lamin C) that are located in the nuclear lamina, a proteinaceous layer apposed to the inner nuclear membrane (Hutchison et al., 2001). The nuclear lamina is composed of a family of proteins, the lamins (A, B, and C), which are highly conserved evolutionarily. During mitosis, lamins are phosphorylated in concert with the dissolution of the nuclear lamina and nuclear membrane. The proteins are subsequently dephosphorylated after mitosis as the membrane and lamina reform.

The lamin A/C gene spans 24 kb and contains 12 protein-coding exons. Alternative splicing in exon 10 generates two mRNA species that give rise to the two different isoforms, A and C. Both isoforms are expressed in terminally differentiated cells in the heart as well as in other tissues. The protein has three predicted domains: a head, a central rod region,

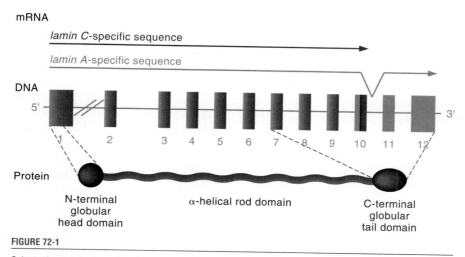

FIGURE 72-1

Schematic structural model of lamin A/C gene. At the top, the messenger RNA (mRNA) is alternatively spliced to generate two different proteins, lamin A and C. In the center, the genomic structure of LMNA is composed of 12 exons. The alternative splice occurs in exon 10. At the bottom, the protein, a member of the intermediate-filaments family, has a small globular head, a central rod domain, and a terminal globular tail.

and a tail. These regions share homology with other intermediate filament protein families. The mature proteins are able to associate with each other to form filamentous structures.

Clinical Features

As a greater number of *LMNA* mutations are reported in FDC families, as well as in families with the other *LMNA*-associated diseases, the phenotype of patients harboring *LMNA* mutations is becoming more clearly defined (Table 72-2). The disease is usually familial and inherited in an autosomal dominant pattern of transmission, but autosomal recessive and sporadic forms have also been described (Mestroni et al., 1999). The penetrance (the proportion of carriers who manifest the disease) is not complete, and some mutation carriers may be clinically unaffected. Furthermore, the disease is adult onset in nature and patients generally manifest the disease in the third or fourth decade (referred to as *age-dependent penetrance*). This is a common feature observed also in other forms of FDC, in which only 20% of patients have developed symptoms by age 20 (Mestroni et al., 1999). *LMNA*-associated DCM is typified by a progressively worsening ventricular dilation and systolic as well as diastolic dysfunction. Conduction system disease may be prominent and can even precede evidence of systolic dysfunction. Pacemaker placement is common in affected patients, and a number of individuals require cardiac transplantation. There are no described ethnically at-risk groups reported to date, and both males and females are at risk to develop the disease phenotype.

In addition to contributing to myocardial disease, mutations in *LMNA* have been associated with autosomal dominant and recessive Emery-Dreifuss muscular dystrophy (EDMD2: OMIM#181350 and EDMD3: OMIM#604929, respectively), limb-girdle muscular dystrophy (LGMD 1B: OMIM#159001), and the Dunnigan-type familial partial lipodystrophy (FPLD: OMIM#151550). Overlap between these diseases has been described, and a number of patients with *LMNA* mutations suffer from a combination of cardiac muscle, cardiac conduction, and skeletal muscle phenotype (Table 72-2). This variable expressivity is evident even among members of the same family (who share the identical mutation), with some members displaying only cardiac muscle disease while others have both cardiac and skeletal components to their illness (Brodsky et al., 2000). In patients ascertained from the standpoint of FDC, the skeletal muscle involvement can range from severe symptomatic weakness and disability to subtle abnormalities evidenced only by mild elevations in creatine kinase or abnormal muscle biopsy histology. Myopathic changes include variability of fiber size, with both atrophic and hypertrophic fibers; increase in internal nuclei; signs of degeneration and regeneration; and increase in endomysial connective tissue. Some patients have normal clinical and histologic skeletal muscle features (Brodsky et al., 2000; Fatkin at al., 1999). To date, familial partial lipodystrophy is more distinct from the cardiac and skeletal phenotypes. Muscle weakness or cardiac involvement has not been clearly described in these patients.

Genetics

In the few short years since the discovery of an association between *LMNA* mutations and DCM with or without muscular dystrophy, a number of mutations have been described throughout the gene. The majority of the described mutations are missense mutations, and segregation, when present through pedigrees, follows an autosomal dominant pattern. Almost all of the mutations described to date are *private* (unique), whereas recurrent mutations in unrelated families have been reported in only a handful of cases. The mutations discovered so far are scattered along the rod domain and the carboxyl-tail domain of the protein. There is no clear phenotype-genotype correlation known at present, except for the mutations identified in the exon 8, typically causing familial partial lipodystrophy (Sackleton et al., 2000). Further investigation will be required to

TABLE 72-2

PHENOTYPES ASSOCIATED WITH LAMIN A/C GENE MUTATIONS

Dilated cardiomyopathy (Brodsky et al., 2000)	Isolated heart disease Atrial and ventricular arrhythmia, sudden death Familial Autosomal dominant transmission Frequent restrictive pattern Normal serum creatine kinase
Conduction disease with dilated cardiomyopathy (Fatkin et al., 1999)	Atrial arrhythmia, sinus node dysfunction, atrioventricular block, pacemaker, sudden death Frequent progression to DCM Familial Autosomal dominant transmission Normal to mildly increased serum creatine kinase
Emery-Dreifuss muscular dystrophy (Bonne et al., 2000)	Mild to severe muscular dystrophy Early contractures of elbows, Achilles tendons, and neck extensor muscles Frequent heart involvement (frequent conduction defects, possible congestive heart failure) Familial or sporadic Autosomal dominant or recessive Normal to severely increased serum creatine kinase
Limb-girdle muscular dystrophy (Muchir et al., 2000)	Slowly progressive proximal muscle weakness and wasting Absence of contractures Myopathic changes on muscle biopsy Atrial arrhythmia, sinus node dysfunction, atrioventricular block, pacemaker, sudden death Normal to mildly increased serum creatine kinase
Familial partial lipodystrophy, Dunnigan type (Sackleton et al., 2000)	Absence of adipose tissue sparing the face Skeletal muscle hypertrophy Insulin resistance, hyperlipidemia, acanthosis nigricans Specific mutations in exon 8
Non-specific muscular changes (Brodsky et al., 2000)	Seen in young gene mutation carriers Minimal muscle weakness Difficulty in climbing stairs, running quickly

determine what genotype-to-phenotype relationships exist in these diseases. The notable intrafamilial variability in penetrance and expression that characterizes the known *LMNA* mutations argues that other modifier genes can influence the phenotype.

Clinical Implications

This new understanding of DCM genetics has relevant clinical implications. The high frequency of familial forms of DCM indicates that clinical screening for *LMNA* and other DCM gene mutations should play a significant role in clinical practice. Familial screening activities permit genetic counseling and offer the possibility of early or presymptomatic identification of patients at risk, who may need early therapeutic interventions. With respect to *LMNA*, clinical evaluations should include a thorough assessment of the skeletal muscles (including measuring serum creatine kinase) and testing for cardiac conduction system disease. An individual with DCM and pathology of either the skeletal muscles or conduction system represents a reasonable candidate for harboring a mutation in *LMNA*. Importantly, there are examples of *LMNA* mutation-carrying individuals who do not manifest complex phenotypes, and thus all patients with FDC or idiopathic DCM represent potential candidates for genetic analysis.

The identification of genetic contributions to cardiac illness represents a new frontier in the study of DCM, and yet another example of the recent impact that gene discovery has on adult-onset illnesses. The further elucidation of the roles of *LMNA* and other important DCM genetic loci will continue to shape the understanding of inherited cardiomyopathies. In the near future, molecular genetic testing will likely become routine in the clinical evaluation of DCM. Ultimately, continued investigation into the genetics of DCM may suggest novel approaches to therapeutics and lead to meaningful reductions in the morbidity and mortality caused by this serious condition.

REFERENCES

Bonne G et al: Clinical and molecular genetic spectrum of autosomal dominant Emery-Dreifuss muscular dystrophy due to mutations of the lamin A/C gene. Ann Neurol 48:170, 2000

Brodsky GL et al: A lamin A/C gene mutation associated with dilated cardiomyopathy with variable skeletal muscle involvement. Circulation 101:473, 2000

Fatkin D et al: Missense mutations in the rod domain of the lamin A/C gene as causes of dilated cardiomyopathy and conduction-system disease. N Engl J Med 341:1715, 1999

Hutchison CJ et al: Lamins in disease: Why do ubiquitously expressed nuclear envelope proteins give rise to tissue-specific disease phenotype? J Cell Sci 114:9, 2001

Mestroni L et al: Familial dilated cardiomyopathy: Evidence for genetic and phenotypic heterogeneity. J Am Coll Cardiol 34:181, 1999

Muchir A et al: Identification of mutations in the gene encoding lamins A/C in autosomal dominant limb girdle muscular dystrophy with atrioventricular conduction disturbances (LGMD1B). Hum Mol Genet 9:1453, 2000.
    OMIM: Online Mendelian Inheritance in Man: *http://www.ncbi.nlm.nih.gov/entrez/query.fcgi?db-OMIM*

Sackleton S et al: LMNA, encoding lamin A/C, is mutated in partial lipodystrophy. Nat Genet 24:153, 2000

EFFECT OF ANEMIA IN SEVERE CONGESTIVE HEART FAILURE

Donald S. Silverberg, Dov Wexler, & Adrian Iaina

Anemia is known to cause congestive heart failure (CHF) even in patients with no underlying heart disease, and correction of the anemia with transfusions can correct CHF (Anand et al., 1993). What is less appreciated is that many patients with CHF *and* underlying heart disease are also frequently anemic (Silverberg et al., 2000). Thus it seems that in CHF, a vicious circle is set in motion wherein CHF causes anemia and the anemia acts to worsen the CHF. It is possible that one reason for the high mortality, morbidity, and rate of rehospitalization seen in CHF is that the associated anemia is usually not treated.

Why Should CHF Patients Become Anemic?

The anemia of CHF could be due to several factors (Silverberg et al., 2000):

1. *Iron deficiency*—caused by poor intake, malabsorption, or chronic blood loss from, for example, use of prophylactic aspirin

2. *The anemia of chronic renal failure* (CRF)—CRF occurs frequently seen in CHF. The anemia of CRF is due to a combination of many factors, of which the most important is the reduced erythropoietin (EPO) production in the kidney.

3. *The use of angiotensin-converting enzyme (ACE) inhibitors*—these may interfere with both EPO production in the kidney and EPO activity in the bone marrow.

4. *The increased activity of cytokines such as tumor necrosis factor (TNF)*—TNF-α levels are markedly elevated in CHF and interfere with the action of EPO on the bone marrow and with the release of iron from the reticuloendothelial system for use in the bone marrow.

How Common Is Anemia in CHF?

Many studies of CHF have shown that the mean hemoglobin (Hb) level in patients is about 12 g/dL (Silverberg et al., 2000). Since the lower limit of normal (the 95th percentile) for Hb for men is 13.5 g/dL and for women is 12 g/dL, this would suggest that at least one-half of patients with CHF are anemic. In a study of 142 consecutive cases of CHF seen in one special CHF outpatient clinic, the mean Hb level was 11.9 g/dL and 55% had a Hb <12 g/dL (Silverberg et al., 2000). The prevalence and severity of the anemia increased with increased severity of the CHF. The mean Hb level fell from 13.6 g/dL in New York Heart Association (NYHA) class 1 patients to 10.9 g/dL in NYHA class 4 patients. The percentage of patients with anemia (Hb <12 g/dL) was 9.1%, 19.2%, 52.6%, and 79.1% for NYHA classes 1 to 4, respectively. In those resistant CHF patients who did not respond to CHF medication, the mean Hb level was even lower: 10.2 g/dL.

How Can Anemia Cause CHF?

Anemia of any cause likely produces CHF in the manner depicted in Fig. 73-1. Vasodilatation caused by the accompanying tissue hypoxia lowers arterial pressure, thus activating the sympathetic nervous system. This causes peripheral vasoconstriction and tachycardia, which are needed to maintain arterial pressure. The associated renal vasoconstriction activates the renin-angiotensin-aldosterone system. The high angiotensin II levels further increase renal and peripheral vasoconstriction and increase aldosterone production. The resultant reduction in renal blood flow and glomerular filtration rate (GFR) can cause renal ischemia and fluid retention. The renal insufficiency thus produced may also cause anemia

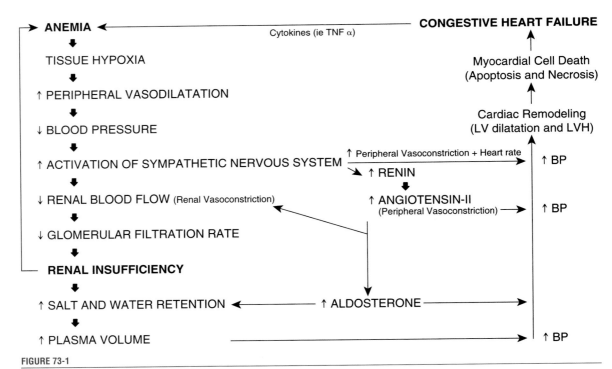

FIGURE 73-1

The vicious circle of anemia, chronic renal failure, and congestive heart failure.

through reduced EPO production and bone marrow utilization. The increased amount of aldosterone further increases the fluid retention. Thus there is a marked increase in plasma and extracellular volume, which can manifest itself as ventricular dilation and central and peripheral edema. The long-term effects of all these factors on the heart can be deleterious. On the one hand, the heart is faced with an increased workload with increased heart rate and stroke volume; on the other hand, the oxygen-carrying capacity of the blood is reduced by the anemia itself. The heart undergoes remodeling with ventricular dilation and left ventricular hypertrophy (LVH). Both the sympathetic nervous system and renin-angiotensin-aldosterone system contribute to this remodeling. Eventually, the left ventricular dilation and hypertrophy lead to myocardial cell death (apoptosis), cardiac fibrosis, cardiomyopathy, and further CHF. The CHF, by way of increased secretion of cytokines such as TNF-α, can also cause anemia, closing the vicious circle.

In patients with coronary artery disease, the effects of anemia on the heart may be even more severe than in normal individuals because of the greater cardiac ischemia caused by blockage of the coronary arteries by plaques and by the failure of associated vasodilatation of the coronary arteries due to endothelial dysfunction (Wahr, 1998). In the heart with cardiac damage, ischemia can occur at a higher Hb level than with a normal heart. While patients with normal hearts undergoing surgery can tolerate low Hb levels without increasing cardiovascular risk, those with coronary heart disease are more likely to have cardiovascular complications at low Hb levels, and animal studies have confirmed these clinical findings (Wahr, 1998). They have demonstrated that (1) reducing the diameter of coronary arteries in healthy animals can cause CHF; (2) CHF occurs at a higher Hb level in animals with coronary stenosis than it does in animals with normal coronaries; and (3) in the animals with stenosed coronary arteries who developed CHF when anemia was produced, the CHF disappeared when the anemia was corrected.

Is Anemia Important in CHF?

All the above points argue for a role of anemia in the production or worsening of CHF. But how clinically relevant is this in CHF? Judging from the literature, anemia in CHF is not considered an important contributor to this condition. In the recent U.S. guidelines on diagnosis and treatment of CHF, anemia is not even mentioned. Studies looking at exacerbating causes of CHF list anemia either as a rare or nonexistent factor (Silverberg et al., 2000). But is this really the case?

It could be argued that the anemia is a beneficial factor because it would be associated with reduced viscosity of the blood and, therefore, might allow the blood to flow more easily through the peripheral circulation. However, a recent preliminary report analyzed the effect of anemia in CHF on mortality in the SOLVD study, a prospective study of treatment of CHF patients with ACE inhibitors (Al Ahmad et al., 2000). The mortality rate was found to increase with increasing severity of the anemia, and the anemia was found to be an independent risk factor for this increased CHF mortality.

Lessons Learned from the Use of EPO in the Correction of Anemia for the Prevention and Treatment of CHF in Patients with CRF before and while on Dialysis

With the advent of EPO 15 years ago there has been a revolution in the treatment of anemia. This agent, produced in the kidney, stimulates bone marrow production of red blood cells (RBCs). Originally, EPO was used primarily in hemodialysis and CRF predialysis patients, where it was shown to have great benefits (Silverberg et al., 2001b). The improvement of anemia in these patients has been associated with a reduction in ventricular dilation and left ventricular mass and hypertrophy. Anemia was also found to be an independent risk factor for LVH, and recurrent CHF, and cardiac mortality in patients on dialysis. In addition, many studies in patients on dialysis have shown that the greater the level of Hb, the lower the risk of hospitalization and death (Silverberg et al., 2001b). With the improvement in Hb levels with EPO treatment, quality of life has improved dramatically, with improved cognitive function, exercise capacity, depression, social relationships, sexual function, sleep, appetite, and nutritional status (Silverberg et al., 2001b). It is even possible that what is called "cardiac cachexia" is, in many instances, nothing more than untreated anemia.

In addition, correction of anemia is associated with an increase in aerobic metabolism, less anaerobic metabolism and lactate production, improved peak oxygen utilization, improved skeletal muscle function, an improvement in angina pectoris, improved cerebral blood flow, improved amino acid metabolism, improved glucose metabolism, improved endothelial cell function, and improved blood rheology. The high levels of 2,3-DPG in these young RBCs produced by EPO improves the uptake of oxygen from the lungs and its release in the tissues. The RBC has many systems for handling oxidation radicals so that these damaging substances are reduced with correction of anemia. This reduces lipid peroxidation, a key step in the production of atherosclerosis (Silverberg et al., 2001b).

EPO has a very low incidence of side effects and is easily administered subcutaneously once every 1 to 2 weeks in doses of 4000 to 10,000 IU. In these relatively low doses, hypertension is rarely caused or worsened. However, even if blood pressure does become elevated because of EPO use, it is almost always easily controlled with slight changes in antihypertensive medications. All of this experience in renal failure patients suggests that EPO may be an ideal agent for the correction of anemia in CHF patients.

Is Correction of Anemia Useful in CHF Patients?

Two recent reports detail experiences in the treatment of anemia in patients seen in an outpatient CHF clinic who were resistant to maximally tolerated

levels of CHF medications including ACE inhibitors, one of three beta blockers (bisoprolol, metoprolol, or carvedilol), aldospirone, nitrates, digoxin, and oral and intravenous furosemide, (Silverberg et al., 2000, 2001b). In a prospective trial subcutaneous EPO and intravenous iron (Venofer-iron sucrose) were administered to 26 patients who had severe CHF and anemia (Hb <12 g/dL) and were resistant to the maximally tolerated therapy for CHF. Mean duration of the treatment was 7.2 months. It was found that the mean Hb level increased from 10.2 g/dL to 12.1 g/dL, and this increase was associated with an improvement in cardiac function [an increase in the mean left ventricular ejection fraction (LVEF) from 27.7 to 35.4 %] and a decrease in the mean NYHA functional class from 3.7 to 2.7. Furthermore, prior to the intervention, the GFR had been deteriorating at a mean rate of 0.95 mL/min per month. During treatment, the mean GFR increased by a mean of 0.85 mL/min per month. In addition, the number of hospitalizations fell from a mean of 2.7 in the months before the trial to 0.2 for the same period of time after the anemia was corrected—an improvement of 92%. Particularly striking was the fact that this improvement took place despite a marked reduction in the dose of oral and intravenous furosemide. The doses of the other CHF agents were kept constant.

In a subsequent controlled study, the anemia was treated in the same manner as above in 16 severe resistant CHF patients (group A) but not in 16 patients of a control group (group B) over a mean of 8.2 months (Silverberg et al., 2001a). In group A, the Hb level was raised from a mean of 10.3 g/dL to 12.9 g/dL. Four patients in group B died of CHF-related illnesses and none died in group A. The mean NYHA class improved by 42.1% in group A and worsened by 11.4% in group B. The LVEF increased by 5.5 in group A and decreased by 5.4 in group B. The serum creatinine did not change in group A and increased by 28.6% in group B. The need for oral and intravenous furosemide decreased by 51% and 91%, respectively, in group A and increased by 29% and 28.0%, respectively, in group B. The number of days spent in hospital compared to the same period of time before entering the study decreased by 79% in

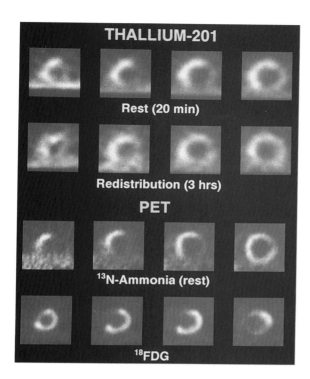

THALLIUM-201

Rest (20 min)

Redistribution (3 hrs)

PET

¹³N-Ammonia (rest)

¹⁸FDG

COLOR PLATE 5 (Figure 34-2)

Concordance between thallium SPECT and PET is demonstrated in this patient example. Rest-redistribution short-axis thallium tomograms (top 2 rows) and ¹³N-ammonia and FDG PET images (lower 2 rows) are displayed from a patient with coronary artery disease. There are extensive thallium abnormalities in the lateral and inferior regions on the initial rest images that are partially reversible on 3- to 4-h redistribution images, suggestive of viable myocardium. The corresponding ¹³N-ammonia and FDG PET images (acquired after an overnight fast) show severely reduced ¹³N-ammonia uptake in the lateral and inferior regions at rest (similar to the initial thallium images) with enhanced FDG uptake (mismatch pattern), suggestive of viable myocardium. [From V Dilsizian (ed): *Myocardial Viability: A Clinical and Scientific Treatise.* Armonk, NY, Futura Publishing, 2000.]

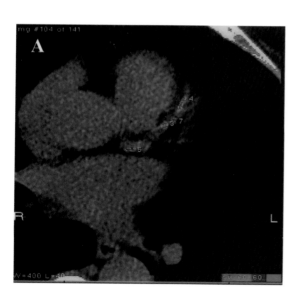

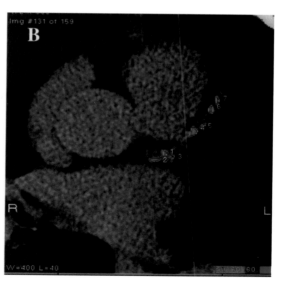

Volume =	179.8	216.7
Score =	142.1	257.7
Percentile =	47	58

COLOR PLATE 6 (Figure 36-5)

Rapid increase of calcium volume in the same patient after one year of follow-up. The initial volume score of 179.8 increased to 216.7. The age-sex percentile has increased from 47th to 58th.

Extra Thoracic MIDCAB Approaches

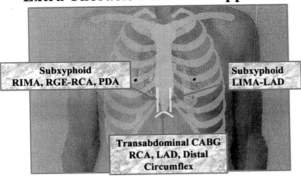

Subxyphoid
RIMA, RGE-RCA, PDA

Subxyphoid
LIMA-LAD

Transabdominal CABG
RCA, LAD, Distal
Circumflex

COLOR PLATE 7 (Figure 44-1)

Extrathoracic MIDCAB approaches. Extrathoracic incisions (without cutting the sternum or spreading the ribs) used to approach right coronary artery (RCA), posterior descending (PDA), and posterolateral branches of right coronary, left anterior descending (LAD), and distal circumflex branches. LIMA, left internal mammary artery.

Thoracic MIDCAB Approaches

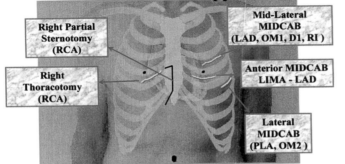

Right Partial
Sternotomy
(RCA)

Mid-Lateral
MIDCAB
(LAD, OM1, D1, RI)

Right
Thoracotomy
(RCA)

Anterior MIDCAB
LIMA - LAD

Lateral
MIDCAB
(PLA, OM2)

COLOR PLATE 8 (Figure 44-2)

Thoracic MIDCAB approaches. Thoracic incisions used for minimally invasive direct coronary artery bypass grafting (MIDCAB) involving right coronary artery, left anterior descending (LAD) and its diagonal branches, ramus intermedius branch, and obtuse marginal (OM) and posterolateral branches of the circumflex artery.

Anterior MIDCAB PostOP

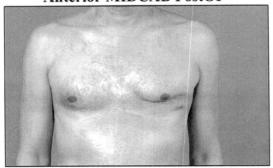

COLOR PLATE 9 (Figure 44-3)

Anterior MIDCAB postoperatively. Healed incision of anterior minimally invasive direct coronary artery bypass grafting surgery.

group A and increased by 58% in group B. The results of these two studies suggest that the treatment of even mild anemia can have a profound effect on cardiac and renal status in CHF patients.

Use of Intravenous Iron as a Supplement to EPO for Anemia in CHF

Intravenous iron has been used in addition to EPO in the treatment of anemia. This regimen is based on studies indicating that the effect of EPO is markedly reduced if intravenous iron is not added (Silverberg et al., 1996). EPO stimulates the rapid production of erythrocytes in the marrow. If the iron supply is inadequate, the RBCs produced are extruded from the marrow with low levels of Hb. Intravenous iron prevents or overcomes this functional iron deficiency. The oral route of iron administration usually does not supply enough iron to the EPO-stimulated bone marrow to produce the increased amount of Hb needed for the increased number of red blood cells produced. The new intravenous iron preparations, such as iron sucrose and iron gluconate, are very safe and have been approved for use all over the world. In contrast, iron dextran, which was for years the main intravenous preparation used, frequently causes serious, adverse side effects.

Impact of CHF on CRF

Studies also indicate that the correction of anemia and the subsequent improvement in CHF are often associated with a slowing or stopping of the

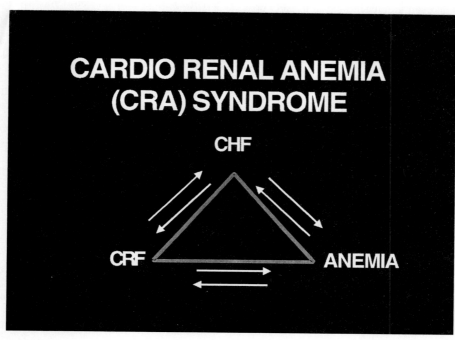

FIGURE 73-2

The cardio-renal anemia (CRA) syndrome.

progression of the CRF. There is a dose-response relationship between the severity of CHF and the frequency and severity of CRF. In the study of 142 patients attending the special outpatient CHF unit mentioned previously (Silverberg et al., 2000), the mean serum creatinine level was within the normal range (1.2 mg/dL) in those with the mildest form of CHF, NYHA class 1, but increased steadily as CHF class rose, reaching 2.0 mg/dL in the patients with the most severe disease (NYHA Class IV). The percentage of patients with serum creatinine >1.5 mg/dL increased from 18.2% in the NYHA class 1 group to 58.2% in the NYHA class IV group. The slowing of deterioration in renal function that the authors observed in two intervention studies (Silverberg et al., 2000, 2001a) is likely due to the improved cardiac function causing increased renal blood flow and GFR. A vicious circle is created in CHF, wherein both CHF and CRF cause anemia that further worsens the CHF—which in turn further worsens the CRF, which causes an even greater reduction in EPO production, and so on. The authors have termed this lethal combination of CHF, CRF, and anemia the *cardio-renal anemia (CRA) syndrome* (Figs. 73-1 and 73-2). The good news is that the cycle can be disrupted at multiple sites by the combined approach of using CHF medications in the recommended doses and by correcting the anemia with subcutaneous EPO and intravenous iron administration. Thus the control of the anemia and the CHF may reduce the need for dialysis in many patients with heart disease.

SUMMARY

Anemia is frequently seen in CHF, and, without correction, a large number of these patients will not benefit from standard CHF therapy. The administration of EPO with intrevenous iron supplementation is very efficient in the correction of this anemia and is associated with a remarkable improvement in the clinical status of these patients.

REFERENCES

Al Ahmad A et al: Anemia and renal insufficiency as risk factors for mortality in patients with left ventricular dysfunction. J Am Soc Nephrol 11:137A, 2000

Anand IS et al: Pathogenesis of edema in chronic anemia: Studies of body water and sodium, renal function, haemodynamics and plasma hormones. Br Heart J 70:357, 1993

Packer M, Cohn J. Consensus recommendations for the management of chronic heart failure. Am J Cardiol 83 (Suppl 2A):1A, 1999

Silverberg DS et al: Intravenous ferric saccharate as an iron supplement in dialysis patients. Nephron 72:413, 1996

Silverberg DS et al: The use of subcutaneous erythropoietin and intravenous iron for the treatment of the anemia of severe, resistant congestive heart failure improves cardiac and renal function, functional cardiac class, and markedly reduces hospitalization. J Am Coll Cardiol 35:1737, 2000

Silverberg DS et al: The effect of correction of mild anemia in severe, resistant congestive heart failure using subcutaneous erythropoietin and intravenous iron: A randomized controlled study. J Am Coll Cardiol 37:1775, 2001a

Silverberg DS et al: The pathological consequences of anaemia. Clin Lab Haematol 23:1, 2001b

Wahr JA: Myocardial ischemia in anaemic patients. Br J Anaesth 81(Suppl):10, 1998

SEQUENTIAL RADIAL TO OM1&OM2

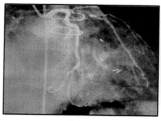
PreOp

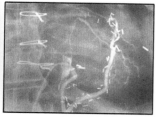
PostOp

Lateral MIDCAB

Sequential radial to obtuse marginal (OM)1 and OM2 (lateral MIDCAB). *(Left)* Lesion in the circumflex artery (reoperative). *(Right)* Patent radial artery graft sequentially anastomosed to first and second obtuse marginal branches of circumflex artery.

TransAbdominal MIDCAB PostOP

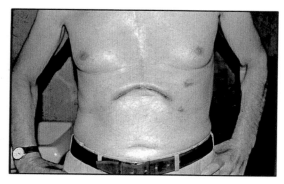

Transabdominal MIDCAB postoperatively. Healed incision after transabdominal approach for MIDCAB.

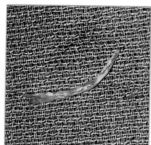
Endarterectomy

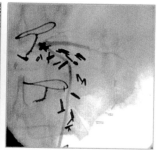
PostOp Angio

TransAbdominal CABG

Transabdominal CABG. (Left) Endarterectomized segment from diffusely diseased posterior descending coronary artery (PDA). (Right) Postoperative angiogram of patent right gastroepiploic (RGEA) to PDA graft done by transabdominal approach in the same patient.

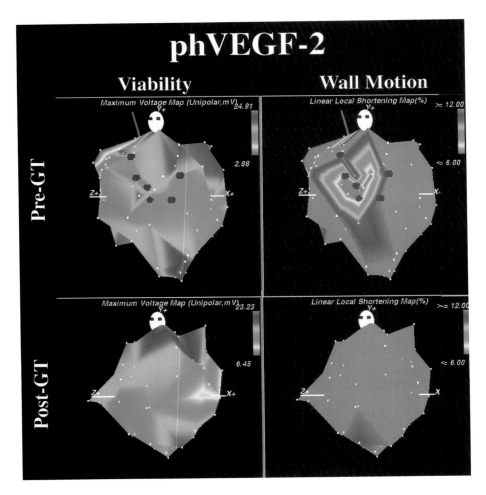

COLOR PLATE 13 (Figure 40-1)

NOGA Left ventricular electromechanical mapping performed in 64-year-old male. NOGA images in left anterior oblique (LAO) projection before gene transfer (pre-GT) show unipolar voltage (UpV) and linear local shortening (LLS) maps; red zone, depicting abnormal wall motion, on LLS map (*upper right*) together with preserved viability (purple/pink/blue/green) on UpV map (*upper left*) constitute focus of electromechanical uncoupling that suggests ischemic or hibernating myocardium (arrow) in anterolateral wall. UpV and LLS maps in same projection 90 days post-GT (*lower left, lower right, respectively*) disclose complete resolution of anterolateral ischemic zone (2.3 cm^2 pre-GT vs. 0 cm^2 post-GT). Circular brown icons in upper panels represent sites of phVEGF-2 injection. Vertical and horizontal axes (X, Y, and Z) are presented by white lines. Red line represents long axis through the apex.

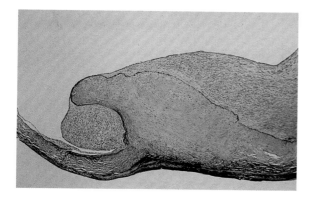

COLOR PLATE 14 (Figure 56-1)

Valve leaflet in a patient with carcinoid heart disease. The leaflet is covered with plaque consisting of an amorphous ground substance infiltrated with spindle-shaped cells.

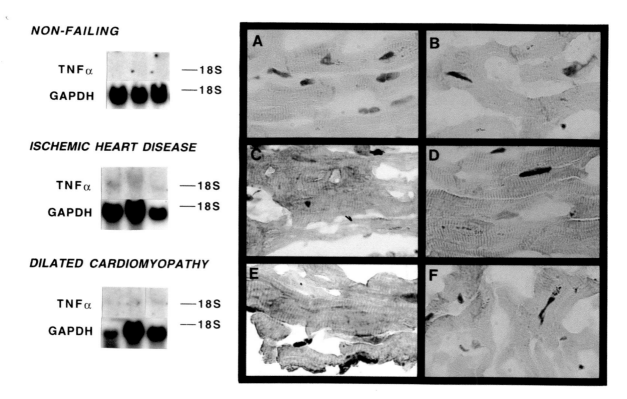

COLOR PLATE 15 (Figure 71-2)

Tumor necrosis factor (TNF) mRNA and protein in nonfailing and failing myocardium. The left-hand side of this figure shows representative northern blot analyses from nonfailing and failing myocardium. As shown, there was no evidence for TNF mRNA in the nonfailing hearts ($n = 3$), whereas TNF mRNA was present in the hearts for ishemic heart disease and dilated cardiomyopathy patients. The right-hand side of the figure shows immunohistochemical staining for TNF in nonfailing and failing myocardium. Panels *A, C,* and *E* show the results obtained with primary and secondary antibody, whereas panels *B, D,* and *F* show the results obtained with secondary antibody alone (control). There was no evidence for TNF immunostaining in nonfailing myocardium (*A*), whereas there was obvious TNF immunostaining of the cardiac myocytes in the hearts from ishemic heart disease (*C*) and dilated cardiomyopathy patients (*E*). There was no evidence for nonspecific staining of the secondary antibody in hearts from normal subjects (*B*), or patients with ischemic heart disease (*D*). (reproduced from Y Seta et al: J Card Fail 2:243, 1996, with permission.)

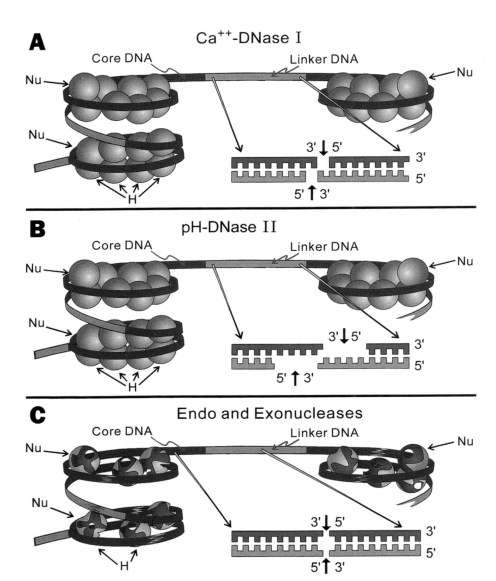

COLOR PLATE 16 (Figure 70-1)

Schematic representation of chromatin structure and DNA damage associated with apoptosis (*A* and *B*) and necrosis (*C*). Panels *A–C* each illustrate three nucleosomes (Nu) connected by linker DNA. Each nucleosome consists of a histone (H) core surrounded by two full turns of double-stranded DNA (Core DNA). A sequence of nucleotides present in the linker DNA is shown in the lower part of panels *A* and *B*. A similar sequence of nucleotides pertaining to the linker or core DNA is depicted in the lower part of panel *C*. (*A*) DNA damage mediated by activation of Ca^{2+}-dependent DNase I characterized by staggered ends in the DNA with single base 3′ overhangs (solid arrows in the sequence of nucleotides). This type of DNA injury is identified by a PCR-generated *Taq* polymerase probe, which possesses complementary structures; this probe interacts only with damaged DNA exhibiting single base 3′ overhanges. (*B*) DNA damage mediated by activation of pH-dependent DNase II characterized by staggered ends in the DNA with one or more, up to four, bases 3′ overhangs (solid arrows in the sequence of nucleotides). This type of DNA injury is identified by the terminal deoxynucleotidyl transferase (TdT) assay that links labeled nucleotides to 3′ overhangs and the generated sequence can be visualized by fluorescence. (*C*) DNA damage associated with cell necrosis. Loss of plasmamembrane integrity and the release of lysosomal proteases lead to degradation of histones in the nucleosomes (Nu), which results in the loss of DNA protection and its exposure to endonucleases and exonucleases. Endonucleases produce double-strand cleavage of the DNA with recessed 3′ ends or 3′ overhangs, whereas exonucleases remove terminal nucleotides leading to a form of damage with blunt DNA ends (solid arrows in the sequence of nucleotides). This type of DNA injury is identified by a PCR-generated *Pfu* polymerase probe, which possesses complementary structures; this probe interacts only with damaged DNA exhibiting blunt ends.

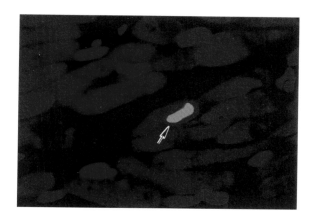

COLOR PLATE 17 (Figure 70-2)

Human heart affected by end-stage ischemic cardiomyopathy. Confocal image illustrating an apoptotic myocyte by yellow fluorescence (arrow). The myocyte nucleus shows positive staining for terminal deoxynucleotidyl transferase assay. Red fluorescence of nuclei corresponds to propidium iodide staining, and red fluorescence of myocyte cytoplasm corresponds to -sarcomeric actin antibody labeling. Confocal microscopy, × 800.

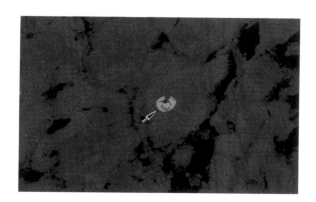

COLOR PLATE 18 (Figure 70-3)

Heart failure in a patient affected by diabetes. Confocal image illustrating a necrotic myocyte by yellow fluorescence (arrow). The myocyte nucleus shows positive staining for *Pfu* polymerase probe. Red fluorescence of myocyte cytoplasm corresponds to -sarcomeric actin antibody labeling. Pink fluorescence reflects nitrotyrosine localization in the myocardium. Confocal microscopy, × 650.

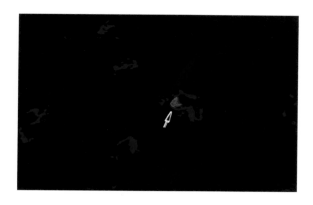

COLOR PLATE 19 (Figure 70-4)

Heart failure in a patient affected by diabetes and hypertension. Confocal image illustrating an apoptotic endothelial cell nucleus by green fluorescence (arrow). The apoptotic nucleus shows positive staining for *Taq* polymerase probe. Red fluorescence of endothelial cell cytoplasm corresponds to factor VIII antibody labeling. Pink fluorescence reflects nitrotyrosine localization in endothelial cells. Blue fluorescence corresponds to nitrotyrosine in the myocardium. Confocal microscopy, × 650.

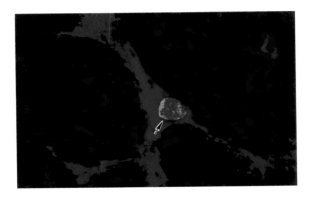

COLOR PLATE 20 (Figure 70-5)

Heart failure in a patient affected by diabetes. Confocal image illustrating a necrotic fibroblast nucleus by green fluorescence (arrow). The necrotic nucleus shows positive staining for *Pfu* polymerase probe. Red fluorescence of fibroblast cytoplasm corresponds to vimentin antibody labeling. Pink fluorescence reflects nitrotyrosine localization in fibroblasts. Blue fluorescence corresponds to nitrotyrosine in the myocardium. Confocal microscopy, × 1300.

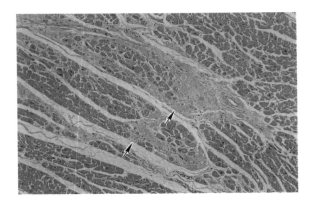

COLOR PLATE 21 (Figure 70-6)

Human heart affected by end-stage dilated cardiomyopathy. Small foci of replacement fibrosis (arrows) are visible within the myocardium. Hematoxylin and eosin staining, × 175.

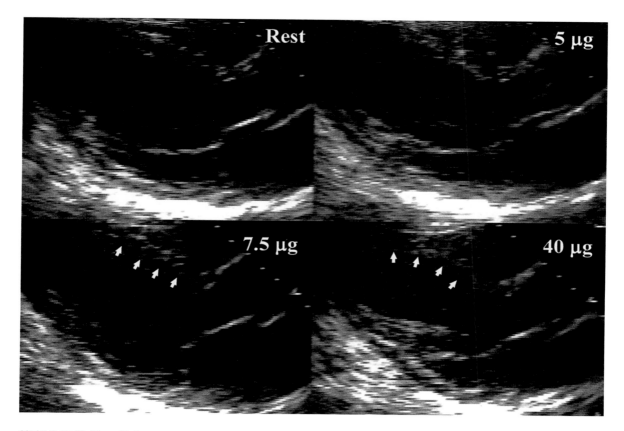

COLOR PLATE 22 (Figure 81-1)

End-systolic echocardiographic images from the parasternal long axis view in a patient evaluated for myocardial viability. A biphasic response is demonstrated in this patient during dobutamine infusion. The anterior septum was akinetic at rest, had significant improvement in wall motion and thickening at 7.5 μg/kg per min of dobutamine. Worsening of wall motion and dyskinesis occurred at 40 μg/kg per min as shown by arrows.

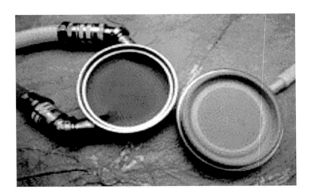

COLOR PLATE 23 (Figure 84-1)

Heartmate LVAD. The inflow cannula on the left and the inside of the pump are made of scintered titanium, while the diaphragm is textured polyurethane.

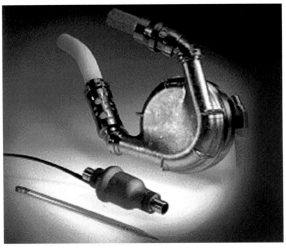

COLOR PLATE 24 (Figure 84-3)

Heartmate II. This small rotary pump is shown opposite the current implantable device.

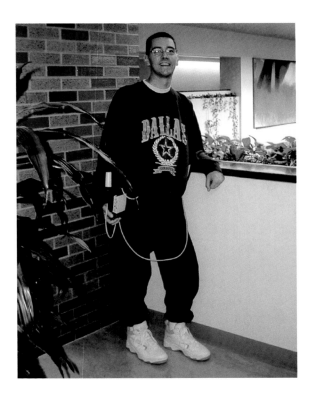

COLOR PLATE 25 (Figure 84-4)

Awaiting Transplants. The lightweight batteries allow nearly normal activity. The driveline must not be submerged, so bathing and swimming are not permitted.

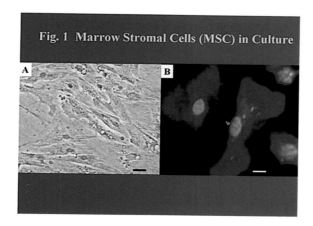

Fig. 1 Marrow Stromal Cells (MSC) in Culture

COLOR PLATE 26 (Figure 87-1)

The morphology of rat MSCs in culture. A. Phase contrast photomicrograph of MSCs just before implantation. Most adherent MSCs are fibroblastic in appearance. B. MSCs were labeled with 49, 6-diamidino-2-phenylindole (DAPI) to trace after implantation. Scale bars represent 60 mm in A and 30 mm in B.

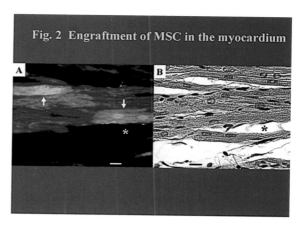

Fig. 2 Engraftment of MSC in the myocardium

COLOR PLATE 27 (Figure 87-2)

MSC grafts in isogenic rat recipient heart 4 weeks after implantation. A. DAPI epifluorescence (blue fluorescence) photomicrograph. Incorporation of DAPI-labeled cells with the host myocardium. B. Hematoxylin and eosin stain. Consecutive section to that shown in A. Labeled MSC-derived cells have the same structure as the surrounding cardiomyocytes. Asterisks (*) show corresponding cross-section of a blood vessel in this pair of images. Scale bars represent 30 mm.

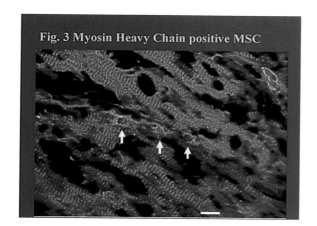

Fig. 3 Myosin Heavy Chain positive MSC

COLOR PLATE 28 (Figure 87-3)

Expression of sarcomeric myosin heavy chain molecules of MSC-derived donor cells in specimen taken 6 weeks after implantation. Combined DAPI and Texas Red images. Arrow shows DAPI-labeled cell is positively stained. Scale bar represents 15 mm.

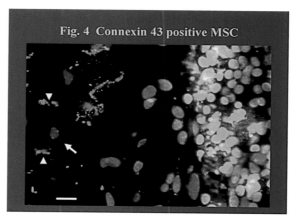

Fig. 4 Connexin 43 positive MSC

COLOR PLATE 29 (Figure 87-4)

Expression of connexin 43 in MSC-derived donor cells in a specimen 6 weeks after implantation. Combined DAPI and fluorescein (green fluorescence) image. Positive connexin 43 staining (arrowheads) is found at the interfaces between DAPI-labeled cell (arrow) and neighboring nonlabeled cells (host cardiomyocytes) and between nonlabeled cells. Scale bar represents 15 mm.

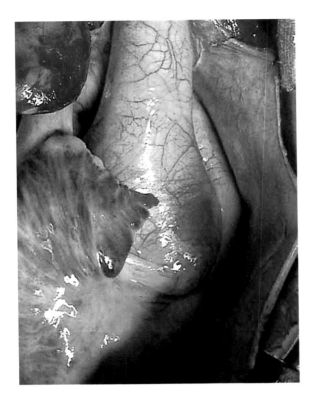

COLOR PLATE 30 (Figure 93-1)

An intraoperative photograph depicting a typical aortic root aneurysm in a 15-year-old male with Marfan's syndrome.

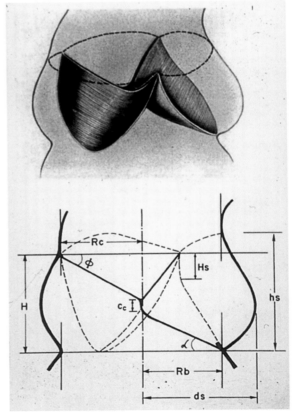

COLOR PLATE 31 (Figure 93-2)

A schematic of the normal aortic root in cross section depicting general anatomical relationships.

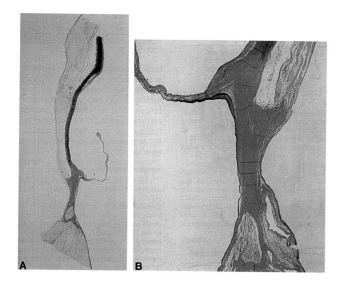

COLOR PLATE 32 (Figure 93-3)

A. A cross-sectional photomicrograph depicting the annulus, valve tissue, sinotubular junction, and ascending aortic tissue. Note that the annulus and valve tissue is relatively devoid of elastin compared to the ascending aorta (black-stained tissue). *B.* A higher power photomicrograph of the confluence of the aortic annulus, sinus of valvsalva, and aortic valve cusp.

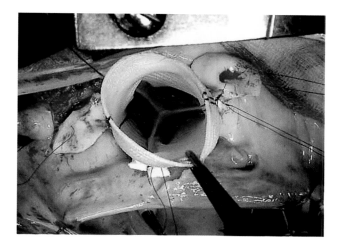

COLOR PLATE 33 (Figure 93-5)

Intraoperative photograph depicting the Dacron-replaced sinuses and coapted native leaflets during a Yacoub valve-sparing reconstruction of the aneurysm shown in Fig. 93-1 in text. The coronary ostial buttons have yet to be implanted.

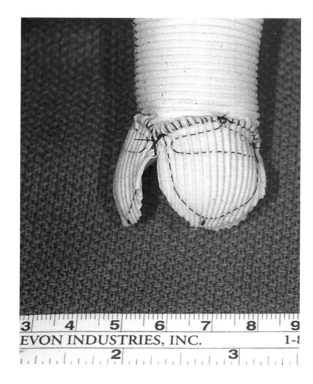

COLOR PLATE 36 (Figure 93-6)

Sinus graft with neosinuses created from Dacron tube graft for aortic root reconstruction.

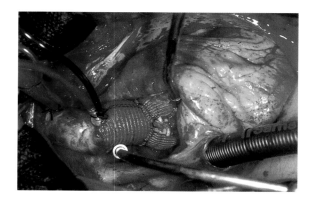

COLOR PLATE 35 (Figure 93-7)

Intraoperative photograph depicting aortic root reconstruction using a sinus graft. Note the normally bulging noncoronary and right neosinuses of Valsalva.

B-TYPE NATRIURETIC PEPTIDE (BNP) LEVELS: A POTENTIAL NOVEL "WHITE COUNT" FOR CONGESTIVE HEART FAILURE

Alan Maisel

Finding a simple blood test that aids in the diagnosis and management of patients with congestive heart failure (CHF) would clearly have a favorable impact on the staggering costs associated with the disease. Imagine the difficulty of diagnosing and then managing a life-threatening infection without the use of a white blood cell count or the problems associated with the diagnosis and treatment of prostate cancer without the benefit of a PSA level. Yet there is no currently accepted blood test to aid in the diagnosis and management of patients with CHF.

B-Type Natriuretic Peptide

B-type natriuretic peptide (BNP) is a 32-amino-acid polypeptide containing a 17-amino-acid ring structure common to all natriuretic peptides (Grantham, Burnett, 1997). Unlike atrial natriuretic peptide (ANP), whose major storage sites include the atria and ventricles, the major source of plasma BNP is cardiac ventricles. This suggests that BNP may be a more sensitive and specific indicator of ventricular

disorders than other natriuretic peptides (Yandle, 1994). BNP release appears to be in directly proportional to ventricular volume expansion and pressure overload (Maeda et al., 1998). BNP is an independent predictor of high left ventricular (LV) end-diastolic pressure and is more useful than ANP or norepinephrine for assessing the mortality in patients with chronic CHF (Tsutamoto et al., 1997).

BNP Levels in Normal Patients and in Those with CHF

As can be seen in Figure 74-1, BNP levels in normal subjects rise with age. This is not unexpected, as the left ventricle stiffens over time, offering a likely stimulus to BNP production. Females without CHF tend to have somewhat higher BNP levels than do males of the same age group. There are no significant differences in BNP levels between patients with either hypertension or diabetes and age-matched controls [U.S. Food and Drug Administration (FDA) submission data on file with Biosite Diagnostics]. Patients with lung disease may have somewhat higher levels

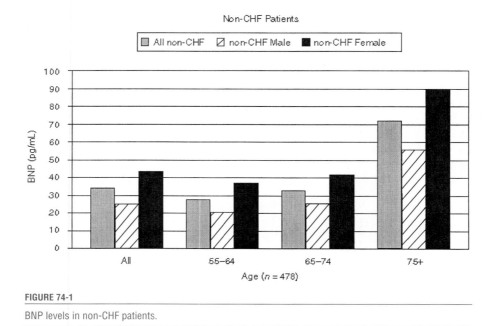

FIGURE 74-1

BNP levels in non-CHF patients.

of BNP than patients without lung disease, in part because many patients with end-stage pulmonary disorders have concomitant right ventricular (RV) dysfunction, another source of BNP release. BNP is elevated in late (predialysis) stages of renal failure and is elevated in virtually every patient on dialysis.

BNP and New York Heart Association Classification

While New York Heart Association (NYHA) classification correlates with symptoms as well as mortality in patients with heart failure, the fact that such a subjective classification is still the major means used to describe the clinical condition of patients with CHF underlies the need for more objective surrogates. Because BNP levels correlate with elevated LV end-diastolic pressure, and since this pressure correlates closely with the chief symptom of CHF, dyspnea, it is not surprising that BNP levels correlate closely with NYHA classification (Fig. 74-2).

What Should Be the Cutoff for BNP to Diagnose CHF?

Receiver-operated characteristic (ROC) curves (data on file, Biosite Diagnostics) suggest that a BNP cutoff point of 100 pg/mL allows for the increased levels seen with advancing age and provides an excellent ability to discriminate CHF from non-CHF subjects. This level shows an overall sensitivity of 82.4% for CHF to over 99% for NYHA class IV. The BNP test specificity exceeds 95% when comparing non-CHF to all CHF patients, and 93% in all subsets studied. A level of 100 pg/mL is high enough to avoid "BNP disease"—that is, a group of patients who are mistakenly said to have CHF because of falsely elevated BNP levels. In practice, though, it is likely that both a high and a low cutoff will be used—a high one (likely around 100 pg/mL) for its specificity and positive predictive value and a low one (40 to 60 pg/mL) for its high sensitivity and negative predictive value.

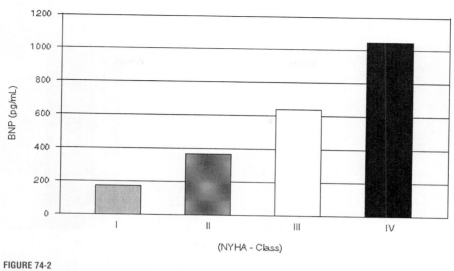

FIGURE 74-2

BNP levels in patients with CHF.

Point-of-Care Testing of BNP in the Emergency Department Setting

Point-of-care testing allows diagnostic assays to be performed in locations such as the emergency department (ED) or intensive care unit where treatment decisions are made and care is delivered based on the results of the assays. A pilot study was completed using a recently approved rapid BNP immunoassay (Triage Cardiac, Biosite Diagnostics, San Diego, CA) to assess 250 patients presenting to the San Diego VA Healthcare system urgent care area with the chief complaint of dyspnea (Dao et al., 2001).

Patients diagnosed with CHF ($n = 97$) had a mean BNP concentration of 1076 ± 138 pg/mL, while the non-CHF group ($n = 139$) had a mean BNP concentration of 38 ± 4 pg/mL (Fig. 74-3). The sicker the patient (based on severity and admission to the hospital), the higher the BNP level. Of crucial importance was the fact that patients with the final diagnosis of pulmonary disease had lower BNP values (86 ± 39 pg/mL) than those with a final diagnosis of CHF (1076 ± 138 pg/mL; $p < .001$).

BNP at a cutoff point of 80 pg/mL was found to be highly sensitive (98%) and specific (92%) for the diagnosis of CHF. The negative predictive value of BNP values <80 pg/mL was 98% for the diagnosis of CHF. Multivariate analysis revealed that after all useful tools for making the diagnosis were taken into account by the ED physician (history, symptoms, signs, radiologic studies, and laboratory findings), BNP levels continued to provide meaningful diagnostic information not available from other clinical variables. Thus, the measurement of the BNP concentration in blood appears to be a sensitive and specific test for identification of patients with CHF in acute care settings. At the very minimum, it is likely to be a potent, cost-effective addition to the diagnostic armamentarium of acute care physicians.

BNP as a Screen for Left Ventricular Dysfunction

While echocardiography, the most commonly utilized method to diagnose LV dysfunction, is one of the fastest growing procedures in cardiology, the

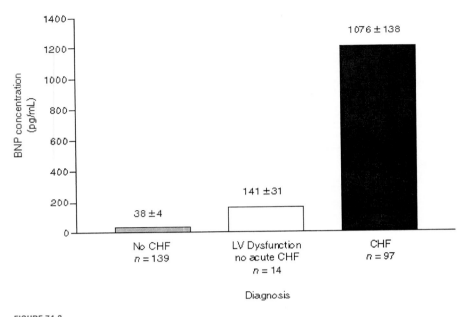

FIGURE 74-3

BNP levels in patients whose dyspnea was due to CHF, non-CHF causes, or baseline LV dysfunction but non-CHF causes.

expense of echocardiography and its limited access in community settings where it may be needed most may not make it the best screening test for patients, especially in those with low probability of LV dysfunction.

Patients who had both echocardiography and BNP levels measured have recently been characterized (Maisel et al., 2001). Among the patients with no documented history of CHF and no past determination of LV function, 51% had abnormal echocardiographic findings. In this group, BNP levels were significantly higher (328 ± 29 pg/mL) than in the 49% of patients with no history of CHF and a normal echocardiogram (30 ± 3 pg/mL; $p < .001$). In patients with a known history of CHF and previously documented LV dysfunction, all had abnormal findings ($n = 102$) with elevated BNP levels (545 ± 45 pg/mL). BNP levels were elevated in both systolic and diastolic dysfunction, with the highest values being reported in patients with systolic dysfunction plus a decreased mitral valve deceleration time.

Among patients with diastolic dysfunction, those with a restrictive filling pattern had higher BNP levels (428 pg/mL) than patients with impaired relaxation (230 pg/mL). The area under the ROC curve for BNP to detect diastolic dysfunction by echocardiography in patients with CHF and normal systolic function was 0.958. A BNP value of 71 pg/mL was 96% accurate in the prediction of diastolic dysfunction in this setting. BNP levels <57 pg/mL gave a negative predictive value of 100% for the detection of clinically significant diastolic dysfunction. Additionally, multivariate analysis showed that in patients with clinical CHF and normal LV function, BNP was the strongest predictor of diastolic abnormalities seen on echocardiography.

Thus, BNP may be an excellent screening tool for LV dysfunction. Low BNP levels may preclude the need for echocardiography in some patients, especially those who, even though at high risk, have no symptoms of heart failure. Elevated BNP levels, on the other hand, clearly indicate the presence of

LV dysfunction, whether the patient has symptoms or not, warranting further cardiac workup. It is clear that BNP should not replace imaging techniques in the diagnosis of CHF because these methods provide complementary information.

Can BNP Serve as a Surrogate End-point for the Treatment of Heart Failure?

Affecting 2% of the population, CHF is the fourth leading cause of adult hospitalizations in the United States and the most frequent cause of hospitalization in patients over the age of 65 (Stevenson, Braunwald, 1998). While patients who are admitted to the hospital with decompensated CHF often have improvement in symptoms with the various treatment modalities available, there has been no good way to evaluate the long-term effects of the short-term treatment. Indeed, in-hospital mortality and the readmission rate for CHF patients are extremely high. The conventional tests for cardiac function take time and often do not correlate well with symptomatic changes in a patient's conditions. Unlike an infection, where we follow the white blood cell count to gauge adequacy of treatment, a simple and reliable method to assess therapeutic efficacy in patients being treated for decompensated CHF is lacking. Therefore, most patients are discharged when they feel better, which might then preclude further titration of medical therapy.

BNP in Patients Admitted for Decompensated Heart Failure

In a pilot study, the course of 72 patients admitted with decompensated NYHA class III-IV CHF was followed, with measurements of BNP levels on a daily basis (Cheng et al., 2001). The association between initial BNP measurement and the predischarge or premoribund BNP measurement and subsequent adverse outcomes (defined as death and 30-day readmission) were determined.

Of the 72 patients admitted with decompensated CHF, 22 end-points occurred (death, $n = 13$; readmission, $n = 9$). In these 22 patients, BNP levels increased during hospitalization (mean increase, 233 pg/mL; $p < .001$; Fig. 74-4). In patients without end-points, BNP decreased during treatment (mean decrease, 215 pg/mL). Patients who had good outcomes were characterized by decreases in both their NYHA class and BNP levels during hospitalization, whereas those patients who were readmitted within 30 days of discharge had only minimal decreases in their BNP levels during hospitalization, despite improvement in NYHA classification. Finally, subjects who died in the hospital had rising BNP levels and little change in symptoms.

While both admission BNP levels and the change in BNP levels over the period of hospitalization were significant predictors of outcomes, the last measured BNP level was the single variable that was most strongly associated with patients experiencing one of the specified end-points. The mean BNP concentration was significantly greater in patients experiencing end-points (1801 ± 273 pg/mL vs. 690 ± 103 pg/mL) than in patients with successful treatment of CHF ($p < .001$). Patients whose discharge BNP levels fell below 430 pg/mL with treatment had reasonable likelihood of leaving the hospital in good condition and not being readmitted within the following 30 days.

BNP Correlations with Falling Wedge Pressures in Patients Being Treated for CHF

In a pilot study, hemodynamic measurements (pulmonary capillary wedge pressure, cardiac output, right atrial pressure, and systemic vascular resistance) along with BNP levels were recorded every 2 to 4 h for the first 24 h and every 4 h for the next 24 to 48 h in patients admitted for decompensated CHF. Patients were treated at the discretion of the intensive care unit physicians in standard fashion with combinations of intravenous diuretics, vasodilators, and inotropic agents. The initial BNP level in the 15 responders

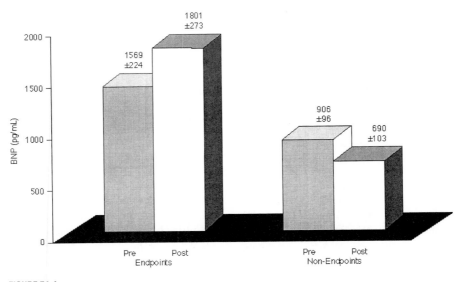

FIGURE 74-4

BNP levels before and after treatment for decompensated CHF based on whether or not the patient developed a subsequent end-point (death or readmission within 30 days).

(patients with a decrease in wedge pressure to <20 mmHg over the first 24 h) was 1472 ± 156 pg/mL. BNP levels had dropped 55% to 670 ± 109 pg/mL 24 h after treatment. There was a significant correlation between percent change per hour in wedge pressure and the percent change of BNP from baseline per hour ($r = 0.73$; $p < .05$), with an average fall of BNP of 33 ± 5 pg/mL per hour. The correlation between BNP levels and other indices of cardiac function—cardiac output (thermodilution), mixed venous oxygen saturation, and systemic vascular resistance—was not significant. In the five nonresponders, there was little change in wedge pressure and only an 8% drop in BNP levels.

Tailored Treatment of Heart Failure—Is There a Role for BNP in the Clinic?

The correlation between a drop in BNP level and a patient's improvement in symptoms (and subsequent outcome) during hospitalization suggests that BNP-guided treatment might make tailored therapy more effective in an outpatient setting such as a primary care or cardiology clinic. Recently, 69 patients were randomized to N-BNP-guided treatment versus symptom-guided therapy (Troughton et al., 2000). Patients receiving N-BNP-guided therapy had lower N-BNP levels along with reduced incidence of cardiovascular death, readmission, and new episodes of decompensated CHF.

Thus, while studies have been limited, it appears that BNP levels may be helpful in guiding therapy in the outpatient setting. Further research is needed in this area.

Conclusions

Finding a simple blood test that aids in the diagnosis and management of patients with CHF would clearly have a favorable impact on the staggering costs associated with the disease. BNP, which is synthesized in the cardiac ventricles and correlates with LV pressure, amount of dyspnea, and the state of neurohormonal modulation, makes this peptide the first potential "white count" for heart failure. The fact that a point-of-care rapid assay for BNP has recently been approved by the FDA gives the clinician an opportunity to explore its potential usefulness. Accumulating data suggest that serial point-of-care testing of BNP will be of immense help in patients presenting to urgent care clinics with dyspnea. Additionally, BNP might serve as a screen for patients referred for echocardiography. A low BNP level makes echocardiographic indices of LV dysfunction (both systolic and diastolic) highly unlikely. BNP might also be an effective way to improve the in-hospital management of patients admitted with decompensated CHF. In some instances, BNP levels may obviate the need for invasive hemodynamic monitoring and, in cases where such monitoring is used, may help tailor treatment of the decompensated patient. Finally, the role of BNP in the outpatient cardiac or primary care clinic may be one of critical importance in titration of therapies as well as in assessing the state of neurohormonal compensation of the patient.

REFERENCES

Cheng VL et al: A rapid bedside test for B-type natriuretic peptide predicts treatment outcomes in patients admitted with decompensated heart failure. J Am Coll Cardiol, 37:386, 2001

Dao Q et al: Utility of B-type natriuretic peptide (BNP) in the diagnosis of CHF in an urgent care setting. J Am Coll Cardiol, 37:379, 2001

Grantham JA, Burnett JC Jr: BNP: Increasing importance in the pathophysiology and diagnosis of congestive heart failure. Circulation 96:388, 1997

Koon J et al: A rapid bedside test for brain natriuretic peptide accurately predicts cardiac function in patients referred for echocardiography. Am Heart J, 141:367, 2001

Maeda K et al: Plasma brain natriuretic peptide as a biochemical marker of high left ventricular end-diastolic pressure in patients with symptomatic left ventricular dysfunction. Am Heart J 135:825, 1998

Stevenson LW, Braunwald E, Goldman L: Recognition and management of patients with heart failure in *Primary Cardiology*. Philadelphia, Saunders, 1998, pp 310–329

Troughton RW et al: Treatment of heart failure guided by plasma amino terminal brain natriuretic peptide (N-BNP) concentrations. Lancet 355:1126, 2000

Tsutamoto T et al: Attenuation of compensation of endogenous cardiac natriuretic peptide system in chronic heart failure: Prognostic role of plasma brain natriuretic peptide concentration in patients with chronic symptomatic left ventricular dysfunction. Circulation 96:509, 1997

Yandle TG: Biochemistry of natriuretic peptides. J Intern Med 235:561, 1994

THERAPY OF DIASTOLIC DYSFUNCTION IN HYPERTENSION AND HYPERTROPHIC CARDIOMYOPATHY

Gretchen Wells & William C. Little

More than 40% of patients with congestive heart failure have a preserved left ventricular ejection fraction (>0.50) (Gandhi et al., 2001; Grossman, 2000). Thus, these patients are presumed to have heart failure due to primary diastolic dysfunction. In the overwhelming majority of these patients, the diastolic dysfunction occurs in patients with hypertension in combination with the normal aging process as well as varying degrees of left ventricular hypertrophy, coronary artery disease, and diabetes. Patients with hypertrophic cardiomyopathy (HCM) also have diastolic dysfunction.

There is much less objective information available concerning the treatment of patients with primary diastolic dysfunction than about the therapy of systolic dysfunction (Little et al., 1997). This relative paucity of objective information is reflected in the American College of Cardiology/American Heart Association (Hunt SA et al., 2001) and the European Society of Cardiology guidelines for the treatment of heart failure (European Society of Cardiology, 2001). A paraphrase of recommendations of these guidelines concerning treatment of diastolic dysfunction is as follows:

1. The goal of therapy of primary diastolic dysfunction is to control symptoms by reducing ventricular filling pressure without reducing cardiac output.
2. Diuretics and nitrates are indicated for symptomatic patients.
3. Calcium channel blockers, beta blockers, and angiotensin-converting enzyme (ACE) inhibitors may be of benefit.
4. positive inotropic agents (including digoxin) are not indicated if systolic function is normal.

Treatment Strategies

Based on the pathophysiology of diastolic dysfunction, there are several potential treatment strategies that may be effective in treating patients with heart failure due to diastolic dysfunction (Little et al., 1997).

Control Systolic Hypertension

The most important strategy to improve left ventricular diastolic performance is the lowering of systolic arterial pressure (Little et al., 1997). Increases in systolic arterial pressure result in an elevation of left atrial pressure. Conversely, lowering of elevated arterial pressure decreases left atrial pressure (Fig. 75-1). The relief of the systolic hypertension allows the left ventricle to eject to a smaller end-systolic volume. Thus the ventricle operates with a smaller diastolic volume and reduced left atrial pressure. Lowering systolic pressure allows the ventricle to relax more rapidly, enhancing early filling. In addition, lowering systolic pressure may reduce or relieve ischemia. Thus, lowering elevated systolic arterial pressure provides a powerful method of acutely improving the diastolic performance of the left ventricle.

Long-term therapy of hypertension can result in regression of left ventricular hypertrophy. This should enhance left ventricular distensibility and improve left ventricular diastolic performance. In the SHEP trial, control of isolated systolic hypertension in elderly subjects was effective in reducing the subsequent development of heart failure (Kostis et al., 1997). Since heart failure in elderly patients is frequently due to primary diastolic dysfunction, it is likely that the treatment of isolated hypertension in these patients reduced the development of symptomatic diastolic dysfunction.

Maintain Sinus Rhythm

Many patients with impaired diastolic performance remain asymptomatic because of the compensatory effect of a vigorous left atrial contraction. If such a patient develops atrial fibrillation, the loss of the atrial contraction may result in an increase in left atrial pressure producing symptomatic diastolic dysfunction. Thus, the maintenance of sinus rhythm is important in these patients.

Avoid Tachycardia

Slowing the heart rate may provide an opportunity to improve diastolic performance (European Society of Cardiology, 2001). With a slower heart rate, there is more time for diastolic filling, allowing filling from a lower left atrial pressure. In patients with mitral stenosis, in whom there is flow across the mitral valve throughout diastole, the left atrial pressure is very sensitive to the heart rate, and pulmonary congestion can be reduced by slowing the heart rate.

In the absence of mitral stenosis, during mid-diastole (diastasis), little or no filling occurs. While slowing the heart rate below 60 to 80 beats/min lengthens the diastolic filling period, it does not actually increase the time of flow across the mitral valve; it just produces a longer period of diastasis. Furthermore, slowing the heart rate reduces the number of stroke volumes ejected, decreasing the cardiac output. Thus, avoiding increases in heart rate may be of benefit to patients with diastolic dysfunction. However, slowing the heart rate below 60 to 80 beats/min may produce little benefit in a patient with diastolic dysfunction without mitral stenosis.

Reduce Venous Pressure

A fourth treatment strategy for diastolic dysfunction is to remove the external restraints on left ventricular filling. An obvious example is a patient with pericardial tamponade with pressurized fluid in the pericardium. Removing the fluid removes the external compression of the ventricle and allows it to fill from a lower pressure. It is important to recognize that the right ventricle forms the external pressure for about one-third of the surface area of the left ventricle. Thus, elevation of right heart dias-

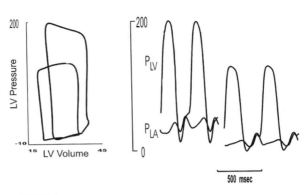

FIGURE 75-1

Recoding of Left Ventricular (LV) and Left Atrial (LA) pressures (P) and LV volume in a conscious animal. The LV compensates for an increase in P by using pre-load reserve (i.e. larger operating volume). Conversely, a reduction in LV P allows the LV to operate at lower volumes and with a lower LA pressure.

tolic pressures can constrain the filling of the left ventricle. Reduction of the right atrial and right ventricular diastolic pressures by diuresis or nitrates may thus unload the septum and improve left ventricular distensibility. This may explain why some patients with diastolic dysfunction can tolerate nitrates or diuretics without a fall in cardiac output. The reduction in right-sided pressures produced by diuresis or nitrates removes some of the external restraints for filling of the left ventricle. This may help offset the reduction in pulmonary venous pressure, preserving left ventricular filling and cardiac output while pulmonary congestion is relieved. However, diuretics and vasodilators must be used with caution in patients with diastolic dysfunction (especially in the absence of systolic arterial hypertension) to avoid a sudden drop in left ventricular filling resulting in a precipitous fall in cardiac output.

Prevention of Ischemia

The earliest effects of myocardial ischemia are to slow the rate of left ventricular relaxation and to increase ventricular end-diastolic pressure (Grossman, 2000). Since ischemia may contribute importantly to diastolic dysfunction, the prevention or relief of

ischemia can provide an avenue for treating/preventing diastolic dysfunction.

Drugs

The drugs that have been suggested for treating primary diastolic dysfunction include diuretics and nitrates, β-adrenergic blockers, calcium entry blockers, and ACE inhibitors and angiotensin II receptor blockers (ARB) (Committee on Evaluation and Management of Heart Failure, 2001; European Society of Cardiology, 2001). These drugs' effects can be classified as direct cardiac effects and indirect (noncardiac) effects (Little et al., 1997) (Fig. 75-2).

Diuretics and Nitrates

Diuretics and nitrates reduce ventricular filling, which has the potential for improving pulmonary congestion, although at the potential cost of a decrease in cardiac output. However, as discussed above, diuretics and nitrates may also reduce external compression, allowing a decreased filling pressure without a reduction in cardiac output. Patients with primary diastolic dysfunction who do not have systolic arterial

Primary Diastolic Dysfunction
Drug Effects

	Cardiac Effects	Indirect Effects
Diuretics/Nitrates	NO Improves Relaxation	Reduce Filling Reduce External Compression
Ca++ Entry Blockers	Negative Inotrope Slow Relaxation Slow Heart Rate ↓LVH	Lower BP
Beta Blockers	Negative Inotrope Slow Relaxation Slow Heart Rate ↓LVH	Lower BP
ACE-Inhibitors *AII Blockers*	Lower Diastolic Pressure Speed Relaxation ↓LVH	Lower BP

FIGURE 75-2

Effects of drugs used to treat heart failure due to diastolic dysfunction. No = nitric oxide; BP = arterial blood pressure; LVH = left ventricular hypertrophy

hypertension may be most prone to a drop in cardiac output and blood pressure. Thus, diuretics and nitrates must be used with caution in these patients.

Diuretics have no direct effect on the left ventricular myocardium, while nitrates, by releasing nitric oxide, may enhance diastolic distensibility.

Calcium Entry Blockers and β-Adrenergic Blockers

The calcium entry blockers are arterial vasodilators that lower systolic arterial blood pressure, thus indirectly improving diastolic performance. However, the direct effects of most calcium entry blockers on normal myocardium, including negative inotropic action and slowing of the rate of left ventricular relaxation, are potentially detrimental to diastolic function.

Similarly, the β-adrenergic blockers have an indirect effect of lowering systolic pressure, which is effective in improving diastolic performance. Their acute direct cardiac effects, however, are potentially detrimental. β-Adrenergic blockers prevent the positive inotropic effect of catecholamines and slow the rate of left ventricular relaxation. Both of these effects impair diastolic performance. β-Adrenergic blockade also slows the heart rate, which could be a benefit if the heart rate is excessively elevated or if the patient has mitral stenosis. Chronic β-Adrenergic blockade may result in regression of left ventricular hypertrophy and improved left ventricular relaxation and distensibility.

Thus, the acute beneficial effects of beta blockers and calcium blockers in patients with diastolic dysfunction may result from their effects on systolic blood pressure rather than their direct effects on the myocardium. Short-term treatment with verapamil may improve exercise tolerance in selected patients with primary diastolic dysfunction. β-Adrenergic blockers and calcium entry blockers may also improve diastolic performance by preventing or relieving ischemia.

ACE Inhibitors and Angiotensin II Receptor Blockers

The ACE inhibitors and ARBS lower systolic pressure, thus indirectly enhancing diastolic performance. In addition, a potential advantage of these agents is that they may speed the rate of left ventricular relaxation. Angiotensin II slows left ventricular relaxation both indirectly, by increasing systolic blood pressure, and by a direct effect that slows relaxation in hypertrophic as well as in failing myocardium. Thus, blunting the generation of angiotensin II or blocking its receptors may result in a direct improvement in left ventricular diastolic function. A recent non randomized study suggests that patients hospitalized with heart failure due to primary diastolic dysfunction have a better outcome if they are discharged on an ACE inhibitor. In addition, a small randomized crossover study demonstrated that 2 weeks of treatment with the ARB losartan improved exercise tolerance in patients with mild diastolic dysfunction and a hypertensive response to exercise (Warner et al., 1999).

Positive Inotropic Agents.

It is generally agreed that positive inotropic agents are not of benefit in the treatment of primary diastolic dysfunction (Committee on Evaluation and Management of Heart Failure, 2001). However, most positive inotropic agents enhance the rate of left ventricular relaxation, which could be beneficial in some patients. Digoxin has been considered to be contraindicated in patients with primary diastolic dysfunction. However, in a substudy of the DIG Trial, patients with heart failure and preserved systolic function had similar survival on digoxin and placebo and a nonsignificant trend towards fewer hospitalizations on digoxin.

Hypertrophic Cardiomyopathy

Diastolic dysfunction is an important manifestation of HCM and is presumed to be the cause of exertional dyspnea in these patients. Beta blockers are first-line therapy for patients with HCM (Spirito et al., 1997). Exertional dyspnea and chest pain are usually improved with beta blockade, probably due to a reduction in exercise-induced tachycardia. In addition, beta blockers can decrease the outflow tract gradient and lessen myocardial oxygen requirements.

The calcium-entry blocker verapamil is also effective in improving symptoms in HCM (Spirito et al., 1997). However, adverse effects occur with calcium entry blockers in some patients with HCM. These problems include atrioventricular block with verapamil and worsening pulmonary congestion, most frequently occurring in patients with outflow tract gradients greater than 50 mmHg. Marked hypotension can also occur. Thus, calcium entry blockers should be used with caution in patients with HCM with pulmonary congestion and/or large gradients across the left ventricle outflow tract. Therapy with disopyramide can reduce the outflow gradient in patients with HCM but does not appear to alter the diastolic dysfunction.

The diastolic dysfunction in patients with HCM can be improved in some, carefully selected patients with surgical resection of the left ventricle outflow tract. A new, promising alternative to this surgical procedure is localized ventricular septal infarction by infusion of ethanol into a major septal perforator branch of the left anterior descending coronary artery. This results in a reduction of the outflow tract gradient, regression of left ventricular hypertrophy, and lessening of symptoms (Mazur et al., 2001).

Conclusion

Treatment of diastolic dysfunction is most effective when it is associated with hypertension. Reduction of systolic arterial pressures acutely reduces pulmonary congestion and ischemia and chronically may lead to regression of left ventricular hypertrophy. Patients with primary or predominant left ventricular diastolic dysfunction in the absence of hypertension are very difficult to treat. They are prone to develop severe hypotension in response to diuretics or nitrates.

REFERENCES

European Society of Cardiology: The Task Force of the Working Group on Heart Failure: Guidelines for the diagnosis and treatment of chronic heart failure. Eur Heart J 22:1527, 2001

Gandhi SK et al: The pathogenesis of acute pulmonary edema associated with hypertension. N Engl J Med 344:17, 2001

Grossman W: Defining diastolic dysfunction. Circulation 101:2020, 2000

Hunt SA et al: ACC/AHA Guidelines for the evaluation and management of chronic heart failure in the adult: Executive Summary Report of the American College of Cardiology/American Heart Association Task Force on Practice Guidelines (Committee on Evaluation and Management of Heart Failure). Circulation, 104:2996, 2001

Kostis JB et al: Prevention of heart failure by antihypertensive drug treatment in older persons with isolated systolic hypertension. SHEP Cooperative Research Group. JAMA 278:212, 1997

Little WC et al: Treatment of heart failure due to diastolic dysfunction. Contemp Treat Cardiovasc Dis 2:71, 1997

Mazur W et al: Regression of left ventricular hypertrophy after nonsurgical septal reduction therapy for hypertrophic obstructive cardiomyopathy. Circulation 103:1492, 2001

Spirito P et al: The management of hypertrophic cardiomyopathy. N Engl J Med 336:775, 1997

Warner JG Jr et al: Losartan improves exercise tolerance in patients with diastolic dysfunction and a hypertensive response to exercise. J Am Coll Cardiol 33:1567, 1999

THE ROLE OF ALDOSTERONE IN HEART FAILURE–RESULTS OF THE RALES TRIAL

Peter Liu & Bertram Pitt

General Biologic Role of Aldosterone

Aldosterone, the most potent mineralocorticoid hormone responsible for systemic fluid and electrolyte balance, is synthesized by the zona glomerulosa cells of the adrenal glands. The primary effects of aldosterone at the distal renal tubular level are the retention of sodium and water and the loss of potassium and magnesium through the induction and recruitment of sodium pumps (Horisberger and Rossier, 1992). Excessive aldosterone production leads to volume expansion and edema formation. (See also Chap. 3, this volume.)

More recently, studies have also demonstrated that aldosterone plays an important role in tissue repair and remodeling (Slight et al., 1998). Increased local concentration of aldosterone can stimulate nuclear factor NF- κB and AP-1 signaling pathways and activate osteopontin, cytokines, and growth factors such as transforming growth factor β_1. These effects result in microvascular inflammation damage and perivascular and interstitial fibrosis (Blasi et al., 2001; Sun et al., 2000; Fiebeler et al., 2001). Aldosterone also causes an increase in myocardial mass independent of its effect on fibrosis and blood pressure (Schlaich et al., 2000), and it has been suggested that this increase in ventricular mass relates to an increase in intramyocardial calcium concentration (Benitah et al., 1999). The action of aldosterone is complementary to that of angiotensin II in that both hormones induce vasoconstriction, sodium retention, tissue fibrosis, and ventricular hypertrophy. However, despite their independent production and regulation, there is a significant degree of synergy in their biologic interaction. Indeed, the stimulation of aldosterone production is in large part mediated by the AT1 subtype of the angiotensin receptor family, and part of the aldosterone tissue action is mediated through an upregulation of the AT1 angiotensin receptors (Robert et al., 1999; Silvestre et al., 1999). Aldosterone has also been shown to increase activity of angiotensin-converting enzyme (ACE) in tissue, resulting in a positive feedback loop (Harada et al., 2001).

The sources of aldosterone can be both systemic and local. Aldosterone is released into the circulation from adrenal gland synthesis by low intravascular volume leading to increased levels of angiotensin II. Aldosterone production is also stimulated by high serum potassium levels and other factors such as ACTH; these mechanisms are independent but synergistic with the angiotensin II–stimulated mechanism (Okubo et al., 1997). In addition to adrenal production, there is now evidence that the cells of the cardiovascular system can express genes responsible for the formation of both aldosterone and corticosterone and are capable of producing these steroids (Takeda et al., 1995). Vascular endothelial and smooth-muscle cells express CYP11B1 and CYP11B2, genes of 11β-hydroxylase and aldosterone synthase, respectively, which are enzymes in the final stages of aldosterone synthesis (Takeda et al., 1995). Adrenalectomy paradoxically leads to higher tissue levels of aldosterone production in compensation. Similar enzyme systems for aldosterone production have also been identified in the myocardium. Cardiac aldosterone and glucocorticoid production can be directly enhanced by angiotensin II and adrenocorticotropin infusion in isolated heart preparation (Silvestre et al., 1999). There is also a consistent dissociation of local tissue levels of aldosterone with that found in the circulation, suggesting a locally regulated steroid production system.

Increased Aldosterone Levels in Heart Failure and the "Aldosterone Escape" Phenomenon

In the setting of heart failure, circulating levels of aldosterone can be markedly elevated in concert with an increase in the other neurohormones found in heart failure, such as angiotensin, norepinephrine, endothelin, and cytokines. The levels of aldosterone confer prognostic significance, with increased incidence of death and heart failure deterioration associated with higher levels of aldosterone (Swedberg et al., 1990). The sources of aldosterone in heart failure may be either systemic or local. The circulating levels of aldosterone in heart failure are increased because of increased production in the adrenal gland secondary to elevated levels of angiotensin II and decreased clearance of aldosterone in the liver due to hepatic congestion (Pitt et al., 1999; Packer et al., 1996; Weber, 1999). The

local production is a response to local tissue injury, such as that found following myocardial infarction or longstanding hypertension. Local tissue injury is associated with the rapid induction of endogenous tissue growth factors and cytokines (Irwin et al., 1999), which in turn is partially responsible for the induction of aldosterone in the cardiovascular tissue. This leads to local induction of aldosterone conversion enzymes as well as actual production of myocardial aldosterone via paracrine and autocrine pathways, again closely interacting with the tissue angiotensin AT1 receptors (Silvestre et al., 1999; Slight et al., 1998). The local levels of aldosterone directly lead to increased tissue fibrosis and scar formation, which can be blocked by an aldosterone receptor antagonist such as spironolactone (Silvestre et al., 1999).

Previously, it was assumed that the administration of ACE inhibitors in the setting of heart failure would effectively decrease aldosterone levels. However, more recent data suggest that the aldosterone levels remain elevated in patients with heart failure despite inhibition of angiotensin II formation by ACE inhibitors; this is termed the *aldosterone escape* phenomenon (Pitt, 1995; Struthers, 1996; Zannad, 1993). Aldosterone escape has been associated with the ACE DD genotype (Cicoira et al., 2001) but may also result from the lower doses of ACE inhibitors frequently used in the clinical setting, sodium loss from salt restriction, diuretic usage that may be associated with increased angiotensin II levels, and angiotensin-independent mechanisms of aldosterone production (Weber, 1999). Thus, despite the presence of ACE inhibitors and/or AT1 receptor blockers, the patient with heart failure is continually being exposed to the biologic influences of increased aldosterone.

The Potential Role of Aldosterone in the Progression of Heart Failure

Aldosterone production is increased in the setting of heart failure and may play an important role in cardiac remodeling and heart failure progression.

Initially, this is an adaptive response to cardiac injury, with aldosterone facilitating the expansion of volume to maintain cardiac output and promotion of healing through scar formation. However, chronic elevation of aldosterone without physiologic modulation leads to pathologic remodeling of the heart and peripheral circulation, leading to progressive maladaptation and ultimately a clinical course characterized by decompensation and finally death. Indeed, during earlier stages of heart failure, the elaboration of atrial natriuretic peptide and nitric oxide can serve to modulate the production of aldosterone (Szalay et al., 1998).

The direct tissue effect of increased aldosterone production is increased fibroblast proliferation, leading to the local production of collagen. Proliferation of the fibroblasts and collagen production lead to increased passive stiffness of the ventricle, with initial diastolic and ultimately systolic dysfunction, and decreased arterial compliance. Clinically, there is an inverse relationship between the levels of aldosterone and arterial compliance in heart failure patients (Duprez et al., 1998). In addition, increased fibrosis around individual myocytes will increase the oxygen and nutrient delivery distance, impede cell-cell communication, and ultimately compromise cell survival. This setting provides the classic substrate for the triggering of ventricular arrhythmias and myocyte apoptosis/necrosis, setting the stage for sudden death and progressive ventricular dilatation (Liu, 1996). In the situation of myocardial infarction, the direct local myocardial levels of aldosterone are increased, accompanied by an increase in collagen deposition. The latter is reversible with the administration of an aldosterone receptor blocker in both animal models and patients (MacFayden et al., 1997; Silvestre et al., 1999; Zannad et al., 2000). Aldosterone may also play a role in the endothelial dysfunction found in patients with heart failure, in that spironolactone has been shown to improve endothelial function significantly in patients with mild to moderate heart failure treated with an ACE inhibitor (Farquiharson et al., 2000). Aldosterone may also play a role in fibrinolysis; when adminis-

tered in conjunction with angiotensin II, it increases plasminogen activator inhibitor levels (Brown et al., 2000).

Aldosterone also decreases the uptake of norepinephrine into the myocardium, increases the circulating levels of norepinephrine in the setting of heart failure and can depress baroreceptor function (Barr et al., 1995; Wang, 1994). The administration of the aldosterone receptor antagonist spironolactone in patients with heart failure decreases heart rate and increases parasympathetic activity (MacFayden et al., 1997). These mechanisms, along with an increase in serum potassium levels, may also contribute to a decrease in ventricular arrhythmias and, possibly, sudden death.

In view of the aldosterone escape phenomenon outlined above, the use of an aldosterone antagonist in combination with an ACE inhibitor has an attractive conceptual basis. Indeed, Barr and colleagues studied 42 patients with heart failure already on ACE inhibitors and randomized them to either spironolactone or placebo (Barr et al., 1995). They found that the patients on the combination of spironolactone and an ACE inhibitor had better preserved norepinephrine uptake in the myocardium and a reduction in ventricular arrhythmias on Holter ECG monitoring.

The Clinical Impact of Aldosterone Receptor Blockade on the Outcomes of Heart Failure (the RALES trial)

To determine the clinical impact of an aldosterone receptor antagonist on the major end-points of morbidity and mortality in heart failure, a landmark multicenter clinical trial was completed (Pitt et al., 1999). The Randomized Aldactone Evaluation Study (RALES) enrolled 1663 patients with class III/IV heart failure with left ventricular ejection fraction $\leq 35\%$, serum creatine < 222 $\mu mol/L$ (<2.5 mg/dL), and a serum potassium level <5 mmol/L, who were already on an ACE inhibitor as tolerated, diuretics, and/or digoxin.

The patients were randomized to spironolactone (25 mg/d, *n* = 822) or placebo (*n* = 841) and clinical events were followed, with total mortality being the primary end-point. The average does of spironolactone ultimately used was 26 mg/d.

The RALES trial was terminated prematurely after 2 years of follow-up because of significant benefit on total mortality in the active treatment group. The patients who were treated with spironolactone had an overall 30% reduction in mortality (*p* < .001) due to both a reduction in death from progressive heart failure and sudden cardiac death, with

a baseline mortality of 46% in the placebo group at the end of 2 years (Fig. 76-1). The benefit was observed across all major subgroups examined and across all geographic boundaries. In addition, there was a 31% reduction in deaths due to cardiac causes, and a 35% reduction in hospitalizations for heart failure. There was also a significant improvement in symptoms of heart failure in terms of NYHA classification. There was no worsening of creatinine levels in the treatment group. The average potassium level rose <0.3 mmol/L, and there was no significant increase in serious hyperkalemia (K ≥ 6.0 mmol/L),

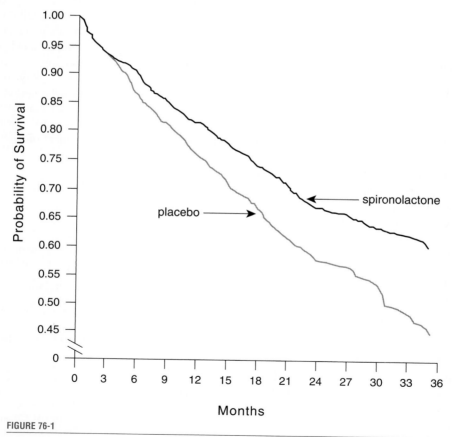

FIGURE 76-1

Data from the RALES trial. Black line, spironolactone; gray line, placebo. RR, 0.70; 95% CI (0.60-0.82); *p* < .001.

attesting to the safety of spironolactone at this dose. The only side effect was an increase in gynecomastia and breast pain in male patients. With the cost of spironolactone being relatively low in many parts of the world, this is indeed the most cost-effective treatment for heart failure to date.

Future Implications of Aldosterone Receptor Blockade in Heart Failure and Cardiovascular Disease

The RALES trial demonstrated that aldosterone antagonism in the setting of severe heart failure has an important therapeutic benefit in terms of both morbidity and mortality. The large impact it showed supports the concept that aldosterone antagonism should now join the strategies of ACE inhibition and beta-receptor blockade as the major cornerstone of therapy in patients with heart failure. Although the beneficial effects of aldosterone receptor antagonists on mortality have been demonstrated only in patients with severe chronic heart failure, it is possible that it may also be useful in patients with less severe heart failure due to systolic left ventricular dysfunction, diastolic heart failure, or heart failure after myocardial infarction. Because previous studies have suggested that ACE inhibitors do not adequately suppress aldosterone production, the patient is still at risk for its adverse remodeling influences (Duprez et al., 1998; Struthers, 1996). The RALES trial therefore also established the important new paradigm of combination neurohumoral blockade in the treatment of heart failure and the inadequacy of single-agent therapy in treating a complex disease such as heart failure. Since the dose of spironolactone used is relatively low, it also suggests that the mechanism of ventricular remodeling and fibrosis promoted by aldosterone is an important detrimental mechanism contributing to the progression of heart failure.

The RALES trial data suggest that class III/IV heart failure patients who are already treated with ACE inhibitors and diuretics, and who have normal renal function [creatinine < 222 μmol/L (<2.5 mg/dL)] and serum potassium levels (<5.0 mmol/L), should be initiated on spironolactone at 25 mg/d with a target dose not exceeding 50 mg/d. Serum electrolytes and creatinine should be closely monitored during the initiation and titration phases. If, at any time, serum potassium exceeds 5.0 mmol/L, the dose of spironolactone should be decreased to 25 mg every other day, with careful adjustment of other medications that may also contribute to hyperkalemia. Spironolactone can also be used with the other classes of diuretics indicated in heart failure to achieve a reduction of the total dose of the diuretics needed.

A new specific aldosterone receptor antagonist, eplerenone, is currently undergoing clinical trials in hypertension and heart failure post infarction (de Gasparo et al., 1987; Pitt et al., 2001) It has minimal cross-reactivity with the androgen and prostagen receptors and confers a lower incidence of side effects such as gynecomastia and changes in libido. Thus, aldosterone antagonism may represent the rediscovery of a new therapeutic option for patients with asymptomatic left ventricular dysfunction or following myocardial injury to prevent adverse remodeling and the development of heart failure and sudden cardiac death.

REFERENCES

Barr CS et al: Effect of adding spironolactone to an angiotensin-converting enzyme inhibitor in chronic congestive heart failure secondary to coronary artery disease. Am J Cardiol 76:1259, 1995

Benitah JP et al: Aldosterone upregulates Ca^{2+} current in adult rat cardiomyocytes. Circ Res 85:1139, 1999

Blasi ER et al: Aldosterone/salt-induced myocardial injury: A vascular inflammatory disease. Am J Hypertens 14:8A, 2001

Brown N et al: Aldosterone modulates plasminogen activator-1 and glomerulosclerosis in vivo. Kidney Int 58:1219, 2000

Cicoira M et al: Failure of aldosterone suppression despite angiotensin-converting enzyme (ACE) inhibitor administration in chronic heart failure is associated with ACE DD genotype. J Am Coll Cardiol 37:1808, 2001

de Gasparo M et al: Three new epoxy-spironolactone derivatives: Characterization in vivo and in vitro. J Pharmacol Exp Ther 240:650, 1987

Duprez DA et al: Inverse relationship between aldosterone and large artery compliance in chronically treated heart failure patients. Eur Heart J 19:1371, 1998

Farquiharson CAJ et al: Spironolactone increases nitric oxide bioactivity, improves endothelial vasodilator dysfunction, and suppresses vascular angiotensin I/angiotensin II conversion in patients with chronic heart failure. Circulation 101:594, 2000

Fiebeler A et al: Mineralocorticoid receptor affects AP-1 and nuclear factor-κB activation in angiotensin II-induced cardiac injury. Hypertension 37:787, 2001

Harada E et al: Aldosterone induces angiotensin-converting-enzyme gene expression in cultured neonatal rat cardiocytes. Circulation 104:137, 2001

Horisberger JD, Rossier BC: Aldosterone regulation of gene transcription leading to control of ion transport. Hypertension 19:221, 1992

Irwin M et al: Tissue expression and immunolocalization of tumour necrosis factor-alpha in post infarction dysfunctional myocardium. Circulation 99:1492, 1999

Liu P: The path to cardiomyopathy: Cycles of injury, repair and maladaption. Curr Opin Cardiol 11:291, 1996

MacFayden RJ et al: Aldosterone blockade reduces vascular collagen turnover, improves heart rate variability and reduces early morning rise in heart rate in heart failure patients. Cardiovasc Res 35:30, 1997

Okubo SN et al: Angiotensin-independent mechanism for aldosterone synthesis during chronic extracellular fluid volume depletion. J Clin Invest 99:885, 1997

Pitt B: "Escape" of aldosterone production in patients with left ventricular dysfunction treated with an angiotensin converting enzyme inhibitor. Cardiovasc Drugs Ther 9:145, 1995

Pitt B et al. The effects of spironolactone on morbidity and mortality in patients with severe heart failure. NEJM 341:709,1999

Pitt B et al: The EPHESUS Trial: Eplerenone in patients with heart failure due to systolic dysfunction complicating acute myocardial infarction. Cardiovasc Drugs Ther 15:79, 2001

Robert V et al: Angiotensin AT1 receptor subtype as a cardiac target of aldosterone: Role in aldosterone-salt-induced fibrosis. Hypertension 33:981, 1999

Schlaich MP et al: Impact of aldosterone on left ventricular structure and function in young normotensive and mildly hypertensive subjects. Am J Cardiol 85:1199, 2000

Silvestre JS et al: Activation of cardiac aldosterone production in rat myocardial infarction: Effect of angiotensin II receptor blockade and role in cardiac fibrosis. Circulation 99:2694, 1999

Slight SH et al: Inhibition of tissue repair by spironolactone: Role of mineralocorticoids in fibrous tissue formation. Mol Cell Biochem 189:47, 1998

Struthers AD: Aldosterone escape during angiotensin-converting enzyme inhibitor therapy in chronic heart failure. J Card Fail 2:47, 1996

Sun Y et al: Local angiotensin II and transforming growth factor-1 in renal fibrosis of rats. Hypertension 35:1078, 2000

Swedberg K et al: Hormones regulating cardiovascular function in patients with severe CHF and their relation to mortality. Circulation 82:1720, 1990

Szalay KS et al: Interaction between ouabain, atrial natriuretic peptide, angiotensin-II and potassium: Effects on rat zona glomerulosa aldosterone production. Life Sci 62:1845, 1998

Takeda Y et al: Production of aldosterone in isolated rat blood vessels. Hypertension 25:170, 1995

Wang W: Chronic administration of aldosterone depresses baroreceptor reflex function in the dog. Hypertension 24:571, 1994

Weber KT: Aldosterone and spironolactone in heart failure (editorial). N Engl J Med 341:753, 1999

Zannad F: Angiotensin-converting enzyme inhibitor and spironolactone combination therapy. New objectives in congestive heart failure treatment. Am J Cardiol 71:34A, 1993

Zannad F et al: Limitation to excessive extracellular matrix turnover may contribute to survival benefit of spironolactone therapy in patients with congestive heart failure: Insight from the randomized aldactone evaluation study (RALES). Circulation 102:2700, 2000

INOTROPIC INFUSIONS IN HEART FAILURE

Carl V. Leier

Principal Indication

Intravenously administered inotropic drugs are primarily approved for the short-term management of decompensated, systolic dysfunction, low-output, congestive heart failure (CHF). The typical patient is one who experienced recent myocardial injury (e.g., infarction, myocarditis) or decompensation of chronic cardiac failure, resulting in marked systolic dysfunction (reduced ejection fraction), reduced stroke volume and cardiac output, systemic hypotension, and hypoperfusion in the face of elevated ventricular diastolic (filling) pressures.

The hemodynamic profiles of the agents most commonly used for acute positive inotropic support are presented in Table 77-1, and Table 77-2 presents the position of the intravenous inotropic agents within the therapeutic spectrum for systemic hypoperfusion and organ dysfunction caused by depressed ventricular systolic function, stroke volume, and cardiac output and elevated ventricular filling pressures.

Intravenously Administered Inotropic Agents

Catecholamines-Catechols

These agents act primarily by stimulating adrenergic receptors, with a consequent rise in intracellular cyclic AMP (ACC-AHA Committee, 1995; Leier et al, 1977; Leier, 1991; Leier and Binkley, 1998).

Dobutamine

This synthetic catechol is the drug most commonly employed for acute inotropic support. Dobutamine, by stimulating β_1-and, to a lesser extent, β_2-and α-adrenergic receptors, augments cardiac contractility and effects vasodilatation to a mild extent. Dobutamine is administered as a continuous infusion, starting at 2 to 3 μg/kg per min and gradually increased by increments of 1 to 2 μg/kg per min until the desired clinical or hemodynamic responses are achieved. The average maintenance infusion dose ranges from 5 to 10 μg/kg per min with an upper dose rarely higher

TABLE 77-1

GENERAL HEMODYNAMIC PROFILES OF AGENTS MOST COMMONLY USED TO DELIVER SHORT-TERM, PARENTERAL POSITIVE INOTROPIC SUPPORT[a]

	Dobutamine	Dopamine		Milrinone	Norepinephrine
		Low Dose	Higher Dose		
Contractility	↑↑↑	↑	↑↑	↑	→↑
Cardiac output	↑↑↑	↑	↑	↑↑↑	→↑
Heart rate	→↑	→↑	↑↑	→↑	→↑
LV filling pressure	↓↓	↓	→↑	↓↓↓	→↑
Systemic blood pressure	→↑	→	↑↑	→↓	↑↑↑
Systemic vascular resistance	↓↓	→	↑↑	↓↓↓	↑↑↑
Pulmonary vascular resistance	↓↓	→	→↑	↓↓↓	↑↑

[a]See text for additional information about these drugs.   → = no change.

than 20 μg/kg per min. Under proper patient and dose selection, dobutamine will increase stroke volume, cardiac output, systemic systolic and pulse pressures, and peripheral perfusion with a reduction in systemic and pulmonary vascular resistances and ventricular filling pressures. Untoward effects, generally related to excessive administration or enhanced adrenergic sensitivity, include tachycardia, cardiac dysrhythmias, inordinate shifts in blood pressure, angina/myocardial ischemia, headaches, and, rarely, nausea and vomiting. The ability of high-dose dobutamine to evoke tachycardia and ventricular hypercontractility forms the basis of the dobutamine stress test.

Dopamine

Dopamine, a naturally occurring (i.e., endogenous) catecholamine, has a more modest effect on cardiac contractility (β_1- and β_2- adrenergic agonism) with more dramatic vascular properties (dopaminergic and α-adrenergic agonism). At lower doses (<5 μg/kg per min), dopamine causes a mild to moderate increase in stroke volume and cardiac output with some reduction in vascular resistance. In this dose range, renal vascular resistance tends to fall, with consequent rise in renal blood flow; for this reason, dopamine is often employed to enhance renal function when hemodynamically impaired. At doses >6 μg/kg per min, dopamine delivers much of its effects via α-adrenergic vasoconstriction. In these doses, dopamine is primarily employed as a vasopressor agent, with some positive inotropy as a second-tier objective. Untoward effects can include tachycardia, cardiac dysrhythmias, excessive vaso-constriction, nausea, and vomiting. Infiltration at the intravenous site can cause local tissue necrosis.

Norepinephrine and Epinephrine

Both norepinephrine and epinephrine are naturally occurring catecholamines. Norepinephrine is primarily an α-adrenergic agonist and, as such, it is used for its vasoconstrictor-vasopressor properties. Norepinephrine is employed after dopamine has failed with vasopressor doses (up to 20 to 25 μg/kg per min) to adequately raise systemic blood pressure. High-dose norepinephrine can evoke digital ischemia and necrosis and local necrosis at the infiltration site.

Epinephrine stimulates all adrenergic receptors. Its use is primarily directed at improving overall

TABLE 77-2

THERAPEUTICS OF LV SYSTOLIC DYSFUNCTION, REDUCED CARDIAC OUTPUT AND PERIPHERAL PERFUSION, AND ELEVATED LV FILLING PRESSURES [a]

Systemic Blood Pressure	First-Line Therapy	Alternative or Supplemental Therapy
Marked hypotension, cardiogenic shock; systolic BP <70 mmHg	Dopamine >5 μg/kg per min	1. Add dobutamine or milrinone if BP ↑ with dopamine 2. Add norepinephrine or mechanical assist (IABP, VAD) if BP and perfusion do not improve
Mild to moderate hypotension; systolic BP 70–110 mmHg	Dobutamine 2–15 μg/kg per min	1. Add vasodilators or milrinone if BP ↑ but hypoperfusion does not improve adequately 2. Add dopamine or mechanical assist if BP and perfusion ↓
Normotension or hypertension; systolic BP >110 mmHg	Vasodilators: IV nitroglycerin, nitroprusside, or nesiritide	Add dobutamine or dopamine if BP and perfusion ↓

[a] The clinical application of IV positive inotropic agents is directed at patients with systemic hypotension and hypoperfusion secondary to LV systolic dysfunction. Most of these patients have elevated LV filling pressures; low ventricular filling pressures (≤12 mmHg) in the setting of low cardiac output, systemic hypotension, and hypoperfusion are initially approached with intravenous fluid administration (to increase LV filling pressure ≥15 mmHg if monitored). In the clinical setting of reduced systolic function, cardiac output, systemic blood pressure, and perfusion in the face of acceptable or elevated ventricular filling pressures (>15 mmHg), systemic systolic blood pressure becomes the determining factor for drug selection.
ABBREVIATIONS: BP, systemic blood pressure; IABP, intraaortic balloon counterpulsation; LV, left ventricular; VAD, ventricular assist device.

hemodynamics immediately after open-heart surgery and as first-line treatment of anaphylaxis.

Phosphodiesterase Inhibitors

Through phosphodiesterase blockade, phosphodiesterase inhibitors increase intracellular cyclic AMP by preventing its metabolism (ACC-AHA Committee, 1995; Anderson, 1991; Leier, 1991; Leier and Binkley, 1998; Mehra et al., 1997).

Milrinone

This agent is the most commonly employed phosphodiesterase inhibitor in cardiovascular medicine. It also augments cardiac contractility but evokes considerably more systemic and pulmonic vasodilatation compared to dobutamine or low-dose dopamine. At a starting dose of 0.2 μg/kg per min with incrementation to 0.7 μg/kg per min, milrinone reduces ventricular filling pressures, pulmonary artery pressure, and vascular resistances, and increases stroke volume, cardiac output, and peripheral perfusion—generally with little change or some reduction in systemic blood pressure. Milrinone is particularly effective in reducing elevated pulmonary artery pressure and pulmonary vascular resistance (Givertz, et al., 1996). A more rapid onset is achieved with bolus loading, 25 or 50 μg/kg over 10 to 15 min, followed by the maintenance infusion. Untoward effects of excessive dosing include hypotension, tachycardia, cardiac dysrhythmias, and angina/myocardial ischemia.

A congener (amrinone) is principally a vasodilating agent that offers no advantage over milrinone as a positive inotropic drug.

Other Intravenously Delivered Positive Inotropic Agents (See Leier and Binkley, 1998)

Digitalis

Digoxin, ouabain, and cedilanid are digitalis compounds that can improve cardiac function following administration. This approach to positive inotropic therapy is limited by a wide variation in patient and drug response, a complex clinical situation (e.g., electrolyte shifts), an ill-defined dosing schedule, and nonideal pharmacokinetics in critical care. Intravenous digoxin can be used to control ventricular rate during atrial fibrillation or flutter.

Calcium

Calcium is administered intravenously to reverse problematic cardiodepressant effects of calcium channel blockers (e.g., verapamil, diltiazem).

Calcium-Sensitizing Agents

This drug group is being investigated as a means of improving cardiac contraction without increasing adrenergic stimulation or intracellular cyclic AMP. Levosimendan, currently under clinical investigation, delivers some of its cardiac effects via this mechanism (Slawsky et al., 2000).

Standard Clinical Application

Intravenous inotropic agents are used primarily to improve and stabilize hemodynamics and the clinical condition of patients with acutely decompensated heart failure secondary to recent loss of ventricular systolic function (ACC-AHA Committee, 1995; Leier, 1991; Leier and Binkley, 1998). The usual setting is one of acute myocardial infarction or acute cardiomyopathy. Intravenous inotropic therapy is employed until the underlying condition has sufficiently improved or the patient is advanced into definitive intervention (e.g., revascularization of occlusive coronary artery disease, valvular repair or replacement) or mechanical sup-

port [e.g., intraaortic balloon counterpulsation, ventricular assist device (VAD)].

Intravenous inotropic agents are commonly used to improve hemodynamics and the clinical condition of patients with chronic CHF and acute or recent decompensation, systemic hypotension, and hypoperfusion. Most of these patients have elevated ventricular filling pressures and depressed cardiac outputs. In this setting, inotropic therapy is continued until the condition improves and the oral medication plan reassessed and readjusted, a period typically ranging from 24 to 96 h.

Intravenous inotropic agents are an effective means of stabilizing and maintaining adequate hemodynamic function in chronic CHF patients experiencing a recent threatening illness (e.g., pneumonia) or undergoing a potentially stressful procedure (e.g., major surgery).

Other Applications

Assessment of Pulmonary Hypertension and Vasoreactivity

Milrinone, with its vasodilating properties, is employed by some transplant programs to determine the reversibility of pulmonary vasoconstriction and pulmonary hypertension in CHF patients undergoing evaluation for their candidacy and listing for heart transplantation (Givertz et al., 1996; Leier and Binkley, 1998).

Inotropic Infusions in Chronic CHF

The primary application of intravenous inotropic therapy in patients with chronic CHF is hemodynamic and clinical stabilization during periods of decompensation and during a potentially stressful or threatening event or procedure.

Intravenous inotropic therapy must on occasion be infused continuously as part of good standard management and care. Patients with severe, end-stage CHF who remain clinically decompensated and unstable despite optimal orally administered therapeutic intervention often require continuous intravenous inotropic infusions simply to keep them alive and reasonably comfortable until cardiac transplantation or VAD placement. For the patients who are not eligible for transplantation or VAD placement, a continuous infusion of an inotropic agent may be the only avenue for discharge from the hospital in-patient setting. Portable infusion pumps allow many of these patients to function beyond the basic activities of daily living. While this approach is not on the list of approved indications for intravenous inotropic agents, few options are available for these uncommon but rather desperate clinical situations. If and when the patient's clinical condition improves to the point where the infusion can be safely discontinued, this should be done.

The use of intermittent infusions (several-hour infusion, one to three times a week) of an inotropic agent (e.g., dobutamine, milrinone) in chronic CHF has evoked considerable controversy. None of these agents has ever been approved for this particular application. This approach is not a recent development. It has its roots in the era *prior* to the use of vasodilators, angiotensin (ACE) inhibitors, and beta blockade for chronic CHF: a time when only digitalis and diuretics were available to manage CHF. Digitalis and diuretics could control symptoms in patients with mild to moderate CHF but were usually inadequate in the moderately severe to severe stages of CHF.

A 1977 report published the unexpected observation that about two-thirds of patients with severe, end-stage CHF experienced clinical improvement following a 72-h dobutamine infusion (Leier et al., 1977). Follow-up studies showed that the clinical improvement might last from 2 to 3 weeks to several months (Leier, 1991; Leier and Binkley, 1998). The mechanisms proposed for the sustained improvement following a ≥72-h infusion are multiple, including an increase in subendocardial blood flow with reversal of ischemia and myocyte dysfunction of this region (in both ischemic and nonischemic dilated cardiomyopathy), conditioning of skeletal muscle and vasculature, and improved function and responsivity of peripheral vasculature (Leier, 1991; Leier and Binkley, 1998; Patel et al.,

1999). Ironically, the mechanisms underlying the sustained clinical and hemodynamic improvement probably have little to do with positive inotropy, per se.

Subsequent studies employing shorter infusions (4 to 12 h) on a weekly basis also demonstrated clinical and laboratory improvement over time in patients with severe CHF (Leier, 1991; Leier and Binkley, 1998; Mehra et al., 1997). The relatively small patient population and/or less than optimal protocol design have blunted the lasting impact of these studies. Nevertheless, these observations brought the concept of inotropic infusion therapy into the outpatient setting with intermittent administration. However, it was at this point (early to mid-1980s) that the introduction of vasodilator and ACE inhibitor therapy into CHF therapeutics greatly reduced the need for intermittent inotropic infusions. In addition, the results of a controlled trial (albeit poorly designed) showed that intermittent dobutamine infusions (48 h/week) significantly increased mortality over that noted for conventional CHF therapy (Leier, 1991; Leier and Binkley, 1998). The preliminary results of the OPTIME CHF trial (Gheorghiade, 2000) showed that 48-h infusions of milrinone did little to improve the clinical course or survival of decompensated functional class III or IV CHF patients while evoking more side effects (hypotension, atrial fibrillation) compared to the placebo-treated control group.

More recently, the introduction of beta blockade to an ever-expanding knowledge- and experience-base of CHF therapeutics virtually eliminates the need to resort to intermittent inotropic infusions.

Nevertheless, this approach has persisted and may be growing in popularity in certain areas. The infusions may render some benefit to the end-stage CHF patient who is not eligible for cardiac transplantation and who remains decompensated despite *optimal* CHF therapy. For this very small subset of CHF patients, intermittent inotropic infusions are generally delivered under the rationale of reducing symptoms, hospitalization, and medical costs, even at the risk of an increased mortality. Inotropic infusions should not be employed in inappropriate CHF populations (functional classes II and III) or in CHF patients not receiving optimal medical management with available orally administered agents; there is no evidence that inotropic infusions are of benefit to these CHF patients, and there is enough information to raise concern that this approach is accompanied by an unacceptable risk of increased mortality.

REFERENCES

ACC-AHA Committee for the Evaluation and Management of Heart Failure: Guidelines for the evaluation and management of heart failure. J Am Coll Cardiol 26:1376, 1995

Anderson JL: Hemodynamic and clinical benefits with intravenous milrinone in severe chronic heart failure: Results of a multicenter study in the United States. Am Heart J 121:1956, 1991

Gheorghiade M: Outcomes of a prospective trial of intravenous (IV) milrinone for exacerbations of chronic heart failure (OPTIME-CHF). J Am Coll Cardiol 36:321, 2000

Givertz MM et al: Effect of bolus milrinone on hemodynamic variables and pulmonary vascular resistance in patients with severe left ventricular dysfunction: A rapid test for reversibility of pulmonary hypertension. J Am Coll Cardiol 28:1775, 1996

Leier CV: Acute inotropic support, in *Cardiotonic Drugs,* 2d ed, CV Leier (ed). New York, Marcel Dekker, 1991, pp 63–105

Leier CV, Binkley PF: Parenteral inotropic support for advanced congestive heart failure. Prog Cardiovasc Dis 41:207, 1998

Leier CV et al: The cardiovascular effects of the continuous infusion of dobutamine in patients with severe cardiac failure. Circulation 56:468, 1977

Mehra MR et al: Safety and clinical utility of long-term intravenous milrinone in advanced heart failure. Am J Cardiol 80:61, 1997

Patel MB et al: Sustained improvement in flow-mediated vasodilation after short-term administration of dobutamine in patient with severe congestive heart failure. Circulation 99:60, 1999

Slawsky MT et al: Acute hemodynamic and clinical effects of levosimendan in patients with severe heart failure. circulation 102:2222, 2000

PACEMAKER THERAPY FOR REFRACTORY HEART FAILURE

Vineet Kaushik / Teresa De Marco / Leslie A. Saxon

Heart failure (HF) affects 4.5 million persons in the United States; it is now the most frequent diagnosis on admission for those hospitalized older than age 65. Over the past 20 years, significant advances have been made in pharmacotherapy that have led to reductions in morbidity and mortality in this population. Despite these advances, HF remains progressive in most cases. As the U.S. population ages, the number of patients with advanced HF refractory to optimal medical therapy will continue to increase. Although cardiac transplantation remains the best treatment option for appropriate candidates, the limited availability of donor hearts restricts its role. This has led researchers to investigate new approaches to the treatment of HF. The purpose of this chapter is twofold: (1) to review the literature and history of pacing for HF, including promising advances that have been made with biventricular or left ventricular stimulation to achieve cardiac resynchronization; and (2) to discuss the future role of device-based therapies capable of multiple functions in the management of HF patients who remain symptomatic on optimal medical therapy.

Dual-Chamber (DDD) Pacing with Short AV Delay

The initial interest in utilizing cardiac pacing to improve HF involved an attempt to optimize the sequence of atrioventricular (AV) contraction. Conduction abnormalities are not uncommon in patients with HF. Nearly 30% of patients with advanced HF have first-degree AV block. This delay in contraction could result in a decrease in cardiac output due to (1) suboptimal left atrial contribution to left ventricular filling, and (2) increasing diastolic mitral regurgitation (MR). Thus, it was hypothesized that dual-chamber pacing with a shortened AV delay could improve cardiac output by resynchronization of atrial and ventricular contraction.

In healthy subjects, atrial transport contributes 15 to 30% to resting cardiac output. However, acute studies have shown that in patients with HF, the importance of atrial contribution may be quite variable. First, atrial mechanical contraction may be ineffective in patients with HF. Second, pacing studies investigating the effect of loss of atrial contraction in patients with HF demonstrate a range of responses. Patients with advanced HF and normal left ventricular (LV) filling pressures demonstrate a significant improvement in cardiac output with DDD pacing with a short AV delay compared to ventricular pacing. In contrast, patients with advanced HF and elevated LV filling pressures (as is often the case with refractory HF patients) demonstrate no significant change in cardiac output between DDD and ventricular pacing alone. The reason for this variable response in hemodynamics can be explained by the Frank-Starling curve. Patients with relatively low LV filling pressures are on the steep portion of the curve and thus respond to additional preload from atrial contraction by increasing cardiac output. In contrast, in patients with high LV filling pressures, the left ventricle is operating on the flat portion of the curve and gains much less improvement in stroke volume with atrial contraction.

Clinical Trials

A decade ago, these observations led researchers to investigate the effects of chronic DDD pacing with shortening of the AV delay as a means to improving hemodynamics in patients with HF. Hochleitner and colleagues were among the first to show a beneficial effect of cardiac pacing with a short AV delay in patients with HF (Hochleitner et al., 1990). In this study, 16 patients with end-stage idiopathic dilated cardiomyopathy and no bradycardia indications for a pacemaker implant underwent DDD pacemaker implant with a shortened AV delay of 100 ms. Both acutely and chronically, this resulted in a dramatic improvement in New York Heart Association (NYHA) symptom class of HF and left ventricular ejection fraction (LVEF).

This initial success led to a series of acute and chronic studies (Tables 78-1 and 78-2) assessing the effect of shortening the AV delay in patients with impaired ventricular function. Most of these studies were uncontrolled and showed mixed results. Three well-designed and randomized studies (one acute, two chronic) by Gold (1995), Innes (1994), and Gilligan (1998) failed to show any consistent

improvements in HF with shortening of the programmed AV delay.

Conclusions

Although initial reports of acute and chronic success with DDD pacing with a shortened AV interval in patients with advanced HF were generally encouraging, subsequent controlled studies failed to demonstrate a clear benefit. It is clear from these studies that certain subsets of patients do indeed benefit from shortening the AV delay, specifically those with a marked prolongation of the PR interval and/or diastolic MR at baseline. However, there is no "universal" short programmed AV delay that results in significant improvement in this subgroup. Thus, the indiscriminate use of DDD pacing with shortened AV delay in patients with advanced HF is not supported by the literature at present.

Cardiac Resynchronization Therapy with Biventricular or Left Ventricular Stimulation

Large observational studies performed in patients with advanced HF have demonstrated that right ventricular (RV) pacing for traditional bradycardia indications results in worsening HF symptoms and long-term outcome. This may be due to the development of RV pacing–induced left bundle branch block resulting in intra- and interventricular dyssynchrony, with resultant further worsening of LV and RV systolic and diastolic function. An analogous phenomenon is seen in patients with advanced HF and bundle branch block (BBB). Indeed, the majority of patients with advanced HF have interventricular conduction delay (IVCD), and up to 50% have manifest BBB caused by direct pathologic involvement of specialized conduction and/or scarring of the myocardium causing inhomogeneous spread of excitation wavefronts. The BBB is left sided in 70 to 80% of patients. The presence of BBB introduces contractile inefficiency and dyssynchrony, causing further diminishment of ventricular function. When LV conduction delay is superimposed upon ventricular

TABLE 78-1

ACUTE STUDIES WITH DDD PACING AND SHORT AV DELAY

Study	Patient number	AV interval, ms	NYHA class, LVEF, %	Result
Hochleitner et al., (1990)	16	100	III-IV, 16	Dramatic improvements in symptoms, LVEF, and systolic blood pressure
Brecker et al., (1992)	12	Optimized per patient (6–31)	Not specified	Increased cardiac output, less TR/MR duration, increased LV filling time
Nishimura et al., (1995)	15	Optimized per patient (60–240)	III-IV, 19	Increased cardiac output, less MR, and increased LV filling time in patients with baseline PR interval >200 ms. No change in patients with PR interval >200 ms
Shinbane et al., (1997)	9	Optimized per patient (50–200)	IV, LVEF not specified	No change in CO/PCWP pressure or systolic and diastolic function
Innes et al., (1994)[a]	12	60 and 100	III-IV, 21	No change in CO at 100 ms, decreased CO/stroke volume at 60 ms

[a]Randomized, cross-over study.
ABBREVIATIONS: CO, cardiac output; PCWP, pulmonary capillary wedge pressure; LV, left ventricle; TR, tricuspid regurgitation; MR, mitral regurgitation; LVEF, left ventricular ejection fraction.

dysfunction, it appears to be a marker of disease severity, predicting an increased risk of both HF progression and susceptibility to ventricular arrhythmias. Thus, pacemakers with the ability to stimulate the left and right ventricles simultaneously could theoretically resynchronize ventricular contraction in patients with HF and BBB. It is in this context that researchers started to investigate the effects of biventricular stimulation to achieve cardiac resynchroniza-tion in patients with advanced HF. Early acute and chronic studies performed in patients with advanced HF and BBB used direct epicardial pacing to stimulate the left ventricle which required a thoracotomy and resulted in significant morbidity. Currently, transvenous approaches are used in which the left ventricle can be stimulated by placement of a pacing lead in a coronary sinus ventricular branch vein (Cazeau et al., 2001, Gold et al., 2000) (Figs. 78-1, 78-2).

TABLE 78-2

CHRONIC STUDIES WITH DDD PACING AND SHORT AV DELAY

Study	Patient number	AV interval, ms	NYHA class, LVEF, %	Follow-up	Result
Hochleitner (1992)	17	100	III-IV, 15	Up to 5 years; only 3 patients survived 5 years	Improved symptoms and LVEF
Guardigli (1994)	4	Optimized per patient (80–200)	III-IV, LVEF not specified	2 months	Increased stroke volume and LVEF
Linde (1994)	10	Optimized per patient (50–150)	III-IV, 16	1, 3, 6 months	No change in symptoms, CO/stroke volume, or LVEF
Gold (1995)[a]	12	Optimized per patient (100–200)	III-IV, 20	4–6 weeks	No change in symptoms or LVEF
Gilligan (1998)[a]	17	"Optimal" (ms not specified)	?class, 25	6 weeks	No improvement in symptoms

[a]Randomized, cross-over study
ABBREVIATIONS: CO, cardiac output; LVEF, left ventricular ejection fraction.

Clinical Trials

The first clinical report of biventricular pacing was reported by Cazeau et al., in 1994. A 54-year-old man with NYHA functional class IV HF on intravenous inotropes and left BBB with a QRS duration of 200 ms was implanted with a four-chamber pacemaker for atrial and ventricular stimulation. This resulted in a dramatic acute increase in cardiac output and decrease in pulmonary capillary wedge pressure. At 6 weeks of follow-up, the patient improved from class IV to class II HF and had a 17-kg weight loss with resolution of peripheral edema. This study was followed by a series of uncontrolled studies demonstrating marked acute improvements in hemodynamics and symptoms with biventricular stimulation. (Table 78-3).

The two largest studies in Europe, the In Sync Study an uncontrolled trial (Gras et al., 1998) and the controlled trial MUSTIC (2000), have yielded consistently positive results. In patients with NYHA functional class II-IV HF, 3, 6, and 12 months of continuous stimulation of chronic biventricular stimulation result in significant improvements in exercise capacity, NYHA functional class, and quality-of-life (QOL) score. Hospitalization rates for HF exacerbations are also decreased. The QRS interval is not always decreased in those patients who benefit from biventricular stimulation, suggesting ventricular resynchronization can be obtained in the absence of QRS narrowing. Resynchronization devices have been approved in Europe since 1998 (Leclerq et al., 1998, Saxon et al., 1998, Saxon et al., 2000).

RAO   **LAO**

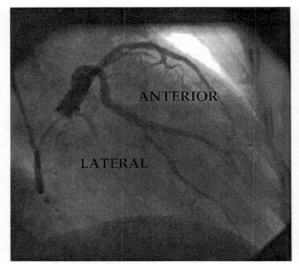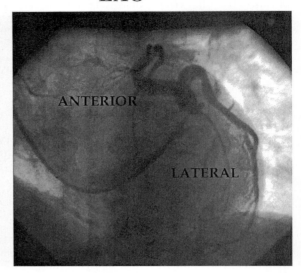

FIGURE 78-1

Coronary sinus branch venography. RAO, LAO, right, left anterior oblique view.

RAO   **LAO**

FIGURE 78-2

Coronary sinus lead placement for left ventricular stimulation. RAO, LAO, right, left anterior oblique view. The LV lead is in a lateral and apical position.

TABLE 78-3

CLINICAL TRIALS OF BIVENTRICULAR STIMULATION

Study	Patient number	NYHA class, LVEF	Duration	Result
Cazeau (1994)	1	IV, LVEF not specified	Acute and 6 weeks	BiV stimulation resulted in marked improvement in symptoms and hemodynamics (increased CO and decreased PCWP)
Cazeau (1996)	8	IV, 22%	Acute	BiV stimulation resulted in increased CO and decreased PCWP
Saxon (1997)	11	I-IV, 36%	Acute	Improved global LV systolic function and LV segmental wall motion activation
Blanc (1997)	23	III-IV, 27%	Acute	LV and BiV stimulation better than RV apex and RVOT stimulation. Decreased PCWP, V-wave amplitude and increased systolic blood pressure
Kass (1997)	18	III-IV, 19%	Acute	LV and BiV stimulation improved dP/dt_{max} and pulse pressure compared to RV pacing. LA better than BiV stimulation
Leclerq (1998)	18	III-IV, 19%	Acute	BiV stimulation better than "optimal" RV pacing with increased CO and decreased PCWP
Gras (1998)	68	III-IV, 21%	Chronic, 1 and 3 months	BiV stimulation improved NYHA class, QOL score, 6-min walk distance
Aurrichio (1999)	27	III-IV, 21%	Acute	LV > BiV > RV stimulation with increased dP/dt_{max} and pulse pressure
Aurrichio (NASPE 2000) PATH-CHF I	15	II-IV, EF not available	Chronic, 1 month	Improved exercise tolerance, quality-of-life score, ventricular function, and heart rate variability
Cazeau[a] MUSTIC Trial	58	III, 22%	Chronic, 3 months	Increased exercise tolerance, improved quality-of-life score, decreased number of hospitalizations for CHF
Bakker (2000)	12	III-IV, LVEF 15%	Chronic, 1 year	Improved NYHA class, increased LVEF and dP/dt, decreased mitral regurgitation, less restrictive LV filling pattern

[a]Randomized clinical trial.

ABBREVIATIONS: BiV, biventricular; CO, cardiac output; PCWP, pulmonary capillary wedge pressure; LV, left ventricle; RV, right ventricle; RVOT, right ventricular outflow tract.

Currently, resynchronization therapy is on the cusp of regulatory approval in the United States. The results of the recently completed MIRACLE and CONTAK CD trials have been presented in abstract form. The MIRACLE trial studied biventricular stimulation in 500 HF patients with predominantly NYHA class III HF and BBB. Significant improvements were noted in exercise time, QOL score, and left ventricular ejection fraction (Abraham, 2002). Preliminary results from this trial and others note reductions in echocardiographic measures of LV size and dimension after as little as 3 months of continuous resynchronization therapy. This suggests that the resynchronization may favorably impact the remodeling process in HF. The CONTAK CD trial studied resynchronization therapy in predominantly NYHA class II-III HF patients with IVCD and an indication for an implantable cardioverter defibrillator (ICD). The study was underpowered to meet its primary composite end-points of morbidity/mortality, hospitalization, and reduction in episodes of ventricular tachycardia/fibrillation. Nonetheless, all results trended toward benefit. Those patients with more advanced symptom class demonstrated marked improvement in exercise time and peak oxygen consumption measured on cardiopulmonary exercise testing (Cannon, 2001). Further large randomized,

controlled studies are underway in the United States; these trials are listed in Table 78-4.

Currently, there are more than 5000 patients enrolled in the U.S. trials of resynchronization therapy. The only trial sufficiently powered to assess total mortality and hospitalization as an end-point is the COMPANION trial (Bristow et al., 2000). This study is the first to randomize advanced HF patients with BBB to standard medical therapy vs. resynchronization therapy vs. resynchronization therapy plus an ICD. The study has randomized approximately 1300 patients and requires 2200 patients to complete enrollment. The PAVE trial is the first controlled study to evaluate the benefits of resynchronization therapy in patients with advanced HF and chronic atrial fibrillation following AV node ablation.

Future Devices in HF

Devices are now available, on clinical protocol, that can be programmed to achieve resynchronization with LV or biventricular stimulation, provide early diagnosis and treatment of atrial arrhythmias, and provide real-time hemodynamic data. Left ventricular stimulation is now achieved reliably and safely using a coronary sinus branch vein. These added features, including the defibrillation capability, offer many potential advantages to the HF patient who remains at significant risk of hospitalization or death on standard drug therapies.

Conclusions

Despite significant advances in the medical management of HF, a large number of patients continue to exhibit refractory symptoms. Preliminary chronic data indicate that cardiac resynchronization achieved with biventricular or LV stimulation is a promising modality for improving NHYA functional class, quality of life, and exercise duration in the subset of HF patients with BBB. The results of ongoing clinical trials will further define the role of ventricular resynchronization and help identify which additional device features, such as defibrillation capability, should be present in the "ideal" HF device.

TABLE 78-4

CONTROLLED CLINICAL U.S. TRIALS WITH RESYNCHRONIZATION THERAPY

Study	
VIGOR CHF	1996–1998
VENTAK CHF/CONTAK CD	1998–2001
MIRACLE	1998–2001
MIRACLE ICD	1998–2001
Re-Le-Vent	1999–
COMPANION	1999–
PAVE	1999–

REFERENCES

Abrahan WT et al: Cardiac resynchronization in chronic heart failure. NEJM 346:1902, 2002

Aurrichio A et al: Effect of pacing chamber and atrioventricular delay on acute systolic function of paced patients with congestive heart failure. Circulation 99:2993, 1999

Brecker SJD, Xiao HB, Sparrow J, et al: Effects of dual-chamber pacing with short atrioventricular delay in dilated cardiomyopathy. Lancet 340:1308, 1992

Bristow MR et al: Heart failure management using implantable devices for ventricular resynchronization: Comparison of medical therapy, pacing and defibrillation in chronic heart failure (COMPANION) trial. J Card Fail 6:276, 2000

Cannon D: Report of the CONTAK CD clinical trial results. Presentation at Guidant Symposium at the 22nd Annual Scientific Session of the North American Society of Pacing and Electrophysiology (NASPE), 2001

Cazeau S et al: Four chamber pacing in dilated cardiomyopathy. Pacing Clin Electrophysiol 17:1974, 1994

Cazeau S et al: Effects of multisite biventricular pacing in patients with heart failure and intraventricular conduction delay. N Engl J Med 334:873, 2001

Gold MR et al: Pacing in patients with heart failure, in *Clinical Cardiac Pacing and Defibrillation,* K Ellenbogen et al (eds). Philadelphia, Saunders, 497-507, 2000

Gras D et al: Multisite pacing as a supplemental treatment of congestive heart failure: Preliminary results of the InSync Study. Pacing Clin Electrophysiol 21 (pt2):2249, 1998

Hochleitner M et al: Usefulness of physiologic dual-chamber pacing in drug-resistant idiopathic cardiomyopathy. Am J Cardiol 66:198, 1990

Hochleitner M, et al. Long-term efficacy of physiologic dual-chamber pacing in the treatment of end-stage idiopathic dilated cardiomyopathy. Am J Cardiol 70:1320-1325, 1992

Innes D, Leitch JW, Fletcher PJ. VDD pacing at short atrioventricular intervals does not improve cardiac output in patients with dilated heart failure. PACE 17:959, 1994

Kass DA et al: Improved left ventricular mechanics from acute VDD pacing in patients with dilated cardiomyopathy and ventricular conduction delay. Circulation 99:1567, 1999

Leclerq C et al: Acute hemodynamic effects of biventricular DDD pacing in patients with end-stage heart failure. J Am Coll Cardiol 32:1825, 1998

Nishimura RA, Hayes DL, Holmes DR Jr, Tajik AJ: Mechanism of hemodynamic improvement by dual-chamber pacing for severe left ventricular dysfunction: an acute Doppler and catheterization hemodynamic study. J Am Coll Cardiol 25:281-288, 1995

Saxon LA: Permanent pacemaker therapy for improvement of cardiac function in advanced heart failure, in *Management of End Stage Heart Disease,* EA Rose, Stevenson L (eds). Philadelphia, Lippincott-Raven 105-113, 1998

Saxon LA et al: Heart failure and cardiac resynchronization therapies: U.S. experience in the year 2000. Ann Noninvasive Electrocardiol 5:188, 2000

Shinbane J, Chu E, De Marco T, et al: Evaluation of acute dual chamber pacing with a range of atrioventricular delays on cardiac performance in refractory heart failure. J Am Coll Cardiol 30:1295-1300, 1997

WHEN TO USE IMPLANTABLE CARDIOVERTER DEFIBRILLATORS IN HEART FAILURE

Bartolomeo Giannattasio / Mark Carlson

Heart failure (HF) is a syndrome defined by functional and clinical markers that are associated with increased mortality. Approximately 5 million people in the United States have heart failure. The risk for death is 5 to 10% per year. In the Framingham study, survival for patients with congestive HF was 50% at 5 years. In the United States, approximately 250,000 individuals die each year of HF, 100,000 of these due to sudden cardiac death (SCD). SCD is usually caused by ventricular tachyarrhythmias but may occur as a result of a bradyarrhythmia in up to 10% of individuals. In patients with HF, SCD may also be caused by pulseless electrical activity, which can occur regardless of the heart rhythm.

The development and use of the implantable cardioverter defibrillator (ICD) during the past two decades has markedly changed treatment and improved survival for patients with SCD (See also Chap. 69, this volume). The ICD continuously monitors the heart rhythm and automatically detects and rapidly terminates ventricular tachycardia (VT) and ventricular fibrillation (VF). The device consists of an impulse generator and electrode leads for sensing, pacing, and shocking.

In this chapter, we discuss the risk for SCD in HF, the influence of conventional therapy and antiarrhythmic drug therapy on mortality and SCD, and the role (proven and potential) of the ICD in patients with HF.

Factors Influencing the Risk for Sudden Cardiac Death

A variety of factors that cause or are associated with HF have been examined as potential risk factors for mortality in the syndrome. Left ventricular ejection fraction (LVEF), functional status, and nonsustained VT have been correlated with SCD risk and with outcome of therapy. Abnormal autonomic control, as evidenced by increased heart rate and decreased baroreflex activity, has been correlated with an increased risk for SCD in patients with myocardial infarction (MI), many of whom had HF. Although more than one may exist in an individual patient, these factors represent independent risk factors for total mortality and SCD.

Impairment of left ventricular systolic function has been recognized as a risk factor for mortality following MI since 1983 (Multicenter Post-Infarction Research Group). The risk for death increases exponentially as the LVEF decreases. In patients with LVEF <0.30, the risk for death in the first year after MI is >20%. Low LVEF is associated with increased mortality in nonischemic cardiomyopathy as well. In survivors of SCD, decreased LVEF is associated with increased recurrence and increased mortality.

Functional status and left ventricular systolic function are related but distinct entities. Not all patients with reduced LVEF have heart failure; 10 to 20% of patients with HF do not have left ventricular systolic dysfunction. Declining functional HF status is an independent risk factor for total mortality and possibly for SCD. The risk of death per year varies from about 5 to 20% in mild HF with NYHA class I-II to >40% in class IV patients. In the Cooperative North Scandinavian Enalapril Survival Study (CONSENSUS) trial, SCD accounted for 30% of the deaths in NYHA class IV patients.

Ventricular arrhythmias are common in HF; premature ventricular beats occur in 70 to 90% of patients and nonsustained VT occurs in 30 to 80% of patients. Ventricular ectopy has long been recognized to be associated with an increased risk for mortality and SCD following MI. The combination of left ventricular systolic dysfunction and ventricular ectopy is associated with a greater mortality risk than either factor alone following MI and in patients with HF.

Effects of Drug Therapy

Any discussion of the role of the ICD in HF must also consider the influence of drug therapy on mortality. Some drugs have shown a beneficial effect, others have had a neutral effect, and others cause increased mortality. Although drug treatment may improve mortality in patients with HF, the risk of SCD remains high.

Drugs that decrease mortality in HF include β-adrenergic receptor antagonists, angiotensin-converting enzyme (ACE) inhibitors, and probably angiotensin II receptor blocker and spironolactone. Drugs that have a neutral effect on mortality include digoxin and certain calcium channel blockers. Drugs that increase mortality in heart failure include positive inotropic agents, class I antiarrhythmic drugs,

certain class III antiarrhythmic drugs (d-sotalol), and certain calcium channel blockers. Amiodarone has shown mixed effects depending on the trial.

β-Adrenergic receptor antagonists decrease mortality by approximately 15% during the first year after MI with half of the benefit due to reduction of SCD. Three of these drugs have been shown to decrease mortality in HF (Table 79-1).

ACE inhibitors reduce mortality following MI. The reduction in mortality is greatest in patients with reduced LVEF (20% in patients with LVEF <0.40). ACE inhibitors confer a survival benefit of 10 to 40% in patients with HF. In a recent meta-analysis, the survival benefit of ACE inhibitors was dependent on NYHA functional class: 20, 25, 31, and 40% in classes I to IV respectively. Most ACE inhibitor trials have examined total death rather than arrhythmic death. However, in the Veterans' Administration Cooperative Heart Failure Trial, the beneficial effect of enalapril was due mostly to a reduction in SCD.

Both beta antagonists and phosphodiesterase inhibitors (milrinone) are associated with increased total and arrhythmic mortality. Most antiarrhythmic drugs are associated with an increased risk for proarrhythmia and, in certain circumstances, increased mortality. In the Cardiac Arrhythmia Suppression Trial (CAST), antiarrhythmic drugs were associated with increased mortality when administered after MI. The mortality risk was greatest in patients with low LVEF. In the Stroke Prevention in Atrial Fibrillation (SPAF) trial, antiarrhythmic drug therapy was associated with increased mortality in patients with heart failure but not in patients without HF. Whereas amiodarone has been shown to decrease mortality in patients with HF due to nonischemic cardiomyopathy, no trial has shown the drug to benefit patients with ischemic-cardiomyopathy. The combination of amiodarone with β-adrenergic receptor antagonists may impart additional survival benefit as compared to either drug alone.

Effects of the ICD on SCD

Since they were approved for use in 1985, ICDs have undergone considerable improvement. The initial models used large generators and were

TABLE 79-1

EFFECT OF β-ADRENERGIC RECEPTOR ANTAGONISTS ON HF MORTALITY

Study	Drug	Degree of heart failure	Reduction in total mortality, %	Statistical significance
MDC	Metoprolol	Mild-moderate	34 (death-transpl.)	No
RESOLVD	Metoprolol	Mild-moderate	54	No
MERIT-HF	Metoprolol	Moderate-severe	35	Yes
CIBIS I-II	Bisoprolol	Moderate-severe	20–34	Yes
New Zealand–Australian Study	Carvedilol	Mild-moderate	23	Yes
United States (combination of four studies)	Carvedilol	Moderate-severe	65 (combined studies)	Yes

ABBREVIATIONS: MDC, Metoprolol in Dilated Cardiomyopathy; RESOLVD, Randomized Evaluation of Strategies for Left Ventricular Dysfunction; MERIT-HF, Metoprolol CR/XL Randomized Intervention Trial in Heart Failure; CIBIS, Cardiac Insufficiency Bisoprolol Study

implanted in the abdomen. The initial shocking leads required thoracotomy and epicardial implant. Endocardial leads that can be implanted transvenously became available in 1992. Generators have become progressively smaller (the smallest is now 35 mL) and can be implanted subcutaneously in the subclavicular area of the chest wall. Dual-chamber pacing defibrillators became available in 1998. Monitoring and information storage capabilities of new ICDs allow for arrhythmia diagnosis and determination of therapeutic efficacy.

Indications for the ICD have expanded since the U.S. Food & Drug Administration (FDA) approved the ICD in 1985 for patients with a history of sustained VT or VF. In 1991, the American College of Cardiology (ACC) and the American Heart Association (AHA) recommended ICDs for patients with prior documented hemodynamically unstable VT/VF in whom electrophysiology study or Holter monitor either could not be used or failed to show suppression of tachycardia by antiarrhythmic drugs. Syncope with inducible VT was considered to be a class II indication. The 1998 ACC/AHA guidelines significantly extended the indications to include patients with nonsustained VT, prior MI, low LVEF, and inducible sustained VT/VF that is not suppressed by an antiarrhythmic drug. The guidelines recommended ICD for patients with the same substrate, syncope, and inducible VT or VF as well.

Factors that favor the ICD over antiarrhythmic drug therapy include (1) the potential proarrhythmic effect and lack of a survival advantage from many antiarrhythmic drugs, (2) the low risk of nonthoracotomy ICD implants, (3) the poor prognosis of patients with CHF when treated with conventional therapy alone, (4) the demonstration that ICD implant is better than conventional therapy for secondary prevention of SCD, and (5) the mortality benefit associated with ICD implantation in certain primary prevention trials.

ICDs reduce total mortality and SCD in survivors of cardiac arrest regardless of the degree of left ventricular dysfunction. Several studies, including the Antiarrhythmics Versus Implantable Defibrillator (AVID) trial, Canadian Implantable Defibrillator Study (CIDS), and Cardiac Arrest Study in Hamburg (CASH), have also shown that ICDs reduce mortality to a greater extent than antiarrhythmic drug therapy in SCD survivors (Table 79-2).

Many of the patients in these trials had left ventricular systolic dysfunction and H.F. The mean LVEF in the CASH study was 0.40. In the AVID

TABLE 79-2

ICD VS. ANTIARRHYTHMICS IN THE SECONDARY PREVENTION OF SCD

Study	Therapy modality	Average EF,%	Death decrease with ICD, %	Inclusion criteria
AVID	Antiarrhythmic (mostly amiodarone) vs. ICD	32 (CHF class I-III)	30 (statistically significant)	SCD, symptomatic VT with EF < 40%
CASH	Metoprolol or propafenone vs. ICD	46	39 (statistically significant)	SCD
CIDS	Amiodarone vs. ICD	34	20 ($p = .07$)	SCD, EF < 35% and symptoms of slow VT, syncope, and monitored or induced VT

ABBREVIATIONS: ICD, implantable cardioverter defibrillator; EF, ejection fraction; SCD, sudden cardiac death; AVID, Antiarrhythmics Versus Implantable Defibrillators; CASH, Cardiac Arrest Study in Hamburg; CIDS, Canadian Implantable Defibrillator Study; CHF, congestive heart failure; VT, ventricular tachycardia.

trial, the mean LVEF was 0.30 ± 13. HF was present in 60% of AVID patients (50% had NYHA class I or II; 10% had class III heart failure). The survival benefit of ICDs was greatest in patients with LVEF < 0.35. In fact, a subgroup of patients with normal LVEF was identified that did not benefit from the ICD as compared to amiodarone therapy. A meta-analysis of the AVID, CASH, and CIDS trials confirmed that patients with LVEF ≤ 0.35 derived greater benefit from the ICD.

These studies indicate that ICDs improve survival and are superior to antiarrhythmic drugs for secondary prevention (treatment after an initial event) of sustained VT or VF. Furthermore, the benefit of the ICD is greatest in patients with reduced LVEF. Subanalysis of the AVID trial has been used to assess markers of poor outcome and increased SCD risk in HF. Of these, one relevant to the use of ICD in HF is atrial fibrillation. Atrial fibrillation is an independent marker of increased mortality and risk of SCD in HF and may possibly be involved in the pathogenesis of HF and SCD. In addition to standard dual-chamber pacing, some ICDs now may include pacing and shocking algorithms for prevention, detection, and termination of atrial fibrillation.

Only 10 to 20% of patients survive an episode of SCD. Therefore, 80 to 90% of individuals who experience a life-threatening ventricular tachyarrhythmia do not survive to benefit from an ICD. Because of this, the concept of the ICD for primary prevention of SCD has received considerable attention.

Trials of ICD Therapy

The Multicenter Automatic Defibrillator Implantation Trial (MADIT) randomized patients with prior MI and several risk factors for SCD to receive an ICD or antiarrhythmic drugs. This was the first trial to show that the ICD reduces mortality in high-risk patients prior to an episode of SCD. Criticisms of MADIT have included the following:

1. Although 7% of patients with ICDs also received amiodarone, 55% of patients in the conventional therapy limb were not taking the drug at the time of last contact.
2. There was no control group that received no antiarrhythmic therapy.
3. The percent of patients on beta blockers in the ICD group was much higher, 27% vs. 5% in the conventional therapy group.

4. Patients were referred to the study following a Holter monitor that showed nonsustained VT, raising concerns that patients were truly asymptomatic.

5. The study was terminated early on the basis of a relatively novel statistical analysis that demonstrated significant mortality reduction in the ICD group.

6. The size of the reduction in total deaths was small.

7. There was a reduction in cardiac nonarrhythmic deaths in the ICD group, for which there was no apparent reason.

The MADIT results have influenced the use of the ICD for patients at risk for SCD. In fact, the FDA has approved ICDs for MADIT-type patients. The MADIT results are also reflected in the 1998 AHA/ACC guidelines for implantation of pacemakers and ICDs. Furthermore, many experts do not consider it necessary to demonstrate that antiarrhythmic drugs do not suppress induction of sustained VT. These individuals advocate ICDs for patients with prior MI, LVEF ≤ 0.35, nonsustained VT and inducible sustained VT.

The Multicenter Unsustained Tachycardia Trial (MUSTT) lends support to the conclusions of the MADIT. Patients with coronary artery disease, LVEF ≤ 0.40 and nonsustained VT, and inducible sustained VT were randomized to receive conventional therapy (ACE inhibitor and β-adrenergic receptor antagonist) or conventional therapy in addition to antiarrhythmic therapy (drugs or ICD). The reduction in total mortality in patients who received antiarrhythmic therapy guided by electrophysiologic study (EPS) was borderline significant ($p = .06$). Arrhythmic mortality was significantly lower in patients who received EPS-guided antiarrhythmic therapy. The decrease in mortality was almost completely explained by a beneficial effect of the ICD.

The Coronary Artery Bypass Graft (CABG)-Patch trial is the only primary prevention trial to date in which the ICD did not confer a survival benefit. In the CABG-Patch trial, patients with prior MI, LVEF < 0.36, and a positive signal-averaged electrocardiogram (ECG) who were undergoing coronary artery bypass graft surgery were randomized to receive or not to receive a thoracotomy-implanted ICD. After 4 years, total mortality was similar in the two groups: 23 and 24% in the control and ICD groups, respectively.

The MADIT, MUSTT, and CABG-Patch trials indicate that the ICD may be effective for primary prevention of SCD but that patient selection is key. Several factors can impact on the effectiveness of the ICD: (1) the all-cause and arrhythmic mortality rates in the absence of ICD, (2) the magnitude of the ICD effect on arrhythmic death, (3) the ICD effect on nonarrhythmic death, and (4) effects of other therapies on mortality. Several of these factors may have been partially responsible for the differences in the MADIT and CABG-Patch trial outcomes (Table 79-3).

The total and arrhythmic mortality rates were greater in the MADIT trial than in the CABG-Patch trial. However, the proportion of deaths that were arrhythmic in both trials was similar. The ICD-associated reduction in arrhythmic mortality was greater in MADIT than in the CABG-Patch trial. For reasons that are not clear, the ICD decreased cardiac nonarrhythmic death in the MADIT trial but did not affect cardiac nonarrhythmic death in the CABG-Patch trial. The ICD had no effect on noncardiac death in MADIT but increased noncardiac death in CABG-Patch, possibly because of perioperative complications. Coronary artery revascularization may have decreased the risk for arrhythmic death and the potential for ICD to benefit patients in the CABG-Patch trial.

A lesson to be learned from both the MADIT and the CABG-Patch trials with respect to the use of the ICD in HF patients is the time-honored adage "do no harm." The benefit of the therapy should exceed the risk. In the CABG-Patch trial, the risk of ICD implantation exceeded the potential for benefit from the device. The challenge for advocates of the ICD as primary prevention of SCD in HF is to identify patients in whom the risk for SCD exceeds the risk of ICD implantation.

Inherent difficulties in defining the timing (sudden vs. nonsudden) and mode of death make it difficult to accurately determine the proportion of deaths that are likely to be sudden in patients with HF.

TABLE 79-3

COMPARISON OF MADIT AND CABG-PATCH

	MADIT	CABG-Patch
Control group total mortality	39% (27/101 pts)	21% (79/454 pts)
Arrhythmic death in controls	12.9% (13/101, pts) 48% of deaths	6.2% (28/454 pts) 35% of deaths
Reduction of arrhythmic death by ICD	76% (control 13/101, ICD 3/95)	45% (control 28/454, ICD 15/446)
ICD effect on cardiac nonarrhythmic death	40% decrease (control 13.8%, ICD 8.4%)	20% increase (control 10.1%, ICD 12.7%)
ICD effect on noncardiac deaths	29% decrease (control 5.9%, ICD 4.2%)	66% increase (control 3.7%, ICD 5.6%)

ABBREVIATIONS: MADIT, Multicenter Automatic Defibrillator Implantation Trial; CABG-Patch, Coronary Artery Bypass Grafting Patch; ICD, implantable Cardioverter defibrillator.

Furthermore, the proportion of sudden deaths that are due to tachyarrhythmias in HF is also not clear. Many investigators believe that electromechanical dissociation (which does not respond to ICD therapy) is a common cause of death in HF. Analysis of stored ECGs from ICDs has shown that the device terminates ventricular tachyarrhythmias with similar efficacy in patients with class I, II or III HF. Few studies have evaluated patients with class IV. In these patients, ICD implant is under consideration as a "bridge" to transplant. In this regard, the 1998 AHA/ACC expert panel recommends that ICDs not be implanted in patients with life expectancy less than 6 months or with class IV HF.

Primary Prevention of SCD in HF

Two trials that address the role of the ICD for primary prevention of SCD in HF, the Sudden Cardiac Death in Heart Failure Trial (SCD-HeFT) and the Multicenter Automatic Defibrillator Implantation Trial II (MADIT II), are underway.* Table 79-4

summarizes ongoing trials evaluating the use of ICD in SCD primary prevention.

The SCD-HeFT trial tests the hypothesis that either amiodarone or the ICD or both improves survival compared to placebo in patients with HF. Patients with ischemic or nonischemic cardiomyopathy, NYHA class II or III HF, and LVEF < 36% are randomized to receive one of these therapies. All patients receive best conventional HF treatment, including ACE inhibitor therapy. β-Adrenergic receptor antagonists are strongly encouraged for all patients.

The project enrolled 2521 patients between October 1997 and June 2001 and is now in the follow-up phase. The sample size is based on a projected 2-year mortality rate of 25% during a minimum of 2.5 years follow-up. Of the patients enrolled through February 2001, 52% had coronary artery disease and 48% had nonischemic cardiomyopathy. Most patients (70%) were NYHA class II; 30% were NYHA class III HF at enrollment.

Based on the favorable results of the MADIT trial, the MADIT II trial was designed and began enrolling patients in January 1998. The objective of MADIT II is to determine if the ICD reduces mortality in patients with prior MI and decreased left ventricular systolic function. The belief is that Holter monitoring and EPS may not be necessary to

* MADIT II was recently terminated due to improved survival in the ICD Group. See addendum

identify MADIT-eligible patients who benefit from an ICD. Patients with prior MI and LVEF ≤ 0.30 are randomized to ICD or no ICD therapy.

SCD-HeFT and MADIT II are trials that evaluate the use of ICD in SCD prevention based on low LVEF and/or class I-III HF. Other means to identify SCD risk (such as the results of EPS) are not required for enrollment but will be evaluated at the conclusion of the studies. Other ongoing SCD primary prevention trials, such as DEFINITE, DYNAMIT, and ABCD, will evaluate the role of additional markers for SCD also (Table79-4).

Both MADIT II and SCD-HeFT will yield important information regarding the role for ICDs in the primary prevention of SCD. Whereas the MADIT II relies on ejection fraction as an enrollment criterion, the SCD-HeFT trial is a true HF trial, requiring symptomatic HF for enrollment. MADIT II is limited to patients with coronary artery disease; SCD-HeFT includes patients with ischemic and nonischemic car-

diomyopathy. Whether the risk for arrhythmic death in the MADIT II and SCD-HeFT is great enough to warrant ICD therapy remains to be determined. Some experts believe that additional factors (i.e., nonsustained VT or inducible VT) are required to identify patients whose risk is great enough to benefit from therapy. Furthermore, the cost of implanting ICDs in the patient populations defined by the MADIT II and SCD-HeFT may be significant. Whether society is willing or able to support these costs also remains to be determined.

Biventricular Pacing

Bundle branch block and intraventricular conduction abnormalities occur in one-third of HF patients and can further reduce cardiac output by causing asynchronous contraction of the right and left ventricles. Atriobiventricular pacing (cardiac resynchro-

TABLE 79-4

ONGOING TRIALS EVALUATING THE USE OF ICD IN SCD PRIMARY PREVENTION

Study	EF	Cardiomyopathy	HF	Comments
SCD-HeFT[a]	<35%	Ischemic and nonischemic	Class I-III	Study has terminated enrollment
MADIT II[b]	<30%	Ischemic	Class I-III	Study will also evaluate the value of EPS
DEFINITE	<35%	Nonischemic	Class I-III	Inclusion is based on the presence of NSVT
DYNAMIT	<40%	Ischemic	Class I-III	Inclusion is based on decreased heart rate variability
ABCD	<40%	Ischemic	Class I-III	Inclusion is based on NSVT Inclusion is based on implant on EPS or T-wave alternans

[a]Heart Failure (HF) and low ejection fraction (EF) are the only inclusion criteria. [b]Trial completed; see addendum
ABBREVIATIONS: EPS, electrophysiologic study; NSVT, nonsustained rentricular tachycardia.

nization therapy) has been used in HF patients alone or in combination with an ICD to resynchronize ventricular contraction. Short-term studies in animals and patients with HF and prolonged QRS duration show that biventricular pacing improves cardiac output and hemodynamics. On the basis of these studies, clinical trials have been performed or are underway. In the European Multisite Biventricular Pacing Trial in Patients with Heart Failure and Intraventricular Conduction Delay (MUSTIC) trial patients, biventricular pacing improved exercise tolerance and quality of life. Whether cardiac resynchronization therapy improves survival and the role of biventricular pacing in patients with ICDs are the subjects of ongoing clinical trials.

Conclusions

SCD accounts for a significant proportion of total mortality in patients with HF. Conventional therapy, including ACE inhibitors and β-adrenergic receptor antagonists, improves survival and may, to a limited extent, decrease arrhythmic mortality in these patients. Antiarrhythmic drugs have limited potential to improve survival in patients with HF. Patients with HF who have survived an episode of sustained VT or VF will benefit from an ICD. The MADIT and MUSTT trials indicated that HF patients with previous MI, nonsustained VT, and certain additional risk factors also benefit from an ICD. Factors that may affect the success of therapy include (1) the rate of reversible arrhythmic mortality, (2) the ICD effect on arrhythmic death, (3) the ICD effect on the nonarrhythmic death, and (4) the effect of other therapies on mortality.

There is no conclusive evidence that ICDs benefit patients with HF in the absence of other risk stratification modalities. However, the ability of conventional therapy to prevent SCD in these patients is limited. Available evidence from SCD primary and secondary prevention trials indicates that many HF patients benefit from an ICD. Many patients in the MADIT and AVID trials had low ejection fraction, prior MI, syncope, and nonsus-

tained VT—risk factors that are often present in HF patients. The CABG-Patch trial, however, showed that the ICD does not produce a survival benefit if the antiarrhythmic effect is small or if the risk of death associated with the ICD implant is too great.

The impact of functional status of HF as an independent risk factor of sudden arrhythmic death and the benefit of ICD implant in this condition are being investigated in patients with either ischemic or nonischemic cardiomyopathy. Two clinical trials (SCD-HeFT and MADIT II) are ongoing to evaluate the effect of ICD implant vs. conventional therapy in patients with HF class II-III NYHA. These trials may either extend the indication for ICD implant in HF patients or indicate the need for further risk stratification.

Addendum

Since this chapter was prepared, the Multicenter Automatic Defibrillator Trial (MADIT) II results were reported (Moss AJ et al, 2002). In this trial, 1232 patients with prior myocardial infarction (>1 month before entry documented by a Q wave on ECG) and left ventricular ejection fraction < 0.30 were randomized to receive conventional therapy and an implantable defibrillator (742 patients) or conventional medical therapy alone (490 patients). During an average followup of 20 months, mortality rates were greater in the conventional therapy group than in the defibrillator group (19.8% vs. 14.2%, p = 0.007). The authors noted that implantation of defibrillators in 3 to 4 million patients in the United States who have coronary artery disease and advanced left ventricular dysfunction would be associated with substantial costs. Nonetheless, the authors expressed the hope that market forces will drive down costs and concluded that prophylactic defibrillator implantation is recommended in these patients.

REFERENCES

Bigger IT: Risk stratification and survival after myocardial infarction. N Engl J Med 309:331, 1983

Bigger IT: Prophylactic use of implanted cardiac defibrilla-tors in patients at high risk for ventricular arrhythmias after coronary artery bypass graft surgery (CABG-Patch trial). N Engl J Med 337:1569, 1997

Bigger IT et al: Mechanisms of death in the CABG-Patch trial. Circulation 99:1416, 1999

Cappato R: Secondary prevention of sudden death: The Dutch study, the Antiarrhythmic Versus Implantable Defibrillator trial, the Cardiac Arrest Study in Hamburg, and the Canadian Implantable Defibrillator Study. Am J Cardiol 83:68D, 1999

Cazeau S et al: Effect of multisite biventricular pacing in patients with heart failure and intraventricular conduc-tion delay. N Engl J Med 334:873, 2001

Connolly SJ et al: Meta-analysis of the implantable cardioverter defibrillator secondary prevention trials. AVID, CASH, and CIDS studies. Antiarrhythmics vs Implantable Defibrillator study; Cardiac Arrest Study in Hamburg; Canadian Implantable Defibrillator Study. Eur Heart J 21:2071, 2000

Farre J et al: Amiodarone and "primary" prevention of sud-den death: Critical review of a decade of clinical trials. Am J Cardiol 83:55D, 1999

Garg R, Yusuf S: Overview of randomized trials of angiotensin converting enzyme inhibitors on mortality and morbidity in patients with heart failure. Collabora-tive group on ACE inhibitor trials. JAMA 273:1450 1995

Gregoratos G et al: ACC/AHA guidelines for implantation of cardiac pacemakers and antiarrhythmia devices. A report of the American College of Cardiology/American Heart Association Task Force on practical guidelines (commit-tee on pacemakers implantation). J Am Coll Cardiol 31:1175, 1998

Higgins SL et al: Biventricular pacing diminishes the need for implantable defibrillator therapy. J Am Coll Cardiol 36:824, 2000

Klein H: New primary prevention trials of sudden cardiac death in patients with left ventricular dysfunction: SCD-HeFT and MADIT-II. Am J Cardiol 83:91D, 1999

Moss AJ et al: Improved survival with an implanted defibril-lator in patients with coronary disease at high risk for ventricular arrhythmia. The Multicenter Automatic Defibrillator Implantation Trial Investigators. N Engl J Med 335:1933, 1996

Moss AJ et al: Prophylactic implantation of a defibrillator in patients with myocardial infarction and reduced ejection fraction. NEJM 246:877, 2002

Naccarelli G et al: A decade of clinical trial developments in post-myocardial infarction, congestive heart failure, and sustained ventricular arrhythmia patients: From CAST to AVID and beyond. Cardiac Arrhythmic Suppression Trial. Antiarrhythmic Versus Implantable Defibrillators. J Cardiovasc Electrophysiol 9:864, 1998

Packer M, Cohn J: Consensus recommendations for the man-agement of chronic heart failure. Am J Cardiol 83:2A, 1999

Pinski S et al: Determinants of outcome in patients with sus-tained ventricular tachyarrhythmias: The antiarrhythmics versus implantable defibrillators (AVID) study registry. Am Heart J 139:804, 2000

Stevenson W et al: Improving survival for patients with atrial fibrillation and advanced heart failure: Future directions. J Am Coll Cardiol 28:1458, 1996

Stevenson W et al: Prevention of sudden cardiac death in heart failure. J Cardiovasc Electrophysiol 12:112, 2001

The Antiarrhythmic versus Implantable Defibrillator (AVID) Investigators: A comparison of antiarrhythmic drug ther-apy with implantable defibrillators in patients resusci-tated from near-fatal ventricular arrhythmia. N Engl J Med 337:1576, 1997

PACING IN HYPERTROPHIC CARDIOMYOPATHY

David A. Kass

Introduction

Therapeutic approaches to hypertrophic cardiomyopathy center around beta receptor and calcium channel blockade and agents such as disopyramide (Spirito et al., 1997). All three depress systolic function, while the first also limits chronotropic responses and the second improves relaxation. Several nonpharmacologic approaches have also been developed including surgical resection of the proximal septum (myotomy/myectomy) (Robbins and Stinson, 1996), intracoronary ethanol injection (Faber et al., 2000), and dual-chamber ventricular pacing (Fananapazir et al., 1994; Nishimura et al., 1996; 1997; Pak et al., 1998; Kass et al., 1999; Maron, 1999; Kappenberger et al., 1997). Of these, surgical resection and intraseptal artery ethanol injection both aim to reduce the mass of the proximal septal muscle either by direct resection or by induced tissue damage.

Dual-chamber cardiac pacing with atrial sensing and premature ventricular activation (VDD mode) provides a third nonpharmacologic approach. Pacing can be applied to patients with disproportionate proximal septal hypertrophy as well as to those with more concentric disease involving the distal chamber (Pak et al., 1998). The dominant mechanism by which a pacemaker is thought to provide benefit relates to its capacity to generate discoordinate contraction by premature activation. Typically, the atrial sinus rate is sensed by one lead, and the right ventricular apex is stimulated in advance of native His-Purkinje conduction by setting an electronically determined atrioventricular (AV) interval shorter than that for native conduction. This creates an "out-of-tune" ventricle, much like an automotive engine with intentionally badly timed cylinders, where some portion of cavity blood is essentially transferred from the early activated to late activated regions during systole, with the net effect being diminished ejection performance.

Since preexcitation typically requires shortening the AV delay time to assure that stimulation precedes intrinsic His-Purkinje conduction, this acutely increases left atrial pressure and may also reduce mitral regurgitation in patients with this abnormality. The second effect from premature stimulation is the alteration of contraction pattern. The paced region shortens prematurely, followed by late activation of the remote territory and late-systolic stretch of the paced muscle.

Figure 80-1 shows regional pressure-volume loops in the apical territory of a patient with hypertrophic cardiomyopathy (HCM) with and without right ventricular (RV) apical pacing. The baseline loop is normal (boxlike shape) with the loop moving in a counter-clockwise direction. During pacing, however, there is marked discoordination—resulting in an S-shaped loop, much as one might observe with ischemia. This altered contraction pattern results in blood volume redistribution into the apical region during systole, and this is the source for a rise in end-systolic volume. This also prevents cavity obliteration, since the heart muscle no longer squeezes on itself to generate high distal chamber pressures, and reduces instantaneous intracavitary pressures in these patients (Fig. 80-2). A potential consequence of a diminution in cavity obliteration is that internal myocardial work (i.e., related to the heart muscle squeezing on itself with virtually zero

chamber blood volume) is reduced. This may contribute to improved regional blood flow and a decline in the chest pain symptom that often accompanies hypertrophic disorders.

Figure 80-3 displays global pressure-volume data from patients with either familial HCM (FHC) or hypertrophic disease associated with hypertension and distal cavity obliteration. The results are similar, displaying a net rightward shift of the end-systolic pressure-volume relation. While relatively small, this shift is still much larger than would be achieved in these hearts under basal conditions and is sufficient to prevent cavity obliteration.

In contrast to potent effects on systolic function and workload, VDD pacing has no significant effect on chamber diastolic stiffness or on the time constant of relaxation (Pak et al., 1998). Thus, acute pacing intervention depresses systolic ejection while reducing overall cardiac energy demand

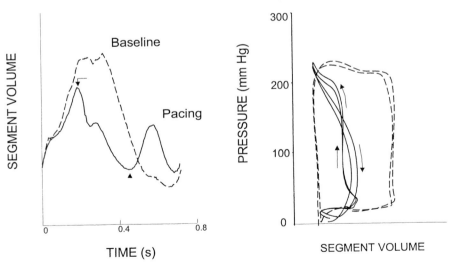

FIGURE 80-1

Regional discoordination induced by right ventricular apex pacing, measured in a patient with hypertrophic cardiomyopathy. Left ventricular apical volume (left) displays filling and ejection under normal sinus conditions (dashed line). With pacing, contraction starts early (arrow) and finishes early. Then this same region is subject to restretch (second arrow) as the remote myocardium is initiating contraction. The net result on the pressure-volume loop is shown to the right. The control loop has a normal appearance, indicating positive external work. The loop with pacing is narrow, s-shaped, and has minimal effective work (area of loop) and paradoxical wall motion.

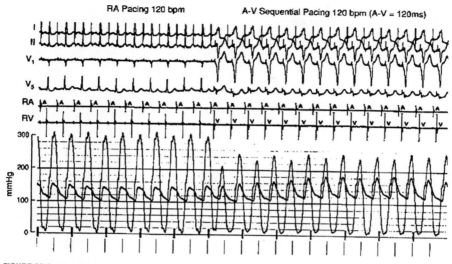

FIGURE 80-2

Effect of atrioventricular (AV) sequential pacing on ventricular pressure gradient. Upper tracings show surface electrocardiograms (leads I, II, VI, and V5), and intra atrial (RA) and ventricular (RV) electrograms demonstrating the changes with pacing initiation. Lower tracings show marked basal difference in systolic ventricular vs. aortic pressures, which is diminished by pacing. (From L Fananapazir et al: Circulation 85:2149, 1992, with permission.)

but has little direct effect on diastolic chamber properties.

These characterizations have all been derived from acute pacing studies. However, as the intervention is applied chronically, it remains possible that additional changes may accrue. For example, some studies have suggested chronic remodeling may occur with pacing, with patients no longer demonstrating intracavitary pressure gradients at rest even when the pacemaker is transiently turned off (Fananapazir et al., 1994). Other studies, however, have not observed similar changes (Maron; 1999). Pacing therapy was first applied to HCM patients with marked asymmetric septal thickening, systolic anterior motion of the mitral valve, and outflow tract obstruction, all presumed to be of genetic origin. However, the effect of pacing on discoordinate wall motion does not depend upon a specific geometry or etiology but is predictable in virtually any heart.

Pacing Therapy and Familial Hypertrophic Cardiomyopathy

Initial studies reporting acute and chronic efficacy for VDD pacing applied the therapy to patients with assymetric septal hypertrophy. All patients had evidence of pressure gradients at rest or with modest provocation. Many had chest pain as well as exertional dyspnea. Examination of the four prominent trials reveal several important features of this therapy. First, there is a major placebo effect, limiting the value of studies lacking appropriate controls or therapy blinding. Second, while many, if not most, patients demonstrate an acute decline in intracavitary pressure gradients when pacing is initiated, there is little to no correlation between the magnitude of this effect and clinical improvement.

The first chronic study reported on 84 patients chronically paced at the RV apex, with a 1-year follow-up (Fananapazir et al., 1994). Pacing reduced

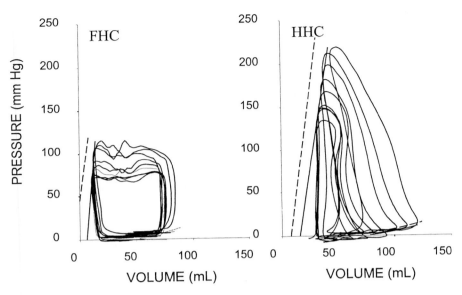

FIGURE 80-3

Net pacing effect on global cardiac function depicted by pressure-volume loops. Two examples are shown (FHC, familial hypertrophic cardiomyopathy; HHC, hypertensive hypertrophic cardiomyopathy). In each instance, the baseline systolic pressure-volume relation is displayed (dashed line), along with data measured during RV apical pacing. The effect of discoordinate apical wall motion induced by pacing is a rightward shift of the systolic pressure-volume relation, i.e., a net increase in end-systolic volume at any systolic pressure. This shift reflects the discoordination, and is the primary mechanical effect from pacing, central to the decline in pressure gradients.

intracavity pressure gradients and substantially improved NYHA function class in nearly all patients (90% had symptomatic improvement). There was an overall correlation between initial gradient reduction and ultimate efficacy, although this was very weak and suggested minimal predictive value regarding acute hemodynamic responses. An important caveat was that this chronic study was neither blinded nor placebo-controlled.

Far less consistent or favorable results have been reported in several subsequent trials in which both controls were applied. In one study, patients were randomly assigned to either pacing on or pacing off, with either setting maintained for 3 months, and then switched for an additional 3-month period (Nishimura et al., 1997). Many patients experienced symptomatic improvement with VDD-mode pacing; however, this was also observed during the period of pacing off, confirming a potent placebo effect. Exercise duration was only modestly improved (414 vs. 342 s) and maximal oxygen consumption unaltered. Importantly, both pacing on and off periods had similar responses. Long-term follow-up data in 38 patients has been reported from the Mayo Clinic (Erwin et al., 2000). At an average of 24 ± 14 months, subjective improvement was found in 47%, but there was no statistical difference in maximal oxygen consumption between this follow-up and the period of placebo (AAI) pacing.

A subsequent multicenter European trial (PIC trial) reported on results from 82 patients, using a similar study design, and again found symptomatic improvement but no significant objective functional improvement overall (Kappenberger et al., 1997). In a post-hoc analysis, a 21% improvement in exercise duration was observed only in patients with reduced baseline capacity (<10 min maximal exercise time). As with the prior studies, ventricular pressure gradients declined about 50% in most patients, regardless of their exercise capacity changes. One-year follow-up data were subsequently reported and found sustained >50% reductions in the resting left ventricular outflow pressure gradient, as well improved heart failure function class and quality of life (Kappenberger et al., 1999). This indicated benefit in a substantial number of patients that appeared to extend well beyond the time of implantation and pointed to an effect beyond placebo.

Maron's team followed with the largest multicenter placebo-controlled U.S. trial employing a study design similar to that of the preceding trials, and also with a 6-month chronic pacing-on period (non-blinded) following the initial 3-month on vs. off double-blind randomized crossover phase (Maron, 1999). These investigators studied 48 patients and again found symptomatic improvement, but this was indistinguishable between the placebo and treatment arms. There was also no change in exercise capacity or metabolic performance nor, in this study, any evidence of echocardiographic changes in wall thickness, mass, or function during pacing. These investigators also examined data by post-hoc analysis and reported that in the responder group (12% of the total study sample), patients were all >65 years of age and demonstrated significantly lower maximal oxygen consumption on exercise testing (12.4 mL O_2/kg per min vs. 17.1 in the other patients). This suggested either that the pathophysiology was different in older individuals or that the benefits of pacing were more evident in patients for whom basal dysfunction and levels of physical activity were possibly more modest.

The cumulative evidence from these trials leaves considerable uncertainty regarding the appropriate role of pacing therapy for the treatment of FHC. Clearly, some patients derive marked benefit, but such individuals are hard to identify prospectively and may in fact be a relative minority among individuals with the disease. Many have argued that as this mode of therapy does not directly benefit diastolic dysfunction, it is not surprising that it would prove both variable and modest in its chronic efficacy. However, as discussed in the next section, responses in patients with hypertensive left ventricular hypertrophy (LVH) and supranormal ejection—many of whom are also thought to have diastolic dysfunction—appear both more consistent and substantial. This suggests that specific features of FHC and/or the dosing efficacy of a pacing may underlie the specific response. At the present time, this approach should be considered in older individuals with FHC refractory to medical therapy and/or in those in whom anatomy or other risk factors preclude the use of myotomy/myectomy or alcohol ablation.

Pacing Therapy and Hypertensive Left Ventricular Hypertrophy

A subgroup of patients with chronic hypertension and LVH commonly present with paroxysmal severe dyspnea and pulmonary edema, associated with marked hypertension and ejection fractions >80%. In a recent small study, patients with this disorder were chronically treated with pacing, using a similar study design to the earlier placebo-controlled trials (Kass et al., 1999). However, the results were far more consistent and striking. Exercise duration prolonged 82% and maximal oxygen consumption increased 24% only during the pacing period. Nearly all patients felt better during the initial 3 months, regardless of whether the pacemaker was on or off, so there was also a substantial placebo effect. However, here was an instance where perception and performance were disparate, as metabolic exercise data did not mirror reported symptom improvement unless pacing was on.

After 1 year of pacing, diastolic heart function was unaltered, but systolic reserve assessed by dobutamine stimulation test improved significantly. For example, cardiac output rose nearly twice as much with the same dobutamine dose (2.4 vs. 4.8 L/min) after 1 year of pacing. This likely relates to the rise in end-systolic volumes generated by pacing, and thus restoration of some systolic reserve (these volumes can once again decrease to enhance ejection).

The difference between pacing responses in earlier FHC trials and this study in patients with hypertensive HCM and cavity obliteration may relate to greater homogeneity in the latter group and an improved capacity to deliver the pacing effect (i.e., discoordinate wall motion) to the relevant region of the heart (i.e., distal cavity). In patients with proximal septal hypertrophy, pacing efficacy likely depends more on delaying septal contraction by spread of the pacing stimulus from the apex. This timing is difficult to control and likely varies with underlying conduction properties, myocardial structure (i.e., fibrosis, fiber disarray), and chamber geometry. In the patients with distal cavity obliteration, pacing at the apex more directly interferes with hypercontraction in this region.

SUMMARY

Patients with FHC and HCM associated with hypertension can benefit from VDD pacing, but responses are more heterogeneous and less impressive in the former group. In both patient groups, therapy should be considered only after optimal medical management has failed. In patients with FHC, pacing may be offered to individuals who do not want to undergo surgery (myotomy/myectomy) or have medical conditions that might increase their surgical risk. New alternative treatments such as ethanol septal ablation also appear promising. Identification of those patients most likely to benefit from VDD pacing remains difficult at present. In FHC patients, age may provide a clue to better therapy response, with older patients receiving greater benefit. This may relate to more modest demands from the therapy in this age group while still conveying meaningful symptomatic improvement. Our understanding of pacing treatment remains limited relative to most drug therapies, in that only a single dose has ever been tested since the pre-excitation stimulus was always delivered by a single pacing lead using conventional technology. However, experimental data suggest that the greater the discoordination induced by premature excitation, the greater the net mechanical effect. Pacing leads might be designed to stimulate larger territories or several regions simultaneously to generate more discoordination and thus greater effect. Also, the site of pacing has not been well studied. While RV apical pacing is likely better than septal pacing, the potential of left heart pacing to improve on this effect has not been tested, but might be efficacious. Whether alterations in delivery might yield more consistent results in both FHC or other forms of HCM remains to be determined.

REFERENCES

Erwin JP III et al: Dual chamber pacing for patients with hypertrophic obstructive cardiomyopathy. A clinical perspective in 2000. *Mayo Clin Procs* 75: 173, 2000

Faber L et al: Percutaneous transluminal septal myocardial ablation for hypertrophic obstructive cardiomyopathy: Long term follow up of the first series of 25 patients [see comments]. *Heart* 83:326, 2000

Fananapazir L et al: Long-term results of dual-chamber (DDD) pacing in obstructive hypertrophic cardiomyopathy. Evidence for progressive symptomatic and hemodynamic improvement and reduction of left ventricular hypertrophy. *Circulation* 90:2731, 1994

Kappenberger L et al, for the PIC Study Group. Pacing in hypertrophic obstructive cardiomyopathy: A randomized crossover study. *Eur Heart J* 18:1249, 1997

Kappenberger LJ et al, for the Pacing in Cardiomyopathy (PIC) Study Group: Clinical progress after randomized on/off pacemaker treatment for hypertrophic obstructive cardiomyopathy. *Europace* 1:77, 1999

Kass DA et al: H. Ventricular pacing with premature excitation for treatment of hypertensive-cardiac hypertrophy with cavity-obliteration *Circulation* 100:807, 1999

Maron BJ: New interventions for obstructive hypertrophic cardiomyopathy: Promise and prudence [editorial; comment]. *Eur Heart J* 20:1292, 1999

Nishimura RA et al: Effect of dual-chamber pacing on systolic and diastolic function in patients with hypertrophic cardiomyopathy. *J Am Coll Cardiol* 27:421, 1996

Nishimura RA et al: Dual-chamber pacing for hypertrophic cardiomyopathy: A randomized, double-blind, crossover trial. *J Am Coll Cardiol* 29:435, 1997

Pak PH et al: Mechanism of acute mechanical benefit from VDD pacing in hypertrophied heart: Similarity of responses in hypertrophic cardiomyopathy and hypertensive heart disease. *Circulation* 98:242, 1998

Robbins RC, Stinson EB: Long-term results of left ventricular myotomy and myectomy for obstructive hypertrophic cardiomyopathy. *J Thorac Cardiovasc Surg* 111:586, 1996

Spirito P et al: The management of hypertrophic cardiomyopathy. *N Engl J Med* 336:775, 1997

81

ECHOCARDIOGRAPHY TO DETERMINE VIABILITY IN HEART FAILURE

William A. Zoghbi

Since the mid 1970s, there has been an increased realization that chronic systolic ventricular dysfunction does not necessarily imply irreversible myocardial injury. *Hibernating myocardium* refers to a state of chronic ventricular dysfunction associated with severe coronary artery disease (CAD) that exhibits complete or partial recovery of function after revascularization. While angina and the absence of Q waves on the electrocardiogram help alert the clinician to the presence of hibernating myocardium, these findings are not sensitive enough for detection of residual viable myocardium in patients with CAD and heart failure.

Several modalities have been used for the identification of viable myocardium. These currently include assessment of myocardial contractile reserve to inotropic stimulation using echocardiography or magnetic resonance imaging, evaluation of membrane integrity with radionuclide techniques, and residual myocardial metabolic activity with positron emission tomography. This chapter focuses on the role of echocardiographic techniques in the detection of viable myocardium and its relevance

with regard to prognosis and selection of patients for revascularization.

Myocardial Hibernation

It is postulated that in some patients with CAD the myocardium may respond to chronic hypoperfusion by downregulating contractile function, thereby reducing cardiac energy demands (Rahimtoola, 1989). Myocardial hibernation describes such a state in patients with chronic ischemic heart disease, whereby restoration of coronary flow allows recovery of ventricular contractile function. Early studies suggested that resting coronary blood flow in this condition is reduced. Recent data, however, indicate that resting coronary flow may be normal or only moderately reduced, with a disproportionate decline in contractile function, implying that myocardial hibernation may involve at least in part an element of repetitive myocardial stunning (Vanoverschelde et al., 1997).

The cellular and molecular mechanisms involved in myocardial hibernation remain incompletely

515

understood, partly because of the inadequacy of experimental models of chronic hibernation. Data from transmural left ventricular biopsies in patients with hibernation undergoing coronary artery bypass surgery show a variety of histologic changes, including depletion of contractile apparatus, glycogen accumulation, and loss of organized endoplasmic reticulum (Vanoverschelde et al., 1997). Dedifferentiation of cardiac myocytes and regression to the fetal phenotype are also described. More recently, alterations in α- and β-adrenergic receptors have also been implicated in the downregulation of resting function in the hibernating myocardium (Shan et al., 2000). The severity of histologic changes may be dependent upon the duration of hibernation, with progression towards irreversibility with time, further stressing the importance of increased awareness of this syndrome and its early detection.

Echocardiographic Techniques in the Evaluation of Myocardial Viability

Echocardiography allows the assessment of myocardial structure in realtime and is well suited to evaluate global and regional ventricular function. Echocardiographic imaging has been combined with inotropic agents, such as dobutamine, for the evaluation of contractile reserve and detection of myocardial ischemia. More recently, myocardial thickness alone or in combination with contractile reserve was also shown to be a valuable indicator of viability. Lastly, among new developments, myocardial contrast echocardiography (MCE) has shown promise for detecting viable myocardium by assessing residual microvascular integrity.

Dobutamine Stress Echocardiography

It is currently well established that hibernating myocardium exhibits contractile reserve in response to inotropic stimulation. This was documented clinically as early as the 1970s in the cardiac catheterization laboratory and more recently with dobutamine

stress echocardiography (DSE). Incremental infusion of dobutamine in low doses, up to 10 to 20 μg/kg per min, elicits an augmentation of regional function in dysfunctional segments that is predictive of recovery of function after revascularization. Sensitivity for recovery of function ranges between 74 and 88%, with specificity between 73 and 87% (Bax et al., 2001). Sensitivity in akinetic segments is lower than in hypokinetic segments (69% vs. 88%).

Contractile reserve, although prevalent, is limited in myocardial hibernation. An increase in inotropic stimulation leads to depletion of energy stores, resulting in ischemia. The use of high-dose (up to 40 μg/kg per min), in addition to low-dose dobutamine in patients with suspected viability unmasks differences in contractile reserve that have significant implications for the prediction of recovery of function after revascularization (Afridi et al., 1995). Dysfunctional myocardium shows one of four characteristic responses to dobutamine: (1) biphasic response—augmentation of function at low dose followed by deterioration at higher doses; (2) sustained improvement response—improvement in function at low dose that persists or further improves at higher doses; (3) no change in function; and (4) worsening of function, without contractile reserve. An example of a patient with a biphasic response during DSE is shown in Color Plate 22, Figure 81-1. During a biphasic response to dobutamine, maximal augmentation of function is most often seen between 7.5 and 10 μg/kg per min of dobutamine, while deterioration of function is observed at higher doses. The highest predictive value for recovery of function after revascularization is demonstrated in myocardial regions that exhibit a biphasic response to dobutamine (72%) (Fig. 81-2). Combination of the types of responses to dobutamine (e.g., any contractile reserve) increases the sensitivity of DSE, with a slight decrease in specificity for recovery of function (Afridi et al., 1995).

Radionuclide imaging techniques have been used extensively for the evaluation of myocardial viability in the setting of chronic CAD and myocardial dysfunction. Individual comparative studies in the same patients and recent pooled data analysis (Bax et al., 2001) have confirmed a higher sensitivity

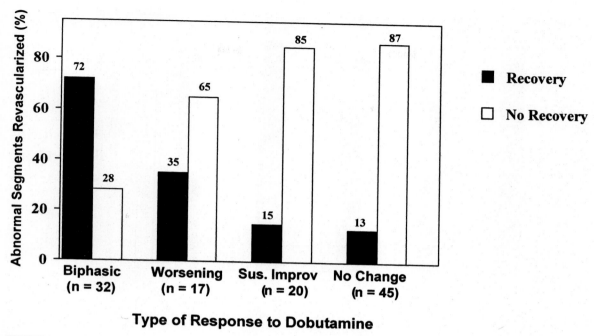

FIGURE 81-2

Prediction of recovery of segmental ventricular function after revascularization by the type of wall motion response to dobutamine prior to revascularization. Sus. Improv. sustained improvement. (From I Afridi et al: Circulation 91:663, 1995, with permission.)

(90% vs. 84%) and lower specificity (54% vs. 81%) of rest-redistribution ^{201}Tl compared to DSE in predicting functional recovery after revascularization.

Several factors play a significant role in determining the contractile response of viable myocardium to dobutamine, including severity of coronary stenosis, coronary reserve, extent of collaterals, cellular degeneration, metabolism, and tethering. Radionuclide myocardial uptake and, more recently, myocardial thickening at low-dose DSE have been shown to relate to the extent of fibrosis evaluated from myocardial biopsies at surgery (Nagueh et al., 1999). Discordances between inotropic reserve and radionuclide uptake in predicting recovery of function occur mostly in areas of myocardium with an intermediate level of fibrosis (Nagueh et al., 1999). Whether revascularization of myocardium with evidence of viability but without subsequent recovery of resting function has beneficial implications for heart failure

and ventricular remodeling, electrical instability, and survival remains to be determined.

End-Diastolic Wall Thickness as an Indicator of Viability

Early pathologic studies have demonstrated that myocardial thinning occurs in areas of myocardial necrosis in chronic transmural infarction. Furthermore, it has long been recognized that the presence of myocardial thinning detected with echocardiography is a marker of chronic myocardial infarction. In a recent study (Cwajg et al., 2000), myocardial end-diastolic wall thickness measured with echocardiography was evaluated as a possible marker of myocardial viability and compared to DSE and rest-redistribution thallium scintigraphy. Overall, myocardial segments that did not recover function after revascularization were thinner compared to

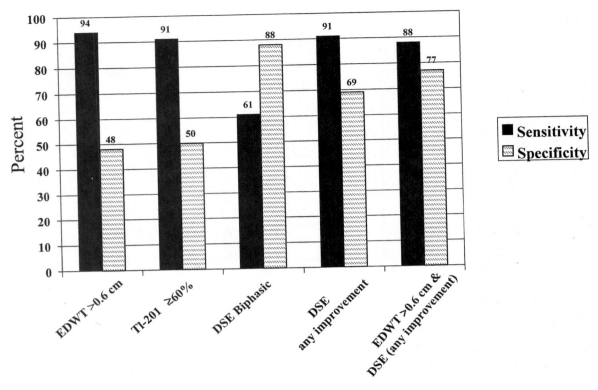

FIGURE 81-3

Sensitivity and specificity for recovery of function after revascularization using end-diastolic wall thickness (EDWT), rest-redistribution thallium uptake, and dobutamine echo (DSE) responses. (From JM Cwajg et al: J Am Coll Cardiol 35:1152, 2000; with permission.)

those that recovered function (0.67 ± 0.22 cm vs. 0.94 ± 0.18 cm). The diagnostic accuracy of end-diastolic wall thickness was similar to that of thallium scintigraphy (Fig. 81-3). An end-diastolic wall thickness of >0.6 cm had a sensitivity of 94%, specificity of 48%, and a high negative predictive value of 93% for recovery of function. Thus, segments with ≤0.6 cm of thickness have a very low likelihood of recovery of function after revascularization. The combination of contractile reserve during DSE and myocardial thickness in the same setting yielded the best diagnostic accuracy for echocardiography in predicting recovery of function (Fig. 81-3). These data are further corroborated with recent observations from magnetic resonance imaging.

Myocardial Contrast Echocardiography

Contrast echocardiography is one of the latest advances in the field of echocardiography. The injection of tiny amounts of microbubbles, which have a similar rheology to red blood cells, can enhance the ultrasound signal in the cardiac cavity and in the myocardium, thus allowing the assessment of myocardial perfusion noninvasively. Initial studies using *intracoronary* administration of contrast agents have demonstrated the utility of this technique in the detection of myocardial viability. The overall sensitivity of MCE and DSE in the prediction of recovery of contractile function was similar. However, the specificity for predicting recovery of function with

MCE was lower than that of DSE (52% vs. 73%) (deFilippi et al., 1995). In a study comparing contrast echocardiography with rest-redistribution thallium scintigraphy, a high concordance was observed between the two modalities, with a high sensitivity and low specificity for prediction of recovery of function (Nagueh et al., 1997). New *intravenous* contrast agents allow the noninvasive quantitation of myocardial blood flow with contrast echocardiography. Preliminary investigations with this technique reveal that MCE may have additive value to that of dobutamine echocardiography in evaluating myocardial hibernation (Shimoni et al., 2001).

Significance of Myocardial Viability in Heart Failure

Left ventricular function is one of the strongest predictors of outcome in patients with CAD. Reduced left ventricular function in patients with heart failure carries a poor prognosis. Patients with ischemic heart disease and congestive heart failure, however, may have a significant component of myocardial hibernation whereby recovery of systolic function may occur after revascularization. Improvement in ventricular function in these patients relates in part to the extent of myocardial viability and translates into amelioration of exercise capacity, heart failure symptoms, and overall prognosis.

Observational data suggest that viable myocardium that is not revascularized is a marker of further ischemic events and higher overall mortality. Early experience with positron emission tomography has shown a cardiac event rate of 50% in patients with depressed left ventricular function and evidence of myocardial hibernation. Corroborative studies on the prognostic impact of viability detected with DSE have recently emerged from several investigations. In a recent study (Afridi et al., 1998), 318 patients with severe ventricular dysfunction who underwent DSE were followed for 18 ± 10 months. Patients were divided into four groups depending on the presence or absence of viability, with or without revascularization (Fig. 81-4).

The mortality rate in the revascularized patients with known viability was 6% and was less than a third of that seen in each of the other three groups. The medical treatment of patients with viability or the absence of viability demonstrated by DSE was an independent predictor of mortality, in addition to the conventional risks of decreased ventricular ejection fraction and age (Afridi et al., 1998).

Clinical Implications

The presence of myocardial viability has consistently appeared as an important prognostic marker in patients with heart failure. Several features of viable myocardium may explain the benefits derived from its revascularization. Ventricular dysfunction, which contributes directly to reduced exercise tolerance and increased mortality, may be reversed. Progression from severe ischemia to necrosis may further worsen ventricular remodeling and prognosis if revascularization is not performed. Lastly, viable myocardium that is repetitively ischemic may be a potential source of electrophysiologic instability.

In approaching a patient with heart failure and ischemic heart disease, several factors are involved in the decision-making process for revascularization. These include, among others, the presence and severity of angina or ischemia, severity and extent of CAD at angiography, adequacy of target vessels for revascularization, severity of ventricular dysfunction and functional class, and overall risk of revascularization, particularly with bypass surgery. Patients with significant angina, multiple-vessel CAD, and ventricular dysfunction benefit from revascularization. Data from DSE, radionuclide perfusion techniques, and positron emission tomography, albeit in retrospective studies, demonstrate that the presence and extent of myocardial viability in patients with heart failure is an important determinant of prognosis. More recently, diastolic function parameters showing compensated heart failure also predicted residual viability and better prognosis (Yong et al., 2001). Such patients clearly benefit from revascularization, highlighting the importance

Dobutamine Echo
Mortality in Patients with LV Dysfunction

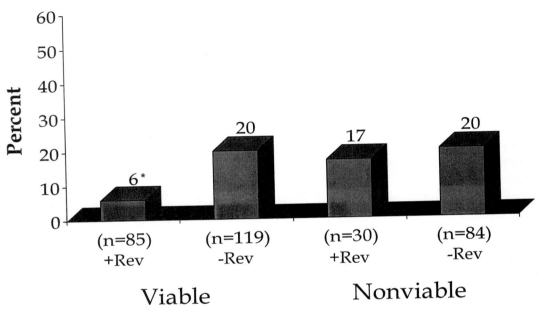

FIGURE 81-4

Mortality rates in patients with chronic left ventricular dysfunction, grouped by the presence of viability by DSE and by whether or not they underwent revascularization (Rev). *p = .01 vs. others. (From I Afridi et al: J Am Coll Cardiol 32:921, 1998, with permission.)

of testing for viability, particularly in advanced heart failure. The best therapeutic approach to patients without significant demonstrable viability remains unclear. Although the effect of revascularization on prognosis in this population appears less pronounced, it is not yet well elucidated. With current advances in both medical treatment for heart failure and interventional techniques for CAD, whether the absence of myocardial viability is best treated medically or with coronary interventions remains to be determined in a large prospective, randomized trial.

REFERENCES

Afridi I et al: Dobutamine echocardiography in myocardial hibernation. Optimal dose and accuracy in predicting recovery of ventricular function after coronary angioplasty. Circulation 91:663, 1995

Afridi I et al: Myocardial viability during dobutamine echocardiography predicts survival in patients with coronary artery disease and severe left ventricular systolic dysfunction. J Am Coll Cardiol 32:921, 1998

Bax JJ et al: Sensitivity, specificity and predictive accuracies of various techniques for detecting hibernating myocardium Curr Prob Cardiol 26:141, 2001

Cwajg JM et al: End-diastolic wall thickness as a predictor of recovery of function in myocardial hibernation: Relation to rest-redistribution Tl-201 tomography and dobutamine stress echocardiography. J Am Coll Cardiol 35:1152, 2000

deFilippi CR et al: Comparison of myocardial contrast echocardiography and low-dose dobutamine stress echocardiography in predicting recovery of left ventricular function after coronary revascularization in chronic ischemic heart disease. Circulation 92:2863, 1995

Nagueh SF et al: Identification of hibernating myocardium: Comparative accuracy of myocardial contrast echocardiography, rest-redistribution thallium-201 tomography and dobutamine echocardiography. J Am Coll Cardiol 29:985, 1997

Nagueh SF et al: Relation of the contractile reserve of hibernating myocardium to myocardial structure in humans. Circulation 100:490, 1999

Rahimtoola SH: The hibernating myocardium. Am Heart J 117:211, 1989

Shan K et al: Altered adrenergic receptor density in myocardial hibernation in man: A possible mechanism of depressed myocardial function. Circulation 102:2599, 2000

Shimoni S et al: Quantitative myocardial contrast echocardiography improves the detection of hibernating myocardium that lacks contractile reserve with dobutamine echocardiography. J Am Coll Cardiol 37:451A, 2001

Vanoverschelde JJ et al: Chronic myocardial hibernation in humans. From bedside to bench. Circulation 95:1961, 1997

Yong Y et al: Deceleration time in ischemic cardiomyopathy: Relation to echocardiographic and scintigraphic indices of myocardial viability and functional recovery after revascularization. Circulation 103:1232, 2001

82

SURGICAL ALTERNATIVES FOR THE FAILING HEART

Patrick M. McCarthy & Katherine J. Hoercher

Heart failure is a rapidly expanding problem. It is the most common DRG diagnosis for those over 65 years old and is the fourth leading cause of hospitalization in the United States. Congestive heart failure (CHF) is a chronic progressive disease, and a common central element involves remodeling of the cardiac chamber with ventricular dilatation. Multiple new approaches are being investigated for this pervasive problem. In addition to the standard medical therapies including digoxin, diuretics, and angiotensin-converting enzyme inhibitors, chronic beta-blocker administration (carvedilol) may stabilize patients and slow the progression of chamber remodeling. Aside from transplantation or mechanical assistance to aid the end-stage heart, heretofore surgical interventions in patients with advanced failure were contraindicated. However, new knowledge and evolving strategies are showing significant promise. In addition, patients can be managed with surgical therapies to improve cardiac function, and then state-of-the-art medical therapy for CHF can be intensified. From this combination of medical and surgical approaches, heart failure centers have developed as well as a new subspecialty within cardiology whose focus is the management of heart failure patients.

Coronary Artery Bypass

The most common operation performed for heart failure is coronary artery bypass grafting (CABG). It is recognized that patients with severe left ventricular (LV) dysfunction before CABG, and especially those with a history of heart failure, are at higher risk for perioperative events and decreased late survival (Yau et al., 1999). In the authors' series from the Cleveland Clinic, severe LV dysfunction and a history of CHF were significant risk factors for late death ($p < .001$). However, new strategies for preoperative evaluation and perioperative management have significantly decreased the perioperative mortality. Using a combination of dobutamine echocardiography, position emission tomographic scans, and magnetic resonance imaging, patients can be selected who have hibernating or ischemic myocardium (Marwick 1999). CABG is offered to most patients with compensated heart failure, assuming that there are adequate "targets" for grafting. The impact of other operative strategies, such as off-pump coronary bypass surgery (beating heart surgery), may further decrease the perioperative risk. With the use of new strategies for cardioplegia and perioperative selection and management, operative mortality for most patients would be approximately 2% (Luciani et al. 2000; Mickleborough et al., 1995).

Valve Operations

Other conventional operations for patients with CHF are usually focused on valve dysfunction. As the ventricle dilates, the papillary muscles are displaced, the coaptation of the mitral valve leaflets is decreased, and a central jet of mitral regurgitation will appear (Fig. 82-1). Previous reports of a prohibitive operative mortality for mitral valve replacement in patients with end-stage cardiomyopathy in the 1970s and early 1980s led to the clinical position that patients with severe LV dysfunction and mitral regurgitation were denied surgery for mitral valve correction. As experience with this operation increased, we have come to understand the importance of conservation of the subvalvular apparatus in the preservation of

systolic function. This concept has been applied successfully in patients who undergo mitral valve surgery with severe LV dysfunction, and there is now an increasing body of evidence demonstrating low operative mortality, good long-term survival, and freedom from readmissions for CHF. In most instances, mitral valve repair has become the surgery of choice, thereby avoiding the complications of long-term anticoagulation and the risks of prosthetic valve failure in late follow-up. As part of our mitral valve repair strategy, the authors have incorporated an "edge-to-edge" approximation of the anterior and posterior leaflets in their mid-portion (Alfieri repair) (Fig. 82-2). This simple suture plication creates a double orifice appearance of the mitral valve and significantly reduces the central jet of mitral regurgitation that occurs when mitral regurgitation is advanced. In addition, the authors use a very small mitral valve ring (typically 26 mm) to significantly reduce the posterior annulus to improve coaptation of the mitral valve leaflets.

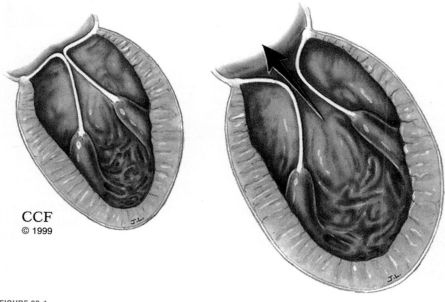

CCF
© 1999

FIGURE 82-1

Ventricular dilatation displaces the papillary muscles, decreases coaptation of the mitral leaflets, and leads to a central jet of mitral regurgitation recognizable on echocardiography.

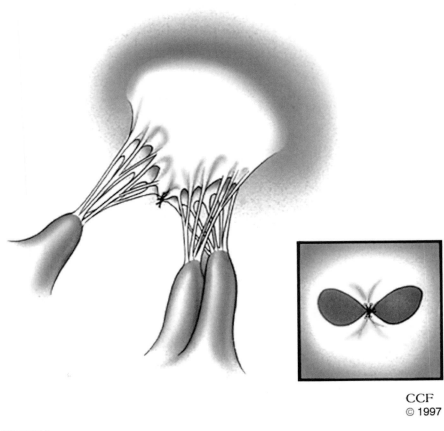

CCF
© 1997

FIGURE 82-2

Edge-to-edge approximation of the mitral leaflets increases coaptation and reduces the central jet of mitral regurgitation. The resultant double-orifice mitral valve does not create mitral stenosis, assuming the mitral leaflets are pliable, as with ischemic or idiopathic dilated cardiomyopathy.

Between 1990 and 1998, 44 patients with mitral regurgitation and a LV ejection fraction EF < 35% underwent isolated mitral repair ($n = 35$) or replacement ($n = 9$) at the Cleveland Clinic. All patients had been hospitalized one to six times for management of CHF (mean 2.3 ± 1.5 hospitalizations). The 1-, 2-, and 5-year survival rates were 89, 86, and 67%, respectively, with an improvement in NYHA class from 2.8 ± 0.8 preoperatively to 1.2 ± 0.5 at follow-up. Overall, mitral valve surgery in patients with severe LV dysfunction offers improvement of symptoms of CHF and good medium-term survival; in many instances, it provides an alternative to transplantation (Bishay et al., 2000).

Evolving experience with patients with aortic stenosis but severe ventricular dysfunction and low gradients indicates that aortic valve replacement can also be safely performed, especially when using a modern low-gradient prosthesis or homograft aortic valve (Connolly et al., 2000). Between 1990 and

1998, 63 patients from the Cleveland Clinic had aortic valve replacement for EF < 35% and aortic valve gradient < 30 mmHg. This group had a perioperative mortality of 4.8%, with 1- and 5-year survival of 85% and 64%, respectively, which represent significant improvements over past experience.

For patients with chronic aortic regurgitation (AR) with severe LV dysfunction, perioperative and late outcomes from earlier eras have been poor. From 1972 to 1980, 24 patients at the Cleveland Clinic had aortic valve surgery for chronic AR with severe LV dysfunction and had a 24% operative mortality. During the 1990s, 34 patients with severe LV dysfunction underwent aortic valve surgery with a perioperative mortality of 0%. The 5-year survival for such surgery in this setting was 84% in the 1990s vs. 59% for the 1970s.

Today, patients are frequently taken off of the transplant list to undergo aortic valve replacement for aortic insufficiency, mitral valve repair for 4 + mitral

regurgitation from either idiopathic or ischemic cardiomyopathy, and aortic valve replacement for aortic stenosis associated with low gradient.

Left Ventricular Reconstruction for Ischemic Cardiomyopathy

Revascularizing the heart and repairing the valves improves function, but efforts now are also being expanded to improve the ventricular function directly through ventricular surgery. It has been recognized for decades that patients with ventricular aneurysm can have their heart failure symptoms improved following ventricular aneurysmectomy. This concept has recently been expanded from dyskinetic (aneurysmal) ventricles to include akinetic ventricles, which heretofore were thought not to improve following ventricular reconstruction. (Buckberg, 1998; Dor et al., 1998). However, with experience, the type

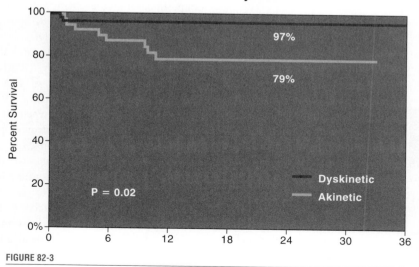

FIGURE 82-3

Survival at 24 months (akinetic vs. dyskinetic) following left ventricular reconstruction for ischemic cardiomyopathy. (ICMP)

of ventricular reconstruction has evolved from linear aneurysm repairs (that simply involve removing the freewall of the anterior left ventricle) to more complicated repairs that exclude the infarcted septum and freewall. Currently, our technique of LV reconstruction has evolved from the experience of Jatene, Dor, and Cooley. Since July 1997, 131 patients have undergone LV reconstruction following an anterior infarct. This surgery is frequently associated with CABG (85%) and often with mitral valve repair (50%). With a mean follow-up of 12 ± 8 months, there is a low perioperative mortality (1.5%), and survival at 24 months is 79% for the akinetic group and 97% for the dyskinetic group (Fig. 82-3). Using three-dimensional intraoperative echocardiography measurements, LV end-diastolic volume indices averaged 99 ± 40 mL/m^2 preoperatively and decreased by $32 \pm 16\%$ ($p < .05$) (Fig. 82-4). There was a significant improvement in LVEF from a mean of $29 \pm 11\%$ to $43 \pm 13\%$ ($p < .01$) (Qin et al., 2000). Importantly, these improvements were sustained at follow-up. Patients are considered candidates for this surgery if they have a discreet transmural LAD infarct with dyskinesia or akinesia. Most also have critical coronary artery disease or mitral valve disease requiring surgery.

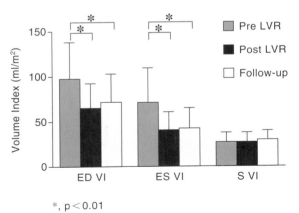

**, p < 0.01*

FIGURE 82-4

Comparison of volume indices before left ventricular reconstruction and at follow-up. Volume indices decreased; however, stroke volume remained unchanged. LVR = left ventricular reconstruction; EDVI = left ventricular volume index; ESVI = end-systolic volume index; SVI = stroke volume index

Partial Left Ventriculectomy

Surgical LV reconstruction for dilated cardiomyopathy, or partial left ventriculectomy (PLV), attempted to create a more normal volume, a more elliptical shape, and decreased wall tension for the left ventricle. Popularized by Randas Batista, this operation gained worldwide attention. The operative technique consists of excision of the lateral LV wall, usually between the papillary muscles, or with papillary muscle transection and reimplantation. If needed, mitral valve repair was also performed. At the Cleveland Clinic, 62 patients with nonischemic cardiomyopathy underwent PLV between May 1996 and December 1998. Preoperatively, mean LVEF was 14%, mean peak oxygen consumption was 10.8 ml/kg per min, and 61% were in NYHA class IV, indicating the disease severity of this cohort. Operative mortality was low—3.2%. Although some patients derived a significant benefit and continue with a sustained response at ≥5 years the authors observed a high early failure rate and an event-free survival at 36 months of only 26%. Overall, the PLV operation was abandoned at The Cleveland Clinic Foundation because of the unpredictable early failures and late return to heart failure; also, experimental studies of new therapies were underway. (McCarthy et al., 1998; Starling et al., 2000; Franco-Cereceda et al., 2001).

The encouraging results of LV reconstruction for ischemic cardiomyopathy (ICM) and the somewhat disappointing results of PLV initially seem to be contradictory outcomes of LV reconstruction. The major differences between the two are with respect to the underlying disease processes. ICM, being a patchy disease (discreet infarcted areas, other areas with normal function), allows for reconstruction to exclude the nonfunctional areas. For dilated cardiomyopathy, the presence of diffuse extracellular fibrosis may account for erratic early and late results. In the authors' opinion, the experience with PLV was not a dead end and provided a great deal of insight into the concept of reverse remodeling and LV shape change and has spawned the development of new surgical strategies to treat the failing heart.

New Concepts and Experimental Options to Reverse Left Ventricular Remodeling

Novel surgical devices specifically targeted at reversing or inhibiting LV remodeling represent newer solutions to this problem. The concept behind both the Acorn Wrap and the Myosplint were developed from surgeries involving direct surgical reconstruction of the left ventricle. The Myosplint (Myocor, Inc., Plymouth, MN) was developed to change LV shape, decrease LV wall stress, and improve LV function and efficiency. The Myosplint implant consists of two epicardial pads and a transventricular tension member. The two pads are located on the surface of the heart with the load-bearing tension member passing through the ventricle connecting the pads and drawing the ventricular walls toward one another. Three Myosplints are placed to create the appropriate shape change along the length of the left ventricle and thereby reduce the LV radius (Fig. 82-5). Experimental studies documented reduced wall stress and increased ejection fraction (McCarthy et al., 2001)

The Myosplint device is easily applied on a beating heart, with minimal localized bleeding and no sustained arrhythmia. The device itself occludes ventricular needle holes, and the epicardial pads tamponade bleeding. This device is currently in early clinical trials in Europe, used alone or as an adjunct for patients needing mitral valve repair or

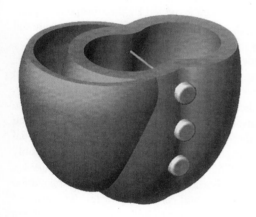

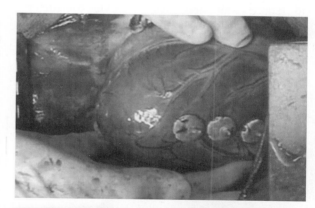

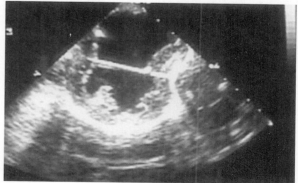

FIGURE 82-5

Three transventricular splints are placed to bisect the ventricle (far left), and epicardial pads are used to tighten the Myosplint device to the desired diameter (upper right). Echocardiography (bottom right) demonstrates the bisected bilobular left ventricular shape change.

bypass surgery. In 16 European patients, there have been no perioperative device-related complications such as bleeding, thromboembolism, or vascular damage. From the European experience, the study design and selection criteria were developed to conduct the safety trial in the United States, which is just beginning.

The Acorn Cardiac Support Device is a custom-made meshlike polyester jacket that is surgically placed around the ventricles of the heart (Fig 82-6). While the Myosplint concept was born from the Batista experience, the concept of the Acorn was developed from the earlier work with dynamic cardiomyoplasty, which demonstrated that the benefit gained from the procedure may have been as a consequence of the girdling effect of the latissimus dorsi muscle. The Acorn device is intended to reduce wall stress and myocyte overstretch during end-diastole and periodic volume overload conditions by supporting the heart. By limiting or

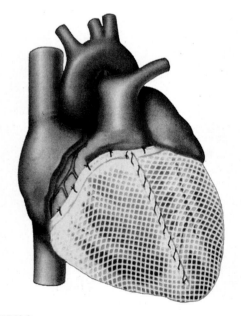

FIGURE 82-6

The Acorn Cardiac Support Device is a preformed polyester mesh–like device surgically placed over the ventricles.

reducing these key remodeling stimuli, the remodeling process may be halted or reversed without an adverse effect on myocardial compliance. The advantages of this device, as opposed to dynamic cardiomyoplasty, are the simplicity of use and the low surgical risk.

The initial safety study was done on a cohort of 29 patients treated with the Acorn device in Berlin, Germany. Ten patients, five of whom had concomitant MV repair and five treated with the device only, have reached 12 months of follow-up. Improvements in LV function and reverse remodeling were initially noted at 3 months and were sustained at 1 year. Acorn therapy was associated with a significant reduction in LV end-diastolic diameter, a significant increase in ejection fraction, and decrease in mitral regurgitation.

From this initial safety study the selection criteria were developed to conduct the randomized clinical trial in North America (Raman et al., 2000). In the United States, 20 patients have been enrolled to date (August 2001), 5 at the Cleveland Clinic; there have been no device-related adverse events to date. Although the data provided by the European experience are encouraging, it is too early to determine the efficacy of this device.

Aside from devices, advances in molecular biology and gene transfer techniques have resulted in new developments in the field of tissue engineering, which includes gene therapy and cell transplantation.

Transplantation of muscle cells into the damaged myocardium as an adjunct to CABG is a potential therapeutic strategy that could augment and possibly heal the failing heart (Weisel et al., 2001; El Oakley et al., 2001). Earlier research with the transplantation of fetal and neonatal cardiac myocytes demonstrated the ability of these cells to integrate with and augment the function of the failing human heart. The widespread clinical application of this approach is currently limited, however, due to the ethical dilemma with the use of human and fetal tissue. Adult bone marrow is another fertile prospect for harvesting autologous stem cells. Skeletal muscle cells can be recovered from the recipient's own body, with the advantage of being a readily available and unlimited source, without the risk of rejection. A phase I trial using skeletal muscle cells has just commenced at the authors' institution and will enroll a total of six patients. A marble-sized section of muscle from the patient's forearm or leg is removed at least 3 weeks prior to the procedure. From this, 10 to 300 million skeletal muscle cells (increasing incremental doses), propagated and genetically modified in vitro, are then implanted into the diseased myocardium.

Direct gene transfer (via intramyocardial injection) of naked DNA encoding vascular endothelial growth factor (VEGF) is another exciting approach for myocardial repair. Early trials, performed primarily to address safety concerns, were conducted on patients with chronic myocardial ischemia. In follow-up, stress single-photon emission computed tomography myocardial imaging demonstrated that mean perfusion-defect scores for both stress and rest images were significantly decreased at day 60, suggesting substantial improvement. Clinical trials to evaluate the efficacy of VEGF gene transfer to allow for a left ventricular assist device (LVAD) as a bridge to recovery as an alternative to cardiac transplantation will be started in the near future. Also, gene therapy for heart failure is being actively investigated in the laboratory.

Mechanical Support

Implantable pulsatile LVADs have evolved to become standard therapy as a bridge to transplant. The current LVADs approved by the U.S. Food and Drug Administration provide excellent hemodynamic support, low need for right ventricular support, and freedom from device failure (Kasirajan et al., 2000; Stevenson et al., 2001). The portable battery-powered devices allow the majority of patients to be discharged from the hospital after they are rehabilitated, typically while waiting for heart transplant. In the authors' experience with almost 300 LVADs since December 1991, survival to transplantation has been 70%. The major clinical problem with the current pulsatile devices continues to be infection. Future strategies for prevention of LVAD-associated bloodstream infections are directed at eliminating the portal of entry: the transcutaneous drive line. The new continuous-flow pumps (Jarvik 2000, Micromed DeBakey), with smaller transcutaneous drive lines, currently in clinical trials, may provide the key for true destination therapy or long term support as a bridge to recovery.

LVAD as bridge to recovery represents an intriguing phenomeneon as therapy for advanced heart failure, and work in this area is expanding. It is thought that combining mechanical support with pharmacologic agents known to optimize unloading and promote reverse LV remodeling may lead to myocardial recovery. The Harefield experience under the direction of Sir Magdi Yacoub has demonstrated improved cardiac function without the support of LVADs and improvement in exercise capacity with the administration of clenbuterol, a beta agonist known to have an effect on skeletal and myocardial cells. Five patients in this study have undergone successful device explantation (Yacoub et al., 2001).

The area of bridge to recovery poses a formidable challenge, but as the donor crisis escalates, research in this area should continue.

Transplantation

Human heart transplantation is used only for the "tip of the iceberg" of patients with end-stage cardiac disease. The short- and long-term success of heart transplantation is limited by the severe shortage of donor organs; only 2300 human heart transplants per year are performed in the United States, far below the anticipated 20,000 to 30,000 patients per year who could benefit from this therapy. The authors' experience using "marginal" donors and older donors (who have no evidence of coronary artery disease by coronary angiogram) is very encouraging. This has allowed us to take older donors (up to age 68 years) and transplant older recipients. Currently with 63 patients over 65 years of age, 1- and 2-year survival rates for this selected older transplant recipient group are 87% and 83% ($p = $ ns vs. younger patients with 88% and 87% 1- and 2-year survival). With the use of older donors and those previously considered marginal, the authors have been able to increase the number of transplants performed. However, transplantation still does not address the epidemiologic problem of CHF, and the long-term effects of immunosuppression and chronic rejection continue to be problematic for many recipients.

Conclusions

The surgical options for CHF are a part of a larger paradigm shift in management. Viable and effective surgical options other than cardiac transplant and ventricular assist devices clearly exist and are applicable to a large portion of patients with CHF. The rapidly evolving therapies for altering the LV remodeling that underlies CHF progression are an exciting and quickly evolving area. These therapies are the foundation of the new discipline of CHF surgery within cardiovascular surgery.

REFERENCES

Bishay ES et al: Mitral valve surgery in patients with severe left ventricular dysfunction. Eur J Cardiothorac Surg 17:213–21, 2000

Buckberg GD: Defining the relationship between akinesia and dyskinesia and the cause of left ventricular failure after anterior infarction and reversal of remodeling to restoration. J Thorac Cardiovasc Surg 116:47, 1998

Connolly HM et al: Severe aortic stenosis with low transvalvular gradient and severe left ventricular dysfunction: Result of aortic valve replacement in 52 patients. Circulation 101:1940, 2000

Dor V et al: Efficacy of endoventricular patch plasty in large postinfarction akinetic scar and severe left ventricular dysfunction: comparison with a series of large dyskinetic scars. J Thorac Cardiovasc Surg 116:50, 1998

El Oakley RM et al: Myocyte transplantation for myocardial repair: A few good cells can mend a broken heart. Ann Thorac Surg 71:1724, 2001

Franco-Cereceda A et al: Partial left ventriculectomy for dilated cardiomyopathy: Is this an alternative to transplantation? J Thorac Cardiovasc Surg 121:879, 2001

Kasirajan V et al: Clinical experience with chronic use of implantable left ventricular assist devices: Indications, implantation, and outcomes. Semin Thorac Cardiovasc Surg 12:229, 2000

Kass DA: Surgical approaches to arresting or reversing chronic remodeling of the failing heart. J Card Fail 4:57, 1998

Luciani GB et al: Predicting long-term functional results after myocardial revascularization in ischemic cardiomyopathy. J Thorac Cardiovasc Surg 120: 478, 2000

Marwick TH: Use of standard imaging techniques for prediction of postrevascularization functional recovery in patients with heart failure. J Card Fail 5:334, 1999

McCarthy JF et al: Partial left ventriculectomy and mitral valve repair for end-stage congestive heart failure. Eur J Cardiothorac Surg 13:337, 1998

McCarthy PM et al: Device-based change in left ventricular shape: A new concept for the treatment of dilated cardiomyopathy. J Thorac Cardiovasc Surg 122:482, 2001

Mickleborough L et al: Results of revascularization in patients with severe left ventricular dysfunction. Circulation 92 (Suppl): II73, 1995

Qin JX et al: Real-time three dimensional echocardiographic study of left ventricular function after infarct exclusion surgery for ischemic cardiomyopathy. Circulation, 102 III-101, 2000

Raman J et al: Ventricular containment as an adjunctive procedure in ischemic cardiomyopathy: Early results. Ann Thorac Surg 70: 1124, 2000

Starling RC et al: Results of partial left ventriculectomy for dilated cardiomyopathy: Hemodynamic, clinical, and echocardiographic observations. J Am Coll Cardiol 36:2098, 2000

Stevenson LW et al: Mechanical cardiac support 2000: Current applications and future trial design; a consensus conference report. J Am Coll Cardiol 37:340, 2001

Weisel RD et al: Cell transplantation comes of age. J Thorac Cardiovasc Surg 121:835, 2001

Yacoub MH et al: Bridge to recovery: The Harefield approach. J Congestive Heart Failure and Circulatory Support 2:27, 2001

Yau TM et al: Predictors of operative risk for coronary bypass operations in patients with left ventricular dysfunction. J Thorac Cardiovasc Surg 118:1006, 1999

83

MANAGEMENT OF THE CARDIAC TRANSPLANT PATIENT

Maria Rosa Costanzo

Demographics and Outcome of Cardiac Transplantation

Data from the Registry of the International Society for Heart and Lung Transplantation (ISHLT) show that the number of cardiac transplants (CTs) performed worldwide gradually declined from 1995 to approximately 3000 in 1998 (Hosenpud et al., 1999). The age distribution of CT recipients clusters between 35 and 64 years. Coronary artery disease (CAD) and dilated cardiomyopathy each account for approximately 45% of CTs. The remaining 10% are performed because of valvular or congenital heart disease, retransplantation, or miscellaneous causes.

Over a 15-year period, the overall 1-year survival after CT is 79%. The patient half-life, or time to 50% survival, is 8.8 and 11.5 years, respectively, for the overall population and for the patient surviving the first postoperative year. The fall off in survival is almost a straight line from year 1 to year 15, with a constant mortality rate of 4% per year. Independent risk factors for a poorer survival after CT have been identified among characteristics of both recipient (retransplantation, preoperative requirement for mechanical circulatory or ventilatory assistance, native heart disease other than ischemic or dilated cardiomyopathy, increasing age, and, at 5 years, presence of CAD, and female gender) and donor (length of ischemia time, female gender, and increasing age). A significant interaction has been identified between ischemia time and donor age. By 1 year after CT, the majority of patients are considered to have no functional limitation, yet fewer than 40% are employed. In the first postoperative year, 40% of CT recipients require hospitalization for rejection, infection, or other comorbidities. Later hospitalization rates fall steadily, but approximately 18% of patients still require hospitalization between the third and fourth postoperative year (Table 83-1).

Within the first postoperative year, rejection and infection are the most common causes of death. More than 1 year after CT, CAD of the transplanted heart is the most common cause of deaths. Between 4 and 5 years after CT, nonlymphoid malignancy is the second most common cause of mortality, accounting for 18% of the deaths. More than 1 year after CT, 3 to 4% of deaths each year are caused by lymphomas.

TABLE 83-1

INCIDENCE OF COMPLICATIONS 1 AND 4 YEARS
AFTER CARDIAC TRANSPLANTATION

Morbidity	Year 1,%	Year 4,%
Hypertension	66.9	71.4
Renal dysfunction	20.5	23.9
Creatinine > 221 μmol/L		
(> 2.5 mg/dL)	7.9	7.4
End-stage renal disease	1.2	1.9
Hyperlipidemia	39.3	56.3
Diabetes	19.5	17.5
Malignancy	3.9	8.5
Lymphoma	31.8	12.1
Skin	34.3	54.5
Other	26.9	30.3
Not reported	6.9	3.0

Selection of Candidates for Cardiac Transplantation

In the United States alone, at least 40,000 heart failure patients progress to end-stage disease each year. The fact that only 3000 CTs are performed each year underscores the severe discrepancy between the number of potential CT candidates and that of patients fortunate enough to receive a suitable donor organ. It also demonstrates the crucial need to restrict the option of CT to the patients who have heart failure refractory to conventional medical and surgical therapy and are likely to derive the maximum benefit from the procedure. In an effort to achieve this goal, increasing attention has been focused on improving the ability to predict the prognosis of patients with advanced heart failure and to standardize the criteria for listing patients for CT (Costanzo et al., 1995). Uniform criteria for the selection of candidates for CT have been formulated and endorsed by the relevant professional organizations [American Society of Transplantation (AST), American Heart Association, American College of Cardiology, ISHLT, and United Network for Organ Sharing (UNOS)].

Despite the progress made in the standardization of CT candidate selection, serious limitations persist in the ability to risk-stratify heart failure patients. There is no variable (including peak exercise oxygen consumption) that, taken alone, can accurately predict the outcome of heart failure patients. This fact has stimulated attempts to stratify the risk of individual patients according to scores inclusive of multiple independent prognostic variables. Aaronson and colleagues, using a prognostic index based on etiology of heart failure, NYHA functional class, third heart sound, pulmonary artery diastolic pressure, pulmonary artery wedge pressure, mean systemic arterial pressure, and cardiac output, were able to stratify 388 CT candidates into three risk classes. Actuarial survival at 1 year after entry into the CT waiting list was 40% for the patients in the high-risk group, 75% for the 160 patients in the intermediate-risk group, and 95% for the 123 patients in the low-risk group.

A newer study by the same authors prospectively applied and validated in a separate group of patients two prognostic models, one consisting exclusively of variables obtained noninvasively, the other including the measurement of pulmonary artery wedge pressure. Since there was no statistical advantage afforded by the inclusion of invasive measures in the analysis, the authors concluded that the noninvasive index is sufficient to predict the outcome of patients with heart failure. Included in the noninvasive prognostic model were ischemic etiology of heart disease, resting heart rate, left ventricular ejection fraction, mean systemic arterial pressure, peak exercise oxygen consumption, serum sodium level, and presence of a cardioverter defibrillator. The priority listing for CT has recently been changed to reflect the new patient categories created by newer therapeutic opportunities such as outpatient administration of intravenous inotropic agents or the ability to discharge from the hospital patients supported with ventricular assist devices.

The UNOS listing criteria for CT (as of January, 1999) *in descending order of urgency* are as follows:

1. Mechanical circulatory support for acute hemodynamic decompensation

2. Mechanical circulatory support for longer than 30 days and evidence of serious device-related complications
3. Mechanical ventilation
4. Need for continuous hemodynamic monitoring of left ventricular filling pressure *and* for high-dose single or multiple inotropic agents
5. Mechanical assist device implanted for longer than 30 days
6. Continuous infusion of intravenous inotropic agents
7. CT candidates who do not meet the above criteria.

Operative Procedure

The CT procedure developed by Lower and Shumway (biatrial, pulmonary, and aortic anastomosis) is still widely employed. However, in recent years, modifications of this procedure have been described and carried out in the clinical setting. The bicaval anastomosis, as the name implies, consists of the anastomosis of donor superior and inferior venae cavae to those of the recipient. The potential benefits of this procedure include maintenance of the normal relationship between donor right atrium and ventricle, thereby preserving the right atrial contribution to right ventricular cardiac output and reducing tricuspid regurgitation, and preservation of the integrity of the sinus node, thus facilitating restoration of sinus rhythm. A limitation of the bicaval anastomosis procedure is that it requires additional operating time and therefore prolongs ischemia time. A few surgeons have performed a total orthotopic CT procedure, which consists of both bicaval anastomosis and anastomosis of donor and recipient pulmonary veins, thus preserving the anatomic integrity of both right and left atria.

Management of Cardiac Transplant Recipients

During the past decade, numerous important changes have occurred in the management of CT recipients in terms of rejection prophylaxis and treatment and prevention and therapy of immunosuppression-related comorbidities.

Immunosuppression

During the past 10 years, the number of CT centers that use perioperative antilymphocyte therapy with either polyclonal horse antithymocyte globulin (HATG) or murine anti-CD3 monoclonal (OKT3) antibodies has declined significantly. The CT centers that do not routinely use antilymphocyte therapy employ it only in patients in whom cyclosporine (CSA) therapy must be delayed because of preoperative renal dysfunction. More recently, chimeric and humanized anti-interleukin-2 (IL-2) receptor monoclonal antibodies have been studied for rejection prophylaxis. Clinical trials in renal transplant recipients have shown that the perioperative use of anti-IL-2 receptor antibodies significantly decreases the incidence of acute rejection and prolongs allograft and patient survival. One of these, zenapax (Roche), is currently being evaluated in a prospective randomized clinical trial in CT recipients.

A significant expansion has occurred in the armamentarium of drugs that can be used for maintenance immunosuppression. A microemulsion formulation of CSA, neoral (Novartis), has been introduced and subjected to a randomized comparison with the earlier CSA formulation, sandimmune (Novartis), in 380 CT recipients. Compared to sandimmune-treated patients, those given neoral had fewer episodes of rejection requiring anti-T cell therapy (6.4 vs. 16.7%; $p = .002$) and fewer cytomegalovirus infections (11.2 vs. 18.8%; $p = .044$). Compared to sandimmune-treated patients, those given neoral required lower CSA doses to achieve target trough CSA levels and, at 12 months, had higher mean triglycerides, creatinine, and diastolic blood pressure levels.

Tacrolimus (FK506 Fujisawa) also has been compared to CSA in both a U.S. and a European trial. Patients in the two treatment groups had similar rates of rejection, infection, hyperglycemia, and renal function. The tacrolimus-treated patients had lower rates of hypertension requiring pharmacologic therapy in both the U.S. (48 vs. 71%; $p = .05$) and the European trials (59.5 vs. 87.55%; $p = .025$)

To date the largest study conducted in cardiac transplantation is the 3-year, double-blind, randomized multicenter trial comparing the effects of mycophenolate mofetil (MMF) with those of azathioprine in 650 CT recipients treated with CSA and prednisone (Kobashigawa et al., 1998). MMF inhibits de novo purine synthesis by blocking the enzyme inosine monophosphate dehydrogenase. Because lymphocytes lack the *salvage pathway* for purine synthesis, MMF selectively inhibits lymphocyte proliferation. Three-year survival was greater in MMF than in azathioprine-treated patients (88.1 vs. 81.6%; $p = .029$), correlating to a 35% reduction in mortality. Most of the excess deaths in the azathioprine group were due to cardiovascular events, infection, and allograft rejection. In addition, serial evaluation of the allografts' coronary arteries with intracoronary ultrasound (ICUS) has shown a trend for intimal thickening to involve a smaller portion of the vessels' circumference in the MMF than in the azathioprine group.

Long-Term Complications After Cardiac Transplantation

Chronic Rejection: Coronary Artery Disease of the Transplanted Heart

Cardiac transplant CAD is the leading cause of death beyond the first postoperative year. This unique and unusually accelerated type of CAD affects both epicardial and intramural coronary arteries and veins. The vascular injury typical of CT CAD is attributable to many factors including the immune response of the recipient against the allograft; ischemia-reperfusion injury; cytomegalovirus infection; and classic risk factors for CAD, such as hyperlipidemia, hypertension, and insulin resistance. The obstructive vascular lesions are thought to progress through repetitive endothelial injury followed by repair response (Weis and von Scheidt et al., 1997). ICUS imaging has confirmed a dual morphology with donor-transmitted or de novo focal, noncircumferential plaques in proximal segments and/or a diffuse concentric pattern in the distal segments of the

vessels. No correlation has been found between the progression of epicardial and microvascular CAD. Apoptosis and loss of functional vascular remodeling may have a significant role in the development and progression of clinically relevant CAD. New strategies for the prevention and treatment of CT CAD include approaches to block T cell co-stimulation and expression of adhesion molecules and methods to augment endogenous nitric oxyde bioavailability. As noted above, antiproliferative agents, such as MMF and HMG-CoA reductase inhibitors, may slow the progression of CAD. Percutaneous transluminal coronary angioplasty is only a palliative procedure for clinically significant obstructive lesions, but it is associated with high restenosis rates and does not alter prognosis. Experiences with stenting, coronary artery bypass grafting, and percutaneous or transmyocardial laser revascularization are very limited. Currently, the only definitive treatment for CT CAD is repeat transplantation. This approach remains highly controversial, however, because it requires the use of scarce donor organs for patients unlikely to have a postoperative survival as high as that of patients undergoing their first CT; Ensley and colleagues (1992), using data from the ISHLT, showed that even "ideal" candidates for repeat CT (CAD as the cause of allograft failure, longer intervals between transplants, lack of preoperative mechanical assistance, and first transplant after 1985) have a 1-year survival of 64%, which is significantly lower than that achieved after the first CT.

Only the clinical application of strategies that effectively induce tolerance (specific unresponsiveness toward donor tissues without the need for long-term immunosuppression) will significantly decrease the incidence and severity of CT CAD.

Osteoporosis

Recipients of cardiac transplantation have multiple risk factors for the development of osteoporosis (Epstein et al., 1995). Preoperative predisposing factors include impaired renal and hepatic function, use of loop diuretics, and heparin anticoagulation. Postoperatively, the use of glucocorticoids and calcineurin phosphatase inhibitors, such as CSA and tacrolimus, is the main factor in the development of osteoporosis. The most critical period of bone loss is within the first 6 months, with the most dramatic reduction occurring in the first 3 months after CT. Trabecular bone is at the greatest risk, with vertebral fractures occurring most commonly. Recipients of CT should be evaluated by bone densitometry and measurements of vitamin D metabolites, blood urea nitrogen, creatinine, calcium, and phosphate levels. Markers of bone turnover may help in assessing the rate of remodeling. Gonadal function should be ascertained by measurement of serum levels of testosterone in males and estradiol in females. Therapy should be directed toward prevention of bone loss as well as restoration of bone already lost. Calcium, vitamin D, and sex hormone replacement, when indicated, are now begun preoperatively, upon placement of the patients on the CT waiting list, and continued indefinitely. Other antiresorptive agents, such as calcitonin, bisphosphonates, or fluoride, should be used when clinically indicated.

Hyperlipidemia

Potential causes of hyperlypidemia in CT recipients include diet, genetic predisposition, and immunosuppressive therapy. By inhibiting the enzyme 26-hydroxylase, CSA decreases bile acids synthesis from cholesterol and cholesterol transport to the intestines (Ventura et al., 1997). In addition, CSA, by binding to low-density lipoprotein (LDL), increases serum LDL cholesterol levels and, by increasing hepatic lipase and decreasing lipoprotein lipase, reduces the clearance of very low density lipoprotein (VLDL) and LDL. Glucocorticoids affect multiple enzymes involved in lipid metabolism, including HMG-CoA reductase, resulting in increased levels of VLDL, total cholesterol, and triglyceride, and decreased high-density lipoprotein levels. It is not surprising, therefore, that lipid abnormalities are reported in as many as 60 to 80% of CT recipients receiving triple-drug immunosuppression. Hyperlipidemia usually develops at 3 to 18 months postoperatively and slowly decreases as time after CT lengthens.

Studies previously described in the cardiac transplantation section have consistently shown that early control of hypercholesterolemia with statin drugs reduces the incidence of acute rejection and the development and severity of CT CAD. Kobashigawa and colleagues reported that at 1 year after CT, compared to 50 patients given no HMG-CoA inhibitors, 47 CT patients started on pravastatin within 6 weeks of CT had a significant reduction in hemodynamically compromising acute rejection (3 vs. 14; $p = .005$), a lower incidence of angiography or autopsy-proven CT CAD (3 vs. 10; $p = .049$), and a better survival (94 vs. 78%; $p = .025$) (Kobashigawa and Kasiske, 1997). The same investigators recently reported that the benefits of lipid-lowering therapy are maintained at 5 years in terms of freedom from CAD and/or death (64 vs. 55%), and survival (83 vs. 62%; $p < .05$). Based on the results of these studies, the current recommendation is that upon documentation of hyperlipidemia [total cholesterol >5.2 mmol/L (>200 mg/dL) and LDL cholesterol >3.4 mmol/L (>130 mg/dL) on two readings], the American Heart Association step I diet be instituted/continued and a statin drug be started (lovastatin, 10 to 20 mg; pravastatin, 20 to 40 mg; simvastatin, 5 to 20 mg). Cardiac transplant recipients given statin drugs should be carefully monitored for the occurrence of myositis. For those CT recipients with hypertryglyceridemia refractory to diet [>2.3 mmol/L (>200 mg/dL)], fibric acid derivatives appear to be a safe and effective option. The safety and efficacy of combination lipid-lowering therapy awaits further study.

Hypertension

As shown above, the 1- and 4-year incidence of hypertension requiring treatment in CT recipients is 66.9% and 71.4%, respectively. Cyclosporine-based immunosuppression is the major culprit for the development of hypertension in CT recipients. The mechanisms that underlie CSA-induced hypertension include endothelin-mediated vasoconstriction, impaired vasodilatation secondary to reduction in nitric oxide, and altered cytosolic calcium translocation. In addition, other studies have shown that CSA activates the sympathetic nervous and the renin-angiotensin systems and alters prostaglandin metabolism.

Hemodynamic features of CSA-induced hypertension consist of elevated peripheral vascular resistance and ventricular-vascular uncoupling, both of which contribute to the development of left ventricular hypertrophy. The management of CSA-induced hypertension is often very difficult despite the use of multiple drug regimens. Meticulous attention to dietary sodium intake and minimization of CSA and glucocorticoid doses, as well as avoidance of nonsteroidal anti-inflammatory drugs, are critical therapeutic steps. Therapy should also be adjusted based on observations that CT recipients lack the normal nocturnal decline in blood pressure and that early morning blood pressure is often the highest. The first multicenter randomized trial comparing the efficacy of the calcium antagonist diltiazem versus that of the angiotensin-converting enzyme inhibitor lisinopril was recently published by Brozena and colleagues (1996). Of 55 patients randomized to diltiazem, 38% achieved a diastolic blood pressure <90 mmHg, 42% did not respond, and 20% were withdrawn from the study. Of 61 patients given lisinopril, 46% responded, 36% did not, and 18% were withdrawn from the study. Thus both agents achieve blood pressure control in fewer than 50% of CT recipients, underscoring the importance of using multiple antihypertensive agents in patients with CSA-induced hypertension.

Renal Dysfunction

The improved survival after CT has been associated with an increased incidence of CSA-related renal dysfunction. The histopathologic abnormalities occurring in the kidneys of CT recipients treated with CSA have been extensively described. However, the factors that predispose a subgroup of CT recipients to develop severe renal dysfunction, which in some cases progresses to end-stage renal disease, have not been systematically evaluated. In one study, Sehgal and collegues compared 39 CT recipients with serum creatinine levels >212 μmol/L (>2.4 mg/dL) with 41 CT recipients with serum creatinine levels <150 μmol/L (<1.7 mg/dL) (Sehgal et al.,

1995). All 80 patients were followed for an average of 4.7 years after CT. Patients with more severe renal insufficiency tended to be older and to have a lower mean glomerular filtration rate (GFR) before CT. There were no differences in race, gender, or history of hypertension between the two groups. Although both groups experienced an improvement in GFR after CT and a subsequent decline by 6 months after CT, the group with greater baseline renal insufficiency achieved a lower peak GFR and a far lower GFR at 6 months after CT. Only the group with baseline creatinine >212 μmol/L (>2.4 mg/dL) showed a continued decline in GFR beyond 6 months. This group also developed more severe post-CT hypertension, requiring a greater number of medications for control. Lipids levels tended to be higher in the patients with greater renal insufficiency. The two groups were similar in terms of CSA dose and levels throughout the study period. The results of this study suggest that older patients with greater preoperative renal insufficiency and those whose 6-month postoperative GFR is more depressed are at higher risk for the development of progressive renal failure. Effective novel interventions to arrest the progression of chronic renal failure remain elusive.

Who Should Manage Cardiac Transplant Recipients?

The prevalence of managed care in the marketplace and the resultant fiscal constraints imposed on cardiac transplantation has resulted in incentives to send CT recipients back to their primary care physician after CT. The following guidelines have been suggested for the primary physician caring for CT recipients: in the first 3 postoperative months, the patient should be monitored at the CT center; after the first 3 postoperative months, and in the absence of significant CT-related complications, the patient may return to the primary care physician for all general medical care unrelated to the CT. Postoperative care by the CT center usually includes endomyocardial biopsies for rejection surveillance and

TABLE 83–2

CONDITIONS NECESSITATING REFERRAL TO THE CARDIAC TRANSPLANT CENTER

Suspected allograft rejection
  Unexplained fever
  Relative hypotension
  New symptoms of fatigue, dyspnea

Allograft dysfunction

New-onset renal failure

Fever without an obvious source

Complicated infections

Cardiac events (myocardial infarction, congestive heart
  failure, syncope, arrhythmia, sudden death)

Suspected major abdominal disease

Malignancy other than skin cancer

Anticipated intolerance to oral medication and need to
  administer immunosuppressive drugs intravenously

Medication change or intolerance

Possible noncompliance

evaluation of allograft function at intervals that are
<3 months. Optimal post-CT management requires
an understanding of the unique physiologic features
of the transplanted heart, as well as in-depth knowledge of drug interactions with immunosuppressive
agents. Patients are usually instructed not to take
medications unless prescribed or approved by the
transplant team. This policy is aimed at avoiding
bone marrow suppression or renal failure by making
the appropriate adjustments in CSA and/or azathioprine doses, should the patient require medications
such as erythromycin, ketoconazole, diltiazem, or
allopurinol. The instances in which the primary care
physician should consult or refer the CT recipient to
the CT center are summarized in Table 83-2.

REFERENCES

Brozena SC et al: Effectiveness and safety of diltiazem or
  lisinopril in treatment of hypertension after heart
  transplantation. Results of a prospective, randomized,
  multicenter trial. J Am Coll Cardiol 27:1707–12, 1996
Costanzo MR et al: Selection and treatment of candidates for
  heart transplantation. Circulation 92:3593, 1995
Ensley RD et al: Predictors of survival after repeat transplantation. The Registry of the International Society for Heart
  and Lung Transplantation. J. Heart Lung Transplant 11:
  S142–58, 1992
Epstein S et al: Organ transplantation and osteoporosis. Curr
  Opin Rheumatol 7:255, 1995
Hosenpud JD et al: The Registry of the International Society
  for Heart and Lung Transplantation. Sixteenth official
  report. J Heart Lung Transpl 18:611, 1999
Kobashigawa JA, Kasiske BL: Hyperlipidemia in solid organ
  transplantation. Transplantation 63:331, 1997
Kobashigawa JA et al: A randomized active-controlled trial
  of mycophenolate mofetil in heart transplant recipients.
  Mycophenolate Mofetil Investigators. Transplantation
  66:507, 1998
Sehgal V et al: Progressive renal insufficiency following cardiac transplantation: Cyclosporine, lipids and hypertension. Am J Kidney Dis 26:193, 1995
Ventura HO et al: Mechanisms of hypertension in cardiac
  transplantation and the role of cyclosporine. Curr Opin
  Cardiol 12:375, 1997
Weis M, von Scheidt W: Cardiac allograft vasculopathy. A
  review. Circulation 96:2069, 1997

IMPLANTABLE LEFT VENTRICULAR ASSIST DEVICES*

Nicholas G. Smedira

Left ventricular assist devices (LVADs) were first used over 30 years ago as a means of supporting patients after cardiac surgery while they awaited ventricular functional recovery or transplantation. Encouraged by these early successes and generously supported by the National Heart, Lung, and Blood Institute, multiple centers continued the bioengineering quest to develop a circulatory support system for chronic permanent cardiac replacement. Multiple devices were designed and clinically tested and have proven quite successful for temporary cardiac support, but the goal of permanent cardiac replacement has yet to be realized. This chapter will describe the implantable LVADs currently available for circulatory support, review the indications for and results of their use, and preview new devices and applications.

Mechanical Circulatory Support

Mechanical circulatory devices can be categorized in many ways, but a useful organization is to separate the devices by their duration of use and whether the device is implantable. Short-term support is accomplished with extracorporeal life support system (ECLS) or the ABIOMED BVS (Abiomed Inc., Danvers, MA). For longer duration of support, mechanical circulatory support is possible with one of three implantable systems—the Novacor LVAS (World Heart Corp., Ottawa, Canada), the Heartmate Vented Electric System (Thoratec Corporation, Pleasanton, CA) and the CardioWest Total Artificial Heart (CardioWest Technologies, Tucson, AZ)—or with a paracorporeal system (not implanted inside the body)—the Thoratec VAS (Thoratec Corporation, Pleasanton, CA). The Thoratec and CardioWest devices have the advantage over the LVAS of biventricular support but are limited by lack of portability, and, in the case of the CardioWest system, the native heart is no longer available for backup in case of device failure and to allow myocardial recovery.

Implantable Left Ventricular Assist Devices

Two implantable assist devices have been studied extensively and are approved by the U.S. Food and

---

* See also in this volume Chap. 85 on Bridge to Transplantation with Mechanical Assist Devices and Chap. 86 on the Abiomed Total Artificial Heart.

Drug Administration (FDA) for circulatory support as a bridge to cardiac transplantation. The pump is implanted in a preperitoneal or rectus sheath pocket in the abdomen below the left hemidiaphragm (McCarthy et al., 1998). The devices have in common a pump inflow conduit that drains the left ventricle through the apex of the heart and ejects blood into the ascending aorta through Dacron grafts. Porcine inflow and outflow valves ensure unidirectional flow and are less thrombogenic than mechanical valves. The internal design and pumping mechanisms are different for the devices, and these have ramifications in terms of management and potential complications.

Heartmate Vented Electric LVAS

The blood-contacting surfaces are textured, and this encourages the deposition of cells and protein, which form a neointima that lines the pump surface. This unique feature results in minimal thrombus formation in the pump and an impressively low incidence of thromboemboli during support, with only aspirin used for anticoagulation (Color Plate 23, Figure 84-1). One unanticipated host device interaction with this neointima has been the chronic activation of the fibrinolytic and immune systems, which may be responsible for delayed bleeding complications, infections, and HLA sensitization while on support (Spanier et al., 1996).

A. Outflow conduit

B. Pump / Drive unit

C. Inflow conduit

D. Percutaneous lead

E. Reserve power pack

F. Electronic controller

G. Primary power pack

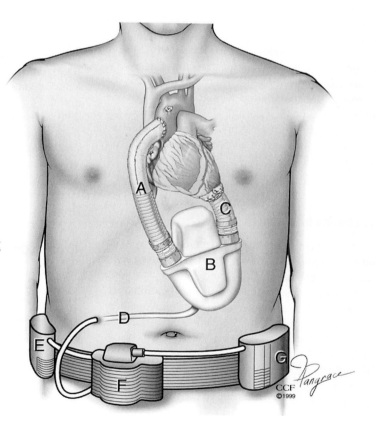

FIGURE 84-2

Novacor LVAS. Portable batteries power the LVAS, and the pump is placed below the diaphragm.

The Heartmate LVAS has a single percutaneous line that connects the pump with the external controller and batteries. It also vents the pump to equalize the air pressure and, in the case of electronic failure, allows emergency pneumatic pump activation. The device can be run in a fixed or automatic mode with a maximum pump flow of 9.6 L/min. The battery packs are lightweight, allowing patients considerable freedom of activity. Most stable patients are now discharged from the hospital to await transplantation.

Novacor LVAS

The Novacor system is an electrically actuated, smooth surface device that was designed for long-term support (Fig. 84-2). The pump has two pusher plates that compress during pump systole and result in ejection of blood. The pump can be run in a number of different modes that may be useful during support where the intent is for myocardial recovery; in this case, retraining the ventricle will likely be necessary. Anticoagulation with coumadin is necessary during support. Like the Heartmate system the device can be run on a battery, allowing ambulatory support while the patient awaits transplantation (See Color Plate 25, Figure 84-4).

Indications for Support

At the present time the implantable devices are approved only for cardiac support while the patient awaits transplantation. It is well known that some acute myopathies, such as acute myocarditis and postpartum and alcohol-related cardiomyopathies, might resolve during support, allowing for device removal. This concept of using the device to bridge to myocardial recovery is being extended to patients with idiopathic dilated cardiomyopathy and with chronic ischemic cardiomyopathy.

Support is indicated in transplant candidates with body surface areas greater than 1.5 m². Ischemic cardiomyopathy, primarily chronic but also after a large acute myocardial infarction; decompensated chronic idiopathic dilated cardiomyopathy; and postcar-

diotomy cardiac failure are the most common indications for support. The majority of patients are on multiple inotropic agents and an intraaortic balloon pump and are often ventilated. Despite this aggressive support, the patient is often hypotensive, and the cardiac output is less than 2.0 L/m² per minute with elevated filling pressures.

In most patients the need for LVAD support is quite obvious. In others, the timing of implant can be quite difficult. Two issues needing careful evaluation are the patient's neurologic status and ruling out possible infection as a cause for decompensation. After cardiac arrest, the possibility of intracerebral injury is increased because of prolonged hypoperfusion with hypoxia and as a result of the administration of potent platelet inhibitors and anticoagulants. Routine neurologic evaluation, including a detailed examination and a CT scan, is indicated. Often the neurologic findings are most consistent with a metabolic encephalopathy that will improve after LVAD support. Acute cardiac decompensation either after an acute myocardial infarction or in the setting of chronic congestive heart failure is often associated with fever and leukocytosis. In some cases the cardiac index is elevated. Line sepsis and aspiration or nosocomial pneumonia must be ruled out, as their presence is associated with a poor outcome after LVAD support (Kormos et al., 1996). Often the cause of the fever is never identified but is thought to be due to myocardial and systemic cytokine release.

LVAD Support and Recovery

Uncomplicated LVAD support is an impressive display of technical advances benefitting the patient. Hemodynamics normalize in the operating room, and over the course of LVAD support norepinephrine and neurohomone levels return to baseline (James et al., 1995). With a focus on nutrition and rehabilitation, most patients' cachexia is slowly reversed and patients are NYHA functional class I prior to transplantation. Despite these impressive improvements, patients supported with implantable LVADs demonstrate a lower functional capacity, as measured by peak oxygen consumption, compared to heart transplant recipients (Jaski et al., 1999).

These findings are in part a result of the maximal output of the devices, which is about 10 L/min.

After the patient has recovered from the surgery and is familiar with the function of the device, he or she is ready for discharge. This freedom is important to the family and can result in significant cost savings for the institution.

Results of Implantable LVADS

The implantable devices have been used clinically since 1984 as a bridge to transplantation. Multiple published series show that survival to transplant ranges from 65 to 80% with most centers having a >90% 1-year survival after transplant. At the author's institution, with over 200 implants, the survival to transplant has been 71% with the Heartmate Device and 67% with the Novacor System. The mean duration of support is 80 days. After transplantation, the survival is 92% and 80% for the Heartmate and Novacor systems, respectively.

Complications During LVAD Support

Complications during support are similar with both implantable devices and have important implications as we approach the use of these devices for cardiac replacement. Bleeding is a common complication after device insertion and occurs in a biphasic pattern. Initially after surgery approximately 20% of the patients will require reoperation for bleeding. This rate is slowly declining with technical improvement, the use of aprotinin, and the selection of patients before multiple organ failure has set in. Late bleeding, including gastrointestinal, pump pocket, and cerebral hemorrhage, is related to the fibrinolytic state of the Heartmate device and the need for anticoagulation with the Novacor system

Thromboemboli are devastating complications of all mechanical devices. The textured surface along with the porcine valves and the short textured inflow cannula of the Heartmate system have resulted in a thromboemboli rate of <10%. The Novacor system has a higher thromboemboli rate, approaching 20%. This rate is declining with modifications to the inflow and outflow cannulas.

Infections of the pump and pump pocket are a major impediment to satisfactory long-term support. The need for a percutaneous line predisposes the patient to colonization of the driveline, pump, and pump pocket. During the author's bridge-to-transplant experience bacteremia occurred in approximately 50% of the patients, while a pump pocket or driveline infection arose in 25%. Intraabdominal placement and antibiotic coating of the driveline may help reduce the incidence of infection, especially in patients in whom the device is permanent, but the solution to this problem is designing a device that is completely implantable. This has recently been accomplished.

Future Applications and Device Advances
Bridge to Recovery

The implantable LVAD has proven quite effective in bridging patients with end-stage heart disease to heart transplantation. However, heart transplantation is limited by the donor pool to about 2500 transplants a year in the United States. Alternatives to transplant are desperately needed. Fueled by this need and the initial experience of the Berlin Heart Institute, there is great interest in using the LVAD to support the patient while the device promotes myocardial recovery (Muller et al., 1997; Mancini et al., 1998). Which type of cardiomyopathy will recover, how long to support the patient before weaning the device so as to promote recovery yet not induce atrophy, and whether the recovery is long lasting are questions remaining to be answered.

Permanent Cardiac Support

Permanent or destination therapy has always been the goal of mechanical circulatory support. The Heartmate device is currently being evaluated in a 2-year randomized trial [Randomized Evaluation of Mechanical Assistance for the Treatment of Congestive Heart Failure (REMATCH) trial] comparing this device to medical therapy in nontransplant patients with end-stage heart failure. Survival and quality of life are two of the end-points of this study.

New Devices

As mentioned earlier the current implantable devices are limited by large size, percutaneous drivelines, and infection complications. Infections will be reduced when the devices are completely implantable. The first totally implanted LVAD (Lion Heart LVD2000 LVAS) was inserted on 10/26/99. The device is derived from the Thoratec pneumatic system and utilizes transcutaneous energy transmission and a compliance chamber to equilibrate pump pressure. Recently, the first totally implantable total artificial heart, the ABIO-COR TAH (Abiomed Inc., Danvers, MA), has been used as a complete heart replacement.

The next generation of pumps will be smaller and use less energy, and some will be totally implantable. An alternative to pulsatile pumps is continuous-flow pumps, one of which is the rotary pump. A rotary pump consists of a turbine that rotates at a very high number of revolutions and can generate flows of 15 L/min. The flow is continuous, therefore inflow and outflow valves are not needed. Due to the small size, the device will fit more patients, require a smaller pocket, and have greater flows than the pneumatic systems (See Color Plate 24, Figure 84-3) (Nose et al., 1998). Many devices are in various stages of development and offer the potential for wider application of mechanical circulatory support with fewer complications, lower cost, and an enhanced quality of life. The Debakey and Jarvik pumps are currently in clinical trials in the United States and Europe as a bridge to transplant. Early experience suggests that continuous flow is well tolerated, and the devices appear to be reliable.

REFERENCES

James KB et al: Effect of the implantable left ventricular assist device on neuroendocrine activation in heart failure. Circulation 92(suppl II): II-191, 1995

Jaski BE et al: Comparison of functional capacity in patients with end-stage heart failure following implantation of left ventricular assist device versus heart transplantation: Results of the experience with left ventricular assist device with exercise trial. J Heart Lung Transplant 18:1031, 1999

Kormos RL et al: Transplant candidate's clinical status rather than right ventricular function defines need for univentricular versus biventricular support. J Thorac Cardiovasc Surg 111:773, 1996

Mancini DM et al: Low incidence of myocardial recovery after left ventricular assist device implantation in patients with chronic heart failure. Circulation 98:2383, 1998

McCarthy PM et al: Cardiopulmonary support and physiology: One hundred patients with the Heartmate left ventricular assist device; evolving concepts and technology. J Thorac Cardiovasc Surg 115:904, 1998

Muller J et al: Weaning from mechanical support in patients with idiopathic dilated cardiomyopathy. Circulation 96:542, 1997

Spanier T et al: Activation of coagulation and fibrinolytic pathways in patients with left ventricular assist devices. J Thorac Cardiovasc Surg 112:1090, 1996

Nose Y et al: Rotary pumps: New developments and future perspectives. ASAIO 44:234–7, 1998

BRIDGE TO TRANSPLANTATION WITH MECHANICAL ASSIST DEVICES*

Jack G. Copeland & Richard G. Smith

In 1969, Cooley first attempted bridge to transplantation with the Liotta total artificial heart (TAH); later, in 1981; he tried with the Akutsu TAH. Oyer, with the Novacor left-ventricular assist system, and Hill, with the Thoratec extracorporeal pulsatile pump, had successful bridges to transplantation in late 1984. The authors had an unsuccessful experience with the Phoenix TAH in early 1985, followed by the first successful bridge with a TAH (Jarvik-7) in mid 1985 (Copeland et al., 1988). Since then, several thousand mechanical assist devices have been used as bridges to transplantation with progressively better results. The U.S. Food and Drug Administration has approved three devices for commercial distribution in the United States, and considerable information has accumulated on the efficacy of and the mortality and morbidity associated with these devices for implantation periods of 1 to 2 years. Estimates of the need for cardiac replacement in the United States have been in the range of 65,000 per year; the donor shortage of hearts (there are about 2500 available annually in the United States) has led

to pressure for alternative replacements. Finally, increasing severity of heart failure in those who are potential cardiac recipients has created more demand for bridge to transplantation.

Description of Devices

As time has passed, the diversity of mechanical assist devices has increased. This has allowed the surgeon to choose a device that is appropriate for the patient. None of the devices is suitable for all situations, and each has particular problems. Options include univentricular and biventricular support, pulsatile and nonpulsatile flow, and implantable or external to the body for a large variety of sizes and shapes.

Nonpulsatile External Centrifugal Blood Pump

A nonpulsatile external centrifugal blood pump (Fig. 85-1) is often used in cardiac surgical operations and in extracorporeal membrane oxygenation support. It is available in most institutions with cardiac surgical programs. In the bridge to transplantation setting, it has most often been used as a "bridge to bridge" temporary support system that maintains life until a

---

* See also in this volume Chap. 84 on Implantable Left Ventricular Assist Devices and Chap. 86 on the Abiomed Total Artificial Heart.

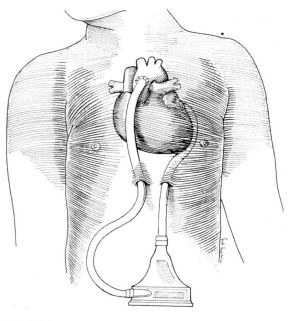

FIGURE 85-1

A centrifugal pump and a LVAD support configuration in a child. Blood is pumped from the left atrium to the aorta through the pump-head. The more common application of this pump-head is in extracorporeal membrane oxygenation support of the patient. This would incorporate an oxygenator and pump blood from the venous to the arterial system via a pump-head and an oxygenator.

longer-term device can be inserted. It is connected to the patient most often by arterial and venous cannulas and requires heparinization and continuous surveillance. It has been very useful as an immediately available, easily inserted support that enables patients to survive cardiac arrest or failure to wean from cardiopulmonary bypass. Physicians and surgeons then have time to assess vital organ function in these patients before proceeding to long-term support.

Recovery of patients with this type of support occurs in 10 to 25% of cases, particularly in those with acute myocardial infarction, acute viral myocarditis, and reperfusion injury after open-heart operations.

Arteriovenous connection with centrifugal pumps can provide a maximal flow of 6 L/min. The problems with this type of support limit its use to less than 1 week in most cases. Full systemic

heparinization is mandatory. Thrombocytopenia is progressive and time- and flow-related. Bleeding is the major complication. Membrane oxygenator malfunction and clotting of the base of the centrifugal pump are common and require change out of components. This support system therefore requires constant vigilance, with 24-h attendance by a perfusionist and intensive management by a physician.

Abiomed Pump

The Abiomed pump (Fig. 85-2) is an extracorporeal pulsatile blood pump that may be used for uni- or biventricular support. It is available in over 450

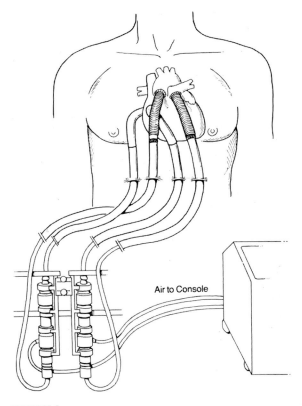

Air to Console

FIGURE 85-2

The biventricular atrial inflow configuration of the Abiomed pump. Blood is taken from the atria and pumped back into the respective great vessels. For left-sided pumping, a left ventricular inflow cannula is often used.

hospitals in the United States. The pumps drain the heart (atrial or ventricular apical connection) by gravity. Each pump consists of a vertical column with a compliant inflow chamber, connected by a polyurethane valve to an outflow chamber that has a rigid outer chamber and a pneumatically powered inner sac. Blood is pumped out through a second polyurethane valve to tubing that connects to a great vessel. This device is typically used in a biventricular configuration, sitting at the bedside, connected by tubing that may be 2 m (6 ft) in length. It is driven with an automatic console that needs no attendance. Maximal flows are limited by inflow tubing size to 6 L/min. The device is most useful in the failure to wean from cardiopulmonary bypass scenario. It is easily inserted. Problems include a tendency to cool the patient because of the long extracorporeal blood pathway, even though tubing insulation has been developed. The patient must be immobile for the duration of support. High afterloads prevent optimal outputs. Systemic anticoagulation limits thromboembolism, but transillumination of the clear plastic outer housing often permits direct visualization of clots that are commonly seen within 1 week of support. The value of this device is therefore its simplicity in rescuing surgical patients and supporting them for short periods of time.

Thoratec

Thoratec (Fig. 85-3) is an extracorporeal, pulsatile, pneumatically driven blood pump that is available commercially. Each ventricle has a rigid outer housing into which air is pumped and from which air is withdrawn. Within the outer housing is a seamless polyurethane bag into which blood flows through a plastic disc valve. Blood is pumped out through a second disc valve. Uni- or biventricular support is possible, and inflow connections can be from the atria or, for higher flows, from ventricular outflow cannulas. The cannulas are short, exiting from the mediastinum-like drainage tubes, allowing the ventricles to rest on the abdomen. The pneumatic console that drives the ventricles is large but mobile and may soon be replaced by a smaller, more portable one. Under

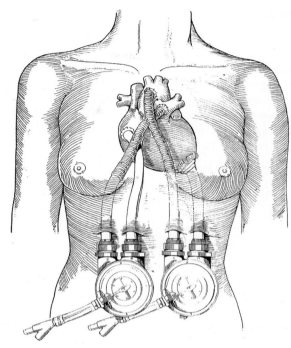

FIGURE 85-3

A biventricular configuration of the Thoratec pump using a left ventricular apical inflow conduit and a right atrial inflow conduit. This device may also be used with two ventricular inflow conduits. As can be seen, the ventricles sit outside the body, the conduits are attached to the ventricles and exit the body much as chest tubes would.

optimal conditions, this device may pump 5 to 6 L/min. It is easily inserted and may be used in patients from 20 to >100 kg. Long-term support of over 1 year has been possible in some patients. Thromboembolism and infection have been uncommon. Because of the possibility of inflow connection from the atrium, bridge to recovery of the native heart is possible. Problems have included lower flows (4 L/min) with atrial cannulation, and flow limitation regardless of cannulation (5 to 6 L/min) that may make resuscitation of very sick and/or large (>1.7 m² body surface area) patients difficult.

Novacor and Heartmate

Novacor (Fig. 85-4) and Heartmate (Fig. 85-5) are both left ventricular assist devices (LVADS) that are pulsatile, implantable (abdominal wall or preperitoneum), electric blood pumps. Both are available commercially. They have a wearable external controller and batteries connected to the device via a combination vent tube and electric cable that passes from the device through a subcutaneous

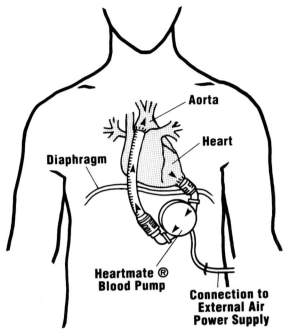

FIGURE 85-5

The Heartmate blood pump, which may connect externally to either an air supply or an electrical power supply. It is generally felt that the electrical device is better in that it is more portable in the long-term application.

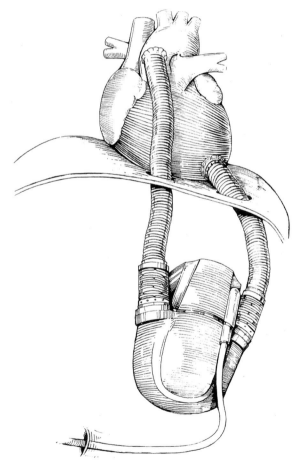

FIGURE 85-4

The Novacor pump, which pumps blood from the left-ventricular apex to the ascending aorta. The electrical venting cable exits near the superior iliac crest.

tunnel. There are significant differences between the two devices in durability, thrombogenicity, inflammatory response, durability, design, and implantation technique (Kormos et al., 1994; Oz et al., 1997), but they also have much in common. These LVADS are connected by an inflow conduit from the apex of the left ventricle that carries blood through a tissue valve into the pumping chamber. Electromechanical systems eject blood through an outflow valve into a conduit anastomosed to the aorta. They are capable of pumping at 6 to 7 L/min under optimal conditions. They completely unload the left ventricle; thus the native aortic valve ceases to open. In some rare instances, this unloading has led to recovery of ventricular function and device removal from patients who had had chronic dilated cardiomyopathies. About 70 to 75% of implanted patients survive to transplantation on the LVADS, and a few have survived over 3 years with Novacor support. Out-of-hospital living is possible with these highly portable, small controllers and batteries, thus dramatically reducing the cost of bridge to transplantation. The possibility of using these wearable devices as destination therapy or alternatives to transplantation and to medical therapy is currently being tested.

Problems with LVADS have included patient selection, durability, stroke, and infection. Patients supported with only a left-sided pump often have right heart failure that carries a significantly increased mortality rate. Also, very sick patients who are decompensating with pulmonary edema, pulmonary hypertension, renal failure, hepatic failure, and sepsis do poorly with support of only the left side. Recent publications have documented a slight increased risk of decreased device durability with Heartmate, increased stroke rate with Novacor, and increased opportunistic infection rate with Heartmate.

CardioWest

CardioWest (Fig. 85-6) is a TAH; it is an orthotopic biventricular pneumatic pulsatile blood pump. It is available in only five centers in the United States as of December 1999. It replaces the native ventricles and utilizes the native atria as inflow chambers. Blood passes from the atria across mechanical valves into polyurethane chambers. A diaphragm driven by air pressure forces blood out of the outflow valve. Counting intraventricular dead space, it has about 1000-mL volume displacement, which means that it will fit into patients with large hearts (>70 mm leftventricular end diastolic dimension), large chests (>10 cm distance from posterior sternum to anterior vertebral column at T-10), or large bodies (>1.6 m² body surface area). The driving console/computer monitor is currently large, but it is mobile; a smaller (camera case size) driver will soon be introduced. This device pumps at 7 to 8 L/min, eliminates arrhythmia problems seen in ventricular assist devices, and has been associated with a >80% survival to transplantation (Copeland et al., 1998). It is useful in very sick

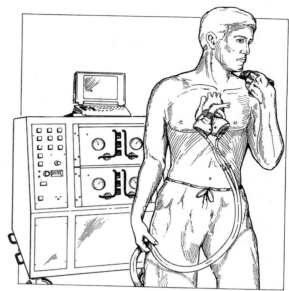

FIGURE 85-6

The orthotopically positioned CardioWest total artificial heart with the current controller driver apparatus. The controller driver has two sets of pumps in case of pump failure and a small computer console that gives continuous outputs and trends as well as the filling curve of the device and the driveline pressures.

patients, in those with right heart failure or recurrent ventricular arrythmias, and for those in whom global cardiac function has been lost (e.g., reperfusion injury, massive infarction, rejection, electromechanical dissociation). Return of renal and hepatic function is commonly seen after several days of support with the TAH. Using an anticoagulation therapy directed at both coagulation proteins and platelets, thromboembolism has been reduced to nearly the same level as is seen with mechanical valves. Major infection has not been a problem; the major problem is fitting the device in the mediastinum.

Miniature Continuous-Flow Pumps

Several very small continuous-flow pumps are under development. The axial flow pumps are cigar-shaped and approximately 15 cm (6 in.) long and 5 to 7.5 cm

(2 to 3 in.) in diameter. They are small electric motors that have an impeller rotating at about 10,000 rpm within a rigid housing. The centrifugal pumps are miniature versions of the larger pumps commonly used in cardiac surgery. Their dimensions are roughly $7.5 \times 7.5 \times 10$ cm ($3 \times 3 \times 4$ in.). Both types of devices are designed for univentricular support and can pump at rates of 4 to 6 L/min. These devices are driven by small controllers connected via transcutaneous leads and are wearable. The most common connection is left ventricle inflow to the pump and outflow into the aorta. The theoretical advantage of these devices is that their small size makes implantation easy and allows the surgeon some creativity in positioning the device to conform to the needs of particular patients. The usefulness of these devices and potential problems are currently being tested in Europe.

Patient Selection and Timing

Selection for bridge to transplantation implies first that the patient is potentially a cardiac recipient (Copeland et al., 1987). Thus, most patients over age 65 and those with active infection, irreversible elevation of the transpulmonary (pulmonary artery–left atrium) gradient (>15 mmHg), and irreversible dysfunction of major organs such as the brain, lungs, kidneys, and liver would not be considered. Patients with other life-limiting conditions such as advanced diabetes mellitus, severe peripheral vascular disease, malignancy, advanced neuromuscular disease, tissue storage diseases, active duodenal ulcer, recent pulmonary embolism, and systemic inflammatory and autoimmune diseases would be excluded. Patients must have failed conventional medical therapy, be dependent upon two or more intravenous inotropic drugs or require intraaortic balloon pump support, or be unable to be weaned from cardiopulmonary bypass. They must also have cardiac indices of <2.2 (L/min)/m^2 and adequate filling pressure, such as a central venous pressure of >17 mmHg.

There are also some device-specific criteria that relate to the size and fit of the device. The Novacor and Heartmate LVADS and the CardioWest TAH were designed for patients with body surface areas of >1.6 m^2 and have typical outputs of 6 to 7 (L/min)/m^2 for the LVADS and 7 to 8 (L/min)/m^2 for the TAH. The Thoratec, an extracorporeal device that can support either ventricle alone (RVAD or LVAD) or both ventricles (BiVAD), may be used in smaller patients but, at best, with biventricular apical cannulation, provides 5 to 6 (L/min)/m^2 flows. Right ventricular failure is a contraindication for LVADS. This is most reliably defined by evaluation of clinical signs of elevated venous pressure in combination with pulmonary artery and wedge pressures.

In addition this basic information, data from several studies may influence selection of patient and device and timing. In the most recent device registry, reporting 184 deaths in over 600 implants, contributing causes of death were bleeding in 59%, renal failure in 46%, and infection in 38% (Mehta et al., 1995). Preoperative parameters correlating with death have been blood urea nitrogen >14.3 mmol/L (>40 mg/dL), urine output <30 mL/h, central venous pressure >16 mmHg (in an LVAD study), and urgency of implantation. In the later study of LVAD implants (Deng et al., 1998), the 30-day mortality rate rose from 5% in the elective group to 33% in the emergency group.

Conclusion

A family of mechanical assist devices will soon be widely available. Each device has associated benefits, risks, and adverse events. The amount of flow, support of one or both sides of the heart, size, ease of implantation and explantation, risk of thromboembolism and infection, availability, and cost are factors to be considered in choosing among current models. All of these devices provide hemodynamic conditions in properly selected patients that are improvements over decompensated heart failure. The challenge of the physician and surgeon is to choose the most appropriate device for his or her patient.

REFERENCES

Copeland JG et al: Selection of patients for transplantation. Circulation 75:2, 1987

Copeland JG et al: Early experiences with the total artificial heart as bridge to transplantation. Surg Clin North Am 68:621, 1988

Copeland JG et al: The CardioWest total artificial heart bridge to transplantation: 1993 to 1996 national trial. Ann Thorac Surg 66:1662, 1998

Deng MC et al: Selection and outcome of ventricular assist device patients: The Muenster experience. J Heart Lung Transplant 17:817, 1998

Kormos R et al: Chronic mechanical circulatory support: Rehabilitation, low morbidity, and superior survival. Ann Thorac Surg 57:51, 1994

Mehta SM et al: Combined registry for the clinical use of mechanical ventricular assist pumps and the total artificial heart in conjunction with heart transplantation. J Heart Lung Transplant 14:585, 1995

Oz M et al: Bridge experience with long-term implantable left-ventricular assist devices. Are they an alternative to transplantation? Circulation 95:1844, 1997

CARDIAC REPLACEMENT THERAPY—DEVELOPMENT OF THE ABIOCOR IMPLANTABLE REPLACEMENT HEART*

Robert D. Dowling & Laman A. Gray

Introduction

Heart transplantation remains the major surgical alternative to the treatment of end-stage heart failure. However, transplantation remains severely limited by the availability of donor organs. In the past 5 years, the number of heart transplants performed in the United States has plateaued at approximately 2400 annually. Multiple efforts are underway to increase the availability of donor hearts but, to date, all have met with minimal success. Transplantation is also limited by strict medical and financial criteria. Currently, the average hospital cost associated with a heart transplant ranges between $85,000 and $100,000. Perhaps more burdensome is the cost of postoperative immunosuppression and other medications as well as other postoperative tests, such as endomyocardial biopsies. The total average cost after transplantation is approximately $2000 to $3000 per

month. The strict financial criterion also limits the eligibility of transplantation to predominantly developed countries. Also, despite major advances in the postoperative care of these patients, the half-life of survival after transplantation is under 9 years. Currently, the major factor that limits long-term survival after transplantation is aggressive allograft coronary artery disease, which is believed to be primarily immune-mediated. One potential option to increase the number of patients who could benefit from cardiac replacement therapy is xenotransplantation. Although significant progress has been made in this field, there still remain very significant immunologic barriers that need to be addressed.

Clearly, there is an acute need for an alternative therapy to address the ever-increasing number of patients with refractory end-stage heart failure who are candidates for cardiac replacement therapy. Replacement of the native heart with a mechanical device that is totally implantable has been under development for decades and, indeed, has been achieved. In addition to providing an alternative for heart transplant candidates, implantation of a total ar-

---

* See also in this volume Chap. 84 on Implantable Left Ventricular Assist Devices and Chap. 85 on Bridge to Transplantation with Mechanical Assist Devices.

tificial heart may be an option for the large cohort of patients that are referred for transplantation but are not deemed appropriate candidates because of strict medical criteria. Another major cohort that could potentially be saved by such a device is the group of patients with acute heart failure in whom all conventional medical and surgical treatments have failed.

The use of mechanical devices to support circulation began in 1966 when DeBakey first used a pneumatic device in a patient with a failing left ventricle. The first attempts at replacement of the native heart with a mechanical device were in the early to mid 1980s with the use of the Jarvik-7 pneumatic total artificial heart. These and other clinical trials demonstrated the ability of these devices to maintain normal circulation with normal end-organ function. However, they were limited by the technology available at the time, which required the use of pneumatic (air-driven) devices and also required percutaneous lines from the artificial heart to the large, bulky control systems.

Beginning in the early 1980s, a number of groups initiated development of devices that would be totally implantable and that could function either as an alternative to transplantation or as an option in patients with end-stage heart failure who do not meet the strict medical and financial criteria for transplantation. The AbioCor implantable replacement heart (ABIOMED Inc., Danvers, MA) is a completely implantable replacement heart that has shown success in animal studies and in the initial clinical trial. Design features of the device eliminate the need for percutaneous access. This chapter summarizes the device design, the animal trials, and the potentials for clinical use.

Device Design

The AbioCor is an electrohydraulically actuated device capable of providing a cardiac output up to 10 L/min and has previously been described (Kung et al., 1993; Parnis et al., 1994; Yu et al., 1993). The device is designed to be totally implanted, with transcutaneous energy transfer (TET) to power the device. The internal components of the device

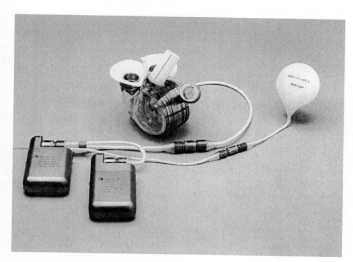

FIGURE 86-1

Internal components of the AbioCor implantable replacement heart. The thoracic unit (top) replaces the patient's heart. The controller (the pack on the left) controls the thoracic unit, monitors system integrity, and communicates with the external system. The battery (the pack on the right) provides operation without the external system. The transcutaneous energy transfer coil receives energy from the external system without penetrating the skin.

(Fig. 86-1) consist of the battery, which will allow the patient to move around untethered for brief periods of time; a controller that contains all of the appropriate drive, monitoring, and control circuitry; a secondary TET coil; and the main thoracic unit itself. The thoracic unit (Fig. 86-2) consists of an energy converter and two blood pumps (left and right ventricles) that approximate the shape and volume of the natural heart. It is implanted in the pericardial space vacated by the excised natural heart. The energy converter is situated between the right and left ventricles and contains an electrically driven centrifugal pump that provides continuous, unidirectional hydraulic fluid motion. A switching valve determines whether the hydraulic fluid moves to the left or to the right, which thereby results in alternate left and right systole. There is a one-to-one correspondence between blood and hydraulic fluid displacement. Design of the device allows for decreased right-sided stroke volume that allows for maintenance of balance between systemic and pulmonary circulation.

All blood-contacting surfaces, including the two blood pumps (stroke volume of ≈ 60 mL) and the four trileaflet valves (24-mm internal diameter) are fabricated from polyetherurethane (Angioflex,

Abiomed, Inc., Danvers, MA). This results in a smooth continuous blood-contacting surface from the inflow cuff to the outflow graft. The thoracic unit is connected to an internal controller, an internal battery, and a secondary TET coil. The internal battery will provide varying durations of operation for up to 45 min of power, potentially providing patients with the ability to shower or perform other activities without being tethered to an external power source. The secondary TET coil is placed in a subcutaneous position and allows for transfer of energy across the skin from a primary TET coil. The primary TET coil may be powered from a conventional AC electrical outlet or from portable, external batteries. The use of batteries that may be carried in a shoulder bag or placed in pockets will allow for unrestricted mobility for prolonged periods of time. Experience with the Jarvik total artificial heart and the current available left ventricular assist devices have clearly demonstrated the need to provide a completely implantable device that can provide unrestricted movement. Also, the elimination of percutaneous lines will dramatically decrease the incidence of infectious complications.

Implant Procedure

Implantation of the AbioCor requires the institution of cardiopulmonary bypass and the excision of the native ventricles just above the annulus of the mitral and tricuspid valves. The left and right atrial cuff of the replacement heart are sewn to the native left and right atrial remnants, respectively. The atrial cuffs consist of Dacron, coated on the external surface with Angioflex. The outflow grafts of the AbioCor device are then sewn end-to-end to the pulmonary artery and aorta. The AbioCor device is placed in the pericardial cavity and rapidly connected to both atrial cuffs and the right and left outflow grafts. After complete de-airing of the device is achieved, the patient is gradually weaned off cardiopulmonary bypass to full AbioCor support. The controller and internal battery are implanted deep to the abdominal musculature, and the secondary TET coil is placed in a subcutaneous position. At the end of the opera-

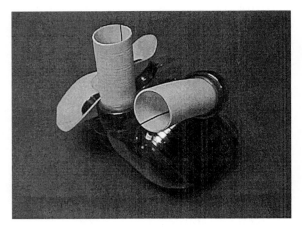

FIGURE 86-2

AbioCor thoracic unit consisting of the left and right ventricles and the energy converter.

tion, function of the AbioCor device is entirely dependent on the internal components with TET. Control of the device is achieved with the internal controller. As noted above, the internal battery will be able to provide energy to the replacement heart to allow for periods of complete freedom of motion.

The initial animal implants of the AbioCor device took place in 1991 at the Texas Heart Institute (THI). In these early prototype models, the group at THI was able to demonstrate the ability of the device to maintain full circulatory support and appropriate balance of the systemic and pulmonary circulation. All of the preclinical implants have been performed in calves approximately 4 months old, weighing 90 to 110 kg. A 108-day survival with a thoracic implant was demonstrated at the THI in 1984. The major limitation of using calves is their rapid growth rate and relatively large cardiac output demands, which quickly exceed the capacity of the device.

Animal (calf) experience with the AbioCor device at the University of Louisville began in 1998. Early efforts were focused on refining and standardizing the operative approach and demonstrating team readiness for clinical trials. In January 1999, a series of experiments began that demonstrated consistent survival. Since then, 41 implants have been performed, with all animals surviving the operative procedure and having normal neurologic and end-organ function. The proposed implant duration in these animals was 30 days — to provide data at elective autopsy and to complement longer duration implants that were concurrently being performed at THI. All animals have had continuous monitoring of left and right atrial pressures, aortic pressure, and pulmonary artery pressure for the entire study duration. All animals have demonstrated normal atrial pressures and normal systemic and pulmonary artery pressures. The left/right balance control mechanism was successful in all animals in maintaining balance of the systemic and pulmonary circulation, as demonstrated by maintenance of normal right and left atrial filling pressures. There was one death on the third postoperative day due to a transfusion reaction. Blood typing is not possible in cows because of the presence of more than 50 different blood group antigens. There was one death on postoperative day 5 of unknown etiology without evidence of device malfunction. All animals have demonstrated normal neurologic activity, and all animals have been able to ambulate either in the halls or on a specially designed treadmill. All animals have demonstrated normal kidney and liver function. There has been no evidence of hemolysis in these animals, and all animals have demonstrated adequate tissue oxygenation as demonstrated by daily assessments of mixed venous oxygen with hematocrits in the low 20s to mid 30s.

Findings at necropsy have demonstrated that the blood pumps have been clean, as have the inflow and outflow tracts. The excised brains and excised kidneys have also appeared normal.

As of the date of this writing (7/12/02), a total of seven AbioCor total artificial heart systems have been implanted. All patients were male with an age range from 51 to 79 years. All patients were in Class IV heart failure and inotrope dependent. Two patients are currently alive in 301 and 238 days after implantation. Two patients have been discharged from the hospital. There have been no significant device problems or malfunctions. There was one intraoperative death due to bleeding, one death due to multisystem organ failure, and one death due to a late retroperitoneal hematoma. There were three cerebro-vascular accidents that were felt to be related to thrombus forming on the atrial strut. These atrial struts were needed for animal implants but have been removed for further human implants. It is hoped that the removal of the atrial struts will result in an acceptable low rate of thromboembolic events.

REFERENCES

Kung RT et al: An atrial hydraulic shunt in a total artificial heart. A balance mechanism for the bronchial shunt. ASAIO J 39:M213, 1993

Parnis S et al: Chronic in vivo evaluation of an electrohydraulic total artificial heart. ASAIO J 40:M489, 1994

Yu LS et al: A compact and noise free electrohydraulic total artificial heart. ASAIO J 39:M386, 1993

STEM CELL THERAPY IN CARDIAC INJURY

Takayuki Saito, Jih Shiuan Wang, and Ray C-J Chiu

Adult mammalian ventricular myocytes have been widely believed to be terminally differentiated and to have lost their ability to multiply. Recently, Beltrami and colleagues challenged this notion, reporting that a small population of surviving cardiomyocytes had the ability to undergo cell division in the myocardium of patients who died of acute myocardial infarction (Beltrami et al., 2001) In this study, they showed a myocyte mitotic index of 0.08% in the myocardium adjacent to an ischemic area. In spite of such claims, it is generally accepted that quantitative deficiency of viable cardiomyocytes as the result of various cardiac diseases often leads to the final common pathway of heart failure. In order to augment the number of cardiac cells that may contribute to improved cardiac function, cellular therapy for heart failure, known as *cellular cardiomyoplasty* (Chiu et al., 1995), is currently undergoing vigorous research and an early clinical trial (Menasche et al., 2001). Several types of donor cells, including fetal and adult cardiomyocytes and even smooth-muscle cells, have been experimentally implanted directly into the myocardium. However, the more promising donor cells are stem cells and progenitor cells, which are capable of

differentiating into mature cardiomyocytes. Some of these cells may also participate in myocardial angiogenesis.

Embryonic and Adult Stem Cells

Stem cells are defined as clonogenic, self-renewing progenitor cells that can generate one or more specialized cell types. In vertebrates, stem cells have been traditionally subdivided into two groups. The first group is the *embryonic stem (ES) cells.* These pluripotent stem cells, which are derived from the inner cell mass of the blastocysts of embryos, are capable of generating all differentiated cell types in the body. ES cells in turn generate the second group of stem cells, which are called *organ-* or *tissue-specific stem cells.* A long-standing concept has held that organ-specific stem cells are restricted to making the differentiated cell types of the tissue in which they reside. In other words, they have irreversibly lost the capacity to generate other cell types in the body. Such restriction fundamentally distinguishes organ-specific stem cells from ES cells. However, many recent studies have demonstrated that these organ-specific stem cells in fact are often quite plastic and may be induced to differentiate into cells of other organs, either in vitro or after transplantation in vivo. For example, Jackson and colleagues demonstrated that a side population of hematopoietic stem cells, if transplanted directly into the injured heart, could differentiate into cardiomyocytes as well as vascular endothelial cells (Jackson et al., 2001). They also demonstrated that skeletal myoblasts can differentiate into hematopoietic cells (Jackson et al., 1999). In addition, Malouf and colleagues have shown that stem cells derived from the liver are capable of differentiating into cardiomyocytes in vivo (Malouf et al., 2001). Although the phenotypes of these cells capable of "switching" lineage have not been precisely characterized, these findings may indicate that stem cells with embryonic characteristics persist throughout life.

Cardiomyogenic Differentiation of Embryonic Stem Cells

At the molecular level, ES cells express a number of transcription factors highly specific for these undifferentiated cells, including Oct-4 and Rex-1. These transcription factors are required for maintaining the undifferentiated phenotype of ES cells and play a major role in determining early steps in embryogenesis and differentiation. Maintenance of human and murine ES cells requires leukemia inhibitor factor (LIF) present in the culture system. When LIF is removed from ES cell cultures and specific growth factors or cytokines are added, differentiation may be induced ex vivo to a number of cell types, including cardiomyocytes (Klug et al., 1996). Because of their extensive differentiating potential, ES cells need to be induced to differentiate down the desired cell lineage before implantation in order to avoid teratoma formation. Klug and colleagues have successfully established cardiomyogenic cell lines from murine ES cells. More recently, spontaneous and guided cardiomyogenesis have also been reported in human ES cells (Kehat et al., 2001). The main advantages of ES cells are that they can be propagated almost indefinitely under laboratory conditions, they can easily be genetically modified,

and they can be induced to differentiate into any desired cell types. However, for clinical application of ES cell–related therapies, there are still problems to be overcome, such as ethical and immunologic rejection issues.

Marrow Stromal Cells as Adult Stem Cells: Cardiomyogenic Differentiation

With the recent advent of stem cell biology, it is now apparent that the so-called marrow stromal cells (MSCs) in bone marrow, which used to be thought to play a supportive role for hematopoietic cells, are pluripotent adult stem cells capable of differentiating into various phenotypes. Since MSCs can be harvested easily from patients' own bone marrow by simple aspiration, can be expanded vastly in culture to provide adequate numbers, and can then be autoimplanted without encountering immunorejection, MSCs have recently been attracting the attention of investigators as a highly promising donor source for cellular cardiomyoplasty. In 1999, Makino and colleagues demonstrated for the first time a cardiomyogenic differentiation of MSCs in culture after treatment with 5-azacytidine (Makino et al., 1999). While the precise mechanism by which 5-azacytidine induces MSCs to differentiate is unknown, it is hypothesized that it involves the hypomethylation of cytosine in the region of the DNA MyoD1, which becomes a transcriptionally active state. In their study, the cells initially showed a fibroblast-like morphology, but about 30% of these cells changed shape after 5-azacytidine treatment and became interconnected with adjoining cells after 1 week, thereafter beginning to beat spontaneously and synchronously. These cells expressed atrial natriuretic peptide—stained positive with antimyosin, antidesmin, and antiactin antibodies. As they were beating, they showed several types of action potentials, such as sinus node-like and later ventricular cell-like action potentials. They also expressed many other genes characteristic of the cardiomyocytic phenotype.

Intramyocardial Implantation of Marrow Stromal Cells

Following the approach of Makino's team, Tomita and colleagues transplanted MSCs pretreated with 5-azacytidine into cryoinjury scars in rat hearts and reported cardiomyogenic differentiation with the expression of myosin heavy chain and troponin I (Tomita et al., 1999). They also reported that local angiogenesis appeared to be enhanced by the implanted cells and that these hearts were smaller and functioned better. At the authors' laboratory, in order to confirm the importance of the microenvironment for implanted MSCs to differentiate into cardiomyocytes, isogenic cultured MSCs (See Color Plate 26, Figure 87-1) were implanted into the left ventricular wall of recipient rats without 5-azacytidine pretreatment (Wang et al., 2000). After 4 weeks, donor MSCs demonstrated myogenic differentiation with the expression of sarcomeric myosin heavy chain, an organized contractile protein in the cytoplasm (See Color Plates 27 & 28, Figures 87-2 & 87-3). These cells were connected to each other or with the host cardiomyocytes by gap junctions, which stained positive for connexin 43 (See Color Plate 29, Figure 87-4) a major component protein in cardiomyocyte junctions known as *intercalated discs*. These results support the hypothesis that signals from the cardiac microenvironment are capable of inducing cardiomyogenic differentiation. In a more recent study, the authors also confirmed that if the therapeutic goal is to repopulate myocardial scar tissue with potentially contractile myogenic cells, preprogramming of MSCs in vitro with agents such as 5-azacytidine may be desirable (unpublished data).

Initiation of Clinical Trials for Cellular Cardiomyoplasty

Following nearly a decade of preclinical experimentation, a phase I clinical trial for cellular cardiomyoplasty was initiated in 2000, using autologous skeletal myoblasts (satellite cells) as the donor cells (Menasche et al., 2001). Satellite cells, which normally lie in a quiescent state under the basal membrane of mature muscle fibers, have several properties that can be exploited for clinical use: autologous origin, ease of expansion in vitro, exclusive differentiation into striated muscle cells, and high resistance to ischemia. Satellite cells were harvested from a patient with refractory heart failure due to ischemia, expanded in cultures for 2 weeks, and then implanted into the infarcted scar of the same patient at the time of coronary bypass surgery. Some 5 months later, they reported evidence of contraction and viable-tissue metabolic activity in the grafted scar segment of the heart. More recently, intramyocardial transplantation of autologous bone marrow cells in a patient has also been reported (Steinhoff et al., unpublished data).

Dawn of a New Therapy for Cardiac Injuries: From Repair and Replacement to Regeneration

To date, the treatment of various cardiac injuries and heart failure consists of palliation using medications and repair or replacement of damaged structures surgically, as in coronary bypass or cardiac transplantation. The advent of cell therapy using stem cells and progenitor cells for neomyogenesis and angiogenesis promises the beginning of an exciting new paradigm of therapy, based on recent rapid progress in stem cell biology and regenerative medicine.

REFERENCES

Beltrami et al: Evidence that human cardiac myocytes divide after myocardial infarction. N Engl J Med. 344: 1750, 2001

Chiu RCJ et al: Cellular cardiomyoplasty: Myocardial regeneration with satellite cell implantation. Ann Thorac Surg 60:12, 1995

Jackson K et al: Hematopoietic potential of stem cells isolated from murine skeletal muscle. Proc Natl Acad Sci USA 96:14482, 1999

Jackson KA et al: Regeneration of ischemic cardiac muscle and vascular endothelium by adult stem cells. J Clin Invest 107:1395, 2001

Kehat I et al: Human embryonic stem cells can differentiate into myocytes with structural and functional properties of cardiomyocytes. J Clin Invest 108:407, 2001

Klug MG et al: Genetically selected cardiomyocytes from differentiating embryonic stem cells form stable intracardiac grafts. J Clin Invest 98:216, 1996

Makino S et al: Cardiomyocytes can be generated from marrow stromal cells in vitro. J Clin Invest 103:697, 1999

Malouf NN et al: Adult-derived stem cells from the liver become myocytes in the heart in vivo. Am J Pathol 158:1929, 2001

Menasche P et al: Myoblast transplantation for heart failure. Lancet 357:279, 2001

Tomita S et al: Autologous transplantation of bone marrow cells improves damaged heart function. Circulation 100(Suppl 2):247, 1999

Wang JS et al: Marrow stromal cells for cellular cardiomyoplasty: Feasibility and potential clinical advantages. J Thorac Cardiovasc Surg 120:999, 2000

CHAPTER

88

VENOUS ULTRASONOGRAPHY IN THE DIAGNOSIS OF PULMONARY EMBOLISM

Clive Kearon / Jeffrey S. Ginsberg

Introduction

Diagnosis of pulmonary embolism is problematic because there are no noninvasive tests that, either alone or in combination, are both sensitive and specific. While pulmonary angiography is sensitive and specific, and consequently has both high positive and negative predictive values, it is invasive, unpleasant for patients, technically demanding to perform, and may be associated with serious side effects. Perfusion lung scanning is sensitive, and a normal scan has a high negative predictive value but is nonspecific; consequently, an abnormal scan has a low positive predictive value. The addition of ventilation scanning, with demonstration of large and/or multiple perfusion defects that are normally ventilated (mismatched defects), increases the specificity and positive predictive value of an abnormal lung scan to a level that allows pulmonary embolism to be diagnosed with confidence in most patients (high-probability scan). However, of patients with suspected pulmonary embolism, only about 25% have a normal perfusion scan and 15% a high-probability ventilation/perfusion scan; consequently, lung scanning is nondiagnostic in over half of patients in whom it is performed (Hull et al., 1983; The PIOPED Investigators, 1990; Wells et al., 1998).

Continuous-volume computed tomography (spiral or helical CT) appears to be more accurate than lung scanning for the diagnosis of pulmonary embolism (sensitivity, 70%; specificity, 90%), but its performance and interpretation are not well standardized and the safety of managing patients according to its findings has not been adequately evaluated in prospective trials.

A frequently encountered clinical problem, therefore, is how to manage patients with suspected pulmonary embolism who have a nondiagnostic ventilation-perfusion lung scan, a group that has an overall prevalence of pulmonary embolism of about 25% (Hull et al., 1983; The PIOPED Investigators; 1990). Management options in these patients include: (1) performing pulmonary angiography; (2) anticoagulation, which will unnecessarily expose the three-quarters of patients who do not have pulmonary embolism to a risk of bleeding; and (3) not treating and not investigating patients further ("doing nothing"), which will expose the one-quarter of patients who have pulmonary embolism to a high risk of recurrence. A fourth option, which is the focus of this chapter, is to use venous ultrasonography to aid with the diagnosis and management of these patients (Kearon et al., 1998a). A discussion of how this might be achieved follows a description of the essential components of ultrasonography in relationship to the diagnosis of venous thromboembolism.

B-mode (brightness modulation) ultrasonography produces a real-time, two-dimensional image of the leg veins. Normally, application of gentle ultrasound probe pressure results in obliteration (full compressibility) of the vein lumen and excludes thrombosis in that venous segment. Inability to fully compress the venous lumen is diagnostic for thrombosis (Kearon et al., 1998b). As venous ultrasound is less accurate in the calf, and isolated calf vein thrombosis is of limited clinical importance (see below), the ultrasound examination is usually confined to the proximal veins, down to and including the point where the calf veins join to form the popliteal vein. For the purpose of detecting asymptomatic proximal deep-venous thrombosis in patients with suspected pulmonary embolism, ultrasound examination that is confined to the common femoral and popliteal venous segments appears to be as accurate as a more extensive examination involving all of the proximal veins of the leg (MacGillaury et al., 2000). Doppler assessment of blood flow (e.g., duplex and color Doppler), as an adjunct to the assessment of venous compressibility, does not improve the accuracy of venous ultrasound for the diagnosis of deep-venous thrombosis (Kearon et al., 1998b).

Role of Venous Ultrasonography in Patients with Nondiagnostic Ventilation/Perfusion Lung Scans

Pulmonary embolism rarely occurs in the absence of preceding proximal deep-venous thrombosis of the legs, an association that can be exploited in two ways in patients with suspected pulmonary embolism and nondiagnostic lung scans (Fig. 88-1). The first relates to establishing the presence of pulmonary embolism at the time that patients present with suggestive symptoms. The second relates to identifying those patients in whom it is safe to withhold anticoagulation without performing pulmonary angiography.

Diagnosis of Pulmonary Embolism Using Ultrasonography

Approximately 70% of patients with pulmonary embolism have deep-venous thrombosis present at the time of presentation, and two-thirds of these thrombi are expected to involve the proximal veins (Hull et al., 1983: Wells et al., 1998). If venous ultrasonography of the proximal veins identifies thrombosis, for which it has a high sensitivity, this establishes the presence of acute venous thromboembolism (and, indirectly, pulmonary embolism) and the need for anticoagulation (Kearon et al., 1998a, 1998b). In practice, about one-third of patients with pulmonary embolism who have a nondiagnostic lung scan are expected to have proximal thrombi detected by bilateral venous ultrasonography. This translates into about 5 to 10% of patients who have nondiagnostic lung scans (Perrier et al., 1996; Turkstra et al., 1997; Wells et al., 1998). If deep-venous thrombosis is not found, it is less likely that the patient has had pulmonary embolism, but this possibility is not excluded and

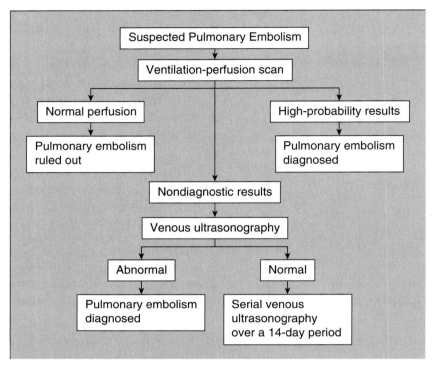

FIGURE 88-1

A diagnostic approach to patients with clinically suspected pulmonary embolism using ventilation-perfusion scanning and venous ultrasonography. In a patient with a high-probability lung scan and a low clinical suspicion for pulmonary embolism, pulmonary angiography should be considered if venous ultrasonography is normal. Abnormal perfusion scan, but not high probability for pulmonary embolism. In patients with a high clinical suspicion for pulmonary embolism, or with a poor cardiopulmonary reserve, supplementary bilateral venography (and/or pulmonary angiography) should be considered at initial presentation.

anticoagulants (or further diagnostic testing) cannot be withheld on the basis of this finding alone.

Withholding Anticoagulants and Pulmonary Angiography on the Basis of Serial Normal Venous Ultrasonography

About 80% of patients with suspected pulmonary embolism, a nondiagnostic lung scan, and a normal proximal venous ultrasound do not have pulmonary embolism (Perrier et al., 1996; Turkstra et al., 1997). The remaining 20% of patients with suspected pulmonary embolism who have a nondiagnostic lung scan and a normal proximal venous ultrasound have had pulmonary embolism and have either small residual thrombi (usually confined to the calf) or no residual thrombus. These patients are at risk of recurrent pulmonary embolism if the small residual thrombi extend or if a new thrombus forms; the highest risk period is within 2 weeks of presentation. However, before they have a recurrent episode of pulmonary embolism, they must first redevelop proximal deep-venous thrombosis.

Performance of serial venous ultrasounds over a 2-week period enables those patients who are progressing toward recurrent pulmonary embolism to be detected and treated prior to recurrent embolism (Wells et al., 1998). In order to detect those patients who are progressing toward recurrent pulmonary embolism, it is necessary to perform serial ultrasonography in all patients with suspected pulmonary embolism, a nondiagnostic lung scan, and a normal initial proximal venous ultrasound, if pulmonary angiography is not performed. With this approach to management, about 2% of patients develop an abnormal ultrasound during serial testing (Hull et al., 1994; Wells et al., 1998). Patients with nondiagnostic lung scans who do not develop an abnormal ultrasound during serial testing are expected to have a very low subsequent risk of symptomatic deep-venous thrombosis or pulmonary embolism (i.e., <2% during 6 months of follow-up) (Hull et al., 1994; Wells et al., 1998).

Limitations

Use of serial venous ultrasonography to manage patients who have suspected pulmonary embolism and a nondiagnostic lung scan is not without limitations. The accuracy of ultrasonography for the diagnosis of thrombosis in patients with suspected pulmonary embolism, but without symptoms of deep-venous thrombosis, appears to be similar to that for the diagnosis of asymptomatic deep-venous thrombosis in postoperative patients (i.e., positive predictive value of about 75%) (Kearon et al., 1998b; Turkstra et al., 1997; MacGillavry et al., 2000). Consequently, treatment of all such patients with an abnormal venous ultrasound will result in inappropriate anticoagulation of about 2% of patients with nondiagnostic lung scans (Turkstra et al., 1997). This risk can be minimized by performing venography and/or pulmonary angiography in patients who are more likely to have a false-positive ultrasound in this setting (Table 88-1).

The use of serial noninvasive testing for deep-venous thrombosis in patients with suspected pulmonary embolism has been inadequately evaluated

---

TABLE 88-1

FACTORS THAT REDUCE THE POSITIVE PREDICTIVE VALUE OF VENOUS ULTRASONOGRAPHY FOR ACUTE THROMBOEMBDLISM

Asymptomatic for deep-venous thrombosis

Low clinical suspicion for pulmonary embolism

Abnormality is confined to a short segment of the proximal veins or to the calf veins

History of previous venous thromboembolism

Other test that is sensitive for deep-venous thrombosis is negative (e.g., D-dimer)

---

in two patient groups. These are patients with very poor cardiopulmonary reserve (Hull et al., 1994) and those with a high clinical suspicion of pulmonary embolism (Wells et al., 1998) [70% prevalence of disease (Hull et al., 1983; The PIOPED Investigators, 1990)]. Therefore, it may not be safe to use the serial testing approach in these patient groups. An alternative is to supplement the serial venous ultrasonography management strategy with the performance of bilateral venography on the day of presentation if the initial ultrasound is normal. Venography will identify a larger proportion of the patients who have had pulmonary embolism. The risk of recurrence in those patients who have had pulmonary embolism and have normal venography should be lower than in the equivalent patients with normal venous ultrasonography, as small residual thrombi will have been excluded.

This chapter has focused on the role of venous ultrasonography in patients with suspected pulmonary embolism who have nondiagnostic ventilation-perfusion lung scans. Although it has yet to be studied, venous ultrasonography can be used in the same way in patients with suspected pulmonary embolism who have nondiagnostic continuous-volume computed tomography (i.e., not diagnostic for pulmonary embolism and no convincing alternative diagnosis revealed).

The authors conclude that venous ultrasonography is a very valuable adjunct for the diagnosis and management of patients with suspected pulmonary embolism. However, in order to utilize venous ultrasonography optimally in this setting, the natural history of venous thromboembolism and the limitations of the technique need to be fully appreciated.

REFERENCES

Hull RD et al: Pulmonary angiography, ventilation lung scanning, and venography for clinically suspected pulmonary embolism with abnormal perfusion lung scan. Ann Intern Med 98:891, 1983

Hull RD et al: A noninvasive strategy for the treatment of patients with suspected pulmonary embolism. Arch Intern Med 154:289, 1994

Kearon C et al: The role of venous ultrasonography in the diagnosis of suspected deep venous thrombosis and pulmonary embolism. Ann Intern Med 129:1044, 1998a

Kearon C et al: Noninvasive diagnosis of deep venous thrombosis. Ann Intern Med 128:663, 1998b

MacGillavry MR et al: Compression ultrasonography of the leg veins in patients with clinically suspected pulmonary embolism: is a more extensive assessment of compressibility useful? Thromb Haemost 84:973, 2000

Perrier A et al: Diagnosis of pulmonary embolism by a decision analysis-based strategy including clinical probability, D-dimer levels, and ultrasonography: A management study. Arch Intern Med 156:531, 1996

The PIOPED Investigators: Value of the ventilation perfusion scan in acute pulmonary embolism. JAMA 263:2753, 1990

Turkstra F et al: Diagnostic utility of ultrasonography of leg veins in patients suspected of having pulmonary embolism. Ann Intern Med 126:775, 1997

Wells PS et al: The use of a clinical model for safe management of patients with suspected pulmonary embolism. Ann Intern Med 129:997, 1998

89

EFFICACY AND COST-EFFECTIVENESS OF LOW-MOLECULAR-WEIGHT HEPARINS FOR TREATMENT OF ACUTE DEEP VENOUS THROMBOSIS

Michael K. Gould

Low-molecular-weight heparins (LMWHs) potentially simplify the initial treatment of acute deep venous thrombosis (DVT). Conventional unfractionated heparin (UFH) is a heterogeneous mixture of polysaccharide chains with a mean molecular mass of 12,000 to 16,000 Da. LMWHs are prepared by depolymerization of UFH chains, yielding heparin fragments with a mean molecular mass of 4000 to 5000 Da. While UFH inhibits factor Xa and thrombin equally, LMWH preparations have greater activity against factor Xa. In addition, LMWHs exhibit less binding to plasma proteins, endothelial cells, and macrophages. As a result, LMWHs have better bioavailability when administered subcutaneously, longer half-lives, and more predictable anticoagulant effects (Weitz, 1997).

The improved pharmacokinetic properties of LMWHs are directly responsible for several practical clinical advantages. First, LMWHs may be administered once or twice daily by subcutaneous injection, in contrast with UFH, which is typically given by continuous intravenous infusion. Second, no monitoring is necessary for most patients who receive LMWH, while UFH use requires laboratory monitoring to achieve and maintain a therapeutic level of anticoagulation. Finally, because dosing is intermittent and monitoring is unnecessary, selected patients may be eligible for outpatient treatment with LMWHs.

Efficacy of LMWHs in Acute Deep Venous Thrombosis

A meta-analysis identified 11 trials that compared a LMWH preparation with UFH for treatment of acute DVT (Gould et al., 1999a). The meta-analysis examined three major outcomes: major bleeding complications during the initial heparin treatment period, recurrent thromboembolic events over 3 to 6 months, and mortality rates over 3 to 6 months.

Major bleeding occurred infrequently in both treatment groups. Only 1.9% of study participants treated with UFH experienced a major bleeding complication during the initial treatment period. Results in seven studies favored LMWHs for this outcome (Fig. 89-1), but the difference was statistically significant for only one study (Hull et al., 1992). For all studies combined, LMWHs reduced the risk of major bleeding by almost 30% (odds ratio, 0.71), but the difference between treatments was not statistically significant. It is not known whether LMWHs might be more effective in reducing the risk of bleeding complications outside of clinical trials, where patients are less highly selected and might receive less intensive monitoring.

Recurrent thromboembolic events were seen in 5.4% of study participants treated with UFH. Recurrent DVT was responsible for >65% of symptomatic thromboembolic events. The results of six studies favored LMWHs for this outcome, while five studies favored UFH (Fig. 89-1). For all studies combined, there was no statistically significant difference between the two treatments in the risk of recurrent thromboembolism.

Of all patients treated with UFH in the 11 studies, 6.8% died. Results in ten studies favored LMWHs

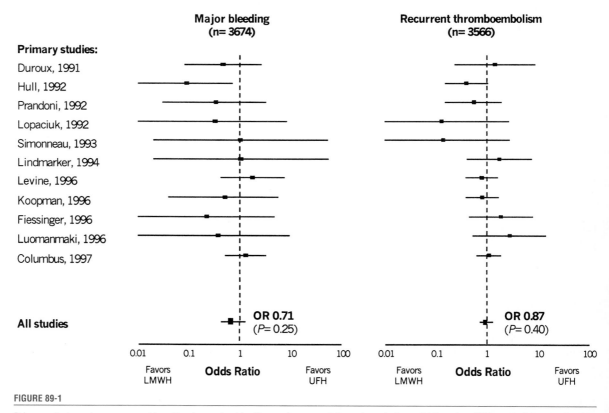

FIGURE 89-1

Primary study and summary odds ratios for major bleeding and recurrent thromboembolism. Odds ratios (OR) are indicated by square boxes. Horizontal lines represent 95% confidence intervals. Odds ratios <1.0 favor low-molecular-weight heparins (LMWHs); odds ratios >1.0 favor unfractionated heparin (UFH). The summary odds ratio for major bleeding favors LMWHs, but this is not statistically significant. The confidence interval for the summary odds ratio for recurrent thromboembolism also crosses 1, indicating no statistically significant difference between the treatments.

(Fig. 89-2), but the difference was statistically significant for only one study (Hull et al., 1992). For all studies combined, LMWHs were found to reduce mortality rates by almost 30% (odds ratio, 0.72; absolute risk reduction, 1.65%; $p = .02$). The number needed to treat to prevent one death was 61.

Only 10% of all deaths were due to confirmed episodes of recurrent thromboembolism, and deaths from bleeding were extremely uncommon. Death rates from documented thromboembolism and/or bleeding were not significantly different in the two treatment groups. The authors concluded that LMWHs reduced mortality rates over 3 to 6 months, but the mechanism responsible for this was uncertain. It is noteworthy that >28% of all deaths occurred in patients reported to have cancer. In this small subgroup, LMWHs reduced mortality from 26 to 17%.

The meta-analysis identified considerable variation in study design and execution. Studies evaluated five different preparations of LMWH— nadroparin, tinzaparin, enoxaparin, dalteparin, and reviparin. Patients with symptomatic pulmonary embolism were eligible for enrollment in four trials.

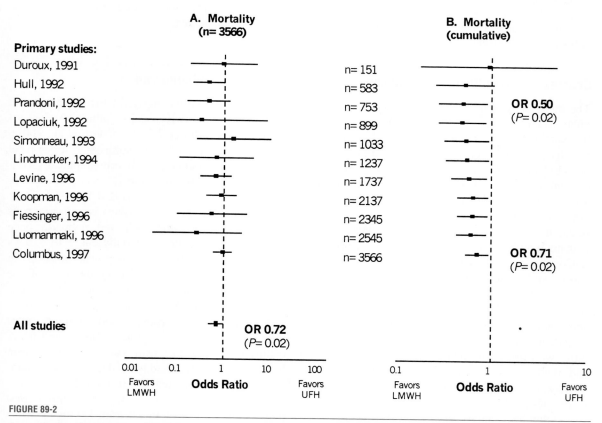

FIGURE 89-2

Conventional and cumulative meta-analysis for mortality rates. *A.* Conventional meta-analysis results showing a statistically significant benefit for low-molecular-weight heparin (LMWH) treatment. *B.* The results of cumulative meta-analysis, in which the summary odds ratio is recalculated after individual studies are added one at a time by year of publication. A statistically significant benefit for LMWH is apparent after the addition of the third study. The direction and statistical significance of the treatment effect remain constant with the addition of each new study, although the magnitude of the effect lessens slightly over time. UFH, unfractionated heparin.

Three studies permitted outpatient treatment with LMWH in selected participants. In seven studies, warfarin was administered on treatment day 1 or 2; in the remaining trials, warfarin was not given until treatment day 7 or later. In five studies, differences between treatments may have been obscured because an unspecified number of participants may have received anticoagulant treatment for up to 48 h prior to randomization. Of the 11 studies, 10 were unblinded or single-blinded. It is interesting to note that statistically significant differences in bleeding complications and mortality rates were seen only in the one double-blind study (Hull et al., 1992). This study compared once daily tinzaparin with UFH in hospitalized patients with venous thromboembolism, 14% of whom presented with symptomatic pulmonary embolism.

Sources of Variability in Study Outcomes

The meta-analysis used statistical models to determine whether variation in treatment outcomes could be explained by one or more of the study-level factors listed above. For death and recurrent thromboembolism, there was little heterogeneity in study outcomes and none of the study-level factors accounted for significant variation. For major bleeding, three significant sources of variation were identified: the type of LMWH studied, whether some patients may have received anticoagulation prior to randomization, and whether outpatient treatment was possible in selected patients.

The type of LMWH significantly influenced the risk of major bleeding, but no single preparation was found to be better or worse than any other preparation. Because the various types of LMWH differ with respect to their mean molecular weights and their ratios of anti-factor Xa:anti-factor IIa activity, it is conceivable that differences in bleeding tendencies might exist.

In the five studies that allowed anticoagulant treatment (usually with UFH) for up to 48 h prior to randomization, bleeding risk was similar in the two treatment groups. In contrast, in trials that did not permit prior anticoagulant therapy, LMWHs reduced bleeding complications by >80% (odds

ratio 0.18). Thus, in some trials, reductions in bleeding risk may have been diluted by allowing 1 or 2 days of UFH treatment in some patients who subsequently would be randomized to receive LMWH.

The treatment setting also appeared to influence the relative risk of bleeding complications. LMWHs reduced bleeding complications by almost 80% (odds ratio, 0.21) in trials in which all participants received inpatient treatment. In contrast, in the three trials that permitted outpatient treatment in selected participants, no significant difference between treatments was observed. This finding should be interpreted with caution, because fewer than half of all patients received outpatient treatment in these trials, and outcomes were not reported separately for inpatients and outpatients.

Frequency of Administration

Two studies recently compared UFH treatment with once daily or twice daily administration of a LMWH (Breddin et al., 2001; Merli et al., 2001). In the Breddin study, a multicenter, open-label study, 1137 participants with venographically confirmed, proximal thrombosis were randomly assigned to treatment with UFH delivered by continuous infusion for 5 to 7 days or subcutaneous administration of weight-adjusted reviparin once daily for 28 days or twice daily for 5 to 7 days (Breddin et al., 2001). Both regimens of reviparin were more effective in reducing the size of the thrombus at the time of repeat venography 3 weeks after enrollment. Major bleeding complications were extremely uncommon, and mortality rates were similar in all three groups. There were fewer confirmed episodes of recurrent thromboembolism in the group that received twice daily reviparin compared with the group that received UFH.

The other multicenter study randomized 900 participants to receive enoxaparin, 1.0 mg/kg twice daily; enoxaparin, 1.5 mg/kg daily; or UFH. Rates of recurrent thromboembolism, major bleeding complications, and death did not differ between the UFH group and either of the LMWH groups (Merli et al., 2001).

Based on these and other studies, once daily treatment with enoxaparin, reviparin, tinzaparin (Hull et al., 1992), or dalteparin (Lindmarker et al., 1994) appears to be as safe and effective as conventional treatment with UFH.

Outpatient Treatment of Deep Venous Thrombosis

Several trials have examined the feasibility of outpatient treatment with LMWHs. In an unblinded, multicenter Canadian trial, Levine and colleagues randomized 500 patients with acute proximal venous thrombosis to receive either enoxaparin, 1 mg/kg subcutaneously twice daily, or UFH by continuous infusion (Levine et al., 1996). Of note, 610 out of 2230 screened patients were excluded from participation because they were not eligible for outpatient treatment due to the presence of coexisting conditions. Of the participants assigned to receive LMWH, almost half were never admitted to the hospital. The mean length of stay in the remaining participants was 2.2 ± 3.8 days, compared with 6.5 ± 3.4 days for those who received UFH.

Koopman and co-workers enrolled consecutive patients with acute proximal venous thrombosis irrespective of their potential eligibility for outpatient treatment. In this unblinded, multicenter international trial, 400 participants were randomized to receive either twice-daily subcutaneous nadroparin or conventional UFH. Of the participants who were assigned to receive LMWH, 36% were never admitted to the hospital and 40% were discharged early (Koopman et al., 1996).

Another unblinded multicenter international study (Columbus Investigators, 1997) randomly assigned 1021 patients with symptomatic venous thromboembolism to receive either twice-daily subcutaneous reviparin or intravenous UFH. In this trial, >25% of participants presented with symptomatic pulmonary embolism. Mean hospital stay was reduced by 3 days in the LMWH cohort, primarily because 27% of these patients were not admitted to the hospital and 15% were discharged within the first 3 days of treatment.

In order to treat DVT outside of the hospital safely and effectively, an organized multidisciplinary approach is necessary. Four essential components of an outpatient treatment program have been identified: appropriate patient selection, patient education, careful follow-up, and access to care (Dunn and Coller, 1999). In many hospitals, anticoagulation clinics serve as coordinating centers for the efforts of emergency department physicians, primary care providers, pharmacists, patient educators, social workers, and visiting nurses. The relative contraindications to outpatient treatment are listed in Table 89-1 (Dunn and Coller, 1999; Yusen et al., 1999). In addition, many patients will not be eligible for outpatient treatment because hospitalization is indicated for some other reason. A retrospective review of 195 hospitalized patients with confirmed proximal lower extremity DVT found that fewer than 20% of patients were eligible or possibly eligible for outpatient care (Yusen et al., 1999). However, 70% of the patients were already hospitalized at the time of diagnosis. In this study, no complications or deaths occurred in the

TABLE 89-1

RELATIVE CONTRAINDICATIONS TO OUTPATIENT TREATMENT WITH LOW-MOLECULAR-WEIGHT HEPARINS

Symptomatic pulmonary embolism

Active bleeding

Increased risk of hemorrhage

Recent surgery

Recent spinal or epidural anesthesia or lumbar puncture

Recent stroke

Severe renal or hepatic dysfunction

Pregnancy

Heparin allergy

History of heparin-induced thrombocytopenia

Limited cardiopulmonary reserve

36 patients who were considered eligible for outpatient treatment.

Cost-effectiveness of Low-Molecular-Weight Heparin Treatment

Hull and colleagues performed an economic analysis of inpatient LMWH treatment, using cost and outcomes data from a single randomized, controlled trial (Hull et al., 1992, 1997). They recorded costs for administering initial and long-term therapy, costs for diagnosing and treating thromboembolic recurrences, and costs for managing bleeding complications. The total cost over 3 months for 100 patients treated with UFH was $375,836, while the total cost for 100 patients who received LMWH treatment was $335,687. Thus, LMWH treatment resulted in net cost savings of roughly $400 for each patient treated.

Gould and co-workers developed a decision model that allowed them to examine the cost-effectiveness of LMWHs in both the inpatient and outpatient treatment settings (Gould et al., 1996). They compared lifetime health care costs and health outcomes for two hypothetical cohorts of patients with acute, proximal venous thrombosis. One cohort received UFH via continuous intravenous infusion in a monitored hospital setting. The other cohort received twice-daily subcutaneous injections of LMWH (enoxaparin). The authors estimated costs using a variety of secondary data sources, including Medicare reimbursement and a proprietary cost accounting system. Probabilities for early treatment complications were derived from results of a meta-analysis (Gould et al., 1999a), and estimates for other model parameters were based on literature review.

In the base case analysis, the authors assumed that all patients in the LMWH cohort received inpatient treatment. Initial treatment costs were $3402 per patient for the UFH group and $3638 per patient for those treated with LMWH twice daily. The difference of $236 per patient was partially offset by reduced costs for early complications in the LMWH cohort. Per patient costs for late complications and unrelated future health care costs were assumed to

be equal for the two cohorts. Total lifetime health care costs were $26,361 for the UFH group and $26,516 for the LMWH patients, yielding a difference of $155 per patient treated. LMWH treatment improved quality-adjusted life expectancy by 0.02 years. Thus, for a small additional cost, LMWH inpatient treatment yielded a small improvement in quality-adjusted survival. The incremental cost-effectiveness ratio was $7820 per quality-adjusted life year gained, indicating that LMWH treatment represented a good value relative to other commonly employed health care interventions. The authors concluded that LMWH was highly cost-effective for inpatient treatment of acute DVT. Sensitivity analysis indicated that LMWH treatment became cost-saving when its pharmacy cost was reduced by 31% or more or when it reduced the yearly incidence of late complications by at least 7%.

In a secondary analysis, the authors assumed that 30% of patients in the LMWH cohort received outpatient treatment and that 25% were discharged after an abbreviated 3 day hospital stay. The authors assigned outpatient costs for phone calls, office visits, and home care by an aide or family member. Costs for monitoring and administering UFH were also included, although time costs for nurses and other personnel were not modeled. Under the assumptions of this analysis, LMWH use reduced total health care costs by $762 per patient treated. When the authors assumed that all LMWH patients received outpatient therapy, the total cost savings amounted to almost $1900 per patient treated. Thus, outpatient treatment with LMWH was associated with considerable cost-savings.

Summary

LMWHs are at least as effective as UFH for treating acute DVT and are more convenient to use. Current evidence indicates that LMWH treatment reduces mortality rates following venous thrombosis, although the mechanism for this is not clear. In the inpatient setting, LMWH treatment represents a very good value in health care spending. While decisions about resource utilization are always subject to budgetary constraints and competing needs, it is reasonable to prescribe LMWHs for all eligible hospitalized patients with DVT. Outpatient therapy with LMWH saves $1900 per patient treated and is likely to be preferred by many patients. Outpatient treatment should be strongly considered in patients with uncomplicated DVT who do not have an increased risk of bleeding or severe underlying comorbidity.

More information is needed to determine the safety and efficacy of outpatient treatment of uncomplicated pulmonary embolism with LMWHs.

REFERENCES

Breddin HK et al: Effects of a low-molecular-weight heparin on thrombus regression and recurrent thromboembolism in patients with deep-vein thrombosis. N Engl J Med 344:626, 2001

Columbus Investigators: Low-molecular-weight heparin in the treatment of patients with venous thromboembolism. N Engl J Med 337:657, 1997

Dunn AS, Coller B: Outpatient treatment of deep vein thrombosis: Translating clinical trials into practice. Am J Med 106, 660, 1999

Gould MK et al: Low-molecular-weight heparins compared with unfractionated heparin for treatment of acute deep venous thrombosis: A meta-analysis of randomized, controlled trials. Ann Intern Med 130:800, 1999a

Gould MK et al: Low-molecular-weight heparins compared with unfractionated heparin for treatment of acute deep venous thrombosis: A cost-effectiveness analysis. Ann Intern Med 130:789, 1999b

Hull RD et al: Subcutaneous low-molecular-weight heparin compared with continuous intravenous heparin in the treatment of proximal-vein thrombosis. N Engl J Med 326:975, 1992

Hull RD et al: Treatment of proximal vein thrombosis with subcutaneous low-molecular-weight heparin vs. intravenous heparin: An economic perspective. Arch Intern Med 157:289, 1997

Koopman MM et al: Treatment of venous thrombosis with intravenous unfractionated heparin administered in the hospital as compared with subcutaneous low-molecular-weight heparin administered at home. The Tasman Study Group. N Engl J Med 334:682, 1996

Levine M et al: A comparison of low-molecular-weight heparin administered primarily at home with unfractionated heparin administered in the hospital for proximal deep-vein thrombosis. N Engl J Med 334:677, 1996

Lindmarker P et al: Comparison of once-daily subcutaneous Fragmin with continuous intravenous unfractionated heparin in the treatment of deep vein thrombosis. Thromb Haemost 72:186, 1994

Merli G et al: Subcutaneous enoxaparin once or twice daily compared with intravenous unfractionated heparin for treatment of venous thromboembolic disease. Ann Intern Med 134:191, 2001

Weitz, J: Low-molecular-weight heparins. N Engl J Med 337:688, 1997

Yusen RD et al: Criteria for outpatient management of proximal lower extremity deep venous thrombosis. Chest 115, 972, 1999

THE ANKLE BRACHIAL INDEX IN THE EVALUATION OF PERIPHERAL ARTERIAL DISEASE

Mary McGrae McDermott

Lower extremity peripheral arterial disease (PAD) is a common, chronic condition among older men and women and is associated with an increased risk of cardiovascular mortality and walking impairment. Clinicians and researchers have traditionally associated PAD with classic intermittent claudication. *Intermittent claudication* is defined as exertional calf pain that subsides with rest and does not begin at rest. However, more recent data show that only a minority of men and women with PAD have classic symptoms of intermittent claudication (Table 90-1). Thus, relying on intermittent claudication to identify PAD will result in significant underdiagnosis.

PAD can be accurately and noninvasively diagnosed with the ankle brachial index (ABI), a ratio of Doppler-recorded systolic pressures in the lower and upper extremities. The normal ABI is 0.9 to 1.5. An ABI < 0.9 is 95% sensitive and 99% specific for angiographically documented PAD. Lower ABI levels are associated with increasing PAD severity. Using the ABI as a screening tool, PAD has been shown to affect 12% of community-dwelling men and women age 65 and older (Newman et al., 1993) and 18% of

men and women age 55 and older in general medicine practices (Leng et al., 1996).

Peripheral Arterial Disease and Cardiovascular Mortality

Both in hospital and in community settings, individuals with an ABI < 0.9 have a three- to sixfold increased risk of mortality due to cardiovascular disease and coronary heart disease as compared to individuals with an ABI between 0.9 and 1.5. The relationship between ABI and cardiovascular events is independent of previous history of heart disease or stroke and independent of coronary heart disease risk factors. ABI < 0.9 has been shown to be a better predictor of future risk of heart disease and stroke than traditional coronary heart disease risk factors such as increased cholesterol level, hypertension, age, or cigarette smoking.

Among PAD patients, the lower the ABI value, the greater the risk of mortality. McDermott and colleagues studied the relationship between ABI

TABLE 90-1

PREVALENCE OF INTERMITTENT CLAUDICATION AMONG MEN AND WOMEN WITH
NONINVASIVELY DIAGNOSED PERIPHERAL ARTERIAL DISEASE

Population studied	Prevalence of peripheral arterial disease based on noninvasive testing, %	Prevalence of intermittent claudication among peripheral arterial disease patients %
Community-dwelling men and women, mean age 66[a]	11	20
Men and women age ≥ 55 years in a general medicine practice with no prior history of peripheral arterial disease[b]	12	4
Men and women age ≥ 55 years in a noninvasive vascular laboratory with peripheral arterial disease[b]	100, by definition	32

[a]MH Criqui et al: Circulation 71:516, 1985.
[b]MM McDermott et al: JAMA 286:1317, 2001.

value and mortality in a population of persons with PAD identified from a noninvasive vascular laboratory (McDermott et al., 1994). In this study, men and women with an ABI < 0.3 had the poorest survival, while those with an ABI of 0.6 to < 0.9 had the best survival over 4.3 years of follow-up.

The Ankle Brachial Index as a Measure of Walking Ability in Peripheral Arterial Disease

The ABI also predicts walking endurance and walking velocity in individuals with PAD. As shown in Fig. 90-1, men and women with an ABI < 0.4 have slower walking velocity and walking endurance when compared to those with an ABI between 0.4 and 0.9 and those with normal ABI values. These relationships between ABI, walking endurance, and walking velocity are independent of age, sex, comorbidities, and leg symptoms (McDermott et al., 1998). Among community-dwelling older persons, those with a slower walking velocity have an associated greater

future risk of mobility loss and nursing home placement as compared to those with faster walking velocity.

Measurement

Arterial pressures normally increase with increasing distance from the aorta. Individuals without PAD have higher pressures in their dorsalis pedis and posterior tibial arteries than in their brachial arteries; consequently, their ABI is > 1.0. Individuals with impairment in lower extremity arterial perfusion have associated decreases in lower extremity arterial pressures, resulting in an ABI < 0.9 when lower extremity arterial obstruction reaches 70% stenosis or more.

Before measuring the ABI, the patient should lie supine for at least 5 min. Appropriately sized blood pressure cuffs are placed around each brachial artery and above each ankle. Using a hand-held 5- or 10-MHz Doppler probe, systolic pressures in each brachial artery and in each dorsalis pedis and posterior tibial arteries are measured. When the dorsalis pedis and posterior tibial artery pressures are both

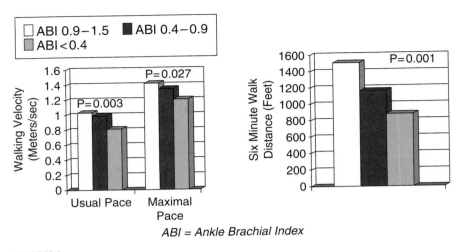

FIGURE 90-1

Age-adjusted walking endurance and walking velocity by ankle brachial index category among men and women age 55 and older.

measured, the highest pressure in each lower extremity is used to calculate the ABI for that leg. However, a study of individuals living in the community showed that measuring the posterior tibial artery pressure alone (rather than both the dorsalis pedis and posterior tibial arteries) is 89% sensitive and 99% specific for diagnosing PAD (Feigelson et al., 1994).

The ABI is calculated for each leg by dividing the lower extremity arterial pressure in each leg by the brachial artery pressure. The brachial artery pressure is determined by averaging the brachial artery pressures in the right and left arms. If the right and left brachial artery pressures differ by 10 mmHg or more, then brachial artery stenosis should be suspected in the limb with the lower pressure and the higher of the two brachial artery pressures should be used to calculate the ABI.

Limitations

Calcification of lower extremity arterial vessels, more commonly associated with diabetes mellitus and older age, may result in poorly compressible arteries, elevated lower extremity pressures, and an ABI > 1.5. In these individuals, lower extremity arterial perfusion cannot be accurately assessed with the ABI. Pulse-volume waveforms, typically performed in a noninvasive vascular laboratory, can diagnose PAD in patients with calcified, noncompressible lower extremity arteries. Another limitation in the ABI measurement described above is that arterial pressure measurements at the ankle do not allow one to identify the specific arterial segments affected by atherosclerosis. Arterial segments affected by atherosclerosis can be determined by performing serial pressure measurement and pulse-volume waveforms in the lower extremities, as typically done in a noninvasive vascular laboratory.

Diagnosing Peripheral Arterial Disease from the History and Physical Examination

The history and physical examination are much less accurate than the ABI in diagnosing PAD. Pulse palpation is not particularly sensitive or specific for PAD. In a study of nonhospitalized men and women, mean age 66 years, of whom 11% had PAD, the sensitivity of any abnormal pulse for PAD was 77%, while the specificity of normal pulses for absence of PAD was 86% (Criqui et al., 1985).

Atypical Symptoms and Absence of Symptoms

Table 90-1 shows the prevalence of intermittent claudication among men and women with PAD according to the population studied. Of PAD patients without classic intermittent claudication, some patients have exertional leg symptoms other than intermittent claudication, while others have no exertional leg symptoms. Thus, as in coronary artery disease, PAD may be asymptomatic or may be associated with atypical symptoms. Older age, male sex, and diabetes mellitus are independent predictors of PAD unaccompanied by exertional leg symptoms. In these patients, screening with the ABI may be particularly important in the diagnosis of PAD.

Conclusion

The ABI is a simple, noninvasive screening tool that accurately diagnosis PAD, provides prognostic information about future risk of total mortality and cardiovascular mortality, and correlates with walking velocity and walking endurance. An ABI < 0.9 is a more powerful predictor of cardiovascular mortality than many traditional risk factors for atherosclerosis. Patients with an ABI < 0.9 should be targeted for intensive treatment of coronary heart disease risk factors. They should also be targeted for interventions to maintain and improve their walking ability. Supervised exercise programs improve walking ability in those with PAD and intermittent claudication but have not been assessed in patients with an ABI < 0.9 who are asymptomatic or have exertional leg symptoms other than intermittent claudication.

REFERENCES

Criqui MH et al: The sensitivity, specificity, and predictive value of traditional clinical evaluation of peripheral arterial disease: Results from noninvasive testing in a defined population. Circulation 71:516, 1985

Feigelson HS et al: Screening for peripheral arterial disease: The sensitivity, specificity, and predictive value of noninvasive tests in a defined population. Am J Epidemiol 140:526, 1994

Leng GC et al: Use of ankle brachial pressure index to predict cardiovascular events and death: A cohort study. BMJ 313:1440, 1996

McDermott MM et al: The ankle-brachial index as a predictor of survival in patients with peripheral vascular disease. J Gen Intern Med 9:445, 1994

McDermott MM et al: The ankle brachial index independently predicts walking velocity and walking endurance in peripheral arterial disease. J Am Geriatr Soc 46:1355, 1998

McDermott MM et al: Leg symptoms in peripheral arterial disease: Associated clinical characteristics and functional impairment. JAMA 286:1317, 2001

Newman AB et al: Ankle-arm index as a marker of atherosclerosis in the Cardiovascular Health Study. Circulation 88:837, 1993

91

CILOSTAZOL AND PENTOXIFYLLINE IN THE MANAGEMENT OF INTERMITTENT CLAUDICATION

David L. Dawson

Intermittent claudication is the first recognizable symptom of peripheral arterial disease (PAD). Intermittent claudication is described as pain, aching, cramping, or fatigue in the muscles of the affected limb, occurring during or after walking, relieved with rest. Patients with claudication symptoms are much more commonly encountered than those with critical limb ischemia (ischemic rest pain, ulceration, or gangrene).

While claudication is not an immediate threat to life or limb, the symptoms can be functionally disabling. In addition, many PAD patients who do not recognize or report "classic" symptoms of exertional leg pain may have impaired walking performance (McDermott et al., 1999a). Such patients walk slower and for shorter distances. Careful questioning may identify the diagnosis of PAD

(McDermott et al., 1998, 1999b). A decrease in functional capacity is correlated with the severity and extent of PAD. Further, the presence of PAD is an important marker for increased risk of cardiovascular mortality and morbidity (Dormandy and Rutherford, 2000; Hirsch, 2001; Hiatt, 2001).

Principles of Pharamacotherapy

Drug therapies for patients with intermittent claudication are directed toward (1) slowing atherosclerosis progression; (2) reducing the risk of myocardial infarction, stroke, and cardiovascular death in this population; and (3) alleviating claudication symptoms (Hiatt, 2001).

Patients with PAD are at increased risk for future cardiovascular events, and lifelong antiplatelet therapy, unless specifically contraindicated, is appropriate (Dormandy and Rutherford, 2000; Hess et al., 1985; Goldhaber et al., 1992; Antiplatelet Trialists'

*The views expressed herein are those of the author and do not reflect the official policy of the Department of Defense or other departments of the United States government.

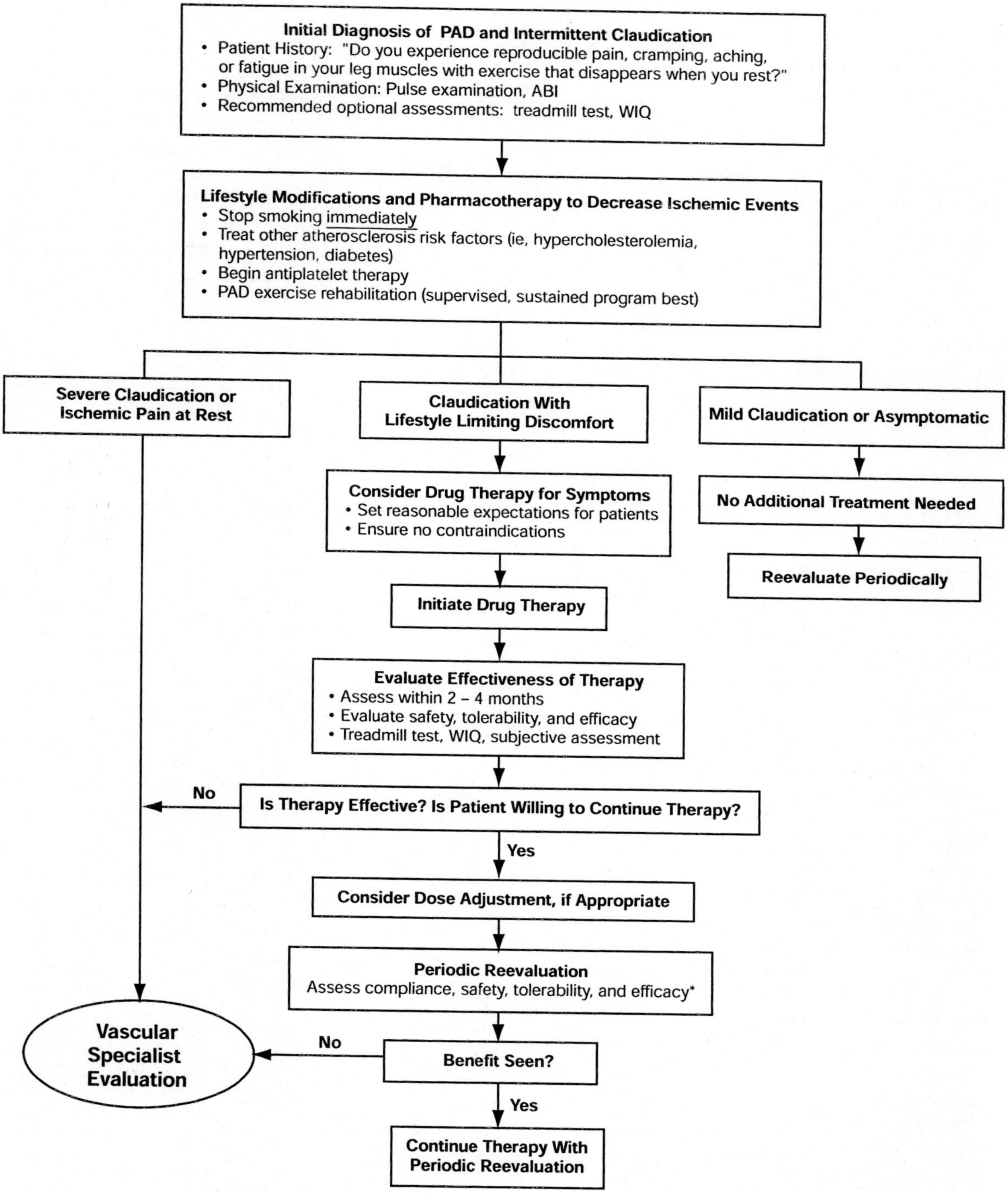

Initial Diagnosis of PAD and Intermittent Claudication
- Patient History: "Do you experience reproducible pain, cramping, aching, or fatigue in your leg muscles with exercise that disappears when you rest?"
- Physical Examination: Pulse examination, ABI
- Recommended optional assessments: treadmill test, WIQ

Lifestyle Modifications and Pharmacotherapy to Decrease Ischemic Events
- Stop smoking immediately
- Treat other atherosclerosis risk factors (ie, hypercholesterolemia, hypertension, diabetes)
- Begin antiplatelet therapy
- PAD exercise rehabilitation (supervised, sustained program best)

Severe Claudication or Ischemic Pain at Rest

Claudication With Lifestyle Limiting Discomfort

Mild Claudication or Asymptomatic

Consider Drug Therapy for Symptoms
- Set reasonable expectations for patients
- Ensure no contraindications

No Additional Treatment Needed

Initiate Drug Therapy

Reevaluate Periodically

Evaluate Effectiveness of Therapy
- Assess within 2 – 4 months
- Evaluate safety, tolerability, and efficacy
- Treadmill test, WIQ, subjective assessment

No ← **Is Therapy Effective? Is Patient Willing to Continue Therapy?**

Yes

Consider Dose Adjustment, if Appropriate

Periodic Reevaluation
Assess compliance, safety, tolerability, and efficacy*

Vascular Specialist Evaluation

No ← **Benefit Seen?**

Yes

Continue Therapy With Periodic Reevaluation

PAD= peripheral arterial disease; ABI=ankle–brachial index; MWD=maximal walking distance; PFWD=pain-free walking distance, WIQ=walking impairment questionnaire.
*The efficacy of any claudication intervention can be assessed by use of the patient history or use of more formal walking impairment questionnaires, treadmill tests, or objective quality-of-life evaluations.

FIGURE 91-1

Algorithm for the Management of Peripheral Arterial Disease

Collaboration, 1988, 1994; CAPRIE Steering Committee, 1996; Weitz et al., 1996), as are therapies for atherosclerosis risk factors (e.g., hyperlipidemia, hypertension, diabetes) (Dormandy and Rutherford, 2000; Hiatt, 2001; Weitz et al., 1996; McNamara et al., 1998; Carman and Fernandez, 2000).

Figure 91-1 provides a general algorithm for the general management of PAD. Drug therapy, when directed toward symptom relief, should be used as part of a comprehensive management plan that includes nonpharmacologic treatments such as exercise rehabilitation therapy, weight loss, and smoking cessation. Cilostazol and pentoxifylline are the only two drugs with U.S. Food and Drug Administration (FDA) approval for the treatment of claudication. Table 91-1 summarizes recommended

TABLE 91-1

PHARMACOTHERAPY FOR SYMPTOMS OF INTERMITTENT CLAUDICATION

FDA - approved drugs (recommended options)
   Cilostazol
   Pentoxifylline

Other established drugs with potential benefit for claudication (not currently available in the United States)
   Buflomedil
   Naftidrofuryl

Therapies with minimal or no claudication-relieving benefit (not recommended for use for symptom relief)
   Antiplatelet drugs (aspirin, clopidogrel)
   Aminophylline
   Anticoagulation (warfarin)
   Cinnarizine
   Defibrotide
   Dextran
   Ginkgo biloba
   Isosuprine
   Isovolemic hemodilution
   Ketanserin
   Nicotinic acid derivatives
   Vasodilators
   Verapamil (and other calcium channel blockers)
   Vitamin E

Medications under investigation, with potential benefit (not yet FDA-approved)
   Beraprost sodium
   L-arginine
   Propionyl-L-carnitine
   Prostaglandins and prostanoids
   Protein kinase C inhibitors
   Vascular endothelial growth factor (VEGF)
   Basic fibroblast growth factor (bFGF)

NOTE: FDA: United States Food and Drug Administration
SOURCE: Adapted from recommendations of the TransAtlantic Inter-Society Consensus, reported by J Dormandy and R Rutherford: J Vasc Surg. 31:S1, 2000.

and nonrecommended pharmaceutical agents for claudication, as well as several drugs currently under investigation in clinical trials.

Evaluation of Treatment Efficacy

Treadmill walking tests are the best way to assess the severity of claudication in PAD patients objectively, and treadmill tests are the standard means for evaluating efficacy of new drug therapies. Testing can be performed with either a fixed or variable workload, but both techniques are valid if repeated measures use the same methodology. The distance walked when claudication symptoms are first reported is termed the *pain-free walking distance* (PFWD), or *initial claudication distance*. The distance walked when the symptoms become severe enough to cause the patient to stop is the *maximal walking distance* (MWD), or *absolute claudication distance*.

The functional benefit of treatment should also be considered. Measurable and statistically significant increases in walking distance on treadmill testing do not necessarily equate with clinically relevant benefit. Patients' perception of their impairment may be measured by other methods, including use of standardized questionnaires that assess walking impairment or perceived quality of life.

have been published (Dawson et al., 1998, 2000; Money et al., 1998; Elam et al., 1998; Beebe et al., 1999). These studies, 12 to 24 weeks in duration, showed that cilostazol increased both the PFWD and MWD on standardized treadmill testing; the percent mean change from baseline was 28 to 100%, while the percent change in the comparable placebo groups was −10 to 30%. A dose-response effect was noted, with a greater effect seen with cilostazol dosed at 100 mg twice daily compared to 50 mg twice daily. This positive treatment effect was independent of sex, age, race, smoking status, coexisting diabetes, or use of beta blockers or calcium channel blockers.

A quality-of-life survey instrument, the Medical Outcomes Study, Short Form 36, was used in six of the U.S. trials. This widely used general health questionnaire found that cilostazol therapy was associated with improvement in several aspects of patient-reported well-being. Scores for Bodily Pain, Physical Function, Role-Physical, Physical Summary, and Vitality were significantly improved compared to placebo-treated patients. These data suggested that cilostazol improved the physical (but not the social or emotional) aspects of quality of life for patients with intermittent claudication. Also, in analyses of pooled data, cilostazol-treated patients reported improvements in walking speed and distance, as assessed by the Walking Impairment Questionnaire.

Cilostazol

Cilostazol, an inhibitor of type III phosphodiesterase, inhibits platelet activation (aggregation and secretion) and relaxes vascular smooth muscle. Other cilostazol effects include inhibition of vascular smooth-muscle cell proliferation, lowering of serum triglyceride levels, and increasing high-density lipoprotein cholesterol levels.

FDA approval of this drug was based on the results of a series of eight trials, involving 2702 patients, that enrolled PAD patients with moderate to severe claudication (Anonymous, 1999). To date, five of the randomized, placebo-controlled trials

Pentoxifylline

Pentoxifylline, a tri-substituted xanthine derivative, is classified as a hemorrheologic agent. The drug and its metabolites are thought to improve the flow properties of blood by decreasing viscosity, increasing erythrocyte membrane deformability, and by decreasing platelet and leukocyte aggregation.

Pentoxifylline has been extensively evaluated for claudication, but most of the reported trials were small and many were compromised by design shortcomings, such as the lack of an adequate placebo-treated control group or failure to use treadmill testing to assess walking ability objectively.

The only U.S. pentoxifylline study was reported by Porter and Bauer in 1982. This study enrolled 128 patients. The differences in walking distance between the placebo- and drug-treated groups were statistically significant. Pentoxifylline-treated patients increased their PFWD by 59%, and there was a 38% increase in MWD. However, the differences in percent change from baseline PFWD and MWD, when considered at week 24, were not significant. In part, this reflects the magnitude of the observed placebo effect in this study: a 36% increase in PFWD and a 25% increase in MWD.

In the Scandinavian Study Group's trial, pentoxifylline-treated patients had an 80% increase in PFWD and a 50% increase in MWD at the end of 24 weeks. There was no statistically significant difference between the treatment ($n = 76$) and control ($n = 74$) groups, however (Lindgärde et al., 1989). This again reflects a large observed placebo effect, as placebo-treated patients had a 60% improvement in PFWD and 29% improvement in MWD.

One group performed a meta-analysis of results from 11 randomized, placebo-controlled, double-blind trials that used treadmill testing as an endpoint (Hood et al., 1996). Evaluating a combined group of 612 patients with moderately severe claudication, they found that the weighted mean improvement in MWD with pentoxifylline therapy was 48.4 m (95% confidence interval 18.3 to 78.6 m). Considering these pooled data, it appeared that pentoxifylline was statistically significantly better than placebo. Despite this fact, lackluster results in broad clinical use and critical reviews of the available data have left many skeptical about its efficacy. For example, other reviewers pointed out that study sample size and pentoxifylline response are inversely correlated (Cameron et al., 1988; Radack and Wyderski, 1990), suggesting a publication bias. Studies reporting the most favorable responses to pentoxifylline therapy were small, often with 20 or fewer treated patients completing therapy.

Direct Comparison of Cilostazol and Pentoxifylline

A multicenter, prospective trial that directly compared the safety and efficacy of cilostazol, pentoxifylline, and placebo for the treatment of intermittent claudication found cilostazol to be superior (Dawson et al., 2000). This study, with 698 patients randomized to three treatment groups, is the largest single trial of drug therapy for claudication that has been reported. Further, as this study randomized 232 patients to treatment with pentoxifylline and 239 to placebo, it was more than three times the size of the largest previous study of pentoxifylline efficacy.

Patients in each treatment group demonstrated a progressive increase in walking distances over time, but the greatest improvement was observed in the patients who received cilostazol (Figs. 91-2 and 91-3). At 24 weeks, cilostazol-treated patients' mean improvement in PFWD was 94 m, and the increase in MWD averaged 107 m. Pentoxifylline increased PFWD by 74 m and MWD by 64 m. In this study population, cilostazol improved treadmill walking performance more than either pentoxifylline or placebo. Pentoxifylline was equivalent to placebo.

Both cilostazol and pentoxifylline were generally well tolerated, though fewer patients (15.8%) in the cilostazol treatment group withdrew due to adverse events compared to the pentoxifylline group (18.5%). The commonly reported side effect after starting cilostazol therapy were headache, diarrhea, and abnormal stools, but these symptoms were generally mild to moderate in severity and self-limited.

Use of Cilostazol and Pentoxifylline for Management of Intermittent Claudication

General recommendations for standardized, evidence-based management approaches for PAD have been published (Dormandy and Rutherford, 2000). The TransAtlantic Inter-Society Consensus (TASC) recommendations were developed through a 3-year

Maximal Walking Distance

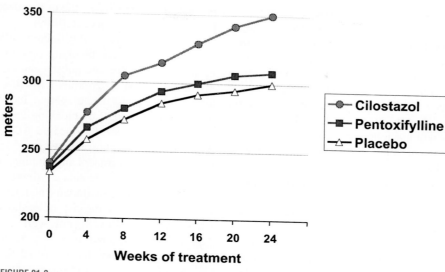

FIGURE 91-2

Comparison of cilostazol, pentoxifylline and placebo on maximal walking distance

Pain Free Walking Distance

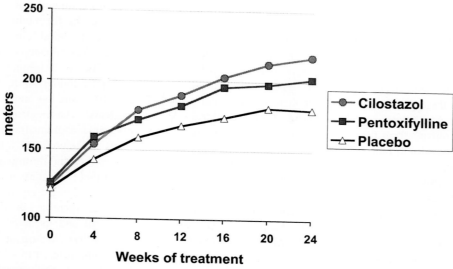

FIGURE 91-3

Comparison of cilostazol, pentoxifylline and placebo on pain free walking distance

collaborative effort involving North American and European vascular professional societies, including cardiology, vascular medicine, radiology, and surgery societies. The TASC report did not endorse any particular choice of pharmacotherapy for patients with intermittent claudication, and it stressed that drug therapy is not a replacement for exercise programs and other life-style adjustments. Drugs, the TASC concluded, "have a place as adjunctive treatment where invasive therapy is not indicated, in those who cannot or will not follow exercise therapy or in those who have not sufficiently benefited from it" (Dormandy and Rutherford, 2000).

Drug therapy for symptom relief is an appropriate and established part of the management of PAD patients with intermittent claudication. Cilostazol is more likely to be effective than pentoxifylline. Still, it only provides appreciable benefit to about half of treated patients. Cilostazol treatment should be initiated on a trail basis, and response to therapy assessed after 3 to 6 months before considering long-term drug administration. If no clinical benefit is noted after 6 months, the drug can be discontinued.

While clinical trial data suggest that pentoxifylline has limited efficacy, there may be a subset of claudication patients who do respond to pentoxifylline therapy. For patients who perceive benefit from chronic pentoxifylline therapy, a trial of drug discontinuation should be considered. Most will have not recrudesence of symptoms when the drug is stopped (Johnson et al., 1994). Those who do can resume pentoxifylline without ill effect. At best, pentoxifylline should be considered a second-line therapy, to be tried only if there is no response after an adequate trial of cilostazol. A summary of prescribing information for cilostazol and pentoxifylline is provided in Table 91-2.

Neither cilostazol nor pentoxifylline has been studied for its effect on the risk cardiovascular events in properly designed clinical trials. The largest single drug trial to look at reduction of cardiovascular morbidity and mortality in PAD patients was the Clopidogrel versus Aspirin in Patients at Risk of Ischaemic Events (CAPRIE) trial, which involved 6452 patients with PAD treated with either aspirin or clopidogrel (CAPRIE Steering Committee, 1996). CAPRIE, however, did not consider whether aspirin or clopidogrel affected clopidogrel affected claudication symptoms. Antithrombotic drugs (including antiplatelet agents), as a group, have little or no effect on walking performance (Girolami et al., 1999).

Clopidogrel irreversibly inhibits platelet aggregation by selectively blocking binding of ADP to its platelet receptor and subsequent ADP-mediated activation of the glycoprotein IIb/IIIa complex. It also inhibits platelet aggregation induced by agonists other than ADP by blocking the amplification of platelet activation by released ADP. Clopidogrel does not inhibit phosphodiesterase activity. Concomitant use of cilostazol and clopidogrel is thought to be safe, but available data are limited.

Though cilostazol inhibits platelet aggregation, its efficacy for reducing risk of cardiovascular mortality and morbidity is not well established. In Japan, where cilostazol is used to treat cerebrovascular disease, studies have verified the antiplatelet activity of cilostazol in these patients, with a 42% reduction in secondary stroke risk (Gotoh et al., 2000). Monotherapy with cilostazol, however, cannot yet be recommended for PAD management. PAD patients should also receive an antiplatelet agent other than cilostazol.

Information about the safety of coadministration of aspirin and cilostazol is limited, but available data suggest that it is safe. In the eight randomized, placebo-controlled, double-blind clinical trials of cilostazol, aspirin was coadministered with cilostazol in 201 patients. The most frequent doses and mean durations of aspirin therapy were 75 to 81 mg daily for 137 days (107 patients) and 325 mg daily for 54 days (85 patients). The incidence of bleeding complications was low. Coadministration of aspirin with cilostazol does not significantly change prothrombin time, activated partial thromboplastin time, or bleeding time, but there is a measurable decrease in ADP-induced platelet aggregation and a small, but clinically insignificant, increase in plasma concentrations of cilostazol and its active metabolites (Mallikaarjun et al., 1999). Aspirin or clopidogrel, therefore, should be administered in addition to any therapy directed at the claudication symptoms.

Unfortunately, there are no reliable criteria to predict response to therapy for either cilostazol or

TABLE 91-2

SUMMARY OF PRESCRIBING INFORMATION

	Cilostazol	Pentoxifylline
Trade name	Pletal	Trental
Manufacturer	Otsuka Pharmaceutical, Ltd	Aventis
Usual dose and route of administration	100 mg orally	400 mg orally (sustained-release tablet)
Frequency of administration	Twice daily, 1 h before or 2 h after meals	Three times daily with meals
Alternative dosing regimen	50 mg orally twice daily as initial dosing for patients receiving CYP3A4 inhibitors (such as ketoconazole, erythromycin, or diltiazem) or CYP2C19 inhibitors (such as omeprazole)	Lower dose, 400 mg orally twice daily, may be tried if patient experiences side effects
Contraindications	Congestive heart failure	Recent cerebral or retinal hemorrhage; history of methylxanthine intolerance
Most common side effects	Headache, palpitation, diarrhea, or abnormal stools	Dyspepsia, nausea, vomiting, dizziness, headache

SOURCE: Compiled and adapted from manufacturers' FDA-approved labeling information.

pentoxifylline. One problem is that no specific drug action has been clearly implicated in defining how these drugs affect walking performance. As improvement is seen over a period of several weeks, it is unlikely due to acute effects on platelet function, erythrocyte membranes, or vasodilation. How these drugs affect endothelium-mediated vascular tone or skeletal myocyte function has yet to be explored.

Cilostazol's apparent superiority awaits confirmation by broader clinical experience and other controlled trials. Findings from two multicenter trials comparing pentoxifylline, cilostazol, and placebo (one in the United States and one in Britain) have yet to published. Additional studies will be also be required to show clinical benefit for the antiplatelet effects or lipid-lowering actions of cilostazol. Concomitant treatment with aspirin, clopidogrel, or other antiplatelet agents should be considered until outcome studies demonstrate that cilostazol can reduce the risk of cardiac events and stroke in PAD patients.

REFERENCES

Anonymous: Cilostazol for intermittent claudication. Med Lett Drugs Ther 41:44, 1999

Antiplatelet Trialists' Collaboration: Secondary prevention of vascular disease by prolonged antiplatelet treatment. Br Med J (Clin Res Ed) 296:320, 1988

Antiplatelet Trialists' Collaboration: Collaborative overview of randomised trials of antiplatelet therapy—I: Prevention of death, myocardial infarction, and stroke by prolonged antiplatelet therapy in various categories of patients. Br Med J 308:81, 1994

Beebe HG et al: A new pharmacological treatment for intermittent claudication: Results of a randomized, multicenter trial. Arch Intern Med 159:2041, 1999

Cameron HA et al: Drug treatment of intermittent claudication: A critical analysis of the methods and findings of published clinical trials, 1965–1985 [see comments]. Br J Clin Pharmacol 26:569, 1988

CAPRIE Steering Committee: A randomised, blinded, trial of clopidogrel versus aspirin in patients at risk of ischaemic events (CAPRIE). Lancet 348:1329, 1996

Carman TL, Fernandez BB Jr: A primary care approach to the patient with claudication. Am Fam Physician 61:1027, 1034, 2000

Dawson DL et al: Cilostazol has beneficial effects in treatment of intermittent claudication: Results from a multicenter, randomized, prospective, double-blind trial. Circulation 98:678, 1998

Dawson DL et al: A comparison of cilostazol and pentoxifylline for treating intermittent claudication. Am J Med 109:523, 2000

Dormandy JA, Rutherford RB: Management of peripheral arterial disease (PAD). TASC Working Group. TransAtlantic Inter-Society Concensus (TASC). J Vasc Surg 31 (1 Pt 2): S1, 2000

Elam MB et al: Effect of the novel antiplatelet agent cilostazol on plasma lipoproteins in patients with intermittent claudication. Arterioscler Thromb Vasc Biol 18:1942, 1998

Girolami B et al: Antithrombotic drugs in the primary medical management of intermittent claudication: A meta-analysis. Thromb Haemost 81:715, 1999

Goldhaber SZ et al: Low-dose aspirin and subsequent peripheral arterial surgery in the Physicians' Health Study. Lancet 340:143, 1992

Gotoh F et al: Cilostazol stroke prevention study: A placebo-controlled double-blind trial for secondary prevention of cerebral infarction. J Stroke Cerebrovasc Dis 9:1, 2000

Hess H et al: Drug-induced inhibition of platelet function delays progression of peripheral occlusive arterial disease.

A prospective double-blind arteriographically controlled trial. Lancet 1:415, 1985

Hiatt WR: Medical treatment of peripheral arterial disease and claudication. N Engl J Med 344:1608, 2001

Hirsch AT (ed): *An Office-Based Approach to the Diagnosis and Treatment of Peripheral Arterial Disease*. Primary Care Series: *Peripheral Arterial Disease and Intermittent Claudication*. Hillsborough, NJ, Excerpta Medica, 2001

Hood SC et al: Management of intermittent claudication with pentoxifylline: Meta-analysis of randomized controlled trials. Can Med Assoc J 155:1053, 1996

Johnson WC et al: Pentoxifylline therapy for chronic claudication: Are patients dependent on therapy? Surgery 115:735, 1994

Lindgärde F et al: Conservative drug treatment in patients with moderately severe chronic occlusive peripheral arterial disease. Scandinavian Study Group. Circulation 80:1549, 1989

Mallikaarjun S et al: Interaction potential and tolerability of the coadministration of cilostazol and aspirin. Clin Pharmacokinet 37(Suppl 2):87, 1999

McDermott MM et al: The ankle brachial index independently predicts walking velocity and walking endurance in peripheral arterial disease. J Am Geriatr Soc 46:1355, 1998

McDermott MM et al: Exertional leg symptoms other than intermittent claudication are common in peripheral arterial disease. Arch Intern Med 159:387, 1999a

McDermott MM et al: Leg symptoms, the ankle-brachial index, and walking ability in patients with peripheral arterial disease. J Gen Intern Med 14:173, 1999b

McNamara DB et al: Pharmacologic management of peripheral vascular disease. *Surg Clin North Am* 78:447, 1998

Money SR et al: Effect of cilostazol on walking distances in patients with intermittent claudication caused by peripheral vascular disease. J Vasc Surg 27:267; discussion, 274, 1998

Porter JM, Bauer GM: Pharmacologic treatment of intermittent claudication. Surgery 92:966, 1982

Radack K, Wyderski RJ: Conservative management of intermittent claudication. Ann Intern Med 113:135, 1990

Weitz JI et al: Diagnosis and treatment of chronic arterial insufficiency of the lower extremities: A critical review [published erratum appears in Circulation 102:1074, 2000]. Circulation 94:3026, 1996

92

UROKINASE OR VASCULAR SURGERY IN THE TREATMENT OF ACUTE ARTERIAL OCCLUSION: THE TOPAS TRIAL

Kenneth Ouriel

Acute arterial occlusion is associated with a substantial risk of limb loss and death, either of which may occur in spite of early operative intervention (Blaisdell et al., 1978). Percutaneous, catheter-directed infusion of thrombolytic agents is presently in widespread use as an alternative to open surgery in such cases. Thrombolysis can restore arterial flow by dissolving the occluding thrombus and can be followed by a percutaneous or simple open surgical procedure to correct any unmasked lesions. Instead of a complex open procedure, a smaller elective procedure is performed under optimal conditions.

Despite the theoretical advantages of thrombolysis, its safety and efficacy remain controversial (Ricotta, 1991). Restoration of arterial flow may be slower than primary surgical intervention, and tissue ischemia may progress to infarction before recanalization occurs. Hemorrhage is also a potential complication; the balance between benefits and the risk of untoward effects can only be assessed through large, controlled trials. The Thrombolysis or Peripheral Arterial Surgery (TOPAS) trial was a randomized, multicenter study designed to answer this question,

comparing the safety and efficacy of catheter-directed recombinant urokinase (r-UK) to primary operation as initial treatment in patients with acute peripheral arterial occlusion (Ouriel et al., 1996, 1998).

Methods

The TOPAS trial was organized into two stages. Stage 1 (Ouriel et al., 1996) was a randomized comparison of three different doses of r-UK and primary operation for the treatment of limb-threatening lower extremity arterial occlusion. Over a 6-month period ending in August of 1993, 79 participating centers enrolled 213 patients into this study and r-UK was administered through a catheter-directed approach to eligible patients. Such patients included those with class II (reversible limb-threatening) ischemia as defined by the Society for Vascular Surgery/International Society for Cardiovascular Surgery. Symptoms were required to be less than 14 days in duration. Patients with thrombotic or embolic causes were eligible, as were patients with native artery or bypass graft involvement. Patients were excluded when a contraindication to surgical or thrombolytic therapy was present. Eligible patients were assigned to a treatment group by a centralized randomization center, contacted at the time of patient enrollment via telephone.

Aspirin was administered orally to each patient enrolled in the study, and heparin therapy was begun after arterial cannulation. The activated partial thromboplastin time was maintained between 1.5 and 2.0 times control. The three r-UK treatment protocols differed in the rate of administration during the initial 4-h infusion period: 2000 IU/min, 4000 IU/min, or 6000 IU/min. Thereafter, administration of r-UK was fixed at a rate of 2000 IU/min in all three groups. Infusions of r-UK were terminated when complete lysis was achieved, when complications occurred, or after 48 h of therapy. Successful r-UK therapy was followed by surgical or endovascular intervention when a lesion was unmasked that was deemed responsible for the occlusive process. Warfarin therapy was begun in patients who required prosthetic bypass grafts to infrapopliteal arteries, in patients with occlusions of embolic cause, and in patients with presumed hypercoagulable syndromes. Mandatory heparin therapy was discontinued during the conduct of stage II of TOPAS. Because of a higher-than-anticipated rate of hemorrhagic complications, investigators were instructed to refrain from aspirin or therapeutic heparin anticoagulation.

The primary end-point of stage I of TOPAS was arteriographic assessment of complete (>95%) clot lysis after 4 h of infusion. This particular time-point was chosen because the three r-UK groups differed in the rate of infusion for the first 4 h only, each converging to 2000 IU/min thereafter. The dose for stage II of the trial was chosen by the steering committee, blinded to the dose for each of the three thrombolytic groups. Stage II of TOPAS was a head-to-head comparison between the best r-UK dose and primary operation (Ouriel et al., 1998). This stage was conducted over an 18-month period ending in December of 1994. The primary end-point of this stage was amputation-free survival 6 months following randomization.

Results

Stage I

No statistically significant differences were found in the rate of recanalization or in the frequency of complete clot lysis between the three r-UK dose regimens. There were, however, trends toward improved recanulization in the 4000 IU/min group. Moreover, there were trends toward improved in-hospital mortality and amputation-free survival in the 4000-IU/min group. These data, combined with reduced severe or life-threatening hemorrhage, were responsible for the steering committee choosing the 4000-IU/min dose as the dose with which to continue in stage II of the TOPAS trial.

Stage II

The head-to-head comparison between recombinant urokinase (4000 IU/min for 4 h followed by 2000 IU/min) vs. primary operation comprised 544 patients suitable for intent-to-treat data analysis. Amputation-free survival rates 6 months after randomization were 71.8% in the r-UK and 74.8% in the operative group ($p = .43$; 95% confidence interval for the difference between treatments, -10.5 to 4.5 percentage points). There was also no significant difference in the rates of amputation-free survival at discharge from the hospital or in the rate of mortality at the time of discharge. At the end of 6 months, Kaplan-Meier analyses showed that 31.5% of the patients in the r-UK group had only percutaneous procedures. By contrast, the vast majority (94.2%) of the patients randomized to primary operation underwent open surgery, a rate that was not unexpected due to the design of the trial. The median length of hospitalization was 10 days in both treatment groups, among patients who survived to discharge. Among patients who were randomly assigned to initial thrombolysis, those with occlusions in bypass grafts had better clinical outcomes and rates of clot dissolution, concurrent with lower rates of major hemorrhagic complications.

Major hemorrhage complications occurred in 32 patients (12.5%) in the r-UK group, as compared with 14 patients (5.5%) in the surgery group ($p =$ .005). Patient age, duration of infusion, and activated partial thromboplastin times at baseline were unrelated to the risk of bleeding. Intracranial hemorrhage occurred in four patients in the r-UK group (1.6%), one of whom died. By contrast, there were no instances of intracranial hemorrhage in the surgery group. The risk of bleeding was significantly greater when therapeutic heparin was utilized as compared to when it was not ($p =$ .02 by Fisher's exact test). In 102 patients who received therapeutic heparin, bleeding occurred in 19 patients (19%). By contrast, in the 150 patients in whom therapeutic heparin was not utilized, bleeding occurred in only 13 patients (9%). Use of therapeutic heparin accounted for an increase in the risk of bleeding with a relative risk ratio of 2.19 (95% confidence interval 1.13 to 4.24, $p =$ .02).

Distal embolization of partially dissolved material occurred 41 times in 36 patients treated with r-UK. The emboli were dissolved in 19 of the 26 cases treated only with continued thrombolytic therapy. Amputation or death during the initial hospitalization occurred in 19% of the patients with emboli and 16% without emboli.

Discussion

For several decades, thrombolysis with agents such as streptokinase, urokinase, and recombinant tissue plasminogen activator has been investigated in uncontrolled trials as a therapeutic alternative to operation for acute peripheral arterial occlusion (McNamara and Fischer, 1985; Sullivan et al., 1991). More recently, several randomized trials have been published comparing thrombolysis with operation for arterial occlusion. The first trial, the Rochester study, randomly assigned 57 patients with acute limb-threatening ischemia to thrombolysis with urokinase or to immediate operation (Ouriel et al., 1994). At 1 year, the amputation-free survival rates were 75 and 52%, respectively, a statistically significant difference.

In the multicenter Surgery versus Thrombolysis for Ischemia of the Lower Extremity (STILE) study

(1994), 393 patients were randomly assigned to surgery or to thrombolysis with either recombinant tissue plasminogen activator or urokinase. Clinical outcomes for both thrombolysis groups were similar, so their data were combined for the overall comparison of thrombolysis with surgery. Post hoc stratification of patients into two subgroups on the basis of the duration of symptoms before enrollment ($>$14 days vs. $\leq$14 days) showed that among patients with symptoms of longer duration, the surgical group had lower amputation rates than the thrombolysis group at 6 months (3 vs. 12%, $p =$ .01). In contrast, among patients with symptoms of shorter duration, patients assigned to thrombolysis had lower rates than surgical patients (11 vs. 30%, $p =$ .02). In the preliminary r-UK dose-ranging study (TOPAS stage 1), the 1-year amputation-free survival rate in the group assigned to receive 4000 IU of urokinase per min (52 patients) was 74.6%, as compared with 66.9% in the surgical group (58 patients) ($p =$ .38) (Ouriel et al., 1996).

The TOPAS results differ from those in the Rochester study. In this study, initial thrombolytic therapy was not superior to operative intervention with respect to the major end-points of survival limb salvage. The TOPAS trial patients differ from those in the Rochester trial, however. The TOPAS patients were less acutely ill than those in the Rochester series, as manifested by the duration and magnitude of limb ischemia, age differences, and the incidence of coronary artery disease. It should be noted that, in the TOPAS trial, a 12.5% incidence of major bleeding was documented with r-UK, with an increase in the risk of hemorrhage when patients received concurrent heparin (Ouriel et al., 1998). Although the potential for significant clinical hemorrhage in patients undergoing thrombolysis remains a concern, present data suggest that the risk of hemorrhage at sites distant from the catheter can be reduced by restricting the concomitant use of heparin. The TOPAS data demonstrated that an initial strategy of thrombolysis, as compared with primary operation, reduced the number of required open procedures. The use of thrombolysis with r-UK allowed some patients to avoid surgical intervention all together, without a significant increase in mortality, amputation rate, or duration of hospitalization.

In summary, the substitution of thrombolysis and close procedure for surgery should be attractive to patients as well as health care providers. In many instances, thrombolysis can offer patients definitive treatment with less accompanying trauma than major surgery. Concurrent with similar rates of amputation and mortality, these results suggest that thrombolytic therapy should be considered in patients with acute limb ischemia secondary to native artery or bypass graft thrombosis.

REFERENCES

Blaisdell FW et al: Management of acute lower extremity arterial ischemia due to embolism and thrombosis. Surgery 84:822, 1978

McNamara TO, Fischer JR: Thrombolysis of peripheral arterial and graft occlusions: Improved results using high-dose urokinase. Am J Roentgenol 144:769, 1985

Ouriel K et al: A comparison of thrombolytic therapy with operative revascularization in the initial treatment of acute peripheral arterial ischemia. J Vasc Surg 19:1021, 1994

Ouriel K et al: Thrombolysis or peripheral arterial surgery: Phase I results. TOPAS Investigators. J Vasc Surg 23:64, 1996

Ouriel K et al: A comparison of recombinant urokinase with vascular surgery as initial treatment for acute arterial occlusion of the legs. N Engl J Med 338:1105, 1998

Ricotta J: Intra-arterial thrombolysis. A surgical view. Circulation 83(Suppl 2):I120, 1991

STILE Trial Investigators: Results of a prospective randomized trial evaluating surgery versus thrombolysis for ischemia of the lower extremity. The STILE trial. Ann Surg 220:251, 1994

Sullivan KL et al: Efficacy of thrombolysis in infrainguinal bypass grafts. Circulation 83(Suppl 2):I99, 1991

93

ANNULOAORTIC ECTASIA AND THE MARFAN SYNDROME: FROM GENETICS TO MANAGEMENT

Kenton J. Zehr

Aneurysms of the aortic root involving the sinuses of Valsalva, the sinotubular junction, and the ascending aorta have been termed *annuloaortic ectasia* (See Color Plate 30, Figure 93-1). The appearance is typically a bulb-shaped dilatation of the aortic root and the proximal portion of the ascending aorta. The pathology lies in the medial layer of the aorta. The tunica media contains large amounts of elastic tissue concentrically oriented, which forms the largest portion of the aortic wall. In addition to the elastic tissue, there are smooth-muscle cells and ground substance made up of proteoglycans. Patients with annuloaortic ectasia exhibit loss and disorganization of the elastic fibers by histologic evaluation. As the medial degeneration progresses, the smooth-muscle cells drop out and the fragmentation of elastic lamina becomes so advanced that the pathologic term is *medial necrosis*. This medial degeneration is the defining pathologic feature of annuloaortic ectasia. The loss of medial integrity contributes to the development of aortic dissection in approximately one-third of patients with aortic root aneurysms. Annuloaortic ectasia results in ascending aortic dissection and severe aortic regurgitation. These are the hallmark catastrophic vascular conditions seen in various connective tissue diseases.

The Marfan Syndrome

The classic Marfan syndrome is the most common heritable connective tissue disease resulting in annuloaortic ectasia. The genetic abnormality renders the elastic layers of the aortic media weak and predisposed to dilation. The prevalence of the syndrome is 1 in 20,000 live births in the United States, and it is inherited as an autosomal dominant trait. Until recent decades, the life expectancy of a Marfan's patient diagnosed in childhood was the third decade of life. As knowledge of varying phenotypes and understanding of the molecular basis of the disease have increased, we now know that there are extreme differences in the manifestation of the vascular effects of this disease. Many patients express a Marfan's phenotype with a milder cardiovascular effect and can present in late adulthood. Molecular study has revealed many mutations of the Marfan's genotype resulting in variable expression.

The Marfan syndrome was first described in 1896 by Antoine Marfan, a Parisian pediatrician, in the Bulletin of the Medical Society of Paris. He described skeletal and ocular abnormalities in a 5-year-old girl with arachnodactyly. It was not until approximately 50 years later that the cardiovascular manifestations of the Marfan syndrome were described (Etter and Glover, 1943). Details of the syndrome and its wide-ranging effects on multiple organ systems were described in 1955 (McKusick, 1955), but isolation of the gene responsible for Marfan's syndrome would need to await the molecular genetic revolution. In 1990 the gene was isolated to a locus on chromosome 15 (Kainulainen et al., 1990). This linkage study coincided with the identification of abnormal fibrillin, a glycoprotein component of the extracellular microfibril matrix in most patients with the Marfan phenotype (Milewicz et al., 1992). In 1991, Dietz and colleagues described a de novo missense mutation in the fibrillin gene in two patients with the Marfan phenotype (Dietz et al., 1991).

Since these initial discoveries, many missense, nonsense, and deletion mutations in the fibrillin 1 gene have been described in patients exhibiting the Marfan phenotype. The Institute of Genetics at The Johns Hopkins Hospital has recently published a revised genomic organization of the fibrillin-1 gene (Biery et al., 1999). The gene has been found to be 200 kb in size, which is more than twice the size previously thought.

Genetic abnormalities of the fibrillin-1 gene result in various abnormalities in fibrillin production and construction of the extracellular matrix. In Marfan families, each affected member exhibits the same fibrillin abnormality. In one study, approximately 25% of patients contained inadequate amounts of fibrillin within the extracellular matrix, 25% secreted fibrillin inefficiently, 25% incorporated this fibrillin inadequately within the intracellular matrix, and in the remaining 25% the exact metabolic abnormality could not be defined (Milewicz et al., 1992). The importance of fibrillin is to aid in organization of tropoelastin molecules into the mature elastic fibers. To date, more than 137 unique fibrillin-1 mutations

have been identified, and different mutations manifest the Marfan phenotype to varying degrees (Furthmayr and Francke, 1997). Mutations are found throughout the entire gene. A cluster of mutations has been found from exons 24 to 32 resulting in the most severe form of the Marfan syndrome, the neonatal Marfan syndrome. Fibrillin-1 mutations have also been found in patients who do not fulfill clinical criteria for the diagnosis of Marfan syndrome but have related disorders of connective tissue, such as isolated ectopia lentis, familial aortic aneurysm, and Marfan-like skeletal abnormalities; thus, Marfan syndrome may be regarded as one of a range of type 1 fibrillinopathies (Robinson and Godfrey; 2000). Understanding of the global and molecular functions of the fibrillin-containing microfibrils is not yet complete. Therefore, no definitive theory of the pathogenesis of Marfan's syndrome has been put forth. Many fibrillin-1 gene mutations appear to have a significant negative effect. The mutant fibrillin monomers tend to impair the global function of the microfibrils. The result is a variety of phenotypic changes, ranging from lethal forms presenting in the neonate to those diagnosed in adult patients primarily with aneurysmal dilatation of the aorta and only minor other Marfanoid-type features.

There has been some success with classification of various individuals with fibrillin-1 abnormalities into groups with differences in severity and prognosis. However, prospective understanding as to the effects of the various genetic mutations on each individual patient's structural integrity of the aorta is not clear. Specific mutations of the fibrillin gene have not been correlated with the rapidity and extent of dilatation of the aortic root or with the propensity of the aortic root for dissection.

Mechanism of Aortic Regurgitation and Principles of Repair

Aortic valve competence requires the maintenance of several geometric relations within the aortic root. The valve mechanism is a complex three-dimensional structure in the shape of a three-point crown

(See Color Plates 31 & 32, Figures 93-2 & 93-3). The commissural attachments of the valve to the annulus represent the points of the crown and are similar to the columns of a suspension bridge. The three leaflets of the valve are suspended from column to column. The sinotubular junction is made up of the three commissural structures and the encircling ridge of aortic wall tissue at the superior junction of the sinuses of Valsalva and the ascending aorta. Competency of the valve requires that the diameter of the sinotubular junction nearly approximate the length of the free margin of each individual cusp.

In annuloaortic ectasia, the cystic medial degeneration and loss of elastic lamina integrity allow enlargement of the ascending aorta involving the sinuses of Valsalva in the sinotubular junction. As the sinotubular junction diameter increases, the free margins of the aortic cusps become stretched between the commissural attachments. Thus, there is inadequate cusp tissue to coapt in diastole. This results in the central jet as seen by echocardiography.

In the Marfan patient, there is often less aortic regurgitation than would be expected for the degree of sinotubular diameter increase. This is likely due to the increased compliance of the Marfan valve cusp. There is some elongation of the free edges of the cusps, resulting in continued coaptation. Thus, it is not uncommon to find a markedly dilated aortic root with only mild to moderate aortic regurgitation. This likely contributes to the fact that the initial cardiovascular presentation of many patients with the Marfan syndrome is dissection. It has long been known that the valve tissue in patients with Marfan's disease can be friable and have myxomatous changes. The diseased valve tissue has been found to be more compliant in order of magnitude compared to normal valves. This is related to disorientation of collagen fibers and the proliferation of mucopolysaccharides. In one study (Fleischer et al., 1997), fibrillin abnormalities were observed in the mid-portion of the aortic valve, aortic wall, and mitral valve tissues. These abnormalities were seen in all patients with the Marfan syndrome and were most severe in those patients older than 20 years. The surgeon planning reconstruction must bear in mind that the disease process affects all the tissue from the annulus distally, including the aortic valve.

Operative Techniques

Reconstruction of the aortic root affected by annuloectasia and the Marfan syndrome dates back to the early 1960s. Reconstruction techniques used were aortoplasty, graft replacement, and aortic valvuloplasty. Techniques have evolved since then. The development of mechanical valves and synthetic tube conduits allowed Groves' team to replace the valve along with a separate tubular graft replacement of the ascending aorta in patients with the Marfan syndrome (Groves et al., 1964). Another team described a technique that allowed for a near-total replacement, including the sinuses and the sinotubular junction (Wheat et al., 1964). The technique was an advancement, but a significant amount of tissue remained in the region of the coronary ostia. This tissue could dilate, resulting in sinus of Valsalva aneurysms. The Bentall procedure initially described the use of a composite graft incorporating the valve and tubular conduit to replace the entire aortic root (Bentall and DeBono; 1968). Adaptations of the original Bentall technique have become the mainstay of operative technique for aortic root reconstruction in patients with aortic root aneurysms, including albumin-impregnated vascular conduits, reattachment of the coronary ostia by the button technique, and felt buttressing of the coronary buttons. These advancements have decreased formation of false aneurysms at the aortic annulus or at the coronary artery ostia, significant bleeding complications, and dilatation of any unresected aortic tissue.

Although it is well known that the valve tissue itself is also affected by the abnormal fibrillin metabolism, the degree in which this abnormality affects its function is less well known. Despite the observed myxomatous changes in the valve cusps, it appears that their functionality is near normal. Some have advocated preserving the valve in these patients, alleviating the need for anticoagulation. Several successful techniques have been described. One such (Yacoub et al., 1998) was used in a large series of patients dating from 1979 (Fig. 93-4). Sixty-eight of these patients had the Marfan syndrome. The technique involves replacement of the entire ascending aorta, sinotubular ridge, and sinuses

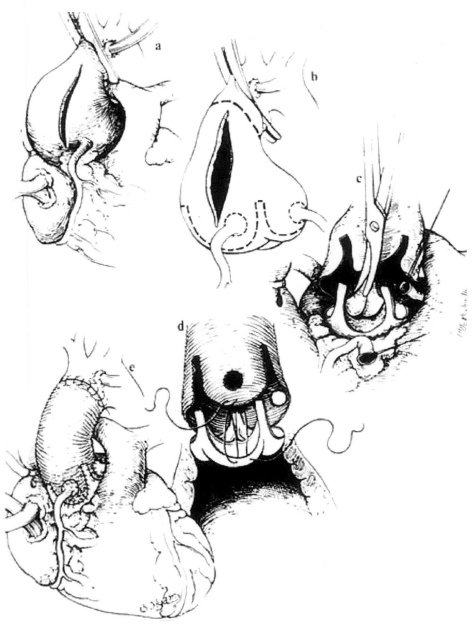

FIGURE 93-4

Steps in a Yacoub valve-sparing procedure. *A.* opening of the aortic root aneurysm after cross clamping the aorta. *B.* Dotted line depicts incision lines. *C.* Transection of the aorta, excision of the coronary sinuses, and dissection of the coronary ostial buttons. *D.* Sewing in the tailored Dacron graft. *E.* The reconstructed aortic root.

of Valsalva with a Dacron tube graft cut into a mirror image of the crown shape of the aortic annulus. The coronary ostia are reimplanted as buttons. In this way the geometry of the natural aortic root is reinstated (See Color Plate 33, Figure 93-5). In a similar type of reconstruction, David described a technique in which the aortic root is reconstructed by resuspending the commissures and annulus within a Dacron tube graft (David, 1997).

The eddy currents occurring within the sinuses of Valsalva in the natural aortic root are considered to be important in the smooth, gradual, and gentle closure of the valve (Robicsek et al., 1999). In 1990, a design of an ascending aortic graft was proposed that had "built-in" sinuses (Robicsek, 1992). Recent studies have established that the compliance of the sinuses is perhaps even more important than the geometry for reducing stress in the leaflets and enhancing valve longevity (Thubrikar, 1990). In accordance with this, a novel Dacron prosthesis with compliant sinuses of Valsalva was made for aortic root replacement (Thubrikar et al., 1999) (See Color Plates 35 & 36, Figures 93-6 & 93-7). These have been implanted in six patients at the Mayo Clinic (Zehr et al., 2000). All had annuloaortic ectasia with cystic medial necrosis, but only two patients had phenotypic Marfan syndrome. A similar idea of creating neosinuses by modifying a Dacron tube with an extension of Dacron oriented longitudinally, allowing expansion of neosinuses after root reconstruction has been reported (De Paulis et al., 2000). This graft has been used in five patients undergoing aortic root reconstructions with good results. These adaptations of the remodeling technique represent an attempt to recreate more perfectly the normal anatomy of the aortic root.

While several centers have had good results using the valve-preserving techniques, others are reluctant to adopt this because of the known histochemical abnormalities within the valve tissue.

Indications

Dissection of the ascending aortic aneurysm requires urgent or emergent repair. Severe aortic regurgitation is also an indication for immediate repair of the aneurysmal root. Elective repair of the aneurysmal root has been shown to carry a markedly lower risk of mortality. Criteria have been presented by several groups as to the appropriate size of the aorta in which to intervene. One group studied the risk of dissection or rupture of ascending aortic aneurysms in relation to size in the Yale database (Coady et al., 1999). They found that the median size in patients suffering these devastating complications was 5.9 cm. The initial size at presentation was 5.2 cm, and the aneurysms were observed to grow at a rate of 0.1 cm per year. In a multivariable regression, a size ≥ 6.0 cm was associated with an increased probability of rupture or dissection of 25.2%. They recommended intervention when aneurysms reached the size of 5.5 cm.

Earlier, another group had suggested operative repair in patients with asymptomatic aneurysms either twice the size of the normal aorta or exceeding 4.7 to 5 cm in diameter (Svensson et al., 1989). This intervention is advised because of their observations of the risk of rupture and dissection in these patients. Yet another group showed that higher systolic blood pressure, increased height and aortic growth rate, and older age were associated with a greater risk of rupture or dissection (Roman et al., 1993). Patients with a sinotubular ridge size of 4 to 6 cm were observed to have a higher rate of complication compared to those with 2.9-cm aortas. In an analysis of 55 patients with aortic dissection, 36% who developed dissection had a maximal aortic diameter of <6 cm (Pyeritz et al., 1992). These studies point to earlier intervention in patients with connective tissue disorders and support surgical repair in an aorta >5 cm in diameter. In high-risk patients, intervention on even smaller aortas should be considered.

Results

The safety and efficacy of elective repair has been well documented by several large series. Of 270 patients undergoing root replacement between 1976 and 1993, 187 had a Marfan aneurysm of the ascending aorta and 53 had annuloaortic ectasia of a nonspecific medial degeneration (Gott et al., 1995). Of the 182 patients undergoing elective root replacement for annuloaortic ectasia, there was no 30-day mortality. Nearly all of these underwent a modified Bentall composite graft repair. Actuarial survival was 73% at 10 years for the overall group.

In a 16-year experience with 168 patients undergoing 172 aortic root replacements, 30 patients had the Marfan syndrome (Kouchoukos et al., 1991). The hospital mortality rate for the overall series was 5%, and no significant differences in the survival rate between varying techniques was observed. However, it was found that the frequency of pseudoaneurysm formation of suture lines and the need for reoperation were less with the open modification of the Bentall technique. Freedom from thromboembolism for the 152 patients who received prosthetic valves was 82% at 12 years. They concluded that continued use of the composite graft technique as a preferred method of treatment was valid. Passek's team presented 52 patients with Marfan syndrome treated surgically between 1964 and 1990 (Passek et al., 1992). Composite grafts were used in 28 patients and other procedures on 24 patients. Early mortality was 7.7%, and late mortality was 27%. Eight of the 14 late deaths were related to cardiovascular complications. Actuarial 5-, 10-, and 15-year survival for the composite graft patients were 87%, 76%, and 57%, respectively, and for those who received other operations were 73%, 53%, and 37%. Passek's team concluded that the composite graft insertion was the operation of choice for patients with ascending aortic disease and/or aortic valve disease in the Marfan syndrome.

In a recent multicenter study, 675 patients with the Marfan syndrome underwent replacement of the aortic root (Gott et al., 1999). The 30-day mortality rate was 1.5% among 455 patients who underwent elective repair. Patients who underwent urgent repair (within 7 days of a surgical consultation) had a mortality rate of 2.6%. The mortality rate rose to 11.7% among the 103 patients who underwent emergent repair (within 24 h after the surgical consultation). Of these patients, 30% had aortic dissection involving the ascending aorta, and 46% of patients with dissection had an aortic diameter of <6.5 cm. This study showed that *elective* aortic root replacement had a low operative mortality. Because of the low elective mortality rate and the high incidence of aortic dissec-

tion in patients with aneurysms of <6.5 cm, it is clear from this study that elective repair should be done in patients with aortic sizes well below this dimension.

Several centers have reported relatively large series of patients undergoing the valve-sparing techniques in patients with annuloaortic ectasia. David's team reported on 120 patients of whom 48 had stigmata of the Marfan syndrome (David et al., 2001). There were two operative deaths. There was one early failure requiring composite replacement, and one failure at 2 years' follow-up. Five late deaths occurred. Follow-up was a mean of 35 ± 31 months. The 5-year actuarial survival was 88 ± 4%. No patients had thromboembolic or endocarditic complications; seven patients had moderate aortic regurgitation. The 5-year freedom from aortic reoperation was 99 ± 1% and from moderate or severe aortic regurgitation was 90 ± 4%. Yacoub's team reported on 158 patients, of whom 68 patients had the Marfan syndrome (Yacoub et al., 1998). Probability of reoperation was 3%, 11%, and 11%, at 1, 5, and 10 years, respectively. At follow-up there was no trivial or aortic regurgitation in 63.6%, mild to moderate in 33.3%, and severe in 3%. Another team reported on 75 patients, of whom 21 had the Marfan syndrome (Harringer et al., 1999). There were no operative and two late deaths. Three patients had progressive aortic regurgitation. All other patients had either none or mild regurgitation at a follow-up of 22 ± 20 months.

At the Mayo Clinic, between October 1994 and October 2000, 72 patients (20 with the Marfan syndrome) underwent aortic root reconstruction with preservation of the aortic valve and replacement of the aortic valve for chronic aneurysm with or without dissection (Burkhart et al., 2001). The reimplantation technique (David) was performed in 52 patients, remodeling technique (Yacoub) in 14, and remodeling with sinus graft root replacement technique in 6 patients. Postoperative echocardiography demonstrated absent to mild aortic insufficiency in 63 patients. Operative mortality was 2.8%. Actuarial survival was 84.1% at 5 years. Freedom from reoperation was 88.8% and 78.7% at 1 and 3 years. Eleven (21.2%) patients repaired by the implantation technique, one (7.1%) patient who underwent remodeling, and one (16.7%) patient who received a sinus graft required aortic valve replacement secondary to aortic valve insufficiency. By univariate analysis, the necessity of aortic cusp repair ($p = .0290$), aortic annulus size >25 mm ($p = .0162$), and male gender ($p = .0101$) were predictors for subsequent aortic valve replacement. This series points out the importance of proper selection in this patient population. The overall results of these series show acceptable early and late mortality rates and acceptable durability of the valve repair procedures.

Summary

The pathophysiology of annuloaortic ectasia is well understood. This has resulted in the ability to both tailor the operative technique and intervene at appropriate time points to effect real change in the prognosis and quality of life of affected individuals. The evolution of understanding of this disease process and its genetic associations should serve as a model toward the understanding and treatment of other cardiovascular diseases.

REFERENCES

Bentall H, DeBono A: A technique for complete replacement of the ascending aorta. Thorax 23:338, 1968

Biery NJ et al: Revised genomic organization of FBN1 and significance for regulated gene expression. Genomics 56:70, 1999

Burkhart HM et al: Valve preserving aortic root reconstruction: a comparison of techniques. Presented at the scientific sessions of the 1st biennial meeting for the Society of Heart Valve Disease, June 15–18, 2001; London

Coady MA et al: Surgical intervention criteria for thoracic aortic aneurysms: A study of growth rates and complications. Ann Thorac Surg 67:1922, 1999

David TE: Aortic root aneurysms: Remodeling or composite replacement? Ann Thorac Surg 64:1564, 1997

David TE et al: Results of aortic valve-sparing operations. J Thorac Cardiovasc Surg 122:39, 2001

De Paulis R et al: A new aortic dacron conduit for surgical treatment of aortic pathology. Ital Heart J 1:457, 2000

Dietz HC et al: Marfan's syndrome caused by a recurrent de novo missense mutation in the fibrillin gene. Nature 352:337, 1991

Etter LE, Glover LP: Arachnodactyly complicated by dislocated lens in death from rupture of dissecting aneurysm of aorta. JAMA 123:88, 1943

Fleischer KJ et al: Immunohistochemical abnormalities of fibrillin in cardiovascular tissues in Marfan's syndrome. Ann Thorac Surg 63:1012, 1997

Furthmayr H, Francke U: Ascending aortic aneurysm with or without features of Marfan syndrome and other fibrillinopathies: New insights. Semin Thorac Cardiovasc Surg 9:191, 1997

Gott VL et al: Aortic root replacement. Risk factor analysis of a seventeen-year experience with 270 patients. J Thorac Cardiovasc Surg 109:536, 1995

Gott VL et al: Replacement of the aortic root in patients with Marfan's syndrome. N Engl J Med 340:1307, 1999

Groves LK et al: Aortic insufficiency secondary to aneurysmal changes in the ascending aorta: Surgical management. J Thorac Cardiovasc Surg 48:362, 1964

Harringer W et al: Ascending aortic replacement with aortic valve reimplantation. Circulation 100(Suppl II): II-24, 1999

Kainulainen K et al: Location on chromosome 15 of the gene defect causing Marfan's syndrome. N Engl J Med 323:935, 1990

Kouchoukos NT et al: Sixteen-year experience with aortic root replacement. Results of 172 operations. Ann Surg 214:308, 1991

McKusick VA: The cardiovascular aspects of Marfan syndrome: A heritable disorder of connective tissue. Circulation 2:321, 1955

Milewicz DM et al: Marfan syndrome: Defective synthesis, secretion, and extracellular matrix formation of fibrillin by cultured dermal fibroblasts. J Clin Invest 89:79, 1992

Passek M et al: Surgical treatment of cardiovascular complications in Marfan syndrome: A 27-year experience. Eur J Cardiothorac Surg 6:149, 1992

Pyeritz RE et al: Abstract, 2nd International Marfan's Symposium, San Francisco, CA 1992

Robicsek F: Ascending aortic prosthesis: United States Patent Number 5139,15. August 18, 1992

Robicsek F, Thubrikar MJ: Role of sinus wall compliance in aortic leaflet function. Am J Cardiol 84:944, 1999

Robinson PN, Godfrey M: The molecular genetics of Marfan syndrome and related microfibrillopathies. J Med Genet 31:9, 2000

Roman MJ et al: Prognostic significance of the pattern of aortic root dilation in the Marfan syndrome. J Am Coll Cardiol 22:1470, 1993

Svensson LG et al: Impact of cardiovascular operation on survival in the Marfan patient. Circulation 80:233, 1989

Thubrikar M. *The Aortic Valve.* Boca Raton, FL; CRC Press, pp. 119–136, 1990

Thubrikar MJ et al: A new aortic root prosthesis with compliant sinuses for valve sparing operations. Circulation 100 (Suppl I):I-461, 1999

Wheat MN Jr et al: Successful replacement of the entire ascending aorta and aortic valve. JAMA 188:717, 1964

Yacoub MH et al: Late results of valve-preserving operation in patients with aneurysms of the ascending aorta and root. J Thorac Cardiovasc Surg 115:1080, 1998

Zehr KJ et al: Clinical introduction of a novel prosthesis for valve-preserving aortic root reconstruction for annuloaortic ectasia. J Thorac Cardiovasc Surg. 120:692, 2000

CATHETER-BASED TREATMENT OF SUBACUTE AORTIC DISSECTION

Christoph A. Nienaber

The management of patients with subacute dissection of the thoracic aorta (i.e., surviving >14 days since the index dissection) is a complex issue with no clear guidelines. Both surgical and medical treatment are imperfect and associated with substantial rates of failure, morbidity, and mortality and with gradual enlargement of the false lumen and formation of aneurysm. While stabilization of the aortic tube remains unpredictable with prevailing rupture and progression under medical treatment, surgical resection carries a risk of both spinal cord injury and death in 14 to 67% of patients (Coselli et al., 1997; Fuster, and Halperin, 1994; Glower et al., 1990). Thus, a new therapeutic strategy for both retrograde and antegrade dissection originating from a tear distal to the subclavian artery is needed; with the advent of nonsurgical reconstruction of thoracic aortic dissection by interventional sealing of the entry site (tear) with stent-grafts, a major therapeutic dilemma is likely to be solved.

Cumulative experience in more than 40 cases suggests that conversion from unstable dissection to a stable reconstructed aorta is feasible through endovascular stent-grafting (Kouchoukos and Dougenis, 1997). Since October 1997, 42 consecutive patients (age 56 ± 12 years) with subacute or chronic type B aortic dissection underwent transluminal endovascular stent-graft placement. Selection criteria were based on anatomical conditions, such as an entry site at or distal to the left subclavian artery and a suitable iliac or femoral access with no major tortuosity; eight patients had previous surgery for type A dissection. The length of the dissecting lamella varied from 15 to 42 cm, with thoracoabdominal extension of the dissection in 17 patients. Transfemoral stent-grafting was offered after identification of a proximal entry to the false lumen, a true lumen diameter of <4 cm, and failure of spontaneous thrombus formation in the false lumen. Dissection extending to the aortic bifurcation, tortuosity, or kinking did not preclude stent-graft placement as long as the iliac artery allowed access of the 22 to 27 F delivery sheath.

Imaging Protocol

Candidates were subjected to spin-echo (anatomical) magnetic resonance imaging (MRI) and three-dimensional MR angiography after bolus injection of gadolinium-DPTA. A fast low-angle shot (FLASH) three-dimensional sequence in breathhold was used to create maximum intensity projections. Imaging of 64 interpolated contiguous slices using 1/2 K-space data acquisition in phase-encoding direction was obtained on a 1.5-tesla MR scanner equipped with an ultrafast gradient system; a body array coil was used for signal transmission and reception. With subvolume multiplanar reconstruction, the dissecting lamella, the exact site of a communication, and false lumen flow were identified in all cases (Fig. 94-1). Morphometric evaluation of MR images and angiograms was used to design each stent-graft prior to implantation. All patients had follow-up MR imaging to document complete closure of the interluminal communication and/or false lumen thrombosis (Fig. 94-2).

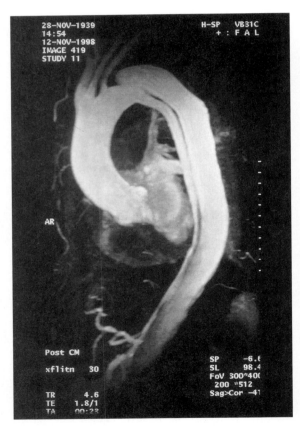

FIGURE 94-1

Three-dimensional MR angiogram (MIP projection in sagittal oblique orientation). Type B aortic dissection after Gd-DTPA bolus. The MR angiogram shows a large entry site distal to the subclavian artery on both a small compressed true lumen and an enlarged false lumen.

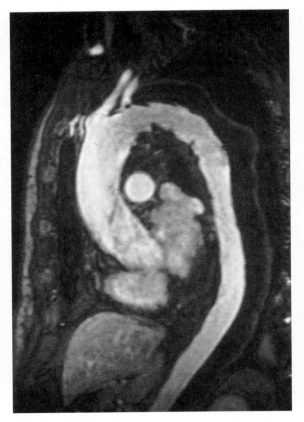

FIGURE 94-2

After sealing of the entry site with an endovascular stent-graft, the true lumen is enlarged to normal diameter and the false lumen is completely thrombosed.

Stent-Graft Implantation

Stent-graft placement was performed in the cardiac catheterization laboratory with patients under general anesthesia and ventilation. The procedure was started by injecting 5000 IE units of heparin and introducing a 6-F pigtail via the left subclavian artery for precise guidance in the acute proximity of the subclavian artery and for intraprocedural angiograms. The femoral or distal iliac artery was surgically exposed and a 0.035-in. guidewire was inserted. When wire position in the true lumen of the aorta was confirmed by fluoroscopy and ultrasound, the sheath with the encroached stent, pusher, and deflated balloon was introduced. The collapsed stent was advanced to the most proximal communication, guided by simultaneous transesophageal color Doppler imaging. With the Dacron shell centered on the communication, the self-expanding stent-graft was launched under ultrasound guidance. To ensure optimal positioning, care was taken to seal the entry and to protect the left subclavian artery with the bare nitinol spring (Kouchoukos and Dougenis, 1997).

Procedural Success

Complete sealing of the entry to the false lumen was documented by color Doppler transesophageal echocardiogram (TEE) and aortography in 39 of 42 patients (93%). Two patients received two stent-grafts, and two others required adjunctive stenting of the ostium of the left renal artery. Initiation of false lumen thrombosis was observed with transesophageal ultrasound during the procedure in 34 patients (81%). None of the patients had a prolonged recovery after stent-graft placement. The length of stay in the intensive care unit was 36 ± 12 h; one patient suffered from embolic stroke 12 h after stent-graft placement. Both intra- and postprocedural outcome was uneventful (Table 94-1). Transient postimplantation syndrome with mild leukocytosis, elevated C-reactive protein levels, and moderately elevated body temperature was seen in 75% of patients; a nonspecific mild to moderate back pain syndrome was described by about one-third of patients and resolved within 12 ± 5 days.

Intraprocedural and Follow-Up Imaging

In addition to repeated contrast angiograms, color Doppler TEE provided useful insight for both exact positioning of the stent-graft and monitoring of entry flow (to the false lumen) by cessation of color flow with stent-graft deployment. Moreover, both angiography and transesophageal ultrasound confirmed true lumen expansion with stent-graft deployment by 28 ± 10 mm (or 51 ± 24% of preimplantation width). Intraprocedural ultrasound also revealed false lumen thrombosis by detection of "smoke" within minutes of sealing the entry in 81%. Moreover, one small endoleak and seven persistent distal communications to the false lumen were also identified.

After 3 months, MRI documented complete thrombosis of the false lumen and patent stent-grafts in all cases (Figs. 94-2 and 94-3). No aortic sidebranch occlusion and no evidence of either stent-graft migration, twisting, or endoleakage were noted. At 3 months, clear evidence of true lumen expansion and false lumen shrinkage from consolidation of thrombosis was documented in all patients, suggesting remodeling of the aortic tube with enlargement of the reconstructed true lumen (Figs. 94-2 and 94-3). All patients with stent-grafts conducted a more active life than a previous group of surgically treated patients; the majority required continuous antihypertensive medication, but none was rehospitalized after interventional stent-graft placement. Conversely, surgery for type B dissection is associated with a 12-month mortality rate of 33% and serious morbidity in 42% (Kouchoukos and Dougenis, 1997). Moreover, both intensive care and hospital stay were markedly longer for surgery patients than for patients subjected to stent-grafting (Table 94-1).

TABLE 94-1

TREATMENT OF TYPE B AORTIC DISSECTION

Variable	Surgery (n = 12)	Stent-Graft (n = 42)	p
Procedure			
General anesthesia	12	40	NS
Duration, h	8.0 ± 2.0	1.4 ± 0.6	<.001
Prosthesis			
Length, cm	22.0 ± 7.4	12.8 ± 4.8	<.001
Diameter, mm	27 ± 2	38 ± 4	<.001
Intensive care, h	92 ± 45	26 ± 10	<.001
Hospital stay, days	40 ± 24	6 ± 7	<.001
Body temperature (>38°C)	6	31	NS
Mortality (n, %)			
Perioperative	1 (8)	0	NS
After 30 days	1 (8)	0	NS
After 1 year	4 (33)	0	.03
Cumulative morbidity (n, %)	5 (42)	4 (10)	.04
Paraplegia	2 (17)	0	NS
Neurologic defect	3 (25)	1 (2.5)	.04
Respiratory complication	5 (42)	2 (5)	.04
Renal failure	3 (25)	0	NS
Physical recovery (n, %)	7 (58)	41 (97.5)	.03

NOTE: NS, not significant.

Endovascular Reconstruction of Aortic Dissection

Nonsurgical reconstruction of aortic dissection constitutes a viable therapeutic option for patients with thoracic dissection originating distal to the subclavian artery with a patent or expanding false lumen and/or recurrent pain. In contrast to thoracic surgery for type B dissection, transfemoral stent-grafting has the potential to reduce mortality and morbidity. Preliminary analysis suggests major cost savings as a result of reduced intensive care and shorter hospital stay. Even though nonsurgical (interventional) techniques have recently been introduced for dilation of congenital aortic stenosis and coarctation and for exclusion of abdominal and thoracic aneurysms, aortic dissection was, for many years, the domain of surgical or medical management—both with disappointing results (Coselli et al., 1997; Fuster and Halperin, 1994). Except for catheter fenestration of occlusive distal flaps, no interventional strategy was useful in managing aortic dissection. While (emergency) surgical repair is life-saving in ascending (type A) aortic dissection (Glower et al., 1990), both emergent and deferred surgery for descending (type B) dissection is associated with a 6 to 67% mortality with no substantial advantage over medical therapy. Accordingly, morbidity (paraplegia/paresis) prevails

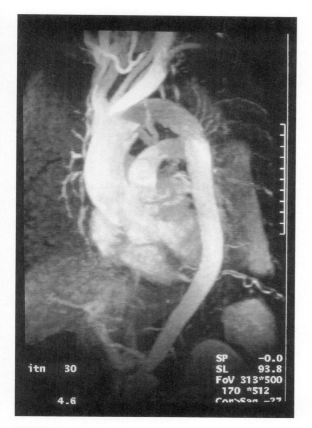

FIGURE 94-3

Follow-up MR angiogram after Gd-DTPA bolus showing successful nonsurgical reconstruction of the thoracic aorta after stent-graft placement to seal the proximal entry to the dissection.

in 7 to 36%, depending on the extent of aortic resection and duration of cross-clamping. Even with intraoperative use of atriodistal bypass, reattachment of all critical intercostal arteries, and permissive use of mild hypothermia, early surgical mortality is 7.1% in chronic and 8.7% in acute type B dissection (Miller, 1993; Nienaber et al., 1999; Nienaber and von Kodolitsch, 1992). Similarly, surgery-related paraplegia/paresis still occurs in 2.9% of chronic and 19% of acute type B dissection, with advanced age, excessive clamp time, and inappropriate reattachment of the great anterior radiculomedullary artery

(Adamkiewicz artery) as predictors of adverse outcome (Nienaber et al., 1993).

In contrast, the procedure of sealing the entry by endovascular stents induces false lumen thrombosis and stable remodeling of the aorta without disturbing the epiaortic integrity (Kouchoukos and Dougenis, 1997).

Although 8% of patients were expected to suffer spinal cord dysfunction with stent-grafts, no neurologic complication was encountered. The preserved integrity of the aorta rather than surgical resection of the dissected segment may be an important mechanism to protect spinal arteries. The use of short stent-grafts of 120 ± 40 mm length and avoidance of T8 to L2 (and the Adamkiewicz artery) further minimizes the risk of paraplegia. Most importantly, the interventional approach takes only 1 h, circumvents circulatory arrest and cross-clamping the aorta with associated ischemia and potential reperfusion injury, and avoids postoperative respiratory failure and prolonged hypotension with the risk of delayed paraplegia.

Aortic Remodeling

Aortic stability results from both thrombosis of the false lumen and the endoprosthesis itself; relatively short stent-grafts can cover the proximal entry and induce false lumen thrombosis over the entire length of the dissected aorta within 3 months (Fig. 94-2). In the patients discussed above, the true lumen revealed substantial expansion from 19 ± 7 mm to 35 ± 3 mm and the diameter of the previous false lumen stabilized by thrombus retraction. Thus, aortic remodeling consists of an active component (stent-induced expansion of the true lumen) and a passive component (thrombus retraction in the false lumen) and mimics the natural healing process, since a thrombosed false lumen was associated with a lower risk for future adverse events and better survival.

Although conceptually promising, management of type B dissection by stent-grafting still lacks long-term follow-up data. Late adverse effects are infrequent. Thrombosis of excluded aneurysms was reported in 95%, with periprocedural mortality of 8% and 6-month mortality of 12%, respectively; paraplegia, stroke, iliac artery avulsion, and proximal dissection occurred in 4, 3, and 2% of patients, respectively. Paraplegia, infection, vascular damage, or endoleakage, however, should become apparent early after placement of stent-grafts. Within 1 year, no such complication occurred in the patients discussed earlier. The author's team now recommends nonsurgical stent-graft placement in type B dissection only for patients with suitable anatomy (accessible proximal entry and at least one femoral artery without dissection and no major tortuosity). Stent-graft placement may constitute a promising nonsurgical therapeutic strategy for type B dissection and thus a better option than surgery or medical management in these high-risk patients. The initiation of the natural healing process (of false lumen thrombosis) by sealing the proximal entry induces both consolidation and remodeling of the aortic wall without side branch occlusion or progression of the dissecting process (Fig. 94-3). Nonsurgical reconstruction of thoracic aortic dissection may emerge as the preferred treatment in selected patients with suitable anatomy.

REFERENCES

Coselli JS et al: Paraplegia after thoracoabdominal aortic aneurysm repair: Is dissection a risk factor? Ann Thorac Surg 63:28, 1997

Fuster V, Halperin JL: Aortic dissection: A medical perspective. J Card Surg 9:713, 1994

Glower DD et al: Comparison of medical and surgical therapy for uncomplicated descending aortic dissection. Circulation 82:IV39,1990

Kouchoukos NT, Dougenis D: Surgery of the thoracic aorta. N Engl J Med 336:1876, 1997

Miller DC: The continuing dilemma concerning medical versus surgical management of patients with acute type B dissections. Semin Thorac Cardiovasc Surg 5:33, 1993

Nienaber CA, von Kodolitsch Y: Meta-analysis of changing mortality pattern in thoracic aortic dissection. Herz 17:398, 1992

Nienaber CA et al: The diagnosis of thoracic aortic dissection by noninvasive imaging procedures. N Engl J Med 328:1, 1993

Nienaber CA et al: Nonsurgical reconstruction of thoracic aortic dissection by stent-graft placement. N Engl J Med 340:1539, 1999

95

ENDOVASCULAR STENT-GRAFT PLACEMENT IN THE TREATMENT OF AORTIC DISSECTION

Gus J. Vlahakes

Introduction

Aortic dissection originating in the descending thoracic aorta is an acute condition that can produce substantial morbidity and mortality. Treatment decision-making has been based traditionally on the prognosis of untreated dissection; therapies, both medical and surgical, have been directed at treating the early and late complications of this lesion. In traditional surgical therapy, major surgical procedures have been indicated by the potential complications of the lesion, as summarized in Table 95-1.

As with other surgical treatment modalities, surgical decision-making is predicated on a risk vs. benefit analysis. Because the surgery for this lesion is often accompanied by substantial risk of morbidity and mortality, in the past it has been reserved for the treatment of the most serious complications of the lesion. Because surgical replacement of the descending aorta involves temporary clamping of the aorta, the circulation to the spinal cord, originating from the lower intercostal arteries, is often at risk. Accordingly, this type of surgery is accompanied by the risk of spinal cord paralysis. Furthermore, for patients undergoing descending aortic resection for aneurysm disease, intercostal arteries are often chronically occluded and the spinal cord blood supply is collateralized, thus reducing the surgical risk of paralysis. In contrast, in cases of acute aortic dissection, descending aortic replacement is more likely to jeopardize critical intercostal vessels. This accounts for the greater surgical risk of spinal cord paralysis in this group of patients; in addition, in the presence of end-organ ischemia, the surgical mortality can exceed 50% (Miller et al., 1984).

Thus, until recently, aortic dissections originating in the descending aorta and not involving the ascending aorta (Stanford classification type B; DeBakey classification type III) have been treated medically by pharmacologic reduction of cardiac contractility and systolic blood pressure. Even with optimized medical therapy, the mortality rate for this disease remains approximately 20% (Elefteriades et al., 1992).

A New Technique

Recent reports have detailed a new treatment modality for both acute as well as subacute

TABLE 95-1

TRADITIONAL INDICATIONS FOR SURGERY IN AORTIC DISSECTIONS ORIGINATING IN THE PROXIMAL DESCENDING AORTA

Uncontrolled pain despite optimized medical therapy

Retrograde dissection resulting in involvement of the ascending aorta

Visceral ischemia (central nervous system and abdominal)

Refractory hypertension

True or false aneurysm formation

Bleeding (aortic rupture)

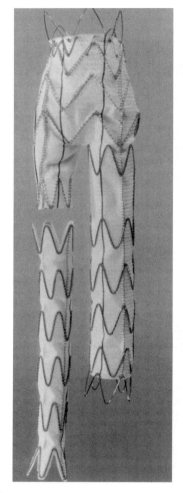

FIGURE 95-1

Examples of stent-grafts used for endovascular arterial stenting. Note the collapsible metal stent that has been incorporated into the fabric grafts. Shown are stent-grafts for use in the aorta, including for placement at the aortoiliac bifurcation.

dissections originating in the descending thoracic aorta: endovascular stent-grafting. This technique involves the percutaneous delivery of an endovascular prosthesis consisting of a collapsible metallic stent covered by prosthetic fabric graft material (Fig. 95-1). The length and expanded diameter of the stent are selected to match the dimensions of the pathologic segment of the aorta, which is being excluded from the lumen. When deployed in the aorta by expansion of the stent, the metallic stent applies the prosthetic graft material to the surface of the aorta, resulting in exclusion of the contained segment of the aorta. In the case of the treatment of aneurysm disease, the aneurysmal segment is excluded, provided there is an appropriate "neck" proximally and distally for seating of the endovascular prosthesis.

Once this technology was developed to a sufficient degree to permit use in patients, reports appeared detailing its use for the treatment of abdominal (Parodi et al., 1991) and thoracic (Dake et al., 1994) aortic aneurysms. With the success of this technique for management of stable aortic aneurysms, it was a natural extension of the method for its use in the treatment of descending aortic dissection. In the case of aortic dissection, seating of the graft by the stent is intended to cover the entrance site of the dissection, hence excluding it from the aortic lumen. Precise imaging techniques,

combining spiral computed tomography or magnetic resonance imaging with angiography, are needed to delineate the surgical anatomy. At least 1 cm of aorta between the left subclavian artery origin and the intimal tear is required for effective seating of the stent-graft.

Dake and colleagues reported the results in 19 patients who underwent stent-graft treatment of acute aortic dissections, originating in the proximal descending aorta, who were not stabilized by medical therapy alone (Dake et al., 1999). Indications for intervention included obstruction of branch vessels, atypical location of the dissection entry tear, acute aortic rupture, and persistent, severe pain. They included patients with Stanford type A dissections (with retrograde involvement of the ascending aorta) as well as those with Stanford type B dissections, which are confined to the descending aorta (± abdominal aortic involvement). In this series, all patients shared the common feature that, irrespective of the regions of the aorta involved, they all had intimal tears located in the proximal descending aorta. They achieved technical success in all 19 patients treated with deployment of the stent-graft in the true aortic lumen. Complete thrombosis occurred in the involved aortic false lumen in 15 patients, and partial thrombosis occurred in the remaining patients (Fig. 95-2). While three patients died in the first month following the procedure, there were no late deaths and no instances of aneurysm formation or aortic rupture up to 13 months after the procedure. Although this series was small, considering the potential morbidity and mortality of both medical and surgical therapy, these preliminary results with this new application of aortic stent-grafting should encourage further work.

In a slightly different setting, another group also published their results with stent-graft treatment of subacute and chronic aortic dissections originating in the descending thoracic aorta (Nienaber et al., 1999). An additional group of 12 patients was used as a comparison cohort and underwent traditional surgical resection and Dacron graft replacement of the aorta. Nienaber and colleagues demonstrated excellent results with no early or intermediate-term mortality in the stent-graft treated patients, with a 25% mortality at 1 year for the patients treated with surgery. Furthermore, they noted that in their experience, there were no instances of paraplegia, a significant potential risk of surgery for this lesion. Stent-grafting preserves the integrity of the aorta and its intercostal branches, whereas surgical resection of the dissected aorta and its associated intercostal arteries predisposes to this complication.

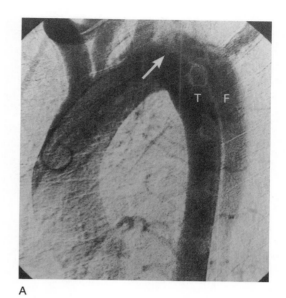

A

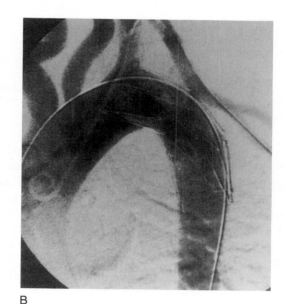

B

FIGURE 95-2

Contrast aortograms. *A.* Contrast aortogram showing an aortic dissection originating in the proximal descending aorta with contrast opacification of the true (T) and false (F) lumens. The angiographic catheter has been advanced through the true lumen. *B.* Repeat contrast aortogram following stent-graft deployment, showing obliteration of the false lumen. Note that the stent-graft is able to flex to accommodate the distal aortic arch.

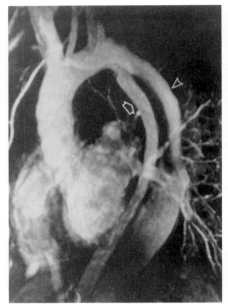 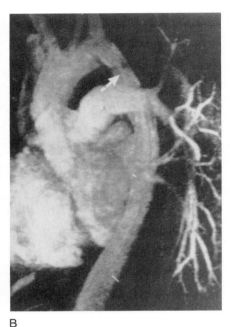

A   B

FIGURE 95-3

MRIs of chronic descending aortic dissection. *A.* Gadolinium-DTPA-enhanced magnetic resonance image of a chronic descending aortic dissection, showing the false lumen (arrowhead) and the true lumen (open arrow). Note the large false lumen and compressed true lumen in the distal descending aorta. *B.* Follow-up magnetic resonance image 3 months following stent-graft placement. Note remodeling of distal descending aorta with obliteration of the false lumen and reexpansion of the true lumen.

Nienaber and colleagues have also suggested that stent-graft treatment of aortic dissection can produce salutary remodeling of the aorta with thrombosis of the false lumen. They were able to demonstrate significant true lumen expansion (Fig. 95-3); obliteration of the false lumen is also associated with improved long-term outcome (Ergin et al., 1994).

While this treatment modality remains novel, the results of these two studies represent a major step forward in the treatment of thoracic aortic dissection. Many questions remain to be answered by future studies of this new approach. These include such issues as the long-term stability of the dissected aorta, the risk of endarteritis with an implanted luminal device, and the risk of stent-graft migration. These issues must be addressed by further clinical trials and close long-term follow-up.

REFERENCES

Dake MD et al: Transluminal placement of endovascular stent-grafts for the treatment of descending thoracic aortic aneurysms. N Engl J Med 331:1729, 1994

Dake MD et al: Endovascular stent-graft placement for the treatment of acute aortic dissection. N Engl J Med 340:1546, 1999

Elefteriades JA et al: Long-term experience with descending aortic dissection: The complication-specific approach. Ann Thorac Surg 53:11, 1992

Ergin MA et al: Significance of distal false lumen after Type A dissection repair. Ann Thorac Surg 57:820, 1994

Miller DC et al: Independent determinants of operative mortality for patients with aortic dissection. Circulation 70(Suppl I):I-153, 1984

Nienaber CA et al: Nonsurgical reconstruction of thoracic aortic dissection by stent-graft placement. N Engl J Med 340:1539, 1999

Parodi JC et al: Transfemoral intraluminal graft implantation for abdominal aortic aneurysms. Ann Vasc Surg 5:491, 1991

PERIPHERAL VASCULAR RADIATION THERAPY (BRACHYTHERAPY) FOR THE PREVENTION OF RESTENOSIS FOLLOWING ANGIOPLASTY

Zvonimir Krajcer

Restenosis

Restenosis is one of the most significant problems limiting the long-term success of percutaneous transluminal balloon angioplasty (PTA) and stenting of the peripheral vessels. Restenosis is mainly due to the process of intimal hyperplasia. The search for a "cure" for intimal hyperplasia has been long but, thus far, unrewarding. Numerous therapeutic strategies, mechanical devices, and various adjunctive pharmacologic approaches have been tested, with little improvement of long-term vascular patency (Dolmath et al., 1995; Martin et al., 1995; Strandness et al., 1989). Restenosis results from neointimal hyperplasia caused by elastic recoil and late vascular contracture. The concept of using local radiation to control smooth-muscle cell proliferation is based on the assumption that ionizing radiation will suppress this proliferation and limit neointimal hyperplasia.

Principles of Radiation Therapy

Intravascular radiation for prevention of restenosis is a relatively new technology emerging from a working hypothesis supported by basic and animal experiments. In 1964, before the angioplasty and restenosis era, Friedman's team reported the use of ^{192}Ir (14 Gy) delivered intraluminally to injured aorta of cholesterol-fed rabbits and demonstrated inhibition of smooth-muscle cell proliferation and intimal hyperplasia in the irradiated arteries (Friedman et al., 1964). Since 1992, numerous radiation platforms have been tried to prevent restenosis after angioplasty. In a pilot study in 1996, Nori and colleagues tried external radiation therapy (Nori et al., 1996). The external radiation beam delivered a uniform dose of 8 to 12 Gy over the entire volume of tissue, with encouraging preliminary results. Unfortunately, long-term follow-up is not available, and the potential long-term consequences of radiation exposure to adjacent tissues are not known.

605

Unlike external radiation, intravascular radiation delivers high doses of radiation directly to the arterial lumen with a fall-off, or attenuation, in dose as a function of distance from the source, thus limiting the exposure of healthy tissue. Intravascular brachytherapy sources are typically radioisotopes that decay by various means producing particulate (gamma and beta particles) and electromagnetic radiation. The most significant issue with intravascular brachytherapy, however, remains unresolved: Which source may be most effective—gamma or beta? While these two radiation sources differ, both have shown potential in significantly reducing the growth of smooth-muscle cells following angioplasty and stenting. Several treatment devices (seeds, wires, or liquids) using a variety of emitters have been tested, and several others are being considered.

Beta emitters deposit a large fraction of their energy locally so they have substantial safety advantages for both the operator and the patient: A lower radiation dose is delivered to the nontargeted tissue; exposure to the catheterization personnel is less; and the source can be shielded using light-weight polymer containers—therefore, supplementary radiation safety procedures, other than those already available in any catheterization laboratory, are not required. Since beta radiation has lower penetration properties and more heterogeneous distribution, it is ideal for smaller arteries (<3 mm).

High-activity gamma-emitting isotopes have been used in clinical studies in the peripheral vasculature. Unlike the coronary circulation, most of the peripheral vessels treated are >3 mm in diameter and many are 7 to 10 mm in diameter. The attenuation for beta-sources is much more rapid than for gamma sources because of increased tissue absorption; hence, centering a beta source in the larger peripheral vessels is much more difficult and can result in an uneven dose distribution, which might lead to suboptimal radiation of subintimal tissue. Asymmetry of the radiation source by as little as 0.5 mm could lead to an error of dosing as much as fivefold. These errors are considerably worse for beta emitters than for the gamma emitters; therefore gamma radiation is necessary in larger vessels so the subintimal tissue can be irradiated.

Beta emitters, however, provide significant advantages over solid sources in dose homogeneity and reduction of the total dose of radiation to healthy tissue. To circumvent the issue of centering, liquid-filled balloon brachytherapy using beta emitters has been tested. The radioisotope-filled balloon also has the advantage of ease of use, although the potential hazard of leakage carries both the life-threatening risk of accidental radiointoxication if balloon rupture occurs and the risk of laboratory contamination after a spill. Recent animal studies, however, using the positron emitter ^{68}Ga, with a half-life of 68 min, achieved biologic efficacy by suppressing neointimal proliferation (Stoll et al., 2001). ^{68}Ga provides an attractive safety profile, with a considerably shorter half-life when compared to other rhenium isotopes with half-lives of ≥ 17 h.

The recent miniaturization of x-ray devices makes possible the use of low-energy, or "soft," x-rays as an ionizing radiation source for intravascular therapy. Unlike gamma and beta sources, the soft x-rays are generated by high-voltage, miniaturized x-ray tubes that may be turned off at will, pose little radiation exposure risk to medical personnel, provide a satisfactory dose profile to the artery, and do not require special-use licensing. Preliminary studies indicate that soft x-rays inhibit cellular proliferation, and this should permit a new therapy to enter the expanding discipline of brachytherapy (Altman et al., 2001).

The investigation for the role of vascular brachytherapy in clinical use presents several very important questions, such as what are the optimal system, accurate dose, and dosimetry. The role of radiosensitizers and their long-term effects also remain unanswered. Numerous studies have demonstrated the ability of ionizing radiation to inhibit vascular smooth-muscle cell proliferation associated with restenosis. However, there is no homogeneous way of defining the target volumes and no uniform way of dose prescription and reporting. It is important to correlate irradiated volume of healthy tissue surrounding the target vessel, whether the target volume received an adequate dose, and whether there are isodose "edge effects" or a "geographical miss" due to insufficient coverage. In a recent study, late arterial responses after ^{32}P beta-emitting stent placement demonstrated sustained intimal suppression at 12 months (Farb et al., 2001). This study also demonstrated impaired arterial healing, characterized by late luminal fibrin deposition, inflammation, incomplete endothelialization, and edge effects present at 6 and 12 months. Late thrombosis was initially reported as high as 10% in patients undergoing coronary irradiation. Late thrombosis events, however, were significantly reduced when prolonged antiplatelet therapy was used (Waksman et al., 2001). The phenomenon of late thrombosis is probably due to incomplete healing and supports the need for prolonged antithrombotic therapy as a potential solution.

Clinical Trials

Liermann and co-workers reported the first human feasibility study of applying intravascular brachytherapy in the peripheral vascular system (Liermann et al., 1994). Schopohl later reported very promising long-term follow-up results (Schopol, 1996). This study involved 29 patients with restenosis after superficial femoral artery stenting. All were treated with ^{192}Ir, and at 6 years' follow-up there was 80% patency in the treated lesions and no adverse radiation-related effects.

Pichler and colleagues treated 24 patients prophylactically with ^{192}Ir after PTA and reported a 60% patency rate at 15 months' follow-up. Liermann's team reported a randomized trial of 40 patients with restenosis in a previously stented superficial femoral artery treated with ^{192}Ir (Liermann et al., 1998). Follow-up was available in 33 of the 40 patients at 2 years. None of the treated patients developed clinical restenosis, although one patient developed acute thrombosis 3 months after restenting, and one developed a new stenosis proximal to the previous stent.

Pokrajac and colleagues reported a randomized trial (Vienna-2) between PTA and brachytherapy for superficial femoral artery lesions: Restenosis at 12 months was 54% in PTA alone versus 28% for PTA plus brachytherapy (Pokrajac et al., 2000).

The PARIS (Peripheral Artery Radiation Investigational Study) multicenter trial, which will randomize in a double-blind fashion, is currently underway studying 300 patients following balloon angioplasty of the superficial femoral artery stenosis using a gamma-radiation ^{192}Ir source. The feasibility study for PARIS (40 patients) demonstrated that ^{192}Ir radiation delivered via a centering catheter is feasible and safe. Restenosis at 6 months for the first 27 patients treated with radiation was 11%. The objectives of this study are to determine angiographic evidence of patency and a reduction of over 30% in the restenosis rate of the treated lesion. A secondary end-point is to determine the clinical patency at 6 and 12 months by treadmill exercise time, improvement in ankle-brachial index by 0.01 compared to preangioplasty values, and the absence of repeat interventions to the treated vessel.

Conclusions

Intravascular brachytherapy for the treatment of peripheral vascular disease is still evolving. The long-term efficacy, the target tissue toxicity, and the dose required are not fully established. Intravascular brachytherapy sources include gamma- and beta rays and more recently, soft x-rays. Further long-term studies are needed to assess the significance of late arterial responses such as sustained neointimal suppression, incomplete healing, inflammation, and fibrin deposition.

At the present time, various isotopes are being tested in an effort to reduce the radiation exposure to both patients and personnel and to reduce the dose delivery in near field (Liermann et al., 1996; Schopohl et al., 1998; Waksman et al., 1998; Pichler et al., 1999; Pokrajac et al., 2000). Balloons have been designed that center the catheter-based isotope within the lumen of the vessel in spite of eccentric plaque. This improves the depth of dose delivery, especially for larger vessels.

Novel techniques, such as the use of high-voltage miniaturized soft x-rays and radioactive liquid- or gas-filled balloons that improve dose delivery, are currently being tested in the femoral arteries (Stoll et al., 2001). Future potential sites for brachytherapy include tibial-peroneal arteries, the hepatic vascular system (transjugular intrahepatic portosystemic shunts), arteriovenous dialysis grafts, renal arteries, and carotid arteries.

REFERENCES

Altman JD et al.: Soft x-rays: Intravascular soft x-rays inhibit cellular proliferation. Cardiovasc Radiat Med 2(1):57, 2001

Dolmath BL et al: Treatment of anastomotic bypass graft stenosis with directional atherectomy: Short-term and intermediate results. J Int Radiol 6:105, 1995

Farb A et al: Late arterial reponses (6 and 12 months) after ^{32}P β-emitting stent placement: Sustained intimal suppression with incomplete healing. Circulation 103:1912,2001

Friedman M et al: The antiatherogenic effect of ^{192}Ir upon cholesterol-fed rabbit. J Clin Invest 43:185, 1964

Liermann D et al: Prophylactic endovascular radiotherapy to prevent intimal hyperplasia after stent implantation in femoropopliteal arteries. Cardiovasc Intervent Radiol 17:12, 1994

Liermann D et al: Brachytherapy with iridium-192 HDR to prevent restenosis in peripheral arteries: An update. Herz 23:394, 1998

Martin EC et al: Multicenter trial of the Wallstent in the iliac and femoral arteries. J Vasc Intervent Radiol 6:843, 1995

Nori D et al: Management of peripheral vascular disease: Innovative approaches using radiation therapy. Int J Radiat Oncol Biol Phys 36:847, 1996

Pichler LJ et al: Endovascular brachytherapy for the prevention of recurrence after PTA. Radiologie 39:118, 1999

Pokrajac B et al: Intra-arterial ^{192}Ir high-dose-rate brachytherapy for prophylaxis of restenosis after femoropopliteal PTA: The prospective randomized Vienna-2 trial radiotherapy and risk factor analysis. Int J Radiol Oncol Biol Phys 48:923, 2000

Schopohl B: ^{192}Ir endovascular brachytherapy for avoidance of intimal hyperplasia after transluminal angioplasty and stent implantation in peripheral vessel: 6 years experience. Int J Radiat Oncol Biol Phys 36:835, 1996

Stoll H-P et al: Liquid-filled balloon brachytherapy using ^{68}Ga is effective and safe because of the short half-life: Results of a feasibility study in the porcine coronary overstretch model. Circulation 103:1793,2001

Strandness DE et al: Indiscriminate use of laser angioplasty. Radiology 172:945, 1989

Waksman R et al: Intravascular radiation for prevention of restenosis after angioplasty of narrowed femoral-popliteal arteries: Preliminary six-month results of a feasibility study. Circulation 98:I:66, 1998

Waksman R et al: Prolonged antiplatelet therapy to prevent late thrombosis after intracoronary γ-radiation in patients with in-stent restenosis: Washington Radiation for In-stent Restenosis Trial Plus 6 months of Clopidogrel (WRIST PLUS). Circulation 103:2332, 2001

MANAGEMENT OF ATHEROEMBOLIC DISEASE

John E. Scoble

Atheroembolic disease was first comprehensively described in 1945 by Flory. Since then, its recognition in clinical practice has increased. The difficulty with the diagnosis is that the condition mimics many others. Importantly, the combination of rash, impaired renal function, hypertension, eosinophilia, and hypocomplementemia has been attributed to a systemic vasculitis caused by the use of immunosuppressive drugs. Renal atheroembolic disease has been described as the Cinderella of renal disease because the clinical features and the diagnosis are rarely associated (Scoble, O'Donnell, 1996). At the same time, the known precipitating factors are increasing in the at-risk population: older members of our society. These include patients undergoing invasive intravascular procedures or thrombolysis. Specifically, the over-60-years age group constitutes an important group of patients receiving arterial surgery, intraarterial instrumentation, and anticoagulation/thrombolysis.

Two separate clinical syndromes have been described. The first is a catastrophic illness following some form of arterial intervention (Gaines et al., 1988). The second and less well-recognized syndrome is that of a slow and insidious decline in renal function. The best illustration of this is the early work of Thurlbeck and Castleman (1957). They showed that in autopsies of patients with significant aortic atherosclerotic disease, there was a significant incidence of cholesterol embolization to the kidneys. This was increased in patients who had abdominal aortic aneurysms prior to death. However, if the patients had had surgery for their aortic aneurysm, then this incidence increased to 75% of patients who had cholesterol emboli in the kidney. This illustrates that in the general population with atheromatous aortic disease, there is atheroembolic disease in the kidneys and, probably less clearly, in the peripheral circulation, and that following intervention, the incidence of atheroembolic renal disease can increase. The postmortem studies also show that the most common organ to be affected is the kidney (Phinney and Smith, 1995). More recent studies have shown that even transplanted kidneys are not spared this problem. It is clear that atheroembolic disease at the time of harvesting, leading to immediate graft nonfunction, is associated with a very poor graft outcome; it is also clear that atheroembolic disease in the transplant kidney has a much better prognosis.

Treatment

The management of atheroembolic disease can be seen as a mirror image of the causes of atheroembolic disease. Avoidance of the factors that precipitate this syndrome has to be at the heart of any protocol. This has recently been addressed by a Paris group (Belenfant et al., 1999), who have made two important advances. The first is that they have defined that, for the most important complication of atheroembolic disease, which is renal failure, there is no need for a renal biopsy if there is a predisposing factor for atheroembolic disease, acute renal failure, and some other manifestation such as skin changes, e.g., live do reticularis. They have also shown that, in patients who have had the condition of atheroembolic renal failure diagnosed, the prognosis is dramatically improved over all published series by a simple regime of avoiding precipitating factors (Table 97-1). This involves avoidance of further surgery or angiography/angioplasty, whatever the indication, and any anticoagulation even for hemodialysis, accompanied by simple supportive measures such as adequate nutritional support on dialysis. There are anecdotal reports regarding the use of statins in this syndrome. This has some theoretical support in that the most important effect of these agents on cardiovascular mortality has probably been in plaque stabilization. In the context of atheroembolic disease, it would appear that, at any time, there may be ulcerated lesions in at-risk patients in the aorta, which are then stabilized by thrombus formation. If these ulcerated lesions could be avoided by stabilization of the underlying atheromatous plaque, then there could be no release of the cholesterol crystals within the lesion.

Conclusion

The treatment of atheroembolic disease is to avoid the precipitating factors and then exclude them from any further therapy. This is difficult in patients with extensive atherosclerotic disease. However, this syndrome will increasingly be recognized in the future as a cause of mortality and morbidity in older atherosclerotic patients.

REFERENCES

Belenfant X et al: Supportive treatment improves survival in multivisceral cholesterol crystal embolism. Am J Kidney Dis 33:840, 1999

Dahlberg PJ et al: Cholesterol embolism: Experience with 22 histologically proven cases. Surgery 105:737, 1989

Fine M et al: Cholesterol crystal embolization: A review of 221 cases in the English literature. Angiology 38:769, 1987

Flory CM: Arterial occlusions produced by emboli from eroded aortic atheromatous plaques. Am J Pathol 21:549, 1945

Gaines PA et al: Cholesterol embolisation: A lethal complication of vascular catheterisation. Lancet 1:168, 1988

TABLE 97-1

OUTCOME IN RENAL ATHEROEMBOLIC DISEASE

Author	Year	Patients	Angiography/ Angioplasty, %	A/C,%	CV Surgery, %	Mortality (1-Year), %
Fine	1987	221				>81
Dahlberg	1989	14	64	29	50	64
Thadhani	1995	52	96	37	41	87
Belenfant	1998	67	85	76	36	21

A/C, anticoagulant; %, percentage of patients with precipitating factor

Phinney MS, Smith MC: Atheroembolic renal disease, in *Renal Vascular Disease,* A Novick et al (eds). London, Saunders, 1995

Scoble JE, O'Donnell PJO: Renal atheroembolic disease: The Cinderella of nephrology? Nephrol Dial Transplant 11:1516, 1996

Thadhani RI et al: Atheroembolic renal failure after invasive procedures. Medicine 74:350, 1995

Thurlbeck WM, Castleman B: Atheromatous emboli to the kidneys after aortic surgery. N Engl J Med 257:442, 1957

CHAPTER

98

PRACTICAL GUIDELINES FOR SMOKING CESSATION

Carolyn M. Dresler & Saul Shiffman

That smoking is unhealthy is no longer a question, except perhaps in the minds of a few recalcitrant tobacco executives. On a regular basis, information is published about the many adverse health effects of both primary and secondary tobacco smoke. Admittedly this information is mostly disseminated in the developed world, which already was fairly well informed about the dangers of tobacco smoke. However, despite this large and growing body of information, smoking remains the number one cause of preventable death and disease in our society.

Why? Nicotine, the substance inhaled while smoking tobacco, is one of the most addictive substances known. And, inhalation of nicotine is the *most* effective delivery method to establish the addiction, partly because it delivers nicotine to the brain so rapidly—within 10 seconds of inhaling. Cigarette smoking therefore is a legal and efficient system to deliver one of our society's most addictive drugs. The development of the habit begins in the teen and pre-

teen years, with the average age of smoking initiation being between 12 and 13 years, in both boys and girls. The serious health-related effects are usually not apparent to the smoker for 20 to 30 years, by which time the habit is very well entrenched. The actual addiction however, may be evident early, within a few years of initiation.

How do we decrease the number of people smoking? Prevention is of course critically important and, if successful, cessation would become progressively less of an issue. However, because approximately 45 million adult Americans still smoke, even if prevention were effective, smoking cessation efforts will still be required for the next 20 to 30 years in order to affect the health of those currently smoking.

Significant progress has been made in recent years in smoking cessation methodologies. Research is continuing to uncover the complicated mechanisms involved in nicotine addiction and reward responses in the brain. Behavioral and pharmaceutical interventions are showing increasing success rates in smoking cessation programs. Breaking the addiction to tobacco will never be easy, but we are beginning to elucidate methodologies that work.

In June 2000, the U.S. Department of Health and Human Services published a smoking cessation guideline, based on extensive review of the literature. Guidelines for the physician and brochures for patients are available free of charge. (U.S. Department of Health and Human Services, Agency for Health Care Policy and Research, 2101 East Jefferson Street, Suite 501, Rockville, MD 20852; 1-800-358-9295); (Fiore et al., 2000.)

The "5 As" in Table 98-1 have been recommended as a simple, brief, and complete method to address smoking. Thus, in addition to simply identifying the addiction and recommending cessation, physicians should be knowledgeable about cessation techniques and medications. Physicians should be familiar with the stages-of-change model as shown in Table 98-2. By identifying the stage in which the patient resides, physicians are able to modify their advice and interventions. The goal is to move the smoker to contemplation and then to action.

Physician Intervention

A key to promoting cessation is the use of the physician as a counselor. Disappointingly, most smokers say that they have never been advised to quit by their doctor. Although doctors are well aware that cigarette smoking is the number one cause of preventable death, they often are not as aggressive in smoking cessation interventions as they are, for example, with an anti-hyperglycemic intervention. Perhaps this is because they feel that they are not well trained or comfortable in conducting behavioral counseling, or that the recidivism rates of a cessation attempts are too frustrating, or that they are not reimbursed for their efforts. In reality, advice from a physician to quit can increase quitting by 65% and more intensive physician counseling doubles quit rates, although the absolute success rates are very modest (Silagy and Ketteridge, 1998).

Intervention on smoking must become routine. Michael Fiore, MD, chair of the Smoking Cessation Guidelines Panel, has recommended that smoking status become a "vital sign" along with pulse, blood pressure, and respiratory rate. The addition of smoking status to every clinical record stresses its importance both to the physician and the patient. Just as a tachycardia or hypertensive result should lead to an evaluation and intervention, so should the presence of a positive smoking status.

TABLE 98-1

THE 5 "As"

1. **ASK**—The physician should ask whether each patient smokes. It would be optimal if the physician also determined the extent of the tobacco exposure as measured in pack-years smoked.

2. **ADVISE**—This is the critical physician intervention: tell patients why it is paramount to their health and well-being to stop smoking. Personalize the message to match the patient's medical condition.

3. **ASSESS**—Determine the patient's motivation to stop smoking. An unmotivated patient will not be receptive to smoking cessation advice or attempts. The goal is to move the smoker into a motivated state.

4. **ASSIST**—Recommend pharmacotherapy; smoking cessation guidelines suggest first-line drugs such as bupropion or one of the nicotine replacement therapies, which have been shown to at least double the quit rates over unassisted attempts. Recommend a behavioral support program.

5. **ARRANGE**—Schedule a follow-up contact to assess progress, to provide encouragement and advice for either continuing success or addressing problems.

TABLE 98-2

THE STAGES OF CHANGE

PRECONTEMPLATION – Not thinking of quitting

CONTEMPLATION – Thinking of quitting

ACTION – Ready to quit, already attempting a quit

MAINTENANCE – Maintained abstinence

RELAPSE – Prolonged resumption of smoking after a quit attempt

Source: From JO Prochaska, CC DiClemente: J Consult Psychol 51:390; 1983.

Nicotine Replacement Therapy

Nicotine replacement therapy (NRT) is an effective method for smoking cessation. It is currently available in a gum, nasal spray, inhalator, transdermal patch, and sublingual tablet (although not in the United States as of mid-2001). The gum and patch are available over the counter (OTC) in the United States. The intent of NRT is to replace the nicotine received via the cigarette in order to help wean the patient off smoking and then gradually to decrease the NRT until the patient is free of nicotine.

There remains significant concern in both professional and lay persons about the safety of NRT. Nicotine does stimulate the sympathetic nervous system, resulting in slightly increased heart rate and blood pressure. Tolerance occurs to nicotine, thus ameliorating these effects. However, much of nicotine's effect depends on its delivery mechanism. Cigarette smoking delivers a large arterial boost, with rapid delivery of nicotine to the brain, much different than that from the medicinal nicotine nasal spray, gum, or patch. The slower delivery of nicotine from noncigarette sources allows more time for tolerance to develop (Benowitz, 1998). Studies have demonstrated the safety of transdermal nicotine patch therapy in patients with cardiovascular disease (Joseph et al., 1995; Mahmarian et al., 1997). In particular, the use of NRT by the patch in the Mahmarian study demonstrated a decrease in exercise-induced myocardial ischemia com-

pared to that occurring in individuals who continued to smoke (Mahmarian et al., 1997).

The safety of NRT in pregnant or nursing women, diabetics, patients with stomach ulcers, etc. has not been thoroughly studied. At present, each of these conditions are currently required by the FDA to be listed as "Warnings" on NRT products, with recommendations that such patients see their doctors prior to using the products. In each of these cases, on-going smoking is undoubtedly harmful for patients, but specific studies demonstrating the safety of NRT have not been carried out.

The choice of which NRT product to use is somewhat dependent on the needs of the patient. Nicotine polacrilex gum has been available since 1984 by prescription and from 1996 as an OTC product. The gum is available in 2 mg, for smokers of fewer than 24 cigarettes per day, and 4 mg for those smoking more than 24 cigarettes per day. The recommended dose is one piece of gum every 1 to 2 h, up to a maximum of 24 per day. Use of adequate amounts of gum (≥ 9 pieces per day) is important for success. Patients may prefer using the gum product if they smoke at irregular intervals (such as more in the evening), feel the need to chew or do something with their hands, or want more control of the amount of nicotine they use.

If patients smoke at regular intervals, prefer once/day dosing, or do not like gum, they may prefer the nicotine patch. Several patch systems are on the market and are available OTC. Most of the patch products have different doses for heavier or lighter smokers. The patches also differ in their constructions, thus differing in their pharmacokinetics and the total amount of nicotine delivered. Patches are recommended to be placed on the skin upon arising in the morning and left in place for 16 to 24 h. Patients who suffer morning cravings for nicotine (the majority of smokers) should leave the patch on for 24 h to help ameliorate the morning cravings. After patients have stopped smoking for a period of time (6 to 12 weeks), they are discontinued from the NRT patch.

The inhalator is available by prescription and delivers up to 4 mg nicotine per cartridge to oropharyngeal (not pulmonary) tissue. The inhaler may be used at a rate of up to 16 cartridges/day for 6 months. The inhalator is "puffed" on similarly to a cigarette, requiring approximately 20 min and many puffs to extract the 4 mg of nicotine.

A nicotine nasal spray is available by prescription and delivers nicotine faster than the gum, patch, or the inhalator. The recommended dose is 1 to 2 doses per hour for 3 months.

Although the use of any of the nicotine replacement products alone approximately doubles the successful quit rate as compared to "cold turkey," for the patient who will accept additional therapy, NRT should ideally be used with a behavioral modification program to further enhance success rates. Using a personalized behavioral modification program can double the rate of successful quitting. Such programs may be available through community hospitals and service groups such as the American Lung Association, American Heart Association, or American Cancer Society. In addition, smoking cessation and behavioral intervention programs have been developed by an increasing number of hospitals for both inpatients and outpatients.

Nonnicotine Therapy

Bupropion HC1, which is also used as an antidepressant, is available by prescription as the first nonnicotinic medication for smoking cessation. The mechanism of action for smoking cessation of bupropion is unclear, but it is believed to increase levels of serotonin, norepinephrine, and dopamine in the brain. Bupropion (300 mg/d) has demonstrated abstinence rates of 23% at 1 year, compared to 12% for placebo (Hurt et al., 1997). Bupropion is started at 150 mg/d for 3 days and then increased to 150 mg bid for 7 to 12 weeks. Patients should stop smoking within the first 2 weeks of treatment, usually in the second week. The dose and dosing interval (at least 8 h between doses) are suggested to minimized the risk of seizures. There is a small (1/1000) dose-related risk of seizure (doses >300 mg/d should not be used for smoking cessation) and is related to patient characteristics (past head injury, heavy drinking,

etc; see labeling). Bupropion should also be used with a behavioral modification program.

Other Interventions

Acupuncture, hypnosis, upper airway stimulation, anxiolytics, herbal products, lobeline, mecamylamine (a nicotine antagonist), and other interventions have not been demonstrated to reliably increase successful smoking cessation rates. Specific behavioral treatment has been demonstrated to help. Research is ongoing in many areas, with a variety of drugs to attempt to ease the craving and withdrawal effects from nicotine that are the cause of smoking relapses.

It is important to remember that behavioral, social, and psychological support are critical not only for a successful quit attempt but also for this quit to be translated to long-term cessation. Physicians can be critical in the cessation process, but it requires their willingness to intervene. The first step is to just ASK.

REFERENCES

Benowitz NL: Cardiovascular toxicity of nicotine: Pharmacokinetic and pharmacodynamic considerations, in Benowitz NL (ed.) *Nicotine Safety and Toxicity.* New York, Oxford University, 1998, pp 19–27

Fiore MC et al: *Treating Tobacco Use and Dependence. Clinical Practice Guideline.* Rockville, MD: US Department of Health and Human Services, Public Health Service, June 2000

Hurt RD et al: A comparison of sustained-release bupropion and placebo for smoking cessation N Engl J Med 337:1195, 1997

Joseph AM et al: The safety of transdermal nicotine as an aid to smoking cessation in patients with cardiac disease. N Engl J Med 335:1795, 1995

Mahmarian JJ et al: High reproducibility of myocardial perfusion defects in patients undergoing serial exercise thallium-201 tomography. Am J Cardiol 30:125, 1997

Prochaska JO, DiClemente CC: Stages and process of self-change of smoking. J Consult Psychol 51:390, 1983

Silagy C, Ketteridge S: Physician advice for smoking cessation (Cochrane Review). In: The Cochrane Library, Issue 4, 1998. Oxford:Update Software.

LUNG TRANSPLANTATION FOR PULMONARY HYPERTENSION

Thomas L. Spray / Nancy D. Bridges

Lung transplantation is employed as a "last or only" therapy for patients with pulmonary hypertension: it is considered when all other therapies have failed or none is available. The availability of epoprostenol has dramatically changed the prognosis for patients with primary pulmonary hypertension (Barst et al., 1996), and other medical therapies will soon be available (Channick et al., 2001; Olschewski et al., 1996; Rabinovitch, 1998; Saji et al., 1996). Nevertheless, many (if not most) patients with pulmonary hypertension, regardless of etiology, eventually become refractory to currently known medical therapies and eventually consider lung or heart-lung transplantation. As is the case with other therapies for the disease, thoracic organ transplantation should be considered palliative rather than curative.

Pretransplant Evaluation

An international committee with representation from the American Society for Transplant Physicians, The American Thoracic Society, The European Respiratory Society, and the International Society for Heart and Lung Transplantation has published guidelines for selection of lung transplant candidates (Maurer et al., 1998). Contraindications to transplantation are defined at individual transplant centers; guidelines from the authors' own program are listed in Table 99-1. Specific to lung transplantation are considerations related to prior thoracic surgery. While prior chest surgery per se is not a contraindication to lung transplantation, the combination of prior thoracotomies plus chronic cyanosis has, in the authors' experience, been associated with uncontrollable surgical bleeding.

In addition to establishing that no contraindications are present, the goals of the evaluation are to determine that there are no other interventions (such as calcium channel blockade, epoprostenol, or surgical correction of a cardiac lesion) that might be offered to the patient with some expectation of improvement and to provide enough information to the patient and his or her family that they can make an informed choice about transplantation.

Given that lung transplantation will be offered only after all other therapies have failed, it is to be expected that many of these patients will be quite ill. In general, lung transplantation offers a survival advantage to patients with pulmonary hypertension

TABLE 99-1

CONTRAINDICATIONS TO LUNG TRANSPLANTATION AT THE CHILDREN'S HOSPITAL IN PHILADELPHIA

- Local or systemic disease that will severely limit survival or functional outcome, regardless of the outcome of thoracic organ transplantation

- Irreversible renal or hepatic failure

- Multiorgan system failure

- Profound neurologic impairment[a]

- Invasive aspergillosis

- Absence of an identified, safe home environment[b]

- Residence in a location where immunosuppressive drugs are not reliably available

- Prior bilateral thoracotomies in addition to chronic cyanosis

- Fibrosing mediastinitis

[a]Moderate developmental delay, for example as seen in trisomy 21, is not a contraindication to thoracic organ transplantation.
[b]For example, residence in a public shelter.

only when offered to those with advanced disease. Thus, poor nutritional status and some degree of general debilitation are not contraindications to the procedure but rather are common characteristics of appropriate candidates by the time organs become available. However, if these characteristics are present at the time that the patient is first referred for evaluation, the likelihood of that patient surviving until organs become available is remote. One-third or more of patients with pulmonary hypertension are referred for lung transplantation when there is no realistic hope that they can survive long enough to receive organs (Bridges et al., 1996).

Timing of Listing and Transplantation

The appropriate time to list a patient for lung or heart-lung transplantation is determined by his or her expected duration of survival without transplantation and the expected waiting time (Nootens et al., 1994), as well as the expected duration of survival after transplantation. None of these can be known with any degree of certainty.

Death from pulmonary hypertension is, in most cases, due to progressive right heart failure and low cardiac output, perhaps exacerbated by an event such as exertion or a medical intervention. Two predictive models using hemodynamic data have been published—one based on a prospective cohort of adults with primary pulmonary hypertension (D'Alonzo et al., 1991) and the other on a retrospective cohort of children with either primary or secondary pulmonary hypertension (Clabby et al., 1997).

Waiting time for lungs or heart and lungs varies with age and location, and the regulations governing allocation of these organs change with time. Median waiting times for lung and heart-lung recipients as recorded by the United Network for Organ Sharing (UNOS) are shown in Table 99-2 (Annual Report of the U.S. Scientific Registry, 2000). The number of pediatric recipients is quite small; thus, waiting times for pediatric heart-lung recipients are not available on a yearly basis from UNOS. Median

TABLE 99-2

MEDIAN WAITING TIME IN DAYS FOR LUNG AND HEART-LUNG RECIPIENTS

Age, years	Lung recipients		Heart-lung recipients	
	UNOS, 1997, median	CHOP, 1995–1999, median (range)	UNOS, 1997, median	CHOP, 1995–1999, median (range)
<1	120	34 (1–116)	NA	30 (2–57)
1–5	189	43 (13–190)	NA	122 (11–208)
6–10	781	92 (4–745)	NA	176 (137–214)
11–17	830	245 (30–325)	NA	NA
18–34	815	NA	NA	NA
35–49	712	NA	824	NA
50–64	526	NA	918	NA
>65	404	NA	NA	NA

NOTE: UNOS, United Network for Organ Sharing; CHOP, Children's Hospital of Philadelphia; NA, data not available.

waiting times for pediatric lung and heart-lung recipients in the authors' program between 1995 and 1999 are therefore also listed in Table 99-2.

In general, a patient should be listed for lung transplantation when the probability of 2-year survival is about 50%. A patient listed at this time has a reasonable chance of surviving long enough to get organs and has a prognosis without transplantation consistent with obtaining a survival advantage from transplantation (Bush DM et al., 2000).

Preoperative Management

Patients with end-stage pulmonary hypertension (i.e., those with right heart failure and systemic or suprasystemic pulmonary artery pressure and who have become refractory to medical therapy) are hemodynamically quite unstable. Many will be hospitalized and receiving intravenous pressor support while awaiting transplantation, and most will have undergone creation of an atrial septal defect (Kerstein et al., 1995; Nihill et al., 1991; Rich et al., 1997; Rothman et al., 1999). The risk of sudden circulatory collapse and cardiac arrest in these patients is considerable. Events that might precipitate a crisis include sedation for procedures, noxious procedures performed without sedation, passage of nasogastric tubes, administration of agents that reduce systemic afterload or increase pulmonary resistance, or hypoventilation. Clinical indications of impending cardiac arrest in these patients include episodes of bradycardia, increasing frequency of ventricular dysrhythmias, increasingly abnormal liver function tests, sudden increase in the prothrombin time or international normalization ratio (INR), and general signs of low cardiac output. Successful resuscitation of a patient with end-stage pulmonary hypertension after complete cardiac arrest requiring chest compressions is unusual; although normal rhythm and adequate circulatory performance may be restored, there is almost inevitably severe brain injury due to inability to maintain adequate cerebral perfusion with cardiopulmonary resuscitation.

Choice of Transplant Procedure

Heart-Lung vs. Lung

The transplantation of both heart and lungs en bloc has a distinct advantage in patients with structurally abnormal hearts or complex venous and arterial connections. However, strict size constraints and limited availability of these organ blocks limit the applicability of this choice. The number of heart-lung transplantations in the United States has progressively declined to approximately 70 per year; very few of these are in children (Boucek et al., 1999; Hosenpud et al., 2000).

The range of donors who can be considered for a recipient of lungs alone can be expanded by downsizing donor lungs and by using lobes for whole-lung transplantation in children and small adults (Starnes et al., 1994); moreover, relatively smaller lungs may be used in larger recipients as the lungs will expand in the chest cavity. There is less flexibility in the size matching of heart-lung blocks; the size match between donor and recipient must be very accurate to prevent pulmonary tamponade of the heart by oversized lungs or inadequate cardiac output from use of a very small heart.

While heart-lung transplantation has the advantage of replacing all the abnormal organs with normal organs (and, in many cases, is a less complex operation), preservation of the patient's own heart has the advantage of avoiding the risk of cardiac rejection or transplant graft vasculopathy. Radley-Smith and colleagues reported finding important coronary artery vasculopathy in 1 of 10 heart-lung blocks examined after explantation or death resulting from obliterative bronchiolitis (Radley-Smith et al., 1995).

Allocation of organs to the greatest possible number of recipients is the most compelling argument against the routine use of heart-lung transplant when lung transplantation alone would be sufficient.

Single vs. Bilateral Lung

In the presence of pulmonary hypertension, single-lung transplantation will result in the entire cardiac output being diverted to the transplanted lung. This can result in mildly elevated pulmonary artery pressure postoperatively and can also be associated with early hemodynamic instability if cardiac repair is additionally required or if reperfusion injury or edema compromise the function of the transplanted lung (Pasque et al., 1992). Therefore, if the option of cardiac repair and isolated single-lung transplantation is selected in patients with pulmonary hypertension, it is important that the cardiac lesion be amenable to accurate and complete repair, and a single lung with the largest potential size be selected. Use of living-donor lobar transplantation is also a desirable option in this circumstance, as the ischemic time for the donor lung can be brief. Whether there is a long-term benefit to bilateral vs. single-lung transplant in patients with pulmonary hypertension remains controversial (Bando et al., 1994; Gammie et al., 1998; Sundaresan, 1998).

Bilateral rather than single-lung transplantation is generally preferred in young children, in order to preserve normal distribution of blood flow to the lungs and to provide maximal lung parenchyma for growth and development. Experimental data suggest that lungs do grow in the recipient, with addition of alveolar number and volume in addition to mass (Binnis et al., 1997a), and experience in children indicates that posttransplantation airway growth is normal (Ro et al., 2000). However, it is unclear whether in small recipients a single lobe from a larger donor will provide adequate alveolar volume for subsequent growth.

Living Donors

The use of living donors requires that two adults each donate one lower lobe for transplantation. Living-donor lobar transplantation for patients with pulmonary hypertension and congenital heart disease has been performed infrequently (Starnes et al., 1997). However, this option does permit the scheduling of elective operation, and the ischemic time for the donor lungs is likely to be quite short. Thus, the technique may have great desirability in patients who are of adequate size to accept the implantation of an adult lobe as a single lung (Binnis et al., 1997 a & b). Unfortunately, the use of this technique is generally limited to patients above 11 to 12 years of age due to the size differences in lobes of adults placed in small pediatric thoracic cavities.

Intraoperative Considerations

Lung transplantation for pulmonary hypertension with or without congenital heart disease generally requires the use of cardiopulmonary bypass. The support of the heart during the procedure is necessary not only for cardiac repair but also for decompression of the heart and circulatory support during pulmonary implantation. If bilateral sequential transplantation is to be performed, generally both lungs are removed prior to implantation of the recipient lungs. This speeds the operation and decreases the ischemic time for the second lung. The bilateral transverse thoracosternotomy incision as described by Pasque and colleagues is useful for patients who have had multiple previous operations and in whom chest adhesions may be problematic, as it offers good access to the posterior mediastinum for control of bleeding and better exposure of the phrenic nerve to avoid injury during dissection (Pasque et al., 1990). However, the incision is associated with sternal instability; therefore, if heart-lung implantation is used or the patient has not had previous surgery, a median sternotomy incision may be preferable (Meyers et al., 1999).

Cardiac repair, if necessary, is usually performed with a short period of cardioplegic arrest prior to implantation of the lungs; in this manner, reperfusion of the myocardium can be permitted during lung implantation. In some cases, with the patient on cardiopulmonary bypass, both recipient lungs can be removed prior to cardiac repair in order to improve exposure of the heart for the cardiac operation. Generally, absorbable suture is used for the suture lines in young children and infants in hopes of maximizing potential growth of the anastomoses.

Simple congenital heart lesions such as atrial septal defect, ventricular septal defect, and patent ductus arteriosus may be repaired in the usual fashion prior to lung implantation. In some cases of more complex disease, the cardiac repair must be modified to permit lung implantation in the most favorable fashion. Patients who have had a previous arterial switch procedure will have the pulmonary arteries anterior to the aorta; the donor pulmonary arteries are connected anterior to the aorta in this circumstance. Anomalous pulmonary venous return is simple to repair with lung implantation because the old pulmonary veins can be ligated or excised and the new veins implanted in the normal anatomic location. Abnormalities of visceral or atrial situs are not a problem for lung implantation as they do not significantly affect the hilar pulmonary anatomy.

Postoperative Management

Moderate levels of positive end-expiratory pressure are used to help preserve alveolar distention and decrease the tendency for fluid accumulation in the newly transplanted lungs. This is particularly important in patients who have undergone single-lung transplant for pulmonary hypertension, in whom increased pulmonary blood flow to the transplanted lung is present. Thoracic epidural catheters are routinely placed to aid in pain management of patients who have had a bilateral transsternal thoracotomy.

An important perioperative complication of lung transplantation for pulmonary hypertension is the development of dynamic right ventricular outflow tract obstruction (Aeba et al., 1993; Fricker et al., 1992; Kirshbom et al., 1996). Treatment with beta-blocking agents, avoidance of inotropic agents, and, on rare occasion, surgical relief of right ventricular outflow tract obstruction have been successful in dealing with this complication. An additional concern with single-lung transplantation in severe pulmonary hypertension is infarction or thrombosis of the non-transplanted lung, which receives little cardiac output and is dependent upon bronchial flow for viability.

Occasionally, reperfusion injury of the transplanted lungs can be significant, requiring increasing oxygen administration, and can be associated with severe bronchorrhea. Generally, this resolves within the first 24 h after transplant, and if the patient can be stabilized through this period, significant improvement in lung function can often be seen over the next 3 to 5 days. Edema of the lungs with chronic proteinacious drainage from the chest tubes is occasionally seen, often requiring prolonged chest drainage.

Outcomes

Data from the Registry of the International Society for Heart and Lung Transplantation (ISHLT) indicate that the current survival rates after bilateral lung transplantation are 77% at 1 year and 44% at 5 years (Hosenpud et al., 2000). Characteristics associated with increased risk of death (odds ratio, >2) among adult lung recipients include the need for preoperative mechanical ventilation, a congenital diagnosis, and history of prior lung transplantation. Risk factors for pediatric lung transplantation are not well defined. Those patients undergoing lung or heart and lung transplantation very early in life—that is, before age 6 months—may have a higher mortality risk. In addition, certain preoperative characteristics, including a diagnosis of congenital heart disease and requirement for mechanical ventilatory assistance, are associated with a longer postoperative length of stay.

Beyond the period of immediate postsurgical risk, morbidity and mortality after lung or heart-lung transplantation are the result of problems related to immunosuppression—not enough, too much, or both. The vast majority of lung recipients are maintained on triple immunosuppression (a calcineurin inhibitor, an antimetabolite, and prednisone). In the authors' experience, the most common cause of early death or graft loss after pediatric lung transplantation is viral pneumonitis and sepsis, particularly with adenovirus but also with parainfluenza or cytomegalovirus (Apalsch et al., 1995; Bridges et al., 1996, 1998). The most common cause of late death or graft loss in all recipients continues to be obliterative bronchiolitis

(OB), which is often complicated by infection, particularly aspergillosis. OB will be diagnosed in about 50% of late survivors of lung or heart lung transplantation. The Registry reports a conditional median survival (among operative survivors) of 6.8 years (Hosenpud et al., 2000).

Late morbidities in lung recipients are those that are common to all solid-organ transplant recipients and include systemic hypertension, diabetes mellitus, renal dysfunction, and lymphoproliferative disease (Boucek et al., 1999; Hosenpud et al., 2000). In addition, reduced lung function due to OB is common and increases over time.

Conclusions

Lung and heart-lung transplantation are imperfect therapies for pulmonary hypertension—as are all other currently available therapies. Nevertheless, when offered to an appropriately selected population, transplantation offers prolongation of and improved quality of life.

REFERENCES

Aeba R et al: Isolated lung transplantation for patients with Eisenmenger's syndrome. Circulation 88:452, 1993

Annual Report of the U.S. Scientific Registry for Transplant Recipients and the Organ Procurement and Transplantation Network: Transplant Data: 1990–1999. U.S. Department of Health and Human Services, Health Resources and Services Administration, Office of Special Programs, Division of Transplantation, Rockville, MD; United Network for Organ Sharing, Richmond, VA, 2000

Apalsch AM et al: Parainfluenza and influenza infections in pediatric organ transplant recipients. Clin Infect Dis 20:394, 1995

Bando K et al: Indications for and results of single, bilateral, and heart-lung transplantation for pulmonary hypertension. J Thorac Cardiovasc Surg 108:1056, 1994

Barst RJ et al: A comparison of continuous intravenous epoprostenol (prostacyclin) with conventional therapy for primary pulmonary hypertension. The Primary Pulmonary Hypertension Study Group. N Engl J Med 334:296, 1996

Binnis OA et al: Mature pulmonary lobar transplants grow in an immature environment. J Thorac Cardiovasc Surg 114:186, 1997a

Binnis OA et al: Use of over-size mature pulmonary lower lobe grafts results in superior pulmonary function. Ann Thorac Surg 64:307, 1997b

Boucek MM et al: The registry of the International Society of Heart and Lung Transplantation: Third Official Pediatric Report—1999. J Heart Lung Transplant 18:1151, 1999

Bridges ND et al: Outcome of children with pulmonary hypertension referred for lung or heart and lung transplantation. Transplantation 62:1824, 1996

Bridges ND et al: Adenovirus infection in the lung results in graft failure after lung transplantation. J Thorac Cardiovasc Surg 116:617, 1998

Bush DM et al: Lung transplantation offers a survival advantage to children with end-stage pulmonary hypertension. J Heart Lung Transplant 19:63, 2000

Channick R et al: Effects of the dual endothelin receptor antagonist bosentan in patients with pulmonary hypertension: A placebo-controlled study. J Heart Lung Transplant 20:262, 2001

Clabby ML et al: Hemodynamic data and survival in children with pulmonary hypertension. Am J Coll Cardiol 30:554, 1997

D'Alonzo GE et al: Survival in patients with primary pulmonary hypertension: Results from a national prospective registry. Ann Intern Med 343:1156, 1991

Fricker FJ et al: Development and resolution of right ventricular outflow tract obstruction after double lung transplantation. Transplant Sci 2:12, 1992

Gammie JS et al: Single- versus double-lung transplantation for pulmonary hypertension. J Thorac Cardiovasc Surg 115:397, 1998

Hosenpud JD et al: The registry of the International Society for Heart and Lung Transplantation: Seventeenth Official Report—2000. J Heart Lung Transplant 19:909, 2000

Kerstein D et al: Blade balloon atrial septostomy in patients with severe primary pulmonary hypertension. Circulation 91:2028, 1995

Kirshbom PM et al: Delayed right heart failure following lung transplantation. Chest 109:575, 1996

Maurer JR et al: International guidelines for the selection of lung transplant candidates. J Heart Lung Transplant 17:703, 1998

Meyers BF et al: Bilateral sequential lung transplantation without sternal division eliminates posttransplantation sternal complications. J Thorac Cardiovasc Surg 117:358, 1999

Nihill MR et al: Effects of atrial septostomy in patients with terminal cor pulmonale due to pulmonary vascular disease. Cathet Cardiovasc Diagn 24:166, 1991

Nootens M et al: Timing of single lung transplantation for primary pulmonary hypertension. J Heart Lung Transplant 13:276, 1994

Olschewski H et al: Aerosolized prostacyclin and iloprost in severe pulmonary hypertension. Ann Intern Med 124:820, 1996

Pasque JH et al: Improved technique for bilateral lung transplantation: Rationale and initial clinical experience. Ann Thorac Surg 49:785, 1990

Pasque MK et al: Single lung transplantation for pulmonary hypertension: Technical aspects and immediate hemodynamic results. J Thorac Cardiovasc Surg 103:475, 1992

Rabinovitch M: Elastase and the pathobiology of unexplained pulmonary hypertension. Chest 144(Suppl):213S, 1998

Radley-Smith RC et al: Graft-vessel disease and obliterative bronchiolitis after heart/lung transplantation in children. Transplant Proc 27:2017, 1995

Rich S et al: Usefulness of atrial septostomy as a treatment for primary pulmonary hypertension and guidelines for its application. Am J Cardiol 80:369, 1997

Ro PS et al: Airway growth after pediatric lung transplantation. J Heart Lung Transplant 19:71, 2000

Rothman A et al: Atrial septostomy as a bridge to lung transplantation in patients with severe pulmonary hypertension. Am J Cardiol 84:682, 1999

Saji T et al: Short- and long-term effects of the new oral prostacyclin analogue, beraprost sodium, in patients with severe pulmonary hypertension. J Cardiol 27:197, 1996

Starnes VA et al: Lobar transplantation: Indications, technique, and outcome. J Thorac Cardiovasc Surg 108:403, 1994

Starnes VA et al: Experience with living-donor lobar transplantation for indications other than cystic fibrosis. J Thorac Cardiovasc Surg 114:917, 1997

Sundaresan S: The impact of bronchiolitis obliterans on late morbidity and mortality after single and bilateral lung transplantation for pulmonary hypertension. Semin Thorac Cardiovasc Surg 10:152, 1998

HEREDITARY HEMOCHROMATOSIS: A RISK FACTOR FOR CARDIOVASCULAR DISEASE

M. Roest / Y.T. van der Schouw / J.J.M. Marx

Hereditary hemochromatosis (HH) is the most common autosomal recessive disorder, with prevalences ranging from 1:200 to 1:400 in populations with European origin. Patients with HH have a disturbed absorption of iron by intestinal mucosal cells and excessive iron deposition in parenchymal cells of the liver and other organs. Clinical symptoms include damage and impaired function of the liver, pancreas, heart, and the pituitary. HH can be diagnosed by a combined measurement of ferritin and transferrin iron saturation. If not treated, some HH patients may die from liver cirrhosis, liver cancer, or cardiomyopathy. The major symptoms of HH are arthralgia, fatigue, and abdominal pain. Phlebotomy has proven to be a successful treatment to reduce the risk of early mortality and to prevent clinical symptoms.

HFE C260Y

The mutation coding for the most common variant of HH is a G → A mutation, located at position 845 of the *HFE* gene on the short arm of chromosome 6.

This mutation is responsible for a cysteine to tyrosine transition at position 260 of the protein (formerly described as *HFE* C282Y). Both the *HFE* gene and the C260Y mutation were described for the first time in 1996. (Feder et al., 1996). More than 83% percent of HH patients are homozygous for this mutation, meaning that the *HFE* gene in both chromosomes 6 contains the C260Y mutation.

Normal HFE (wild type) is an HLA class 2 protein that is involved in the modulation of iron uptake in the small intestine. The mechanism by which HFE regulates iron homeostasis is not yet fully understood, but HFE is active only when bound to β_2-microglobulin, as shown in β_2-microglobulin knock-out mice, which develop symptoms similar to those of HH patients (Santos et al., 1996). Furthermore, HFE is involved in modulation of iron homeostasis via the transferrin receptor. The mechanism by which *HFE* C260Y leads to HH remains to be elucidated. It has been suggested that HFE is needed to express the transferrin receptor on the basolateral membrane in the crypts of Lieberkühn in the small intestine, which enhances the iron uptake needed for cell proliferation (Waheed et al., 1999).

Impairment of this function caused by *HFE* gene mutations could provide a paradoxical signal in crypt enterocytes that programs the differentiating enterocytes to absorb more dietary iron when they mature into villus enterocytes.

HH Carriers

An individual is called an *HH carrier* when only one chromosome 6 contains a C260Y mutation in the *HFE* gene while the other chromosome 6 contains the wild type *HFE* gene. The prevalence of HH carriers is 7 to 10% in populations with European origin. HH carriers do not develop clinical symptoms of HH but express slightly higher levels of serum iron, serum ferritin, and transferrin saturation in comparison to non-HH carriers, indicating that HH carriers are exposed to moderate excessive iron throughout their entire life (de Valk et al., 2000). HH carriers therefore provide a unique opportunity to study genetically determined increased iron exposure in large population studies. Unlike plasma markers, genes have the advantage of being fixed at conception and do not change until death; genetic markers are therefore not subject to confounding by disturbing variables.

HH and Cardiovascular Disease

Two large independent population studies on the relationship between HH carriership and cardiovascular disease have been published (Roest et al., 1999; Tuomainen et al., 1999). In a Dutch cohort study of 12,239 postmenopausal women who were followed for cardiovascular mortality for up to 18 years (182,976 follow-up years), it was found that HH carriers had a 1.6-fold (95% CL: 1.1 to 2.4) increased risk of death from any kind of cardiovascular disease (Roest et al., 1999). More specifically: the HH polymorphism is predictive of a 1.5-fold (95% CL: 0.9 to 2.5) increased risk of death from myocardial infarction (MI); a 2.4-fold (95% CL: 1.3 to 3.5) increased risk of death from cerebrovascular disease, and a 1.2-fold (95% CL: 0.7 to 2.3) increased risk of death

from any other form of cardiovascular disease (Table 100-1). The population-attributable risks of HH heterozygosity for mortality from MI, cerebrovascular disease, and from any other form of cardiovascular disease were 3.3%, 8.8%, and 1.4%, respectively. This means that 3.3% of deaths from MI in the entire population were attributable to the HH mutation and 8.8% of the cerebrovascular mortality in the entire population was attributable to the HH mutation. The second cohort study comprised 1150 Finnish men who were followed for up to 12.8 years for incidence of MI. HH carriers had a 2.3-fold (95% CL: 1.1 to 4.8) higher risk of developing acute MI than wild types (Tuomainen et al., 1999). Recently, a similar relationship between HH carriership and increased risk of cardiovascular disease incidence was found in a third cohort study (Rasmussen et al., 2001), whereas a nonsignificant increased risk of cardiovascular disease was found in a multicenter case control study (Hetet et al., 2001). A pooled analysis of the relationship of HH genotype to occurrence of symptomatic cardiovascular events is presented in the upper half of Table 100-1. The HH polymorphism was associated with a 1.7-fold (95% CL: 1.4 to 2.0) increased risk of symptomatic cardiovascular events.

At present, three studies have been published on the relationship between HH polymorphism and the prevalence of severe luminal narrowing of the coronary arteries (lower half of Table 100-1). In contrast to symptomatic cardiovascular events, no relationship was found between HH genotype and severe luminal narrowing of the coronary arteries (0.7; 95% CL: 0.4 to 1.1).

Interaction with Smoking and Hypertension

The pathophysiology of cardiovascular disease is influenced by multiple interacting factors. This was also found in the Dutch cohort study, in which the relationship between HH carriership and cardiovascular mortality was stronger when women were also exposed to other cardiovascular risk factors (Roest et al., 1999). The relationship between HH genotype and cardiovascular mortality was expressed most strongly in women who were smoking and hypertensive. Risk profiles of HH carriership (yes/no), hyper-

TABLE 100-1

POOLED ANALYSIS OF ALL STUDIES ON HFE GENOTYPE AND CARDIOVASCULAR DISEASE (CVD) INCIDENCE AND PREVALENCE OF CORONARY STENOSIS

Subgroup	Case definition	Cases		Controls		Risk ratio (95% CL)
		HH carrier	Wild type	HH carrier	Wild type	
CVD incidence						
Roest et al, 1999	Cardiovascular mortality	56	474	40	512	1.6 (1.1–2.4)
Tuomainen et al, 1999	Myocardial infarction	8	60	60	1022	2.3 (1.1–4.8)
Rasmussen et al, 2001	CVD incidence	24	219	32	535	1.6 (0.9–2.9)
Hetet et al, 2001	CVD incidence	234	1092	190	1060	1.2 (1.0–1.5)
Total		322	1845	322	3129	1.7 (1.4–2.0)
Prevalence of coronary stenosis						
Franco et al, 1998	Lumen diameter	22	508	38	506	0.6 (0.3–1.0)
Battiloro et al, 2000	Lumen diameter	4	170	3	184	1.4 (0.3–6.5)
Calado et al, 2000	Lumen diameter	7	153	7	153	1.0 (0.3–2.9)
Total		33	831	48	843	0.7 (0.4–1.1)

tension (yes/no), and smoking (yes/no) in relation to cardiovascular mortality were determined as demonstrated in Fig. 100-1. Smoking, hypertension, and the HH mutation are all moderate risk factors for cardiovascular mortality, with a single relative risk of <2. However, a strongly increased cardiovascular mortality risk was observed when all three risk factors were present: women who were smokers, hypertensive, and HH carriers have a 21-fold (95% CL: 9.16 to 47.48) higher risk of cardiovascular mortality during follow-up than women who were nonsmokers, were not hypertensive, and were HH wild type. HH carriership plays an important role in this statistical interaction, because women who were smokers and hypertensive but not HH carriers had a 2.1-fold (95% CL: 1.4 to 3.2) increased risk of cardiovascular mortality in comparison to women who were nonsmokers and not hypertensive but were HH

wild type. In women with normal blood pressure who did not smoke, HH carriership appeared to play a minor role in the cardiovascular mortality risk; the relative risk was 1.2 (95% CL: 0.5 to 2.6).

Iron and Cardiovascular Disease

The finding that HH is associated with an increased risk of symptomatic cardiovascular events is direct evidence for the hypothesis that iron is involved in cardiovascular disease. Until recently, this hypothesis was based on observations that premenopausal women have a much lower risk of developing cardiovascular disease than do postmenopausal women or men (Sullivan, 1999). A plausible explanation for this difference is that the reduced risk of cardiovascular disease in premenopausal women is a consequence of

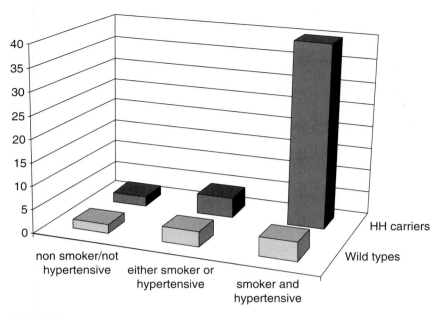

FIGURE 100-1

Cardiovascular mortality, mortality from myocardial infarction, cerebrovascular mortality, and all other forms of cardiovascular mortality in subgroups: HH carrier/not HH carrier by (1) not hypertensives and non smoker, (2) either hypertensive or smoker, and (3) both hypertensive and smoker. Smoking was defined as reported to be current smoker in the baseline questionnaire. Hypertension was defined as diastolic pressure >95 and/or systolic pressure >160 mm Hg.

monthly iron loss during menstruation. A further indication that iron reduction protects against cardiovascular disease is the finding that blood donors have a lower risk of developing MI than nondonors (Salonen et al., 1998). Furthermore, (1) excessive iron intake via red meat is associated with an increased risk of cardiovascular disease; (2) the ratio between plasma levels of transferrin receptor and ferritin is associated with a reduced risk of cardiovascular disease; and (3) plasma ferritin levels, serum iron levels, or total iron binding capacity may be associated with increased risk of cardiovascular disease (reviewed by de Valk and Marx, 1999).

HH, Iron, and Pro-oxidative State

The proposed mechanism of HH and iron's involvement in cardiovascular disease is a multistep process that may be represented in the following way:

$$\text{HH mutation} \xrightarrow{1} \text{increased iron} \xrightarrow{2} \text{oxygen radical formation} \xrightarrow{3} \text{cardiovascular disease}$$

The relationship between the HH mutation and moderately increased iron stores (step 1) is established in several clinical and epidemiologic studies (reviewed by de Valk et al., 2000). HH carriership might lead to moderately increased deposition of iron in sensitive cells and generation of catalytically active, labile forms of iron. Iron is a major pro-oxidant that is involved in the hydroxyl radical formation (OH·, step 2) via the Haber-Weiss reaction:

$$O_2^- \cdot + Fe^{3+} \rightarrow O_2 + Fe^{2+}$$
$$Fe^{2+} + H_2O_2 \rightarrow Fe^{3+} + OH^- + OH\cdot$$
$$O_2^- \cdot + H_2O_2 \rightarrow O_2 + OH^- + OH\cdot$$

Excessive and labile iron may lead to increased hydroxyl radical formation and hence local tissue damage or other detrimental processes. Population studies have shown that the pro-oxidative state is predictive of an increased risk of cardiovascular disease (step 3). The pathway of oxygen radical formation leading to cardiovascular disease remains to be elucidated. The recent finding that the HH mutation is directly predictive of an increased risk of cardiovascular morbidity and mortality (steps 1 + 2 + 3) completes the causal chain.

Mechanism

The mechanism by which iron overload is involved in cardiovascular disease pathophysiology remains to be established. It has been proposed that excessive amounts of iron are associated with increased oxygen radical formation and peroxidation of low-density lipoprotein (LDL), leading to the formation of minimally modified LDL (MM-LDL). MM-LDL may initiate inflammation of the arterial wall or may further oxidize to oxidized LDL (ox-LDL). Ox-LDL can be recognized by the scavenger receptor and taken up by macrophages in the intima of the arterial wall, leading to transformation of tissue macrophages into foam cells, the most important cells of the fatty streak. However, the observation that the HH genotype is not associated with the presence of atherosclerotic coronary luminal narrowing (Table 100-1) suggests that iron is involved in a nonatherogenic process of cardiovascular disease. Potential nonatherogenic actions of iron in relation to cardiovascular disease are described below.

Iron-induced oxygen radicals may attack the fibrous cap of the atherosclerotic plaque. This may lead to destabilization and rupture of the atherosclerotic plaque and hence induce an occlusive infarction (Libby, 2000). Alternatively, iron may play a role in the sensitivity of organs to ischemia, because iron-mediated free radicals are generated after restoration of blood flow to ischemic myocardium. These radicals may induce so-called reperfusion injury (Ferrari, 1995). Furthermore, recent evidence suggests that iron availability contributes to impaired nitric oxide action in atherosclerosis and may therefore contribute to endothelial dysfunction (Duffy et al., 2001).

Summary and Conclusions

The discovery of the HH mutation was an important step forward in the research into the role of iron in cardiovascular disease. The HH mutation represents a unique opportunity to study inherited lifelong exposure to moderately elevated iron levels in relation to cardiovascular morbidity and mortality in large prospective studies. The findings of these studies provide direct evidence that iron is involved in cardiovascular disease etiology. The HH mutation is a human genetic model of disturbed iron metabolism, which facilitates research into the mechanism by which HH and iron are involved in cardiovascular disease. It is expected that this mechanism will soon be better understood.

REFERENCES

Battiloro E et al: Haemochromatosis gene mutations and risk of coronary artery disease. Eur J Hum Genet 8:389, 2000

Calado RT et al: HFE gene mutations in coronary atherothrombotic disease. Braz J Med Biol Res 33:301, 2000

Duffy SJ et al: Iron chelation improves endothelial function in patients with coronary artery disease. Circulation 103:2799, 2001

Feder JN et al: A novel MHC class 1 - like gene is mutated in patients with hereditary hemochromatosis. Nat Genet 13:399, 1996

Ferrari R: Metabolic disturbances during myocardial ischemia and reperfusion. Am J Cardiol 76:17B, 1995

Franco RF et al: Prevalence of hereditary haemochromatosis in premature atherosclerotic vascular disease. Br J Haematol 102:1172, 1998

Hetet G et al: Association studies between haemochromatosis gene mutations and the risk of cardiovascular diseases. Eur J Clin Invest 31:382, 2001

Libby P: Coronary artery injury and the biology of atherosclerosis: Inflammation, thrombosis, and stabilization. Am J Cardiol 86(Suppl 2):3, 2000

Rasmussen ML et al: A prospective study of coronary heart disease and the hemochromatosis gene (HFE) C282Y mutation: The Atherosclerosis Risk in Communities (ARIC) study. Atherosclerosis 154:739, 2001

Roest M et al: Heterozygosity for the hereditary hemochromatosis gene is associated with cardiovascular mortality in women. Circulation 100:1268, 1999

Salonen JT et al: Donation of blood is associated with reduced risk of myocardial infarction. The Kuopio

Ischaemic Heart Disease Risk Factor Study. Am J Epidemiol 148:445, 1998

Santos M et al: Defective iron homeostasis in β_2-microglobulin knockout mice recapitulates hereditary hemochromatosis in man. J Exp Med 184:1975, 1996

Sullivan JL: Iron and the genetics of cardiovascular disease. Circulation 100:1260, 1999

Tuomainen TP et al: Hemochromatosis gene HFE Cys282Tyr polymorphism is associated with two-fold increased risk at acute myocardial infarction in men. Circulation 100: 1274, 1999

de Valk B, Marx JJ: Iron, atherosclerosis, and ischemic heart disease. Arch Intern Med 159:1542, 1999

de Valk B et al: Biological expression of heterozygous hereditary hemochromatosis. Eur J Intern Med 11:317, 2000

Waheed A et al: Association of HFE protein with transferrin receptor in crypt enterocytes of human duodenum. Proc Nati Acad Sci USA 96:1579, 1999

INDEX

Index

Page numbers in *italics* denote figures; those followed by "t" denote tables.

POLITICAL PARTIES
OF ASIA AND THE PACIFIC

POLITICAL PARTIES OF ASIA AND THE PACIFIC
A Reference Guide

Editors: D. S. Lewis and D. J. Sagar

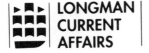

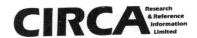

POLITICAL PARTIES OF ASIA AND THE PACIFIC

Published by Longman Group UK Limited, Westgate House,
The High, Harlow, Essex CM20 1YR, United Kingdom.
Telephone (0279) 442601
Telex 81491 Padlog
Facsimile (0279) 444501

Distributed exclusively in the United States and Canada by Gale Research Inc.,
835 Penobscot Building, Detroit, Michigan 48226, USA.

ISBN 0-582-098114

A catalogue record for this publication is available from the British Library.

Printed and bound in Great Britain by
William Clowes Limited, Beccles and London

Contents

Introduction

The aim of this volume is to provide accurate and detailed information on the political parties currently operating in Asia and the Pacific. The book is divided into country entries arranged alphabetically, each of which includes essential background information on the constitutional structure, franchise and electoral system of the country concerned, as well as information on recent elections. The party by party data is divided to differentiate between major and minor parties; in both cases basic data is provided on party title, address, leadership, and political orientation. In the case of major parties the book also seeks to show their historical evolution and to provide information on electoral performance, internal structure, membership and international affiliation. Information is included on defunct parties where they are considered sufficiently important to be of continuing relevance to the contemporary politics of a country. There are also entries on major guerrilla organizations.

The dividing line between a political party and a protest movement or pressure group is necessarily imprecise, and varies in accordance with the context in which an organization operates. For the purposes of this volume the editors have tended to accept self-definition as the starting point for inclusion but, inevitably, editorial judgements have had to be made on a case-by-case basis. This has been true also in deciding whether a party is of sufficient size and importance to warrant inclusion, and whether it should be classified as a major or minor organization. In all cases the editors have used their regional expertise to adjudicate, attempting to provide the broadest possible range of information, while maintaining standards of consistency and accuracy.

A common problem of any reference book is that some of its information may become outdated in the period between going to press and publication. A volume on political parties—which deals with thousands of entities which are, by definition, continually evolving through mergers, schisms and realignments—is particularly prone to this weakness. The editors have attempted to ensure that the information contained in the volume is correct as of the end of June 1992. Moreover, by providing details of the evolution and context of parties the editors hope that the book will remain a valuable reference aid for anyone interested in the politics of Asia and the Pacific for years to come.

The editors wish to thank all of those who made the compilation of this volume possible. This includes the parties themselves, many of which provided invaluable information, but also the government departments, high commissions and embassies, specialist agencies, libraries, journalists and academics who helped with the information-gathering process. The editors are also grateful to the resources provided by the editorial offices of CIRCA Research and Reference Information. Finally, they would like to thank Farzana Shaikh for her assistance and advice on the entries for the Indian sub-continent and to acknowledge their debt to the individual contributors to this volume—Tanya Joseph, Brian MacDonald, Corrine Richeux and Wendy Slater.

D. S. Lewis
D. J. Sagar
London, October 1992

Editors

D. S. Lewis is a regional editor for CIRCA. He has been a contributor to numerous books, and is the author of *Illusions of Grandeur: Mosley, Fascism and British Society 1931-81* (Manchester University Press, Manchester, 1986) and editor of *Korea: Enduring Division?* (Longman UK, Harlow, 1988).

D. J. Sagar is a regional editor for CIRCA. He has contributed to many books, is the author of *Major Political Events in Indo-China 1945-1990* (Facts on File, New York, 1991), and is a major contributor to *Cambodia: A Matter of Survival* (Longman UK, Harlow, 1989).

CIRCA Research and Reference Information Limited specializes in reference works on international politics and current affairs, and is responsible for researching, writing and editing the monthly *Keesing's Record of World Events*.

Contributors

Tanya Joseph, who worked on some of the material relating to the Indian sub-continent, is a regional editor for CIRCA. She is a contributor to *The World's News Media* (Longman UK, Harlow, 1992), and to *Islam and Islamic Groups* (Longman UK, Harlow, 1992).

Brian MacDonald, who wrote many of the Pacific and Pacific rim entries, is a recent graduate of the London School of Economics and is a specialist in the field of international relations.

Corrine Richeux, who wrote the entries for the Indian sub-continent, is a recent graduate of Pembroke College, Cambridge. She is currently working as a research assistant to Dr Joseph Needham at the Needham Research Institute in Cambridge.

Wendy Slater, who wrote entries covering central and east Asia is a regional editor for CIRCA. She is also a contributor to *The World's News Media* (Longman UK, Harlow, 1992), and to *Islam and Islamic Groups* (Longman UK, Harlow, 1992).

Afghanistan

Capital: Kabul   **Population: 16,600,000 (1990)**

The modern Afghan state was built at the end of the 19th century by Amir Abdur Rahman Khan who conquered and united the region's many disparate and warring tribes and created a monarchy. While the tribes have continued to resist integration into a formal modern federation, the unity achieved was sufficient to resist Britain's three incursions in the Anglo-Afghan wars of 1877, 1905 and 1921. A Constitution was introduced in 1964 by King Mohammad Zahir, but the monarchy was overthrown in 1973 by a military coup led by Lt.-Gen. Mohammad Daoud Khan, who became President of the new Republic of Afghanistan. His military dictatorship was in turn overthrown by the People's Democratic Party (PDPA) in the "Saur Revolution" of 1977 which renamed the country the Democratic Republic of Afghanistan.

Fierce tribal opposition to the new communist regime led to armed insurrection, quelled by the Soviet invasion of 1979 which brought a new pro-Soviet faction of the PDPA to power. In spite of the massive Soviet military presence, the government continued to be unable to impose unity due to continued guerrilla resistance by the *mujaheddin* ("holy warriors"), a loose and often feuding alliance formed in 1978 from numerous opposition groups within the country and in Pakistan and Iran. The *mujaheddin* maintained control of most of the countryside, and were aided and abetted, financially and militarily, by the United States, the United Kingdom and the People's Republic of China between 1984 and 1989.

In an attempt to put an end to the civil war, the new PDPA leader, Najibullah, urged by the Soviet leader Mikhail Gorbachev, announced at the end of 1986 a programme of "national reconciliation" which largely failed, due to the refusal of the *mujaheddin* to co-operate with the government without the prior complete and unconditional withdrawal of the Soviet forces. The National Assembly in November 1987 passed a new Constitution which restored the country's name to the Republic of Afghanistan, legalized the official existence and participation in politics of political parties other than the PDPA and adopted a more conciliatory policy towards religion. In 1988 Gorbachev announced the phased withdrawal of Soviet troops, which was completed in 1989.

These events in Afghanistan were paralleled by the formation in Peshawar (Pakistan) in February 1989 of an Afghan Interim Government, composed of representatives from seven Pakistan-based Sunni *mujaheddin* groups, and led by Seghbatullah Mujaddedi, head of the Afghan National Liberation Front. The legitimacy of this interim government was called into question by *mujaheddin* groups operating within Afghanistan and by the Iran-backed Shia alliance, the Islamic Coalition Council of Afghanistan, later renamed the Islamic Unity Party of Afghanistan. It did, however, receive recognition from the Islamic Conference Organization (ICO) as the legitimate government of Afghanistan.

The completion of the withdrawal of Soviet troops and the continuing civil war led to the declaration of a state of emergency and to various superficial government reforms, including the renaming of the PDPA in June 1990 as the Homeland Party (*Hezb-i Watan*). The reforms failed to appease the *mujaheddin* and fighting continued and intensified throughout 1991. In April, the *mujaheddin* achieved a victory with the capture of Khost. A UN peace plan proposing the sharing of power between the *mujaheddin* and the government won the approval of the Afghan and Pakistan governments and of some of the more moderate *mujaheddin* factions, but fighting nevertheless intensified around Kabul. In September 1991 talks between the Soviet Union and the USA produced an agreement to halt arms sales to both sides in the civil war. The intransigence and infighting of the *mujaheddin* lost them international support, and

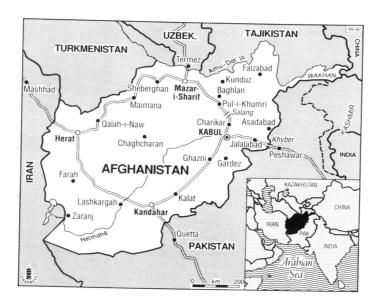

Recent elections

The first two general elections in the history of Afghanistan took place in the years 1965 and 1969 respectively; they were on a non-party basis and elected a 215-member lower house and one-third of the 84 seats in the upper house of the new bicameral parliament. Parliament was dissolved after the 1973 coup, and no elections were held until April 1988, as required by the 1987 Constitution. By this time there were five officially recognised political parties, all of which put forward candidates for election to the National Assembly. Moderate members of the *mujaheddin* were also invited to contest for seats, but both they and the Shi'ite Muslim opposition boycotted the election. According to official statistics 1,547,000 people voted, and elections took place in 184 of the 234 constituencies. Of the remaining 50 seats in the Council of Representatives, 48 were reserved for the opposition; two seats were not filled due to the cancellation of elections in two constituencies because of "violations" and "non-organization". Senatorial elections were held in 51 out of 128 constituencies, 45 senators were directly appointed by the President and the remaining 32 seats were reserved for the opposition. The PDPA gained a majority in both houses.

Najibullah was elected President of the Republic and Commander-in-Chief of the Armed Forces by the *Loya Jirga* in November 1987. There have been no elections since the overthrow of the Najibullah regime.

the USA reduced aid to the *mujaheddin* by one-third, but Pakistan and Saudi Arabia continued to supply arms. In mid-November, talks between the Afghan Interim Government and the Soviet Union resulted in the Soviet Union denouncing the 1979 invasion and agreeing to end its support for the Najibullah regime. A joint statement was issued envisaging the handover of power to an interim Islamic government which would rule for two years before elections under UN and ICO auspices.

In March 1992, Najibullah announced that he was prepared to resign, but his government was overthrown a month later when two *mujaheddin* forces, led by Ahmed Shah Massud and Gulbuddin Hekmatyar respectively, closed in on Kabul. Various *mujaheddin* groups continued to fight over the leadership of the newly created Islamic State of Afghanistan, and as of the time of writing (mid-1992) Kabul was being torn apart by fighting *mujaheddin* factions, in particular those of Hekmatyar and Massud, now Defence Minister in the new Islamic *Jihad* Council. In the main, local militias surrendered peacefully to local *mujaheddin* units. The removal of Najibullah also prompted the return of large numbers of refugees from Iran and Pakistan to Afghanistan.

The new Islamic *Jihad* Council was formed of 51 members from six parties (excluding the Hekmatyar faction of the Islamic Party) under the leadership of Seghbatullah Mujjaddedi, leader of the Afghan Interim Government in Peshawar. The new regime, although dominated by Pashtun Sunni groups, also included representatives from minority ethnic groups, and in early June was given the support of the predominately Shia Muslim coalition, the Islamic Unity Party of Afghanistan. According to an agreement reached in Peshawar before the return of the exiled *mujaheddin* groups, the presidency was transferred in June to Burhanuddin Rabbani, leader of the Afghan Islamic Association, but the situation as of mid-1992 was far from stable.

Constitutional structure

The communist revolution replaced the 1977 Constitution with the Basic Principles of the Democratic Republic of Afghanistan in 1980. The "national reconciliation" programme of 1986 led to the ratification in November 1987 of a new Constitution, which was then amended in May 1990. This Constitution allowed for the formation and participation in national elections of political parties with at least 500 members which applied for and were granted official registration, providing that they complied with the Constitution and laws of the country. In practice, power remained concentrated in President Najibullah's National Front, a coalition of his supporters, the political wing of which was the Homeland Party. Islam was the official religion of Afghanistan and theoretically the basis of the laws of the country. However, after the *mujaheddin* takeover many "un-Islamic" laws were abolished, alcohol was banned and women required to observe the Islamic dress code. The structure of the communist regime was entirely dismantled, including the cabinet, the National Assembly, the state security apparatus and the Homeland Party, and by mid-1992 there was no new constitution.

Electoral system

Under the communist Constitution, the executive President was both elected by and accountable to the Grand National Assembly or Supreme Council (*Loya Jirga*). The President, who had to be a Muslim, was elected for a seven-year term, renewable only once. The President appointed the Prime Minister, who in turn appointed the Council of Ministers, both subject to approval by the *Loya Jirga*. The council of ministers was responsible for the formulation and implementation of domestic, foreign and economic policy and for ensuring public order. The 10-member Constitutional Council, entrusted with ensuring the conformity of laws with the Constitution, was appointed by the President.

The *Loya Jirga* was a nationwide traditional gathering of tribal and other leaders, chaired by the President, and the highest manifestation of the will of the people of Afghanistan. Legislative authority was vested in the bicameral National Assembly (*Meli Shura*), comprising a 234-member fully elected lower house (the Council of Representatives—*Wolosi Jirga*) and a 192-member upper house (the Senate or House of the Elders—*Sena* or *Meshrano Jirga*) which was partly elected, and partly appointed by the

President.

As of mid-1992 the Islamic state of Afghanistan was under the leadership of an interim government, the Islamic *Jihad* Council whose structure was unclear.

Evolution of the suffrage

The principle of universal suffrage was first introduced into Afghanistan in the 1964 Constitution, which gave all citizens of at least 20 years of age the right to vote. This principle was revived in the 1987 Constitution with the voting age amended to 18 years. Laws on suffrage in the new Islamic state are as yet unknown.

PARTY BY PARTY DATA

The main political parties of Afghanistan can be divided into three types as follows: (i) the many different *mujaheddin* groupings, whose compositions and affiliations change constantly especially at the present time (mid-1992) in their bloody contest for the leadership of Afghanistan; (ii) the Shia Muslim groups; (iii) the now defunct communist party and the other left-wing parties legal under the communist regime since 1987 and probably also defunct under the new regime.

Groups currently active

Afghan Islamic Association
Jamaat-i-Islami Afghanistan
Leadership. Burhanuddin Rabbani (l.).
Founded. 1970.
Orientation. The creation of an Islamic state in Afghanistan (on lines less rigid than those of the Islamic Party). Member of the Islamic Union of Afghan *mujaheddin*.
History. This Tajik-dominated group has a large following among non-Pashtun nationalities, most notably the *mujaheddin* of the Panjsher Valley associated with Ahmed Shah Massud. On Jan. 27, 1980, it took part in the formation of the Islamic Alliance for the Liberation of Afghanistan, of which Ghulam Abdur Rasoul Sayaf (the deputy leader of the party, who had spent six years in prison) became leader on March 19, 1980.

At a meeting in Washington on June 16, 1986, Rabbani urged US President Ronald Reagan to sever diplomatic relations with the Afghan government and extend full diplomatic recognition to the *mujaheddin*. Prof. Rabbani also met with the French Prime Minister, Jacques Chirac, on June 23.

The Association's offices in Peshawar, Pakistan, were bombed on Feb. 19, 1987, when at least 14 persons were killed.

Rabbani has opposed the Soviet-backed offer to restore the King, stating that the monarchy was responsible for the present condition of Afghanistan. Prior to the overthrow of the Najibullah regime, Rabbani stated a willingness to negotiate directly with the Soviet Union, but not with the regime in Kabul, and said that no other power would be allowed to establish bases in Afghanistan after a Soviet withdrawal.

Ahmed Shah Massud (known as the Lion of Panjsher), the group's military commander who wrested control of the Panjsher Valley from Soviet Forces in 1979, was thought to have been instrumental in forging the Tajik-Pashtun anti-government alliance which finally toppled the Najibullah regime in April 1992. In May 1992, he was appointed Defence Minister in the Islamic *Jihad* Council.

Rabbani took over the leadership of the Islamic *Jihad* Council in June 1992 and thus at time of writing (mid-1992) was de facto leader of the country.
Membership. 20,000 (reported mid-1987).
Publications. *Afghan News* (printed in English).
International affiliations. The movement has been supported by the *Jamaat-i-Islami* of Pakistan, a component of the Pakistan National Alliance, members of which held posts in the government of President Zia ul-Haq.

Afghan National Liberation Front
Jahb-i-Nejat-i-Melli Afghanistan
Leadership. Imam Seghbatullah Mujjaddedi.
Founded. 1979.
Orientation. Moderate.
History. On March 12, 1979, this Front—which also embraced a faction of the Islamic Party—called for a *jihad* (holy war) against the Kabul regime. On Jan. 27, 1980, it took part in the formation of the Islamic Alliance for the Liberation of Afghanistan. On June 1,

1981, however, it formed (together with the National Islamic Front of Afghanistan and the Movement for Islamic Revolution) the Islamic Union of Afghan *mujaheddin*.

Following the fall of Najibullah, Seghbatullah Mujjaddedi, a traditional Islamic scholar and head of the Naqshbandiyyah Sufi order in Afghanistan, became President of the Afghanistan Interim Government and subsequently head of the Islamic *Jihad* Council until June 1, 1992, when Rabbani took over.
Membership. 35,000.

Islamic Alliance for the Liberation of Afghanistan (IALA) (also known as the National Alliance)
Ittehad-i-Islami
Leadership. Prof. Ghulam Abdur Rasoul Sayaf (l.), Ahmad Shah (deputy l.).
Founded. Jan. 27, 1980.
Orientation. Militant Wahhabi Sunni fundamentalist.
History. This Alliance was formed at an extraordinary meeting of the Foreign Ministers of the Islamic Conference Organization (ICO) in Islamabad, Pakistan, by representatives of Afghan rebel organizations—the Afghan Islamic Association; the Movement for Islamic Revolution; the Afghan National Liberation Front; the Afghan Islamic and Nationalist Revolutionary Council; and both factions of the Islamic Party; the Hekmatyar faction, however, withdrew in March 1980 because of disagreement over representation on a proposed Supreme Revolutionary Council.

At the 11th session of the Foreign Ministers of the Organization of the Islamic Conference, held in Islamabad on May 17-22, 1980, Rasoul Sayaf presented a list of demands which included the severance of diplomatic relations with the Soviet Union and Afghanistan, the recognition of the insurgent organizations as the sole legitimate representatives of Afghanistan and their acceptance as a member of the ICO. The meeting, however, adopted a resolution providing for the establishment of a three-member committee to seek "ways and means for a comprehensive solution of the crisis with respect to Afghanistan". (The ICO had suspended Afghanistan's membership in January 1980 and a number of its member states, among them Saudi Arabia, had provided funds "to assist Afghan insurgents and refugees".)

Talks between the three-member ICO committee and an IALA delegation, led by Sayaf, in Switzerland on June 20-21, 1980, ended inconclusively. The committee assured the IALA of the moral and political support of the Islamic nations and restated its aim of seeking a peaceful solution to the conflict on the basis of "immediate, total and unconditional withdrawal of Soviet troops from Afghanistan" in order to restore to that country political independence, sovereignty, nonalignment, an Islamic identity, and freedom to choose its own form of government as well as its political, social and economic system. The IALA delegation restated its refusal to negotiate with the Afghan or Soviet governments, called for the withdrawal of Soviet troops, demanded the recognition of the *mujaheddin* as the sole legitimate representatives of the Afghan people and their own participation in the committee in this capacity, and pledged that under their leadership Afghanistan would pursue a policy of "active nonalignment" and would decide on its own future freely and without super-power interference. The delegation also called (i) for special UN and Islamic meetings to be held on Afghanistan; (ii) for the Islamic nations to re-examine their relations with the Soviet Union; and (iii) for the opening of a special Afghan resistance fund financed partly by members of the Organization of Petroleum Exporting Countries (OPEC).

The IALA was by this time, however, deeply divided. The Hekmatyar faction of the Islamic Party had left the IALA in March 1980. A moderate faction consisted of the Afghan National Liberation Front, the Movement for Islamic Revolution and the Afghan Islamic and Nationalist Revolutionary Council (later known as National Islamic Front of Afghanistan). Another faction embraced two Muslim fundamentalist groups—the Afghan Islamic Association and the Khales faction of the Islamic Party.

Sayaf, noted for his preference for a military solution to the Afghan problem, on July 17, 1987, rejected the coalition initiatives of the Kabul government, stating that only a *mujaheddin* government would be acceptable.

The IALA was given five seats on the new Islamic *Jihad* Council.
Membership. 15,000.

Islamic Party
Hizb-i-Islami
This major Sunni fundamentalist *mujaheddin* party has two factions led respectively by (i) Gulbuddin Hekmatyar and (ii) Mohammad Yunus Khales. Before the split over personal differences in 1979, the party announced in Islamabad, Pakistan, on July 30, 1978, that it had launched guerrilla attacks against the communist government and was the following year reported to

seek the restoration of the monarchy in Afghanistan.

Hekmatyar Faction

Leadership. Gulbuddin Hekmatyar.

Founded in 1979, after a split in the Islamic Party, its aims included the creation of a strict Islamic state in Afghanistan. It was reputed to be the largest and best-organized fundamentalist Islamic Party, and joined the Islamic Alliance for the Liberation of Afghanistan, formed on Jan. 27, 1980. Instigated a strike by shop-keepers in Kabul, later joined by civil servants and office workers, on Feb. 21-27, 1980. This led to the imposition of martial law and a curfew in the capital on Feb. 22 and to demonstrations on the same day, when at least 300 civilians and an unknown number of Soviet and Afghan troops were reported killed, and many thousands arrested. Parallel strikes took place in several regional towns.

A member of the Islamic Union of Afghan *Mujaheddin*, it withdrew from the Afghan Interim Government in 1989 and after the overthrow of Najibullah's regime refused to co-operate with the *mujaheddin*-dominated Islamic *Jihad* Council. It is now one of the major factions in the bitter fight for leadership in Kabul.

Membership. 35,000.

International Affiliations. Has close links with the *Jamaat-i-Islami* of Pakistan and sections of the Pakistani army and intelligence services dealing with Afghan affairs.

Khalis Faction.

Leadership. Mohammad Yunus Khales.

Founded in 1979, after a split in the Islamic Party, it shares with the Hekmatyar faction the belief that only devout Muslims should rule Afghanistan. On Aug. 11, 1979, this faction of the party joined the Afghan National Liberation Front and (along with the other faction) joined the Islamic Alliance for the Liberation of Afghanistan formed on Jan. 27, 1980. The group is reported to have a wide following among Afghan refugees in Pakistan and to have received substantial assistance from the US Central Intelligence Agency (CIA). A member of the Islamic Union of Afghan *Mujaheddin* the faction quit the Afghan Interim Government in May 1991, accusing it of complicity with the Kabul-based government.

Membership. 20,000.

Islamic Union of Afghan Mujaheddin (also known as Islamic Unity of Afghan Mujaheddin)

Ittehad-i-Islami Afghan Mujaheddin

Address. Formerly Peshawar, Pakistan. Now Kabul.

Leadership. The organization has a rotating leadership which changes every three months.

Founded. May 1985, Peshawar, Pakistan.

Orientation. Sunni Islamic.

History. Formed as an alliance representing seven major *mujaheddin* groups, both moderate and fundamentalist, as follows: the two factions of the Islamic Party, two factions of the Islamic Afghan Association, two factions of the Movement for Islamic Revolution, and the Afghan National Liberation Front.

The union, based in Pakistan, issued a joint statement at a rally on Jan. 17, 1987, firmly rejecting the Afghan government's ceasefire and its proposals for a government of national reconciliation. It subsequently became the kernel of the Pakistan-based Afghan Interim Government, and consequently of the Islamic *Jihad* Council. Disagreement over the nature of these two organizations, however, meant that the Hekmatyar faction of the Islamic Party withdrew from the alliance.

Membership. 100,000.

Movement for Islamic Revolution

Harakat-i-Inqilab-i Islami

Leadership. Mawlawi Muhammad Nabi Muhammadi (traditional Islamic scholar known for his anti-Shia views).

Orientation. Moderate *mujaheddin*.

History. On Jan. 27, 1980, this movement joined the Islamic Alliance for the Liberation of Afghanistan, and on June 1, 1981, it formed (together with the Afghan National Liberation Front and the National Islamic Front) the Islamic Union of Afghan *Mujaheddin*.

Membership. 20,000.

National Islamic Front of Afghanistan

Mahaz-i-Melli-i-Islami

Leadership. Pir Sayed Ahmed Gailani.

Orientation. A small but visible moderate Pashtun-dominated organization (dubbed "Gucci *mujaheddin*" by the Western media). Liberal and pro-monarchist.

History. It took part in the formation of the Islamic Alliance for the Liberation of Afghanistan in January 1980. It was originally known as the Afghan Islamic and Nationalist Revolutionary Council. After the adoption of its new title it formed (together with the Afghan National Liberation Front and the Movement for Islamic Revolution) the Islamic Union of Afghan *Mujaheddin*. A spokesman for the organization was quoted on July 5, 1982, as saying that the Soviet military forces in Afghanistan were turning the country into a forward military base for possible moves into South-West Asia by (i) developing a major air-base at Shindand (western Afghanistan); (ii) building a bridge across the Amu Darya River (on Afghanistan's border with the Soviet Union) and starting a railway line from the frontier to Kabul; and (iii) by annexing (in 1981) the Wakhan corridor (in north-east Afghanistan, bordering on Pakistan, China and the Soviet Union). (This annexation would deprive Afghanistan of its frontier with China and would give the Soviet Union a common frontier with Pakistan.)

Gailani, head of the Sufi Qadiriyyah sect in Afghanistan, has consistently favoured the return to Afghanistan of ex-King Zahir Shah, and envisaged a role for him in a transitional government. On July 18, 1987, he rejected Najibullah's offer of a power-sharing role. *Membership.* 20,000.

Shia Groups

Afghani Nasr Organization (*Sazmane Nasr*); Abdul Karim Khalili (l.). The largest Iran-based Shia organization; part of Islamic Unity Party of Afghanistan; claims a membership of 50,000.

Afghanistan Party of God (*Hezbollah-i-Afghanistan*); Alhaj Shaikh Ali Wosoqusalam Wosoqi (ch.). Founded in 1990. An Islamic party founded in Kabul and approved under the communist regime. Member of Islamic Unity Party of Afghanistan.

Da'wa Party of Islamic Unity of Afghanistan (*Da'wa-i-Ittehad-i-Islami Afghanistan*); a Shia group with support in Ghazni province; member of the Islamic Unity Party of Afghanistan.

Guardians of Islamic Jihad of Afghanistan (*Pasdaran-i-Afghanistan*); led collectively by 10-member council. A Shia organization which is a member of the Iran-based Islamic Unity Party of Afghanistan.

Islamic Force of Afghanistan (*Nahzat-i-Afghanistan*); collective leadership concentrated in a three-member council. A Shia group; a member of Islamic Unity Party of Afghanistan with a wide following in the Jogore area.

Islamic Movement of Afghanistan (*Harakat-i-Islami Afghanistan*); led by Ayatollah Aseh Mohseni. This Shia movement seeks the establishment of an Islamic Republic of Afghanistan on the model of that of Iran. Its precise relationship to the Islamic Unity Party of Afghanistan is unclear. Some reports, observing its closeness to the Iranian government, infer membership while others note the anti-Iranian stance of its leader, reportedly the only Afghan Shia leader with headquarters in Peshawar, Pakistan. It has 20,000 members.

Islamic Struggle for Afghanistan (*Narave Islami Afghanistan*); the group's most prominent member is Zaidi Mohazzizi. A Shia organization; member of the Islamic Unity Party of Afghanistan.

Islamic Unity Party of Afghanistan (IUPA) (*Hizb-i-Wahdat-i-Afghanistan*); formerly known as the Islamic Coalition Council of Afghanistan (Teheran); Rehmat Ullah Mutazawi (l.). Founded in June 1990. An Iran-backed alliance of Islamic Shia groups in Teheran. Members: the Afghan Nasr Organization, the Guardians of Islamic *Jihad* of Afghanistan, United Islamic Front of Afghanistan, the Islamic Force of Afghanistan, the Da'wa Party of Islamic Unity of Afghanistan, the Islamic Movement of Afghanistan, the Afghanistan Party of God, the Party of God, the Unity Council and the Islamic Struggle for Afghanistan. It refused to acknowledge the legitimacy of the Afghan Interim Government in Pakistan but has now been given eight seats and the control of three government ministries in the present Sunni-dominated Islamic *Jihad* Council.

Party of God (*Hezbollah*); leadership: Qari Ahmed (also known as Qari Yakdasta). A militant Shia group; member of Islamic Unity Party of Afghanistan.

Peoples' Islamic Party of Afghanistan (Kabul); leadership: Alhav Maulvi Ruhollah Abed. Founded in 1987. This Islamic party was the only "religious" party with official status under the communist government at the time of the 1987 elections. Its present status is unclear.

Union of the Companions of the Prophet (*Ittehad-i-Ansarollah*); leadership: Haji Zafar Muhammad Khadem. Founded in 1988. Islamic party legal under former communist government.

United Islamic Front for Afghanistan (*Jabhe Muttahid-i-Afghanistan*); collective leadership. Shia organization with strong following among ethnic Hazara; member of Iran-based Islamic Unity Party of Afghanistan.

Unity Council (*Shura-i-Ittefaq*). Largest and most organized Shia organization with broad-based support but concentrated mainly in the Hazarajat area; member of the Islamic Unity Party of Afghanistan.

Defunct parties

Afghan National Movement Party (Kabul); leadership: Abdol Aziz Aziz. Founded in 1989 as Young Workers's Organization of Afghanistan, name changed 1991.

Afghanistan Peace Front (replaced National Front); Abd Al-Hakim Tawana (ch.); Nur Akbar Paiesh (Sec.-Gen.). Founded in 1990.

Homeland Party (*Hezb-i Watan*) (formerly known as the People's Democratic Party of Afghanistan (PDPA)—*Jamiyat-e Demokratiki Khalq-e Afghanistan*); leadership: Najibullah (ch. and gen. sec.), Suleiman La'eq, Farid Ahmad Mazdak, Abdul Mobin. Founded in 1965, abolished in 1992. Initially theoretically Marxist-Leninist and subservient to the Soviet line, although it later advocated a mixed economy leaving light industry and trade mostly in public ownership. From 1979 on, the party claimed to be the ruling party in a country undergoing the "national democratic stage of revolution", not a socialist party, and in the early 1980s it engaged in nationalization and the establishment of co-operatives. Latterly under the "national reconciliation" programme private enterprise and land-ownership were revived and religion shown greater tolerance.

The party was founded as an illegal organization by Nur Mohammed Taraki. In 1966 it was divided into two wings—the *Khalq* (People's) group led by Taraki and the *Parcham* (Flag) group led by Babrak Karmal. The *Khalq* group advocated the overthrow of the monarchy as a first step to socialism; after this overthrow had been carried out by left-wing officers in 1973 the *Khalk* group refused to abide by a Soviet directive to give wholehearted support to the regime of President Daoud, whereas the *Parcham* group co-operated with that regime. In July 1977 the two groups were reunited in the *Khalq* Party under Taraki's leadership with a view to building a Communist mass party.

The party came to power with the overthrow of President Mohammad Daoud by a Revolutionary Council in April 1978 (the "Saur Revolution"), when Taraki became Prime Minister and Babrak Karmal (known as a pro-Moscow hardliner) one of three Deputy Prime Ministers. The latter was, however, dis-

missed in July 1978 from his posts of Vice-President of the Revolutionary Council and of Deputy Prime Minister. In March 1979 Taraki surrendered the premiership to Hafizullah Amin (hitherto a Deputy Prime Minister and Minister of Foreign Affairs), and in September 1979 the latter replaced Taraki as President of the Republic and party leader. It was later revealed that Taraki had been killed in the takeover. It appeared that Hafizullah Amin did not enjoy Soviet support (as Taraki had), and in late December 1979 a further change of regime occurred when Soviet troops entered the country and brought about the installation of Babrak Karmal as head of state and PDPA leader.

The new Soviet-backed government and PDPA politburo were drawn mainly from the *Parcham* faction, although the *Khalq* faction was also represented in both. Conflict between them nevertheless continued, with several of Amin's ministers and associates being executed in 1980 and *Khalqis* being purged from the army, the administration and the party leadership. A party congress scheduled for March 1982 was downgraded to a conference, which lasted only two days, apparently because of factional disagreements over the election of delegates.

In an attempt to conciliate public opinion, in 1981-82 the regime drastically modified the radical agrarian reform programme (introduced in 1978), established the National Fatherland Front (NFF) as a broad alliance of political parties, trade unions, mass organizations and religious and tribal bodies, and emphasized its respect for Islam and traditional customs.

By 1985 a military stalemate had been reached in the civil war, with Soviet and Afghan government forces controlling the towns and *mujaheddin* guerrillas most of the countryside. In May 1986, apparently at Soviet instigation, Karmal was replaced as PDPA general secretary by Najibullah, also a member of the *Parcham* faction. At the end of the year, following an announcement that Soviet forces would begin a phased withdrawal as soon as conditions permitted, Najibullah launched a programme of "national reconciliation" and offered the *mujaheddin* a ceasefire. This process culminated in the approval in November 1987 of a new Constitution providing for a measure of multiparty representative democracy under which the PDPA ceased to have a monopoly of power, although in practice it remained the dominant force within the National Front (as the NFF had been renamed in January 1987).

These changes, which included the appointment to the government of representatives of other political organizations, had earlier been approved at the PDPA's second national conference held on Oct. 18-20, 1987, immediately prior to which a number of Karmal supporters had been removed from the party's central committee.

In April 1988 the PDPA won fewer than one-quarter of the seats in a general election for the newly formed bicameral National Assembly (*Meli Shura*); many of the other members, however, were from organizations in the NFF or were pro-regime independents. The maximum landholding of 15 acres was raised to 50 acres, and former landlords who had fled abroad were invited to return and reclaim expropriated property. The government claimed that the private sector now accounted for over 90 per cent of the economy. The civil war continued, however, as did the feuding between the factions within the party, and defections thinned the leadership's ranks.

In December 1989 there was an attempted coup against Najibullah by *Khalqi* members of the armed forces, who disapproved of attempts to conciliate the regime's opponents. Among the 127 people arrested were 11 generals, but they were subsequently released following a three-day strike by the *Khalqi* army commander, Lt.-Gen. Tanai. In early March 1990 Tanai himself launched a coup against Najibullah, which was again defeated after bitter fighting, which included loyal and dissident air force pilots bombing each others' positions in Kabul, with large numbers of civilian casualties. Tanai briefly fled to Pakistan, before returning to Afghanistan and making common cause (under Pakistan pressure) with one of the leading Islamic guerrilla organizations, the Islamic Party.

Najibullah took advantage of these events to purge half of the Political Bureau. Tanai's successor was another *Khalqi* (after the attempted coup Najibullah claimed that Tanai had been a member not of the *Khalq* faction but of the Zarghonist sub-faction), the former Interior and Defence Minister, Lt.-Gen. Mohammad Aslam Watanjar.

The guerrillas continued to demand Najibullah's resignation as a precondition for any truce. In January 1990 he declared that he would accept the verdict of genuinely free elections, but the *mujaheddin* called instead for their own national Grand Assembly (*Loya Jirga*).

Najibullah finally offered his resignation in April 1992, and was removed after elements of his party, with the help of the military, carried out what was effectively a low-key coup. Najibullah attempted to flee the country, but was prevented from reaching the airport by troops under the command of Gen. Abdul Rashid Dostam, an Uzbek military leader previously employed by the government against Pashtun *mujaheddin* groups who had switched alliance to Massud. Najibullah was forced to take refuge in a UN office in Kabul, where he reportedly remained as of late April.

Najibullah was replaced by Abdorrahim Hatef, a vice-president of the party who became acting president only in name and only temporarily, as Kabul was now under the control of the *mujaheddin*, who abolished the Homeland Party on taking power in May.

National Fatherland Front (NFF); founded in 1981 as an umbrella organization of political parties, trade unions, mass organizations and religious and tribal bodies supportive of the communist regime. In January 1987 it changed its name to the National Front.

Peasants' National Unity (PNU—*Bazgari Meli Ittehad*) (formerly Peasants' Justice Party of Afghanistan); leadership: Abd Al-Hakim Tawana (ch.). Founded 1987, changed name 1990. One of the five main parties which contested the 1987 elections.

Solidarity Movement of Afghan People; leadership: Mohammad Sarwar Lemach. Founded in 1988.

Supreme Revolutionary Council; leadership: Mohammad Babrak Zai. The council was formed in May 1980 as a provisional government at a special tribal meeting (*Loya Jirga*) in Peshawar, Pakistan, attended by delegates from all areas of Afghanistan. The meeting passed a number of "fundamental resolutions" designed to form the basis of a future constitution for Afghanistan, and it is also decided that all treaties signed after April 1978, notably the Soviet-Afghan treaty of friendship under which Soviet troops had entered the country, would be considered void.

Toilers' Organization of Afghanistan; leadership: Hamidollah Gran. A left-wing party; one of the five main official parties who contested the 1987 elections.

Toilers' Revolutionary Organization of Afghanistan; leadership: Mahbubullah Koshani; Muhammad Bashir Baghlani; Muhammad Eshaq Kawa. Founded in 1968. A left-wing party; one of the five main official parties who contested the 1987 elections.

Unity of Strugglers for Peace and Progress in Afghanistan (*Etafaq-e Mabarezan-e Solha wa taraqi Afghanistan*). Founded in 1990.

Australia

Capital: Canberra   **Population: 17,414,300**

Australia is a parliamentary democracy with a federal constitution dating from January 1901. Originally colonized by the British, Australia is currently an independent member of the Commonwealth. The head of state is the British sovereign, represented by a Governor-General. Since 1945 the country has essentially operated a two-party system with the Australian Labor Party (ALP) being opposed by an alliance between the Liberal Party and the smaller Nationalist Party. In recent years the Australian Democrats have developed into a significant third force but have yet to make serious inroads into the legislature. In the general election of March 1990 the ALP was returned by a narrow margin for a fourth successive term. In December 1991 its veteran leader Bob Hawke was replaced by Paul Keating.

Constitutional structure

Under the federal constitution adopted in 1901, executive authority is in the hands of a Prime Minister who governs with the assistance of an appointed Cabinet all of whom must be members of, and are responsible to, the legislature. Legislative authority within the Commonwealth of Australia is vested in a bicameral parliament. This consists of (i) a 76-member Senate, with 12 seats apportioned to each of the country's six states and two each for the Northern Territory and the Australian Capital Territory (the state members sit for six-year terms, with half being renewed every three years, and the territorial members serve for three-year terms); and (ii) a more powerful 148-member House of Representatives elected for three years. Seats within the House are distributed among the states on the basis of population, but each state must have at least five seats. The Senate acts as a reviewing chamber and may veto legislation or return it to the House for amendment. It may also initiate legislation other than money bills. In the event of deadlock between the two chambers the Prime Minister may seek a dissolution of both houses. Double dissolutions occurred in 1974, 1975 and 1983.

The federal government is responsible for national matters such as foreign policy, defence, immigration, customs and excise duties, external trade and commerce, communications and tax collection. Those powers not specifically allocated to the federal government are in the hands of individual states. Each state also has its own legislature (all except Queensland are bicameral), government and constitution. State governments have wide powers in areas such as education, transport, law enforcement, health services and agriculture.

Electoral system

Voting is by secret ballot and is compulsory for all citizens aged 18 years and over in federal and state elections, except for electors living overseas, working in the Antarctic or defined as itinerant. Those failing to vote without good reason are liable to fines. Anyone entitled to vote is eligible to stand as a candidate.

Members of the House (and members of the lower houses of all state legislatures except Tasmania, which uses proportional representation) are elected to single member constituencies under the alternative vote system. If no candidate achieves more than 50 per cent of first preference votes the lowest scoring candidate is eliminated and his second preferences re-distributed among the remaining contestants. This

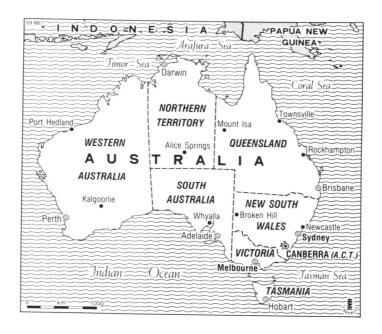

Recent elections

Date	Winning Party
Sept. 28, 1946	Australian Labor Party (ALP)
Dec. 10, 1949	Country-Liberal Parties
April 28, 1951	Country-Liberal Parties
May 29, 1954	Country-Liberal Parties
Dec. 10, 1955	Country-Liberal Parties
Nov. 22, 1958	Country-Liberal Parties
Dec. 9, 1961	Country-Liberal Parties
Nov. 30, 1963	Country-Liberal Parties
Nov. 26, 1966	Country-Liberal Parties
Oct. 25, 1969	Country-Liberal Parties

Date	Winning Party
Dec. 2, 1972	ALP
May 18, 1974	ALP
Dec. 13, 1975	Country-Liberal Parties
Dec. 10, 1977	Country-Liberal Parties
Oct. 18, 1980	Country-Liberal Parties
March 5, 1983	ALP
Dec. 1, 1984	ALP
July 11, 1987	ALP
March 24, 1990	ALP

General election, July 11, 1987

Party	House of Representatives		Senate	
	Percentage	Seats	Percentage	Seats
ALP	45.8	86	41.6	34
Liberal Party	34.3	43	43.1	29
National Party	11.5	19	5.3	4
Australian Democrats	6.0	—	6.3	6
Others	2.4	—	3.7	3

General election, March 24, 1990

Party	Seats won	
	House of Representatives	Senate
ALP	78	32
Liberal Party	55	27
National Party	14	6
Australian Democrats	—	7
Others	1	4

process is repeated until a candidate exceeds the winning threshold. Vacancies are filled through by-elections.

Senators are directly elected on a proportional basis by the population of a state or territory voting as a single multimember constituency. A quota is determined by dividing the total number of formal votes by the number of Senate vacancies for that constituency, plus one. A candidate who receives a number of first preference votes equal to or greater than the quota is elected. If an elected candidate has a surplus of votes, these are transferred to the remaining candidates, on the basis of second preferences. The process continues until the required number of senators is elected. Senators serve for six years with one-half liable for re-election every three years. Territorial senators serve a maximum of three years. If a seat becomes vacant the appropriate state legislature chooses a replacement to hold the office until the expiration of the term or a until new a new election can be held.

Evolution of suffrage

Universal suffrage for those over 21 years of age was introduced in 1902 in accordance with the practice already in existence in many of the country's constituent states. The voting was reduced to 18 prior to the 1974 elections. Compulsory voting was adopted in 1924.

PARTY BY PARTY DATA

Australian Democrats

Address. 6 Muir Street, Hawthorn, Victoria 3122, Australia.

Leadership. Senator J. R. Coulter (parl. leader).

Orientation. Centrist. The party's constitution commits it to "achieve and defend effective participatory democracy and open government by appropriate constitutional, parliamentary and governmental reforms". Its policy objectives include increased education and social welfare provisions; the reduction of poverty; opposition to gender or racial discrimination; opposition to the proliferation of nuclear weapons; and the protection of civil liberties.

Founded. 1977.

History. The party was formed by people disillusioned with the existing two-party political system. It drew heavily from disaffected members of the Liberal Party and from those previously associated with the Australia Party, a democratic group which grew up in the 1960s in opposition to the Vietnam War. From the outset the Democrats portrayed themselves as qualitatively different from the old parties because they were associated with neither the trade union movement nor the business community. The party also prided itself on its level of democracy, with its office-holders and its policies being determined by postal ballots of the entire membership.

The Democrats polled 9.4 per cent of the vote in the 1977 elections, and although they failed to win any seats in the House of Representatives, they won two seats in the Senate. In the federal election of 1980 the party gained a further three Senate seats, thereby giving it the balance of power in the upper chamber. In the 1984, 1987, and 1990 elections the party won seven seats in the Senate.

Structure. The party has divisional offices in each state and territory, with local branches based usually on federal electoral districts. The national executive is the main governing body of the party and comprises a national president, two deputy presidents and six office holders (all of whom are elected by a postal ballot of all members), and representatives from each state and territory who are elected by members in their divisions. Each division has a considerable degree of autonomy in the running of election campaigns, development of local policy and the management of divisional finances. Similar principles of autonomy apply to local branches.

Publications. The *National Journal*, a monthly publication mailed to each member which serves as a forum for the discussion of policy issues.

Australian Labor Party

Address. PO Box E1, Queen Victoria Terrace, ACT 2600.

Leadership. Paul Keating (parl. leader).

Orientation. Social-Democratic. The party is committed to "the democratic socialization of industry, production, distribution and exchange to the extent necessary to eliminate exploitation and other anti-so-

cial features". Specific policy aims include the restoration of full employment; the abolition of poverty;
greater equality of distribution for wealth and income;
equal rights; and a greater provision of educational and
social welfare services.

Founded. 1901.

History. The Australian Labor Party (ALP) was created from the separate labour parties formed in the
Australian states in the 1890s prior to federation. In the
first national elections, in 1901, the ALP gained 16
seats in the House and eight in the Senate. The first
federal ALP government came to power as a minority
administration in 1904, under John Watson, but remained in office for only three months.

In October 1907 Watson was succeeded as leader by
Andrew Fisher, who in the same month formed the
second minority ALP administration, which lasted
until June 1909. In the election of April 1910 the party
gained an outright majority in both chambers of Parliament. It was defeated in May 1913, but was returned
to power at elections in September 1914. In October
1915 Fisher resigned to become High Commissioner
in the United Kingdom, and was succeeded by W. M.
Hughes.

The party was severely damaged by World War I,
and in particular by the issue of conscription, which
was supported by the ALP leadership but strongly
opposed by much of the trade union movement.
Hughes and 23 of his ALP parliamentary colleagues
eventually left the party and joined the opposition to
form a nationalist government.

The ALP remained out of office until the election of
1929 when its leader, J. H. Scullin, became Prime
Minister. His government was immediately engulfed
in the Great Depression, however, and was defeated in
1931. The defeat was the signal for further splits within
the party and renewed factional fighting between the
political and industrial wings of the ALP.

In 1935 Scullin was succeeded as federal leader by
John Curtin, who gradually reconstructed the party and
restored its electoral appeal. Curtin served as Prime
Minister between October 1941 and his death in July
1945. He was succeeded by J. B. Chifley who was
defeated in December 1949. Chifley died in June 1951
and was succeeded by H. V. Evatt, under whose leadership the ALP lost three consecutive elections. During
this period the party was weakened by fierce internecine fighting resulting from a campaign by those determined to resist the growth of communist influences
within the trade union movement. The conflict led
ultimately to several splits within the party and the

formation of the Democratic Labor Party of Australia
[see below].

In the late 1960s the ALP began to recover under
the leadership of Gough Whitlam, who pushed through
an ambitious programme of policy and administrative
reform. The rejuvenated party narrowly lost the 1969
election, but won in 1972, securing 67 seats in the
125-member House. Whitlam's administration made
a number of important advances but was constantly
frustrated by an opposition majority in the Senate.
Eventually he called for a double dissolution and, in
May 1974, attempted to win overall majorities in both
houses. Although he retained power in the House with
a reduced majority (winning 66 of the 127 seats), he
failed to achieve a majority in the Senate, winning 29
of the 60 seats.

The Whitlam government continued its programme
of socialist reform until October 1975, when the opposition in the Senate blocked its budget in an effort to
force an early general election. The political impasse
which followed was broken when Governor-General
Sir John Kerr dismissed the ALP government and
appointed an opposition minority administration as a
caretaker government pending fresh elections. The
ALP was decisively defeated at the subsequent election of 1975 and again in 1977, winning 36 and 38 seats
respectively. Bill Hayden was elected leader of the
party in 1977 and undertook a comprehensive policy
and administrative review in a bid to restore the party's
morale and standing with the electorate. The ALP
narrowly failed to achieve power in the election of
1980, securing 45.1 per cent of the vote and 51 seats
in the 125-member House.

Hayden was replaced as leader in February 1983 by
Bob Hawke, a charismatic former president of the
Australian Council of Trade Unions. The Hawke years
were characterized by the discarding of many of the
ALP's traditional values and policies, particularly in
the economic sphere, where Treasury Minister Paul
Keating pursued a relentless course of deregulation,
privatization and austere monetary control. Under
Hawke's leadership the party won an unprecedented
four consecutive election victories in 1983, 1984, 1987
and 1990. In 1983 the ALP secured 75 seats in the
House and 30 in the 64-member Senate. In the 1984
elections the party won 47.7 per cent of the vote in the
lower house elections and secured 82 seats in the newly
expanded 148-member House, and 34 in the 76-mem-
ber Senate. In 1987 its share of the vote fell to 45.8 per
cent but the party won 86 seats in the House and 32 in
the Senate. In 1990 its vote declined but it retained its

overall majority, winning 78 seats in the House.

Not only did the ALP achieve an unprecedented fourth consecutive federal election victory, but by the middle of 1991 it was also in control of every state government except New South Wales, where it had lost power in 1988. Superficially, the party's position looked unassailable, and commentators repeatedly suggested that, under Hawke's leadership, the ALP had been transformed into the natural party of government. Careful analysis of the 1990 electoral results, however, showed that the ALP's narrow victory had been achieved through skilful targeting of marginal constituencies and preference voters. Within weeks of the election victory, both Hawke and his party were recording high levels of public dissatisfaction in opinion polls, increased by the growing popularity of new Liberal-National parliamentary coalition leader John Hewson, who replaced Andrew Peacock after the election.

By the end of 1990 Australia was also in the depths of a serious economic recession and the Hawke government began 1991 some 18 percentage points behind the opposition in opinion polls, raising questions concerning Hawke's future as leader. This speculation was exacerbated by the stance of Keating, who made no secret of his ambition to be Prime Minister.

On June 3 the rivalry between the two men culminated with a challenge by Keating to Hawke's leadership. Hawke won the ballot by 66 votes to 44, but the allegations concerning his judgment and honesty— Keating alleged that Hawke had promised to stand down in his favour after the election—left him politically damaged. On Dec. 19 a renewed challenge by Keating unseated Hawke by 56 votes to 51, and ended his tenure as Prime Minister.

Despite the leadership change the ALP continued to record high levels of unpopularity in the opinion polls in the first half of 1992. The party was also in trouble in all states except Queensland, where it continued to benefit from reaction to the Fitzgerald inquiry into the corruption associated with the former National Party government, which had been in power for 30 years until defeated in 1989. In Tasmania the increasing friction between the minority ALP administration and the Green Party legislators on whose support it depended led to a premature election in December at which the ALP was defeated. In Victoria the opinion polls also suggested that the ALP would be defeated at the next election. State Premier Joan Kirner had inherited office when John Cain was forced to resign in August 1990 after a Royal Commission inquiry into

the collapse of the merchant banking arm of the state bank, Tricontinental, revealed a record of financial mismanagement, but she had been unable to reverse the consequent unpopularity of her party. In South Australia another Royal Commission had raised doubts concerning the judgement of ALP Premier John Bannon, the national party president, who was forced to provide an A$970 million rescue package for the state bank only months after he had assured the legislature that he had every confidence in the bank. In Western Australia, the state government was forced to establish a Royal Commission to examine claims of corrupt links between politicians, bureaucrats and businessmen.

Following his ejection from the leadership, Hawke retired from politics. On April 11, 1992, the ALP suffered a humiliating defeat when it lost the Melbourne federal constituency in the subsequent by-election to a local Australian rules football coach running as an independent. The party scored only 29 per cent of first preference votes, down almost 20 per cent on its 1990 showing.

Structure. The ALP has local and state branches. The latter enjoy a high degree of autonomy, conducting their own election campaigns and determining their own state policies. The party's national organization is responsible for federal election campaigns and national policies. The supreme governing authority of the party is its National Conference, which usually meets every two years and includes delegations drawn from all of the states and territories of the party. Between conferences authority is in the hands of a 28-member national executive, which includes federal leaders, state and territory delegations and 10 members elected by the national conference. In addition to individual membership of the party, trade unions are also directly affiliated to the ALP.

International affiliations. Socialist International.

Liberal Party of Australia

Address. PO Box E13, Queen Victoria Terrace, ACT 2600.

Leadership. John Hewson (parl. leader).

Orientation. Centre-right. The Liberal Party is the major non-socialist party in Australian politics, and is strongly committed to the promotion of free enterprise and individual independence and initiative. It is opposed to large-scale government intervention and spending, and believes in rewarding individual enterprise through low levels of taxation.

Founded. 1944.

History. The Liberal Party was formed after Robert Menzies called conferences in Canberra and Albury in order to unify the various anti-ALP organizations into a single federal party. As such the party was derived from the various anti-labour organizations of the late 19th and early 20th centuries, particularly the Fusion Party led by Andrew Deakin from 1909, although the first government generally accepted to have been "Liberal" was that of Joseph Cook in 1913. The line of Liberal succession evolved through the Nationalist Party from 1917 and the United Australia Party (UAP) from 1931. These parties formed administrations (usually, after 1922, in coalition with the Country Party, later the National Party) from 1917 to 1929 and from 1932 to 1941.

In 1941 the UAP lost office to the ALP. In 1943 Menzies assumed the leadership of the party and began rejuvenating non-ALP forces which lay outside the immediate sphere of the UAP. As opposition leader he drew together 18 separate organizations which shared a belief in "liberal, progressive policy and are opposed to socialism with its bureaucratic administration and restriction of personal freedom." At a conference in Canberra in October 1944 it was decided to form the Liberal Party of Australia.

Liberal governments were formed in Western Australia, South Australia and Victoria in 1947. In 1949 the party came to power at federal level in alliance with the Country Party. The Liberals won 39.4 per cent of the vote and 55 seats in the House while the Country Party won 10.8 per cent and 19 seats. It was the beginning of a long period of hegemony, with Menzies remaining in office at the head of the Liberal-Country coalition until his retirement in 1966. Throughout the 1950s the Liberals consistently secured around 55 seats in the House (apart from the 1954 election when the party won only 47) but were given a comfortable majority in the 122-member chamber by the Country Party which consistently won between 15 and 20 seats. In the 1961 election the coalition was almost defeated as the Liberal vote fell to 33.6 per cent and its number of seats was reduced to 45. Although the ALP won 60 seats, once again Menzies was kept in office by the 17 members of the Country Party. In 1963 Menzies increased his majority (the Liberals winning 52 seats and the Country Party 20), and in November 1966 the Liberals succeeded in winning an outright majority with 61 seat and 40.1 per cent of the vote.

In January 1966 Menzies retired and was succeeded by Harold Holt. On Dec. 17, shortly after the party's 1966 election triumph, Holt disappeared while swimming in heavy surf. His death sparked a bitter feud for the leadership with both John Gorton and William McMahon serving periods as Prime Minister. Weakened by the internal dissension the party lost power in 1972. The Liberal-Country coalition used its majority in the Senate to frustrate the ALP government and, following an impasse between the two chambers in 1975, Governor-General Sir John Kerr dismissed the Australian Labor Party (ALP) government and invited the opposition coalition to form a minority government. In the subsequent election, in December 1975, the coalition won a majority under its new leader Malcolm Fraser. Fraser's government was returned to power in 1977 and 1980, the Liberals winning 67 and 54 seats with 39.6 and 37.4 per cent of the vote respectively.

The Senate's rejection of several pieces of legislation led Fraser to seek a dissolution of both the House and the Senate in 1983. In the elections which followed, the party was decisively defeated, winning only 33 seats in the House, its poorest result since 1949, and 24 seats in the Senate. Fraser immediately resigned and was succeeded by Andrew Peacock. The party recovered somewhat in the 1984 election, winning 45 seats with 34.2 per cent of the vote, but failed to oust the ALP administration of Bob Hawke. The defeat led to a bitter leadership contest which resulted in Peacock's replacement in September 1985 by John Howard.

In 1987 the Liberal-National coalition collapsed as a result of the leadership ambitions of the Queensland National Party Premier Sir Johannes Bjelke-Petersen [see under National Party]. Capitalizing on the opposition's disarray the ALP won a third election in 1987. Although the Liberal vote remained almost constant, its number of seats fell to 43. The alliance between the two parties was re-established after the defeat of Sir Joh's leadership challenge, and in May 1989 Howard was replaced by Peacock as Liberal leader.

The Liberals continued to suffer from the tension between Peacock and Howard. In the 1990 elections the party won 55 seats in the House, but once again failed to dislodge the Hawke administration. Peacock immediately resigned and was replaced by John Hewson. Capitalizing on the unpopularity of the ALP government, by mid-1992 Hewson and the Liberals were recording opinion poll ratings considerably higher than the ALP.

Structure. The party has divisions in each of the states and in the Australian Capital Territory. Each has its own constitution and enjoys a large measure of autonomy in formulating state policy, raising funds and conducting state election campaigns. At divisional and federal level there is an autonomous Young Liberal Movement for those aged 16-30, and there are state women's councils which are represented in the federal women's committee and on federal bodies. At national level the party's governing body is the annual federal council which includes delegates from all divisions, and also leaders from the state and federal legislatures. Between meetings of the council the management of the federal structure is in the hands of the federal executive, comprising the division presidents, the federal president and vice president of the Young Liberals, the chair of the federal women's committee, federal parliamentary leaders and federal office holders including the president, two vice presidents and the treasurer.

National Party of Australia

Address. PO Box E265, Queen Victoria Terrace, ACT 2600.

Leadership. Tim Fischer (Parl. leader).

Orientation. Right-wing agrarian. In addition to emphasizing traditional conservative concerns such as national security, free market economics, and "family values", the party was acknowledges a "fundamental concern for the welfare of rural dwellers".

Founded. 1916.

History. The National Party (the party is almost never referred to by its full title) was founded as the Country Party (a name retained until 1975) in 1916 as a coalition between farmers' associations from New South Wales, Victoria, Western Australia and Queensland. In 1923 the party joined the federal government as the junior partner of the Nationalist Party and then the United Australia Party, the forerunners of the Liberal Party. During the decades which followed, the Country Party held between 10 and 20 seats in the House, and between 1966 and 1977 it always held more than 20 seats. During this period the party was led by Earle Page (1921-39); A. G. Cameron (1939-40); Arthur Fadden (1940-58); John McEwen (1958-71); and Doug Anthony (1971-83).

The alliance with the Liberals broke down temporarily in 1972-74 when the ALP was in government. The relationship was reformed in 1975 and the coalition returned to power in December of that year. In 1975 the party changed its name to the Country-National Party, and in October 1982 became the National Party.

The party suffered a severe defeat in 1983, winning only 17 seats, its lowest figure since 1961. Following the election Ian Sinclair became party leader in January 1984. In the election of that year the party increased its representation in the House to 21 seats with 10.8 per cent of the vote.

In 1987 the alliance with the Liberals broke down once again as the National Party's veteran Queensland Premier Sir Johannes Bjelke-Petersen attempted to take control of the coalition at federal level. Although the challenge was beaten off by Sinclair, the party fared badly at the election winning only 19 seats with 11.5 per cent of the vote.

In May 1989 Ian Sinclair was replaced as federal leader by Charles Blunt. The party suffered a disastrous result in the 1990 election, however, winning only 14 seats, its lowest figure since 1934. Blunt lost his seat and resigned immediately. He was replaced on April 10 by Tim Fischer. The National Party's poor showing in the elections came despite the economic problems affecting much of rural Australia. As such, its loss of support was part of the continuing legacy of the Fitzgerald inquiry into corruption within the Queensland government, where the Nationals had been in power for 30 years until defeated in 1989. The inquiry had been established in 1987 by Bjelke-Petersen as a sop to the opposition, but gradually developed into a thorough examination of institutionalized corruption within the state. By mid-1991 more than 200 people—including police officers, judges, businessmen and former members of Bjelke-Petersen's Cabinet—had been charged with criminal offences.

In early August 1991 former police commissioner Sir Terence Lewis was sentenced to 14 years' imprisonment. The trial of Bjelke-Petersen himself ended in October, in highly controversial circumstances, with the jury unable to agree upon a verdict. The foreman was discovered to be a National Party member and a prominent support of the former state premier.

Structure. The party has more than 1,400 branches throughout the country, but is concentrated in Queensland. A federal council, which meets at least once a year, is responsible for managing party affairs at national level. The council consists of the federal president, the federal parliamentary leader, the leader in the Senate, the parliamentary leader in each state, plus one representative of the federal parliamentary party from each state, three representatives elected by the Central Council of each state organization, one women's representative from each state, one representative form the Young National Party from each state, the immediate past federal president, the federal secretary and treasurer, the president of the Women's Federal Council and the president of the Young National Party. Between Council meeting power is exercised by a Federal Management Committee appointed by the Council.

Membership. 130,000.

Minor Parties

Communist Party of Australia (CPA); collective leadership (Brian Aarons and Dennis Freney are spokesmen). Founded in 1920, the CPA grew during the depression of the 1930s, particularly within the trade union movement. Banned in 1940 because of its anti-war stance, it was legalized in 1942 and had more than 22,000 members by 1944. The party declined in the post-war period in the face of increasing harassment by the authorities. An act banning the party was passed in 1950 but declared unconstitutional, and a referendum proposing an alteration of the Constitution to prohibit the party was defeated in the following year. The party was also weakened by splits which included the formation in 1963 of the Communist Party of Australia (Marxist-Leninist), which was aligned with China, and the establishment in 1971 of the Socialist Party of Australia, which remained closely aligned with the Soviet Union. The CPA has never held any seats in the federal legislature.

Communist Party of Australia (Marxist-Leninist) *see under* **Communist Party.**

Democratic Labor Party of Australia (DLP); 82 Huxley Avenue, Mulgrave, Victoria, 3170. The party was formed by right-wingers who split from the Australian Labor Party (ALP) in Victoria in 1955 and formed the Australian Labor (Anti-Communist) Party. Opposed to the alleged penetration of the trade union movement by communists, the party advocated a strong anti-communist stance on foreign and defence matters, but retained policies similar to the ALP in most other areas. Originally the party confined its activities to Victoria, but following an ALP split in Queensland in 1957, it began organizing on a national basis and adopted its current name. Although the party failed to win any federal seats, it polled over 7 per cent in the House of Representatives elections of 1958, 1961, 1963, and 1969. Thereafter its vote declined, falling to less than 2 per cent in 1974 and 0.3 per cent in 1980.

The Greens; Wellspring Centre, 483 Crown Street, Wollongong, NSW 2500; Senator Jo Valentine (parl. leader). The Greens are a loose federation of autonomous groups including the ACT Green Alliance; Central Coast Greens; Cowper Greens; Eastern Suburb Greens; Green Alliance Senate—New South Wales; Greens in Lowe; Illawarra Greens; Richmond Green Alliance; South Sydney Greens; Sydney Greens; Green Party South Australia; The Greens (WA) Inc.; Victorian Green Alliance; and the Western Suburbs Greens. The party is concerned with environmental protection generally, and is strongly antinuclear. It advocates international nuclear disarmament, the maintenance of Australia as a nuclear-free area, and opposition to uranium mining and civil nuclear power. Valentine was originally elected to the Senate as a member of the Nuclear Disarmament Party (NDP) [see below] in 1984, but left in 1985 and founded the Nuclear Free Australia Party. She was re-elected to the Senate in 1987.

Nuclear Disarmament Party; GPO Box 414, Canberra ACT 2601. The party was founded in June 1984 on a platform of opposition to foreign military bases within Australia, the stationing or passage through Australia of nuclear weapons, and the immediate termination of the mining and export of uranium. In the 1984 election it succeeded in winning a seat in the Senate for Jo Valentine. At its first national congress in April 1985 some 30 per cent of delegates, including Valentine, walked out in protest over the alleged infiltration of the party by members of the Socialist Workers' Party. The party won a single Senate seat in 1987.

Socialist Party of Australia (SPA). *see under* **Communist Party.**

Defunct parties

Country Party *see under* **National Party.**

Nationalist Party (1917-31), a forerunner of the Liberal Party.

United Australia Party (1931-1944), a forerunner of the Liberal Party.

Major guerrilla groups

Australia has no significant guerrilla organizations.

Australian external territories

Christmas Island

Capital: None   **Population: 2,800**

Christmas Island, which lies 1,400 km off the north-west coast of Australia, was annexed by Britain in the late 19th century, and transferred to Australian administration in 1958.

Constitutional structure

Executive authority lies with a resident Administrator appointed by the Governor-General of Australia and responsible to the Australian government. An elected Christmas Island Assembly was created in 1985 to advise the Administrator, but was dissolved in 1987 and its functions assumed by the Administrator.

Electoral system

The nine members of the Christmas Island Assembly were elected for one-year terms. There is no current electoral system.

Evolution of suffrage

Elections were held on the basis of universal adult suffrage.

Recent elections

No elections have been held since 1987.

PARTY BY PARTY DATA

There are no political parties on Christmas Island.

Major guerrilla groups

There are no guerrilla groups operating on Christmas Island.

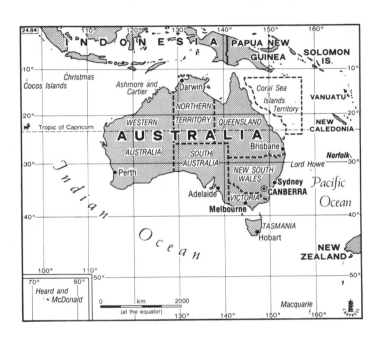

Norfolk Island

Capital: Kingston   **Population: 2,175 (1981)**

Norfolk Island lies off the east coast of Australia, and was uninhabited when discovered by the British in 1774. Originally used as a penal colony, Norfolk Island was resettled in the mid-19th century by people from Pitcairn. Administrative control of the territory was passed to the Australian government in 1913.

Constitutional structure

Under the terms of the Norfolk Island Act of 1979, executive authority lies with a resident Administrator, appointed by the Governor-General of Australia, who is responsible to the Australian government. There is an elected nine-member Legislative Assembly, from which is drawn an Executive Council, the members of which exercise a form of Ministerial authority. Both bodies are presided over by the President of the Legislative Assembly. Legislation approved by the Assembly only becomes valid with the Administrator's assent.

The 1979 Act was amended in 1985 in order to transfer to the territory a wider range of legislative and executive powers, as part of a progression towards eventual internal self-government for the territory.

Electoral system

The members of the Legislative Assembly are elected for up to three years under a system of proportional representation. The Adminstration has the authority to call fresh elections at any time.

Evolution of suffrage

The territory operates on the basis of universal adult suffrage.

Recent elections

In May 1989 the nine seats in the legislature were contested by 16 candidates. The most recent elections were in May 1992, following which the new assembly chose John Brown as its President.

PARTY BY PARTY DATA

There are no political parties in Norfolk Island.

Major guerrilla groups

There are no guerrilla groups operating in Norfolk Island.

Torres Strait Islands

Capital: Thursday Island (administrative centre)   **Population: 4,837 (1986 census)**

The Torres Strait Islands number more than 70, and lie between Papua New Guinea and Australia. Although the international border passes through the group, the islands constitute a single Australian possession. A further 21,541 Torres Strait Islanders are resident in Queensland.

Constitutional structure

The Torres Strait Islands are administered as part of Queensland. An Executive Officer and Assistant Executive Officer of the Department of Community Services, together with subsidiary staff, are based on Christmas Island. Extensive local power is devolved to four elected regionally based Islander Community Councils. There is also an Island Co-ordinating Council which represents all of the islands and meets regularly to discuss issues of regional importance.

Electoral system

Islander Community Councils are usually elected for three years.

Evolution of suffrage

Those aged 18 years and over are entitled to vote.

Recent elections

Elections have been held regularly in recent years.

PARTY BY PARTY DATA

There are no political parties in the Torres Strait Islands.

Major guerrilla groups

There are no guerrilla groups operating in the Torres Straits Islands.

Cocos (Keeling) Islands

Capital: None   **Population: 555 (1981)**

The 27 Cocos (Keeling) Islands, which lie 2,7460 km off the north-west coast of Australia, were colonized by Britain in the 19th century, and transferred to Australian administration in 1955. Since 1975, executive authority has been exercised by a resident Administrator, appointed by the Governor-General of Australia and responsible to the Australian government. An elected Cocos (Keeling) Islands Council was created in 1979 to administer a wide range of local responsibilities. In an April 1984 referendum on the territory's future status, a large majority of the population voted for total integration with Australia. There are no political parties or guerrilla groups operating in the Cocos (Keeling) Islands.

Lord Howe Island

Capital: None   **Population: 270 (1987)**

Administered as a dependency of New South Wales, the territory comprises a land area of 14.5 sq km. The island is administered by an appointed Administrative Officer and a small Lord Howe Island Board. There are no political parties or guerrilla groups operating on Lord Howe Island.

Bangladesh

Capital: Dhaka   **Population: 107,992,140 (1991)**

The eastern and predominantly Muslim section of Bengal was included in Pakistan when India was partitioned in 1947, being known as East Bengal until 1955 and subsequently as East Pakistan. The Awami League (AL) won a huge majority of the East Pakistan seats in the 1970 elections, but its demands for the autonomy of East Pakistan were rejected by President Yayha Khan. Civil war broke out in 1971 after the Pakistan army occupied Dhaka, and the Awami League declared Bangladesh an independent republic. The war ended in December with the intervention of the Indian army, and the People's Republic of Bangladesh was established as an independent state within the Commonwealth.

The AL formed a government in Bangladesh with Sheikh Mujibur first as Prime Minister and, after January 1975, as President, when he attempted to create a single-party state. He was overthrown and murdered in a military coup on Aug. 15, 1975, and after two further coups in November Gen. Ziaur Rahman (Zia) took control as Chief Martial Law Administrator, assuming the presidency in 1977. Presidential elections were held in 1978, when Zia was elected with a large majority. Parliamentary government was restored in 1979, when elections were held, but in 1981 President Zia was murdered in an attempted coup. After a brief period of civilian government, Lieut.-Gen. Hussain Mohammad Ershad seized power in 1982 and dissolved parliament, and in the following year proclaimed himself President. The country was placed under martial law between March 1982 and November 1986. In a general election in March 1988 Ershad's National Party won 252 of the 300 elective seats.

In October 1990, the Ershad regime faced nationwide student protests. An attempt to suppress further political unrest by imposing a state of emergency and ordering the arrest of the country's principal opposition leaders failed, and Ershad was forced to resign as President in early December 1990. Control of the government was handed over to Chief Justice Shehabuddin Ahmed, who had been nominated as acting President by the main opposition alliances.

After a general election in February 1991, a new government led by the Bangladesh Nationalist Party (BNP) was formed in March and Begum Khaleda Zia (widow of the assassinated President) was sworn in as the country's first woman Prime Minister. Various constitutional amendments, including the restoration of parliamentary democracy, restored the political credibility of the government, and members of the former government of President Ershad were arrested and tried on charges of corruption and abuse of power. Ershad was sentenced to 10 years' "rigorous imprisonment".

Constitutional structure

The Constitution of the Independent Republic of Bangladesh, approved in November 1972, a year after secession from Pakistan, was initially based on the principles of nationalism, socialism, democracy, secularism and guaranteed freedom of religious worship. In 1977 a constitutional amendment replaced secularism with Islam and a further amendment in 1988 established Islam as the state religion. A nationwide referendum in September 1991 overwhelmingly endorsed new constitutional provisions restoring a parliamentary form of government and full powers to the *Jatiya Sangsad*, Bangladesh's unicameral parliament. Under the amended Constitution, the President has a largely ceremonial role.

Executive power is vested in the Prime Minister, appointed by the President, who also appoints, on the Prime Minister's recommendation, the Council of Ministers.

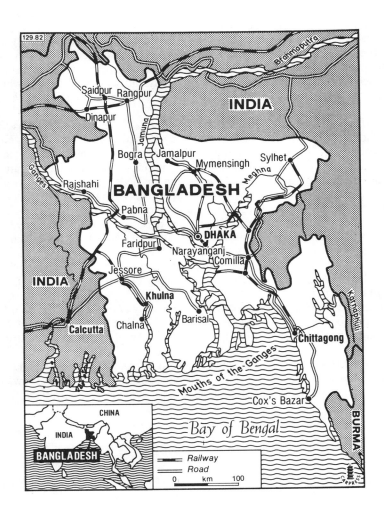

Recent elections

The first parliamentary elections in independent Bangladesh were held in March 1973, and were fully competitive, although the left-wing opposition to the dominant Awami League was too fragmented to be effective. The authenticity of the results of the three elections of 1979, 1986 and 1988 is highly questionable due to the repressive military regime.

The 1979 election was called and won by Gen. Zia who had established the Bangladesh Nationalist Party (BNP--*Bangladesh Jatiyatabadi Dal*) after the military coup which brought him into power in 1976. While there were no great electoral abuses, the BNP benefited from access to state patronage and from the fact that martial law was in effect.

Demonstrations and calls to boycott preceded the postponed 1986 parliamentary elections, held on May 7. They proceeded amidst allegations of intimidation and violence, with voting suspended in 284 centres and official reports of 12 people killed. The elections were boycotted by seven parties, headed by the BNP which refused to participate in any elections under martial law and while Ershad was in power. The National Party (*Jatiya Dal*) formed by Ershad at the beginning of the year, won by a narrow margin.

After the presidential elections of 1978, won by Gen. Zia, there were no presidential elections until October 1986, the presidency having been assumed by Ershad in 1983 without an election. The 1986 presidential elections were boycotted by the opposition, who claimed that only 3 per cent of those eligible actually voted. Prior to the elections, full martial law was reinstated, anti-election rallies banned, 2,000 political agitators arrested and the leaders of the AL and the BNP placed under house arrest. There were also allegations of pre-marked ballots and the forging of voting registers. Since a constitutional amendment in 1991, the president has been elected by parliament.

The 1988 parliamentary elections were held after the dissolution of parliament by Ershad in response to general strikes and demonstrations. The National Party won a landslide victory mainly due to the lack of preparation of the opposition and low voter turnout.

The forced resignation of Ershad at the end of 1990 led to a general election on Feb. 27, 1991, which was won by the Bangladesh Nationalist Party (BNP) under Begum Zia. Although the BNP fell short of an absolute majority (subsequently obtained in by-elections in September), it was able to secure pledges of support from smaller parties, notably the Islamic Assembly (*Jamaat-e-Islami Bangladesh*--JIB). The elections were described as the most peaceful in Bangladesh's history, although 15 people died in campaign-related clashes. By-elections in September 1991 gave the BNP an absolute majority, with 169 of the 330 seats.

Parliamentary elections on Oct. 8, 1991, elected Abdur Rahman Biswas as President, replacing Chief Justice Shehabuddin Ahmed, Acting President since the resignation of Ershad. Biswas received 172 of the 264 votes cast. The other candidate, Badrul Haider Chowdhury, obtained 92 votes.

General elections 1973-1991

Date	Winning Party
1973	Awami League
1979	Bangladesh Nationalist Party
1986	National Party
1988	National Party
1991	Bangladesh Nationalist Party

1988 general election

Party	Elective seats
National Party	251
*Combined Opposition Group	18
Others/Independents	31
Total	300

* Consisting of 76 groups and parties.

1991 general election*

Party	Elective seats[+]
Bangladesh Nationalist Party	142
Awami League	91
National Party	35
Islamic Assembly	18
Communist Party	5
Jatiya Samajtantrik Party (Shahjahan Siraj)	1
Bangladesh Workers Party	1
National Awami Party (Muzaffar)	1
Others	3
Independents	3
Total	300

*Held on Feb. 27; repolling in three constituencies followed immediately, leaving at that stage three elective seats still to be decided. By-elections were held in 11 constituencies on Sept. 11, when the BNP won five seats, the National Party four seats and the Awami League two seats. The distribution of seats as given above is as at June 1992.

[+]Of the additional 30 non-elective seats, allocated to women, the Bangladesh Nationalist Party was awarded 28 and the Islamic Assembly two.

Electoral system

Prior to 1991, the president was elected by universal suffrage for a five-year term and was executive leader of the country. Now he is appointed by the parliament (*Jatiya Sangsad*) with powers reduced to a titular role. The *Jatiya Sangsad* consists of 300 of directly elected members, and 30 women members who are appointed by the other members.

Evolution of the suffrage

Universal suffrage, introduced in Bangladesh during its period as East Pakistan, was maintained under the 1972 Constitution. The minimum voting age is 18.

PARTY BY PARTY DATA

There are believed to be well over 100 political parties in Bangladesh, many consisting of only a handful of individuals. Many are factions which have broken off from another party.

Awami League (AL)

Address. 23 Bangabandha Avenue, Dhaka.

Leadership. Sheikh Hasina Wazed (pres.); Begum Sajeda Chowdhury (gen.sec.).

Orientation. Moderate socialist, secular, nationalist, pro-Indian and pro-Soviet.

Founded. 1949.

History. Founded as the Awami (People's) Muslim League by left-wing Bengali nationalists opposed to the right-wing orientation of the Muslim League after the 1947 partition, the party headed coalition governments in what was then East Pakistan in 1956-58 and was represented in Pakistan governments in 1956-57 and in 1958. In 1957 a leftist faction, led by Maulana Abdul Hamid Khan Bhashani and opposed to the leadership's alleged failure to condemn Pakistan's Western-oriented foreign policy, broke away to form the National Awami Party.

In elections held in 1970 the League won 151 of the 153 East Pakistan seats in the Pakistan National Assembly on the basis of a six-point charter presenting the demands of Bengali nationalism. Under the leadership of Sheikh Mujibur Rahman it headed the successful movement for independence from Pakistan and became the ruling party in Bangladesh from 1971. In January 1975 Mujibur introduced a presidential form of government and moved to a single-party system by creating the Bangladesh Peasants' and Workers' Awami League (Bangladesh *Krishak Sramik Awami* League (BKSAL)), within which all existing political tendencies were required to operate.

After the overthrow and murder of Sheikh Mujibur in August 1975, the League was temporarily banned and its new leader, Abdul Malek Ukil, was imprisoned in April 1977. Meanwhile, the 1976 Political Parties Regulation had enabled the League to resume political activity under the leadership of Sheikh Mujibur's daughter, Sheikh Hasina. It was the strongest of the five parties of the Democratic United Front which unsuccessfully campaigned for Gen. Mohammed Ataul Ghani Osmani in the June 1978 presidential elections, which were won by Gen. Zia of the Bangladesh Nationalist Party (BNP).

In the February 1979 parliamentary elections the League won 40 of the 300 elective seats, while in the November 1981 presidential elections the League's candidate, Kamal Hossain, was officially credited with 25.35 per cent of the vote. He challenged the result on the grounds of alleged irregularities and the League boycotted the swearing-in of the victorious BNP candidate.

Following the military coup of March 1982 and the suspension of political parties, the League was in the forefront of the campaign for a return to democracy and the 1972 Constitution, participating in the launching of a 15-party opposition alliance in January 1983 and also, from September 1983, in the broader Movement for the Restoration of Democracy (MRD), which included the main current of the BNP and its allies. Leftist elements of the League, led by its then general secretary Abdur Rassaq, broke away in July 1983 to form the Peasants' and Workers' Awami League.

Over the next two years the MRD maintained pressure on the Ershad regime for a resumption of constitutional rule, achieving partial success when the ban on political activity was lifted in January 1986 and parliamentary elections were called for May 1986. However, the MRD formations split on whether adequate concessions had been made by the government, with the Awami League and seven allied parties deciding to contest the elections (on a joint list of candidates), whereas the BNP and other opposition groups declared a boycott of the electoral process.

Allegations of widespread irregularities in the conduct of the elections were endorsed by the League, whose share of the 300 elective seats was eventually determined at 76. Although its elected members were sworn in, the League and other opposition groups boycotted the opening of the new Parliament on July 9, 1986, in protest against the slow progress of democratization, and set up a "people's parliament", of which Sheikh Hasina was elected leader. The League then joined with the BNP-led alliance in boycotting the presidential elections held on Oct. 15.

Conciliatory gestures by Ershad's government persuaded the League and other opposition parties to attend Parliament in late January 1987, but they quickly resumed their boycott in protest against government moves to institutionalize the political role of the armed forces.

Over the following months the League participated in a series of mass demonstrations and general strikes in support of a call for Ershad's resignation, culminating on Nov. 10, 1987, in the "siege of Dhaka" in which the opposition sought to immobilize the government by assembling some 2,000,000 supporters in the capital.

Sheikh Hasina was placed under house arrest on Nov. 11, emerging a month later to condemn the state of emergency declared by Ershad on Nov. 27 and to reiterate the League's demand for his immediate resignation. The League also announced that, together with other opposition parties, it would boycott the parliamentary elections which the government had called for March 1988, claiming that they would be a "farce" as long as Ershad remained in power.

Since the overthrow of Ershad, the Awami League has been the main opposition group to the ruling BNP; it gained 32 per cent of the vote in the 1991 elections, the same percentage of the vote as the BNP, but only 85 seats as compared with the 138 of the BNP. (Later it won three of the six re-polled seats.)

Structure. The Awami League is a mass party directed by a 12-member presidium elected by the party council. It has integral women's, peasants', workers', students' and youth organizations.

Membership. 1,025,000. (est.).

Bangladesh Nationalist Party (BNP)

Bangladesh Jatiyatabadi Dal

Address. Sattar House, 19/A, Road No. 16, Dhanmondi R/A, Dhaka 9.

Leadership. Begum Khaleda Zia (ch.); Prof. A. Q. M. Badruddoza Chaudhury (vice-ch.); Abdus Salam Talukdar (gen. sec.).

Orientation. Centrist, Islamic, democratic and nationalist. The party favours multiparty democracy, presidential government and a mixed economy.

History. The BNP was formed by the then President, Gen. Ziaur Rahman (Zia) on the basis of the *Jatiyatabadi* Front which had successfully campaigned for his election in June 1978. Headed by the Nationalist Democratic Party, the Front also included factions of the Muslim League, the National Awami Party, the Popular Unity Party, the Labour Party and an organization representing the Hindu minority. Other factions of most of these constituents continued to operate as independent parties.

In the parliamentary elections of February 1979 the BNP obtained 49 per cent of the votes and a two-thirds majority of seats on a platform of inscribing faith in Islam into the Constitution and pursuing social justice rather than socialism. Martial law and the state of emergency were lifted in the course of 1979. However, Zia was assassinated on May 30, 1981, in an apparent attempted military coup and was succeeded by the Vice-President and senior BNP vice-chairman, Justice Abdus Sattar. In presidential elections held in November 1981, Abdus Stattar, the BNP candidate, was elected, being officially credited with 65.8 per cent of the votes. Begum Khaleda Zia (widow of the late President) succeeded Sattar as leader of the mainstream of the BNP in January 1984.

After the military takeover of March 1982, the BNP and six allied formations in September 1983 joined with the Awami League and its associated parties to launch the Movement for the Restoration of Democracy (MRD), whose subsequent pressure on the Ershad regime produced a partial resumption of legal political activity from January 1986 and the calling of parliamentary elections for May 1986. In the event, however, the MRD formations became divided over whether adequate concessions had been made by the government, with the result that BNP and its allies boycotted the elections, whereas the Awami League and its major associated parties decided in favour of participation.

Shortly after the May 1986 elections the BNP resumed co-operation with the Awami League in pressing for speedier progress towards democratization, with both groups and their allies boycotting the October 1986 presidential elections. Over the next 12 months the BNP was in the forefront of a series of mass demonstrations and strikes calling for President Ershad's resignation, culminating in the "siege of Dhaka" on Nov. 10, 1987, in which the opposition sought to immobilize the government by assembling some 2,000,000 supporters in the capital. On Nov. 27 President Ershad declared a state of emergency. On her release on Dec. 11 from one month's house arrest Begum Khaleda Zia reiterated the party's demand for the immediate resignation of the government and announced that the BNP would not participate in the new parliamentary elections called for March 1988.

In July 1988, a group of dissidents led by a former secretary general, A. K. M. Obaidur Rahman, formed a rival faction.

In the parliamentary elections which followed the overthrow of Ershad, the BNP won a substantial victory (in terms of seats rather than percentage of the vote), and Begum Zia became the country's first woman Prime Minister. By-elections in September of the same year gave the party an absolute majority.

Structure. The BNP is based on a number of sectional organizations for women, students, youth, peasants, workers, volunteers (*Jatiyatabadi Sechchasebak Sangathan*) and cultural pursuits.

Communist Party of Bangladesh (CPB)

Address. 21/1 Purana Paltan, Dhaka 2.

Leadership. Saifuddin Ahmed Manik (pres.); Nurul Islam Nahid (gen. sec.).

Orientation. An orthodox pro-Soviet Marxist-Leninist party, the CPB advocates secularism and "scientific socialism" taking account of the economic backwardness of Bangladesh. It pursues a policy of supporting "pro-people patriotic governments" to achieve economic self-reliance and social progress.

Founded. 1948.

History. Originally the East Pakistan section of the Communist Party of Pakistan (CPP), itself descended from the Communist Party of India, the party was illegal for most of its early history, although it had several members elected to the East Pakistan Assembly in 1954 as candidates of a four-party United Front. Driven underground by the promulgation of martial law in October 1958, the CPP virtually ceased to exist as an organized force in West Pakistan and was further weakened by the breakaway of its pro-Chinese wing in the mid-1960s. In 1968 the pro-Soviet wing in the East formed the independent Communist Party of East Pakistan, which became the Communist Party of Bangladesh after independence in 1971.

Under the 1971-75 Awami League government the CPB became legal. It unsuccessfully contested four seats in the 1973 elections, subsequently forming an alliance with the League and the pro-Soviet wing of the National Awami Party to combat terrorism and corruption. Banned again in 1977, it was legalized in 1978 but was still constrained under a December 1978 decree which banned all parties which received foreign financial assistance, were affiliated to any overseas organization, propagated views detrimental to the sovereignty or security of the state or maintained an armed underground organization. The party did not present candidates under its own banner in the 1979 elections. In April 1980 the party's then general secretary, Mohammed Farhad, and 52 other leading CPB members were arrested for sedition, although Farhad was released on bail on July 29, 1980.

In the wake of the March 1982 coup, the CPB joined the 15-party alliance of left-wing opposition groups headed by the Awami League and participated actively in the campaign for the restoration of democracy. It was one of the eight parties of this alliance which decided to contest the May 1986 parliamentary elections on a joint slate of candidates, its eventual seat tally of six (including one independent who later joined the CPB) marking the first time that the party had secured national parliamentary representation in its own name.

Thereafter the party remained closely allied to the Awami League in the continuing campaign for a full restoration of democracy, and joined other opposition parties in declaring a boycott of new parliamentary elections called for March 1988.

The party won five seats in the 1991 elections.

Structure. Organized on "democratic centralist" lines, the CPB has a congress as its highest body, a central committee and a presidium.

Membership. 2,500 (est.).

Freedom Party

Address. House No.48, Road No. 15/A, Dhanmondi Residential Area, Dhaka.

Leadership. Lt.-Col. Sayed Faruq Rahman (chair); Lt.-Col. Khandaker Abdur Rashid (dep. leader).

Orientation. Islamic, conservative, opposed to Awami League.

Founded. August 1987.

History. Rahman and Rashid were two of the three

principal leaders (the "majors") of the August 1975 coup in which the Awami League government was overthrown and Sheikh Mujibur Rahman and members of his family were killed. Following their own overthrow in November 1975 they were allowed to seek exile in Libya. Rahman returned to Bangladesh in 1985 and, after a period of detention, was a candidate in the October 1986 presidential elections, officially coming third with just over 1,000,000 votes.

Following the formation of the Freedom Party, clashes took place between its supporters and those of the Awami League, whose leader, Sheikh Hasina Wajed, had consistently demanded that the "majors" should be brought to trial for her father's murder.

Islamic Assembly (JIB)

Jamaat-e-Islami Bangladesh

Address. 505 Elephant Road, Bara Maghbazar, Dhaka, 1217.

Leadership. Abbas Ali Khan (Acting Amir - ch.).

Orientation. Islamic fundamentalist.

Founded. 1941.

History. Founded by Maulana Abul Ala Maududi, the JIB opposed the creation of a separate Muslim state from British India as being contrary to the basic principles of Islam, while at the same time it was anti-Hindu and anti-Indian. After partition in 1947 the organization's main strength was in West Pakistan, and it was led in East Pakistan by Golam Azam. Opposed to the secularism and Bengali nationalism of the Awami League, it campaigned actively against the Bangladesh independence movement in 1970-71 and was banned following the creation of the new state, Golam Azam being deprived of his citizenship for alleged collaboration with the Pakistani forces.

Following the overthrow of Sheikh Mujibur Rahman in August 1975, the JIB regained legal status in 1976 and became an active component of the Islamic Democratic League. Divisions in the latter led to the relaunching of the JIB as an independent organization in 1979 under its present leadership. After the March 1982 Ershad takeover, the JIB maintained its distance from the main opposition alliances, although it made similar calls for the restoration of democratic rule. In the May 1986 parliamentary elections it fielded 76 candidates, of whom 10 were elected.

From 1978 on the JIB was led by Azam, who had returned secretly from Pakistan. In December 1991 Azam's election as Amir was met with widespread calls for his trial over his leadership of the JIB, which, since he was a foreign national, was illegal. After a

"mock-trial" attended by more than 100,000 people in the capital, the government agreed in April 1992 to bring formal charges.

Muslim League

Address. Allahwala Building. 109 Motijheel C/A, Dhaka.

Leadership. Alhaj Kazi Abdul Kazer (pres.); M. A. Matin (gen. sec.).

Orientation. The League is a conservative party standing for "Muslim nationalism", parliamentary democracy, a welfare state which retains traditional sociopolitical institutions, and the separation of the judiciary from the government administration.

Founded. 1947.

History. Having supported Pakistan in the independence struggle, the League was banned on the establishment of an independent Bangladesh in 1971. It returned to legality in 1977 but was further weakened the following year when its dominant liberal wing joined President Zia's newly formed Bangladesh Nationalist Party (BNP). Moreover, a number of other breakaway groups were formed, several of them calling themselves Muslim League.

An alliance between the Muslim League and the Islamic Democratic League (IDL—later known as Islamic Unity Movement) won 20 seats in the 1979 election.

The Muslim League led by Alhaj Kazi Abdul Zazer presented 103 candidates in the May 1986 parliamentary elections, four of them being successful.

National Awami Party (Muzaffar) (NAP—Muzaffar)

Address. 20 Dhanmondi Hawkers Market, Dhaka 5.

Leadership. Muzaffar Ahmed (pres.); Pankaj Bhattacharya (gen. sec.).

Orientation. The pro-Soviet NAP stands for progressive nationalism, democratic socialism and observance of religious rites. Its immediate programme advocates a corruption-free mixed economy, job-creation measures, unemployment benefit and radical land reform in favour of peasants.

Founded. 1957/1967.

History. Founded in 1957 by Awami League dissidents, the NAP in 1967 itself split into a larger pro-Soviet party led by Muzaffar and a pro-Chinese party led by Maulana Abdul Hamid Khan Bhashani. The former opposed the Pakistan government of Ayub Khan and also favoured autonomy for East Pakistan, taking an active part in the 1971 independence struggle and thereafter adopting a position of "constructive opposition" to the Awami League government of Sheikh Mujibur Rahman.

In the 1973 parliamentary election the party obtained some 1,600,000 votes but no seats; in that of 1979 it secured nearly 500,000 votes and one seat. Following the Ershad military takeover of March 1982, it joined the 15-party opposition alliance led by the Awami League and was one of the eight opposition organizations which contested the May 1986 parliamentary elections, presenting 10 candidates and winning two seats. Those elections were also contested by a group known as the NAP (Bhashani/United) whereas various other factions descended from the original NAP, including several calling themselves NAP (Bhashani), did not participate.

Membership. 500,000.

National Party
Jatiya Dal
Address. 104 Road No. 3, Dhanmondi R/A, Dhaka/1A; Road No. 79, Gulshan, Dhaka.
Leadership. Mohammed Mizanur Rahman Chowdhury (acting ch.); Shah Moazzam Hossain (gen. sec.).
Orientation. The National Party claims to seek the promotion of national unity on the basis of the following five fundamental principles: (i) independence and sovereignty; (ii) faith in Islam combined with respect for all religions: (iii) Bangladeshi nationalism; (iv) democracy; and (v) social progress aimed at economic emancipation.
Founded. Jan. 1, 1986.
History. Moves to create a political base for Lt.-Gen. Hossain Mohammed Ershad following his seizure of power in a bloodless military coup on March 24, 1982, led initially to an announcement in November 1983 by the President installed by Ershad, Justice A. F. M. Assanuddin Chowdhury, that a new People's Party (*Jana Dal*) had been created, fusing various elements of both the Awami League and the Bangladesh Nationalist Party (BNP), the two main opposition groups. The following month Ershad declared himself to be President and Chowdhury became "convener" of the People's Party, but prospects of early democratic elections receded amid deadlock between the regime and the opposition parties on the means of ending martial law. In June 1984 the People's Party was joined by the then Prime Minister, Ataur Rahman Khan, leader of the National League.

In July 1985 the People's Party became the principal component of a broader pro-government National (*Jatiya*) Front, which also included the United People's Party, the Democratic Party and breakaway factions of the BNP and the Muslim League. On Jan. 1, 1986, the Front was converted into the National Party, it being disclosed that all government ministers had joined the new party. It was stated that President Ershad, while at that stage having no formal position in the party, had nevertheless inspired its formation.

In the May 1986 parliamentary elections the National Party presented candidates for all 300 elective seats and, after re-runs, by-elections in August and shifts of party allegiance, secured 180 seats, added to which it took all 30 of the seats reserved for women. Having resigned his post as Chief of Army Staff on Aug. 28, 1986, President Ershad on Sept. 1 announced his decision to join the National Party and the following day was elected chairman. On Sept. 17 he was nominated as the party's candidate for the presidential elections scheduled for Oct. 15, 1986, and was duly elected with (according to official results) 83.6 per cent of the votes (the main opposition parties having declared a boycott).

In late 1987, the main opposition parties launched protests to force Ershad's resignation, whereupon he declared a state of emergency. After the 1988 election victory his government was paralysed by renewed agitation in October 1990 with student activists in the forefront. His declaration of a state of emergency failed to restore order as opposition groups defied curfews, and academics and civil servants joined the protesting students. Violent clashes with the security forces ensued. Opposition leaders rejected his offers of concessions, and without the backing of the military, Ershad was forced to resign in December 1990.

Ershad and many of his supporters were arrested and put on trial, but the party continues to operate under new leadership. On Jan. 1, 1991, a spokesman said that the party would contest the coming parliamentary elections, and that it "begged forgiveness" from the people adding that "if we have done anything wrong, we are ready to rectify ourselves". They won 35 seats and over 10 per cent of the vote in the 1991 general election, including Ershad's own seat in his home district of Rangpur.

Structure. Directed by a 57-member national committee, the National Party is based on numerous affiliated organizations, including the National Student Society (*Jatiya Chhatra Samaj*), National Youth Solidarity (*Jatiya Jubo Sanghati*), National Women (*Jatiya Mahila*), National Peasants (*Jatiya Krishak*), National Workers (*Jatiya sramik*) and National Volunteers

(*Jatiya Sechehasebak*).

National Socialist Party (Rab) (JSD-Rab)

Jatiya Samajtantrik Dal (Rab)

Address. 115 Fakirapook, Dhaka.

Leadership. Nur-e-Alam Ziku (pres.); Humayun Kabir (gen. sec.).

Orientation. Advocating "scientific socialism", the party maintains that Bangladesh has a ruling capitalist class which is connected with imperialism and is maintaining a "monopolistic grip" on power through "controlled democracy" and "fascism". It seeks to use the democratic process to achieve "bourgeois democracy" as a step towards the establishment of socialism. It also regards the armed forces in developing countries as having a legitimate role to play in the struggle for national independence from imperialism.

Founded. October 1972/January 1984.

History. The JSD was formed by a breakaway group of young militants of the then ruling Awami League dissatisfied with the latter's "non-scientific socialism". Its founders were Abdur Rab and Shajahan Siraj, then both student leaders of the underground Bangladesh Communist League; Sirajul Alam Khan was also influential in creating the new party. It quickly gained a substantial urban following for its militant opposition to the Awami League government, which suppressed the party and its Revolutionary People's Army (*Biplobi Gana Bahini*) in 1975 after an alleged attempt to seize power.

The JSD in August 1975 welcomed the overthrow of the Awami League government (but not the murder of Sheikh Mujibur Rahman) and played a prominent role in the November 1975 military and popular uprising which brought Gen. Zia to effective power. Zia (who assumed the presidency in April 1977) nevertheless disowned the JSD, whose leaders were arrested and subsequently sentenced in July 1976 on charges of attempting to overthrow the government, one of them being executed.

In October 1977 the JSD was officially dissolved, but from November 1978 it was again allowed to operate. Over 300 JSD members were released from prison in February 1979, when the party took part in parliamentary elections, winning nine of the 300 seats. The JSD's military wing was again accused of involvement in political murders in the first half of 1981. In the November presidential elections the JSD candidate, Maj. M. A. Jalil, forfeited his deposit.

Following the Ershad military takeover in March 1982, factional strife within the JSD intensified, leading in January 1984 to the formation of a breakaway party by three of its most prominent leaders (Abdur Rab, Sirajul Alam Khan and Maj. Jalil), while Shajahan Siraj and his followers maintained what they claimed to be the historic JSD. The JSD-Rab participated in the Movement for the Restoration of Democracy and joined the Awami League and some other opposition parties in contesting the May 1986 parliamentary elections, fighting 138 of the 300 elective seats; four of its candidates were elected. Thereafter the JSD-Rab joined the opposition boycott of Parliament and was prominent in the campaign for Ershad's resignation, while at the same time acknowledging that the armed forces had a significant political role to play in an under-developed country like Bangladesh.

National Socialist Party (Siraj) (JSD-Siraj)

Jatiya Samajtantrik Dal (Siraj)

Address. 23 D. I. T. Road, Malibagh, Dhaka/ 11, Bangabandhu Avenue, Dhaka.

Leadership. Shajahan Siraj (pres.); A. B. M. Shajahan (gen. sec.).

Orientation. Advocating "scientific socialism", the party contends that Bangladesh is under the domination of capitalism, imperialism and fascism; it regards electoral participation under "bourgeois democracy" as one method of advancing towards its eventual goals.

Founded. October 1972.

History. This organization claims to represent the original JSD following the formation of the breakaway JSD-Rab in January 1984 [see previous entry, where the earlier history of the JSD is summarized]. It participated in the Movement for the Restoration of Democracy campaigning against the Ershad government and also in the eight-party alliance (headed by the Awami League) which decided to present a joint list of candidates in the May 1986 parliamentary elections. Of the 14 JSD-Siraj candidates, three were elected.

Thereafter the party participated in the opposition boycott of Parliament and in the renewed campaign for Ershad's resignation. However, it withdrew from the eight-party alliance in protest against what it described as the "atrocities, undemocratic attitude and selfish activities" of the Awami League.

International affiliations. The party's labour organization (*Jatiya Sramik Jote*) is affiliated to the Prague-based World Federation of Trade Unions.

Membership. 5,000.

Peasants' and Workers' Awami League
Krishak-Sramik Awami League (BKSAL)
Address. 91 Nawabpur Road, Dhaka.
Leadership. Abdur Razzak (gen. sec.); Mohuddin Ahmed (ch.).
Orientation. Claiming descent from the front organization of the same name created by Sheikh Mujibur Rahman shortly before the overthrow of the Awami League government in August 1975, the BKSAL stands for "scientific socialism", Bengali nationalism, secularism and democracy. It advocates nationalization, radical land reform and an "anti-imperialist" foreign policy based on strengthened ties with "progressive and friendly Muslim countries, socialist and democratic countries".
Founded. October 1983.
History. The party effectively came into being with the expulsion from the Awami League (on July 31, 1983) of its left-wing general secretary Abdur Rahman, following a bitter power struggle in which he and his supporters challenged what they regarded as the non-socialist orientation of Sheikh Hasina's leadership. The Razzak faction formally established itself as the BKSAL in October 1983.

The party participated in the Movement for the Restoration of Democracy and was one of the eight parties (headed by the Awami League) which decided, in alliance, to contest the May 1986 parliamentary elections. Although the BKSAL leadership eventually rescinded this decision (in protest against the "arbitrary" manner in which the Awami League had drawn up the joint list of candidates), six BKSAL candidates nevertheless stood, three of them being elected. Thereafter the BKSAL joined the opposition boycott of Parliament and participated in the renewed campaign for the resignation of President Ershad.
International affiliations. The BKSAL's labour organization is affiliated to the Prague-based World Federation of Trade Unions.

Peasants' and Workers' Party (Solaiman)
Krishak Sramik Dal
Address. Sonargaon Bhaban, 99 South Kamalapur, Dhaka 19.
Leadership. A. S. M. Solaiman (pres.)
Orientation. Conservative socialist, eschewing revolutionary approaches to social and economic problems.
Founded. 1914, renamed 1953.
History. The party is descended from the All-Bengal *Praja Samity* founded under British rule by Shere Bangla A. K. Fuzlul Huque as Bengal's first political party for peasants. It adopted its present name in December 1953 and in 1954-62 participated in coalition governments with the Muslim League and other organizations. In opposition after 1982 to the Ershad regime, in 1984 the party joined the National Unity Front headed by Khandaker Moshtaque Ahmed's Democratic League, but withdrew when a majority of the Front decided to boycott the May 1986 parliamentary elections. The party presented 25 candidates in that contest, none of whom were returned. However, the party won four seats in the 1991 elections.
Membership. 125,000.

Workers' Party (Menon)
Address. 31/E-F Topkhana Road, Dhaka.
Leadership. Rashed Khan Menon (gen. sec.); Abul Bashar (pres.).
Orientation. Marxist-Leninist, seeking a "people's democratic revolution to achieve socialism" and unity in the international communist movement. Its immediate objectives include a decentralized administration run by people's representatives, ownership of the land by peasants, a strengthened state-owned industrial sector and an independent and neutral foreign policy based on close relations with the socialist countries.
History. Having contested the February 1979 parliamentary elections (and secured the election of Menon), this group rejected participation in those of May 1986 and accordingly withdrew from the 15-party left-wing opposition alliance headed by the Awami League. This step led to the creation of a breakaway Workers' Party under Nazrul Islam, which favoured participation in the elections. Subsequently, the Menon party joined a five-party alliance of left-wing groups opposed to electoral politics so long as President Ershad remained in power.

Workers' Party (Nazrul)
Leadership. Nazrul Islam (ch.).
Orientation. Marxist-Leninist, seeking the reunification of the international communist movement.
History. This grouping originated as an offshoot of the Workers' Party led by Rashed Khan Menon [see previous entry]. Whereas the Menon party rejected electoral participation under the Ershad regime, the Nazrul faction argued that given the existing disorganization of the people such participation was necessary to mobilize them at grass-roots level. It described the Menon party as "petit-bourgeois revolutionaries" who failed to understand objective conditions.

The Nazrul party participated in the May 1986 parliamentary elections witin the eight-party alliance headed by the Awami League, three of its four candidates being elected.

Minor parties

None of the parties described below obtained representation in the 1991 parliamentary elections, although some of them presented candidates. As the listing shows, a feature of the proliferation of parties in Bangladesh is the frequent occurrence of two or more groupings using the same title, as a result of splits, realignments and factional defections leading to the creation of separate groups. Another feature is the complex and continuing alignment and realignment of individual parties within broader alliances and fronts, which means that some of the parties listed below may by now be defunct.

Awami Islami Party (3/5 Chand Khar Pool Lane, Dhaka 1); leadership: Mohammad Shahjahan (founder-convenor). Founded in July 1986. An Islamic fundamentalist party which, while favouring parliamentary democracy, has advocated that Bangladesh should be run by "the pious Muslim intelligentsia" to stem the tide of "moral erosion".

Awami Ulema Party; 27/28 Mohammadpur, Dhaka; leadership: Maulana Khairul Islam Jashori (pres.); founded in 1980. The party, committed to establishing an Islamic social system, was revived in 1980 by Maulana Jashori, who had led it in the 1970s but had joined the National Party (Huda) in 1978. A supporter of President Zia (until his assassination in May 1981), he became president of the Islamic Unity Movement of 16 Islamic parties in 1984 and unsuccessfully contested the October 1986 presidential elections.

Bangla Communist Party; Sheikh Shaheb Bazaar, Lalbagh, Dhaka; leadership: Mannan Sikdar (ch.); founded in 1972. A Marxist-Leninist, Maoist, pro-Albanian party. Descended from the pre-independence pro-Chinese Communist Party of East Pakistan, this party later became critical of the reformist direction of the Chinese party leadership. Part of a six-party Left Front, the party boycotted the May 1986 parliamentary elections.

Bangladesh Janata Dal; 3/5 Asad Avenue, Mohammadpur, Dhaka; leadership: K. M. Obaidur Rahman.

Bangladesh Nationalist Party (BNP-Aziz) (*Jatiyatabadi Dal Aziz*); 18 Road No. 18, Gulshan, Dhaka; leadership: Shah Azizur Rahman (ch.); Shamsul Alamin (gen. sec.). A centre-right, moderate Islamic party founded in January 1986. Shah Azizur Rahman, who had been Prime Minister under Gen. Zia, was expelled from the main Bangladesh Nationalist Party (BNP) in July 1985 for leading a dissident group which favoured participation in the new National Front inspired by President Ershad. However, when the Front was converted into a unified party in January 1986, Shah Aziz declined to join and maintained his grouping as a distinct party, which subsequently became the main component of a national front.

Bangladesh Nationalist Party (Dudu) (BNP-Dudu); 55 Satmasjid Road, Dakha; leadership: Khalequzzaman Dudu (ch.); Maj. (retd.) Muslim Uddin (gen. sec.). A centre-right, moderate Islamic party founded in 1983. This version of the BNP arose from a split in the party in April 1983, when some elements opposed Begum Khaleda Zia's policy of confrontation with the Ershad regime.

Caliphate Movement (*Jhelafat Andolang*); 314/2 Lalbagh, Fort Bend; leadership: Maulana Mohammed Ullah Hafezji Huzur (founder and Amir); founded in November 1981. An Islamic fundamentalist movement, advocating the rule of God as revealed in the Koran and late Sunni Muslim texts and as practised under the Rashidite Caliphates. Maulana Hafezji Huzur, a noted religious teacher, entered politics in 1952 when he initiated the creation of the *Nezam-e-Islam* Party and thereafter played an influential role in Islamic political circles. He established the Caliphate Movement to support his candidature in the November 1981 presidential elections (in which he came third with some 387,000 votes). He stood again in October 1986 (at the age of 88) and came second, being officially credited with some 1,500,000 votes. Meanwhile, the Movement had fielded 43 candidates in the May 1986 parliamentary elections, none of them being elected.

Prior to the parliamentary elections, divisions in the Caliphate Movement had led to the formation of a breakaway group led by Azizul Huq. The latter continued to recognize Maulana Hafezji Huzur as leader, while claiming that his sons and sons-in-law were isolating him from his disciples. Both factions continued to participate in the broader Joint Caliphate Movement Council, of which Maulana Hafezji Huzur was the spiritual head.

Communist Party *(Samyabadi Dal)*; there are two factions of this revolutionary Marxist-Leninist grouping, the first led by Nani Dutta was formed by elements dissatisfied with the lack of commitment to Marxist-Leninist unity in other revolutionary Communist parties; the second led by Badruddin Umar has operated in clandestinity, concentrating on organizing peasant resistance to oppression.

Communist Party of Bangladesh, Marxist-Leninist (CPB-ML) *(Bangladesher Samyabadi Dal)*; 43/1 Joginagar Lane, Dhaka 3; leadership: Mohammed Toaha (ch.); founded in 1971. Formerly pro-Chinese, the party later inclined to a pro-Soviet stance. The CPB-ML is descended from the Communist Party of East Pakistan, Marxist-Leninist (CPEP-ML), which was formed in 1966 by the pro-Chinese wing of the Communist Party of Pakistan. In compliance with Chinese government policy, the CPEP-ML opposed the secession of Bangladesh from Pakistan in 1971, whereupon a section of the party led by Toaha formed what became the CPB-ML, which conducted guerrilla operations against Pakistani forces and attempted unsuccessfully to seize the leadership of the liberation movement. It aims at a democratic revolution based on the "marginal peasantry", pending which it is prepared to use "bourgeois instruments" such as parliamentary elections to prepare the ground for revolution.

After independence the party waged a militant campaign against the Awami League government, whose overthrow in August 1975 was followed by the party's legalization. Toaha was a member of Parliament in 1979-82, during which period the party gave support to President Zia's policy of maintaining independence from India and the Soviet Union.

Following the military takeover in March 1982, the party moderated its anti-Indian and anti-Soviet stances and joined the left-wing opposition alliance headed by the Awami League. It participated in the May 1986 parliamentary elections with six candidates (two of them on the joint opposition list), but failed to win representation.

Democracy Implementation Council *(Ganotantra Bastobayon Parishad*—GBP); 53 Road No. 3/A, Dhanmondi R/A, Dhaka 9); leadership: Maj. (retd.) Mohammed Afsaruddin (pres.); Khondakar Mahtabuddin (gen. sec.); founded in September 1985. A progressive, nationalist and moderate Islamic group,

the GBP advocates democratic government, workers' participation in ownership and management, and peasant co-operatives. It was founded by Afsaruddin to support his candidacy in the October 1986 presidential elections, in which he received a negligible vote. He had previously been vice-chairman of Rahman's Bangladesh Nationalist Party and before that leader of the Justice Party until its dissolution in 1984.

Democratic League; 68 Jigatola Road, Dhaka 9; leadership: Khandaker Moshtaque Ahmed (ch.); founded in 1976. Following the overthrow of the Awami League government in August 1975, Khandaker Moshtaque Ahmed was briefly President of Bangladesh. He founded the conservative, moderate Islamic Democratic League on the resumption of legal political activity late in 1976, but he was charged with corruption and abuse of power and given a five-year prison sentence in February 1977. The League itself was banned in October 1977 for involvement in "terrorism, foreign infiltration and conspiracy", although the ban was lifted in 1978.

Having initially adopted a co-operative attitude towards the Ershad military regime which took power in March 1982, Ahmed subsequently became leader of a National Unity Front of conservative groups and participated in the campaign for a return to constitutional rule. After some initial uncertainty, the League eventually decided to boycott the May 1986 parliamentary elections, although some other constituents of the front did not follow suit. Two splinter groups broke off from the main (Ahmed) faction of the Democratic League in the mid-1980s. One group, led by Oli Ahad, broke away from the main Democratic League in 1984 in protest against Ahmed's alleged "aversion to movement" and co-operative attitude towards the Ershad military regime. The other, led by Abdur Rouf Chowdhury, joined the seven-party centre-right opposition alliance headed by Begum Khaleda Zia's Bangladesh Nationalist Party, within which it called unsuccessfully for full participation in the May 1986 parliamentary elections.

Democratic Party (Islam) *Ganotantrik Dal (Islam)*; 19/A Anwara Bhaban, East Rajabazar, Dhaka; leadership: Tajul Islam (sec.); founded in January 1986. The party seeks "to free the state machinery from the clutches of the comprador-bureaucratic capitalist class and its close ally, the feudal class" and to carry through radical land reforms and the creation of an industrial infrastructure. This faction of the Democratic Party (itself founded in 1980) opposed the decision to merge into the new ruling National (*Jatiya*) Party.

Gano Azadi League; 30 Banagram Road, Dhaka; leadership: Alhaj Abdus Samead (gen. sec.); founded in 1976. The League was founded by Maulana Abdur Rashid Tarkabagish (who died in August 1986) as a moderate left-wing party, standing for Bengali nationalism, parliamentary democracy, the rule of law, a welfare-oriented balanced economy and freedom of religion. It participated in the five-party Democratic United Front (headed by the Awami League) which unsuccessfully campaigned for Gen. Mohammed Ataul Ghani Osmani in the June 1978 presidential elections won by Gen. Zia. After the Ershad military takeover in March 1982 it joined the 15-party left-wing opposition alliance led by the Awami League and followed the latter in deciding to contest the May 1986 parliamentary elections. Its sole candidate (Alhaj Abdus Samad) was defeated. In 1991, the party joined the Patriotic Democratic League.

Hindu Oikyo Front; 170 Free School Street, Dhaka 5; leadership: Manindra Nath Sarker (ch.). The Front combines its efforts to protect the interests of the minority Hindu community with co-operation with Muslim parties on issues affecting the national interests of Bangladesh. The Front participated in the National United Front led by Khandaker Moshtaque Ahmed of the Democratic League but withdrew when the main components of the National Unity Front eventually decided against participation in the May 1986 parliamentary elections. Its four election candidates were all unsuccessful.

Islahul Muslemif; Darbar Sharif, East Nakhalpara, Dhaka; leadership: Alhaj Maulana Abul Bashar a *pir* (Muslim saint) who has campaigned for the establishment of Islam in all spheres of life. The party provides financial assistance to the poor.

Islami Oikyo Jote; 44/1 Purana Paltan, Dhaka; leadership: Alhaj Md. Obaidul Haque.

Islamic Party (Hossain); 1st floor, 124/1 New Kakrail Road, Dhaka; leadership: Sheikh Ashraf Hossain (pres.). Islamic fundamentalist party which is an offshoot of the main Islamic Party led by M. A. Malek.

Islamic Party (Malek); 27/4 Aminbagh Road, Dhaka; leadership: M. A. Malek (pres.). An Islamic fundamentalist party, but committed to democracy, it was founded in April 1979 by Malek who was formerly a member of the Islamic Democratic Party. A member of the Nationalist Front headed by Shah Azizur Rahman's Bangladesh Nationalist Party, the Islamic Party refused to participate in the May 1986 parliamentary elections.

Islamic Unity Movement (previously Islamic Democratic League) (*Islami Oikyo Andolang*); 84 Prubo Testuri Bazaar, Tejgaon, Dhaka 15; leadership: Maulana Abdur Rahim (ch.); founded in November 1984 as an Islamic fundamentalist party, advocating an "Iranian-style Islamic revolution" in Bangladesh. A veteran Islamic fundamentalist activist, Maulana Rahim was a member of the pre-independence East Pakistan Assembly and was elected to the Bangladesh Parliament in 1979 as a candidate of the Islamic Democratic League, which became the Islamic Unity Movement in November 1984. It is a member of the Joint Caliphate Movement Councils.

Jana Shakti Party; 13/B Road No. 10/11. Mirpur, Dhaka; leadership: Abdullah Al-Naser (pres.). Fatema Khatun (gen. sec.). A moderate Islamic, nationalist party, favouring a free market economy. It was founded in March 1984 and later joined the Nationalist Front headed by Shah Azizur Rahman's Bangladesh Nationalist Party.

Labour Party; 27 Purana Paltan, Dhaka; leadership: Maulana Abdul Matin (pres.); founded in November 1969 as a moderate Islamic and anti-nationalist party which also advocates the emancipation of the poor. A noted author of religious books, Maulana Matin was detained under the 1971-75 Awami League government for protesting against the publication of works which he regarded as derogatory to Islam. Released in late 1975, he became a supporter of President Zia, although he declined to join the latter's Bangladesh Nationalist Party (BNP) when it was created in September 1978. The Labour Party subsequently became a member of the Nationalist Front headed by Shah Azizur Rahman's group, the Bangladesh Nationalist Party (Aziz) (founded after he was expelled from the original BNP). A dispute between two leadership groups split the party, with the other faction led by Abdul Mutalib Sikdar.

Muslim League Factions. As well as the Muslim League listed under the major parties above, there are several factions including those led by Abu Ali Chowdhury; Alhaj Mohammed Shamsul Huda; Kamruzzaman Khan; and Syed Kutub Uddin.

Muslim Nationalist Party (*Muslim Jatiyatabadi Dal*); 4th floor, Bikrampur House, 47/3 Toynbe Circular Road, Dhaka 3; leadership: Sirajul Huq Gora (pres.). A Muslim nationalist party, committed to the creation of an Islamic republic. Having earlier been a member of the National Awami Party, Sirajul Huq Gura joined the Progressive Democratic Force in 1981. He subsequently led a breakaway faction called the Progressive Nationalist Party, which was renamed the Muslim Nationalist Party in 1983.

National Awami Party (Bhashani) (NAP-B). Claiming to represent the political principles of the NAP's founder, Maulana Abdul Hamid Khan Bhashani, the NAP-B stands for Bengali nationalism, democracy, secularism and socialism. It advocates the emancipation of the working class form domestic and foreign exploitation, an independent national economy, priority for agro-based industrial projects and promotion of a state-owned heavy industrial sector. It was formed as a result of a split in the NAP (Muzaffar) in 1967.

Having not participated actively in the Bangladesh independence struggle, the NAP (Bhashani) had by 1974 fallen under the influence of right-wing Muslim elements and was openly anti-Indian and anti-Hindu as well as in opposition to the Awami League government. Maoist elements deserted or were expelled and Mashiur Rahman, a right-wing leader, became head of the party's organizing committee. After being suppressed under martial law in August 1975, it became legal at the end of 1976 and in June 1978 backed the *Jatiyatabadi* Front in its successful campaign for the election of Gen. Zia as President, whereupon Mashiur Rahman was appointed a senior minister in the government.

Meanwhile, the death of Maulana Bhashani in November 1976 had precipitated a series of splits, producing a number of groups calling themselves the NAP (Bhashani) accompanied by a complex series of realignments and mergers involving the various NAP factions as well as other groups. Following the Ershad military takeover in March 1982, some NAP (Bhashani) groups gravitated towards the seven-party alliance headed by the Bangladesh Nationalist Party (BNP) and followed the BNP in boycotting the May 1986 parliamentary elections. Others joined with a

dissident section of the main NAP (led by Muzaffar) and other leftist elements to contest the elections as the NAP (Bhashani/United), presenting 10 candidates and winning five seats. These include factions led by: Abu Nasser Khan Bhashani (the National Awami Party (Bhashani/United) (NAP-BU)); Gazi Shahidullah; M. A. Hannan; A. K. M. Fazlul Huq; Abdul Khaleque; Shakwat Matin; and Mir Abu Zafar.

National Congress; 38 Topkhana Road, Dhaka; leadership: Mohammed Mofizur Rahman Dhali (pres.); S. M. Alam Faridi (gen. sec.). The Congress advocates a free market economy and secularism. Dhali, a former official of the Awami League, was later a member of the Bangladesh Nationalist Party before launching the National Congress.

National Democratic Party (NDP); 3/4 Purana Paltan, Dhaka; leadership: Salahuddin Qader Chowdhury (sec.-gen.).

National Democratic Party (Jagpa) (*Jatiya Ganotantrik Party*); 33 Captain Bazaar, Dhaka; leadership: Shafiul Alam Prodhan; founded in April 1980. Centre-right party, opposed to nationalization. Prodhan was leader of the Awami League's student wing in the early 1970's and was later convicted of involvement in terrorist violence. Freed by President Zia in 1977, he gravitated to the right and founded Jagpa as an anti-socialist party.

National Democratic Peasant Party *Jatiyatabadi Ganotantrik Chashi Dal (Jaagchad)*; 20/Gha, Katasur, Master Bari Mohammadpur, Dhaka 7; leadership: Afazuddin Chowdhury (ch.). A moderate Islamic party. A former member of the Democratic Party, Chowdhury contested the February 1979 parliamentary and November 1981 presidential elections, in each case without success. The party initially decided to contest the May 1986 parliamentary elections, but later reversed this decision.

National Hindu Council (*Jatiya Hindu Parishad*; leadership: Prem Ranjan Devwas (pres.). The Council seeks to protect and further the interests of the minority Hindu community. Before independence Devwas was a member of the pro-Chinese Communist Party of East Pakistan, Marxist-Leninist; he was later associated with the National Awami Party (Bhashani) and was also a member of Gen. Zia's Bangladesh Nationalist Party.

National (*Jatiya*) **League**; 27/1 Elephant Road, Dhaka 5/500A Dhamandi R/A. Road 7, Dhaka; leadership: Giauddin Ahmed Chowdhury (convener). Moderate Islamic party, advocating a free market economy. Founded in 1970 as Pakistan National League, renamed 1972. Dating from the pre-independence period, the League was relaunched in 1976 under the leadership of Ataul Rahman Khan and won two seats in the 1979 parliamentary elections. In 1984-85 Rahman Khan served as Prime Minister under President Ershad and in June 1984 joined the pro-government People's Party (*Jana Dal*), the forerunner of the later ruling National Party. A section of the League led by Chowdhury opposed the merger with the government party and maintained the League as an independent party.

National Party (Begum) (*Jatiya Dal* (Begum)); 71 Bara Mogh Bazaar, Dhaka; leadership: Amena Begum (pres.). A conservative party founded in November 1976. Having been a senior officer of the pre-independence Awami League, Amena Begum in 1970 transferred her allegiance to the newly formed National League. On the resumption of political activity in November 1976 she led a faction of the League into a merger with a faction of the Democratic Party to create the National Party (her party subsequently remaining distinct from the government party of the same name created in January 1986).

National People's Party (Asad) (*Jatiya Janata Dal*) (JJD-Asad); 1st floor, 67 Sultangonj Rald, Rayer Bazaar, Dhaka; leadership: Sheikh Mohammed Asad (convenor). A centrist progressive grouping which is descended from the party founded in September 1976 by Gen. (retd.) Mohammed Ataul Ghani Osmani, who had commanded Bangladeshi forces during the 1971 War of Independence. Backed by the JJD-instigated Democratic United Front (which also included the Awami League), Gen. Osmani obtained some 4,400,000 votes in the June 1978 presidential elections (won by Gen. Zia), although in the November 1981 presidential elections (won by Abdus Sattar) his support slumped to only 300,000 votes. Following his death in 1985, the JJD split into four factions, each claiming to represent his ideals. The three other faction are led by Suzat Ahmed Chowdhury; Rear Adml. (retd.) H. M. Khan; and Khan Mohammed Anwarul Wadud.

National Socialist Party (Inu) ((*Jatiya Samajtantrik Dal--Inu*) (JSD-Inu); Allahwalah Building, 108 Motijheel C/A, Dhaka 2; leadership: Hasanul Huq Inu. Advocating "scientific socialism", this faction of the JSD (originally formed in 1972 by left-wing elements of the Awami League) opposed participation in the May 1986 parliamentary elections, whereas they were contested by the party's two main factions.

National United Front; leadership: Khandaker Moshtaque Ahmed (chair); founded 1991. An alliance of 23 nationalist and Islamic groups; calls for a representative government and economic emancipation.

Patriotic Democratic Front; founded 1991. An alliance of the following four left-wing political parties: the Bangladesh Communist Party; the Gano Azadi League; the National Awami Party (Muzaffar faction); the Communist Party—Marxist-Leninist.

Nezam-e-Islamic (Ali); 5/6 Shayesthakhan Road, Lalbagh, Dhaka; leadership: Maulana Ashraf Ali (pres.). An Islamic fundamentalist party founded in 1952 at the instigation of Maulana Hafezji Huzur (later leader of the Caliphate Movement), this group opposed Bengali nationalism and the creation of an independent Bangladesh in 1971. It was revived in 1976 under the leadership of Syed Manzoorul Ahsan. His death in 1986 precipitated the division of the party, of which there are three other main factions, led by Maulana Mohammed Abdur Rahman Azad; Maulana Abdul Jabbar Badarpuri; and Khwaja Sayeed Shah.

People's League A centre-left grouping which supports parliamentary democracy. It is split into three factions lead by Syed Mahbub Hossain; Nur Mohammed Kazi; and Garib Newaz.

Peasants' and Workers' Emancipation Movement *Krishak Sramik Mukti Andolan*; 41 Greenway, Bara Moghbqazar, Dhaka 17; leadership: Mohammed Sadeq (pres.); Fakhruddin Ahmed (gen. sec.). The party seeks to promote the interests of peasants and workers through a more equitable distribution of wealth.

People's Party (Huq) (*Jana Dal (Huq)*); 126 Motijheel C/A, Dhaka; leadership: Mohammed Abdul Huq (ch.); founded in January 1986. The conservative People's Party was originally created in 1983 as a pro-government party and was a major component of the new ruling National (*Jatiya*) Party launched in

January 1986. Elements of the People's Party opposed the merger, however, and maintained the party in being, although it quickly split into two factions [see next entry]. The Huq faction presented 34 candidates in the May 1986 elections, but all were defeated.

People's Party (Shahidullah) (*Jana Dal* (Shahidullah)); 30 Road No. 4, Dhanmondi R/A, Dhaka; leadership: Sheikh Shahidullah (ch.); founded in 1986. One of two factions of the original People's Party which rejected merger into the new ruling National Party, this grouping did not participate in the May 1986 parliamentary elections.

Progressive Democratic Force (*Progotishil Ganotantrik Shakti* (Progosh)); 34 Free School Street, Hatirpool, Dhaka; leadership: Lt.-Col. (retd.) Shariar Rashid Khan (pres.), one of the "majors" who led the military overthrow of Sheikh Mujibur Rahman in August 1975.

Sarbajara Party (Kabir); leadership: Anwarul Kabir (ch.). Revolutionary Marxist-Leninist Maoist party, which is one of two factions claiming descent from the movement led by the militant revolutionary Siraj Sikdar, who was killed under the 1971-75 Awami League government. It is allied with the Communist Party (Dutta) and the Revolutionary Communist League.

Sarbajara Party (Ziauddin); leadership: Lt.-Col. (retd.) Ziauddin (ch.). Revolutionary Marxist-Leninist party, critical of Maoist precepts. Led by a fugitive army officer, this faction of the Sarbahara Party is allied with the Revolutionary Communist Party.

Socialist Party (Bhuiyan) *Samajtantrik Dal (Bhuiyan)*; 23/2 Topkhana Road, Dhaka; leadership: Khalequzzaman Bhuiyan (ch.). A radical socialist party which was formed in November 1980 by former student leaders who broke away from the National Socialist Party in protest against its leadership's alleged revisionism and involvement in "bourgeois politics". The two factions into which the Socialist Party later split both participated in the 15-party left-wing opposition alliance headed by the Awami League and they were both among those elements which refused to follow the League in contesting the May 1986 parliamentary elections. The other faction is led by A. F. M. Mahbubul Huq.

United People's Party (UPP-Khan); 1st floor, 10/C Asad Avenue, Dhaka 7; leadership: Shamsul Arefin Khan (ch.). Originally founded in May 1974 by a left-wing dissident faction of the National Awami Party (Bhashani), the UPP later aligned itself with President Zia and participated in government under him. Following the Ershad military takeover of March 1982, a majority of the UPP participated in the creation of a pro-government party, but the eventual decision to merge the UPP into the new ruling National Party was opposed by a minority, which maintained the UPP in being and continued to adhere to the seven-party opposition alliance headed by the Begum Khaleda Zia's Bangladesh Nationalist Party.

United People's Party (UPP-Rahman); 100 Fakirapool Bazaar, Dhaka; leadership: Miah Sadequr Rahman (ch.); founded in April 1983. This progressive UPP faction also resulted from a split over the leadership's policy of co-operation with the Ershad regime. Like the UPP-Khan, it formed part of the opposition alliance headed by the Bangladesh Nationalist Party.

Principal illegal organizations

Chittagong Autonomists *(Shanti Bahini)*. Autonomist aspirations had already been expressed at the time of the East Pakistan government (overthrown in 1971) by tribal people (mainly Buddhist, Christian or Hindu) of the Chittagong Hill Tracts, who lived on a traditional "slash and burn" basis. Since 1947 the government had encouraged the tribal people to take up settled farming and had moved in (mainly Muslim) Bengalis. This process was speeded up in 1978-79 with the result that the proportion of Bengalis in the area rose from 11.6 percent in 1974 to 39 per cent in 1981.

Guerrilla warfare by Chittagong Hill Tracts tribes began in 1975 under the leadership of Manabendra Larma (a former independent member of the *Jatiya Sangsad*) after appeals for regional autonomy had met with no response from the government.

Since 1975 there have been widespread atrocities committed by guerrillas on Bengali settlers, thousands of arrests, and allegations of reprisal massacres carried out by the Bangladesh army on tribal people. In December 1980 the government adopted a Disturbed Areas Bill (with implied reference to the Chittagong Hill Tracts situation), giving police officers and army non-commissioned officers unlimited authority to fire upon a person or to make arrests without a warrant. Government figures in December 1986 put the number of people killed in tribal warfare since 1975 at 1,000.

In October 1983 the government offered a general amnesty, a cash reward, free rations and a plot of land to all guerrillas who surrendered by Feb. 25, 1984 (extended to April 26), but only 200-300 of an estimated 3,000 active guerrillas were reported to have given themselves up.

Representatives of the Chakma tribe have reported that Buddist tribespeople face virtual genocide unless they convert to Islam. The number of refugees fleeing to the neighbouring Indian states of Tirpura and Mizoram between April 1986 and January 1987 was estimated at 24,000. Reports of alleged army brutality against refugees included one of up to 200 people shot and killed after being lured into a narrow defile.

Bhutan

Capital: Thimpu

Population: 1,500,000 (1990)

The region that is today Bhutan came under Tibetan rule in the 16th century. The British extended their influence to the region in the 19th century, finally establishing a monarchy in 1907 and a British protectorate in 1910. Bhutan became independent in 1949 and at the same time entered into the Indo-Bhutan Treaty of Perpetual Peace and Friendship, which made it an associated state of India. While other Himalayan states were absorbed by the large Asian powers, namely Tibet by China and Sikkim by India, Bhutan managed to negotiate compromises on formal sovereignty in the areas of defence and foreign affairs, first with Britain and then with India, into a lasting and secure independence.

The Code of Conduct (*Driglam Namzha*) programme, initiated in 1990 to revitalise (Buddhist) Drukpa culture, has had the effect of seriously alienating the (Hindu) Nepalese minority, relatively recent arrivals who have contributed to the development of the southern mountainous regions. Among other cultural and social restraints, the Code requires all citizens to adopt Bhutanese traditional dress and be schooled in the Dzongkha language. Various parties and groups were established in 1989 to oppose the programme and call for democratic reforms, the most influential of which was the Bhutan People's Party (BPP). Tensions increased markedly at the end of 1990, reaching a peak in September, with reports of violence carried out against Bhutanese citizens by ethnic Nepalese and other dissident elements. Schools and richer homes were looted.

In October 1990, King Jigme Singye Wangchuck expressed his willingness to enter into dialogue with the dissidents. He admitted that the current mode of representation in the *Tsogdu* (National Assembly) was imperfect since it gave the Nepalese-dominated districts in the South only 16 seats out of a total of 151. In September 1991 he was reported to have stated that he did not consider monarchy to be the best form of government.

The unrest took a new turn in October 1991 when the King threatened to abdicate if no solution were found, and when he later stated that he was unable to attend a meeting of the heads of state of the South Asian Association for Regional Co-operation (of which Bhutan is a member) it was seen as an indication of the level of instability in the country. There were reports of cross-border raids into India to pursue members of the BPP. India gave assurances in September 1991 that it would not permit anti-Bhutanese activities by ethnic Nepalese who had fled into West Bengal and Assam.

Constitutional structure

In 1907 the *Tsonga Penlop*, governor of the eastern province of Tsonga, was elected as the first hereditary maharajah of Bhutan. The monarch's Bhutanese title is *Druk Gyalpo* (Dragon King), but he is generally referred to as the King of Bhutan. The monarchy is hereditary, and the present King, Jigme Singye Wangchuk, ascended to the throne in 1972.

The Kingdom of Bhutan has no formal constitution. The King is the highest executive and judicial authority, but his powers are limited by a code of written and unwritten rules and procedures. He is advised by an eight-member Royal Advisory Council (RAC—*Lodoi Tsogdu*). The RAC is composed of two monastic representatives from the Central and District Rabdeys (monastic bodies), respectively; six people's representatives; and a chairman, or *Kalyon*, nominated by the King, all of whom serve five-year terms. The Council of Ministers serves in the capacity of a cabinet, with all of its members appointed and removable by the King, who is its chair, with the consent of the National Assembly.

The 151-member unicameral National Assembly, or *Tsogdu*, is the principal legislative body and was established in 1953. In addition to enacting laws, the National Assembly also advises on constitutional issues and is the forum for debates on all matters of national importance. Since 1969, the Tsogdu has been required to pass a vote of confidence in the King by a two-thirds majority every three years, and is empowered to replace the monarch.

The state religion is Buddhism, and the importance of Buddhism in Bhutan is seen by the roughly equal status given to the King and the Buddhist spiritual leader, the *Je Khempo*, nominated by a central organization of Buddhist monks with the approval of the King. Buddhist monks hold a variety of positions at all levels of government.

Electoral system

The National Assembly consists of 106 members who are directly elected for three-year terms from 18 multi-member districts; 10 members indirectly elected by various religious organizations; one member elected by the Bhutan Chamber of Commerce and Industry; 18 members who are the leaders, or *Dzongdas*, of Bhutan's 18 district governments; and 16 members nominated by the government who usually come from the two Councils. There are no legal political parties, and candidates for election to the National Assembly must run as individuals.

The six people's representatives to the Royal Advisory Council are nominated by the village assemblies and elected by the National Assembly for five-year terms.

Evolution of the suffrage

There is universal adult suffrage for the elections of members of the National Assembly.

Recent elections

Elections to the National Assembly are on a non-party basis with candidates running as individuals.

PARTY BY PARTY DATA

There are no legal political parties. Listed below are three of the many newly formed illegal opposition groups, mostly based in Katmandu, Nepal.

Bhutan People's Party (BPP); leadership: R. K. Budathoki (pres.); D. K. Rai (gen. sec.); founded in 1990. Made up mostly of Nepalese Hindus, the group calls for democratic reform from hereditary monarchy to constitutional monarchy; judicial reform; freedom of religion, speech and the press; equal rights for all ethnic groups; and the release of all political prisoners. It claims not to be anti-monarchist but anti-corruption. The most influential of the new political groups

formed in 1989 and 1990, the BPP organized a series of large demonstrations in Southern Bhutan in September 1990 to protest against *Drukpa* domination and to demand political reform. Many of the demonstrators were Nepalese who had crossed from India into southern Bhutan. The demonstrations were broken up by the security forces and according to some unsubstantiated BPP sources, some 300 people were killed during the security operation.

United Liberation People's Front; leadership: Balaram Poudyal.

People's Forum for Human Rights; leadership: Gopal Sharma (l.); Vikay Thapa (l.).

Brunei

Capital: Bandar Seri Bagwan

The Sultanate of Brunei, which had been a British protectorate since 1888, gained full internal self government in 1971 and became a fully independent sovereign state in 1984. Sultan Hassanal Bolkiah rules the country primarily by decree.

Population: 250,000 (1989 est.)

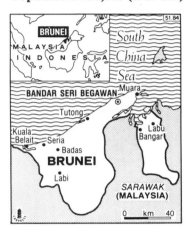

Constitutional structure

Under the terms of the 1959 Constitution, the Sultan, as head of state, is assisted and advised by a Council of Cabinet Ministers, a Privy Council and a Religious Council. The Constitution also provides for a Council of Succession. A state of emergency has been in force, and the Sultan has ruled by decree since 1962, when a large-scale revolt resulted in the suspension of sections of the Constitution.

PARTY BY PARTY DATA

Political parties were proscribed in 1988, and the parties listed below have all formally been dissolved; some may operate clandestinely.

Brunei National Democratic Party (*Partai Kebangsaan Demokratik Brunei*) (PKDB); moderate; pro-parliamentary democracy; advocated principals based on Islam and liberal nationalism; founded 1985. Following independence in 1984 the Sultan seriously considered introducing a party political system and hence in 1985 he allowed Abdul Latif Hamid and Abdul Latif Chuchu to form the PKDB. The party's moderate pro-democratic stance received little support from a public apparently content with Brunei's incomparable state welfare system. In 1988 the party allegedly issued a call for democratic elections, an end to the state of emergency and the resignation of the Sultan as head of the government. The Sultan responded by dissolving the party and arresting the two Latifs.

Brunei National United Party *Partai Perpaduan Ke-*

bangsaan Brunei (PPKB); pro-government; founded 1986. The PPKB was formed by Awang Hatta Zainal Abiddin as a moderate breakaway faction of the Brunei National Democratic Party. The party found little support and was de-registered shortly afterwards.

Brunei People's Party *Partai Rakyat Brunei* (PRB); left wing; founded 1956. The PRB was founded by A. M. N. Azahari and was modelled on the left wing Malaysian People's Party. While professing loyalty to the Sultan, the PRB advocated self-government for Brunei as part of a unitary state to include the adjacent British territories of Sarawak and North Borneo (Sabah). The Sultan excluded the PRB from negotiations with the British which resulted in the promulgation of the 1959 Constitution. Nevertheless, in mid-1962 the party won all elective seats in the Legislative Council. At the end of the year a rebellion was launched by the PRB-backed "North Borneo Liberation Army" with the object of preventing Brunei's entry into the then proposed Federation of Malaysia. With the encouragement of Indonesia, Azahari proclaimed a "Revolutionary State of North Kalimantan", but within a few weeks the revolt was suppressed with the help of a British task force. The PRB was banned and hundreds of its members arrested, while Azahari was granted political asylum in Malaysia. In 1990 the final group of PRB prisoners were released in Brunei.

Brunei People's National United Party *Partai Perpaduan Kebangsaan Rakyat Brunei* (PERKARA); founded 1968. This party was founded in 1968 but had little political impact.

People's Independence Front (*Barisan Kemerdeka'an Rakyat*) (BAKER); moderate; pro-parliamentary democracy; founded 1966. BAKER was established as an amalgamation of all the existing political parties in Brunei. The party pressed for a fully elected legislature and a full ministerial system but received little public support. It was de-registered because of inactivity in 1985.

Parties in conflict with the government

About 100 members and supporters of the Brunei People's Party are reported to operate in exile in Indonesia and Malaysia.

Cambodia

Capital: Phnom Penh   **Population: 8,200,000 (1990)**

The Kingdon of Cambodia gained independence from France in 1953 and for the next 17 years Prince Norodom Sihanouk was the dominant political force in the country. After Sihanouk's overthrow by rightists led by Lon Nol and Sirik Matak in 1970, the country was renamed as the Khmer Republic (Khmer being the predominant ethnic group in Cambodia). Cambodian communists (dubbed *Khmers Rouges* by Sihanouk) toppled the Lon Nol regime in 1975 and the following year they renamed the country Democratic Kampuchea (DK). The DK regime was itself toppled in 1979 by *Khmer Rouge* rebels backed by troops from neighbouring Vietnam. A new pro-Vietnamese government was established and the country was renamed as the People's Republic of Kampuchea (PRK, renamed as the State of Cambodia—SOC—in 1989). A civil war ensued between the PRK government, based in Phnom Penh and backed by Vietnamese troops, and *Khmer Rouge* and Sihanoukist guerrillas, based on the Thai border and backed by China and the West.

Vietnam withdrew its forces from Cambodia in 1989 and in October 1991 the warring factions signed a peace agreement in Paris. Under the terms of the agreement a UN Transitional Authority in Cambodia (UNTAC) would: (i) administer the country until the election of a Legislative Assembly and the formation of a government; (ii) supervise the partial demobilization of the warring factions' armed forces; and (iii) enforce a ceasefire. The Supreme National Council (SNC) formed by all the factions in September 1990 was to embody Cambodia's "independence, sovereignty and unity" and represent the country at the UN, while the Chair of the SNC, Sihanouk, was to serve as the country's head of state. As of mid-1992, the day-to-day running of the country remained largely in the hands of the SOC government.

Constitutional structure

The National Assembly approved a new Constitution in 1981, replacing that introduced by the *Khmer Rouge* regime in 1976. In 1989 the Assembly endorsed several major constitutional amendments, including changing the name of the country from the People's Republic of Kampuchea to the State of Cambodia. Under the 1981 Constitution, the National Assembly is the supreme organ of state power. A Council of State serves as the Assembly's standing organ and the Chair of the Council is Supreme Commander of the Armed Forces and Chair of the National Defence Council. A Council of Ministers, headed by a Chair, is the governing body responsible to the Assembly.

With the signing of the October 1991 peace accord, the Constitution remained in place, but its was envisaged that the United Nations would play a major role in the governance of the country during the period leading up to general elections in 1993.

Electoral system

Voting for the National Assembly takes place in multi-member constituencies where the number of candidates exceeds the number of seats. In the 1981 elections, all candidates were nominated by the Kampuchean United Front for National Construction and Defence.

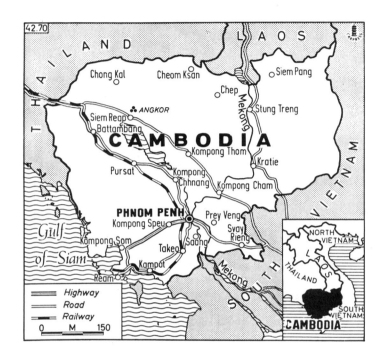

Recent elections

A general election was held in May 1981 when 117 National Assembly seats were contested by 148 candidates. According to official government figures, 99.17 per cent of the 3,417,339 electors had taken part in the vote. In 1986 the Assembly voted to prolong its first five-year term for another five years. In mid-1987, supplementary elections were held in six provinces increasing the membership of the Assembly to 123.

Evolution of the suffrage

Under the 1981 Constitution, Cambodian citizens who are at least 18 years of age have the right to vote.

PARTY BY PARTY DATA

Cambodian People's Party

Address. Phnom Penh.

Leadership. Chea Sim (ch.); Hun Sen (vice-ch.).

Orientation. Former communist party; officially supports multiparty system and free market economy.

Founded. 1951.

History. A Cambodian organization known as the Kampuchean People's Revolutionary Party (KPRP), *Kanak Pracheachon Padevat Kampuchea*) was founded in 1951. Ideologically, the party was closely aligned to the Vietnamese Workers' Party, which had re-emerged from dissolution that same year. The KPP carried out small-scale guerrilla activities against the French, the colonial power in Cambodia. Following the granting of independence in 1953 and the holding of the Geneva Conference on Indo-China the following year, the armed struggle virtually ceased and the party pursud a policy of legal opposition, under the name of People's Group (*Krom Pracheachon*). Despite serious harrassment from the ruling Sihanouk regime, the Group competed in elections in 1955 and 1958, but with little success.

The party convened in secret in Phnom Penh in 1960, a meeting clouded in controversy. According to one party faction (the Pol Pot faction), the meeting constituted the inaugural meeting of the Workers' Party of Kampuchea (*Pak Polakor Kampuchea*, renamed as the Communist Party of Kampuchea (CPK)—*Pak Kommunis Kampuchea*—in 1966). According to the opposing faction (the faction currently in control in Phnom Penh), the meeting was in fact the party's second congress, the first having been held in 1951.

It was agreed at the meeting to abandon the policy of legal opposition to the Sihanouk regime and adopt a policy of violent, guerrilla opposition. Tou Samouth was elected as the party general secretary and other members elected to leading posts included Saloth Sar (Pol Pot), Ieng Sary and Son Sen, all members of a group of young, radical intellectuals who had returned from university in Paris in the early 1950s. Tou Samouth was killed in 1962, possibly by rivals within the party, and Pol Pot was elected as general secretary at a congress held early the next year. Shortly after the

congress, the party leadership (including Pol Pot, Ieng Sary and Son Sen) went into hiding in the Cambodian countryside and their names were not mentioned in any Cambodian press reports until the early 1970s. However, Pol Pot was thought to have made visits to Hanoi and Beijing in 1965-66. Party members (often described by now as *Khmer Rouge, Khmer Vietminh* or *Khmer Hanoi*) launched a major peasant revolt in north-western Cambodia in 1967, in which they were joined by a number of Cambodian communists who had remained in Phnom Penh during the mid-1960s, including Khieu Samphan. The uprising was brutally repressed by the government, but the party managed to retain control of large sections of the countryside.

Prince Sihanouk's neutralist regime was toppled by pro-US rightists led by Lon Nol in 1970. The Prince fled to China where he entered into coalition with the CPK, forming the *Gouvernement Royale de l'Union National de Kampuchea* (GRUNK) in opposition to Lon Nol's regime.

In 1973 Pol Pot began to purge the CPK of its pro-Vietnamese elements, and when in April 1975 GRUNK forces finally gained control of the whole of Cambodia, the dominant political organization in the country was a pro-Chinese, anti-Vietnamese CPK, whose members were drawn entirely from Pol Pot's supporters. However, it was not until September 1977 that it was officially disclosed that the ruling organization in Democratic Kampuchea (as the country had been renamed under its new 1976 Constitution) was the CPK led by Pol Pot.

At the time of the disclosure, violent factionalism within the party had developed into virtual civil war and coincided with the eruption of full-scale border warfare between Cambodia and Vietnam. Hence, in late 1978 a pro-Vietnamese Kampuchean National United Front for National Construction and Defence (KNUFNCD) was formed in the "liberated" eastern zones and began working towards the overthrow of the Pol Pot regime. The KNUFNCD leader, Heng Samrin (a CPK official), took effective control of the country when, with the aid of Vietnamese forces, the Pol Pot government was overthrown in early 1979. A CPK "reorganization" congress was immediatly held by the new leadership and it was decided to revert to the name of Kampuchean People's Revolutionary Party (KPRP), to distinguish it from the Pol Pot faction of the party which established itself along the Thai-Cambodian border. Pen Sovan was elected as the new general secretary of the party, at the head of a new central committee, politburo and secretariat. In late 1981 Pen Sovan was replaced as general secretary by Heng Samrin in what appeared to be the outcome of an internal power struggle. The KPRP held its fifth congress in 1985, at which a number of technocrats replaced military cadres on the central committee.

At an extraordinary congress held in October 1991, in the aftermath of the signing of the Paris peace accords, the KPRP changed its name to the Cambodian People's Party (CPP), and officially renounced its communist policies, announcing its support for a multiparty system and free market economy. At the same time the party removed the hammer and sickle from its emblem and renamed the politburo as the standing committee of the central committee. Chea Sim, the powerful Chair of the National Assembly and, according to many western commentators, a relative hardliner, was appointed as Chair of the standing committee, thereby replacing Heng Samrin as leader of the party. Heng Samrin was appointed as the party's honorary Chair, a purely cosmetic post. Premier Hun Sen, leader of the party's liberal faction, was named as Chea Sim's deputy.

Structure. Central committee and central committee standing committee.

Publications. Pracheachon.

Khmer People's National Liberation Front

Address. KPNLF cantonment, Phnom Penh.

Leadership. Son Sann (pres.).

Orientation. Centre-right, nationalist and anti-communist.

Founded. 1979.

History. The Khmer People's National Liberation Front (KPNLF) was established in France by Son Sann, a former Cambodian Premier under Prince Norodom Sihanouk, with the avowed object of uniting all non-communist resistance to the Vietnamese-backed regime in Phnom Penh. Along with the Sihanoukist and *Khmers Rouges* groups, the KPNLF established military bases along the Thai-Cambodian border and waged a guerrilla war against the Vietnamese and Phnom Penh forces. In 1982 the KPNLF, the *Khmers Rouges* and the Sihanoukists formed the Coalition Government of Democratic Kampuchea (CGDK) in an attempt to co-ordinate diplomatic and military actions against Vietnam and Phnom Penh. Son Sann was appointed as CGDK Prime Minister. However, the formation of the CGDK did little to improve the military impact of the three constituent armies on the Vietnamese forces and the KPNLF suffered serious military setbacks in the period between 1983-85, losing most of its military bases. These reversals were compounded by serious internal divisions within the KPNLF in 1985-86, which further reduced its already largely ineffectual military capabilities. Following the withdrawal of Vietnamese troops from Cambodia in 1989, rebel radio broadcasts tended to stress the military prowess of the KPNLF and the Sihanoukists (the other non-communist faction of the CGDK) in what was widely regarded as an attempt to minimize the dominance of the *Khmers Rouges*. However, analysts were generally agreed that the *Khmers Rouges* were by far the dominant military force in the coalition and that the KPNLF was a poor fighting force.

A Cambodian Supreme National Council (SNC) was formed in 1990 as part of a nascent UN peace plan. The SNC was composed of members from all four warring factions, the KPNLF, the *Khmers Rouges*, the Sihanoukists and the Phnom Penh government, and was intended to represent Cambodian sovereignty while the UN would assume most aspects of government, pending a general election. The KPNLF had two seats on the 12-member SNC, filled by Son Sann and Ieng Muli. In October 1991 the KPNLF, along with the other Cambodian factions and various foreign powers, signed a comprehensive UN peace agreement. Under the terms of the agreement, the KPNLF was installed in a cantonment in Phnom Penh pending demobilization and the beginning of UN supervised elections.

Party of Democratic Kampuchea

Khmers Rouges

Address. PDK cantonment, Phnom Penh.

Leadership. Khieu Samphan (pres.); Son Sen (vice-pres.).

Orientation. Communist party; extreme nationalist and anti-Vietnamese.

Founded. 1960.

History. The Party of Democratic Kampuchea (PDK), more commonly known as the *Khmers Rouges*, is one of two factions of the Cambodian communist movement, the other faction being the Cambodian People's Party (CPP, see CPP entry for history of both factions from the early 1950s until the late 1970s). The PDK faction, led by general secretary Saloth Sar (Pol Pot) and Ieng Sary, Son Sen and Nuon Chea, dates its existence from a founding congress in Phnom Penh in 1960. After years of civil war, the party came to power in 1975 and inaugurated a radical social, political and economic programme based loosely on earlier Chinese communist policies. The party also pursued an extreme nationalist line that manifested itself noticeably in its antagonism towards the (communist) government and people of neighbouring Vietnam. Upon its assumption of power the party was deeply factionilized and Pol Pot only maintained control by carrying out numerous brutal purges. The party's fanatical anti-Vietnamese line manifested itself in the form of border skirmishing in 1977 and developed into serious warfare the following year.

At this time, Vietnam began working with anti-Pol Pot elements within the party from the country's eastern regions (bordering Vietnam) towards establishing a more accessible government in Phnom Penh. In late 1978 Vietnamese forces, supported by anti-Pol Pot elements within the party, launched a full scale invasion of Cambodia and toppled the Pol Pot government. In early 1979 Vietnam established the anti-Pol Pot faction, headed by Heng Samrin, in power. This faction altered its name from the Communist Party of Kampuchea (CPK) to the Kampuchean People's Revolutionary Party (KPRP), to differentiate itself from the ousted Pol Pot faction which was forced to flee to the Thai border. The Pol Pot faction announced the creation of a Patriotic and Democratic Front of the Great National Union of Kampuchea, the purpose of which was to rally all elements opposed to the Vietnamese-backed government in Phnom Penh. From its bases along the Thai border, the Pol Pot faction organized a guerrilla war against its rival Vietnamese-backed faction in Phnom Penh.

The central committee of the Pol Pot faction announced in December 1981 that it had been decided at a congress held in September to dissolve the party "in order to conform with the new strategic line which does not pursue socialism and communism". However, most commentators agreed that the announcement of the dissolution was false and that the exercise was part of Chinese and Western efforts to garner support for the Pol Pot faction (by now commonly known as the *Khmers Rouges*, but officially described as the Party of Democratic Kampuchea) which had been widely criticized on account of its poor human rights record. Towards this end, in 1982 the *Khmers Rouges* joined with the two other groups opposing the Phnom Penh regime (the Khmer People's

National Liberation Front and the Sihanoukists) in the Coalition Government of Democratic Kampuchea (CGDK). Military activities against the Phnom Penh regime were henceforth carried out under the auspices of the CGDK, although most of the fighting was performed by *Khmer Rouges* troops. The CGDK also provided a credible front, especially in the person of Prince Norodom Sihanouk who presided over the coalition, for the diplomatic manouvering which accompanied the fighting.

The notorious *Khmer Rouges* government's human rights record meant that the party's leading role within the coalition was often concealed and attempts were constantly made to improve its international image. Hence, in 1985 it was announced that Son Sen, a relatively unknown party figure, had replaced Pol Pot as Chair of the party's Supreme Military Commission. In 1989 it was announced that Pol Pot had resigned his last official *Khmer Rouges* post as director for the Higher Institute for National Defence. At the same time it was announced that Ta Mok (Chhit Choeun), one of the most powerful and infamous *Khmer Rouges* officials, had retired. Commentators reacted to such announcements with great scepticism, maintaining that Pol Pot, in particular, continued to exercise considerable political and military influence and probably maintained the general secretaryship at the head of the party's clandestine structure.

With the withdrawal of Vietnamese forces from Cambodia in 1989, diplomatic efforts to resolve the civil war accelerated, but were also accompanied by a fresh *Khmer Rouges* offensive. However, in 1990, UN efforts to broker a comprehensive peace plan bore fruit with the creation of a Supreme National Council (SNC), a reconciliation body uniting the warring Cambodian factions. Khieu Samphan, Vice-President in the CGDK, and Son Sen, were chosen to represent the *Khmer Rouges* on the SNC, which also included officials from the Phnom Penh regime and the rival wing of the communist party. In October 1991 a UN peace agreement was finally signed providing for massive UN involvement in Cambodia prior to the holding of general elections scheduled for 1993. Under the terms of the agreement the *Khmer Rouges*, along with the Khmer People's National Liberation Front (KPNLF) and Sihanoukists, were officially established in cantonments in Phnom Penh prior to demobilization and the start of the political process leading to the holding of the elections.

An attempt in late 1991 by Khieu Samphan and Son Sen to return to Phnom Penh and establish the cantonment was briefly delayed when demonstrators attacked them. The *Khmer Rouges*, under the banner of the Party of Democratic Kampuchea, is expected to contest the forthcoming elections. According to some analysts *Khmer Rouges* cadres had infiltrated Cambodian villages and established political cells in preparation for the elections even prior to the signing of the UN peace agreement.

United Front for the Construction and Defence of the Kampuchean Fatherland

Address. Phnom Penh.

Leadership. Chea Sim (ch. of national council); Heng Samrin (ch., presidium); Ros Chhun (sec.-gen.).

Orientation. Mass organization which supported the policies of the former Kampuchean People's Revolutionary Party.

Founded. 1978.

History. Created (as the Kampuchean National United Front for Salvation) by members of the anti-Pol Pot wing of the Communist Party and with the support of Vietnam, the organization supported Vietnam's 1978 invasion of Cambodia. Four of the 14 members of the central committee were included in the People's Revolutionary Council, established as a provisional government in Phnom Penh following the overthrow of Pol Pot. At the Front's third congress held in 1981 it was renamed as the Kampuchean United Front for National Construction and Defence; the Front adopted its present name in 1989.

Structure. 89-member national council and seven-member honorary presidium.

United National Front for an Independent, Neutral, Peaceful and Co-operative Cambodia

Address. FUNCINPEC cantonment, Phnom Penh.

Leadership. Prince Norodom Rannarit (l.).

Orientation. Monarchist, nationalist and anti-communist.

Founded. 1982.

History. Prince Norodom Sihanouk announced the formation of United National Front for an Independent, Neutral, Peaceful and Co-operative Cambo-

dia (FUNCINPEC) in March 1982, as an apparent successor organization to his Confederation of Khmer Nationalists. The group effectively served as the political wing to the Prince's own armed forces, the Sihanoukist National Army (*Armee nationale sihanoukiste*, ANS; also known as the National Army of Independent Cambodia), which were part of the tripartite anti-Vietnamese Coalition Government of Democratic Kampuchea (CGDK) formed in 1982, with Sihanouk as its president. Militarily, the ANS was perhaps the weakest of the three constituent CGDK members and it had little success against forces loyal to the Vietnamese or Phnom Penh government.

Prince Sihanouk resigned as FUNCINPEC and ANS leader following his appointment in 1990 as head of the Supreme National Council (SNC), the all-faction body established to provide momentum to a UN peace plan for Cambodia. Sihanouk's position as FUNCINPEC leader was taken by his son, Prince Norodom Rannarit. However, despite Sihanouk's official declarations of neutrality as SNC Chair, FUNCINPEC remained a Sihanoukist organization, loyal to its founder and former leader. With the signing of the UN peace agreement in October 1991, FUNCINPEC was officially installed in Phnom Penh as one of the main political organizations expected to contest the UN supervised elections scheduled for 1993.

Parties in conflict with the government

The Sihanoukists, Khmer People's National Liberation Front and *Khmers Rouges* formed the **Coalition Government of Democratic Kampuchea** (CGDK) in 1982 in opposition to the Vietnamese-backed State of Cambodia (SOC) regime in power in Phnom Penh. The CGDK was renamed as the **National Government of Cambodia** (NGC) in early 1990. In September all three groups joined, along with the SOC government, a Supreme National Council. With the formation of the SOC and the signing of a comprehensive peace treaty between the four warring factions in October 1991, the NGC was effectively terminated.

China

Capital: Beijing **Population: 1,139,100,000 (1990 UNFPA estimate)**

The last Chinese imperial dynasty, the Manchu, was overthrown in the revolution of 1911-12 led by the nationalist party, the *Kuomintang* (KMT) [see entry for Taiwan]. A confused period of civil war followed, during which the country was fragmented between rival generals and the KMT government. The Japanese invasion of 1937-1945 temporarily dampened the conflict between the KMT and the growing Communist Party. Following Japan's defeat, however, the civil war continued and on Oct. 1, 1949, the People's Republic of China was proclaimed following the victory of the Communist Party forces.

Constitutional structure

Under the 1982 Constitution (China's fourth), China is "a socialist state under the people's democratic dictatorship". The highest body of state power is the National People's Congress (NPC), which convenes annually and, together with its permanent body, the 155-member Standing Committee, exercises legislative power. Executive power is vested in the State Council, appointed by the NPC. The 1982 Constitution restored the office of President of the Republic (head of state).

Although the 1982 Constitution makes no reference to the Chinese Communist Party (CCP) in its articles, its preamble proclaims the "leadership of the CCP and the guidance of Marxism-Leninism and Mao Zedong Thought". Effective political power is thus held by the CCP, despite the nominal participation of "democratic parties and people's organizations" in "a broad patriotic front" led by the CCP.

Electoral system

The 2,970 deputies of the NPC are indirectly elected for a five-year term by the People's Congresses of China's 22 provinces, five autonomous regions and three municipalities, and by the People's Liberation Army (PLA), which unites all armed services. The NPC elects the Standing Committee from among its members and also elects the President of the Republic. All candidates for the NPC are approved by the CCP.

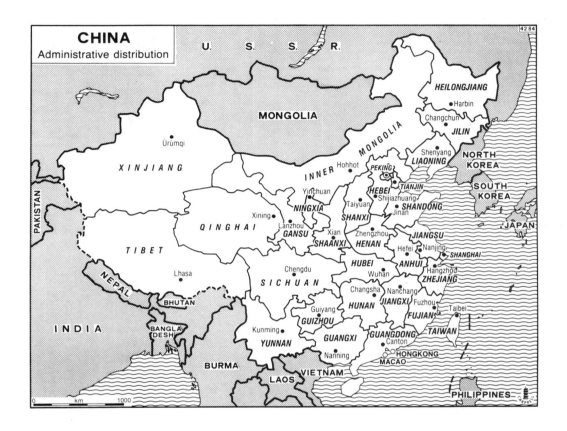

CHINA
Administrative distribution

42 84

U. S. S. R.

MONGOLIA

HEILONGJIANG

• Harbin

Changchun

JILIN

Ürümqi

XINJIANG

INNER MONGOLIA

Hohhot

PEKING

Shenyang

LIAONING

NORTH KOREA

SOUTH KOREA

JAPAN

PAKISTAN

Yinchuan

NINGXIA

HEBEI

TIANJIN

Taiyuan

Xining •

QINGHAI

Lanzhou

GANSU

SHANXI

Shijiazhuang

SHANDONG

Jinan

Xian

SHAANXI

Zhengzhou

HENAN

JIANGSU

Hefei

Nanjing

SHANGHAI

TIBET

Lhasa

Chengdu

SICHUAN

HUBEI

Wuhan

ANHUI

Hangzhou

ZHEJIANG

NEPAL

BHUTAN

Changsha

Nanchang

JIANGXI

Fuzhou

INDIA

BANGLA DESH

Guiyang

HUNAN

GUIZHOU

Kunming •

YUNNAN

Nanning

GUANGXI

GUANGDONG

Canton •

FUJIAN

Taibei •

TAIWAN

HONGKONG

MACAO

BURMA

LAOS

VIETNAM

PHILIPPINES

0   km   1000

Recent elections

Elections to the NPC were held between September 1987 and March 1988. Non-CCP candidates or members of Democratic Parties accounted for 18.2 per cent of the total elected deputies (540).

Evolution of the suffrage

All persons over 18, except the mentally ill and those stripped of their political rights, may vote.

PARTY BY PARTY DATA

Chinese Communist Party (CCP)

Zhongguo Gongchan Dang

Address. c\o CCP Central Committee, Beijing.

Leadership. Jiang Zemin (gen. sec); standing committee of the Politburo: Li Peng; Qiao Shi; Yao Yilan; Jiang Zemin; Song Ping; Li Ruihuan.

Orientation. Ruling party; its ideology centres on Marxism-Leninism—Mao Zedong Thought. The CCP's current core task remains economic construction while retaining tight political control.

Founded. July 1921.

History. The CCP was founded in 1921 at a conference in Shanghai attended by 11 delegates, representing 57 members. Among the delegates was Mao Zedong. Chinese students in France, including Zhou Enlai, simultaneously formed a Chinese Communist Party there. Encouraged by the 1917 Bolshevik revolution in Tsarist Russia, the CCP also drew support from China's patriotic "May 4th Movement", which had originated in the protests within China at the 1919 Treaty of Versailles ceding the German-leased port of Qingdao to Japan. The CCP initially put forward the programme of "science and democracy"; the popularization of Chinese culture; and the abolition of feudalism.

During the period following the revolution against the Manchu dynasty, led by the Nationalist Party (*Kuomintang*—KMT), co-operation between the KMT and CCP enabled CCP members to join the KMT as individuals. The KMT was at this time in receipt of Soviet aid, perceived as the protagonist of China's "bourgeois revolution". However, by the end of 1927, the CCP had 10,000 members, and, fearing its strength, the KMT's second leader, Gen. Chiang Kai-shek, ended inter-party co-operation and in March 1927 sanctioned the massacre of at least 5,000 workers in Shanghai. The workers, under CCP leadership, had taken the city from the Chinese warlords then fighting for control of the country. The CCP subsequently suffered attacks from KMT forces in five "bandit extermination campaigns" which were carried out between 1929 and 1935.

During the fifth campaign, the CCP, blockaded by KMT troops, was forced to break out of the "Chinese Soviet republic" which it had established on the Hunan-Jiangxi border, on what became known as the "Long March". Some 100,000 men, women and children marched for over a year to reach north Shaanxi, but only about one-fifth arrived.

A CCP conference held during the Long March in January 1935 elected Mao Zedong as party chair—a post he retained until his death on Sept. 9, 1976. Mao had become leader of the "Chinese Soviet Republic" in 1931. During the 1920s, power struggles in the CCP had centred on the role of the peasantry. As head of the party's peasant department since 1926, Mao suggested that China's peasantry formed a considerable revolutionary force, whereas the more orthodox Marxist views held by CCP General Secretary Chen Tu-hsiu considered the industrial proletariat to be the leaders of socialist revolution. However, Chen was removed from his post in August 1927, and support among the peasantry for the CCP, and concurrently for Mao, increased.

The Japanese invasion of China in 1937 forced the KMT to declare a "united front" with the CCP. The CCP had in fact declared war on Japan as early as 1932, after the Japanese had overrun Manchuria, although this was more a propaganda exercise than a serious challenge. Chiang Kai-shek was keener to fight the CCP than the Japanese and co-operation between the two parties collapsed in 1941. At the end of the Second World War, the CCP controlled the north of China, and, despite United States efforts at mediation, civil war again broke out between the CCP and KMT forces in 1946. Victory for the CCP in what was largely a guerrilla war against militarily superior forces came in 1949. Subsequently the People's Republic of China (PRC) was proclaimed in Beijing and KMT forces fled to the offshore island of Taiwan. In the newly formed PRC, Mao Zedong became head of state and Zhou Enlai Prime Minister.

The new leadership pursued policies which centred on economic reconstruction after the ravages of invasion and civil war. This gained popular support for the CCP. Land reforms redistributed land equally and a system of mutual aid and then co-operatives soon developed in the agrarian sphere. Meanwhile, China's involvement in the Korean War (1950-53), while intensifying the country's economic problems, also raised the government's prestige. China's first five-year plan (1953-57) concentrated on the development of heavy industry along the lines of Soviet economic practice: although agriculture had been collectivized, industry had remained in the private sphere. Joint state-private ownership over enterprises was introduced in 1956, and a more rapid collectivization of agriculture was then introduced, at the insistence of Mao.

The more moderate approach of the early years of CCP rule changed in the late 1950s when, in 1958, the "Great Leap Forward" (GLF) was launched. Cancelling the programmes of the Second Five Year Plan adopted the previous year, the GLF embodied Mao's belief that inspired leadership by the CCP would encourage the population to increase economic output, without the need for capital investment. Mao appeared to believe that this putative revolutionary enthusiasm would bring greater economic success than the more bureacratized Soviet system. However, the economic disaster precipitated by the GLF has been estimated to have caused as many as 37,000,000 deaths through famine. Economic production statistics were inflated to an even greater extent than the normal "figure padding" endemic to a planned economy because of CCP cadres' desire to compete for high output figures. In December 1958 the Central Committee adopted a resolution admitting that there had been mistakes in the implementation of the GLF. Nevertheless, the policy continued into 1959, and in July 1959, Minister of Defence Marshal Peng Dehuai, who had severely criticized the "Great Leap", was dismissed on Mao's insistence.

A brief interlude of intellectual openness had preceded the GLF when Mao, in a speech in May 1956, called for open criticism of the CCP. The "Hundred Flowers" movement took its name from Mao's slogan "Let a hundred flowers bloom, let a hundred schools of thought contend". The policy had been influenced by the Soviet Communist Party's criticism of their recently deceased leader Josef Stalin in Nikita Khrushchev's "secret speech" of 1956. In early 1957, the Chinese campaign took its ideological justification from Mao's distinction between "antagonistic" contradictions between "ourselves and the enemy" and "non-antagonistic" "contradictions among the people" which could be resolved by popular involvement in politics. After a slow start because of fears that the campaign to criticize the CCP would be reversed, the

enthusiastic response did indeed reverse the policy, and in June 1957 an "anti-rightist" campaign against critics of the regime was initiated. Over 1,000,000 CCP members intellectuals were expelled or reprimanded.

Meanwhile, internal CCP manoeuvring in this period had sought to reduce Mao's political power. The new CCP constitution adopted at the eighth party congress in 1956 omitted the references to "Mao Zedong Thought"; the post of General Secretary (vacant since 1937) was resuscitated for Deng Xiaoping and the Standing Committee of the Politburo was created to function as a collective leadership.

Mao withdrew from domestic policy in 1958-59, ostensibly to concentrate on ideological matters, chief among which was the Sino-Soviet dispute. Soviet aid to China was withdrawn in 1960 and relations between them were broken off in 1966. Meanwhile Deng Xiaoping, Zhou Enlai and Liu Shaoqi, Mao's successor as head of state, directed economic recovery from the disaster of the "Great Leap Forward". However, their more liberal policies, together with the 1956 upheavals in eastern Europe and Mao's doubts about the Soviet leadership, encouraged his growing conviction that a country could experience a restoration of capitalism even after a socialist revolution. To combat this, Mao launched the Great Proletarian Cultural Revolution in May 1966.

Mao by this time had the support of the PLA, largely thanks to the policies pursued by Peng Dehuai's replacement as Defence Minister, Marshal Lin Biao. Lin had elevated the study of "Mao Zedong Thought" in the armed forces and emphasised their role as a "people's army" in contrast to the professional forces active in the Soviet Union. Thus the PLA cadres in the early 1960's spread a cult of Mao and his ideology. The Cultural Revolution took the form of a campaign against "party leaders in authority taking the capitalist road" and against the "four olds"—old ideas, customs, culture and habits. This campaign was carried out largely by the Red Guards: units formed of school and university students who were guided by the Cultural Revolution Group of the Central Committee, including Mao's wife, Jiang Qing. The aim of the Cultural Revolution, it was stated at the 11th Plenum of the Central Committee in August 1966, was "to revolutionize people's ideology and as a consequence to achieve greater, faster, better and more economical results in all fields of work". However, the reforms in fields such as public health and education soon disintegrated into virtual anarchy as rival groups fought for the right to be considered true followers of "Mao Zedong Thought", and the casualties included high-level CCP members, such as Liu Shaoqi and Deng Xiaoping. The PLA was the only organization in the country with an effective chain of command, and in September 1967 it was ordered to restore order. The Red Guards were finally disbanded in 1968.

The Cultural Revolution played itself out in factional struggles in the top leadership. The Ninth Party Congress was convened in 1969 as Mao called for a reconstruction of the CCP. Dominated by the PLA, although including also pre-Cultural Revolutionary leaders and newly promoted leaders, the Congress heard Lin Biao deliver the CC report and adopted a new party constitution, naming him as Mao's successor. The new constitution also abolished the post of General Secretary and revived references to Mao Zedong Thought. Lin Biao died in 1971; the improbable official explanation of his death was that his plane had crashed over Mongolia as he was trying to flee to the Soviet Union after plotting a coup against Mao. Lin's death opened the way for the rehabilitation of many leaders disgraced during the Cultural Revolution, chief among them being Deng Xiaoping, who in 1975 became First Deputy Prime Minister and Chief of General Staff, and in effect assumed many of the responsibilities of Zhou Enlai, already terminally ill. After Lin's death, a confusing campaign, led by the radical proponents of the Cultural Revolution, began to vilify the reformist wing.

However, the reformers had support among the population, and when Zhou died in January 1976, public demonstrations in his memory took place in major cities during April, the traditional Chinese festival for commemorating the dead. A serious disturbance in Beijing on April 5 became known as the "Tiananmen incident". Labelled "counter revolutionary" at a meeting of the CC, it was then used to disgrace Deng Xiaoping, who was condemned as the instigator of the disturbance and stripped of his posts. Nevertheless, on Mao's death in September 1976 the cultural revolutionary radicals still in power were left undefended and in October Jiang Qing and three associates in the Politburo (together known as the "gang of four") were arrested, along with six others. They were sentenced in January 1981, most of them to imprisonment and Jiang and Zhang Chinqiao to death. They were not executed, but Jiang committed suicide in May 1991.

Mao was briefly succeeded as CCP Chair and Chair of the Central Military Commission by Hua Guofeng, who had succeeded Zhou as Prime Minister in February 1976. While committed to modernization, Hua could not negate the Cultural Revolution or the verdict of the "Tiananmen incident" without undermining his own position, since he had personally benefited from both events. Citing Mao Zedong as the guiding principle in an attempt to retain prestige, Hua's faction became known as the "whateverists".

Deng Xiaoping had been restored to his former posts in July 1977. In December 1978, at the Third Plenum of the Central Committee of the 11th Congress of the CCP, Deng emerged as the new leader, and the "whateverists" were criticized. Economic reforms were adopted. These were intended to rebalance the economy, severely skewed due to Hua's programme, announced in early 1978, to modernize the country by 1985. The policies adopted at the Third Plenum were still cited in 1992 as having established the guiding principles for China's modernization. The theoretical influences of the Cultural Revolution were countered by policies which elevated "socialist modernization" as the guiding principle to replace "class struggle", while pragmatism or "seeking truth from facts" became the guiding ideology.

However, a popular movement for democracy—"the 5 April Movement" named after the "Tiananmen incident"—which Deng had encouraged before the Plenum, was crushed after Deng had safely assumed leadership as no longer of use to the reformers. In early 1979, Deng proclaimed the "four cardinal principles" which were to serve as the limits of change and tolerance of popular demands. Still cited in 1992, despite being extra-Constitutional, these were (i) the leadership of the CCP; (ii) the socialist road; (iii) the dominance of Marxism-Leninism and Mao Zedong Thought; and (iv) the people's democratic dictatorship or the dictatorship of the proletariat. Further exorcism of the Cultural Revolution took the form of a revision of CCP history, produced in 1981. Mao was criticized for excessive personal power and "leftism" in his last years, although the final analysis of his life was, naturally, positive. The Cultural Revolution was condemned as a disaster, based on a mistaken theory which took no account of reality.

Meanwhile, Deng Xiaoping's faction assumed leadership; Hua Guofeng was replaced as Prime Minister by Zhao Ziyang in 1980, and in 1981 Hu Yaobang, former Secretary-General of the Politburo, took over as CCP Chairman. Deng took on Hua's post as Chair of the Central Military Commission. Hua was excluded from the Politburo in September 1982. Also in September 1982 the CCP's 12th Congress consolidated the ascendency of Deng's party. The office of CCP Chairman was abolished and Hu Yaobang became General Secretary with increased powers. A Central Advisory Commission was established for leaders with 40 years of CCP membership, thus ending the practice of life tenure for senior posts. A three-year "rectification programme", launched in October 1983, aimed to wipe out the traces of the Cultural Revolution and expose "Maoists" who had benefited from it. The new Constitution was adopted in December 1982, restoring the post of Head of State (abolished in 1975). In September 1985 the first CCP national delegate conference for 40 years was held with the aim of rejuvenating the central leadership. The result was the appointment of some younger and better educated Central Committee members, believed to support Deng Xiaoping, who retained all his posts, despite his advanced age.

Although economic reform was relatively successful in the 1980s, producing an average annual growth of about 10 per cent, institutional modernization was less so. The continued commitment to socialism and continued central guidance and political control of enterprises was at odds with the shift to market forces in economic reform. The CCP found difficulty in adapting to the new social conditions generated by greater prosperity and a less centralized economy. Corruption and nepotism, prevalent in all levels of the CCP, also undermined its authority. In 1986 intellectuals began to question the policies and ways of working of the CCP, even to the extent of calling for a more Western-style democracy in China. Student demonstrations in late 1986 in major cities demanded greater democracy. However, the CCP launched a campaign against "bourgeois liberalization" in 1987 and prohibited the demonstrations as a threat to public order. The sixth plenary session of the 12th CCP Central Committee in September 1986 had defined "bourgeois liberalization" as "the negation of the socialist system in favour of capitalism", and one of the first casualties of the new campaign was Hu Yaobang who resigned in January 1987.

However, Prime Minister Zhao Ziyang assumed the post of acting General Secretary, in which he was formally confirmed at the 13th CCP Congress on Oct. 25-Nov. 1, 1987, and the Congress was used as a platform by Deng's reformist group to reaffirm their predominance over the conservatives. Deng was re-elected as Chair of the Central Military Commission, although he resigned from the Politburo's Standing Committee. A younger, better educated Central Committee was appointed. The main speech by Zhao Ziyang formulated the ideological justification for continued economic reforms, while still ensuring the leading role of the CCP. The speech postulated that because China was economically underdeveloped when socialist rule had begun, it still had to undergo forms of economic development experienced by other countries under capitalism. Thus the implementation of market forces and economic co-operation with foreign countries could be justified, while ideological direction by the CCP meant that China would assuredly remain a socialist country.

Economic reform was thereby sanctioned, but the demand for further political reform was not satisfied, and on Hu Yaobang's death on April 15, 1989, student demonstrations began once more, perceiving in Hu a symbol of political liberalism. The demonstrations in Beijing were allowed to grow until a condemnatory editorial was published in the *Renmin Ribao* (People's Daily) on April 26, clearly under the orders of the central leadership. However, the editorial failed to stop the students who were joined by workers and intellectuals in Tiananmen Square in Beijing. This new development represented a more serious challenge to the leadership. Similar demonstrations were held in 21 other Chinese cities. The demonstrations coincided with the visit of Soviet President Mikhail Gorbachev on May 15-18, which marked the normalization of relations between China and the Soviet Union. Gorbachev's presence was important for the demonstrators as a symbol of the political reforms introduced in the Soviet Union under his leadership. On May 30, the demonstrators erected a replica of the Statue of Liberty, naming it the "Goddess of Democracy". On June 3-4 soldiers and tanks of the PLA were ordered to clear the square. Up to 1,000 people are thought to have died.

A conservative backlash followed the crushing of the demonstration. A group of CCP veterans, some of whom no longer held senior party posts yet still voted at "enlarged" Politburo meetings, were believed to have influenced the decision to suppress the pro-democracy movement. At a plenary session of the CCP Central Committee on June 23-24, Zhao Ziyang, who had appeared to show sympthy for the demonstrators' demands, and other prominent reformers were dismissed from their party posts. Jiang Zemin became the new CCP General Secretary, and the Standing Committee of the Politburo was enlarged to six seats. At the fifth Plenary session of the 13th CCP Central Committee on Oct. 30-Nov.3, 1989, Deng resigned from his last official post, that of Chair of the Central Military Commission, to be replaced by Jiang.

The social aftermath of the Tiananmen Square massacre centred on a CCP-led attempt at the reindoctrination of Chinese youth, in addition to political trials and the repression of dissidents which caused condemnation of China by human rights organizations. In the economic sphere, the policies of austerity and retrenchment which initially accompanied the political repression were relaxed in mid-1990 when it was realized that China's fragile economic prosperity was being jeopardized. In 1991, some of the top leadership who had been demoted for their support of Zhao Ziyang, were rehabilitated. Nevertheless, the impact of the massacre was still evident in 1992, when, on the third anniversary of the crushing of the pro-democracy movement, new regulations were published which tightened still further the restrictions on demonstrations, imposed in the immediate aftermath of the Tiananmen Square affair.

However, by 1992 there were signs that at least in the economic sphere, the reformers were once more gaining strength. The most prominent indication of this was a tour of southern China which Deng Xiaoping made during January—his first public appearance for over a year. An enlarged meeting of the Politburo on Feb. 12, 1992, heard Jiang Zemin read out the speeches made by Deng during his January tour. By the end of February, the speeches had been consolidated into a document for study among CCP work groups.

The CCP document codifying Deng's speeches effectively followed the line adopted by the Third Plenum of the 11th CCP Central Committee in 1978 [see above]. In the political sphere, the response to the "turmoil" (the pro-democracy movement) had been correct, for had the leadership "failed the test" of June 4, 1989 "there would have been a chaotic situation which might have led to a civil war". However, the country remained stable after the "4th June incident" because "reform and opening" had "improved the people's livelihood". On ideology, Deng insisted that China should "mainly guard against leftism" and should "seek truth from facts" rather than in formalism and ideology. "Rightism", however, was also a danger, as the "turmoil", which was "a rightist thing", had exemplified. Deng's four cardinal principles limiting political reform, first codified in 1979 [see above] must still be observed. Economic reform should centre on "building socialism with Chinese characteristics", but Deng gave explicit approval to absorbing the economic methods and institutions traditionally associated with capitalism in order to boost "the development of the socialist productive forces". As part of this, the special economic zones (SEZ) should be used as an engine to drive the economy of other areas. Asia's "four little dragons" were countries which China should seek to emulate and surpass. On the succession to the leadership, Deng noted: "As long as we, the older generation, are still around and still carry weight, the hostile forces know they cannot change things". However, "if problems should arise in China they will come from within the Communist Party". The training and recruiting of cadres was therefore of great importance.

In the first six months of 1992, Deng's reformist line appeared to be carrying the day against the anti-reform faction led by economist Chen Yun, although not without a struggle. The lack of unanimity among the leadership was demonstrated at the NPC session in March-April 1992, when Prime Minister, Li Peng, delivered the government's work report. He warned of the potential for an "ideological trend towards bourgeois liberalization". However, in a speech relayed to the public on June 14, Jiang endorsed the economic reforms championed by Deng and criticized "leftists" (conservatives) for using revolutionary slogans to "confuse the people".

Structure. Primary cells exist in the workplace, the armed forces and in the place of residence. CCP organizations are then structured in a pyramid, rising to the National Congress. Nominally meeting every five years, this elects the Central Committee (CC), which consisted of 175 full members and 108 alternate, ie.non-voting, members in 1988. The Politburo exercises plenary powers of the CC when the latter is not in session. The CC appointed 17 full members and one alternate member to the Politburo in 1988. Within the Politburo, a standing committee is considered to be the collective leadership of the party. The post of General Secretary applies only to the CC and not the whole party, in contrast to the now defunct Soviet Communist Party.

Membership. 50,320,000.

Publications. Renmin Ribao (People's Daily) circulation 5,000,000; *Guangming Ribao* (Enlightenment Daily) circulation 1,500,000; *Beijing Ribao* (Beijing Daily); *Jiefang Ribao* (Liberation Daily), *Nanfang Ribao* (Southern Daily): regional newspapers for Beijing, Shanghai and Guangdon areas, each with a circulation of 1,000,000; *Ban Yue Tan* fortnightly magazine, published by CCP propaganda department; *Qiushi* (Seek Truth) theoretical, monthly.

Other parties

Other parties in China exist on a "united front" basis together with the CCP. Officially, they are recognized as having co-operated with the CCP in the "war of resistance" against Japan (1937-1945) and the "war of liberation" against the *Kuomintang* and as having participated in negotiations over the formation of the PRC in 1949. They were accepted by Mao Zedong's policy of "long-term coexistence and mutual supervision" between the CCP and other parties. They were, however, suppressed during the Cultural Revolution.

The "democratic parties" are essentially powerless: although customarily about 7 per cent of seats in the NPC are held by "democratic parties'" representatives, all candidates for the NPC must be vetted by the CCP. The parties are officially characterized as "political alliances of socialist workers" and "patriots who support socialism". The "bourgeoisie", the "intelligentsia" and "other patriotic people" are said to form the social base of the "democratic parties".

China Association for Promoting Democracy (CAPD)
Zhongguo Minzhu Cujin Hui
Address. 98 Xinanli Guloufangzhuangchang, Beijing 100009.
Leadership. Lei Jiequiong (ch.); Chen Yiqun (sec.-gen.).
Orientation. The CAPD "devotes itself to building China into a socialist country with its own characteristics" and believes that "education should take priority in economic development strategy".
Founded. 1945.
History. The Association's membership is drawn mainly from literary and cultural circles and workers in education. Its sixth National Congress, held on Nov. 19-28, 1988, was attended by over 500 delegates and adopted a new party constitution.
Structure. A national congress elects a central committee and its chair. There is an honorary chair and nine vice-chairs of the central committee.
Membership. 40,000.

China Democratic League (CDL)
Zhongguo Munzhu Tongmeng (Minmeng)
Address. 1 Beixing Dongchang Hutong, Beijing 100006.
Leadership. Fei Xiaotong (ch.); Wu Xiuping (sec.-gen.).
Orientation. To "promote socialist democracy" and to

work closely with the Chinese Communist Party (CCP).
Founded. 1941.
History. The CDL is the reorganized League of Democratic Parties and Organizations of China, which united intellectuals against the *Kuomintang*'s policies and fought against the Japanese with CCP support. It was forcibly dissolved in China in 1947. Currently its membership consists of intellectuals engaged in science, education and culture. The sixth National Congress was held on Oct. 8-16, 1988, attended by 880 delegates. CDL chair, Fei Xiaotong, is deputy chair of the National People's Congress Standing Committee. In September 1988, the CDL proposed establishing a multi-ethnic economic development zone in the upper Yellow river region in north-west China.
Structure. A five-yearly National Congress elects a Central Committee, which elects the CDL chair. There are 14 vice-chairs.
Membership. 80,000.
Publications. *Popular Voice* monthly.

China National Democratic Construction Association (CDNCA)
Zhongguo Minzhu Jianguo Hui
Address. 93 Beiheyan Dajie, 100006 Beijing.
Leadership. Sun Qimeng (ch.); Feng Kexu (sec.-gen.).
Orientation. Co-operation with the Chinese Communist Party (CCP); "the reunification of the motherland"; to "strive to turn China into a modern socialist country".
Founded. 1945.
History. The Association's membership is drawn mainly from industrialists and businessmen. The fifth national congress was held on June 16-28, 1988. Reporting on recent work, Sun Qimeng said that the CDNCA had offered an information service to enterprises, helped to introduce advanced technology into China and strengthened contacts with overseas Chinese. It had witnessed rapid growth in recent years.
Structure. A quinquennial national congress elects a central committee and its chair. There is an honorary chair of the CDNCA and nine deputy chairs of the national congress.
Membership. 42,000.

Party for Public Interests (PPI)
Zhongguo Zhi Gong Dang
Address. Beijing.
Leadership. Dong Yinchu (ch.); Wang Songda (sec.-gen.).

Orientation. "Reform and construction under the banner of socialism and patriotism". Fights for the "reunification" of China.

Founded. 1925.

History. Inaugurated in San Francisco in 1925, the PPI was reorganized in 1947 in Hong Kong when its members, mostly overseas Chinese, were re-registered. The ninth National Congress was held on Dec. 12-18, 1988. The report by Dong Yinchu said that over 1,500 party members had served as deputies to legislative bodies since 1983.

Structure. A national congress elects a central committee, which in turn elects a chair and deputy chairs (currently six, one of whom is the Secretary General).

Membership. 8,000.

Chinese Peasants' and Workers' Democratic Party (CPWDP)

Zhongguo Nonggong Minzhudang

Leadership. Lu Jiaxi (ch.); Zhang Shiming (sec.-gen.).

Orientation. Co-operation with the Chinese Communist Party (CCP); active in the fields of health and education reform.

Founded. 1930.

History. The CPWDP was founded as the Provisional Action Committee of the nationalist party, the *Kuomintang* (KMT), and took its present name in 1947. In the interim it was called the Action Committee for the Liberation of the Chinese Nation. It failed to overthrow KMT leader Chiang Kai-shek, and its founder was murdered in 1931. In 1935, the CPWDP abandoned its aim of founding a republic led by the bourgeoisie and collaborated with the Chinese Communist Party (CCP) in the Chinese revolution. Its membership consists mainly of senior doctors, scientists and professors.

Structure. A quinquennial national congress elects a central committee and its chair. There is an honorary chair and currently eight deputy chairs, one of whom is the secretary-general.

Membership. 46,000.

Revolutionary Committee of the Chinese Kuomintang (RCCK)

Zhongguo Guomindang Geming Weiyuanhui

Leadership. Zhu Xuefan (ch.); Peng Quingyuan (sec.-gen.).

Orientation. The RCCK aims "to promote the peaceful reunification of the motherland".

Founded. January 1948.

History. The Committee was formed in Hong Kong by

Kuomintang (KMT) members opposed to the policies of Chiang Kai-shek and in support of Chinese Communist Party (CCP) resistence to the Japanese invasion. Its membership embraces former KMT members and workers in health, finance, culture and education. A new constitution adopted at the seventh national congress on Nov. 12-20, 1988, described the RCCK as a "democratic party. . . carrying forward Dr. Sun Yat-sen's patriotic and revolutionary spirit in leading RCCK patriots at home and abroad in striving for a united and vibrant China".

Structure. A quinquennial national nongress elects a central committee and its chair. There are currently eight deputy chairs of whom one is the secretary general, and an honorary chair.

Membership. 38,000.

Publications. Unity, biweekly.

Taiwan Democratic Self-Government League (TDSGL)

Taiwan Minzhu Zizhi Tongmeng

Leadership. Cai Zimin (ch.); Pan Yuanjing (sec.-gen.).

Orientation. To promote contact between China and Taiwan and work for China's "reunification".

Founded. 1947.

History. The TDSGL was founded by Chinese from Taiwan who had gone to Hong Kong. Cai Zimin was elected chair of the central committee (CC) presidium at the second plenum of the fourth CC on Dec. 12-18, 1988, replacing Lin Shengzhong. The TDSGL hosts delegations from Taiwan and aims to attract investment from Taiwanese enterprises.

Structure. A quinquennial national congress elects a central committee. The chair of the CC presidium heads the party.

Jiusan (September 3) Society

Leadership. Zhou Peiyuan (ch.); Zhao Weizhi (sec.-gen.).

Orientation. Improve the development of science and technology and the education system.

Founded. 1946.

History. Originally the Democracy and Science Forum, established by scholars in Sichuan, the Society was renamed in commemoration of the victory over Japan (Sept. 3, 1945). The fifth national congress on Dec. 31, 1988-Jan. 8, 1989, approved a new constitution which emphasised the Society's role as a political party for the intelligentsia. Its membership is drawn principally from scientists and technologists in all fields. The eighth central committee elected four honorary chairs.

Structure. A quinquennial national congress elects a central committee, the chair of which heads the party.

Major guerrilla organizations

There are no guerrilla organizations in China.

Federated States of Micronesia

Capital: Pohnpei Island   **Population: 91,440 (1985)**

The Federated States of Micronesia (FSM) comprises more than 600 islands spread 2,900 km across the Caroline Islands' archipelago. Originally one of the four constituent elements of the UN Trust Territory of the Pacific created in 1947, the FSM signed a Compact of Free Association with the USA in 1982 which gave the country internal self-government and US economic aid in return for continuing US control of its defence and foreign policies. The US declared the Trusteeship terminated in 1986, but this was not endorsed by the Security Council until Dec. 22, 1990. With the termination of Trust status, the FSM became an independent state. It joined the United Nations in September 1991.

Constitutional structure

The FSM has four constituent states—Chuuk (formerly Truk), Kosrae, Pohnpei and Yap—each of which has its own government. Executive authority is vested in a President, who is elected by the 14-member federal legislature, and an appointed Cabinet. Legislative authority is vested in the unicameral National Congress of the Federated States of Micronesia, composed of 10 senators elected for two-year terms, and four at-large senators (one from each state) who are elected for four years.

Each of the country's four states has its own constitution providing for an elected Governor and a unicameral state legislature, the members of which are elected for a four-year term.

Electoral system

Members of the federal and state legislatures are popularly elected. Both President and Vice-President are elected by the National Congress from among the four at-large senators and, therefore, cannot come from the same sate.

Evolution of suffrage

Since independence the FSM has functioned on the basis of universal adult suffrage.

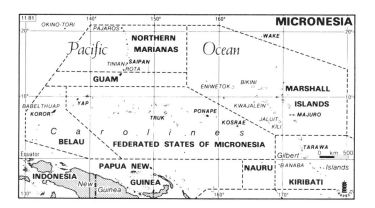

Recent elections

Legislative elections were held on March 5, 1991, when John R. Haglelgam, who had been president since 1987, failed to secure re-election as the at-large Senator for Yap. The country's vice president, Hirosi Ismael, was also defeated in his bid to win re-election as the at-large Senator for Kosrae.

The National Congress met on May 11, 1991, and unanimously elected Bailey Olter, 59, a native of the state of Pohnpei to the presidency. Jacob Nena, 49, of Kosrae, was elected Vice President.

PARTY BY PARTY DATA

There are no formally constituted political parties in the Federated States of Micronesia. Political allegiances tend to derive from family or geographical ties.

Major guerrilla groups

There are no guerrilla groups operating in the FSM.

Fiji

Capital: Suva

Population: 800,000 (1990 UNFPA est.)

Discovered by Europeans in the 17th century, Fiji became a British possession in 1874, and an independent country within the Commonwealth in 1970, under a constitution which provided that the head of state was the British sovereign, represented by a Governor-General, who would appoint the Prime Minister and Cabinet in accordance with the wishes of the bicameral Fijian Parliament. The Alliance Party (which represented the native Melanesian population) governed the country from independence, but was defeated in the general election of April 1987. The new government was composed from an alliance between the multiracial Fiji Labour Party, and the National Federation Party, which was closely allied to the interests of those of Indian extraction who slightly outnumbered the Melanesian population.

On May 14, 1987, there was a coup led by Lt.-Col. (subsequently Maj.-Gen.) Sitiveni Rabuka, and supported by the (predominantly Melanesian) armed forces, which involved the detention of the new government and the establishment of a military regime. Although civilian government was later restored, Rabuka and his supporters remained influential within the Council of Advisors which was established as an interim administration by the Governor-General, *Ratu* Sir Penaia Ganilau. An agreement in September to create a racially bipartisan administration, as a prelude to returning the country to full democracy, prompted Rabuka to stage a second coup on Sept. 25. On Oct. 1 he announced that the constitution had been revoked and on Oct. 6 declared the Republic of Fiji. Queen Elizabeth II accepted the resignation of *Ratu* Ganilau on Oct. 15, and thereby ceased to be Fiji's head of state. The country was returned nominally to civilian rule on Dec. 5, when *Ratu* Ganilau was sworn in as President, and in January 1990 the last Army officers, including Rabuka, left the administration. A new constitution which guaranteed Melanesian control of the legislature was promulgated in July 1990, and elections were held in May 1992.

Constitutional structure

Under the constitution promulgated on July 25, 1990, Fiji is described as a "sovereign, democratic republic". Executive power is vested in a President who is appointed by the Great Council of Chiefs—*Bose Levu Vakaturaga*, a traditional structure consisting of some 100 Melanesian leaders which constitutes the country's traditional forum of Melanesian authority—for a five-year term, and who serves as head of state and commander-in-chief of the armed forces. A Presidential Council advises the President, who is also equipped with wide emergency powers. The President appoints as Prime Minister (who must be of Melanesian race), the party leader from among the legislature who is most likely to command a Parliamentary majority. The Prime Minister governs in conjunction with an appointed Cabinet.

Legislative power is in the hands of a bicameral Parliament consisting of an elected 70-member House of Representatives, wherein a majority of seats are reserved for those of Melanesian race, and an appointed Senate containing 34 members (24 of whom must be Melanesians) who are chosen on the advice of the Great Council of Chiefs. The Senate acts as a reviewing chamber, with some powers to initiate legislation but limited influence on financial matters. The maximum duration of a Parliament is five years.

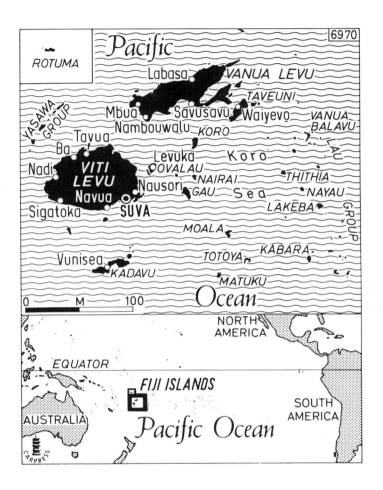

Recent elections

From independence until 1987 elections were held regularly and power was retained by the Melanesian-dominated Alliance Party. The party's monopoly on government was broken at the election of April 1987 by a coalition between the National Federation Party and the Labour Party, but the new government was overthrown by a military coup in May.

Election Date	Winning party
April 1972	Alliance Party
March-April 1977	Alliance Party
September 1977	Alliance Party
July 1982	Alliance Party
April 1987	NFP-Labour Party coalition*
May 1992	Coalition led by Fijian Political Party

*Overthrown by military coup, May 1987.

General election, May 23-30, 1992

Party	Seats won
Fijian Political Party	30
Fijian Nationalist United Front	5
National Federation Party	14
Fiji Labour Party	13
General Voters' Party	5
Independents	3

Electoral system

Of the 70 seats in the House of Representatives, 37 are reserved for, and elected by, Melanesian Fijians. A further 27 are reserved for, and elected by, those of Indian extraction. One seat is reserved for the inhabitants of Rotuma Island, and the remaining five for "General Voters", those members of the electorate—including those of European extraction—who are not covered in any of the other categories. Within the Senate 24 seats are reserved for Melanesians, one for a Rotuman (appointed on the advice of the Rotuma Island Council) and the remaining nine to be appointed at the President's discretion.

The electoral system also weights Melanesian representation disproportionately in favour of the rural communities (dominated by traditional chiefs) as against urban areas. In elections to the House, Melanesians vote in five single-member urban constituencies and 14 multimember rural ones.

Evolution of suffrage

Universal adult suffrage, with a voting age of 21 years, was introduced in 1966. The first women permitted to vote did so in the election of 1963.

PARTY BY PARTY DATA

Fijian Political Party
Soqosoqo ni Vakavulewa ni Taukei (SVT)
Address. c/o House of Representatives, Suva, Fiji.
Leadership. Maj.-Gen. Sitiveni Rabuka (pres).
Orientation. Melanesian supremacist

Founded. June 1990.

History. In March 1990 the Great Council of Chiefs proposed the creation of a Fijian Political Party (FPP), which was designed to unite the native Melanesian vote and thereby exploit the racial bias of the new constitution and secure a majority within the legislature. The leader of the two 1987 military coups, Lt.-Col. Sitiveni Rabuka, immediately expressed his interest in leading the new party. He made no secret of his political ambitions—in July 1991 he left the armed forces when forced to choose between his military and his political careers—nor of his belief that the new FPP offered that best channel through which this ambition might be realised. The majority of the chiefs wanted someone more pliant and more deferential to the traditional hierarchies which the Great Council represented. Nevertheless, at the FPP's first national convention, held at the end of October 1991, Rabuka was elected president of the new party. In the process he defeated two senior chiefs of far greater traditional status: *Adi* Lady Lala Mara, wife of the interim Prime Minister *Ratu* Sir Kamisese Mara, and a chief in her own right, and *Ratu* William Toganivalu.

Rabuka took his new position very seriously and, in accordance with Prime Minister Mara's injunction that serving Cabinet members could not lead political parties, Rabuka resigned as Deputy Prime Minister and Minister of Home Affairs with effect from Dec. 1. Thereafter he concentrated exclusively on his duties as FPP leader. In addition to wooing the Fijian electorate in advance of the elections, Rabuka also struck up a dialogue with a range of other parties and openly acknowledged that it might be necessary to form a coalition government of "national unity". In the event, the FPP stood candidates in all 37 of the seats reserved for Melanesians, and won 30 of them.

Although it was clear that the FPP had won the election, the party's constitution provided for separate posts of party president and parliamentary leader, and so it was not immediately clear that Rabuka would become Prime Minster. In the event he resisted a challenge by Josefata Kamikamica, the Finance Minister in the outgoing Mara government (who was believed to be the preferred choice of both Mara and President Ganilau), and demonstrated to the President that he had the support of 26 of the 30 FPP representatives.

Rabuka was sworn in as Prime Minister in early June, having negotiated the support of the General Voters Party (GVP) and two independents. Although he favoured including the Fijian Nationalist United Front (FNUF) within his coalition, this proposal was rejected by his FPP colleagues. He had also managed to win an endorsement from Fiji Labour Party leader Mahendra Chaudhry, in return for a promise of an early review of the constitution and several other key issues including land tenure and trade union legislation.

Following the agreement, Rabuka stated that "no longer am I promoting the aspirations we had in 1987; now it is for all races in Fiji". His new Cabinet gave two portfolios to the GVP and also included two independents, one of whom was the representative for Rotuma who had been elected unopposed. Kamikamica was not included in the 19-member Cabinet.

Fiji Labour Party

Address. c/o House of Representatives, Suva, Fiji.
Leadership. Mahendra Chaudhry.
Orientation. Social-Democratic and multiracial. The FLP supports a non-aligned, anti-nuclear foreign policy, together with social, economic and land reforms, including the nationalization of some industries.
Founded. 1985.
History. The Fiji Labour Party (FLP) was formed by labour activists, including James Raman, general secretary of the Fijian Trades Union Congress, and the was the successor of the National Labour and Farmers' Party formed in 1982. Under the leadership of Timoci Bavadra (a Fijian of Melanesian descent), the new party quickly grew and acquired representation in the legislature through the defection of three National Federation Party (NFP) members and a member of the Western United Front (WUF). It also polled strongly in the November 1985 Suva city council elections. The FLP allied itself with the NFP and the WUF in late 1986, thereby providing the predominantly Indian NFP with much greater credibility among Melanesian electors. This coalition won 28 of the 52 seats in the election of April 1987, and Bavadra duly became Prime Minister at the head of the country's first predominantly Indian government. The government was overthrown by the first Rabuka coup, in May, and Bavadra and his colleagues were briefly detained by the military.

Having appealed unsuccessfully for international and Commonwealth support for his reinstatement as Prime minister, Bavadra and three former members of his government agreed to participate in a Constitutional Review Committee established in July, and supported a minority report which argued for a return of the 1970 constitution. Despite growing racial attacks by Melanesian nationalists against FLP members, in September, Bavadra participated in talks concerning the formation of an inter-racial government of national unity. These talks were terminated by the second of Rabuka's coups. Thereafter the FLP was excluded from government, although it remained an influential force within many sections of the labour movement,

(particularly among the predominantly Indian sugar-cane workers) where resentment over the coups, together with the imposition of anti-trade union laws, led to numerous labour disputes.

Bavadra died of cancer in 1989, and was succeeded by his widow, *Adi* Kuini Bavadra, although her subsequent remarriage meant that she increasingly distanced herself from FLP activities. In August 1991 she was succeeded by Jokapeci Koroi, a union activist and party vice president. The FLP denounced the new constitution as racist and anti-democratic but prevaricated for some time over whether or not to appear to endorse it by participating in the forthcoming elections. Despite a decision by its coalition partner, the NFP, to participate, a convention of FLP party delegates in September 1991 eventually voted overwhelmingly not to take part. This decision effectively dissolved the alliance with the NFP. At the last moment, however, in April 1992, a special delegates conference of the FLP reversed its decision to boycott the elections. It decided that it would stand candidates—in Melanesian as well as Indian seats—but that it would continue to express its contempt for the constitution by ensuring that none of those who secured election would take up their seats. Attempts to reach a last-minute deal to avoid competing directly with the NFP failed, not least because of FLP demands that successful NFP candidates should also refuse to take their seats.

Despite its commitment to multiracial politics, the FLP's candidates were overwhelmingly drawn from the Indian community, and all of the seats which it won were among the 27 reserved for Indians. In the immediate aftermath of the election the FLP's leader, Mahendra Chaudhry (who had succeeded Koroi), reached an agreement with Rabuka whereby the FLP would support his campaign for the Premiership in return for a commitment by the new Prime Minister for an early review of the constitution, and other key issue of law including land tenure and anti-trade union legislation.

Fijian Nationalist United Front(FNUF)

Address. c/o House of Representatives, Suva, Fiji.
Leadership. Sakeasi Butadroka.
Orientation. Melanesian supremacist. The FNUF seeks to defend the Melanesian community's control of the political process, protect its customs, and maintain its ownership of land.
Founded. 1991.
History. The Fijian Nationalist United Front (FNUF)

was created through the merger of Fijian Nationalist Party (FNP) led by Sakiasi Butadroka and the Fijian Conservative Party (FCP), led by Isireli Vuibau, which had earlier split from the FNP. The FNP had been created in 1974 by Butadroka, who had resigned from the Alliance government in 1973 in protest at what he perceived to be the under-representation of Melanesians under the political system created by the 1970 constitution. The party offered the first serious challenge to the Alliance Party for the allegiance of the Melanesian electorate. Although the FNP won only one seat (that contested by its founder) in the 1977 election, its campaign on the racially-nationalist platform of "Fiji for the Fijians", eroded the Alliance's support. However, by the time of the next general election, six months later, Butadroka had been imprisoned for inciting racial hatred and the FNP failed to win any seats. The party continued openly to promote the interests of Melanesians over Indians, and although it failed to win seats, it had the effect of forcing the Alliance to use tougher pro-Melanesian rhetoric in an effort to prevent the defection of its native Fijian support. The FNP returned to prominence when the issues of race and politics exploded in the 1987 coups. The party supported Rabuka's actions and participated in the subsequent interim governments.

The FNUF was formed prior to the 1992 elections in order to offer Melanesian voters a more uncompromising vehicle for race-based nationalism than that offered by the FPP. In the event the party won five seats, all of which were among the 37 reserved for the Melanesian community. Although FPP leader Lt.-Col. Sitiveni Rabuka wanted to include the party within his coalition government, he was overruled by parliamentary colleagues. Butadroka responded by claiming that the new government was doomed, and indicated that he would seek to mobilize FPP dissidents and Indian representatives in an early vote of no confidence.

General Voters Party

Address. c/o House of Representatives, Suva, Fiji.
Leadership. Leo Smith.
Orientation. Centrist.
Founded. December 1990.
History. The General Voters Party (GVP) was the direct descendent of the General Voters Association (GVA), which had emerged in the 1960s as a vehicle for those members of the electorate descended from European and Chinese immigrants. The GVA gradually lost its separate identity as a result of becoming one racial faction with the Alliance Party, which suc-

cessfully dominated the country's political system from independence until 1987 [see below]. The collapse of the Alliance in the period after the military coups, and the establishment of a new constitution which reserved numbers of seats for various racial categories, led to the creation of the GVP shortly before the 1992 election. The party contested all five seats in the General Voters' category (those whose racial origin was neither Melanesian nor Indian), and won all of them. The party supported the FPP and received two posts in the new Rabuka Cabinet.

National Federation Party

Address. c/o House of Representatives, Suva, Fiji.
Leadership. Harish Chandra Sharma.
Orientation. Indian-dominated, democratic socialist party. Although more successful than the Alliance in attracting support from outside its ethnic base, the NFP has always been closely associated with the Indian community. It opposes discrimination against Indians in politics, land tenure and other areas. It has also tended to support an open, rather than a racially based electoral system, and a non-aligned foreign policy.
Founded. July 1960 (as the Federation Party).
History. The National Federation Party (NFP) was formed as the Federation Party, and emerged from the sugar farmers' association formed in 1959. From the outset it was closely associated with the Indian community, which was descended from indentured sugar cane workers brought to Fiji in the 19th century. In 1963 the party, under the leadership of A. D. Patel, won all nine Indian seats in the colonial Legislative Council. It then merged with the predominantly Melanesian National Democratic Party, led by Isikeli Nadalo and Apisai Tora and adopted its current name. The NFP pursued centre-left policies and sought early independence for Fiji. Patel died in 1969 and was succeeded as party leader by Siddiq Koya who pursued a more accommodating line towards the Alliance government.

In the April 1972 election the NFP won 19 of the 52 seats. This figure increased to 26 in the 1977 contest, but the party was prevented from forming a government by a split between a faction loyal to Koya, and one which supported Jai Ram Reddy. In the election of September 1977 the party representetion was reduced to 15 seats. Among those who failed to gain re-election was Koya, and he was succeeded as party leader by Reddy. Reunited, the party won more than 41 per cent of the vote and 22 seats in the July 1982 elections. Together with the two seats won by its ally, the Western United Front (WUF), the result took the NFP once more to the threshold of power. Reddy was suspended from Parliament in 1983 for refusing to stand while addressing the Speaker, and he then initiated a boycott which was joined by 22 of the other 23 members of the opposition. In May 1984 Reddy resigned his seat, Koya was re-elected as leader, and the opposition boycott was quickly ended.

The return of Koya signalled a renewed bout of internecine fighting, complete with a series of resignations and by-election defeats for the party. Koya resigned as leader in May 1986 and was succeeded by Harish Chandra Sharma. In the run-up to the 1987 election the party, while maintaining its relationship with the WUF, forged an alliance with the newly formed Fiji Labour Party (FLP), and it was this coalition which finally succeeded in breaking the Alliance's grip on government. The coalition won 28 seats and, under the leadership of FLP leader Timoci Bavadra (a Melanesian), the country's first predominantly Indian government was formed with Sharma as Deputy Prime Minister and Reddy as Attorney General. On May 14, however, the government was deposed by a military coup led by Lt.-Col. Sitiveni Rabuka, the then third-in-command of the army, and all 28 government party representatives were detained for a week.

Although the coalition participated in the political talks which followed the first coup, the NFP withdrew from the negotiations over the formation of a government of national unity after several of its members suffered racially motivated attacks. The talks were restarted but were terminated by the second coup. Thereafter, the NFP remained excluded from the political process which culminated in the promulgation of a constitution which sought to maintain a permanent hold on government by the Melanesian community.

In July 1991 the NFP announced that it had decided to contest the elections, despite its criticisms of the racist aspects of the constitution. It called upon the FLP to do the same, and when the FLP voted later that year not to do so, their coalition was dissolved. Although the FLP reversed its decision in April 1992, the two erstwhile allies were unable to agree upon a formula for avoiding competing against each other. In the event the NFP fielded candidates—including two members of the 1987 Bavadra Cabinet—in 25 of the 27 Indian seats, and 14 were successful in securing election.

Minor parties

All Nationals Congress; formed by former Cabinet Minister Apisai Tora in June 1990, the party attempted to create a multiracial grouping. It succeeded in attracting some former members of the defunct Alliance Party, the National Federation Party and the General Voters Party, but its support tended to remain regionally confined to the Melanesian communities of western Viti Levu. It stood some 20 candidates in the 1992 election, few of whom were Indians. All were defeated.

Fiji Indian Congress Party (FICP); launched in mid-1991 by members of the Indian community in Suva on the basis that the unjust nature of the new constitution could be altered only by working within its parameters. The party's president, Ishwari Bajpai, was once a member of Ratu Maras's Alliance Party government.

Fiji Indian Liberal Party (FILP); founded in March 1991 as a "moderate progressive" Indian Party. It was centred upon western Viti Levu, and supported Rabuka's FPP in the run-up to the May 1992 elections.

New Labour Party (NLP); formed on Feb. 25, 1992, by members of the Fiji Labour Party who disagreed with the decision to boycott the elections. It was headed by Michael Columbus, president of the Fiji Trade Union Congress, and was committed to fighting the country's "racist" constitution.

NFP splinter group; formed by a breakaway faction of the NFP, under the leadership of Siddiq Koya, a former Leader of the Opposition and the chairman of the Sugar Cane Growers' Council.

Taukei Solidarity Movement *see under Taukei* **in guerrilla groups (below).**

Western United Front (WUF); created in 1981 as a predominantly-Melanesian organization centred upon Nadroga Province, in western Viti Levu. In the election of July 1982 the party, in alliance with the National Federation Party, won 3.9 per cent of the vote and two seats in the House. One of the WUF representatives defected to the Fiji Labour Party in mid-1986. The party entered the 1987 election in alliance with the NFP and the FLP but failed to win any seats.

Defunct Parties

Alliance Party; formed in 1965 as the main party of the Melanesian community, committed to the preservation of a traditional Fijian cultural and national identity, and to the maintenance of Melanesian ownership of most of the country's land. Nominally it espoused multiracialism and was founded as a coalition of groups representing each of the country's racial communities: the Fijian Association (formed in 1956 and operating in the mid-1960s under the title of the Fijian United People's Party); the Indian Alliance (or Indian National Congress, formed in the 1960s as the political wing of the *Kisan Sangh* farmers' union); and the General Electors Association (formed in the 1940s as the European Electors Association, but revived in the mid 1960s with the incorporation of the newly enfranchised Chinese community). Nevertheless, the Melanesian component was always the dominant one and from an early stage the party was clearly identified with "ethnic Fijians" as opposed to those of Indian extraction. Under the leadership of *Ratu* Sir Kamisese Kapaiwai the party remained in government for 17 years, from independence until the election of 1987. Following both the May and October military coups, *Ratu* Mara and other Alliance members participated in the interim administrations. In December Mara accepted the office of Prime Minister and presided over the process of altering the constitution in a bid to ensure the future hegemony of the Melanesians. The increased racial tension in the after 1987, together with the abandonment of even the pretence of racial equality, destroyed the foundations of the Alliance. Although Mara remained in office until the 1992 elections, the party was eclipsed by political organizations which were more precisely racially focused upon a particular community.

Fijian Nationalist Party (FNP) *see under* Fijian Nationalist United Front.

Major guerrilla groups

There are no guerrilla groups operating in Fiji. However the *Taukei* organization, an extreme Melanesian supremacist movement, has been responsible for racial attacks against the Indian community. The movement seeks to preserve Melanesian culture, and opposes equal rights for Indians and other ethnic groups. It emerged in the mid-1980s as a pressure group (with members in both the Alliance and Fijian Nationalist Party) which campaigned strongly for greater Melanesian political representation and against any alteration of the existing system of land tenure. It strongly opposed the formation of an Indian-dominated government after the April 1987 election, and supported the May and September military coups led by Rabuka. In the poisonous racial atmosphere which followed the coups the *Taukei* was responsible for a campaign of intimidation and racist propaganda. Its leaders also participated in the governments established after the coups. In 1988 the movement went some way towards becoming a formal political party with the establishment of the Taukei Solidarity Movement. The movement was also believed to have members in both the FPP and the FNUF.

French Pacific Territories

France's four Overseas Territories (*territoires d'outre-mer*) are all located in the Pacific: French Polynesia, New Caledonia, the Wallis and Futuna Islands and the French Southern and Antarctic Territories. They are regarded as an integral part of France, although each has a degree of internal self-government. Each (apart from the Southern and Antarctic Territories) elects its own territorial assembly and sends representatives to the French legislature in Paris.

French Polynesia

Capital: Papeete, on the island of Tahiti   **Population: 196,000 (1989)**

The 130 or so islands which comprise French Polynesia were colonized in a piecemeal fashion in the 19th century. Until 1957 the territory was governed by decree; thereafter it became a French Overseas Territory.

Constitutional structure

Legislative power is vested in a Territorial Congress of 41 members, elected by universal suffrage for up to five years. From within its own members the Assembly elects a Territorial President who, with an appointed Council of Ministers, exercises executive authority. The metropolitan French government, represented locally by a High Commissioner, retains control of various spheres of government, including defence, foreign relations and justice. In 1990 the internal autonomy statute of 1984 was modified in order to increase the powers of the President and the Territorial Assembly.

French Polynesia also elects two deputies to the French National Assembly and one representative to the French Senate.

Electoral system

The 41 seats in the Territorial Assembly are distributed as follows: the Windward Islands elect 22 seats; the Leeward Islands eight; the Tuatotu Archipelego and the Gambier Islands five; the Austral Islands three; and Marquesas three.

Evolution of the suffrage

All elections are conducted on the basis of universal adult suffrage.

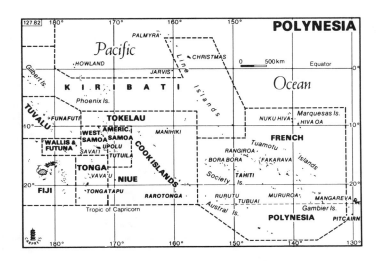

Recent elections

Election date	Winning party
May 1982	*Tahoeraa Huiraatira*/RPR-led coalition
March 1986	*Tahoeraa Huiraatira*/RPR*
March 1991	*Tahoeraa Huiraatira*/RPR-led coalition

*Ousted from power in 1987 following a party split.

Legislative elections, March 17, 1991

Party	Seats won
Tahoeraa Huiraatira/RPR	18
Te Tiarama-Papu Here Ai'a Te Nunaa Ia Ora alliance	14
Ai'a Api	5
Front de Libération de la Polynésie/Tavini Huiraatira	4
Total	41

Following the elections a coalition was formed between the *Tahoeraa Huiraatira*/RPR led by Gaston Flosse and *Ai'a Api*, led by Emile Vernaudon. The latter was elected President of the new Territorial Assembly on March 28, whilst on April 4 Flosse was formally elected as President of the territorial government. In September 1991 Flosse dropped his junior coalition partner in favour of a new alliance with the *Papu Here Ai'a Te Nunaa Ia Ora*.

PARTY BY PARTY DATA

Autonomous Patriotic Party

Te Papu Here Ai'a Te Nuna'a la Ora

Address. BP3195, Papeete.

Leadership. Jean Juventin (pres).

Orientation. Autonomist, favouring a peaceful transition to full independence, but with the country remaining "in association" with France. THe party opposes the continued use of Polynesia as a testing site for French nuclear weapons.

Founded. 1965.

History. The rural-based party, usually known as *Papu Here Ai'a*, or simply *Here Ai'a* (patriotism), was founded by John Teariki, a deputy who had belonged to the radical Democratic Rally of the Tahitian People (*Rassemblement Democratique du Peuple Tahitien—RDPT*, formed in 1949 and banned in 1963). It won seven of the 30 Territorial Assembly seats in 1967, and in 1968 it formed a coalition, Patriotic New Way (*Te E'a Api o Te Here Ai'a*) with the New Way Party [see under United Front]. The autonomist majority thus formed was lost in 1972, when the balance of power went to the independents.

In the 1973 National Assembly elections the revived coalition was named New Way and Patriotic Federation (*Te Amuiraa E'a Api Here Ai'a*). In 1977 *Here Ai'a* won nine of the 14 seats gained by the United Front for Internal Autonomy (*Front Uni pour l'Autonomie Interne*—FUAI), and participated in the resulting coalition administration. Teariki declared his support for independence in 1978, despite opposition from the United Front.

Juventin was re-elected to the French National Assembly in 1981, although in the Territorial Assembly elections in May 1982 the party won only six seats. In September it replaced the *Ai'a Api* as the coalition partner of the ruling *Tahoeraa Huiraatira*. Teariki died in 1983 and replaced as party leader by Juventin. In December 1987 the *Tahoeraa Huiraatira* split, with the breakaway faction led by Alexander Leontieff, forming the core of a new opposition coalition which included the Te Pupu Here Ai'a Numa'a la Ora. Within days the government was forced to resign, with Leontieff replacing Gaston FlosseGaston as President of the Council of Ministers, and Juventin being elected President of the Territorial Assembly. Juventin and Leontieff maintained the alliance between their two parties at the 1991 election, but won only a combined total of 14 seats. In September 1991 the *Pupu Here Ai'a Te Nunaa Ia Ora* joined the government as the junior partner to the *Tahoeraa Huiraatira*/RPR in place of the *Ai'a Api*.

New Land

Ai'a Api

Address. BP 11055, Mahina, Tahiti, French Polynesia.

Leadership. Emile Vernaudon (l.).

Orientation. Centrist.

Founded. 1982.

History. The *Ai'a Api* was established in a major split from the *Te E'a Api* (United Front). It won three seats in the May 1982 Territorial Assembly elections. It subsequently joined the *Tahoeraa Huiraatira*-led government coalition, but went into opposition in September. It contested the 1986 election as part of the centre-left opposition group *Amuitahiraa Mo Porinesia* (Polynesian Autonomists) which won a total of six seats. Following the fall of the *Tahoeraa Huiraatira* government in December 1987, the *Ai'a Api* joined the new government of Alexander Leontieff. In the 1991 election the party won five seats and joined the *Tahoeraa Huiraatira* in a coalition government. In September 1991, however, Gaston Flosse abandoned his junior coalition partner in favour of a new alliance with the *Pupu Here Ai'a Te Nunaa Ia Ora*.

Polynesian Liberation Front

Front de Liberation de la Polynesie (Tavini Huiraatira) (FLP)

Address. Mairie de Faaa, Tahiti, French Polynesia.

Leadership. Oscar Temaru (l.).

Orientation. Pro-independence.

Founded. 1984.

History. The FLP was formed in succession to earlier independence parties, including the Rally for Independence (*Tavini Huira'atiraa—Rassemblement pour l'Independance*), led by Temaru and Henri Hiro, which contested the 1982 territorial elections without success. It organized meetings in Papeete in 1985 in support of the New Caledonian independence movement, and won two seats in the 1986 elections. At the 1991 election the FLP increased its representation to four seats. In the subsequent elections for the post of President of the Territorial Assembly, on March 28, Temaru was defeated by Emile Vernaudon by 37 votes to four.

Power to the People

Ia Mana Te Nunaa

Address. Rue de Commandant Destremau, BP1223, Papeete, Tahiti.

Leadership. Jacques Drollet (sec.-gen.).

Orientation. Socialist and pro-independence.

Founded. 1976.

History. The *Ia Mana Te Nunaa* party was founded to co-ordinate non-violent class struggle against "colonial capitalism" in French Polynesia, and against French nuclear weapons testing in the Pacific. It won three seats in the 1982 and 1986 elections, but lost them all in the 1991 contest, and appeared to have been eclipsed as an independence vehicle by the more hardline FLP.

Publications. *Te Ve'a Hepetoma* (weekly); *Ia Mana* (monthly).

Rally for the Republic

Tahoeraa Huiraatira/Rassemblement pour la Republique

Address. Rue de Commandant Destremau, BP 471, Papeete, Tahiti, French Polynesia.

Leadership. Gaston Flosse (pres. and l.).

Orientation. Conservative. The party supports the enhancement of territorial status, the continuation of nuclear testing and the maintenance of a close relationship with France.

Founded. 1971, as the Tahiti Union-Union for the Defence of the Republic (*Union tahitienne-Union pour la Defense de la Republique*—UT-UDR).

History. The UT-UDR was formed from a number of conservative groups dating back to the 1950s, under the leadership of Flosse. It unsuccessfully contested the 1971 senatorial elections, but temporarily allied itself with the short-lived centre-right Union Party (*Te Autahoeraa*, led by Charles Taufa) to form the largest bloc in the Territorial Assembly after the 1972 elections. It led the Territorial government in 1972-75, and again from 1976. In 1977 the party became the metropolitan section of the French Rally for the Republic (RPR), and by 1979 the party, then known as the *Tahoeraa Huiraatira/Rassemblement pour la Republique*, had become the largest political organization in French Polynesia.

In the 1982 Territorial Assembly elections the party (operating under the name *Partie de l'Union Populaire*—PUP) won 30 per cent of the vote and 13 seats. Flosse formed a coalition government first with the *Ai'a Api* (New Land Party) and, from September, with the *Te Pupu Here Ai'a Te Nuna'a la Ora*. His admin-

istration pursued development-orientated policies and negotiated greater autonomy for the country. A statute in 1984 extended concessions made in 1977 by creating a new post of President of the Council of Ministers, to which Flosse was duly elected on Sept. 14. In the 1986 election the party won 24 seats in the enlarged Territorial Assembly, the first time a majority had been won by a single party. Increasingly, however, there were allegations against Flosse concerning the corrupt use of public funds. In February 1987 he was forced to resign as President of the Territorial Council and was succeeded by Jacques Teuira. Further misfortunes followed for the party, as a group of legislators resigned to form the breakaway *Te Tiarama* (The Flame) under the leadership of Alexander Leontieff. With its legislative majority destroyed, the *Teuira* administration fell from office in December 1987.

Thereafter the party remained in opposition until the 1991 election when it emerged as the largest single group in the new Territorial Assembly. Following the election Flosse formed a coalition government with the *Ai'a Api*, led by Emile Vernaudon. The election for the President of the new Territorial Assembly on March 28 was won by Vernaudon, while on April 4 Flosse was formally elected as President of the Territorial Council. The new government immediately announced a rigorous cost-cutting programme, claiming that the financial position was catastrophic. The proposed introduction of new and increased indirect taxes led to protests in June, and serious rioting in Papeete on July 10. Peace was restored after the government agreed to abandon the tax increases. Shaken by the violence, Flosse retired for a week of reflection on July 12. In September he abandoned his junior coalition partner in favour of a new alliance with the *Pupu Here Ai'a Te Nunaa Ia Ora*, thereby bolstering his majority in the Territorial Assembly.

The Flame

Te Tiarama

Address. c/o Territorial Assembly, Papeete, Tahiti, French Polynesia.

Leadership. Alexander Leontieff.

Orientation. Centre-right.

Founded. 1987.

History. The *Te Tiarama* was established in 1987 by a breakaway group of *Tahoeraa Huiraatira* representatives under the leadership of Leontieff. When the *Tahoeraa Huiraatira* government fell in December 1987, Leontieff formed a new coalition government which remained in power until the 1991 election, which it fought in coalition with the *Papu Here Ai'a Te Nunaa Ia Ora*. The coalition was defeated, winning a combined total of only 14 seats. The coalition broke up later in the year when the *Papu Here Ai'a Te Nunaa Ia Ora* joined the government of Gaston Flosse.

Minor Parties

Taatiraa Polynesia; BP 283, Papeete, Tahiti; Arthur Chung (l.). Founded in 1976, this autonomous party won a single seat in the Territorial Assembly elections of 1982 and 1986, but none in the 1991 election.

Te Pupu Taina/Rassemblement des Liberaux. This liberal party was formed in 1977 by a split from *Te E'a Api/Front Uni*. Its leader, Michel Law, was elected to the Territorial Assembly in 1977, but lost the seat in 1982. The party contested the 1986 elections as part of the *Amuitahiraa Mo Porinesia* (Polynesian Autonomists) but, following the breakup of that coalition, has not been represented in the Territorial Assembly

Defunct Parties

Polynesian Autonomists (*Amuitahiraa Mo Porinesia*); a loose centre-left coalition formed around the *Ai'a Api*, which won six seats in the 1986 elections but disintegrated thereafter.

United Front (*Te E'a Api/Front Uni*). This urban-based party was founded in 1964 as the *Te E'a Api no Polynesia* (The New Way for Polynesia) and was derived from the banned RDPT [see under Autonomous Patriotic Party]. In 1967 the party won 10 seats and, allied with the *Te Pupu Here Ai'a Te Nuna'a la Ora*, became the largest bloc in the Territorial Assembly. In 1972 the alliance between the two parties won 13 seats and retained control of the Assembly. A new version of the alliance, the United Front for Internal Autonomy (FUAI), formed a new territorial government and secured important concessions from France after winning 14 seats in 1977. In 1982 *Te E'a Api* suffered a major split, which led to the creation of the *Ai'a Api*, and in the 1982 election only its leader and founder, Francis Sanford, secured election. Following his retirement from politics in December 1983 the party declined into insignificance.

Major Guerrilla Groups

There are no guerrilla groups operating in French Polynesia.

New Caledonia

Capital: Noumea   **Population: 164,000 (1989)**

The archipelago of New Caledonia became a French possession in 1853, initially as a dependency of Tahiti and then, after 1884, as a separate administration. White settlers quickly obtained possession of much of the territory's land leading to periodic rebellions by the dispossessed Kanaks, the native Melanesian population. A significant degree of self-government was introduced in 1976 but, when pro-independence Kanak parties gained control of the territory's Council of Government in 1978, the French government returned the territory to direct rule. Self-government was re-introduced in 1984, but the inability to find a compromise which encompassed the Melanesian demand for independence and the white community's desire to remain attached to France led to a renewed period of direct rule in 1988-89. This was followed by a new constitutional structure which created three provinces, each with its own local powers and legislative assembly, which together formed the Territorial Congress.

Constitutional structure

Legislative power is vested in a Territorial Congress of 54 members, who serve for up to six years, and who are responsible for the territorial budget and fiscal affairs, infrastructure and primary education. The Territorial Congress is composed of the combined memberships of the three Provincial Assemblies, for the South (32 seats), the North (15 seats) and the Loyalty Islands (seven seats). Each provincial assembly is responsible for local economic development, land reform and cultural issues. Each provincial assembly also elects a President, as does the Territorial Congress. These four office holders assist the High Commissioner (the representative of metropolitan France) in forming a territorial executive. The High Commissioner is responsible for issues such as foreign relations, defence, law and order, and secondary education.

New Caledonia also elects two deputies to the French National Assembly and one representative to the French Senate.

Electoral system

The country's electoral system is based on the territory's three provinces. The Kanak population, a minority of the population as a whole, is in the majority in the North and Loyalty Island provinces, while the South province is dominated by white settlers loyal to France.

Evolution of the suffrage

Voting is conducted on the basis of universal adult suffrage. The first legislature was established in 1956, but effective power remained with the French Governor.

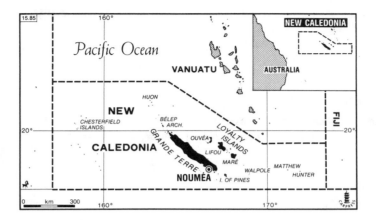

Recent elections

Date	Majority party in Territorial legislature
Sept. 29, 1985	Rassemblement pour la Caledonie dans la Republique (RPCR)
April 24, 1988*	RPCR
June 11, 1989	RPCR

*Boycotted by pro-independence Front de Liberation National Kanak et Socialiste (FLNKS).

Legislative elections, June 11, 1989

Seat distribution in provincial assemblies

Party	North	Loyalty Islands	South
RPCR	4	2	21
FLNKS	11	4	4
Front National	—	—	3
Caledonie Demain	—	—	2
Union Oceanienne	—	—	2
Front Anti-Neacolonialiste	—	1	1

Level of popular support and seats in Territorial Congress

Party	Votes	Percentage	Seats
RPCR	27,777	44.5	27
FLNKS	17,898	28.7	19
Front National	4,204	6.7	3
Caledonie Demain	3,219	5.2	2
Union Oceanienne	2,429	3.9	2
Others	6,943	11.1	1

PARTY BY PARTY DATA

Caledonian Union (UC)
Union Caledonienne
Address. 8-18 rue Gambetta, le Valee du Tir, Noumea.
Founded. 1952.
Orientation and history. See under Kanak Socialist National Liberation Front

Kanak Socialist National Liberation Front
Front de Liberation National Kanak Socialiste (FLNKS)
Address. BP 3553, Noumea.
Leadership. Paul Neaoutyine.
Orientation. Melanesian socialist; Pro-independence.
Founded. 1984.
History. The FLNKS was created in 1984 as a coalition of socialist and social democratic parties in favour of independence from France. It quickly superseded the less radical *Front Independantiste* (FI) [see below] as the primary vehicle for Melanesian nationalism, and soon gained the allegiance of all of the FI's constituent parties except the *Liberation Kanake Socialiste* (LKS).

The largest element in the five-party coalition is the *Union Caledonienne* (UC—Caledonian Union) a pro-independence, socialist movement founded in 1952 by Maurice Lenormand who, in the previous year, had become the first Melanesian to win election to the French National Assembly. The UC was supported not merely by Kanaks, but also by left-wing members of the white community, and the party encouraged a multiracial following with its "two colours, one people" approach. From the first elections to the (relatively ineffective) Territorial Assembly in 1956, until 1972, the UC was the majority party. It lost control in 1972 but was later able to form a coalition government which negotiated a new statute in 1976 conceding some internal powers to a Council of Government chosen by the Assembly. In 1977 and 1979, however, the UC won only nine seats. It was led by Lenormand in 1952-64 and 1969-72, and by Roch Pidjot in 1964-69 (while Lenormand was legally disqualified from office) and in 1972-85. Either Lenormand or Pidjot held a seat in the National Assembly from 1952 to 1986. The assassination on Sept. 19, 1981, of the UC's general secretary, Pierre Declercq, led to communal violence and to the radicalization of the independence movement. In June 1982 the UC was represented in the newly formed FI-FNSC coalition [see Kanak Federal Party]. From the mid-1980s the UC has operated almost exclusively within the framework of the FLNKS.

In January 1985 its general secretary, Eloi Machoro, was shot dead in a confrontation with police, and in 1989 its leader Jean Marie Tjibaou (and also the leader of the FLNKS) was assassinated [see below].

In addition to the UC, the FLNKS includes the *Union Progressiste Melanesienne* (UPM—Melanesian Progressive Union) an agrarian socialist movement formed as a result of a split in the United Kanak Liberation Front (FULK); the *Parti de Liberation Kanake* (Palika—Kanak Liberation Party), a radical independence party formed in 1975, which had been expelled from the FI (and replaced by the Kanak Socialist Liberation—LKS) as a result of its increasing pursuit of independence through extra-parliamentary means; the *Parti Socialiste Caledonien* (PSC—Caledonian Socialist Party), formed in 1975-76 by labour activists; and (until it was expelled in 1990) the *Front Uni de Liberation Kanak* (FULK).

Although more radical than the FI, the FLNKS remained committed to the pursuit of independence through constitutional means. The problem, however, was that the Kanak population constituted only around 43 per cent of the whole population and, particularly after the changes imposed by the French authorities in 1979, the party had little realistic hope of achieving an overall majority in the Territorial Assembly, or of achieving victory in a referendum on the issue of independence. It was partly for this reason that the FLNKS boycotted the Assembly elections of November 1984 and, the next month, proclaimed the formation of a "provisional government of Kanaky" headed by the party's leader, Jean-Marie Tjibaou. The move intensified the independence question and there were increasingly frequent confrontations between the authorities and the Kanak population. A state of emergency was declared on Jan. 12, 1985, which lasted until the middle of the year. A new High Commissioner proposed a rapid transition to "independence association" for the territory, subject to a referendum. The plan was rejected on both sides: by the Kanaks because it gave equal voting rights to all, regardless of their length of residence in the territory, and by the settlers because it offered the possibility of independence as a possible option. The political violence increased, and among those killed was UC secretary general and leading FLNKS member, Eloi Machoro, shot dead by police in highly controversial circumstances.

In 1985 the Fabius plan was considered more acceptable by the FLNKS as it restructured the constitution by dividing the territory into four regions each of which had its own assembly. In the subsequent elections on Sept. 29, the party won majorities in three of the four regions but, due to the concentration of support for the RPCR in the most densely populated southern region, the FLNKS won only 16 of the 46 seats in the Territorial Congress formed from the combined memberships of the four regional bodies. The party boycotted the 1986 elections to the French National Assembly, and the referendum on independence held on Sept. 13, 1987. Around 59 per cent of the registered electorate voted in the referendum, with more than 98 per cent of votes in favour of maintaining New Caledonia as a part of France. In Melanesian dominated areas, however, the abstention rate was as high as 90 per cent.

In mid-1988 the FLNKS participated in constitutional negotiations with the Rally for Caledonia in the Republic (RPCR) which were chaired by newly elected French Prime Minister Michel Rocard at the Hotel Matignon (the French Prime Minister's official residence) in Paris. The resulting Matignon Accord, agreed by Tjibaou and RPCR president Jacques Lafleur, returned administrative control of New Caledonia to Paris for one year, pending the implementation of a new electoral system which divided the territory into three provinces each with devolved powers and its own assembly, the combined sum of which formed a new Territorial Congress. The fact that a majority in the Congress was still likely to be drawn from the political parties of the settlers was offset by the increased powers available to the North and Loyalty Island Provincial Assemblies where the FLNKS was the dominant force. The Matignon Accord was also acceptable to the FLNKS because of its commitment to hold a referendum on the issue of independence in 1998, with a franchise restricted to those resident in the territory at the time the Accord was signed, and their direct descendants.

In May 1989 Tjibaou was murdered by extreme separatists who were alleged to be connected to one of the component parties of the FLNKS, the FULK, which disapproved of the Matignon Accord. Tjibaou was succeeded as leader by Paul Neaoutyine, president of the PALIKA. Despite the assassination, elections under the new structure went ahead in June as scheduled. The FLNKS won majorities in the North and Loyalty Island provinces, and secured a total of 19 seats in the Territorial Congress compared with 27 for the RPCR. After the elections relations between the FLNKS and the RPCR improved substantially. There were suggestions by some members of the settler community that the planned 1998 independence referendum should be abandoned in favour of a form of independence in association with France. Supporters of the plan claimed that it would allow an immediate settlement of the territory's status and therefore end the climate of uncertainty which was adversely affecting foreign investment. In May 1991 Lafleur threw his support behind the idea by calling for a "consensual solution" to the future status of the territory to be adopted prior to 1998. Although Neaoutyine suggested that the pro-independence forces were "open to any discussion", an FLNKS congress in June 1991 reasserted its position that the planned referendum was "a determining stage in New Caledonia's march towards independence".

Structure. The structure of the FLNKS is based on the traditional Kanak regions, with 32 regional committees sending delegates to a national assembly. The party executive, elected at the assembly, considers itself to be the "provisional government of Kanaky".

National Front
Front National
Address. c/o Territorial Congress, Noumea.
Leadership. Guy George.
Orientation. Extreme right-wing, anti-independence; the party is a territorial section of the racist French party of the same name.
Founded. 1984.
History. In elections to the European Parliament in 1984 the *Front National* won 15.7 per cent of the vote, and appeared capable of making serious inroads into the RPCR's position as the representative party of the settler community. In the Territorial Assembly elections in November 1984, however, the party won only 2,379 votes (6.1 per cent). Its one successful candidate was one of its founders, Roger Gailot, Mayor of Thiou. In 1985 the FN only contested seats in the southern region, and won three. In the 1989 elections it polled 4,204 votes (6.7 per cent) and once again won three seats. Although its share of the vote and the seats made it the third largest party in New Caledonia, it remained well behind the RPCR and the FLNKS, and there appeared no immediate prospect of it seriously eroding the core support of the former.

Rally for Caledonia in the Republic
Rassemblement pour la Caledonie dans la Republique (RPCR)
Address. 8 avenue Foch, BP 306, Noumea.

Leadership. Jacques Lafleur.

Orientation. As the main party of the white community the RPCR opposes independence, and advocates retention of a close relationship between New Caledonia and France. The party represents most of the white population—both *"caldoches"* (settlers) and *"metros"* (recent immigrants)—and is affiliated to the metropolitan Rassemblement pour la Republique.

Founded. 1978.

History. The RPCR was created from a coalition of conservative and anti-independence parties which, to some extent, have retained their separate identities and following. The original members were Dick Ukeiwe's *Rassemblement pour la Republique* (RPR—Rally for the Republic) a right-wing party formed in 1977 as an affiliate of the metropolitan French RPR, and the *Rassemblement pour la Caledonie* (RPC—Rally for Caledonia), founded in 1977 by Jaques Lafleur as the successor to the conservative *Entente Democratique et Sociale* (EDS—Democratic Social Accord). Since then the RPCR has been joined by other conservative groupings, including the **Union for the Renaissance of Caledonia** (*Union pour la Renaissance de la Caledonie*); the **Caledonian Liberal Movement** (*Mouvement Liberal Caledonien*—MLC) formed by Jean Lecques in 1971; and the **Christian Social Democrats—Inter Ethnic Accord** (*Sociaux Democrates Chretiens—Entente Toutes Ethnies*), a centre-right party founded in 1979 by Raymond Mura by the merger of two existing parties.

The RPCR won 15 seats in the 1979 Territorial Assembly elections, and Lafleur was re-elected in 1981 as one of the territory's two representatives to the French National Assembly. The party subsequently blocked French plans for greater autonomy, as a result of which its coalition partner the *Federation pour une Nouvelle Societe Caledonienne* (FNSC) [see under Kanak Federal Party] broke away to form a new government with the Independence Front (FI). The RPCR, then the main opposition party, participated in negotiations on a revised statute for the territory but it vigorously opposed the plan put forward by the French authorities. In the 1984 Territorial Assembly elections the RPCR, assisted by a Kanak boycott, won 27,851 votes (70.9 per cent) and 34 of the 42 seats. Lecques was elected president of the Assembly, and Ukeiwe president of the Council of Ministers.

The party resisted all autonomy proposals, and denounced the 1985 Fabius Plan—which divided the territory into four regions, each of which elected its own assembly and which together formed a territorial legislature—on the grounds that it gave too much influence to the Kanak-dominated areas. Nevertheless, the party participated in the 1985 elections under the new Constitution and, by winning 17 of the 21 seats in the southern council together with some seats in the other regions, gained a majority in the new Territorial Congress, whereupon it used its power to reject and delay any further reform. The party also won the March 1986 elections for representatives to the French National Assembly (in a vote which was boycotted by most Kanaks), and retained the seats in 1988.

Under the new Constitution resulting from the Matignon Accord, the party contested seats in all three of the territory's provinces in 1989. Although defeated by the FLNKS in two of the three provinces, the party's victory in the densely populated South province was sufficient to give it a majority in the Territorial Congress. Increasingly, however, the party appeared more flexible in its attitude to the future status of New Caledonia. In 1990 it acknowledged the possibility that the planned independence referendum—scheduled for 1998—could be abandoned in favour of a form of independence in association with France. Supporters of the plan claimed that it would allow an immediate settlement of the territory's status and therefore end the climate of uncertainty which was adversely affecting foreign investment. In May 1991 Lafleur, the RPCR's leader and president of the South province, threw his support behind the idea by calling for a "consensual solution" to the future status of the territory to be adopted prior to 1998.

Minor Parties

Anti-Neocolonialist Front (*Front Anti-Neocolonisaliste*) *see under* Kanak Socialist Liberation.

Caledonian Front (*Front Caledonie*—FC). The FC was founded in 1981 by Justine Guillemard, who defected to the Rally for Caledonia in the Republic in 1983 and was succeeded by Claude Sarran. It is an extremely right-wing, white-racist organization, with close links to the National Front.

Caledonian Liberal Movement (*Mouvement Liberal Caledonien*—MLC) *see under* Rally for Caledonia in the Republic.

Caledonian Republican Party (*Parti Republicain Caledonien*—PRC). An autonomous but anti-independence party founded in early 1979 by Lionel

Cherrier, it is affiliated to the metropolitan French national Republican Party (PR) [see under Kanak Federal Party].

Caledonian Socialist Party (*Parti Socialiste Caledonien*—PSC); M. Violette (l.) *see under* Kanak Socialist National Liberation Front—FLNKS.

Caledonian Youth Union (*Union Jeunesse Caledonienne*—UJC), also known as the *Avenir Jeunesse de la Caledonie*, the party was formed in 1977 by Jean-Paul Belhomme; *see under* Kanak Federal Party.

Caledonie Demain. This right-wing party consists of former supporters of the Rally for Caledonia in the Republic and the National Front; it is currently led by Bernard Marant. In the 1989 Territorial Congress elections it won more than 5 per cent of the vote and two seats, both of which were in the South province.

Christian Social Democrats—Inter Ethnic Accord (*Sociaux Democrates Chretiens—Entente Toutes Ethnies*) *see under* Rally for Caledonia in the Republic (RCPR).

Democratic Union (*Union Democratique*—UD); formed in 1968 by Gaston Morlet *see under* Kanak Federal Party.

Kanak Federal Party (*Parti Federal Kanak*—PFK); 8 rue Gagarine, Noumea. The PFK was founded in 1979 by its current leader, Jean-Pierre Aifa, as the *Federation pour une Nouvelle Societe Caledonienne* (FNSC). It was a coalition of five small parties: Aifa's New Caledonian Union (*Union Nouvelle Caledonienne*—UNC); the Democratic Union (*Union Democratique*—UD); the Caledonian Youth Union (*Union Jeunesse Caledonienne*—UJC); the Caledonina Republican Party (*Parti Republicain Caledonien*—PRC); and the Wallis and Futuna Movement (*Mouvement Wallisien et Futunien*). In the July 1979 Territorial Assembly elections the FNSC won seven of the 36 seats and joined the Rally for Caledonia in the Republic (RPCR) in government. In the 1984 elections it won only a single seat (securing only 4.4 per cent of the vote) and shortly afterwards changed its name to *Union pour la Liberte dans l'Ordre* (Union for Liberty in Order). It adopted its current name in April 1985. In May 1985 its only legislator defected to the Kanak Socialist Liberation (*Liberation Kanake Socialiste*—LKS), since when it has been unrepresented in the

Territorial Congress.

Kanak Liberation Party (*Parti de Liberation Kanake*—Palika); Paul Neaoutyine (l.). PALIKA, a radical independence party, was formed in 1975. After being expelled from the Independent Front for its increasing pursuit of independence through extra-parliamentary means, it won two seats in the 1977 and 1979 Territorial Assembly elections. In 1984 it joined the Kanak Socialist National Liberation Front (FLNKS).

Kanak Socialist Liberation (*Liberation Kanake Socialiste*—LKS). The LKS, led by Nidoish Naisseline, was founded in April 1981 by a split in the Kanak Liberation Party (PALIKA). As a member of the Independence Front (*Front Independantiste*—FI) [see below] it participated in governments formed by the FI and the Kanak Federal Party (*Parti Federal Kanak*—PFK). It declined to join the FI's successor, the FLNKS, when it called for a boycott of the Territorial Assembly elections in 1984. The LKS won 2,879 votes and took six seats, making it the second-largest party in the Assembly. In May 1985 it recruited the sole Assembly representative of the PFK, but soon afterwards it withdrew from the Assembly in protest over the escalating level of political violence within the territory. In the September 1985 election it won 4,594 votes but only one (Loyalty Islands) seat. In 1989 it established the **Anti-Neocolonialist Front** (*Front Anti-Neocolonisaliste*) which, in the Congress elections, won a seat in the Loyalty Islands. Allied with the FULK, the LKS also won 23 per cent of the vote in municipal elections in February 1990.

Melanesian Progressive Union (*Union Progressiste Melanesienne*—UPM); Edmond Nekiriai (l.); Victor Tutugoro (sec.-gen.); formed in 1974 (as the Union Progressiste Multiraciale), adopted current name in 1977; *see under* Kanak Socialist National Liberation Front (FLNKS).

New Caledonian Union (*Union Nouvelle Caledonienne*—UNC); formed in 1977 after a split in the Caledonina Union; *see under* Kanak Federal Party.

Rally for Caledonia (*Rassemblement pour la Caledonie* —RPC); *see under* Rally for Caledonia in the Republic (RPCR).

Rally for the Republic (*Rassemblement pour la Re-*

publique—RPR); *see under* Rally for Caledonia in the Republic (RPCR).

Union for the Renaissance of Caledonia (*Union pour la Renaissance de la Caledonie*); *see under* Rally for Caledonia in the Republic (RCPR).

Union Oceanienne); Michel Hema (l). Formed in 1989 as a result of a split in the RPCR, the party competes with the Wallis and Futuna Movement (*Mouvement Wallisien et Futunien*) for the support of the sizeable community of those from Wallis and Futuna.

United Kanak Liberation Front (*Front Uni de Liberation Kanak*—FULK); Mare, Loyalty Islands. The party was founded in 1977 and led by Yann Celene Ureguei, a member of the Independence Front and later of the Kanak Socialist National Liberation Front (FLNKS). Ureguei, originally a member of the Caledonian Union (CU), had in 1970 formed the Multi-Racial Union of New Caledonia indexMulti-Racial Union of New Caledonia (New Caledonia) (*Union Multiraciale de Nouvelle Caledonie*—UMNC) based in the Loyalty Islands. The UMNC had adopted independence as its goal in 1975, and was superseded by the FULK in 1977. Ureguei won a seat in the Territorial Assembly in the election of 1977 and retained it in 1979, but the FULK boycotted the election of 1984. As the Foreign Affairs spokesman of the FLNKS "provisional government", but acting without its authority, he made a controversial visit to Libya in March 1986, which resulted in his dismissal from the his post in August. Increasingly, in the late 1980s, the FULK found itself at odds with the FLNKS leadership as its advocacy of a total boycott of all French-created institutions appeared increasingly incompatible with the new flexibility of the coalition's leadership. The FULK boycotted the 1989 elections to the Territorial Congress, and the party was expelled from the FLNKS in January 1990. In the municipal elections on Ouvea in February 1990 the FULKS allied itself with the Kanak Socialist Liberation (LKS) [see below]. This coalition won 23 per cent of the vote compared with the 45.4 per cent won by the FLNKS. It was reported in January 1991 that the 22nd congress of the FULK had voted to dissolve the party in order to enable its members to join a planned new Kanak nationalist

organization.

Wallis and Futuna Movement (*Mouvement Wallisien et Futunien*); formed in 1979 and led by Finau Melito, the party represents the less right-wing elements of the migrant worker community from the eponymous French Pacific Territory [see under Kanak Federal Party].

Defunct parties

Independent Front (*Front Independantiste*—FI). The FI was created in 1979 after Kanak nationalist and socialist parties had won a majority in the Territorial Assembly elections of 1978. Its attempt to force concessions from the French government led the French authorities to dissolve the Council of Government and to impose direct rule by the High Commissioner. After electoral reforms which handicapped minor (mostly Kanak) parties, fresh elections resulted in an anti-independence majority, with the FI winning 14 of the 36 seats. In 1982 the FI participated in government by forming a coalition with the *Federation pour une Nouvelle Societe Caledonienne* (FNSC—see under Kanak Fedeeral Party) after the latter's partnership with the Rally for Caledonia in the Republic had broken down. In September 1984, as it became clear that the FLNKS had superseded the party as the main vehicle for Kanak aspirations to independence, the FI dissolved itself.

Major guerrilla groups

Although the territory does not have any guerrilla groups as such, supporters of many of the pro-independence Kanak parties were involved in violent confrontations with the authorities in the latter half of the 1980s, and there was considerable communal violence between the white and the Kanak communities. The most dramatic incident occurred on April 22, 1988, shortly before the French national elections, when a band of Kanaks attacked police quarters on Oueva, in the Loyalty Islands, killing four gendarmes and taking a further 27 hostage, 11 of whom were later released. On May 5 French security forces stormed the cave where the hostages were being held in an operation which cost the lives of 19 Kanaks and two soldiers, but which secured the release of all of the remaining hostages.

Wallis and Futuna Islands

Capital: Mata-Utu   **Population: 12,408 (1983 census)**

The Wallis and Futuna Islands became a French protectorate in the 19th century, but the territory was never formally annexed, nor French law or institutions introduced. In 1959 the territory's traditional Kings and chiefs petitioned for incorporation into the French Republic and, in July 1961, the islands formally became an Overseas Territory. The three traditional kingdoms in the territory (two on Futuna and one on Wallis) have continued to exist.

Constitutional structure

Executive authority is in the hands of the Chief Administrator, who is appointed by the French government. He is assisted by a six-member Council of the Territory, half of which is composed of the territory's three monarchs, and half is chosen by the Territorial Assembly, the 20-member legislature. The Territorial Assembly also elects its own President, and elects one representative to the French National Assembly and one to the Senate.

Electoral system

The Territorial Assembly, elected for up to five years on a common roll, has 20 seats, 13 elected from Wallis and seven from Futuna.

Evolution of the suffrage

Elections take place on the basis of universal adult suffrage.

Recent elections

Date	Winning party
March 1982	Rassemblement pour la République (RPR)
March 1987	RPR coalition government with Union Populaire Locale (UPL)
March 1992	RPR

PARTY BY PARTY DATA

Lua-kae-tahi *see under* **Union for French Democracy.**

Local People's Union

Union Populaire Locale (UPL)

Address. c/o Territorial Assembly, Mata-Utu, Uvea, Wallis Island.

Leadership. Falakiko Gata (l.).

Orientation. Regionalist. The UPL seeks to further the economic and social welfare of the islands by strengthening local control over development funding and obtaining finance for specific projects.

Founded. 1985.

History. The UPL was created by Gata who had been elected to the Assembly in 1982 as a member of the Rally for the Republic (RPR), but who had accepted Union for French Democracy (UDF) support in November 1983 to win the election for president of the Assembly. In the 1987 election his party won six seats, all of them on Futuna, and entered an alliance government with the RPR.

Rally for the Republic

Rassemblement pour la République (RPR)

Address. c/o Territorial Assembly, Mata-Utu, Uvea, Wallis Island.

Leadership. Clovis Logologofolau (l.).

Orientation. Conservative. The Wallis and Futuna RPR is a section of the metropolitan French party of the same name.

History. In the elections of 1982 the RPR won an absolute majority in the Territorial Assembly with 11 of the 20 seats. It gained another representative in late 1982 when a member of the Union for French Democracy (UDF) defected. In November 1983, however, three of its legislators defected to the UDF, depriving the ruling party of both its majority, and the presidency of the Assembly. At the 1987 election both the RPR and the UDF won seven seats, but the former remained in power by forming a coalition with the Local People's Union (UPL). The party retained power at the election in March 1992.

Union for French Democracy

Union pour la Democratie Francaise (UDF—Lua-kae-tahi).

Address. c/o Territorial Assembly, Mata-Utu, Uvea, Wallis Island.

Orientation. Centre-right; a section of the metropolitan UDF.

History. In the elections of 1982 the UDF and its allies won nine of the 20 seats in the Territorial Assembly, losing narrowly to the Rally for the Republic (RPR). Defections from the RPR, however, enabled the UDF to wrest the presidency of the Assembly away from the ruling party in 1983. In the election of 1987 both the UDF and the RPR won seven seats, although the latter was able to form a government after forming a coalition with the UPL. The UDF was once again defeated in the election of March 1992. In Wallisian the party is known as the *Lua-kae-tahi.*

Minor parties

Mouvement des Radicaux de Guache (MRG); a left-wing party without significant support.

Major guerrilla groups

There are no guerrilla groups operating in Wallis and Futuna.

French Southern and Antarctic Territories

Although technically an Overseas Territory, the French Southern and Antarctic Territories are governed by special statute. The territories, which consists of a portion of Antarctica and associated islands, are populated only by members of scientific expeditions.

Hong Kong

Capital: Victoria   **Population: 5,900,000 (1990)**

Hong Kong island was ceded to the UK in 1862 under the Treaty of Nanking. Under the Convention of Beijing concluded in 1860, the UK also acquired the Kowloon peninsula. A 99-year lease on the New Territories was granted by China to the UK in 1898. In 1984, the UK conceded that, on the expiry in 1997 of the lease on the New Territories, the whole of Hong Kong would revert to Chinese sovereignty. The Sino-British Joint Declaration of September 1984 included Chinese guarantees that the capitalist economy of Hong Kong would continue for 50 years after 1997.

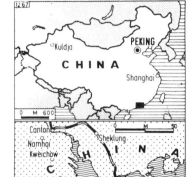

Constitutional structure

Hong Kong is administered by a Governor representing the UK Sovereign. The Governor chairs an Executive Council consisting of four ex officio members and 10 nominated members; and a 60-member Legislative Council (Legco). Since 1991 the composition of the Legco has changed to consist of three of the four Executive Council ex officio members; 18 appointed members; and 39 elected members. The last Governor of Hong Kong, Chris Patten, was appointed in April 1992.

The composition of the Legco had been altered in 1985 to include 24 indirectly elected members, of whom 12 were chosen by electoral colleges from district boards, the Urban Council (Urbco) and the Regional Council (Regco), and 12 from functional constituencies. Two more deputies' seats were added in 1988. In addition, there were ten ex officio members and 20 appointees.

In April 1990 China's legislature, the National People's Congress, promulgated the Hong Kong Special Administrative Region (SAR) Basic Law (a mini-Constitution). Although it was intended to increase the number of directly elected seats in the Legco to one-third of the total by 1997 (i.e. 20 out of 60), and one-half of the total by 2003, the new Basic Law did not guarantee fully representative government.

There are no genuine political parties and voter participation is low. However, some narrowly based political groups do exist, and cover all shades of the political spectrum from liberal to conservative and business interests. Hong Kong also houses covert branches of the Chinese Communist Party and the *Kuomingtang* [see entries for China and Taiwan].

Electoral system

Of the 39 elected members of the Legco in 1991, 18 members were directly elected from double-member constituencies and 21 members were elected as representatives from 15 "functional constituencies" (business, trade and service sector groups).

RECENT ELECTIONS

Legco Elections, Sept. 22, 1988

Of the 26 seats in these indirect elections 13 were uncontested. Moderate or conservative candidates performed best in the nine contested electoral college constituencies, while liberals won the four contested functional constituencies.

Legco Elections Sept. 15, 1991

These were the first direct elections to the Legco. The turnout was low, however, at 39 per cent. There were 54 candidates for the 18 directly elected seats and 40 candidates for the functional constituency seats, of whom 12 stood unopposed. Only two of those elected in functional constituencies were backed by the UDHK.

Party	Seats
UDHK	12
UDHK allies	3
Independents	3

Evolution of the suffrage

Citizens over 21 who have been resident in Hong Kong for seven years have the right to vote. The franchise for the functional constituencies in elections to the Legco includes corporate or individual representatives of major economic, social or professional sectors.

PARTY BY PARTY DATA

There are no genuine Hong Kong political parties, although the current narrowly based groups appear to be developing into political parties. There are covert branches of the Chinese Communist Party (CCP—*see* China) and the *Kuomintang* (KMT—*see* Taiwan).

When China resumes jurisdiction over Hong Kong, it is expected that laws will be enacted prohibiting laws of subversion against the People's Republic of China and that political organizations in the Hong Kong SAR will be prohibited from establishing links with foreign political organizations.

Co-operative/Co-opted Resources Centre (CRC)

Leadership. Allen Lee (ch.).

Orientation. Conservative.

Founded. November 1991.

History. Allen Lee resigned as a senior member of the Legco on Nov. 15, 1991, because of criticism that his leadership of the newly established CRC—a group of mainly conservative councillors—could lead to a conflict of interests. The CRC was intended to act as a counterweight to the liberal members of the Legco, newly elected in September 1991, and consisted of 21 councillors, none of whom were from directly elected constituencies and who were perceived as supporting business and government interests. The CRC was widely expected to evolve into a formal political party.

Democratic Alliance for Betterment of Hong Kong (DABHK)

Leadership. Tsang Yok-sing; Tam Yiu-chung.

Orientation. The DABHK is a pro-People's Republic of China (PRC) group. It calls for the election of all legislature and executive members and the reintegration of Hong Kong with China.

Founded. May 19, 1992.

History. The declaration of the DABKH's foundation was welcomed as bringing pro-PRC interests in Hong Kong into the open. Previously these interests had worked covertly through the Federation of Trade Unions and through business and social organizations. The DABKH's founders admitted that it received financial support from Chinese-owned companies. There were 50 founding members among whom were the current leadership of Tsang Yok-sing, a headmaster of a pro-PRC school, and Tam Yiu-chung, vice-chair of the Federation of Trade Unions. The DABKH's stated aims also included social welfare, human rights, and stability in Hong Kong before and after reversion to Chinese rule.

Structure. 18-member preparatory committee; two spokesmen/leaders.

Liberal Democratic Federation (LDF)

Leadership. Hu Fa-kuang (ch.).

Orientation. Conservative, representing business interests.

History. The LDF contested seven seats in the May 1991 Urbco elections and won three of them.

United Democrats of Hong Kong (UDHK)

Leadership. Martin Lee (ch.); Szeto Wah.

Orientation. Calls for greater autonomy for Hong Kong on its reversion to Chinese rule and more representative democracy.

Founded. April 1990.

History. The UDHK was founded by the colony's main liberal lobby groups, and may be considered Hong Kong's first formal political party. About one-third of the 216 founding members came from three lobby groups: the Hong Kong Affairs Society; Meeting Point; and the Association for Democracy and People's Livelihood. The UDHK represents a total of six liberal political groups. On April 8, 1990, the UDHK published a manifesto and elected an executive committee. Martin Lee was elected UDHK chair. Lee was an outspoken critic of the People's Republic of China (PRC), which had denounced him as a subversive for having organized protests in Hong Kong against the Tiananmen Square massacre in 1989. The UDKH manifesto nevertheless committed the UDHK to supporting the implementation of the 1984 Sino-British Joint Declaration.

Major guerrilla organizations

There are no guerrilla organizations in Hong Kong.

India

Capital: New Delhi Population: 853,100,000 (1990)

India gained independence from the United Kingdom in 1947, when the subcontinent was divided into the new states of India and Pakistan. Since independence politics has been dominated by the Congress Party which has ruled continuously since independence, except for a three-year period in the late 1970s and a 17-month period in the late 1980s and early 1990s.

Constitutional structure

Under the (amended) 1949 Constitution the Union of India is defined as "a sovereign socialist secular democratic republic". The Union is divided into 25 self-governing states and seven union territories. The legislative field is divided between the Union and the states, the former possessing exclusive powers to make laws with respect to matters grouped under 97 headings in the Constitution including foreign affairs, defence, citizenship and trade with other countries.

Executive power is vested in a President and in the Legislative Assemblies of the states. The President appoints a Prime Minister and, on the latter's advice, a Council of Ministers, all of whom are responsible to parliament. Parliament consists of an upper house (*Rajya Sabha*) and a lower house (*Lok Sabha*).

Electoral System

The *Lok Sabha* has 545 members of whom 543 are chosen by direct election through a simple majority system in single-member constituencies (with vacancies being filled by by-elections). The remaining two members are appointed by the President to represent the Anglo-Indian community. The term of the *Lok Sabha* is five years, subject to dissolution or extension by one year in an emergency. The *Rajya Sabha* consists of up to 250 members, at present 245, mostly indirectly elected by the State Assemblies, of whom one-third are elected every two years. The President nominates 12 members on the strength of achievement in culture, science or social service. Office is for six years and not subject to dissolution. The President is elected indirectly for five years by directly elected members of the union and state legislatures.

India possesses a broad array of political parties, alliances and factions at national and regional level. However, parties are characterized by constant splits, defections, realignments and mergers. In 1985 the Anti-Defection Act was passed to curb such activities. The Act specified that members of the national, state and Union Territory legislatures would be disqualified if they gave up membership of the party for which they were elected, or if they voted, abstained or defected contrary to their party direction, unless the defection or split carried one-third of the party members or a merger occurred where at least two-thirds of the original party were in favour.

Evolution of the suffrage

Citizens aged 18 years and over are entitled to vote.

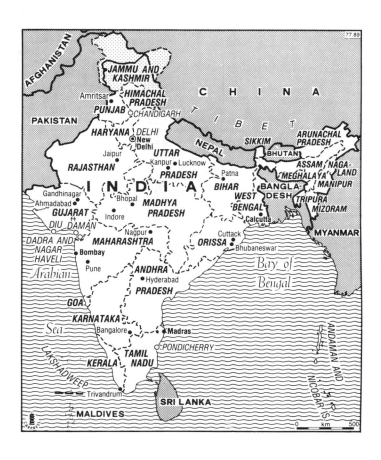

Recent elections

1989 general election

Party	Seats
Congress (I) (and allied parties)	192
*Janata Dal	141
Bharatiya Janata Party	86
+Left-Front parties	51
*Telegu Desam Party	2
*Congress (S)	1
Others	52
Assam and Punjab seats (elections not held)	14
Countermanded	4
Nominated	2
Total	545

*National Front component parties.

+Communist Party of India (Marxist) (32); Communist Party of India (12); Other Left Front parties (7).

1991 general election

Party	Seats
Congress (I)	226
Bharatiya Janata Party	119
*Janata Dal	55
#Communist Party of India (Marxist)	35
*Telegu Desam	14
#Communist Party of India	13
+All India Anna Dravida Munnetra Kazhagam	11
Jharkand Mukti Morcha	6
Samajwadi Janata Party	5
§Shiv Sena	4
#Revolutionary Socialist Party	4
#Forward Bloc	3
+Indian Union Moslem League	2
*Asom Gana Parishad	2
Bahujan Samaj Party	1
Haryana Vikas Party	1
+Janata Dal (Gujarat)	1
+Kerala Congress (Mani)	1
Manipur People's Party	1
Nagaland People's Council	1
+Sikkim Sangram Parishah	1
Congress (S)	1
Countermanded	12
Results withheld	5
Punjab seats (elections not held)	13
Jammu and Kashmir seats (elections not held)	6
Nominated	2
Total	545

+Congress (I) allied parties.

*National Front parties.

#Left Front parties.

§Allied with BJP.

PARTY BY PARTY DATA

Major national parties

Bharatiya Janata Party (BJP)

Indian People's Party
Address. 11 Ashoka Road, New Delhi 110001.
Leadership. Shri Murli Manohar Joshi (pres.); Kushabhau Thakre (gen. sec.); O. Rajopal (gen. sec.); Suraj Bhan (gen. sec.); Govindacharya (gen. sec.).
Founded. 1980.
Orientation. Radical right-wing Hindu communalist; close links with paramilitary *Rastriya Swayam Sewat Sangh* (RSSS—National Union of Selfless Servers).
History. The BJP was formed as a breakaway group from the *Janata* Party (JNP). In the general election to the *Lok Sabha* in November 1989 the BJP won 88 out of 525 seats, and subsequently supported the *Janata Dal*-led National Front coalition government. In October 1990 the BJP withdrew its support on the arrest of BJP president Lal Krishna Advani after he led a controversial procession of Hindu followers to Ayodhya, Uttar Pradesh, to construct a Hindu temple at the site of a disused ancient mosque. Thousands of Hindu activists were arrested following clashes with the police and the storming and siege of the damaged mosque which had lasted several days.

In the June 1991 elections the party won 119 seats, emerging as the main opposition to the new Congress government and reflecting its rising popularity in a period of growth in Hindu fundamentalism and increasing assertiveness of other Hindu groups. The party performed extremely well in the north and was the only party to make a substantial overall gain. As of mid-1992 the party also controlled a number of state legislative assemblies, including those of Uttar Pradesh, Madhya Pradesh, Rajasthan and Himachal Pradesh.
Membership. 3,500,000.

Communist Party of India (CPI)

Address. Ajoy Bhawan, 15 Kotla Marg, New Delhi 110002.
Leadership. Shri Indrajit Gupta (gen. sec.)
Founded. 1925.
Orientation. Advocates unity of "left and democratic forces" against the "reactionary and authoritarian" internal policies of the ruling Congress (I); generally supportive of Congress external policies.
History. Following the 1977 general election the CPI abandoned its policy of co-operation with Congress and conceded that support for emergency rule in 1975-77 had been an error. In alliance with the Communist Party of India (Marxist) (CPI-M) it won 11 seats in the 1980 elections and was represented in CPI-M state governments in Kerala in 1980-82 and again from March 1987, and in West Bengal from 1980. After the 1984-85 general election, when the party suffered its biggest defeat, retaining only six seats and 2.7 per cent of the overall vote, it maintained its policy of opposition to the Congress (I) government, working closely with the CPI-M and other left-wing parties in this framework. In 1989 it joined with other left-wing parties to form a Left Front to oppose the rise of communalism. This Front co-ordinated arrangements so that representatives of the various parties did not stand against each other. As a result the CPI recovered to win 12 seats in the November 1989 elections and the party offered broad support to the shortlived government of V. P. Singh. In the 1991 election it won 14 *Lok Sabha* seats.
Structure. Branches are formed on a residential or workplace basis, and are organized at district and state level. State party conferences elect the state council, which elects its executive committee and secretariat. The party congress, held every three years, elects the 125-member national council, which in turn elects the nine-member central executive council, the secretariat and the general secretary.
Membership. 455,196 (1989).
Publications. *New Age* (weekly central organ); *Party Life* (fortnightly). The CPI also publishes daily newspapers in Kerala, Andhra Pradesh, West Bengal, Punjab and Manipur, as well as more than 20 weeklies in various languages.

Communist Party of India-Marxist (CPI-M)

Address. 14 Ashoka Road, New Delhi 110001.
Leadership. Somnath Chatterjee (parl. l.); Jyoti Basu, M. Basavapunnaiah (l.); Shri Harkishan Singh Surjeet (gen. sec.).
Founded. 1964, as a pro-Beijing breakaway from the Communist Party of India (CPI).
Orientation. The CPI-M's central objective is "to complete the people's democratic revolution in the country, go over to the socialist revolution and ultimately build a communist society". Originally pro-Chinese, the party declared its independence of China in 1968, and in 1976 criticized both Soviet "revisionism" and the Maoist "three worlds theory". The CPI-M

calls for a united front of left-wing parties and co-operation with the democratic "bourgeois" parties against
the Congress (I). In West Bengal the CPI-M-led government has pursued a policy of land reform, village
development, including the provision of roads, schools
and water supply, and the suppression of corruption.

History. Following the 1977 elections the CPI-M
headed left-front state governments in West Bengal,
Kerala and Tripura, but as of mid-1992 it retained
control only of West Bengal. In elections to the *Lok
Sabha* held in 1989 and 1991, the party won 32 and 35
seats respectively, making it by far the largest leftist
grouping in the country.

At the 13th party congress in 1989, only six new
members were elected to the central committee, while
only two new faces were added to the politburo, where
the age of the youngest member is now 61.

Structure. The CPI-M has branches; local, town (*ta-
luka*), district and state committees; and a 65-member
central committee, which elects a 12-member political
bureau including the general secretary. The party has
associated trade union, peasants', agricultural labour,
youth, students' and women's organizations, as well
as various special interest, cultural and professional
affiliated groups.

Membership. 564,000.

Publications. Central committee organs: *People's
Democracy* (weekly, circulation 15,000); *Lok Lahar*
(Urdu weekly, circulation 2,000); *Marxist* (theoretical
quarterly, circulation 4,000). The party also publishes
six daily newspapers (in Andhra Pradesh, Punjab, Kerala, Tamil Nadu, Tripura and West Bengal) with an
aggregate circulation of some 200,000 and eight weeklies in various states with an aggregate circulation of
some 67,000.

India National Congress (Indira)—Congress (I)

Address. 24 Akbar Road, New Delhi 110001.

Leadership. V. P. Narasimha Rao (pres. and parl. l.);
Balram Jakhar (l.) H. K. L. Bhagat, Rajendra Kumari
Bajpai, Jardhan Poojari, Ghulam Nabi Azad, Meera
Kumar (gen. secs).

Founded. January 1978; the original Indian National
Congress was founded in 1885.

Orientation. Traditionally committed to democracy,
socialism and secularism as enshrined in the Indian
Constitution, under Rajiv Gandhi's leadership Congress (I) advocated pragmatic economic and social
policies designed to encourage foreign investment and
private economic initiative. The party remains com-

mitted to non-alignment in external relations.

History. Founded as a breakaway group led by Indira
Gandhi, Congress (I) was confirmed as the official
Congress party in 1981. In October 1984 Indira Gandhi
was assassinated by Sikh extremists and was succeeded both as leader of Congress (I) and as Prime
Minister by her son Rajiv Gandhi. He led the party to
victory in the *Lok Sabha* elections of 1984-85, taking
415 of the 545 seats compared with 339 seats at dissolution. He then proceeded with a radical shake-up of
the party membership. Following Rajiv Gandhi's re-
election, substantial opposition to his leadership developed within the party, leading to the subsequent
expulsion or suspension of several prominent members in 1986. In August 1986 a number of "Indira
loyalists" launched a rival Indian National Congress
(Indira Gandhi) and in 1987 other Congress (I) dissidents founded the National Socialist Congress led by
Pranab Mukherjee. In 1986 agreements were secured
by Congress (I) to absorb factions of the Congress (J)
and Congress (S) parties and the National Democratic
Party of Andhra Pradesh, and in 1988 Mukherjee
announced the reintegration of his faction with the
ruling party.

Meanwhile, however, the Congress (I)'s working
president, K. Tripathi, had resigned in November
1986, criticizing Rajiv Gandhi's leadership. Further
resignations, dismissals and ministerial expulsions followed in 1987, amid intensifying controversy over
various corruption scandals and widespread demands
both inside and outside the party for the Prime Minister's resignation.

Gandhi's authority at the centre was not matched by
similar authority at state level, and his years in office
were marked by increasing friction between the national and state capitals. Local political leaders
resented his attempts to modernize and rejuvenate the
government at local level as well as at the centre. In
addition intercommunal violence and demands for
greater regional autonomy, even separatism—as in the
Punjab—became more frequent. From 1986 onwards
the Rajiv Gandhi government was increasingly
criticized for indecisiveness, or, when it responded by
imposing central rule in an increasing number of states,
for authoritarianism. Then too the administration came
to be tainted with corruption connected with the supply
of munitions by the Swedish Bofors Company.

Those leaving the party included V. P. Singh, an
eminent member of the *Rajya Sabha* and former minister, who in October 1987 launched an anti-corruption
campaign *Jan Morcha*, committed to defeating the

government. In September 1987 Gandhi responded by replacing five of six Congress (I) general secretaries in a further move to consolidate his authority over the ruling party. Meanwhile, a number of opposing parties had formed a National Front to contest the forthcoming general election.

In January 1989, Congress (I) was defeated in the state elections in Tamil Nadu but gained a clear majority in the elections in Nagaland and Mizoram. In July all the opposition members of the *Lok Sabha* resigned, and those of the *Rajya Sabha* protested at alleged government corruption and incompetence; this was followed by an anti-government general strike at the end of August. In October Gandhi attempted to take his opponents by surprise by calling a general election for the following month. In the event he was narrowly defeated, the number of seats won by the Congress (I) falling by half. He was succeeded as Prime Minister by V. P. Singh, now leader of the newly formed *Janata Dal* Party, who presided over a fragile minority coalition administration which had the support of both right-wing and left-wing parties. Congress (I)'s national defeat was compounded in February 1990 when it lost power in eight of 10 State Assemblies which it had hitherto controlled, with increased support for the *Bharatiya Janata* Party (BJP).

In November 1990 the *Lok Sabha* passed a vote of no confidence in the *Janata Dal* government led by Singh. He resigned immediately and the President asked Rajiv Gandhi to form a new government as leader of the single party with the largest number of seats. Gandhi refused the offer in favour of the *Janata Dal* (S) (under the leadership of Chandra Shekhar) which Congress (I) backed.

In December 1990 Gandhi announced that Congress (I) would no longer support *Janata Dal* (S) and in March 1991, the party began a boycott of Parliament. Chandra Shekhar resigned but remained Prime Minister in the interim.

The resulting general election was scheduled to take place over three days in May 1991. On May 21, after the first day's polling had taken place, Gandhi was assassinated in Tamil Nadu, allegedly by the Sri Lankan Liberation Tigers of Tamil Eelam (LTTE), although other separatist groups claimed responsibility. Following the assassination, the final elections were postponed until mid-June. Congress (I), benefiting from a considerable "sympathy" vote, won 226 of the 511 seats contested, and V. P. Narasimha Rao, the party's new president (Rajiv's widow, Sonia Gandhi, having refused the post), became Prime Minister of a new minority government.

The new government's main priority was to solve the country's severe economic crisis, the chief components of which were a huge foreign debt and severe inflation. The new Minister of Finance, Manmohan Singh, launched a reform to dismantle bureaucratic regulations and encourage private and foreign investment.

Structure. The party's leading body is the All-India Congress committee, which co-ordinates the various state and union territory party organizations.

Membership. 4,000,000 (1986).

Janata Dal (JD)

People's Party

Address. 7 Jantar Mantar Road, New Delhi 110001.

Leadership. V. P. Singh (parl. l.); S. R. Bommai (pres.).

Founded. 1988.

Orientation. Advocates non-alignment, the protection of the minorities and the eradication of poverty, unemployment and wide disparities in wealth. The objectives of the broad coalition were to reduce regional and ethnic divisions through a National Integration Council but without bowing to secessionist demands; to devolve further powers to local governments; to continue to reserve jobs for India's lower castes; and to introduce tight fiscal policies thereby enabling the government to finance its deficit through the capital markets instead of placing an embarrassing debt with the IMF.

History. Formed as a merger of parties including the *Jan Morcha*, the *Lok Dal*, and the *Janata* Party. The JD won 141 seats in the November 1989 *Lok Sabha* elections, with its allies winning three—together they formed the National Front (*Rashtriya Morcha*). The Front, with the support of the *Bharatiya Janata* Party (BJP) and communist parties, formed a new government and on Dec. 2, 1989, Singh was sworn in as the new Prime Minister. He appointed Devi Lal, then leader of the *Lok Dal* (B) as Deputy Prime Minister. A few weeks later the Singh government won a vote of confidence (all Congress (I) members abstained), following which all state governors were asked to resign and new ones were appointed by the President.

The coalition government was anchored by Singh's centrist *Janata Dal* party and ranged from the communists on the left to the Hindu revivalist BJP on the right. In July 1990 there was a government protest at the reinstatement of Om Prakash Chautala by his father, Devi Lal, as Chief Minister of Haryana after he had been forced to resign following allegations of corruption. Chautala resigned and Devi Lal was dismissed on the grounds of corruption, nepotism and disloyalty. The Singh government's introduction of a plan to raise the quota of official jobs reserved for the *harijan* (untouchables) and lower castes along with its prevention of the construction of a Hindu temple on the site of a Muslim mosque in Andhra Pradesh led to many violent demonstrations in Northern Indian states, primarily organized by higher caste students. The scheme was temporarily halted in October to curb the violence, but Singh said that he would rather resign than withdraw the scheme. Later that month the *Bharatiya Janata* Party (BJP) withdrew their support for the National Front government.

In November 1990 Chandra Shekhar, the main rival to Singh within the *Janata Dal*, formed his own dissident faction with the help of Devi Lal which became known as the *Janata Dal* (S). Its members were then expelled from the official *Janata Dal*. After a *Lok Sabha* convention, a parliamentary vote of no confidence was passed on Nov. 7 1990, Singh resigned, Rajiv Gandhi was asked to form a new government but refused and a new minority government with Chandra Shekhar as Prime Minister was sworn in on Nov. 10. Following the June 1991 general election the official *Janata Dal* won only 55 seats out of the 545 contested in the *Lok Sabha*, reflecting the considerable decline in its popularity under Singh. A breakaway faction led by Ajit Singh was formed in February 1992.
Membership. 136,000,000.

Samajwadi Janata Party (SJP)

Address. 16, Dr Rajendra Prasad Road, New Delhi.
Leadership. Devi Lal (pres.); Om Prakash Chautala (sec.-gen.).
Founded. 1991.
History. Formed by the merger of the *Janata Dal* (S) and the Janata Party (JNP) in April 1991. The *Janata Dal* (S) had been dissident faction from the *Janata Dal*, formed by Chandra Shekhar with the help of the deposed deputy Prime Minister Devi Lal. When Chandra Shekhar was sworn in as Prime Minister in November 1990, Devi Lal became Deputy Prime Minister and President of the *Janata Dal* (S). Shekhar won a vote of confidence with the backing of Congress (I), but the violence between Hindus and Muslims increased throughout India in December, and the implementation of the Mandal Commission quota scheme that V. P. Singh had tried to introduce in earlier 1990 remained postponed. Following Rajiv Gandhi's withdrawal of

the support of the Congress (I) from the government in March 1991, Chandra Shekhar resigned but accepted the offer to head an interim government until the next general election which was finally held in mid-June. By this time the SJP was formally established with Devi Lal as its president. It won five seats in the general election.

Minor national parties

All-India Forward Bloc (AIFB) (28 Gurudwara Rakab Ganj Road, New Delhi 110001); leadership: Prem Dutta Paliwal (ch.); Chitta Basu (gen.-sec.). Founded in 1939. An independent socialist party which has generally won a small number of *Lok Sabha* and State Assembly seats, usually in its stronghold of West Bengal. However, the party failed to win a single seat in the 1991 general election.

All-India Hindu Association (*Akhil Bharat Hindu Mahasabha* (ABHM) (Hindu Mahasabha Bhawan, Mandir Marg, New Delhi 110001); leadership: Shive Saran (pres); Dewan Chand Tyagi (gen. sec.). Founded in 1915. A right-wing Hindu party which was represented in the *Lok Sabha* from 1952-1967, and has held seats in state Legislative Assemblies.

Bahujan Samaj Party. (5325 Haryana Singh Road, Raigharpura, Karol Pagh, New Delhi 5). Leadership: Kanshi Ram. This party was created to promote the rights of the "untouchables" (Harijans). The party won three Lok Sabha seats in the 1989 general election (two in Uttar Pradesh and one in Punjab) and one seat in the 1991 general election (in Madhya Pradesh). In elections held in Punjab in February 1992, the party won one Lok Sabha seat and nine seats in the Assembly, where it emerged as the second party, having previously held no seats.

Communist Party of India (Marxist-Leninist) CPI (ML). Leadership: Satya Narain Singh (gen.-sec.). Founded in May 1969 by Maoists expelled from the Communist Party of India (Marxist) for their support of the armed revolutionary Naxalite movement. The party organized peasant revolts in West Bengal, Andhra Pradesh and other states. It was banned between 1975-77, after which it adopted policies which included participation in the political process. It has no state or federal representation.

Indian Islamic Society (*Jamaat-i-Islami Hind*, JIH);

leadership: Sayyed Ali Shah Gilani. Fundamentalist religio-political organization, aiming to safeguard the religious and cultural identity of Indian Muslims, with special emphasis laid on a programme of religious education, common defence of Muslim personal law, religious endowments, the Urdu language and Muslim educational institutions. It has no federal or state representation.

Indian National Congress (Socialist)—Congress(S). Founded as a Congress (I) breakaway party in 1981, it failed to win a seat in the 1984 general election. In late 1986 the party split, with one faction rejoining Congress (I). In the 1989 and 1991 general elections the party was a member of the *Janata Dal*-led National Front, winning one seat on both occasions.

Indian Union Muslim League (IUML) formerly All-India Muslim League (Court Road, Calicut 673001, Kerala); leadership: Ibrahim Suleiman Sait (pres.); Panakkad Mohammad Ali Shihab Thangal (pres., Kerala). Founded pre-independence; renamed in 1959. This party seeks to represent the interests of the Muslim ethnic and religious minority, often in alliance with India's left-wing parties. The party gains its support from Muslims in southern India, and particularly Kerala, where it regularly returns two *Lok Sabha* seats. In the 1991 Kerala state assembly elections the party won 19 seats (out of 140) and joined the Congress (I)-led United Democratic Front coalition. The party is also allied with Congress (I) at the national level.

Insaf Party. Leadership: Syed Shahabuddin (l.). Founded in 1990 to protect the interests of Muslims.

Peasants' and Workers' Party of India (PWPI) (Hari Kharude Nivas, Mahatma Phule Road, Naigaum/Dadar, Bombay 400014, Maharashtra); leadership: Dajiba Desai (gen. sec.). Founded in 1948 as a left-wing offshoot of the Indian National Congress, the PWPI won two *Lok Sabha* seats in 1952 and four in 1957, was unrepresented in 1967-77, won five in 1977, was unrepresented in 1980-84, won one seat in 1984, but none in 1989 and 1991. The party has been represented in the Maharashtra state Assembly since 1952.

Revolutionary Communist Party of India (RCPI) (5/1 Rammoy Road, Calcutta 700025, West Bengal); leadership: Sudhin Kumar (sec.-gen). Founded 1934. A small independent Marxist party which has been a member of the West Bengal government since the

1970s.

Revolutionary Socialist Party (RSP) (780 Ballimaran, New Delhi 110006). Leadership: Nani Bhattacharya (parl. l.); Tridib Chaudhuri (gen. sec.). Founded in March 1940 as an independent Marxist-Leninist party. The party contests general elections as part of the Left Front. In the 1989 and 1991 elections it won four Lok Sabha seats, all from West Bengal. It has also won representation in a number of state assemblies, including West Bengal and Tripura.

Socialist Unity Centre of India (SUCI) (48 Lenin Sarani, Calcutta 700016, West Bengal); leadership: Nihar Mukherjee (gen.-sec.). Founded in 1948 as an independent Marxist-Leninist party. It has held a small number of state assembly seats in West Bengal and Orissa.

Society of Indian Scholars (Jamiat-ul-Ulama-Hind JUH); leadership: Maulana Easied Madani (pres.). Founded 1919. Small, orthodox Muslim pro-Congress party.

United Communist Party of India (UCPI); leadership: Shripad Amrit Dange (ch.); Mohit Sen (gen. sec.). Founded 1989. Unlike other factions of the Communist Party, the UCPI has been largely supportive of Congress (I). In the 1989 general election it won one seat in the *Lok Sabha*, a Tamil Nadu constituency. It failed to retain the seat in the 1991 general election and has no state-level representation.

Regional parties

Andhra Pradesh

Telugu Desam (Land Of Telugu) (P. O. Nagar, Moinabad Mandal, Ranga Reddy Distt, Andhra Pradesh, 500171); leadership: Nandamuri Taraka Rama Rao (parl. l.). Founded in March 1982. Telugu being the language of Andhra Pradesh, this formation promotes the interest of the state to which its support is largely confined. The party declared on formation that it would support whichever party was in central power but would pursue its own activities within the state. It has a radical economic programme, including provision of rice subsidies, and campaigns against rural poverty and social prejudice (especially against women).

In the party's first state elections in 1983 it won a

huge majority, gaining 202 of the 294 Assembly seats, and thereupon formed a government. The party remained in government until 1989 when it was defeated by Congress (I). In the 1989 general election *Telegu Desam* was a member of the anti-Congress National Front led by V. P. Singh's *Janata Dal*. Although the Front managed to defeat Congress, *Telegu Desam* itself performed poorly, winning only two *Lok Sabah* seats. The party performed better in the 1991 general election, winning 14 seats; however, on this occasion, the National Front was defeated.

Arunachal Pradesh

People's Party of Arunachal (PPA) (P.O.Naharlagun 791111, Arunachal Pradesh); leadership: Shri Tomo Riba (pres). Founded by Congress (I) rebels in 1977, the party briefly held power in Arunachal in 1979 but recently has had little success.

Assam

Assam People's Council (*Asom Gana Parishad—AGP*) (Gopinath Bordolc Road, Guwahati 781001, Assam); leadership: Thaneswar Boro (pres.). The AGP won power in Assam in 1985, the year of its foundation. However, in late 1989 the federal government imposed President's rule in the state as a result of the activities of separatist groups. Fresh state assembly elections were eventually held in mid-1991 when the AGP was easily defeated by Congress (I). At the federal level, the AGP was a member of the anti-Congress (I) National Front. However, in the 1991 elections the party only managed to win two seats.

Other smaller Assam-based parties include:
Plains Tribal Council of Assam; United Minorities Front; and the **United Tribal Nationalists Liberation Front.**

Bihar

Jharkhand Mukti Morcha (JMM) (Bariatu Road, Ranchi 834008, Bihar). Founded in 1980 to represent the interests of the tribal people of Bihar. In state assembly elections the party generally wins a small number of seats, but has never been in a position to form a government. In the 1989 and 1991 general elections, the JMM won three and six seats respectively.

Goa

Maharashtrawadi Gomantak Party (MGP) (Camila, Old Bus Stand, Panaji 403001, Goa); leadership: Ramakant Dattaram Khalap (pres.). Founded in June 1963. This Hindu-dominated party has long competed with Congress (I) for control of Goa. Its current aims include recognition of Marathi (the dominant language of Goa, Maharashtra and parts of Karnataka) as the official language of the state. The party also campaigned for Goan statehood, which was eventually achieved in 1987.

In terms of representation in the *Lok Sabha*, the party held a seat from 1977 to 1984 and from 1989 to 1991. In April 1990 the party managed to form a state government with the aid of Congress (I) defectors. The government proved unstable, forcing the centre to impose President's rule for a short period in late 1990 and early 1991. However, the party managed to form another, more durable government, again with the help of Congress rebels.

Haryana

Haryana Vikas Party (Kothi No.136/22, Rohtak, Haryana); leadership: Rao Birender Singh (pres.). Founded in 1968. This party gained representation in its state Assembly in 1968 and in 1971 but not subsequently. The party won one *Lok Sabha* seat in Haryana in the June 1991 general election.

Jammu and Kashmir

Jammu and Kashmir National Conference (JKNC-Farooq) (Mujahid Manzil, Srinagar, Jammu and Kashmir); leadership: Farooq Abdullah (pres); Sheik Nazir Ahmed (gen. sec.). Founded in 1931 as the All Jammu and Kashmir National Conference the party was renamed in 1938 and reactivated in 1975. Socialist and opposed to Hindu communalism, the JKNC stands for the maintenance of Kashmir's status as an integral part of the Indian Union but with special constitutional guarantees, in particular on civil liberties. It advocates internal autonomy and self-government.

In the late 1980s the relationship between the Muslim and Hindu community throughout India deteriorated and the worst communal rioting since independence occurred. This was reflected most acutely in the predominately Muslim state of Jammu and Kashmir where a movement for political autonomy rapidly developed into a Muslim religious cause.

By 1989 opposition by Pakistan-backed Kashmiri sep-aratist organizations to the ruling alliance of the JKNC-Farooq and Congress (I) degenerated into a bloody civil war. Farooq resigned in early 1990 and Governor's rule was imposed (President's rule was subsequently imposed). Because of the war the federal government excluded the state from the 1991 general election. Effectively, the party is in a state of paralysis, with no representation at state or federal level and no control over the worsening security situation.

Other state-based parties include: **Jammu and Kashmir National Conference (Khaleda)**, a JKNC off-shoot which ruled the state briefly in the mid-1980s with the support of Congress (I); **Jammu and Kashmir Panthers Party; Jammu and Kashmir People's Conference; Muslim United Front.**

Karnataka

Karnataka-based parties include: **Kannada Nadu**, a *Bharatiya Janata*Party offshoot; **Maharashtra Eki-karan Samati; Revolutionary Front Kranti Ranga.**

Kerala

Kerala Congress (Mani) (Near Fire Station, Kot-tayam 686001, Kerala) K. M. Mani (l.). In the late 1970s the Kerala Congress divided into two main factions, one headed by K. M. Mani and the other by K. C. Joseph. The Joseph faction remerged with Congress (I) in 1985, but the Mani faction remained sep-arate, while supporting Congress (I) at state and federal level. Congress (Mani) won one *Lok Sabha* seat in 1989 and 1991 and participated, with Congress (I), in the United Democratic Front governments which has intermittently ruled the state.

National Democratic Party (Geetha Bhawan, Press road, Trivandrum, Kerala) Kidangoor A. N. Gopalak-rishna Pillai (pres.). Founded in July 1973. Small, pro-Congress (I) party.

Islamic Seva Sangh. This party was founded in 1992 in response to extremist Hindu fundamentalist groups.

Maharashtra

Shiv Sena (Shivsena Bhavan, Gadkari Chowk, Dadar, Mumbai Maharashtra 400028); leadership: Balasaheb Thackrey (pres.). Founded 1967. An extreme right-wing Hindu communalist party which seeks to defend the interests of native Maharashtrians against non-Hindu immigrants from the southern states. The party won four *Lok Sabha* seats (all from Maharashtra) in the 1989 and 1991 elections. It is closely allied with the *Bharatiya Janata* Party.

Other Maharashtra-based parties include: **Bharatiya Congress; Indian Liberal Group; Republican Party of India (Khobragade).**

Manipur

Manipur People's Party (MPP) (People's Road, Paona Bazaar, Imphal 795001, Manipur); leadership: Mohammed Alimuddin (pres.). Founded 1969. The MPP draws support from both Muslims and Hindus for its moderate left-wing policies. Formed by Con-gress dissidents, the MPP won 15 out of 60 state Assembly seats in its first elections in 1972. After this it headed a coalition ministry of non-Congress parties and independents. In 1974 the MPP went into opposi-tion with the Congress, but allied itself with the *Janata* Party in 1977, re-emerging in 1980 as an independent formation. In state assembly elections held in early 1990 the MPP, in alliance with *Janata Dal* and other parties, defeated the Congress (I) government. Raj Kumar Ranbir Singh of the MPP was appointed as the new Chief Minister. In early 1991 the party divided into two factions, but despite the split the coalition managed to remain in power. In the 1991 general election the MPP struck a further blow against Con-gress by taking one of the three Manipur *Lok Sabha* seats. However, in early 1992 the government was dismissed and President's rule was imposed. In April the MPP formed a fresh coalition government with Congress (I).

Other Manipur-based parties include: **Kuki National Assembly; United Democratic Party of Manipur.**

Meghalaya

All-Parties Hill Leaders' Conference (APHLC) (P.O.Tura Chandmari, West Gare Hills, Meghalaya 794002); leadership: Armison Marak (pres.). Founded in 1960 to promote the interests of the tribal peoples of the area. The APHLC was the ruling party during the period immediately following Meghalaya's achievement of full statehood in 1972. During the 1970 and 1980s large sections of the APHLC merged with

Congress (I) and other regional parties. By the early 1990s the party had no state or federal representation.

Hill People's Union (HPU) (Mawlai Nonglum, Shillong 793008, Meghalaya). Founded in 1985 to represent the interests of the tribal hill peoples of Meghalaya. The party incorporates elements of longer established state formations of the same orientation, notably a large faction of the APHLC. In the 1988 state assembly elections the party gained 19 out of 60 seats, only three less than the ruling Congress (I). In March 1990 the Congress (I) government collapsed and a new coalition was formed, which included the HPU. However, dissension within the coalition led to the imposition of President's rule in October 1991. Eventually, in February 1992, a new government was formed when the HPU entered into coalition with Congress (I).

Hill State People's Democratic Party (HSPDP). (Lumsohphoh, Lower Manprem Shillong 793002, Meghalaya); leadership: H. S. Lungdoh (l.); Lambourne Kharlukhi (gen. sec.). The HSPDP was originally founded to seek the establishment of a separate state from the parts of Assam inhabited by the tribesmen of the Khasi, Jaintia Garo Hills, an objective largely achieved with the conferment of full statehood on Meghalaya in 1972. Since then the party has pursued a programme for the preservation of the distinct identity of the tribal peoples of the state and for the protection of their cultural, social and economic interests within the Union of India. The party was a member of the coalition which ruled from March 1990 to October 1991.

Public Demands Implementation Convention (PDIC) (Demth Ring House, Upper Noggthymmai, Shillong 793002, Meghalaya). This party traditionally wins a small number of seats in state elections. It has supported a number of Congress (I) governments.

Mizoram

Mizo National Front (MNF) (Aizawl 796001, Mizoram); leadership: Lalthanhawla (pres.); C. Chawngzuala (vice-pres.); R. Zamawia (gen. sec.). Founded 1961. Having fought underground for the national self-determination of the (largely Christian) Mizo people, the MNF adjusted its program on being legalized (under the August 1986 settlement conferring full statehood on Mizoram) and now seeks to preserve and promote the Mizo people's traditions,

language and culture and to bring all Mizos under "one administrative unit". The creation of Mizoram as a Union territory in 1972 facilitated negotiations between the MNF and the Indian government. However, the 1976 agreement broke down and the MNF was declared an unlawful organization in 1979. With the conferment of statehood on Mizoram in 1986 the MNF was legalized and an interim coalition with Congress (I) was formed. In elections to the new state Assembly in early 1987 the MNF achieved an absolute majority, winning 24 of 40 seats, and formed a ministry of its own, headed by the then MNF president, Laldenga. President's rule was imposed in 1988 when the Laldenga government was no longer able to command a majority in the State Assembly. Fresh elections were held in early 1989 in which the MNF failed to win a majority; the party formed a coalition with Congress (I), headed by the new MNF president, Lalthanhawla.

Democratic Party (formerly People's Conference). (Treasury Square, Aizawl 796001, Mizoram); leadership: Brig. (retd) Thenphunga Sailo (pres.); Kenneth Chawngliana (gen. sec.). Founded in 1977. This party was the most powerful regional force in the 1970s and 1980s, before Mizoram achieved full statehood. In 1984 it lost control of the State Assembly to Congress (I); its position was further weakened with the achievement of statehood in 1986 and the legalization of the MNF, and in the 1987 and 1989 state elections the party won only three seats and one seat respectively.

Nagaland

Nagaland People's Council (NPC) (Nagaland News Review House, New Market, Kohima 797001, Nagaland). Defections from the long-time ruling Congress (I) allowed the NPC, hitherto the main opposition party, to form a government in May 1990. However, the government collapsed after a month and the party was obliged to enter into coalition with Congress (I). In the 1991 general election the NPC won the state's sole seat.

Other Nagaland-based parties include: **Naga National Democratic Party**; **Naga National Party**.

Orissa

Jagrata Orissa (8/SGO-6, Unit 6, Bhubanerwar 751001, Orissa). This small state formation obtained one seat out of 147 in the Orissa State Assembly elections of 1985.

Pondicherry

Pondicherry Maanila Makkal Munnani (36 Monyorsier Street, Pondicherry 6605001); leadership: S. Ramassamy (l.). This small party is committed to promoting the interests of the Tamil (Dravidian) people in the union territory of Pondicherry. It has had little electoral success.

Punjab

Akali Religious Party (*Shiromani Akali Dal*) (House No.4, Sector 8/A, Chandigarh, Punjab); leadership: Simranjit Singh Mann. Founded in December 1920.

As the supreme political organization of India's Sikh community (concentrated in Punjab), the *Akali Dal* advocates autonomy for all states in India, equal rights for all and safeguards for all minorities. Its autonomy demands were set out in the 1973 "Anandpur Sahib resolution", which also called for full recognition of Sikh religious arrangements and practices.

Following serious communal riots in 1981, in which Sikh extremists were involved, the *Akali Dal* in 1982 launched a "holy struggle" (*dharmyudha*) for an autonomous state of Punjab (Khalistan). The few political concessions that were made failed to stop the agitation, which in October 1983 brought about the resignation of the Congress (I) state Ministry and the imposition of President's rule.

With control of the Sikh agitation increasingly passing from the *Akali Dal* leadership to more militant factions, a full-scale crisis developed in June 1984 when government troops forcibly occupied the Sikh's Golden Temple in Amritsar, in the process killing many hundreds of Sikh militants. The assassination of Indira Gandhi by her Sikh bodyguards and the intercommunal violence which followed further delayed any progress being made by the *Akali Dal* leadership in negotiations with the central government. However, following his release from prison in March 1985 (together with other *Akali Dal* leaders), Sant Longowal in July 1985 signed an agreement with Rajiv Gandhi (the new Prime Minister) incorporating certain concessions to the Sikh political demands (including a pledge that Chandigarh would become solely the capital of Punjab rather than of both Punjab and Haryana) but expressly within the framework of the existing Constitution. This agreement was immediately denounced by *Akali Dal* militants as a

"stab in the back" and Sant Longowal was assassinated by Sikh gunmen in the following month.

Nevertheless, elections to the Punjab state Assembly went ahead in September 1985, when the Akali Dal won 73 of the 115 seats. The party accordingly formed a ministry under Surjit Singh Barnala, on whose swearing-in as Chief Minister President's rule was lifted.

The assassination of Sant Longowal in August 1985 exacerbated existing divisions within the Akali Dal, whose more militant members had already set up a breakaway Akali Dal (United) under the leadership of Joginder Singh. Having unsuccessfully tried to establish control over the whole party, this faction boycotted the September 1985 state elections in protest against the Longowal-Gandhi agreement and thereafter opposed the new leadership of Surjit Singh Barnala.

A further split developed in May 1986 after Barnala, as Chief Minister, had ordered Punjabi paramilitary forces into the Amritsar Golden Temple to quell Sikh extremists who had declared an independent "Khalistan". A number of state ministers and senior party figures resigned in protest against this action, the outcome being the formation in July 1986 of the Akali Dal (Badal) under the leadership of Prakash Singh Badal, a former Chief Minister of the Punjab. The Barnala faction, which became known as the Akali Dal (Longowal), remained the largest group in the state Assembly, but was left dependent on the Congress (I) members for a majority.

In a move to repair the breaches in Akali Dal unity, the five Sikh head priests issued a directive in February 1987 ordering the leaders of the various factions to resign to facilitate the formation of a unified party. Joginder Singh and Badal complied immediately, whereupon the priests announce the creation of a new Unified Akali Dal with Simranjit Singh Mann as its president but with a five-member presidium (including Joginder Singh and Badal) acting with equal presidential powers in Mann's absence. However, Barnala declined to comply with the priestly directive and maintained the *Akali Dal* (Longowal), with the support of most of his faction.

In May 1987 President's rule was reimposed in Punjab, the official reason being that the Barnala ministry lacked control so that many areas had plunged into "chaos and anarchy". Despite the imposition of President's rule, violence in the state escalated.

In 1988 the Unified Akali Dal split into two groups, after Badal moved to remove the imprisoned Mann from the presidency. Nevertheless, despite the rifts at leadership level, most of the factions remained committed to a non-violent, non-separatist solution to the Punjab issue. In the elections to the Lok Sabha in late 1989 the Mann faction of the *Akali Dal* won six of the 13 Punjabi seats, with three independents supported by the faction also being elected. Mann himself was elected by a large majority while still in prison; a few months prior to the election he had been charged in connection with the assassination in 1984 of the Prime Minister, Indira Gandhi, but was released later in the year. The success of the Mann faction was seen as a rejection by voters of the more moderate Longowal and Badal factions.

At a meeting in Chandigarh in early 1991, senior *Akali* leaders representing the Mann, Longowal and Badal factions decided to merge as a single *Akali Dal* to be known as *Shoromani Akali Dal*. Mann, as leader of the new grouping, sadi that henceforth no *Akali Dal* would be known after any individual and that "now our aim is one, the right of self-determination for Sikhs". In the weeks prior to the unification meeting, Mann had held talks with the Prime Minister, Chandra Shekhar. Little emerged from the talks, and militants denounced Mann and rejected dialogue with the government. Elections were held in February 1992 in Punjab for 13 seats in the *Lok Sabha* and for the State Assembly. All but one small faction of the *Shiromani Akali Dal* boycotted the election and Congress (I) won 12 of the *Lok Sabha* seats and a clear majority in the Assembly.

Sikkim

Sikkim Revolutionary Forum (*Sikkim Sangram Parishad*, SSP) (Sangram Bhavan, Jewan Theeng Marg, Gangtok 737101, Sikkim); leadership: Nar Bahadur Bhandari (pres). Founded in 1977, the SSP draws particular support from the majority Nepali population of Sikkim. The party was recognized in 1980 as the Sikkim unit of the Congress (I) and has since operated as its close ally. The party has consistently returned Sikkim's one *Lok Sabha* seat for the Congress (I) alliance and maintains a majority in the state Legislative Assembly.

Other Sikkim-based parties include: **Sikkim Congress (Revolutionary)**; **Rising Sun Party**.

Tamil Nadu

All-India Anna Dravida Munnetra Kazhagam (AIADMK—All-India Anna Dravidian Progress Movement) (275 Avvai Shanmugam Salai, Royapettah, Madras 600014, Tamil Nadu); leadership: Jayalalitha Jayaram. Founded in 1972. The party reflects Tamil (or Dravidian) nationalist sentiment, advocating the transfer to the states of all powers not reserved to the central government, abandonment of Hindi as the national language and its replacement by regional languages in each state (with English being the link-language), total prohibition of alcohol throughout India, a ceiling on incomes and the confiscation of "ill-gotten wealth", further nationalization in the banking, industrial and commodity distribution sectors, and power for electorates to "recall" elected representatives.

The AIADMK was founded as a splinter group of the *Dravida Munnetra Kazhagam* (DMK—Dravida Progress Movement), then the ruling party in Tamil Nadu. Originally called the ADMK (the prefix "Anna" signifying the movement's historic leader, C. N. Annadurai, who died February 1969), the breakaway party added "All-India" to its title in 1976. It quickly overtook the parent party, winning 130 seats in the state Assembly in 1977 and forming a ministry with its leader, Marudur Gopala Ramachandran ("M. G. R.", formerly a popular film star), as Chief Minister. The party was returned to power in May 1980 (in alliance with the two main Communist parties and other formations) and again in December 1984, when it won 132 of the 232 seats, this time in alliance with Congress (I), which had abandoned its previous alliance with the DMK.

In elections to the *Lok Sabha*, the AIADMK won 18 seats in 1977 in alliance with Congress but then aligned itself with the victorious *Janata* Party coalition. In the 1980 elections it was reduced to two seats, while the DMK, then allied with the victorious Congress (I), won 16. In the 1984-85 elections the AIADMK had the benefit of alliance with Congress (I), the formation winning 12 and 25 seats respectively of the 39 Tamil Nadu seats, while the DMK was reduced to two.

The death in December 1987 of M. G. Ramachandran generated a political crisis within the AIADMK, culminating in the imposition of President's rule in January 1988. At the heart of the crisis had been a split within the party into factions led by Ramachandran's widow, Janaki Ramachandran, and by his mistress, Jayalalitha Jayaram. With state elections due in January 1989, Congress (I) refused an offer of an electoral alliance with the Jayalalitha faction, and relied instead on intensive personal campaigning by Rajiv Gandhi. In the event this tactic proved counter-productive, and the DMK was elected to office with a two-thirds majority. The two opposing factions of the AIADMK merged in March 1989 to form a united front against the DMK.

The party won 11 seats in the 1989 general election, but its Congress (I) ally was defeated. In early 1991 the DMK government was dismissed and President's rule imposed as a result of increased activity by Tamil militants in the state. In state elections held that June the AIADMK was swept back to power and Jayalalitha became Chief Minister. The party also won 11 *Lok Sabha* seats in the general election held in May-June.

Dravida Munnetra Kazhagam (DMK—Dravidian Progress Movement) ("Anna Arivalayam" 268-269, Anna Salai, Teynampet Madras 600018, Tamil Nadu); leadership: Muthuvel Karunanidhi (pres); K. Anbuzhan (gen. sec.). Founded in September 1949. A Tamil (i.e. Dravidian) communalist group, urging full autonomy for the state of Tamil Nadu within the Union and the recognition of regional languages as state languages (with English becoming the official all-India language). Originally to the right of the breakaway All-India *Anna Dravida Munnetra Kazhagam* (AIADMK) on economic policy, the DMK has recently gravitated to the left and formed alliances with the main Communist parties. The DMK has also voiced strong support for the Tamil struggle in Sri-Lanka, in contrast to the more cautious approach of the AIADMK. It first secured representation in the *Lok Sabha* in 1957 and went on to win 25 seats in 1967 and 23 in 1971. The party split in 1972, with one faction becoming the AIADMK. The DMK was reduced to one seat in 1979, despite being a part of the victorious *Janata*-led coalition, but recovered 16 seats in 1980, when it was allied to the victorious Congress (I). In the 1984-85 elections Congress (I) was allied with the AIADMK and the DMK's *Lok Sabha* representation fell to two seats. The party failed to win any seats in either the 1989 or 1991 general elections. However, in January 1989 the party scored a spectacular victory in state elections, easily defeating the AIADMK to take control of the State Assembly. DMK rule ended in January 1991 when President's rule was imposed; five months later the party suffered a massive defeat at the hands of the AIADMK, winning only one Assembly seat, against 163 for its rival.

Other Tamil Nadu-based parties include: **Gandi Kamaraj National Congress; Indian Farmers and Toilers Party; Pattali Makkal Katchi; Tamil Nadu Congress (Kanaraj); Tamil Nadu Forward Bloc;** and the **Backward and Depressed People's Protection Front**.

Tripura

The main regional parties in Tripura are the **Tripura Tribal Youth Organization** and the **Tripura State Congress for Democracy**.

West Bengal

There is a proliferation of regional left-wing parties in West Bengal. Some support the ruling Communist Party of India (Marxist) at state level; others, like the **Forward Bloc** (with 28 state and three *Lok Sabha* seats) support the CPI (M) at state level and also at federal level as part of the Left Front; others have no state or federal representation. These parties include: **Biplabi Bangla Congress; Bolshevik Party of India; Democratic Socialist Party;** and the **West Bengal Socialist Party**.

Defunct Parties

Janata Party (JP) Founded in 1977. This socialist party was led from the start by Chandra Shekhar. The party won 21 seats in the 1980 elections and 10 in the 1984 election. In 1988 the party merged with other opposition groups to create the *Janata Dal*.

Jan Morcha (People's Front). Founded in October 1987 by Congress (I) rebels led by V. P. Singh, the *Jan Morcha* quickly united a previously divided opposition. It merged with other opposition groups in 1988 to form a single anti-Congress party, *Janata Dal*.

Lok Dal (The People's Party). Founded in 1979 by Charan Singh. The party merged with the Democratic Socialist Party in 1984 to form the *Dalit Mazdoor Kisan*, which went on to win only three seats in elections held later in the year. Following the elections *Lok Dal* re-emerged as a distinct entity, but in 1987 it split into two opposing factions, one led by Ajit Singh (Charan Singh's son) and the other by party president H. N. Bahuguna. In 1988 the Ajit faction merged into the *Janata* Party. Later that year the Bahuguna faction was effectively displaced and the remainder of the party joined with other opposition groups to form the *Janata Dal*.

National Sanjay Organization (*Rashtriya Sanjay*

Manch). Founded in 1983 by Maneka Gandhi, widow of Indira Gandhi's younger son, Sanjay, who was killed in a flying accident in 1980 and who had previously been associated with some of his mother's more controversial policies, particularly sterilisation and the emergency rule of 1975-77. In the 1984 general election Maneka failed to displace her brother-in-law and new Congress (I) leader Rajiv Gandhi from his Amethi constituency. The party failed to win a seat. In 1988 the party merged with the *Janata* Party.

Dalit Mazdoor Kisan Party. Founded in 1984 as a merger between the *Lok Dal* and the Democratic Socialist Party, it won only three seats in the general election held later that year. After the elections *Lok Dal* re-emerged as a separate entity and the party disintegrated.

Indian National Congress (Jagjivan). Founded in as a centre-left party, committed to democracy, secularism and social equality by Jagjivan Ram, leader of the *harijan* (untouchables). With the death of Jagjivan Ram in 1986 the party divided into various factions, none of which contested the 1989 election.

Illegal Parties

Illegal parties are mainly separatist or communal, although guerrilla operations were still being carried out by Maoist Naxalite rebels in some states. Right-wing Hindu extremist groups include: **Vishawa Hindu Parishad; Anand Marg;** the **Rashtriya Swayam Sewak Sangh** (National Union of Selfless Servers); Universal Proutist Revolutionary Front;

The main separatist movements are as follows.
Assam: United Liberation Front of Assam; All Bodo Students' Union.

Bihar: Jharkhand Co-ordination Committee; Hill Tribal Liberation Organization.

Kashmir: Kashmir Liberation Army; Kashmir Liberation Front; Jammu and Kashmir Student Liberation Front; *Hizbullah*; Muslim Crusade Force; *Ikhwan al-Muslimeen*; *Jamaat-i Islami* Jammu and Kashmir; Peoples' League; *Jamaat-i Tulaba*; Students' Islamic Movement of India.

Manipur: People's Liberation Army.

Nagaland: Naga Separatist Movement; National Socialist Council of Nagaland; North-Eastern region Liberation Organization.

Punjab: All India Sikh Student Federation; Dashmesh Regiment; International Sikh Federation; Khalistan Commando Force; National Council of Khalistan; Khalistan National Organization; United *Akali Dal*.

Tripura: Tripura National Volunteers; **West Bengal:** Gorkha National Liberation Front (GNLF).

Indonesia

Capital: Jakarta   **Population: 184,300,000 (1990)**

Indonesia, comprising some 13,700 islands, gained full independence from the Netherlands in 1950. The country is divided into 27 provinces, the most recent (East Timor) having been annexed in 1976. Despite the existence of the necessary elements of constitutional government, the state has been dominated since the installation of the military "New Order" regime in 1966 by President Suharto, whose power is based primarily on the continued support of the armed forces. The dominant political organization, *Sekber Golongan Karya* or *Golkar*, was brought under government control in 1969 to provide a civilian vehicle for the Suharto regime. In 1973 the nine other existing political organizations were ordered by the government to fuse into two new parties, the Indonesia Democratic Party and the United Development Party; the three-party system was consolidated in 1975 by legislation which permitted no other parties to exist. All political organizations are obliged under a law of 1984 to adopt the *Pancasila*, the creed enshrined in the 1945 Constitution, (monotheism, humanitarianism, national unity, democracy by consensus and social justice), as their sole ideological foundation.

Constitutional structure

According to its 1945 Constitution, the Republic of Indonesia is a unitary state with an executive President who governs with the assistance of a Cabinet appointed by him, and who is elected (and can be re-elected) by a 1,000-member People's Consultative Assembly (*Majelis Permusyarawatan Rakyat*), the highest authority of the state. Of the Assembly's members, 500 are from the House of Representatives (*Dewan Perwakilan Rakyat*), the legislature, to which 400 members are elected for a five-year term by direct universal adult suffrage and the rest, mostly representatives of the armed forces, are appointed by the government. The Assembly's other 500 members are government appointees, delegates of regional assemblies, and representatives of parties and groups (appointed in proportion to their elective seats in the House of Representatives).

Electoral system

Candidates for the elective seats in the House of Representatives are returned in multimember constituencies under a system of proportional representation. The People's Consultative Assembly elects the President and Vice-President for a five-year term.

Evolution of the suffrage

All adults aged 17 and over, or younger if married, are entitled to vote, with the exception of members of the armed forces, persons involved in the abortive communist-backed coup in 1965 and other categories of person such as convicted criminals.

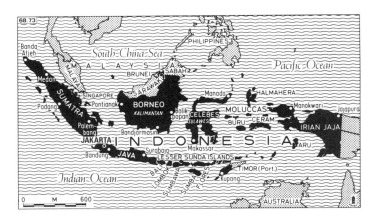

Recent elections

Elections to House of Representatives 1977-1992

Party	Year			
	1977	*1982*	*1987*	*1992*
Golkar	232	246	299	282
Indonesian Democratic Party	29	24	40	56
United Development Party	99	94	61	62
Total elective seats	360	364	400	400

PARTY BY PARTY DATA

Functional Group Centre
Golongan Karya Pusat (Golkar)
Address. Jalan Anggrek Nelimurni, Jakarta 11480.
Leadership. Suharto (ch. of advisor board); Sudharmono (co-ordinator of presidium); Wahono (gen. ch.); Manihuruk (dep. gen. ch.); Rachmat Witoelar (sec.-gen.).
Orientation. Pro-government organization.
Founded. 1964.
History. Technically, Golkar is not a political party but an amalgamation of numerous occupational groups, ranging from farmers and fishermen to civil servants and security personnel. Under Suharto's "New Order" *Golkar* has been lauded as the alternative to traditional political parties, which have been regarded as socially divisive and potentially dangerous. However, in reality, *Golkar* has been used by Suharto and the armed forces as a means of establishing a civilian basis for the regime.

Golkar entered the 1971 elections firmly established as the pro-government organization and won a resounding victory, obtaining 236 out of 360 contested seats and 62.8 per cent of the total votes cast. The introduction of legislation in 1975 consolidating the country's nine opposition parties into two new parties strengthened *Golkar*'s position and in the 1977 election, despite increasing disenchantment with the government's economic policies, it secured another victory, winning 232 out of 360 seats and 62.1 per cent of the vote. *Golkar* increased its representation to 246 seats (out of 364) in 1982 and to 299 (out of 400) seats in 1987, when it gained an overall majority in all 27 provinces. In 1988 *Golkar* held its fourth national congress which was preceded by intensive military manoeuvres aimed at obstructing the re-election of the incumbent general chair, Vice-President Sudharmono, who was perceived by some in the army to have leftist sympathies. In the event, Sudharmono was replaced by a civilian, Wahono, an outcome viewed by many commentators as less than ideal for the military.

Golkar was returned to power with a slightly reduced majority in elections held in June 1992 to 400 seats in the House of Representatives. Although *Golkar* again won an overall majority in all 27 provinces (including the disputed territory of East Timor), its share of the vote fell from 73 per cent in 1987 to 68 per cent in 1992. Analysts appeared unsure whether the result represented a clear mandate for continuity or reflected a growing, if tentative, desire for change.

However, they were generally agreed that *Golkar*'s performance in Java, where it suffered losses, was a cause for some concern within the organization.
Structure. Organizational leadership resides in a five-member national council and an advisory board. There are 13 co-ordinating bodies grouped under five secretaries responsible for the following areas; civil service and labour; cultural and spiritual; economic and production; defence and security; and youth, women's and intellectuals' activities.
Membership. 25,000,000.

Indonesian Democratic Party
Partai Demokrasi Indonesia (PDI)
Address. Jalan Anggrek Nelimurni, Jakarta 11480
Leadership. Soerjadi (gen. ch.); Nico Daryanto (sec.-gen.); Kwik Gian Gee (sec.-gen.)
Orientation. Seeks the restoration of full civilian rule, but remains largely supportive of the Suharto regime.
Founded. 1973.
History. The PDI was formed as a result of the Suharto regime's desire to "simplify" the party system. Hence, the party was created by the merger of five parties, three nationalist and two Christian-based, namely (i) the Indonesian Nationalist Party (*Partai Nasional Indonesia*—PNI); (ii) the Movement for the Defence of Indonesian Independence (*Ikatan Pendukung Kemerdekaan Indonesia*—IPKI); (iii) the People's Party (*Partai Murba*); (iv) the Catholic Party (*Partai Katolik*); and (v) the (Protestant) Christian Party (*Partai Keristen Indonesia*—Parkindo). The PDI seeks a full restoration of civil rule, but its support has not been consistent. In the first general election to the House of Representatives which it contested (in 1977) the PDI gained an overall 8.6 per cent of the total vote and 29 seats. In the next election held in 1982 its share fell to 24 seats and less than 5 per cent of the vote in 14 provinces, less than 10 per cent in another eight provinces, and only 12 per cent in Jakarta (its main centre of support). In the 1987 elections there was a resurgance of support for the party, largely a result of an energetic campaign conducted by high-profile figures such as former President Sukarno's daughter Negawati Sukarno-putri. The party increased its share of the vote to 10.9 per cent and gained 40 seats. In a general election held in June 1992 the PDI performed extremely well, increasing its representation to 56 seats and 15 per cent of the vote, gaining all its extra 16 seats from the ruling *Golkar*. During the campaign the party

had staged large, exhuberant rallies and had even managed to stretch the limits of official tolerance by attacking "nepotism" in high places, a clear reference to the business dealings of President Suharto's family, and by calling for the presidential term to be limited to two years, an implicit criticism of Suharto's long period in office.

United Development Party

Partai Persatuan Pembangunan (PPP)

Address. Jalan Diponegoro 60, Jakarta.

Leadership. Ismael Hassan Metareum (pres.); Mardinsyah (sec.-gen.).

Orientation. Moderate Islamic; supports the Suharto regime in all matters other than religious ones.

Founded: 1973.

History. Government pressure on political organizations to "simplify" the party system resulted in the merger of four Islamic groups into the PPP. The four were (i) the Moslem Scholars' League (*Nahdatul-'Ulama*—NU); (ii) the Indonesian Moslem Party (*Partai Muslimin Indonesia*—PMI); (iii) the Indonesian Islamic Association Party (*Partai Sjarikat Islam Indonesia*—PSII); and (iv) the Islamic Education Party (*Persatuan Tarbijah Islamijah*—Perti). In the 1977 election to the House of Representatives the PPP gained 29.3 per cent of the total vote, and 99 seats, rather more than those obtained in 1971 by the four parties from which it was formed. From the outset the PPP was beset by sectarian and regional differences and in the 1982 elections the party's share of the vote fell to 28 per cent (with 94 seats). However, the results were challenged by the party leadership which claimed, in particular, that it had overwhelming support in Jakarta, where it had won a majority in 1977 but only five seats in 1982 (against six for the ruling Functional Group Centre (*Golkar*) and two for the Indonesian Democratic Party).

The PPP held its first congress in 1984 when it complied with new legislation and formally adopted *Pancasila*, the secularist state creed, as its sole ideological foundation. The congress was characterized by factional wrangling and dissatisfaction was voiced over the leadership of party chair John Naro, who was accused of favouring the PMI faction. At the congress conservative elements within the NU faction, led by Abdurrahman Wahid, called for the party's complete withdrawal from "practical politics". In late 1984 the NU faction withdrew from the party to devote itself to social and religious works. With the withdrawal of the NU, support for the party fell dramatically and in the

1987 elections the party won only 16 per cent of the vote and 61 seats. In 1988 Naro presented himself as a candidate for the vice-presidency, but he withdrew prior to the election thereby allowing *Golkar* chair Lt.-Gen. Sudharmono to be elected unopposed. The party held its second congress in 1989, at which Ismael Hassan Metareum was named as party chair.

In a general election held in June 1992 for 400 seats in the *Dewan Perwakilan Rakyat* the PPP increased its seats from 61 to 62 and its percentage of the vote from 16 per cent to 17 per cent. The one seat gain was made at the expense of the ruling *Golkar*.

Structure. The party has a national executive; the constituent parties exist as "non political associations".

Other legal political organizations

The government sanctioned the formation of two new organizations in 1990-91.

The **Association of Moslem Intellectuals** (*Ikatan Cendikiawan Moslem Indonesia*—ICMI) held its inaugural congress in late 1990, which was attended by President Suharto. The ICMI claimed to be a non-political organization, but many commentators speculated that it would be used by Suharto to build a broad-based, non-military constituency to support his re-election as President in 1993. The ICMI is chaired by Bacharuddin Habibie.

A **Democracy Forum** was formed in April 1991, headed by Abdurrahman Wahid, leader of the *Nahdatul-'Ulama*. Wahid claimed that the Forum aimed to promote a national political dialogue.

Parties in conflict with the government

The **Communist Party of Indonesia** (*Partai Komunis Indonesia*—PKI) was banned in 1966 and as of 1992 was virtually inactive.

The **Petition of 50** (*Petisi 50*) a potent source of opposition to the Suharto regime, is a group of dissident military officers and political activists formed in 1980.

Major guerrilla groups

National Liberation Front of Aceh (also known as the **Free Aceh Movement**) seeks independence for the north Sumatran state of Aceh.

Papua Independent Organization (*Organisasi Papua Merdeka*—OPM) seeks the integration of Irian Jaya into Papua New Guinea [see also Papua new Guinea].

Revolutionary Front for the Independence of East Timor (*Frente Revolucionario de Este Timor Independente*—Fretilin) is the main pro-independence group in East Timor.

Japan

Capital: Tokyo **Population: 123,611,541 (1990)**

Japan is a constitutional monarchy with a stable democratic system. Forcibly opened to Western influences in 1853, Japan soon began a process of military expansion which ended with its defeat in 1945. The US occupation which followed the Pacific War involved a comprehensive revision of Japan's political structure, and included a renunciation of the tradition of imperial divinity.

Elections in Japan have been held regularly since 1890 (including during times of war) in accordance with constitutional requirements. Since its formation in 1955, the conservative Liberal Democratic Party (LDP) has enjoyed an uninterrupted period in office.

Constitutional structure

The current constitution, promulgated by the emperor on Nov. 3, 1946, and effective from May 3, 1947, was a product of the US military occupation which had followed Japan's defeat in the Pacific War. Whereas in the pre-war era the Emperor had been regarded as a god, the 1947 constitution established the principle of popular sovereignty and defined the monarch's function as "the symbol of the state and the unity of the people, deriving his position from the will of the people with whom resides sovereign power". The constitution also enshrines the principle of pacifism, stating that the Japanese people "forever renounce war as a sovereign right of the nation and the threat or use of force as a means of settling international disputes".

Electoral system

Legislative authority is vested in a popularly elected bicameral Diet, defined by the constitution as the "sole law-making organ of the state" and as the "highest organ of state power". The Diet is composed of a 512-member House of Representatives (elected for up to four years) and a House of Councillors (whose 252 members are elected for six years, with half being due for re-election every three years). In the event of a disagreement between the two chambers, the constitution stipulates that the House of Representatives shall take precedence. The Prime Minister (who appoints a Cabinet) is chosen by, and remains responsible to, the Diet.

The 512 lower house seats are divided among 130 multimember constituencies, each of which contains between three and five members. In the upper house 100 members are elected under a system of proportional representation, while the remaining 152 are elected from 47 prefectural electoral districts, each of which has between two and eight seats.

Evolution of the suffrage

From the passage of the first House of Representatives Members Election Law in 1889 until 1900 suffrage was restricted to men aged 25 years or over who paid at least 15 yen in annual direct state taxes. This meant that only 450,000 men (1.1 per cent of the total population) were enfranchised. In 1900 the taxation requirement was reduced to 10 yen per year which increased the electorate to 980,000 men (2.2 per cent of the total). In the same year secret ballots were also introduced. In 1919 the tax threshold was

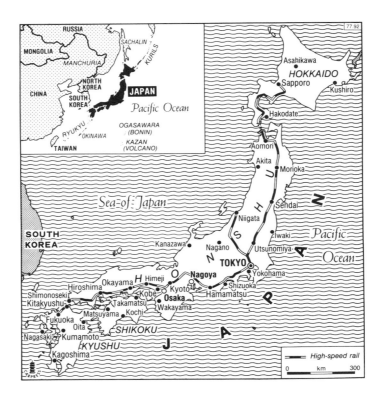

Recent elections

Elections to House of Representatives since 1945

Date	Winning Party	Date	Winning Party
April 10, 1946	Japan Liberal Party*	Jan. 29, 1967	Liberal Democratic Party
April 25, 1947	Socialist Party*	Dec. 27, 1969	Liberal Democratic Party
Jan. 23, 1949	Japan Liberal Party	Dec. 10, 1972	Liberal Democratic Party
Oct. 1, 1952	Japan Liberal Party	Dec. 5, 1976	Liberal Democratic Party*
April 19, 1953	Yoshida Liberal Party*	Oct. 7, 1979	Liberal Democratic Party*
Feb. 27, 1955	Democratic Party*	June 22, 1980	Liberal Democratic Party
May 22, 1958	Liberal Democratic Party	Dec. 18, 1983	Liberal Democratic Party
Nov. 20, 1960	Liberal Democratic Party	July 6, 1986	Liberal Democratic Party
Nov. 21, 1963	Liberal Democratic Party	Feb. 18, 1990	Liberal Democratic Party

*Denotes failure to achieve an overall majority.

Last two lower house elections

Party	1986 Percentage of vote	1986 Seats won	1990 Percentage of vote	1990 Seats won
LDP	49.4	300	46.1	275
JSP	17.2	85	24.4	136
Komeito	9.4	56	8.0	45
JCP	8.8	26	8.0	16
DSP	6.4	26	4.8	14
NLP	1.8	6	—	—
Minor Parties	1.1	4	1.4	5
Independents	5.8	9	7.3	21
Total	100	512	100	512

The LDP maintained an overall majority in the 252-member House of Counsellors (the upper house) from the party's formation in 1955 until the elections of July 23, 1989. As a result of that election the party's strength in the House of Counsellors fell from 142 to 109.

lowered to 3 yen, resulting in an electorate of 3,100,000 (5.5 per cent of the population). Universal male suffrage was introduced in 1925. Following Japan's defeat in 1945 there was sweeping constitutional reform which included the enfranchisement of women and a lowering of the voting age to 20 years.

PARTY BY PARTY DATA

Clean Government Party
Komeito
Address. 17 Minami Motomachi, Shinjyuku-ku, Tokyo 160.
Leadership. Koshiro Ishida (ch.).
Orientation. The political arm of the *Soka Gakkai*, a lay organization affiliated with the *Nichiren Shoshu* sect of Buddhism. In orthodox political terms it is usually classified as centrist.
Founded. November 1964.
History. The *Soka Gakkai* established the Koemei Political League as its political arm in 1961. By the time that the organization became a full political party it already had 15 seats in the Upper House, and some 1,500 local assembly members. Following its first two leaders, Koji Harashima and Takeji Tsuji, Yoshikatsu Takeiri took over as chairman and remained at the head of the party until December 1986.

The *Komeito* won 25 seats in the House of Representatives in the general election of 1967, and increased this figure to 47 seats in 1969. Having fallen back to 29 seats in 1972, it rose to 56 seats in 1976 and 57 in 1979. Its lower house representation fell to 33 in the 1980 election, but rose to 58 in 1983. Since then its representation has fallen to 56 in 1986, and 45 in 1990. Despite maintaining its position as the third largest party in the Diet, *Komeito* has been unable to increase its share of the vote beyond 11 per cent or to challenge the position of the ruling Liberal Democratic Party (LDP) or the Social Democratic Party of Japan (SDPJ).

At the time of its foundation *Komeito* was a religious party, the primary aim of which was to create a coalescence of temporal power and Buddhist law. In the late 1960s, however, the party found that its relationship with the *Soka Gakkai* was the source of difficulties and in 1970 it severed all formal relations with the organization. Nevertheless, close informal links were retained, with most *Komeito* legislators continuing to be *Soka Gakkai* members. *Komeito* redefined itself as "a national political party committed to a centrist ideology based on respect for humanity". It also incorporated "humanitarian socialism", an independent peace-orientated foreign policy, and respect for the constitution and for the parliamentary process. The break was followed by declining electoral support and in the early 1970s the party moved further to the left. At its 1973 convention it expressed vehement opposition to the LDP and the forces of large-scale capitalism, and announced its readiness to co-operate with the Japan Communist Party (JCP).

The alliance with the JCP proved less than harmonious and in October 1975 the *Komeito* annual convention moved the party back towards the right and endorsed the concept of an opposition coalition which would include the Japan Socialist Party (now renamed the Social Democratic Party of Japan—SDPJ) and the Democratic Socialist Party (DSP) but which would exclude the communists. This move to the right culminated in the party's 1978 decision to support the Japan-US security arrangements to which it had previously expressed implacable opposition. The three opposition parties did make attempts to create an effective opposition coalition, particularly after the LDP lost its overall majority in the upper house in 1989, but no stable relationship could be maintained.

In the 1980s the party was damaged by its involvement in a series of scandals, the most infamous of which was the Recruit-Cosmos share scandal which led to the fall of the Takeshita government in 1989. In May 1989 a *Komeito* legislator was among the first two Diet members to be indicted in connection with the Recruit affair. The party's secretary general, Junya Yano immediately resigned as an act of atonement. He was replaced by Koshiro Ishida.

The party was undermined further by the outbreak of a ferocious struggle surrounding *Soka Gakkai*. On Nov. 7, 1991, the clergy of the *Nichiren Shoshu* Buddhist sect, founded in the 13th century, ordered the dissolution of its lay organization. The clergy alleged that *Soka Gakkai* was corrupt and that its leader since 1960, Daisaku Ikeda, was working to undermine the authority of the clergy with a view to creating his own religion. The leadership of *Soka Gakkai* refused to comply with the order and called instead for the replacement of Nikken Abe the chief priest of the Buddhist sect.

The opposition's failure to break the monopoly of

power enjoyed by the LDP, together with the decline of the SDPJ in the early 1990s, saw the fracturing of the opposition coalition and the increasing readiness of *Komeito* to work with the LDP. The party was soundly criticized by its erstwhile opposition allies in when it co-operated with the government in forcing onto the statute books a highly controversial bill to allow Japanese military forces to serve overseas as part of UN peace keeping forces.

Structure. The party's highest decision-making body is its national convention which meets annually and elects a central executive committee.

Membership. 213,000.

Publications. Komei Shinbun (daily); *Komei* (weekly).

Democratic Socialist Party (DSP)

Minshato

Address. 6th Floor, No. 18 Mori Building, 2-3-13, Toranomon, Minato-ku, Tokyo 105.

Leadership. Keigo Ouchi.

Orientation. Right-wing democratic socialist. The party stands for limited public ownership and the maintenance of current constitutional and human rights.

Founded. January 1960.

History. The Democratic Socialist Party (DSP) was created by Suehiro Nishio and other dissidents from the right of the Japan Socialist Party (JSP). The catalyst for the split was the imminent revision of the Japan-US Security Treaty. While the left-wing leadership of the JSP was implacably opposed to any security arrangement with the USA, Nishio and his supporters advocated putting forward concrete proposals for revising the treaty. After being fiercely criticized at the 1959 JSP party convention, the rebels resigned at the end of the year and, in January 1960, founded a new party.

The party modelled itself upon the social democratic movements of Western Europe rather than on the Marxist parties which had heavily influenced the JSP. From the outset, the DSP and its policies reflected pragmatism and a desire to achieve office—Nishio aimed at "seizing power within five years"—rather than any deep ideological commitment. At the election of 1960, however, the party's strength in the lower house fell from 40 to 17 seats. Its representation rose to 23 in 1963, 30 in 1967 and 31 in 1969, but fell back to 19 in 1972. In 1976 the party won 29 seats, in 1979 this rose to 35, but fell to 32 in 1980. Its total of seats increased to 38 in 1983, but fell to 26 in 1986 and to only 14 in 1990. Although the party managed small increases in the percentage share of its vote in 1969,

1979 and 1983, the overall trend during the entire period of its existence was of declining support. Having achieved 8.8 per cent of the vote in 1960, it never again achieved 8 per cent, and in 1990 was reduced to a mere 4.8 per cent.

The party's failure to displace the JSP and establish itself as the main vehicle of opposition to the Liberal Democratic Party (LDP) led it towards a three-party centrist-progressive coalition with *Komeito* and the JSP. This was formally adopted at the party conference of February 1974. Shortly afterwards, under the leadership of Ryosaku Sasaki, this position evolved into a strategy of both working towards an alliance of the non-communist opposition parties, and expressing an interest in working with the LDP. Saburo Tsukamoto inherited this policy when he became leader in 1985, but the LDP's decisive election victory in 1986 and its absorption of the New Liberal Club, reduced the prospect of any immediate alliance with the DSP.

The resurgence of the opposition and the difficulties experienced by the LDP in the late 1980s intensified speculation that the opposition parties might coalesce into a real alternative to the LDP. Little progress was made in this direction, however, and, like *Komeito*, the DSP suffered from its involvement in the Recruit-Cosmos scandal which brought down the Takeshita government in 1989. One of the first casualties of the scandal was Tsukamoto, who resigned in February 1989 because of his involvement in the share scandal. Even after the LDP's loss of its overall majority in the upper house in 1989 there was little effective opposition unity. Like *Komeito*, the DSP frequently co-operated with the LDP to enable the government to ensure the passage of legislation through the upper chamber.

Structure. The party is organized in communities, constituencies, and prefectures, and holds an annual convention which elects a central executive committee.

Membership. 213,000.

Publications. Shukan Minsha (weekly); *Kakushin* (monthly).

International affiliations. Socialist International.

Japan Communist Party (JCP)

Nihon Kyosanto

Address. 4-26-7 Sendagaya, Shibuya-ku, Tokyo, 151.

Leadership. Tetsuzo Fuwa.

Orientation. The JCP has traditionally prided itself on its independence from external influences. In 1976 it abandoned the theory of dictatorship of the proletariat and replaced the term "Marxism-Leninism" with that of "scientific socialism".

Founded. July 1922.

History. The Japan Communist Party (JCP) was an underground organization between 1922 and 1945, and was frequently subjected to intensive persecution by the authorities. The trial and conviction of its senior leaders in 1932 dealt the party a severe blow. The party emerged into the political mainstream in 1945 and held its fourth congress, the first such meeting for 19 years, which was attended both by former political prisoners and by those who had returned from periods of exile in China.

Initially the party adopted a policy of "peaceful revolution under the Occupation". Untainted by the militarism of the pre-war period the party prospered. At the 1949 election it gained 9.8 per cent of the vote and won 35 seats in the House of Representatives. In 1950, however, the peaceful revolution approach was denounced by the Coninform causing the party to split between a hardline "mainstream" faction led by secretary general Kyuichi Tokuda, and a smaller "international" faction. Against the background of the Korean War, the party adopted an uncompromising stance at its 1951 national conference, endorsing a policy of revolution through armed insurrection. Membership declined and the party lost all of its seats in the Diet in 1952, with its share of the vote falling to 2.5 per cent.

Further defeats followed and from the mid-1950s the party began to revise its policies. Unity was restored at the seventh party congress in 1958 under the leadership of Kenji Miyamoto, on the principles of "self-reliance and independence", non-violence, and an acceptance of parliamentary government. Miyamoto repeatedly purged hardline pro-Moscow and pro-Beijing members and revised the party's constitution and policies in order to demonstrate its allegiance to the new principles. He also increased his hold over the party with the creation of the post of chairman of the Presidium in 1970, a position which he himself assumed. Gradually the party recovered and in 1972 it won 10.5 per cent of the vote and 38 seats in the House of Representatives. It maintained this level of support in the elections of 1976 and 1979 winning 17 and 39 seats respectively. Thereafter, the party's strength declined. In 1980 it won 29 seats (9.8 per cent of the vote), while in 1983 and 1986 it achieved 26 seats with around 9 per cent of the vote.

At the 16th congress in July 1982 the leadership was reshuffled, with Miyamoto continuing to exert authority as chairman of the central committee while his appointee, Tetsuzo Fuwa, became chairman of the presidium. Fuwa was succeeded in 1987 by Hiromu Murakami. Despite advocating an opposition coalition against the ruling Liberal Democratic Party (LDP), the JCP was largely ignored by the other opposition parties. Adversely affected by the collapse of the Soviet Union and by its increasing isolation within the Diet, in the 1990 election the JCP's share of the vote fell to 8 per cent and its number of seats declined to 16.

Structure. The JCP has branches on a residential and occupational basis and is organized at district and prefectural level. Its supreme organ is its congress, which elects a central committee, which in turn elects a chairman and a presidium. The latter appoints a permanent bureau and a secretariat.

Membership. 400,000

Publications. *Akahata* (daily); *Gurafu Konnichiwa* (monthly); *Zen'ei* (monthly).

Liberal Democratic Party (LDP)

Jiyu Minshuto

Address. 1-11-23 Nagata-cho, Chiyoda-ku, Tokyo 100.

Leadership. Kiichi Miyazawa (ch.).

Orientation. Conservative. The LDP advocates an unfettered capitalist system as the foundation of democratic government, and supports a continuing close relationship with the USA, and an increase of Japanese influence in Asia.

Founded. November 1955.

History. The Liberal Democratic Party (LDP) was created through the merger of the two main conservative parties of the time, the Liberal Party (led by Taketora Ogata) and the Democratic Party (led by Ichiro Hatoyama, then Prime Minister). The former had been founded in 1945 but had been subject to numerous splits, particulary in the early 1950s. The Democratic Party had been created in 1954 by defectors from the Liberal Party who had been joined by the Reform Party. Both of the constituent elements of the new party were composed of factions based around individuals, and this characteristic became a feature of the LDP. As the party developed, so the role of the factions increased, until they became hugely wealthy and largely autonomous organizations. This process was assisted by the country's multimember electoral system as, with LDP members competing against one another in the same electoral district, candidates came to rely upon factional support for their election.

Initially the leadership of the party was shared by a "presidential caretaker committee". Following Ogata's death, however, Hatoyama became party president in April 1956. Since then almost all LDP leaders have been factional leaders and have been selected as party leader as a result of inter-factional negotiations. Although subject to election by the party, in reality the result of leadership contests has tended to have been determined in advance by back-room brokering. Currently the party's rules allow an individual to serve no more than two two-year terms as LDP president, although in October 1986 Yashuhiro Nakasone was granted a one-year extension at the end of his second term. As the LDP has been in government continuously since its formation, the selection of its leader has been synonymous with the choice of Japan's Prime Minister.

Following the 1955 merger the LDP held 299 seats in the House of Representatives and 118 in the House of Councillors. At the elections of 1958 and 1960 it polled over 57 per cent of the vote and won 287 and 296 seats respectively. In 1963 its vote fell to 54.7 per cent but it retained a comfortable overall majority with 283 seats. In the 1967 election its share of the vote fell to 48.8 per cent, the first occasion that it had ever dropped below 50 per cent, although the party retained 277 seats. In 1969 it increased its number of seats to 288, but polled only 47.6 per cent of the vote.

Hatoyama was succeeded as party leader by Tanzan Ishibashi, but he was forced from office after only 65 days as a result of illness. He was succeeded by Nobusuke Kishi, who governed from 1957 to 1960, and succeeded in renegotiating the Japan-US Security Treaty, although the methods used to gain Diet approval for the new treaty in 1960 led to major protests which ultimately forced Kishi from office. Kishi's resignation in July was followed by 12 years under two Primes Minters: Hayato Ikeda 1960-63 and Eisaku Sato 1964-72. By serving as Prime Minister for seven years and eight months, the latter became the longest continuously serving premier in modern Japanese history.

In July 1972 Kakuei Tanaka won a fiercely contested leadership struggle to succeed Sato. His relative youth—he was 54 when he became Prime Minister—his image as a self-made man, and his reputation for dynamism all made a sharp contrast with the bureaucratic Sato years, and created the impression that he was about to usher in a new age of Japanese politics. Almost immediately he pulled off a spectacular coup by normalizing relations with China. In late 1972 he called a general election and won 271 seats with 46.9 per cent of the poll. After a period of rapid economic expansion in the 1950s and 1960s, the autumn of 1973 saw the Japanese economy—totally dependent on foreign oil—hit by the first oil price crisis. Damaged by the resulting austerity measures and by his growing notoriety as an exponent of "money politics", Tanaka was forced to resign in December 1974 and was succeeded by Takeo Miki.

A further blow to the LDP came in early 1976 with the emergence of the political bribery scandal involving the Lockheed Aircraft Corporation. Miki's forthright approach in uncovering the scandal made him unpopular among many of his party colleagues, particularly after the arrest of Tanaka in July 1976. The Lockheed scandal also caused Yohei Kono and several other Diet members to defect from the LDP in June and form the New Liberal Club (NLC), a party which offered conservatism without the corruption associated with old-style "money politics". At the election of December 1976 the LDP failed to secure an overall majority for the first time in its history, polling 41.8 per cent of the vote and winning 249 seats. Although the party was able to put together a slim majority by attracting a dozen of the independents, Miki resigned almost immediately.

He was succeeded by Takeo Fukuda who lost the party leadership in 1978 to Masayoshi Ohira, a candidate supported by the powerful Tanaka faction. In the general election of 1979 the LDP scored 44.6 per cent of the vote but saw its number of seats reduced to 248. Unable to agree on a candidate for Prime Minister, the party put forward both Ohira and Fukuda to the Diet, with the former narrowly winning after an indecisive first ballot. Tension between the two remained a source of LDP weakness and in May 1980 Ohira was forced to dissolve the Diet after members of the Fukuda and Miki factions failed to defend the government against an opposition vote of no confidence. During the subsequent campaign June 1980 Ohira died, but the party went on to win a decisive overall majorities in both the upper and lower house. In the contest for the lower house the party polled 47.9 per cent and won 284 seats. In July Zenko Suzuki was chosen as party leader, and he served a competent if somewhat undistinguished term.

In 1982 Yashuhiro Nakasone, supported by the huge Tanaka faction, won the election to succeed Suzuki. In 1983 Tanaka was found guilty of accepting bribes from Lockheed and the general election held later that year was conducted in the context of strong opposition criticism concerning the former Prime Minister's continued influence over the party. As a result the LDP suffered a major setback, failing to win an overall majority. Nevertheless, Nakasone retained power by forging an alliance with the NLC. Nakasone retained the leadership in 1984 despite criticism from within the party over his high-profile style of leadership. In July 1986 he timed a lower house election to coincide with that scheduled for the upper house and won majorities in both chambers. His triumph was completed by the decision of the NLC to rejoin the LDP, and by his party's agreement to extend Nakasone's leadership term by a further year.

Nakasone's final year in office was not a happy one. Harassed abroad by the USA and Europe over the size of Japan's trade surplus, at home he was forced to abandon his plans to introduce a sales tax. In late 1987 he was succeeded by his chosen successor, Noboru Takeshita. In 1989, however, a new scandal hit the party when it emerged that numerous senior politicians had between 1984 and 1986 accepted cut-price, unlisted shares in a real estate company as a form of bribery. The Recruit-Cosmos scandal forced the resignation of Takeshita in mid-1989. He was succeeded by Sosuke Uno, one of the few senior members of the party untainted by the scandal. Almost immediately, however, Uno became embroiled in a series of allegations about extra-marital sexual relationships. Against this background the party in July elections lost its overall majority in the upper house for the first time since 1955. On July 24, only 53 days after being confirmed in office, Uno announced his forthcoming resignation.

With the party's most eligible candidates for the leadership still barred by the Recruit affair, Uno's successor was Toshiki Kaifu, an obscure politician who was a member—but not the leader—of the small Komoto faction. Having been elected for the remaining months of the current term, Kaifu was re-elected as party leader in October 1989. Against all expectations his premiership was successful and stable. He led the LDP to victory in February 1990, with the party winning 46.1 per cent of the vote and 275 seats. Ultimately, however, he was brought down by his failure to secure support for (i) his planned constitutional reforms—particularly his desire to reduce the role of "money politics" and party factions by replacing the multimember constituencies with a system based on single members and proportional representation; and (ii) a bill which would have allowed Japanese troops to be dispatched abroad for the first time since 1945 in order to assist with UN peace-keeping operations. Without a basis of personal support within the party, Kaifu was forced to stand down when his term expired in October 1991.

Kaifu was replaced by Kiichi Miyazawa, the leader of the second-largest faction within the LDP, who had been forced to resign as Finance Minister in December 1988 because of his involvement in the Recruit scandal. In addition to the support of his own faction Miyazawa's leadership bid was backed by the large Takeshita faction and by the Komoto group. He polled 285 votes compared with 120 and 87 cast respectively for rival faction leaders Michio Watanabe and Hiroshi Mitsuzuka. Almost immediately Miyazawa's government was plunged into difficulties by a series of financial scandals, by the failure to achieve Diet support for the overseas troops bill which had eluded Kaifu, and by a resurgence of opposition interest in the Prime Minister's precise role in the Recruit affair. His public opinion rating fell from 57 per cent upon taking office to around 20 per cent in early April 1992. By mid-1992, however, the situation had improved somewhat as the powerful Takeshita faction appeared to be making greater efforts to throw its support behind Miyazawa, and he reached an agreement with *Komeito* and the Democratic Socialist Party (DSP) which enabled him to enact the peace-keeping operations bill.

Structure. The most distinctive characteristic of the LDP's structure lies in the existence of its distinct factions. Originally these were composed of Diet members with similar background, bound together by the ties of obligation and debt which have traditionally played a major role in Japanese politics. Today, however, the factions are powerful, profit-making machines which dominate the choice of party president and the subsequent composition of the Cabinet and party official.

Membership. 1,750,000.

Publications. *Jiyu Shinpo* (weekly); *Jiyu Minshu* (monthly); *Liburu* (monthly).

International Affiliations. International Democratic Union.

Social Democratic Party of Japan (SDPJ)
Nippon Shakaito

Address. 1-8-1 Nagata-cho, Chiyoda-ku, Tokyo 100.

Leadership. Makoto Tanabe (ch.).

Orientation. Social-democratic. Traditionally the Social Democratic Party of Japan (SDPJ—known as the Japan Socialist Party (JSP) until Feb. 1, 1991) advocated a style of socialism highly dependent upon Marxist analysis, which included large-scale state ownership, international neutrality, and an absolute opposition to the existence of Japan's Self Defence Forces. From the mid-1980s, however, the party began to abandon much of its Marxist ideology and came to resemble more closely many Western European social democratic parties.

Founded. November 1945.

History. The party was founded as the Japan Socialist Party (JSP) immediately after the Pacific War as a united front for the country's diverse socialist and proletarian movements. From the outset it was divided by issues of ideology and personality. In May 1947 one of the party's founders, Tetsu Katayama, formed a right-wing progressive government through a coalition of the JSP, the Democratic Party and the National Co-operative party. He soon encountered strong opposition from those on the left of the JSP led by Mosaburo Suzuki with the result that the government was forced from power after only eight months. Discord between the wings of the JSP worsened after its crushing defeat in the January 1949 election and, at the fourth party convention in April, Suzuki established a semi-autonomous left-wing leadership. Relations worsened in late 1951 as the left opposed the San Francisco Peace Treaty and the Japan-US Security Treaty. In October the party split between its left and right wings, each claiming to be the country's only legitimate socialist party.

The right-wing party moved increasingly towards Western Christian social democracy, while that of the left adopted an orthodox Marxist-Leninist stance and aligned itself to the communist bloc. In the early days of the schism the right wing socialists outnumbered the left in the Diet, but this balance shifted to the left at the general election of April 1953, in part because of Suzuki's strongly pacifist stance during the Korean War. In the election of February 1955 the left-wing socialists significantly outpolled those of the right, winning 89 seats compared with the 67 won by the right. Thus, when the two parties reunited in October 1955 the left was in the ascendant and the platform of the newly unified party was heavily influenced by Marxist doctrine.

The party continued to move leftwards as it gained seats in the House of Councillors' election in July 1956 and the lower house elections of May 1958 where it won 32.9 per cent of the vote and 166 seats. During this period the JSP was widely regarded as the guardian of the post-war Constitution. As the 1960 revision of the Japan-US Security Treaty approached, the party's uncompromising opposition to the agreement led a significant portion of its right wing to split from the JSP and form the Democratic Socialist Party. The JSP suffered a further blow when, in October 1960, its

chairman, Inejiro Asanuma, was assassinated by a right-wing fanatic. In the lower house elections held later that year, the party polled 27.6 per cent of the vote and won 145 seats. In the 1963 election it scored 28.6 per cent and won 144 seats.

In the early 1960s, against the background of the Sino-Soviet split and rapid Japanese economic development, there was renewed tension between the left and right wings of the party. The leader of the right, Saburo Eda, advocated a new policy based upon the structural reform of capitalism from within. At the party's 1964 convention, however, this revisionist view was rejected in favour of the maintenance of a Marxist revolutionary strategy as contained in a policy document entitled "The Road to Socialism". At the general election of 1967 the party's vote slipped slightly to 27.9 per cent and it won 140 seats. Following the party's loss of further ground in the upper house elections of 1968, it became increasingly apparent that the JSP was entering a period of decline. Chairman Seiichi Katsumata resigned to take responsibility for the losses and thereby established a precedent which was followed by the next four leaders: Tomomi Narita, Ichio Asukata, Masashi Ishibashi, and Takako Doi.

The pattern of decline was confirmed at the 1969 lower house elections when the party's share of the vote fell to 21.4 per cent and it won only 90 seats. In the 1972 election the party won 118 seats but its share of the vote remained low at 21.9 per cent. It fell further in 1976 when the party polled 20.7 per cent, although once again it managed to increase its number of seats to 123. In 1977 the defection and subsequent sudden death of Eda reduced the degree of factional discord in the party. This process was assisted by a split in the left between the pro-Chinese Sasaki faction and the pro-Moscow Socialist Association. It provided an opportunity for Ichio Asukata to begin a rebuilding process which began to cut the party loose from its Marxist heritage. Evidence of this move to the right was provided in early 1980 with its advocacy of participation in a coalition government with the centrist opposition parties, excluding the Japan Communist Party (JCP).

The sacrifice of its hardline socialist perspective did not halt the decline in the party's electoral fortunes, however. In the 1979 election it had polled 19.7 per cent of the vote and won 107 seats and, while it retained this number at the 1980 election, its share of the poll fell to 19.3 per cent. In 1983 this rose fractionally to 19.5 per cent and the party increased its representation to 112 seats in the lower house.

In January 1986, at its 50th convention, the JSP

adopted a new platform entitled the "New Declaration". It represented a historic turning point, for it explicitly rejected much of the Marxist ideology which had been adopted by the 1955 and 1964 policy documents and instead aligned itself with the social democratic model of Western European socialist parties. Ishibashi hoped to use the document to lay the foundations for a gradual JSP recovery, but within six months the party was faced with simultaneous upper and lower house elections. It suffered a comprehensive defeat, taking only 17.2 per cent of the vote in the lower house contest and securing only 85 seats.

Ishibashi resigned immediately and was replaced by Takako Doi, who became the first woman ever to lead a major Japanese political party. She continued the direction of the policy revision which had been initiated under her predecessor, but she also brought a new style of leadership which was flamboyant and charismatic, and contrasted sharply with most of her colleagues in the Diet. She scored early successes against the government by waging an effective campaign against the proposed sales tax, and the JSP made a strong showing in the 1987 local elections. By sheer force of personality she appeared to be able to obscure the fundamental differences which remained within the party over issues such as the constitutional legitimacy of the Self-Defence Forces, nuclear power, and the relationship between Japan and the USA.

In mid-1989 the Liberal Democratic Party (LDP) government of Noboru Takeshita was forced from office by the Recruit-Cosmos scandal, and his successor, Sosuke Uno, was immediately involved in a sex scandal. Against this background upper house elections were held on July 23, with Doi leading the JSP in a skilfully orchestrated campaign. A particularly high profile was given to the increased number of female candidates run by the party, an approach which was popularly dubbed the "Madonna Strategy", with the result the JSP polled particularly well among women voters. The party increased its strength in the upper house from 42 to 66 seats and in so doing denied the LDP an overall majority.

Despite this breakthrough, however, the JSP was unable to create a stable opposition coalition which could present itself as a serious alternative to the LDP. Under the steady leadership of Toshiki Kaifu the LDP recovered some of its lost ground and, in February 1990, was victorious in the lower house elections. By contrast the JSP's campaign was less effective than in 1989, with the party managing to field only 148 candidates for the 512 seats open to election. Doi wanted to put forward more but was opposed by many incumbents within the party who feared that by running more than one candidate per constituency they would split the socialist vote and endanger existing seats. The party polled 24.4 per cent of the vote and won 136 seats.

In the period which followed the JSP continued its revisionist course, and in early 1991 changed the English translation of its name to the Social Democratic Party of Japan (SDPJ), although the Japanese original remained unaltered. The continuing allegiance of the party to many of its former positions was clearly illustrated, however, by its passionate denunciation of the Gulf war. Falling back on old-style pacifism and a denunciation of the USA, the party condemned Japan's financial contribution to the allied war effort and castigated proposals that units from the Self-Defence Forces—which the party continued to view as unconstitutional by their very existence—should be dispatched abroad to provide logistical support for the UN forces being amassed to liberate Kuwait.

In April 1991 the SDPJ lost seats in the local elections and Doi resigned as leader. She was succeeded on July 31 by Makoto Tanabe, a representative of the right wing, who defeated the centre-left candidate Tetsu Ueda in a ballot of the party's membership on July 23. Although Ueda attempted to exploit the fresh LDP difficulties in late 1991 and early 1992, the party's failure to forge a workable alliance with the DSP and *Komeito* rendered such efforts largely ineffective.
Structure. The party used to contain several distinctive factions, but these were disbanded in the late 1970s. Its policies are determined by its annual convention and directed by its central executive committee.
Membership. 130,000.
Publications. Shakai-Shinpo (weekly); *Gekkan Shakaito* (monthly).
International Affiliations. Socialist International.

Minor parties

Japan New Party (JNP) (*Nippon Shinto*). The party was founded in May 1992 by Morihiro Hosokawa who, before serving as Governor of Kunamoto Prefecture for two terms in 1983-91, had served for 12 years as an Liberal Democratic Party member of the Diet. The JNP was designed as a modern, centrist party which would appeal to both salaried workers and rural residents. Its avowed aim is to decentralize a government which Hosokawa claims is "rigid, outmoded and yoked to vested interests". The party believes in free trade and is committed to opening all of Japan's markets. It is also committed to creating a world free of nuclear weapons by the 21st century.

Progressive Party (*Shinpoto*); Matsuzaki Building, 1-2-2, Atago, Minato-ku. Tokyo 105. The party was formed in 1987 by a group from the New Liberal Club (NLC) which objected to the NLC's decision in 1986 to rejoin the Liberal Democratic Party (LDP). The current leader is Seiichi Tagawa. The party polled 0.43 per cent of the vote in the 1990 lower house elections and won one seat.

Rengo-na-Kai is not strictly a political party in that it has no fixed policies and little in the way of an organizational or financial network. As a political organization it amounts to a working relationship between the Social Democratic Party of Japan and the Democratic Socialist Party, the country's two labour-backed social-democratic parties. *Rengo*, led by Akira Yamagishi, is Japan's largest labour organization. It was created in 1989 by the merger of the left-wing *Sohyo* (General Council of Trade Unions) and the right-wing *Domei* (Japan Confederation of Labour). The former, representing public sector workers, was the principal backer of the JSP, while the latter, representing mainly private-sector workers, provided support for the DSP. As a political entity *Rengo* emerged during the upper house election of 1989 and involved standing candidates supported jointly by JSP, DSP, and Social Democratic Federation (SDF) in districts where none of these parties was in a position to challenge the Liberal Democratic Party (LDP) on its own. Eleven of the organizations's 12 candidates were elected in 1989 and formed the *Rengo Sangiin* as a quasi-political party in the upper house. The party increased its representation in the upper house to 13 with two by-election victories in March 1992 which appeared to confirm the emergence of *Rengo* as a potent vehicle for the anti-LDP protest vote. *Rengo Sangiin* is currently led by Tasaburo Furukawa.

Salaried Workers' New Party (*Sarariman Shinto*); Hanzomon Co-op. 608, 2-12 Hayabusa-cho, Chiyoda-ku, Tokyo 102. Founded in 1983, the party advocates a reform of the taxation system. Its current leader is Shigeru Aoki.

Social Democratic Federation (SDF—*Shaminren*). Also known as the United Social Democratic Party indexUnited Social Democratic Party (Japan)(*Shakai*

Minshu Rengo); 2F Top Edogawabashi, 2-6-3 Suido, Bunkyo-ku, Tokyo 112. The party was formed in March 1978 when a number of right-wing members of the Japan Socialist Party defected and joined forces with the Socialist Citizen's League, a coalition embracing a number of socialist citizens' organizations. In the 1990 lower house elections the party won 0.86 per cent of the vote and four seats. Its current president is Satsuki Eda.

Sports Peace Party (*Supotsu Heiwato*); Inue Building 7F, 6-7-13, Minami Aoyama, Minato-ku, Tokyo 107. The party is led by Kanji Inoki.

Taxpayers' Party (*Zeikinto*); House of Councillors, 1-7-1 Nagata-cho, Chiyoda-ku, Tokyo 100. The party is currently led by Chinpei Nozue (sec).

Defunct Parties

Japan Cooperative Party (*Nihon Kyodoto*). Founded in December 1945 the JCP evolved into the National Co-operative Party (*Kokumin Kyodoto*) in March 1947, the National Democratic Party (*Kokumin Minshuto*) in April 1950, the Reform Party (*Kaishinto*) in February 1952, and the Japan Democratic Party (*Nihon Minshuto*) in November 1954, in which form, in 1955, it was one of the constituent elements of the Liberal Democratic Party.

Japan Liberal Party (*Nihon Jiyuto*). The JLP was formed in November 1945. It evolved into the Democratic Liberal Party (*Minshu Jiyuto*) in March 1948 and the Liberal Party (*Jiyuto*) in March 1950, in which form, in 1955, it was one of the constituent elements of the Liberal Democratic Party.

Japan Progressive Party (*Nihon Shinpoto*). The JPP was founded in November 1945, and evolved into the Democratic Party (*Minshuto*) in March 1947, the National Democratic Party (*Kokumin Minshuto*) in April 1950, the Reform Party (*Kaishinto*) in February 1952, and the Japan Democratic Party (*Nihon Minshuto*) in November 1954, as which, in 1955, it was one of the constituent elements of the Liberal Democratic Party.

New Liberal Club (*Shin Jiyu Kurabu*). Formed in June 1976 by Liberal Democratic Party (LDP) members who were disgusted by the Lockheed scandal, the NLC sought to offer conservatism without the corruption and money politics associated with the ruling party.

Initially the party made rapid gains and polled 4.2 per cent of the vote in the 1976 lower house elections, winning 17 seats. Thereafter it was plagued by internal bickering and the lack of a clear identity, and in 1979 its vote fell to 3 per cent and it won only four seats in the lower house. In the following year it retained its share of the poll but increased its representation to 12. Although its vote fell to 2.4 per cent in the 1983 election, its eight members were instrumental securing an overall majority for the LDP. This alliance paved the way for the party's reabsorption into the LDP. In July 1986 the NLC's vote fell to 1.8 per cent and its number of seats to six. In the following month its members voted to rejoin the ruling party.

Major guerrilla groups

Japan has numerous extremist groups of both left and right which have frequently resorted to violence, although none has posed a serious threat to the stability of the state. Recent estimates suggest that there are around 980 extreme right-wing groups, with a total membership of some 120,000. They advocate authoritarian government, often in the form of a revival of the Emperor's powers, as a means of eradicating the corruption, materialism and subservience to foreign powers which they see as the prevailing characteristics of post-war Japanese society. It is estimated that there are around 25 left-wing groups which contain some 14,000 members in total. The majority are Trotskyist in perspective, believing that the violent overthrow of the capitalist order can be hastened through the activities of a revolutionary vanguard. In particular they tend to oppose the continuance of the monarchy—during the 1989 enthronement of Emperor Akihito there were 84 instances of arson, bombing and other violent attacks—and the Japan-US Security Treaty.

Japan Volunteer Army for National Independence (*Nihon Minzoku Dokuritsu Giyungun*); a right-wing group, active since 1983, which has specialized in making attacks on liberal journalists.

Middle-Core Faction (*Chukaku-Ha*). Since its formation in 1960 the *Chukaku-Ha* has come to public attention because of its repeated violent clashes with the rival *Kakumaru-Ha* movement (Revolutionary Marxist Faction); its use of crude incendiary missiles; and its involvement in the epic struggle against the Narita airport project. It is the country's largest leftist group, with an estimated membership of 5,000, some 400 of whom constitute its underground guerrilla squad, the People's Revolutionary Army.

Spiritual Justice School (*Seiki Juku*); a right-wing group which was responsible for the attempted assassination of the Mayor of Nagasaki in 1990, after he had suggested that Emperor Hirohito bore some degree of responsibility for the Pacific War.

United Red Army (*Rengo Sekigun*). Formed in 1969, this left-wing group was responsible for violent incidents inside Japan and for numerous acts of international terrorism—including an attack on Lod airport (Tel Aviv, Israel) in 1972 in which 26 people were killed—in its campaign against Zionism and Japanese imperialism. The group has been largely inactive since the late 1970s.

Kazakhstan

Capital: Alma Ata   **Population 16,793,000 (official est. at Jan 1, 1991)**

The Republic of Kazakhstan, a constituent Union Republic of the Soviet Union since Dec. 5, 1936, declared sovereignty on Oct. 25, 1990 and independence on Dec. 16, 1991. It was a founder member of the Commonwealth of Independent States (CIS), which came into being on Dec. 21, 1991, precipitating the collapse of the Soviet Union.

Constitutional structure

The ex-Soviet Constitution was still in place as of June 1, 1992, although the draft of a new Constitution was under public discussion. The 360-seat Supreme Soviet acts as the legislative body; executive power rests with the President and the government. Until popular presidential elections in December 1991, the Chair of the Supreme Soviet (speaker of parliament) had been head of state.

Electoral system

The 1990 elections to the Supreme Soviet reserved 81 out of 360 seats for official organizations (Communist Party of the Soviet Union, Komsomol, trades unions, etc.), making Kazakhstan the only ex-Soviet republic bar Byelorussia to do so. Voting went to a second round if a candidate, including a candidate for an uncontested seat, failed to win at least 50 per cent of the vote.

The law on presidential elections required candidates to collect 100,000 signatures in order to be registered.

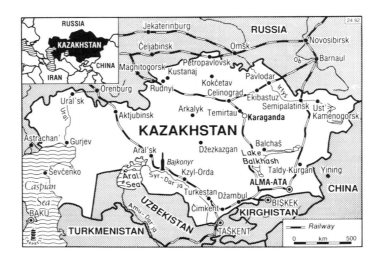

Recent elections

Supreme Soviet elections, March 25, 1990

The Supreme Soviet elections were not contested on a party basis. 1,077 candidates (87.8 per cent of whom were CPSU members) were registered for the 279 seats which were contested. The first round turnout was 83.9 per cent.

Presidential elections, Dec. 1, 1991

Candidate	Percentage
Nursultan Nazarbayev	98.76

PARTY BY PARTY DATA

Alash National Independence Party
Partiya natsionalnoi nezavisimosti Alash
Leadership. Aron Atabek (ch.).
Orientation. Islamic nationalist. The party aims to create a united Islamic Kazakhstan, but adheres to the Turkish solution: a secular state in an Islamic country.
Founded. April 14-15, 1990.
History. The founding congress was designated as the revival of the *Alash-Orda* ("camp of Alash (the mythical ancestor of the Kazakhs)") party, which was a nationalist Kazakh political organization which existed from 1905 to 1920. The new Alash Party organized protest meetings and hunger strikes during the 1990 and 1991 sessions of the Kazakh Supreme Soviet and in December 1991 Alash members occupied the mosque in Alma Ata, forcing the security services to come to the rescue of the *Mufti.* The party, harried by the Kazakh authorities, had to be officially registered as a commercial organization in Moscow.
Structure. The most active members form a 10-15-strong Executive Committee.
Membership. Probably about 100 activists.
Publications. Khak (Truth) newspaper, published in Moscow since late 1991 in Russian.

Communist Party
Kommunisticheskaya partiya
Orientation. Communist, following the defunct Communist Party of the Soviet Union (CPSU).
Leadership. Leonid Korolkov; Askar Kashibekov (co-ch.).
Founded. Dec. 6-7, 1991.
History. The Communist Party (CP), like the Socialist Party of Kazakhstan [see separate entry], claims to be the successor to the Kazakhstan branch of the CPSU, which dissolved itself on Aug. 28, 1991. Its founding congress on Dec. 6-7, 1991, was designated the 19th Kazakh Communist Party Congress. It has provided a forum for many of the ethnic Russian members of the former Kazakh CP, but few party workers have become members and its leadership includes only one member of the former Kazakh CP Central Committee.
Structure. 52-member central committee elected at the congress.
Membership. 10,000.

Jeltoksan National-Democratic Party
Natsionalnaya-demokraticheskaya partiya Jeltoksan
Leadership. Khasen Kozhakhmetov (ch.).

Orientation. Democracy and Kazakh independence.
Founded. May 20, 1990.
History. Jeltoksan ("December") originated as a protest movement aiming to rehabilitate participants in the December 1986 riots in Alma Ata. These were occasioned by the appointment of an ethnic Russian, Gennady Kolbin, to replace the Kazakh incumbent, Dinmukhammed Kunayev as Communist Party First Secretary of Kazakhstan. Kozhakhmetov was himself imprisoned for four years after the riots. At *Jeltoksan's* congress on Jan. 26-27, 1991, the posts of co-chairmen were abolished after disagreements between the incumbents and Kozhazkhmetov. Membership in the party increased when in September 1991, *Jeltoksan* began to pressure the Kazakh government to honour its promise to order an objective investigation into the 1986 protests.

Kozhakhmetov was the only potential alternative candidate to Nazarbayev at the presidential elections, but failed to gather sufficient signatures to stand. In March 1992, the party informed President Nazarbayev that it intended to send volunteers to the ethnic conflict in Azerbaijan and, if necessary, aid the Azerbaijanis.
Structure. The ruling body is a 7-member central political council, elected by the party congress.
Membership. over 2,500.
Publications. Jeltoksan newspaper, issued periodically with a circulation of 3-5,000.

People's Congress Party
Partiya Narodny kongress
Leadership. Olzhas Suleimenov; Mukhtar Shakhanov (co-ch.).
Orientation. Cautious proponent of reform; no ethnic or nationalist element.
Founded. Oct. 5, 1991.
History. The original concept of the People's Congress Party's (PCP) founders and current co-chairmen, both of them activists in the ecological movement and writers, was to create a movement uniting Kazakhstan's informal political groups. The PCP was formed when the *Azat* Movement [see Republican Azat (Free) Party entry] refused to participate in this scheme. The *Edinstvo* Movement (supports the ethnic Russian population) and the *Jeltoksan* Party also refused to join, but the PCP was supported by activists in the anti-nuclear Movement Nevada-Semipalatinsk and by part of *Azat,* as well as by the official creative unions, the *Birlesu* trades union and the semi-official *Kazak*

tili (Kazakh language) society.

Nazarbayev's appearance at the PCP's founding congress and the PCP's support for his political line encouraged civil servants and bureaucrats to join the party.

Structure. 15-strong political executive committee and 5-member multi-ethnic secretariat. A central co-ordinating committee comprises deputies from the Kazakh and ex-Soviet parliaments who have joined the PCP.

Membership. 5,000, including 17 Supreme Soviet members.

Affiliations. Inter-republican Democratic Congress.

Republican Azat (Free) Party
Respublikanskaya partiya Azat

Leadership. Sovetkazy Aktayev (ch.).

Orientation. Kazakh independence, oriented towards Kazakh nationalism.

Founded. Sept. 4, 1991.

History. The Republican Azat (Free) Party (*Azat*) was formed as the political wing of the *Azat* Citizens' Democratic Movement, an informal group founded in April 1990 which then became the main force of the national democratic opposition to the communist regime. However, disagreements over the nationality question meant that the more internationalist section of the *Azat* Movement joined the People's Congress Party [see separate entry], and the Kazakh nationalist wing formed the *Azat* Party. The *Azat* Movement continued to function with neither faction gaining total control.

Structure. 33-member co-ordinating council and nine-member politburo.

Membership. over 3,000 (Jan. 1992), including two Supreme Soviet members.

Publications. Azat Movement's fortnightly paper, *Azat* published in Russian and Kazakh with a total circulation of 40,000.

Affiliations. Democratic Congress.

Social Democratic Party of Kazakhstan
Sotsial-demokraticheskaya partiya Kazakhstana

Leadership. Sergei Duvanov; Dos Kushimov (co-ch.).

Orientation. Multi-ethnic, moderate. "To improve citizens' quality of life through practical political, economic and social reforms."

Founded. May 26-27, 1990.

History. In January 1990, Duvanov and *Jeltoksan* leader Kozhakhmetov [see separate entry], set up a party from among the informal groups active in Alma Ata. Finding the Social Democratic Party of Kazakhstan (SDPK) insufficiently nationalistic, the *Jeltoksan* contingent left it in May of that year. At the second congress on Dec. 2, 1990, a group of radicals also left the party. The third congress on Oct. 18-19, 1991, discussed (inconclusively) a proposal to turn the SDPK into a liberal party. The SDPK's small membership belies its political weight. Its fourth conference held in November 1991 adopted a declaration of the party's principles, and committed itself to agitate for the holding of extraordinary multiparty parliamentary elections, to form a "highly professional parliament capable of creating an effective legislative basis for the switch to a market economy".

Structure. A co-ordinating council unites representatives of 11 regions in Kazakhstan where the SDPK has branches.

Membership. 250 members, all active.

Publications. S-demokrat, published irregularly with a circulation of 10,000.

Affiliations. Inter-republican Democratic Congress.

Socialist Party
Sotsialisticheskaya partiya

Leadership. Anatoly Antonov; Yermukhammed Yertysbayev (co-ch.).

Orientation. Little emphasis on socialist ideology, and a conservative attitude to the market economic reforms promoted by the government.

Founded. Oct. 5, 1991; registered Oct. 21, 1991.

History. The Socialist Party (SP) was founded at the extraordinary 18th Congress of the Communist Party of Kazakhstan (CPK), which had dissolved itself on Aug. 28, 1991, and on the basis of the CPK. Nursultan Nazarbayev, CPK first secretary until Aug. 22, 1991, did not participate in the congress, which was taken as a sign that the SP would not be taking over the CPK's role as ruling party.

Structure. A political executive committee of 65 members has an 11-member buro. Factions are permitted and currently include communist and workers factions.

Membership. 45,000 (at the end of 1991), including 30 Supreme Soviet members. The SP's membership is mainly Kazakh, although Kazakhstan's population included 30 per cent ethnic Russians in 1989.

Publications. Weekly newspapers *Sukhbat* (in Kazakh) and *Pozitsiya* (in Russian).

Kirgizstan

Capital: Bishkek (Frunze until February 1991) Population: 4,422,000 (official est. at Jan. 1, 1991)

The Republic of Kirgizstan was formed on Dec. 5, 1936 as a Union Republic within the Soviet Union (having previously been an autonomous region in the Russian Federation). It declared its sovereignty on Oct. 30, 1990 and independence on Aug. 24, 1991. It was a founder member of the Commonwealth of Independent States, formed on Dec. 21, 1991 after the collapse of the Soviet Union.

Constitutional structure

The highest legislative body is the 350-seat Supreme Soviet. In February 1992, the Executive (the government) was directly subordinated to the President, who is directly elected.

Electoral system

In the 1990 Supreme Soviet elections, voting went to a second round if a candidate failed to win at least 50 per cent of the vote, even for an uncontested seat. A nationally-elected Presidency, introduced in October 1991, is limited to a maximum of two consecutive five-year terms. Previously the head of state was the Chair of the Supreme Soviet, elected by that body.

Evolution of the suffrage

All adults over 18, except prisoners, those in psychiatric institutions and those declared incapable by a court, are entitled to vote.

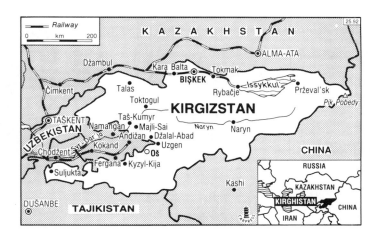

Recent elections

Legislative elections, Feb. 25, 1990

The legislative elections of Feb. 25, 1990 to the 350-seat Supreme Soviet were not contested on a party basis, and 70 seats were contested by a single candidate. On a 92 per cent turnout, 250 seats were filled at the first round, 84 seats were carried over to a second round, and a further 16 were contested on a first round basis.

Presidential elections, Oct. 12, 1991

Candidate	Percentage of vote
Askar Akayev	93.5

PARTY BY PARTY DATA

Asaba National Renaissance Party
Partiya natsionalnovo vozrozhdeniya Asaba
Leadership. Asan Ormushev (ch.).
Orientation. Kirgiz nationalist.
Founded. April 26, 1990.
History. The Asaba National Renaissance Party (Asaba being the name of a Kirgiz military banner) was a member of the Democratic Movement Kirgizstan (DDK—see separate entry) until a conference on Nov. 20, 1990 when, having found the DDK insufficiently nationalist, it became a political party in its own right. The party's membership grew significantly after the attempted Soviet coup of August 1991. The second congress on Nov. 2, 1991 elected the leadership.
Structure. Executive committee of 7.
Membership. Over 3,000.

Ashar Movement
Dvizhenie Ashar
Leadership. Dzhumagazy Usupov (ch.).
Orientation. Kirgiz nationalist, with the specific demand of housing for Kirgiz.
Founded. July 15, 1989.
History. Ashar (meaning "mutual aid") began in June 1989 when young people in Bishkek formed a defence committee and seized land to build on. Disagreements soon followed over whether the movement should become politicized, as the authorities attempted to suppress *Ashar*. In May 1990, *Ashar* became a founder member of the Democratic Movement Kirgizstan (DDK—see separate entry), but retained its individual status as, in April 1991, supporters of dissolving *Ashar* into the DDK were expelled from the movement. *Ashar* remains the largest organization in the DDK and is not always in accord with the leadership. Other organizations of homestead-builders were united with *Ashar* at the third congress on Nov. 16, 1991.
Structure. 10-member governing body; Council representing 18 member organizations.
Membership. 20,000.

Communists of the Republic of Kirgizstan
Kommunistov Respubliki Kyrgyzstana
Leadership. Absamat Masaliyev (first sec.).
Orientation. Communist.
History. The Communist Party of Kirgizstan (CPK) was suspended in August 1991. The then first secretary, Djumgalbek Amanbayev, and others in the leadership underwent investigation, having declared support for the leaders of the attempted August 1991 coup in Moscow. However, in May 1992 Amanbayev was elected a People's Deputy of Kirgizstan, as was a former First Secretary of the CPK, Usubaliyev. On June 22, 1992, *Izvestiya* reported the founding conference of the Communists of the Republic of Kirgizstan, attended by 250 delegates and chaired by former CPK First Secretary, Absamat Masaliyev, whom Amanbayev had replaced in April 1991.

Democratic Movement Kirgizstan
Demokraticheskaya dvizhenie Kirgizstan
Leadership. Kazat Akhmatov (ch.), resigned April 1992.
Orientation. Increasingly Kirgiz nationalist, having previously supported democratization.
Founded. May 26-27, 1990.
History. The Democratic Movement Kirgizstan (DDK) was founded by representatives of virtually all the informal groups active in Kirgizstan in 1990, both Kirgiz and Russian. However, the Kirgiz nationalist wing later took the leading role. Although initially supporting the policies of President Akayev, the DDK disagreed with his moderate line over land ownership, which allowed all ethnic groups of the republic equal rights to land. The first congress on Feb. 9-10, 1991 saw disagreements over whether or not to transform the DDK into a coalition of organizations. The second congress, on Nov. 30, 1991, retained the DDK as a single party and established a leadership structure. It was also decided to issue party cards for active members. However, a news report of April 1992 suggested the DDK might be on the verge of disintegration.
Structure. A co-ordination council represents equally the regional and party organizations comprising the DDK. The Chairman is supported by two deputies.
Membership. 300,000, about 10 Supreme Soviet members.
Publications. Weekly newspaper *Maidan* (Front), with circulation 10,000.
Affiliations. Democratic Congress.

Democratic Party Free Kirgizstan (Freedom Party)
Demokraticheskaya partiya Erkin Kirgizstan
(Partiya Erk)
Leadership. Omurbek Tekebayev (ch.).
Orientation. Liberal economic policy.
Founded. Feb. 9-10, 1991.

History. The party was established during the first congress of the Democratic Movement Kirgizstan (DDK—see above), partly on the basis of the *Atuulduk demilge* (Citizens' Initiative) organization, created in March 1990. It tries to influence government policy by preparing legislation, and it claims businessmen, private farmers and members of the intelligentsia among its membership. The party's second congress was held on Nov. 29, 1991.

Structure. 16-member council; seven-member executive committee.

Membership. 3,000-5,000, two parliamentary deputies.

People's Unity Democratic Movement

Demokraticheskaya dvizheniye Narodnoye Yedinstvo

Leadership. Jumagul Saadanbekov; Abdygan Erkebayev; Yury Razgulyayev (joint chairmen).

Orientation. Internationalist, countering Kirgiz nationalist tendencies; supports mixed economy.

Founded. 26 Oct. 1991.

History. People's Unity Democratic Movement grew out of the parliamentary opposition "group of 114", formed after the Osh riots in June-July 1990, when ethnic clashes between Kirgiz and Uzbeks resulted in at least 200 deaths. In June 1991, government and opposition political leaders, including 144 deputies and Vice-President German Kuznetsov, proposed the creation of People's Unity as a constituent party in the newly established Soviet opposition group, the Democratic Reform Movement. The constituent congress in October elected the leadership, and the party was registered on Dec. 31. People's Unity supports President Akayev's reform policies. Two of its three co-chairs are ex-ministers.

Structure. 70-member co-ordinating council; 17-strong executive committee.

Membership. Over 5,000, including about 100 deputies.

Affiliations. Democratic Reform Movement.

Kiribati

Capital: Bairiki, Tarawa island (administrative centre)   **Population: 63,883 (1985 census)**

The Gilbert Islands, lying astride the equator and scattered over an area of 5,000,000 sq miles of ocean, were discovered by Europeans in the 17th century, and were colonized by the British in 1892. The territory became the independent Republic of Kiribati on July 12, 1979; it is a member of the Commonwealth.

Political parties have slowly emerged, but remain relatively weak and loosely organized. The political process remains dominated by individuals, the most outstanding of whom is Ieremia Tabai, who was President between 1978 and 1989.

Constitutional structure

Legislative power is vested in a unicameral House of Assembly (*Maneaba-ni-Maungatabu*), comprising 39 members, together with the Attorney General as an ex officio member, unless already elected. The Constitution also makes provision for one legislator to be appointed by the Banaban community, the bulk of which is resident in Fiji because of the destruction of Banaba through phosphate mining, and the effects of Japanese occupation during the Pacific War. The leaders of the Banaba community have traditionally failed to nominate a representative in pursuance of their claim for independence from Kiribati.

The head of state and head of government is the *Beretitenti* (President) who is popularly elected from among the members of the Assembly. He governs with the assistance of an appointed Cabinet and is empowered to dissolve the Assembly and to call a general election.

Electoral system

The Assembly, like the President, is popularly elected for four years, with an additional round of voting held in those constituencies where no single candidate receives more than 50 per cent of the vote. Only members of the legislature may stand as presidential candidates. Prior to a presidential election the Assembly is constitutionally bound to nominate not fewer than three and not more then four presidential candidates. A person may serve no more than three terms as President.

Evolution of the suffrage

Since independence Kiribati has functioned on the basis of adult suffrage, a system first adopted in 1971 when an elected Legislative Council was established with limited powers.

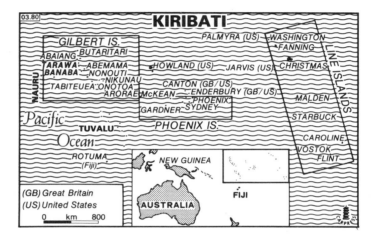

Recent elections

Legislative elections were held in March 1982, January 1983, March 1987 and, most recently, on May 8, 1991, with an additional round of run-off contests on May 15. On each occasion presidential elections were held shortly afterwards. Since independence the political system has been dominated by Ieremia Tabai who served as President from independence until the 1991 elections, when he was succeeded by his chosen successor, Teatao Teannaki.

Presidential elections

Date	Winning candidate
May 1982	Ieremia Tabai
February 1983	Ieremia Tabai
May 1987	Ieremia Tabai*
July 1991	Teatao Teannaki

*Although he had already won the presidential elections of 1978, 1982, and 1983, and was prohibited from serving more than three terms, Tabai fought a successful legal action over his eligibility for the 1987 contest on the grounds that his second term in office had been of less than a year in duration and, therefore, did not constitute a full term.

Presidential elections, May 12, 1987
(Political affiliation in parentheses)

Candidate	Percentage of vote
Ieremia Tabai	50.1
Teburoio Tito (CDP)	42.7
Teatao Teannaki	7.2

Presidential elections July 3, 1991
(Political affiliation in parentheses)

Candidate	Percentage of vote
Teatao Teannaki (NPP)	46.3
Roniti Teiwaki	41.9
Beniamina Tinga	—
Boanareke Boanareke	11.8

PARTY BY PARTY DATA

Christian Democratic Party

Address. c/o Maneaba-ni-Maungatabu, Tarawa, Kiribati.

Leadership. Teburoio Tito.

Orientation. Opposition to the administration of Ieremia Tabai, and specifically its sale of fishing rights to the Soviet Union in 1985-86.

Founded. 1987.

History. The Christian Democratic Party (CDP) was founded in order to give some organizational structure to the opponents of Ieremia Tabai. Initially its strength in the legislature was around 15 members, but this was reduced to around six at the 1987 election. Its first leader, Harry Tong, filed a legal challenge to the validity of Tabai's candidature in the 1987 presidential election, and subsequently attempted to have the results declared void. The party's candidate in the election, Teburoio Tito, finished second to Tabai. Tito's strong showing in the election meant that it was widely predicted that he would be selected as a candidate for the 1991 contest. In the event, however, the poor results of the CDP in the 1991 legislative elections meant that none of its members were among the four candidates selected to contest the July presidential elections.

Kiribati United Party

Address. c/o Maneaba-ni-Maungatabu, Tarawa, Kiribati.

Leadership. Tewareka Teutoa.

Orientation. Liberal.

Founded. 1990.

History. The Kiribati United Party (KUP) was formed during the final years of the last Tabai administration. It was expected that its leader, an outspoken liberal, would be chosen from among the candidates for the 1991 presidential election but, surprisingly, no representative of the party was among the four candidates finally selected.

National Progressive Party

Address. c/o Maneaba-ni-Maungatabu, Tarawa, Kiribati.

Leadership. Teatao Teannaki.

Orientation. Centrist.

Founded. 1974.

History. The National Progressive Party (NPP) was revitalized by supporters of President Ieremia Tabai in response to the creation of the Christian Democratic Party (CDP) by his opponents [see separate entry]. With Tabai constitutionally debarred from a further presidential term, the creation of the loosely-organized NPP allowed him to propel his friend and Vice-President, Teatao Teannaki, into the Presidency in 1991. With Tabai holding his seat in the legislature, the existence of a party structure also assisted him in his desire to continue wielding a considerable degree of influence within the political system.

Minor parties

Voice of the Kiribati People (*Wiia i-Kiribati*); founded in 1982, the *Wiia i-Kiribati* was the first political party to be created in the independent state of Kiribati. Its loose group of members succeeded in forcing the government to resign in December 1982. From the mid-1980s, however, it was eclipsed as a focus for the opposition by the Christian Democratic Party (CDP) and has ceased to be an influential force in the country's political process.

Defunct parties

Democratic Labour Party; established in 1974, the DLP under Tabai constituted the opposition in the pre-independence House of Assembly.

Major guerrilla groups

There are no guerrilla groups operating in Kiribati.

North Korea
(Democratic People's Republic of Korea)

Capital: Pyongyang

Population: 21,800,000 (1990)

In the early 17th century the 1,000-year-old Kingdom of Korea became a vassal state of China. In 1904-5 it was conquered by Japan, and in 1910 it became a Japanese colony. Liberated in 1945, the north of the peninsula was occupied by Soviet troops and the south by US forces. In 1948 separate states were established on either side of the 38th parallel, each of which reflected the ideology of its respective super-power, and each of which claimed jurisdiction over the entire peninsula.

In 1950 the communist North invaded the South and was opposed by US-led United Nations' forces. The war was ended by an armistice in 1953, with the ceasefire line (which became the new de facto border) straddling the 38th parallel. Although initially the North used its dominant share of the peninsula's mineral resources to increase its industrial capacity, its economy began to stagnate in the 1970s and was overtaken by the rapidly developing South. The North Korean political regime also stultified, becoming ever-more internationally isolated and secretive, and encouraging the development of a grotesque personality cult around Kim Il Sung, "The Great Leader".

Constitutional structure

The Democratic People's Republic of Korea was established as an independent communist state in September 1948. Under the terms of the 1972 Constitution, nominal political authority is held by the Supreme People's Assembly (SPA), the nominally-elected unicameral legislature. The SPA elects a standing committee to represent it when not in session. It also elects the President who, in addition to being head of state, holds executive power and governs in conjunction with a Central People's Committee and an appointed State Administrative Council (Cabinet). Effective political control is exercised by the (communist) Korean Workers' Party (KWP), established in 1946.

Since the mid-1970s, the ageing leader of the party and the state, Kim Il Sung, has been grooming his son, Kim Jong Il, as his successor.

Electoral system

The 687 members of the SPA are elected every four years from a single list of candidates. Since the 1960s, official statistics have routinely made the seemingly absurd claim that a full 100 per cent of the electorate had participated in general elections, and had all voted for the KWP-approved candidates on the official list.

Evolution of suffrage

Since its foundation, the North Korean state has practised universal adult suffrage. Voting is compulsory.

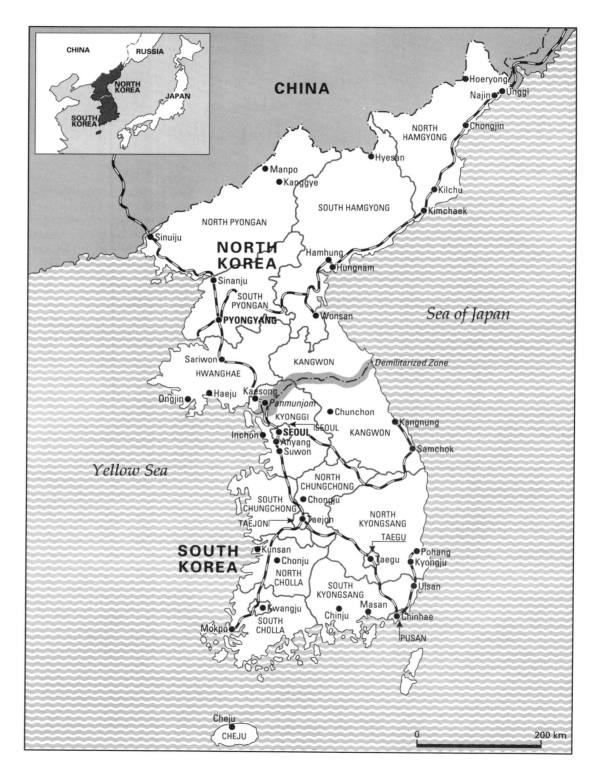

Recent elections

Although national and local elections have been held regularly, North Korea's position as a one-party state has meant that the outcome of any contest has never been in doubt. The most recent legislative elections were held on April 22, 1990, with Kim Il Sung being re-elected as President for a fifth consecutive term on May 24, 1990.

PARTY BY PARTY DATA

Korean Workers' Party

Chosen No-Dong Dang

Address. The Central District, Pyongyang.

Leadership. Kim Il Sung (gen. sec.); members of presidium: Kim Il Sung, Kim Jong Il, Oh Jin Woo.

Orientation. Communist. The party defines its "immediate objective" as "to achieve the complete victory of socialism" in the northern half of the Republic (ie in North Korea), and to liberate the people in the south through a national liberation revolution. In addition to the extraordinary personality cult which has developed around its leader, the KWP differs from other communist parties in its advocacy, since the mid-1950s, of "*Juche*". The term, variously translated as "self-reliance", "self-independence" and "self-image", is an imprecise combination of autarchy, militarism, revolutionary zeal and the primacy of the ruling party.

Founded. 1946.

History. The Korean Workers' Party (KWP) was created through a merger of the Communist Party of North Korea (which had been founded in 1945) and the New People's Party of Korea. Originally called the North Korean Workers' Party, its current name was adopted following its merger with the South Korean Workers' Party in 1949.

Although the party immediately became the sole ruling force in the newly-established North Korean state, it was far from a monolithic force. It was divided into five clearly-identifiable factions. These included the partisan faction (led by Kim Il Sung), which together with the North Korean and Soviet factions had constituted the Communist Party of North Korea. The other main groups were the Yenan faction, which was derived from the New People's Party, and the South Korean faction which had comprised the South Korean Workers' Party. The North Korean faction was the first to be purged by Kim. Following the Korean War the South Korean faction was blamed for the massive destruction suffered by North Korea, and its leaders were purged as pro-Western spies. The final factional struggle occurred in the latter half of the 1950s, as Kim battled to overcome the pro-China Yenan faction and the Soviet faction.

In a speech on Dec. 28, 1955, Kim launched the concept of *Juche* as an ideological foundation for North Korean communism which was distinct from both Stalinism and Maoism, and which he claimed represented the creative application of Marxist-Leninist ideas to North Korean conditions. An imprecise collection of principles which included autarchy, militarism, nationalism, revolutionary zeal and the unquestioned primacy of the ruling party, Juchism provided Kim with a platform from which he could attack the KWP's other factions and elevate himself into a position of complete dominance over the entire party. Later *Juche* was expanded into an all-embracing philosophy which reinforced the personality cult of Kim and became the basis of North Korea's foreign policy by embodying the country's unique geographical and ideological position, and assisting in avoiding becoming the satellite of either the Soviet Union or China.

Kim's opponents attempted to move against him at a plenum of the central committee at the end of August 1956, calling for a more collective form of leadership. In the power struggle which followed Kim quickly routed his adversaries and then destroyed the remaining factions within the KWP, freeing the party from the "ugly historical phenomenon of factionalism". By early 1958 Kim's leadership was undisputed.

In the period following the Korean War, the central economic concern of the KWP was to use Soviet and Chinese aid in an attempt to repair the massive damage which had been inflicted on the country during the war. An initial three-year plan concentrated on repairing the country's infrastructure and heavy industrial base. A five-year plan, formulated in 1956 and implemented in 1957, shifted the focus to the achievement of massive economic growth. The plan coincided with the *Chollima* movement which, like the Chinese Great Leap Forward, sought to overcome concrete constraints through the ruthless application of revolutionary will. The plan was declared fulfilled a year ahead of schedule in 1960.

Although impressive levels of growth and industrialization were achieved in the late 1950s and early 1960s, the problems of a command economy—particularly over-centralization, worker-apathy and a bloated and unresponsive bureaucracy—became increasingly apparent within North Korea. While the party attempted to introduce greater individual incentives in the 1960s, these problems intensified rather than receded. Although subsequent plans—a seven-year plan (1960-67, extended for a further three years), a six-year plan (1971-76), and seven-year plans (1978-84) and (1987-93)—claimed impressive levels of growth, most objective evidence suggested that the North Korean economy was stultified and increasingly inefficient. The policy of attempting to import Western technology, in the early 1970s, and then reneging on the subsequent debt repayments, only exacerbated these difficulties by increasing the country's economic isolation.

The stagnation of the country's economy in recent years has been reflected by the political stagnation within the KWP. The personality cult surrounding Kim Il Sung has by far exceeded that associated with Mao or Stalin, and has stifled any real political debate. Since the mid-1970s the most dominant, although largely unacknowledged, issue within the party has been the issue of the succession. The grooming of Kim's son, Kim Jong Il, the "Dear Leader", for the leadership of the KWP and the state has been accompanied by the growth of a personality cult almost as extravagant as that surrounding his father. Nevertheless, there have been persistent rumours of deep-seated opposition to the younger Kim, both within the KWP and within the armed forces.

Structure. The party has cells, primary party committees and party committees at city, county and provincial level. Its position of dominance throughout the history of the North Korean state has meant that it has become deeply woven into the fabric of the society.

Membership. Estimated to be in excess of 2,000,000.

Publications. Rodong Sinmun (newspaper); *Kunroza* (magazine).

Minor parties

Those minor parties which have been allowed to remain in existence are mere appendages of the KWP.

Ch'ondogyo Yong Friends' Party (CYFP—*Ch'on-dogyo Ch'ong-u-dang*); established in early 1946, the CYFP (also known as the North Korean Youth Fraternal Party) was a successor to an anti-Japanese nationalist party of the same name which had been formed in 1919. Like its forerunner, the CYFP was formed around the *Ch'ondogyo* religious movement (the Teaching of the Way of Heaven) which had been founded in the latter half of the 19th century. Although the party initially enjoyed cordial relations with the ruling communists, this changed with the Korean War as many party members collaborated with the invading UN forces. Subsequently the CYFP's leadership was purged and much of the party's apparatus dismantled. Since the late 1950s the remnants of the party have been thoroughly subservient to the ruling KWP.

Korean Democratic Party (KDP—*Chosun Minju-dang*); founded as the North Korean Democratic party in 1945, the party was the first non-communist organization to be established north of the 38th parallel, and drew its support largely from Christian intellectuals, businessmen and rich peasants. The leadership of the party was eradicated by the communist authorities in 1946, following anti-communist unrest for which the KDP was held responsible. Its apparatus was taken over by communists and thereafter the party became obedient to the KWP. In 1959 and 1960, its provincial and local branches were dissolved by government order.

Major guerrilla groups

There are no known guerrilla organizations in operation in North Korea.

South Korea
(Republic of Korea)

Capital: Seoul   **Population: 42,000,000 (1990)**

In the early 17th century the thousand-year-old Kingdom of Korea became a vassal state of China. In 1904-05 it was conquered by Japan, and in 1910 it became a Japanese colony. After its liberation in 1945, the north of the peninsula was occupied by Soviet troops and the south by US forces. In 1948 separate states were established on either side of the 38th parallel, each of which reflected the ideology of its respective super-power, and each of which claimed jurisdiction over the entire peninsula.

In 1950 the South was invaded by the communist North but was saved from annihilation by a vast US-led UN military intervention. The war was ended by an armistice in 1953, with the ceasefire line (which became the new de facto border) straddling the 38th parallel. Although lacking the mineral resources and industrial base of the North, the South's economy expanded massively in the 1960s and 1970s under a system of rigorous government guidance and control. During this period brief experiments with democracy were invariably destroyed by military intervention in the political process. This pattern appeared to have been broken with the establishment of the Sixth Republic and the election of President Roh Tae Woo in 1988. Roh's accession marked the first occasion in the South Korean history on which there had been a peaceful transfer of authority. In 1990 Roh created the ruling Democratic Liberal Party by merging the governing party with two of the three main opposition groups.

Constitutional structure

The Republic of Korea was established as an independent state in 1948. There were frequent constitutional revisions (1952, 1954, June and November 1960, December 1962, October 1969, December 1972, October 1980) as the country evolved through five republics between 1948 and 1987. The Sixth Republic was formally proclaimed on Feb. 25, 1988, following a revision of the Constitution in October 1987, in the face of massive popular unrest.

Under the terms of the current Constitution executive power is held by the President who is popularly elected for a single five-year term and who governs with the assistance of an appointed State Council (Cabinet) led by a Prime Minister. Legislative authority rests with a unicameral National Assembly whose 299 members serve for four years.

Electoral system

Two-thirds of the members of the National Assembly are elected by popular vote, while the remaining seats are distributed proportionately among parties winning five or more seats in the direct elections. The President is elected by direct popular vote. Parties which win 20 seats or more receive official recognition by being permitted to form a caucus in the National Assembly. Those which fail to achieve 2 per cent of the total vote in legislative elections are subject to dissolution unless they are successful in securing at least one seat.

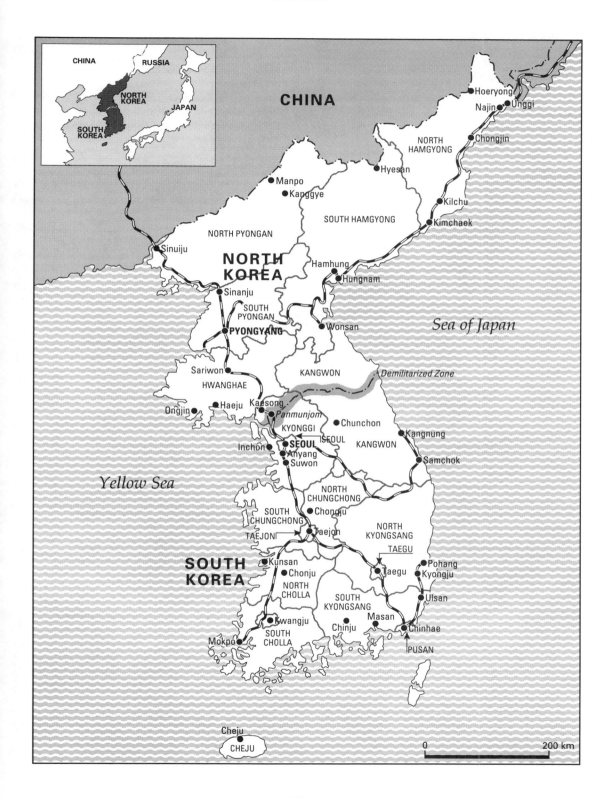

Recent elections

Fifth Republic (1980-88)

Under the constitution of the Fifth Republic political activity was severely circumscribed. Chun Doo Hwan, the leader of the 1979 military coup, was elected President by an electoral college in February 1981. In legislative elections on March 25, 1981, and Feb. 12, 1985, Chun's conservative Democratic Justice Party won majorities in the National Assembly.

Legislative elections, April 26, 1988

Party	Percent- age of vote	Seats won	Proportional seats won	Total
DJP	33.9	87	38	125
PPD	19.3	54	16	70
RDP	23.8	46	13	59
NDRP	15.6	27	8	35
Others	6.0	10	—	10

Legislative elections, March 24, 1992

Party	Percent- age of vote	Seats won	Proportional seats won	Total
DLP	38.5	116	33	149
DP	29.2	75	22	97
UNP	17.3	24	7	31
Others	15.0	22	—	22

Evolution of the suffrage

The South Korean state was founded on the basis of universal suffrage for those aged 21 years or more.

PARTY BY PARTY DATA

Democratic Liberal Party

Minja Dang

Address. 14-8, Youido-dong Youngdung, P'o-gu, Seoul

Leadership. Roh Tae Woo (pres.).

Orientation. Conservative-centrist. The DLP was forged from three separate parties for tactical rather than ideological reasons. It advocates traditional liberal freedoms within the context of stability and order.

Founded. February 1990.

History. The Democratic Liberal Party (DLP) was formed by Roh Tae Woo through the merger of his minority ruling Democratic Justice Party (DJP) with two of the three main opposition parties: Kim Young Sam's Reunification Democratic Party (RDP) and Kim Jong Pil's New Republican Democratic Party (NRDP). Although the DJP was more conservative and had greater associations with the military than did either of its two new partners, all three parties were constructed more around regional and leadership loyalties than ideological considerations. Therefore, Roh's unexpected initiative appeared as a shrewd means of transforming a minority administration into a government which commanded more than two-thirds of the seats in the legislature. It also expanded Roh's electoral power base beyond the DJP's traditional heartland of North Kyongsang province and Taegu city. The RDP had traditionally drawn the bulk of its support from South Kyongsang province (including Pusan), while the NDRP had been based in the north and south Chungchong regions.

The only area where the new party lacked influence was Cholla province and the city of Kwangju, in the comparatively underdeveloped south-west of the country, which remained the preserve of the Party for Peace and Democracy (PPD), led by Kim Dae Jung, the only significant opposition grouping excluded from the new ruling coalition.

The formation of the DLP produced unexpected problems, however, not the least of which was a public backlash against what was widely seen as a cynical manipulation of the electoral system. This view was encouraged by Kim Dae Jung who accused Roh of staging a constitutional coup and characterized the DLP as no more than an attempt to provide a form of constitutional legitimacy for the government's increasing authoritarianism. His claim was given credence by the DLP's use in July 1990 of its legislative majority to enact 26 bills in defiance of normal legislative procedure. In addition to bills to restructure the military leadership and to reorganize the broadcasting media, there was also a particularly sensitive measure to settle the level of compensation for those killed or injured in the government's brutal suppression of the 1980 Kwangju uprising.

The DLP's enactment of the package of legislation provoked fighting within the National Assembly and widespread street protests. It also resulted in a boycott of the legislature by the PPD between July and November.

Public disquiet over the legitimacy of the new ruling party was exacerbated by the personal feuding and factionalism which characterized the DLP almost from the outset. In April 1990 Park Chul Un, Roh's nephew and a key presidential adviser, became involved in a major confrontation with Kim Young Sam over control of the accelerating process of rapprochement with the Soviet Union. Although Park had been largely responsible for South Korea's successful drive to establish diplomatic links with the countries of eastern Europe, Kim had visited Moscow in March and appeared intent on becoming increasingly involved in the process. In the resulting confrontation the threat of Kim withdrawing his former RDP members from the DLP was eventually sufficient to force Roh to side with him. There was a further dispute later in the year over the issue of whether the country should retain its current presidential system of government or should adopt a prime ministerial system.

In May the three former party leaders within the DLP had signed a secret memorandum agreeing to begin moving towards the latter system during 1990. The unpopularity of the planned change, however, led Kim Young Sam to reverse his position and exposed him to subsequent attack by DJP supporters within the ruling party, who leaked his role in the memorandum agreement to the press. Kim denied charges of inconsistency, and characterized the dispute as a further attempt to discredit him. The threat of his withdrawing from the coalition was again sufficient to rally the support of Roh, who was forced to join Kim in disowning the planned constitutional reform.

Combined with the government's unimpressive pace of democratic reform and concerns about the state of the country's economy, the ruling party's level of support dwindled throughout the year, a fact which was translated into several humiliating by-election losses. The situation was made worse when, in May 1991, South Korea experienced the worst popular unrest since Roh had become President as many thousands of students participated in street protests throughout the country. Unlike the protests of 1987 which had ended the Fifth Republic, the 1991 protests, although frequently large and violent, lacked support from the country's middle class. Nevertheless, the protests eventually forced Roh to replace the Prime Minister.

The DLP's internal discord worsened as the presidential elections approached and the different factions struggled to secure the candidacy for Roh's succession. Although Roh's faction—largely composed of former DJP members—remained the largest, there were persistent rumours that Kim Young Sam's agreement to join the new party had been bought with the promise that he would be selected as the party's presidential candidate in 1992. This belief was reinforced as Kim Young Sam, who made no secret of his wish to be Roh's successor, frequently behaved as though the succession was his by right. Although Kim commanded the second-largest faction—former members of the RDP—he was widely distrusted and disliked by many former members of the DJP. The third faction was that grouped around Kim Jong Pil, consisting mainly of former NDRP members.

The DLP did well in the local elections held in 1991, the first to be held in South Korea for 30 years. In the legislative elections of March 1992, however, it suffered a sharp rebuff from the electorate. The DLP won 116 of the 237 seats open to popular election, thereby entitling it to 33 of the 62 seats awarded on the basis of proportional representation, bringing its total in the 299-member Assembly to 149, one seat short of an overall majority. President Roh reacted to the election defeat by stating, on March 25, that "the government and the ruling party should humbly acknowledge the people's will", and should seek to improve its management of the economy. He also suggested that it was imperative that the DLP should put an end to the internal discord. The immediate problem of the DLP's

lost legislative majority was overcome by March 26, when negotiations secured the support of at least two independents. The fact that a significant number of the independents who were elected were DLP sympathizers who had failed to secure party endorsement as candidates, meant that Roh was able to construct a working majority within the new Assembly.

The election's damaging impact on the longer term future of the DLP was less easy to assuage, however, particularly in terms of its effect on the delicate and potentially explosive balance between the three factions, each of which had been damaged by the election results. Roh's faction had suffered the loss of seats in its heartland of North Kyongsang province and Taegu, while that of Kim Jong Pil suffered heavy defeats in its power base—the city of Taejon and the surrounding province of South Chungchong. The faction of Kim Young Sam maintained its dominance in Pusan, but saw many of its candidates defeated in Seoul and elsewhere. As leader of the election campaign for the party as a whole, Kim was also blamed for the losses suffered by the other factions. He rejected calls for his resignation as DLP executive chairman, however, arguing that it was the government's poor economic record rather than the DLP's inadequate election campaign which had cost the party its legislative majority. But with the prospect of renewed factional discord, and with the strength of his faction in the new Assembly reduced from 40 to 22 seats, Kim's ambition to succeed Roh as president appeared to have been badly shaken by the election.

Nevertheless, on May 19, 1991, a 6,713-delegate DLP nominating convention chose Kim Young Sam as its candidate for the 1992 presidential elections. Kim received 4,318 votes (66.6 per cent) compared with 2,214 (33.4 per cent) cast for his only rival for the candidacy, Lee Jong Chan; there were 53 abstentions and 28 spoilt ballots. The decision was greeted by violent demonstrations in Seoul and elsewhere as thousands of students denounced Kim as a traitor and demanded democratic reform and the disbanding of the DLP. Two days before the convention, on May 17, Lee had announced his withdrawal from the nomination contest on the grounds that the result had been determined in advance by a series of backroom deals. Following the formal election of Kim, Lee gave notice of his intention to contest the presidential elections as an independent.

Structure. The party has local and regional branches; it remains subject to deep internal divisions between the three parties from which the DLP was created.

Democratic Party

Minju Dang

Address. 51-55, Yonggang-dong, Mapo-gu, Seoul.

Leadership. Kim Dae Jung; Lee Ki Taek (joint chairmen).

Orientation. The Democratic Party's platform advocates democratic reform and the peaceful and democratic pursuit of Korean reunification. It also supports a market economy, increased taxation for the wealthy, the increased availability of social welfare provision, and the retention of the current system of a directly elected president.

Founded. September 1991.

History. The Democratic Party (DP) was created on Sept. 16, 1991, through the merger of Kim Dae Jung's New Democratic Party (NDP)—itself formed from a merger between the Party for Peace and Democracy (PPD) and the small Party for New Democratic Alliance, in April 1990—and the smaller Democratic Party led by Lee Ki Taek, which was largely composed of members of the Reunification Democratic Party who had chosen not to join the Democratic Liberal Party [DLP—see above]. Although at its formation the party possessed a total of only 77 seats in the National Assembly, its creation was seen as crucial in providing new momentum for the anti-DLP opposition. It appeared to mark the end of the process of fracturing which had characterized the opposition since the split between Kim Dae Jung and Kim Young Sam in the run-up to the 1987 presidential elections.

Whereas the NDP's support had been based almost entirely in the south-western Cholla province, the focus of Li Ki Taek's support was in the south-eastern Kyongsang region. By returning some degree of regional breadth to the opposition forces, the creation of the DP also had the effect of marking a return to two-party politics after several years of fragmentation into three or four groupings divided upon regional lines.

In the 1991 legislative elections the DP dominated its traditional stronghold of North Cholla province, although the DLP unexpectedly captured two seats in this opposition heartland. The DP failed to win any seats in the Kyongsang provinces—as had the opposition in 1988—the traditional base of the governing party, and the new party also failed to win any of the 16 seats in Pusan or the 11 seats in Taegu, the home town of Roh. In the more marginal areas, most notably Seoul and its surrounding Kyonggi province, the DP secured an unexpectedly high level of support. It won 25 of the 44 directly elected seats in the capital, compared with 16 for the DLP and two for the Unification National Party (UNP). The election result improved the presidential chances of Kim Dae Jung who was selected as the DP's candidate on May 26, 1991.

Structure. The party has local and provincial branches. Executive authority is in the hands of the joint chairmen and a 10-member supreme executive council the membership of which is evenly divided between members of the two parties which merged to form the DP.

Unification National Party

Address. c/o National Assembly, Seoul, South Korea.

Leadership. Chung Ju Yung (ex. ch.).

Orientation. Centre-right. The party upholds capitalism, and is committed to reducing corruption and crime. It opposes the record of economic management associated with the administration of Roh Tae Woo, and promises to reduce inflation and to increase levels of economic growth.

Founded. January 1992.

History. The Unification National Party (UNP) was created by Chung Ju Yung, the 76-year-old founder of the giant Hyundai group, the country's second-largest conglomerate. Born in what is now North Korea, Chung was an outspoken advocate of Korean reunification and was the first prominent South Korean businessman to travel to the North to discuss possible joint ventures. He was also an outspoken critic of the Roh adminstration's economic policy, particularly its plans to streamline the *chaebol* system through competition-inducing measures such as requiring chaebol to restrict their business activities to three core areas and to reduce or sell non-core operations. Clumsy attempts by the authorities to harass Hyundai and the Chung family only appeared to spur Chung's determination to make a significant intervention in the 1992 legislative elections.

Drawing upon his massive personal fortune Chung fought a vigorous, centrist, pro-business campaign, which attacked the economic record of the Roh government, and in particular its inability to reduce inflation, currently running at an annualized rate of approximately 10 per cent. The party won 31 seats (24 in direct voting and seven in the national constituency) and, by exceeding the threshold of 20 Assembly seats, was entitled to form a formal negotiating caucus on the floor of the House. Following the strong showing of the UNP, Chung Ju Yung also hinted strongly that he was considering a bid for the presidency.

Minor parties

Conference of Citizens' Coalition for Participation and Autonomy; founded in March 1991 to contest the local elections, it has five co-leaders, and includes many representatives of the intelligentsia and the arts.

Impartial Democratic Party (IDP); 50-2, Sosomun-dong, Chung-gu, Seoul; Kim Sung Ok (spokesman). The IDP contested the 1992 legislative elections but failed to win any seats.

Party for New Political Reform (PNPR); contested the 1992 legislative elections. Although it won less than 2 per cent of the total vote, it escaped dissolution by securing one seat in the legislature. The successful candidate was its leader Park Chan Jong.

Saehan Party; formed in February 1992 through a merger between the existing Saehan Party, led by Kim Tong Kil, and the New Democratic Party, which had been formed by members of the Democratic Korea Party which had been disbanded in 1987.

Defunct parties

Democratic Justice Party(DJP—*Minju Jongui Dang*); founded in January 1981 by President Chun Doo Hwan. Although committed to democracy, justice and a comprehensive welfare system, in reality the DJP was the vehicle of Chun and his military associates who had created the Fifth Republic following their military coup in 1979. It remained the ruling party until 1990 when it merged with the opposition Reunification Democratic Party and the New Democratic Republican Party to create the Democratic Liberal Party.

Democratic Party(DP—*Minju Dang*); formed in June 1990 as an alternative to the Democratic Liberal Party (DLP) and Party for Peace and Democracy, it drew heavily upon those supporters of the Reunification Democratic Party who rejected the decision to join the DLP. The party merged with the larger New Democratic Party (NDP) in September to form the principal source of opposition to the Roh government.

Clean Democratic Party(*Kongmyong*); in accordance with the constitution, the party was dissolved in April 1992 after winning only 0.1 per cent of the vote in the March legislative elections.

Masses Party(*Minjung Dang*); this small party, created in 1990, claimed to be the voice of the country's industrial workers. Concentrating on the southern industrial regions of Masan, Ulsan, and Changwon, the party fielded 51 candidates in the 1992 elections, and fought upon an explicitly socialist platform which included large-scale nationalisation. The party polled 1.5 per cent of the vote, failing to win any seats. It was therefore formally dissolved in April 1992.

New Democratic Party(NDP—Sinmin Dang); formed in 1991 from a merger between Kim Dae Jung's Party for Peace and Democracy and the small Party for New Democratic Alliance. The party fared badly in the local elections of mid-1991 and ceased to exist in September of that year when it merged with the Democratic Party to form the principal source of opposition to the Roh government.

New Democratic Republican Party(NDRP—Shin Minju Konghwa Dang); based on the defunct Democratic Republican Party, the NDRP was founded by Kim Jong Pil as a vehicle for his candidacy in the 1987 presidential elections. In 1990 it constituted the smallest of the three parties which merged to form the Democratic Liberal Party.

Party for Peace and Democracy(PPD—P'yonghwa Minju Dang); created by Kim Dae Jung in November 1987 to serve as a vehicle for his candidacy in the presidential elections. The consequent splitting of the opposition vote was crucial in allowing Roh Tae Woo to win the presidency with less than 36 per cent of the vote. The PPD ceased to exist in April 1991 when it merged with a smaller opposition group and became the New Democratic Party.

Reunification Democratic Party(RDP—*T'ongilmin-judang*); formed in May 1987 when Kim Dae Jung and Kim Young Sam split from the opposition New Korean Democratic Party. The party split in November when both Kims insisted upon contesting the presidency. After Kim Dae Jung and his supporters left the party, the RDP was dominated by Kim Young Sam, and eventually merged with the Democratic Justice Party and the New Republican Party to form the Democratic Liberal Party.

Major guerrilla groups

Although South Korea does not have any groups currently engaged in a serious guerrilla struggle against the state, the years of authoritarian rule and political restrictions mean that there are numerous underground organizations. This is particularly true of student bodies. Throughout the history of South Korea students have played a key role in challenging authoritarian governments, and it was they who ignited the protests which brought down the Fifth Republic in 1987. The continued existence of the country's draconian National Security Law—which bans, among other activities, all unauthorized contact with North Korea—means that, while some former dissidents have been brought into the political mainstream, many radical organizations remain illegal.

Korean Trade Union Congress(KTUC, Chunohyup); radical labour movement which was formed in January 1990 and immediately banned. Despite numerous arrests of its leaders, Chunohyup has been responsible for organizing several large-scale strikes in key sectors.

National Council of University Student Representatives(Chundaehyup); formed in 1987 and consists of some 140 student associations. Chundaehyup opposes authoritarianism (and, in particular, the country's National Security Law), and advocates a nuclear-free Korean peninsula reunified on a confederal basis. It believes in violent confrontation with the Roh government as a continuance of its opposition to the authoritarianism of Fifth Republic. On May 30, 1992, some 50,000 students from throughout the country gathered at Hangyang university in Seoul to celebrate the sixth anniversary of the organization's creation.

National Democratic Alliance of Korea(NDAK, Chunminryun); founded in January 1989 as a successor to Mintongryun (the United People's Movement for Democracy and Unification), the NDAK is a coalition of numerous radical and dissident groups. It opposes the "dictatorship" of the Roh government and advocates the opening of contacts with North Korea.

Laos

Capital: Vientiane

Population: 4,100,000 (1990 UNFPA est.)

The Lao People's Democratic Republic (LPDR) was proclaimed in 1975 after the communist *Pathet Lao* forces had achieved victory at the end of a 25-year civil war. A President, Council of Ministers and Supreme People's Assembly were installed, but effective political power has since been exercised by the leadership of the sole legal political organization, the Lao People's Revolutionary Party (LPRP).

Constitutional structure

The LPDR's first Constitution was unanimously endorsed by the Supreme People's Assembly in August 1991. Under the terms of the Constitution the LPRP is defined as the "leading nucleus" of the political system. The President, the head of state, is elected by a popularly elected legislative organ, the National Assembly, for a five-year term. A Prime Minister and Council of Ministers is appointed by the President, with the approval of the Assembly, for a five-year term.

Electoral system

Under the terms of the 1991 Constitution a National Assembly, the legislative organ, is elected for a five-year term. The number of members of the Assembly is based on the number of citizens throughout the country. One member of the Assembly is elected from every 50,000 citizens. The Lao Front for National Construction is charged with proposing and confirming names of candidates for election.

Evolution of the suffrage

Under the terms of an Election Law promulgated in August 1991, Lao citizens of 18 years of age and over have the right to vote and the right to be elected at the age of 21 and over, except insane persons and persons whose right to vote and to be elected have been revoked by a court.

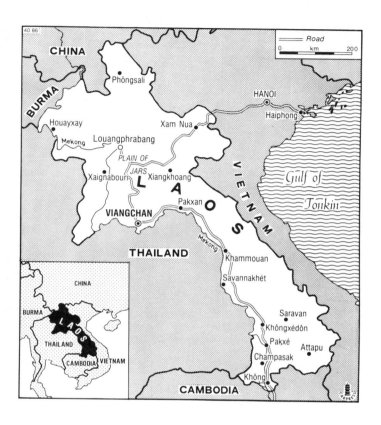

Recent elections

Nationwide elections began during 1988, the first ever held in the LPDR, and took place in three stages. The first of these was elections to district-level People's Councils, which were held in June 1988. The Lao Front for National Construction proposed a total of 4,462 candidates to contest the 2,410 district seats. In November 1988 national elections were held at provincial and municipal level, where 551 candidates were elected from a total of 898. The final stage took place in March 1989 when national elections were held to the Supreme People's Assembly. A total of 121 candidates (of whom up to 70 per cent were reported to be LPRP members) contested the 79 seats.

PARTY BY PARTY DATA

Lao Front for National Construction

Address. Vientiane.

Leadership. Souphanouvong (pres.); Maisouk Saisompheng (ch.); Vongphet Saikeu-Yachongtoua (vice- ch.); Saman Vignaket (sec. of cen. cttee).

Orientation. Aims to foster national solidarity and socialist economic development.

Founded. 1979.

History. The Lao Front for National Construction (LFNC) replaced the Lao Patriotic Front (which had incorporated the Lao People's Revolutionary Party (LPRP) and the *Pathet Lao* forces during the civil war) as the umbrella organization for the country's various political and social groups. The LPRP remained the LFNC's main component. The LFNC's second congress was held in 1987. An extraordinary LFNC plenum was held in September 1991 at which Phoumi Vongvichit and Bolang Boualapha were replaced as chair and vice-chair, respectively, by Maisouk Saisompheng and Vongphet Saikeu-Yachongtoua.

Structure. A 94-member central committee and seven-member standing committee.

Lao People's Revolutionary Party

Phak Pasason Pativat Lao

Address. Vientiane.

Leadership. Kaysone Phomvihane (pres.).

Orientation. Communist party.

Founded. 1955.

History. The Lao People's Revolutionary Party (LPRP) evolved out of the Indo-Chinese Communist Party (ICP), founded by Ho Chi Minh in 1930. The ICP authorized the formation of a separate Lao communist party in 1951 (at the same time that separate communist parties were formed in Vietnam and Cambodia), but it was not until 1955 that the Lao People's Party (LPP) was created. At the time of its formation, and through its subsequent development, the LPP was assisted by aides from neighbouring Vietnam. During its struggle for power the LPP was extremely secretive, operating under the umbrella of the Lao Patriotic Front headed by Souphanouvong. During the years 1963-73, the highest-ranking LPP leaders (Kaysone Phomvihane, Phoumi Vongvichit, Phoune Sipaseuth and Souphanouvong) directed the struggle from a cave complex underground in Sam Neua to protect themselves from the heavy US aerial bombardment. In 1972 the LPP held its second congress in Sam Neua, at which the party's name was changed to the Lao People's Revolutionary Party.

With victory in 1975, the LPRP became more open and its leadership structure was identified. The party held its third and fourth congresses in Vientiane in 1982 and 1986. At the fourth congress the party emulated the new Vietnamese line and initiated a programme of economic restructuring and reform. At the same time a number of younger provincial party officials and military officers were drafted onto the party central committee to replace some of the "old guard" revolutionaries. By the time of the fifth congress in 1991 most of the elements of a market-based economic system were in place. However, in keeping with the Vietnamese reform model, the party resisted mounting international pressure (brought about by the collapse of communism in the Soviet Union and Eastern Europe) to introduce political reforms. Hence, in late 1990 two former deputy ministers were arrested after attempting to form a pro-democracy grouping.

At the fifth congress, Kaysone Phomvihane was elected as "president of the party"; his previous post of party general secretary was left vacant. Kaysone's grip on the party was enhanced by the abolition of the central committee's nine-member secretariat, the organ which had previously conducted party affairs on a day-to-day basis. A central committee advisory board was created to accomodate three "old guard" revolutionaries not re-elected to the politburo: Souphanouvong, Phoumi Vongvichit and Sisomphone Lovansay. The three were replaced by three supporters of Kaysone's economic reform policies, Somlak Chanthamat, Khamphoui Keoboualapha and Thongsing Thammavong, who joined Kaysone, Nouhak Phoumsavan, Khamtay Siphandon, Phoune Sipaseuth, Maychantane Sengmany, Saman Vignaket, Oudon Khattigna and Choummali Saignakong.

Structure. Central committee of 55 full members and four alternate members; 11-member politburo; three-member central committee advisory board.

Membership. 60,000.

Publications. *Aloun Mai* (New Dawn), theoretical and political organ; *Pasason* (The People) and *Valasan Khosana* (Propaganda Journal), central committee organs.

Dissident groups

Resistance to the Lao People's Revolutionary Party's (LPRP) regime and the Vietnamese military presence in the country by right-wing groups has generally taken the form of sporadic and badly organized guerrilla operations. The **United Front for the National Liberation of the Lao People,** a coalition grouping of the major rightist groups, has been in operation since 1980. A potentially more serious source of rebellion has arisen from the Hmong tribespeople, who have been in armed opposition to the LPRP since the 1960s. A major source of concern for the government is the operation from Lao territory of the Vietnamese rebel group, the **National United Front for the Liberation of Vietnam.**

Macao

Capital: Macao City

Population: 500,000 (1990 UNFPA est.)

Macao, which was established by the Portuguese as a trading post with China in 1557, became a Portuguese Overseas Province in 1951. A new statute in 1976 redefined Macao as a Special Territory of Portugal. Negotiations between China and Portugal, which began in 1986, concluded with the signing of the Sino-Portuguese Joint Declaration of April 13, 1987. According to this document, on Dec. 20, 1999, Macao will revert to Chinese administration. Provisions similar to those for Hong Kong, which is scheduled to return to Chinese administration in 1997, allow for a 50-year period in which the future Special Administrative Region, Macao, China will retain its capitalist structures.

Constitutional structure

Under Macao's Constitution, embodied in an Organic Law of Portugal, promulgated on Feb. 17, 1976, and revised in 1990, executive power is invested in the Governor, appointed by the President of Portugal after consultation with the Macanese Legislative Assembly. The Governor is assisted by up to seven Under-Secretaries wielding executive powers. Foreign affairs remain under Portuguese jurisdiction. The Governor presides over the Consultative Council and the Superior Council of Security. The 23-seat Legislative Assembly represents the local population.

Electoral system

The Legislative Assembly of Macao, which has a four-year mandate, comprises seven members appointed by the Governor from residents; eight members elected indirectly by business associations; and eight members elected by direct and universal suffrage. The Consultative Council, also presided over by the Governor, comprises five members appointed by the Governor; four elected on a four-year mandate (two by members of administrative bodies; one by social organizations and one by economic associations); three ex officio members and two nominated by the Governor. Six additional seats to the Legislative Assembly were created by the revised Organic Law of 1990.

Evolution of the suffrage

In August 1984 the franchise was extended from the Macanese (Euro-Asian) minority to include the Chinese majority, regardless of their length of residence in the territory.

Recent elections

Legislative Assembly elections, August 1984: four of the six directly-elected seats went to the Electoral Union. The six indirectly elected members (all Chinese) were returned unopposed.

Legislative Assembly elections, October 1988: the "liberal" grouping of independents increased its representation to the Legislative Assembly from one to three of the directly-elected seats, while the remaining three seats were won by the Electoral Union. The turnout was low at less than 30 per cent.

PARTY BY PARTY DATA

There are no formal political parties in Macao, but a number of civic organizations do exist. Some of these have played a role in pressing for political reform, and have backed candidates for the Legislative Assembly:

Associaçáo para a Defesa dos Interesses de Macao (ADIM); a conservative group established in 1974, whose candidate defeated the *Centro Democrático de Macao* candidate in the April 1975 elections for Macao's representative to the Lisbon Assembly. In July 1976, ADIM won 55 per cent of the votes in the elections to the Legislative Assembly, thanks to the manipulations of the then Governor Col. Garcia Leandro (the total number of votes cast was 2,700).

Centro Democrático de Macao (CDM) was established after the 1974 military coup in Portugal to press for radical political reform and the replacement of leaders connected with the former regime there. The 1976 Legislative Assembly elections returned one CDM member.

Electoral Union (UNE); one of the most influential political organizations, which represents a coalition of pro-China and conservative Macanese (Euro-Asian) groups. It won three of the six directly elected seats to the Legislative Assembly in the 1988 elections.

Grupo Independente de Macao (GIMA).

Pro-Macao and Flower of Friendship and Development of Macao (FADEM); also one of the more influential groups.

Major guerrilla groups

Macao has no guerrilla organizations.

Malaysia

Capital: Kuala Lumpur   **Population: 17,900,000 (1990 UNFPA est.)**

The Federation of Malaysia came into being in 1963, through the merger of the already independent Federation of Malaysia (which had gained independence from the United Kingdom in 1957) with the self-governing State of Singapore and the former British Crown Colonies of Sarawak and Sabah (North Borneo). Singapore's inclusion in the Federation of Malaysia was terminated in 1965. The major political force in Malaysia is the National Front (*Barisan Nasional*), a coalition of parties representing all the country's major ethnic groups, Malay, Chinese and Indian.

Constitutional structure

The current Constitution came into effect in 1957 when the Federation of Malaysia gained independence from the United Kingdom. The constitution codifies a federal system of government under an elective constitutional monarchy. The supreme head of the federation is the paramount ruler (*Yang di-Pertuan Agong*) who exercises the power of a constitutional monarch in a parliamentary democracy. The *Yang di-Pertuan Agong* is chosen for a five-year term by, and from among, the nine hereditary rulers of the Malay States, who, along with the heads of state of Malacca, Penang, Sabah and Sarawak, constitute the Conference of Rulers (*Majlis Raja-Raja*). Executive power is vested in a Cabinet and a Prime Minister responsible to a bicameral legislature consisting of a partially elected 69-member Senate (*Dewan Negara*) and a fully elected 172-member House of Representatives (*Dewan Rakyat*). The administration of the 13 states is carried out by rulers or governors and each state has its own constitution and a unicameral State Assembly which shares power with the federal parliament.

Electoral system

The *Yang di-Pertuan Agong* is elected by the Conference of Rulers for a five-year term. The House of Representatives, consisting of 172 members elected from the 13 states and eight from the Federal Territories of Kuala Lumpur and Lubuan, is elected by all Malaysian citizens for a five-year term. Two members of the Senate are elected for each of the 13 states and a further 43 members are appointed by the *Yang di-Pertuan Agong*. The term of office for a Senate member is three years and a member cannot hold office for more than two terms.

Evolution of the suffrage

Under the terms of the 1957 Constitution, all citizens over the age of 21 can vote in House of Representative and Legislative Assembly elections. A person is disqualified from voting if he or she is detained as a person of unsound mind or is serving a sentence of imprisonment.

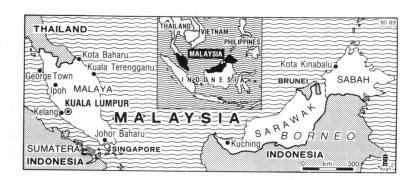

Recent elections

Party	Year		
	1982	1986	1990
National Front			
United Malays National Organization	70	83	71
Malaysian Chinese Association	24	17	18
Malaysian Indian Congress	4	6	6
Malaysian People's Movement	5	5	5
*Sarawak parties	19	22	21
+Sabah parties	10	15	6
Democratic Action Party	9	24	20
Pan-Malaysian Islamic Party	5	1	7
Spirit of '46	—	—	8
United Sabah Party	—	—	14
Independents	8	4	4
Total	154	177	180

*In 1982, 1986 and 1990 the Sarawak parties consisted of the United Traditional *Bumiputra* Party, the Sarawak United People's Party, the Sarawak National Party and the Sarawak Dayak Party.

+In 1982 the Sabah parties consisted of the Sabah People's Union and the United Sabah National Organization (USNO); in 1986 USNO and the United Sabah Party; and in 1990 USNO.

PARTY BY PARTY DATA

Community Coalition Congress
Kongres Penyatuan Masyarakat
Address. 1, Jalan Tambun, 30350, Perak Darul Ridzuan.
Founded. 1987.
History. This small opposition party has never enjoyed state or federal representation.

Democratic Action Party
Address. 24, Jalan 20/9, 46300 Petaling Jaya, Selangor Darul Ehsan.
Leadership. Chen Man Hin (ch.); Lim Kit Siang (sec.-gen.); Sim Kwang Yang (deputy sec.-gen.).
Orientation. The Democratic Action Party (DAP) seeks the establishment by constitutional means of a democratic, socialist pattern of society in Malaysia.
Founded. 1966.
History. Formed as the Malaysian offshoot of the Singapore People's Action Party, the DAP participated in general elections for the first time in 1969, when it won 13 federal and 31 state assembly seats; in 1974 it gained nine federal and 21 state assembly seats; and in 1978, 16 federal and 24 state assembly seats. In 1982, it retained only nine federal seats and 12 assembly seats. It improved its position dramatically in the 1986 election, taking advantage of serious internal dissension within the Malaysian Chinese Association (MCA—the DAP's main rival within the ruling National Front coalition) to win 24 federal seats and 37 assembly seats, including 13 and 10 in Perak and Penang respectively.

Although the DAP has been the main opposition party in the House of representatives since the late 1960s, its activities have been somewhat circumscribed by prosecutions of prominent members on various charges. In 1987, for example, a number of high-ranking DAP officials, including the party secretary-general and official leader of the opposition Lim Kit Siang, were arrested along with numerous other politicians on charges of having provoked racial tension. Lim was given a two-year detention centre, but resumed his position as opposition leader upon his release in 1989.

The party contested the 1990 election as part of the loosely grouped People's Might (*Gagasan Rakyat*) opposition coalition. The DAP won 20 federal seats and maintained its position as the main opposition party. The party also increased its representation in the state assemblies to a total of 45 seats (Penang 14, Perak 13, Selangor 6, Negri Sembilan 4, Johore 3, Malacca 3, Kedah 1 and Pahang 1).
Membership. 12,000.
Affiliations. Socialist International; Asia-Pacific Socialist Organization.

Democratic Malaysian Indian Party
Parti Demokratik Indian Malaysia
Address. 10B, Tingkat 2, Jalan 54, Desa Jaya, 52100 Kuala Lumpur.
Leadership. V. Govindaraj (l.).
Founded. 1985.
History. The Democratic Malaysian Indian Party (DMIP) was founded by dissidents from the Malaysian Indian Congress. The party has no federal or state representation.

Front Malaysian Islamic Council
Barisan Jema'ah Islamiah Semalaysia (Berjasa)
Address. 1618, Jalan Kerbau, 15300 Kota Bahru, Kelantan.
Leadership. Wan Hashim Bin Haji Wan Achmed (pres.); Mahmud Zuhdi Bin Abdul Majid (sec.-gen.).
Orientation. Kelantan based, moderate pro-Islamic party.
Founded. 1977.
History. The party was formed by Muhamad Nasir, who became its chair and who had been expelled from the Pan-Malaysian Islamic Party [see separate entry]. In the 1978 State Assembly elections in Kelantan, Berjasa supported the National Front, with which it subsequently formed a coalition government. The party did not take part in the federal general elections of 1978, but in 1980 it joined the ruling National Front coalition and in the 1982 general election it contested two federal seats unsuccessfully. The party gained no seats in the 1986 elections and subsequently left the National Front to join the opposition Muslim Unity Movement coalition in 1989.

The party won no seats for the Muslim Unity Movement in the federal general election of 1990, but gained one seat in the State Assembly elections held at the same time in Kelantan.
Membership. 50,000.
Publications. Voice of Jama'ah.

Islamic Alliance Party
Ikatan Masyarakat Islam
History. This small Terengganu-based party applied to

join the ruling National Front coalition in 1991, but a decision was deferred. The party has no federal or state representation.

Islamic Front of Malaysia
Hizbul Muslimin Malaysia (Hamin)
Address. 4815D, Tingkat 1, Jalan Dusun Muda, 15200 Kota Bahru, Kelantan.
Leadership. Asri Muda (pres.).
Orientation. The party's leaders had opposed the ascendancy of the "theocratic" element in the Pan-Malaysian Islamic Party [see separate entry].
Founded. 1983.
History. This party was founded by Asri Muda as a breakaway from the Pan-Malaysian Islamic Party, of which he had been president. The split occurred after Asri had opposed efforts to transfer powers held by the party leadership to a Council of Theologians. Asri was joined by four of the five Pan-Malaysian Islamic Party members elected to the *Dewan Rakyat* in 1982, and thus became the second largest opposition party in the House after the Democratic Action Party. The party joined the ruling National Front in 1985, but failed to win a seat in the 1986 federal and state elections. Hamin subsequently left the National Front and in 1989 it joined the opposition Muslim Unity Movement, alongside the Pan-Malaysian Islamic Party, the Malaysian Islamic Council Front and Spirit of 46. The party contested the 1990 federal and state elections as part of the coalition, but won no seats.

Malaysian Ceylonese Congress
Address. 11, Jalan, Emas Batu 3.5, Jalan Sungei Besi, 57100 Kuala Lumpur.
Leadership. N. Arumugasamy (l.).
Orientation. Represents Malaysia's small Sri Lankan population.
Founded. 1958.
History. This small party has no federal or state representatation.

Malaysian Chinese Association (MCA)
Address. 163, Jalan Ampang, 50450 Kuala Lumpur.
Leadership. Ling Liong Sik (pres.); Lee Kim Sai (vice-pres.); Ng Cheng Kiat (sec.-gen.).
Orientation. Chinese-based party; more conservative than the Chinese opposition Democratic Action Party, drawing its support from among the Chinese middle and upper classes. The MCA is a member of the ruling National Front coalition.
Founded. 1949.

History. The MCA was an original partner in the Alliance Party which ruled Malaysia from 1957 until the formation of its successor coalition, the National Front, in 1974. However, the MCA withdrew from the government in 1969 after violent communal rioting in Malaysia and did not rejoin until 1982. In the 1982 general elections, the party returned with 24 seats. However, in 1986 its representation fell to 17 seats, reflecting in part serious factional infighting within the party during 1985 and the controversy surrounding the arrest on fraud charges in January 1986 in Singapore of Tan Koon Swan, the party's president. Shortly after the election Tan was sentenced to two years' imprisonment in Singapore and he resigned the party presidency in favour of Ling Liong Sik. The party was again involved in controversy in 1987 when, after rising tension between the Malay and Chinese communities, Prime Minister Mahathir Mohamad ordered mass arrests under the country's stringent Internal Security Act. Among those arrested were eight MCA members, including party vice-president Chan Kit Chee. In the 1990 general election the MCA won 18 seats. In the new cabinet appointed after the election, party president Ling Liong Sik was Transport Minister and party vice-president Lee Kim Sai was Health Minister.
Membership. 500,000.

Malaysian Indian Congress (MIC)
Address. Bangunan MIC, 1, Jln Rahmat, off Jln Tun Ismail, Kuala Lumpur.
Leadership. S. Samy Vellu (pres.); G. Vadiveloo (sec.-gen.).
Orientation. The main representative of the Indian community in Malaysia. The MIC is a member of the ruling National Front coalition.
Founded. 1945.
History. The MIC was founded to represent the interests of the Indian community in Malaysia. It formed part of the Alliance Party and, after 1973, part of the National Front.

The current president, Samy Vellu, was first elected to the post in 1981. As in 1986 the party gained six seats in the 1990 election. Following the general election, Samy Vellu was reappointed to the Cabinet as Minister of Energy, Telecommunications and Posts.
Membership. 335,000.

Malaysia Indian Muslim Congress
Kongress Indian Muslim Malaysia (KIMMA)
Address. 97-4, Flat Jalan Tun Razak, 50400 Kuala Lumpur.

Leadership. Ahmed Elias (pres.); Mohamed Ali bin Haji Naina Mohamed (sec.-gen.).

Orientation. The party's aim is to unite the Malaysian Indian Muslims, with emphasis on their loyalty to Malaysia, and to improve their harmony and peace with other communities in the country as well as their economic and educational opportunities.

Founded. 1977.

History. KIMMA has gained no representation at state or federal level.

Membership. 25,000.

Malaysian People's Movement
Parti Gerakan Rakyat Malaysia (Gerakan)

Address. 10 and 12, Jalan 1/77b, off Changkat Dollah, Pudu, 551000 Kuala Lumpur.

Leadership. Lim Keng Yaik (pres.); Chan Choong Tak (sec.-gen.).

Orientation. Penang-based social democratic party which attracts the support of Chinese intellectuals. The party upholds the Constitution of Malaysia and advocates "an egalitarian Malaysian society based on humanitarian and democratic principles". The party seeks "to ensure social and economic justice", with "public ownership of the vital means of production and distribution", the "individual ownership of economic lots of land by the peasants and workers and the efficient utilization of land by co-operative and joint management"; it also seeks "equal pay and privileges" for women, and to "eliminate the causes which have made the Malays and other indiginous people economically weak". Gerakan is a member of the ruling National Front coalition.

Founded. 1968.

History. This party was formed by United Democratic Party members, leaders of the moderate wing of the Labour Party and a group of academics, and was strengthened by the accession of a group of former Malaysian Chinese Association reformists. Gerakan captured the Penang state government in 1969 and, having entered into a coalition with the Alliance Party (predecessor to the ruling National Front coalition) in 1972, it remains the major party in that government.

Gerakan gained five seats for the National Front in the 1982 and 1986 federal elections. The party suffered an internal rift in 1988 that resulted in a number of defections to the Malaysian Chinese Association (the party's Chinese rival in the National Front) and the resignation of two of its vice-presidents, Michael Chen and Paul Leong. Despite the internal wrangling, Gerakan still managed to win five seats in the 1990 federal election. Following the elections party president Lim Keng Yaik was reappointed as Minister of Primary Industries.

Structure. Gerakan has branches, divisions, state liaison committees, a central committee and a central working committee.

Membership. 140,000.

Publications. Gerakan Rakyat (People's Movement).

Malaysian People's Party
Parti Rakyat Malaysia (PRM)

Address. 6a, Jalan K-2 Kampong Sekudai Kiri Batu 4/5, Jalan Sekudai 81200 Johor Baharu, Johor.

Leadership. Syed Husin Ali (pres.); Abdul Razak Ahmad (sec.-gen.).

Orientation. Left-wing; one of the country's oldest opposition parties.

Founded. 1955.

History. In the 1959 general elections the party, then known as the People's Party (*Parti Rakyat*), won two seats as part of the Malayan People's Socialist Front (a leftist alliance with the now defunct Labour Party of Malaya). The party also won four State Assembly seats (in Pahang, Selangor and Penang). It adopted the name Malaysian People's Socialist Party (*Parti Sosialis Rakyat Malaysia*) in the late 1960s.

Between 1968 and 1981 the party's leader, Kassim Ahmad, was detained for alleged pro-communist activities, and the party was banned from holding public rallies. The party has had little electoral success since the 1950s, gaining neither federal nor state representation. In 1989 it dropped the word 'socialist' from its name in an attempt to portray a more moderate stance.

Malaysian Punjabi Party
Parti Punjabi Malayasia

Address. Tingkat 3, Bangunan Persatuan, Pekerja Kenderaan, 21, Jalan Barat, 46200 Petaling Jaya, Selangor Darul Ehsan.

Orientation. Represents the Punjabi community in Malaysia.

Founded. 1982.

History. This small party has no federal or state representation.

Malaysian Unity Movement
Parti Perpaduan Anak Malaysia

Address. Suite 903, Tingkat·9, Selangor Complex, Jalan Sultan, 50000 Kuala Lumpur.

Founded. 1986.

History. This small party has no federal or state representation.

Muslim Unity Movement
Angkatan Perpaduan Ummah
Leadership. Tengku Tan Sri Razaleigh Hamzah (Spirit of 46); Fadzil Noor (Pan-Malaysian Islamic Party); Wan Hashim Bin Wan Achmed (Front Malaysian Islamic Council); Asri Muda (Islamic Front of Malaysia).
Orientation. Right of centre opposition coalition.
Founded. 1989.
History. This loose coalition was formed in 1989 by four Malay-based opposition parties (three of them Islamic in orientation), namely Spirit of 46, Pan-Malaysian Islamic Party, Islamic Front of Malaysia and the Front Malaysian Islamic Council. In the 1990 general election the four parties agreed not to put up candidates against each other. The Muslim Unity Movement gained a total of 15 seats in the House of Representatives emerging, therefore, as less of an opposition force than the (Chinese) Democratic Action Party. In the state elections the coalition had more success, winning control of the Kelantan State Assembly from the ruling National Front.

National Front
Barisan Nasional (BN)
Address. Bangunan UMNO, 399, Jalan Tuanku Abdul Rahman Mohamed, 50100 Kuala Lumpur.
Leadership. Abdul Ghafar Baba (sec.-gen.).
Orientation. An essentially conservative alliance within which there is general agreement that Malays should be politically predominant and receive positive discrimination at the economic level.
Founded. 1973.
History. The National Front superceded the earlier Alliance Party, which had been founded in 1952 and held power from independence in 1957. The Alliance Party had consisted of the United Malay National Organization (UMNO), the Malysian Chinese Association (MCA), the Malaysian Indian Congress (MIC) and the Sabah and Sarawak Alliances.

The National Front contests elections as a single political body, with candidates of the constituent parties undertaking not to stand against each other. Since its foundation the National Front has remained in power, winning a majority of seats in five consecutive general elections. In the 1990 general election it won 127 out of a total 180 seats in the House of Representatives. In state elections held in 1990-91 the party won control of all State Assemblies except Kelantan and Sabah.

UMNO is the principal party within the National Front. As of mid-1992 the other 11 member parties were: the MCA, MIC, Malaysian People's Movement, People's Progressive Party of Malaysia, Sarawak United People's Party, Sarawak National Action Party, United Traditional Bumiputra Party, Sarawak Dayak Party, United Sabah National Organization, People's Justice Movement and the Liberal Democratic Party. Of the 12 member parties, only three were not represented in the House of Representatives elected in 1990, namely the Perak-based People's Progressive Party of Malaysia and the Sabah-based People's Justice Movement and Liberal Democratic Party.

Pan-Malaysian Islamic Party
Parti Islam Se-Malaysia
Address. Markas Tarbiyyah, PAS Pusat, Lot 2549/3, Lrg Hj Hassan off Jln Batu Geliga, Taman Melewar, 68100 Batu Caves, Selangor Darul Ehsan.
Leadership. Fadzil Noor (pres.); Abdul Hadi Awang (deputy pres.); Halim Arshat (sec.-gen.).
Orientation. The party seeks the establishment of the Islamic system in society and the nation, including maintenance of the nation's independence and sovereignty, preservation of Malay as the country's national language and Arabic as the second language, and rejection of all "man-made" ideologies.
Founded. 1952.
History. The Pan-Malaysian Islamic Party (PAS) arose out of the Muslim *Ummah* movement led by *Ulema* (Muslim scholars) to fight against "Western imperialism and colonialism". Early *Ulema* organizations in Malaysia included a Higher Islamic Council (formed in 1947), and the *Hizbul Muslimin* (an Islamic political party established in 1948). The party was founded to seek independence based on Islamic principles. In the first elections of the independent Federation of Malaya held in 1959, PAS gained 13 out of 104 seats and also took control of the State Assembly in Kelantan, the party's stronghold. It won nine seats in 1964, 12 in 1969 and in 1973 it joined the ruling National Front coalition and took Cabinet representation. The following year the party lost control of the Kelantan Assembly, winning only two of its 36 seats.

The PAS withdrew from the National Front in 1977 in protest at government threats to impose federal rule in Kelantan. In federal elections held the next year, its representation was reduced to five seats, all of which were retained in the 1982 elections. In the run-up to the 1986 elections, Islamic fundamentalism was a major campaign issue and the possibility of a major PAS revival was viewed with some concern by the National Front. Concern within the ruling coalition was heightened by PAS attempts to recruit converts from the Chinese community. In the event, PAS won only one seat; however, the party lost 19 of the seats which it contested by a margin of less than 1,000 and another 11 seats by less than 500, indicating that in many constituencies the contest had been closer than the formal figures suggested. The National Front also managed to retain Kelantan in state elections held in 1986, defeating PAS by 29 seats to 10.

PAS fought the 1990 general election as part of a loosely based opposition coalition, the Muslim Unity Movement (MUM), alongside the United Malays National Organization splinter party, Spirit of 46, and two other pro-Islamic parties, the Front Malaysian Islamic Council and the Islamic Front of Malaysia. PAS increased its federal representation to seven seats and regained control of Kelantan in concurrent state elections. A PAS government was established in the state headed by Nik Abdul Aziz Nik Mat. The party also made inroads in Terengganu and gained a seat in Kedah, but National Front governments were still established in both states.

Structure. The supreme council of the PAS is its annual general meeting, which elects members of the party's executive committee every two years. There is a state liaison committee responsible for co-ordinating party activities in the states and for implementing party policies at state level. The party is organized in administrative districts or in parliamentary constituencies.

Membership. 300,000.

Publications. Harakah.

Parti Merdeka Malaysia

Address. Lot 2, Tingkat 2, Bangunan Mah Sing, 112-114, Jalan Pudu, 55100 Kuala Lumpur.

Founded. 1988.

History. Small opposition party with no state or federal representation.

Spirit of 46

Semangat 46

Address. 2, Jalan 10E, lembah Jaya Selatan, 68000 Ampang, Selangor Darul Ehsan.

Leadership. Tengku Razaleigh Hamzah (pres.); Rais Yatim (deputy pres.).

Orientation. Right of centre, UMNO splinter grouping; claims to be dedicated to the establishment of Islam "as a way of life . . . while guaranteeing and protecting the freedom of religion".

Founded. 1988.

History. This party was formed by dissidents from the United Malays National Organization (UMNO, see separate entry), which had supported Razaleigh Hamzah's audacious challenge to Mahathir Mohamad's presidency of UMNO in 1987. The party was named after the year in which the original UMNO was launched. Razaleigh was elected as party president at its first congress held in 1989. That year the party was instrumental in the formation of a loose opposition coalition (the Muslim Unity Movement, see separate entry) alongside three pro-Islamic parties, the Pan-Malaysian Islamic Party, the Front Malaysian Islamic Council and the Islamic Front of Malaysia.

In the 1990 general elections the coalition members agreed not to contest each other at federal or state level. At the federal level Spirit of 46 won eight seats, leaving it only the third largest opposition party behind the Democratic Action Party and the Sabah United Party. At the state level, the party was part of the MUM coalition which took control of Kelentan. The party also gained two seats in Trengganu, and one each in Johore, Pahang and Selangor, all National Front controlled states.

United Malays National Organization (*Baru*)

Pertubuhan Kebangsaan Melayu Bersatu (Baru)

Address. Tingkat 8, Menara Dato' Onn, 5048 Kuala Lumpur.

Leadership. Mahathir Mohamad (pres.); Abdul Ghafar Baba (deputy pres.); Abdullah Ahmad Badawi (vice-pres.); Anwar Ibrahim (vice-pres.); Sansui Junid (vice-pres.); Mohamad Rahmat (sec.-gen.).

Orientation. Supports the interests of the numerically dominant Malays, while accepting the rights of all Malaysians to participate in the political, social and economic life of the nation. The party has been the dominant political organization in the country since its formation and is currently the leading component of the ruling National Front coalition.

Founded. 1946.

History. The original United Malays National Organization (UMNO) was founded by Onn Jaafar "to fight for national independence and safeguard the interests of the indiginous people", later including "the interests of all the resident communities". Since the attainment of independence in 1957, UMNO has been the dominant party in Malaysia as the leading partner in successive electoral alliances, namely the Alliance Party, which won a majority of seats in 1959, 1964 and 1969, and the National Front, which similarly won the elections of 1974, 1978, 1982, 1986 and 1990.

Following the 1986 elections, in which the National Front won a landslide victory with UMNO returning 83 of its total 148 seats (out of 177 contested), the party entered a period of unprecedented internal conflict. At UMNO's 38th general assembly held in April 1987, Prime Minister Mahathir Mohamad only narrowly defeated a challenge for the party presidency by one of his key ministers, Razaleigh Hamzah. Razaleigh was only the second individual to challenge for the presidency in the party's history. The resultant intra-party struggle led to UMNO being rendered an "illegal society" in a High Court ruling in early 1988. Mahathir was forced to register UMNO afresh (as United Malays National Organization *Baru—Baru* being the Malay word for new), while Razaleigh and his supporters (who included former Prime Ministers Abdul Rahman and Hussein bin Onn) formed a rival party, the Spirit of 46 [see separate entry].

Despite the period of discord within UMNO, Mahathir led the party to victory in the 1990 elections, winning 71 of the National Front's 127 seats (out of a total of 180). Following his success at the elections Mahathir was unanimously re-elected UMNO president at the party's general assembly in late 1990, the first leadership elections since the Razaleigh challenge of 1987.

Structure. Power lies with the party's general assembly which meets annually. The main policy-making body is the party's supreme council, consisting of elected and nominated members. Below it there are a state liaison committee, divisional committees and branch committees.

Membership. Over 1,000,000.

Publications. Suara Merdeka.

Workers Party of Malaysia
Parti Pekerja-Pekerja Malaysia
Address. 18a, Jalan 13b, 68000 Ampang Jaya, Selangor Darul Ehsan.
Founded. 1978.
History. This small, left-wing party has no federal or state representation.

Regional parties
Perak

People's Progressive Party of Malaysia
Address. 43, First Floor, Jalan Station, Ipoh, Perak.

Leadership. Mak Hon Kam (pres.).

Orientation. This left-wing party draws its support mainly from the poorer Chinese community around Ipoh, the capital of the north-western state of Perak. The People's Progressive Party (PPP) is a member of the ruling National Front coalition.

Founded. 1953.

History. Founded as the Perak Progressive Party by two brothers, S. P. and D. R. Seenivasagam, the party changed to its present name in 1956. The PPP was a vocal opposition party before joining the ruling National Front coalition prior to the 1974 federal election, in which it retained only one of the four seats it had won in 1969. In subsequent elections in 1978, 1982, 1986 and 1990 the party failed to win any federal representation.

Sabah

Liberal Democratic Party
Parti Liberal Demokratik
Address. 5, First Floor, Tg Lipat, Jalan Fuad Stephens, 88300 Kota Kinabalu, Sabah.
Orientation. Chinese party; member of the National Front.
Founded. 1988.
History. The Liberal Democratic Party was the only Sabah-based Chinese party to contest the 1990 State Assembly election, but it was defeated in all nine Chinese-dominated seats by the ruling United Sabah Party. In mid-1991 the party was admitted into the ruling federal National Front.

Parti Bersatu Rakyat Bumiputera Sabah (Bersepadu)
Address. Lot 1, Tingkat 4, Bangunan Natikar, Jalan Padang, 88000 Kota Kinabalu, Sabah.
Leadership. Datuk Pengiran Othman Rauf.
Founded. 1983.
History. This small party has no representation in either state or federal legislature.

People's Justice Movement
Angkatan Keadilan Rakyat
Address. Lot 3, First Floor, Paramount Industrial Centre, Jalan Kolombong, off Mile 5, Jalan Tuaran, 88300 Kota Kinabalu, Sabah.
Leadership. Datuk Mark Koding (l.); Pendikar Amin Haji Mulia (l.); Kalakau Untol (l.).
Founded. 1989.
History. In August 1989 Joseph Pairin Kitingan, the

Chief Minister of Sabah and leader of the ruling United Sabah Party (*Parti Bersatu Sabah*—PBS, see separate entry), dismissed Deputy Chief Minister Mark Koding when he discovered that he was planning to form a splinter party. Within weeks of his dismissal, Koding, along with two former PBS colleagues Pendikar Amin Haji Mulia (the former Sabah Legislative Assembly speaker) and Kalakau Untol (a former deputy minister in the Kitingan government), announced the formation of AKAR. In a late 1989 by-election, Koding failed to regain his vacated State Assembly seat, which returned to PBS control. In mid-1991 AKAR, which had no federal or state level seats, was admitted into the ruling federal Barisan Nasional.

Sabah Chinese Consolidated Party

Parti China Bersatu Sabah (PCBS)

Address. 2, Blok E, Sinsuran Complex, 88000 Kota Kinabalu, Sabah.

Leadership. Johnny Soon (pres.); Chan Tet On (sec.-gen.).

Orientation. The party's aim is "to safeguard and uphold the interests of the Chinese and to work with other political organizations with similar aims".

Founded. 1964

History. Created by the merging of Sabah's Chinese parties, the PCBS was called the Sabah Chinese Association until 1979. It served in the ruling Sabah Alliance for a number of years, but withdrew into opposition in the mid-1970s. The party currently has no federal or state representation.

Structure. The party has a 39-member central executive committee (including 10 officials and four members appointed by the president, the remainder being elected by delegates). Each constituency may form a division, provided there are three branches with 100 members each.

Sabah Chinese Party

Parti China Sabah (PCS)

Address. Tingkat 1, Lot 1, Jalan Pinang, Tanjong Am, Kota Kinabalu, Sabah.

Leadership. Encik Francis Leong.

Orientation. Represents Chinese community in Sabah.

Founded. 1986.

History. This small party has no representation in either state or federal legislature.

Sabah National Momogun Party

Parti Momogun Kebangsaan Sabah (Momogun)

Address. 11a, Jalan Likas Jaya, 88000 Kota Kinabalu, Sabah.

Leadership. Edward Sinsua.

Founded. 1984.

History. This small party represents a revival of the United National Pasok Momogun Party, first formed in 1962 and dissolved in 1967. It has no representation in either the state or federal legislature.

Sabah People's Party

Parti Rakyat Sabah (PRS)

Address. Tingkat 3, Block 3, Wisma KK, 88000 Kota Kinabalu, Sabah.

Leadership. Datuk James Ongkili (pres.).

Founded. 1989.

History. The PRS was founded by James Ongkili, a former leader of the Sabah People's Union. The party had no success in the 1990 State Assembly and federal elections.

Sabah People's Union

Bersatu Rakyat Jelata Sabah (Berjaya)

Address. Blok M, Bangunan Sinsuran, 88000 Kota Kinabalu, Sabah.

Leadership. Haji Mohammad Noor bin Haji Mansoor (pres.).

Orientation. The party's aims are to preserve the integrity, independence and democratic status of the nation and uphold the principles of the *Rukunegara*, i.e. faith in God, loyalty to king and country, and maintenance of the Constitution, the rule of law, good behaviour and morality; to protect the rights and interests of Sabah within the Federation of Malaysia; to safeguard and promote the special position of the natives and the constitutional rights of every citizen in Sabah; to promote national unity, self-respect, self-reliance and a sense of commitment to creating a prosperous. stable and just society; and to protect the freedom of religion.

Founded. 1975.

History. Founded by Tun Mohamad Fuad Stephens to contest the 1976 state elections, the party defeated the United Sabah National Organization (USNO) administration of Tun Datu Mustapha, winning 34 of 54 seats in the Sabah State Assembly. The party subsequently joined the ruling federal National Front. In the 1981 Assembly elections it won all but four of the seats. The party suffered a massive defeat in the 1985 elections at the hands of USNO and a group of Berjaya dissidents who had formed the United Sabah Party (*Parti Bersatu Sabah*—PBS) prior to the elections. Berjaya retained only six Assembly seats and a post-election plan to remain in government in coalition with USNO collapsed and a PBS administration took control of the state. Berjaya withdrew from the National Front prior to the 1986 general elections. The party has subsequently had little success either at federal or state level.

Structure. Berjaya has 48 divisions in Sabah and a congress which meets annually. Party officials elected every three years include the president, the deputy president, seven vice-presidents, the secretary-general and 20 committee members.

Sabah United Party
Parti Bersatu Sabah

Address. Blok M, Lot 4, Tingkat 3, Donggongon New Township, 89500 Penampang, Sabah.

Leadership. Datuk Joseph Pairin Kitangan (pres.); Datuk Bernard Dompok (deputy pres.); Joseph Kurup (sec.-gen.).

Orientation. The Sabah United Party draws its support in the main from the mainly Christian Kadazan and Chinese communities.

Founded. 1985.

History. The party was founded by Pairin and other Berjaya dissidents in the run-up to the 1985 state elections in which the new party won a resounding victory. Pairin formed a new state government and the Sabah United Party was admitted to the ruling federal National Front prior to fresh elections held in mid-1986, when the party was again victorious. The party suffered a division in 1989 when Pairin's deputy, Mark Koding, defected to form the People's Justice Movement [see separate entry]. However, the defection had little impact and the Sabah United Party retained control of the Sabah State Assembly in elections held in mid-1990, winning 36 seats (almost all of them in Kadazan and Chinese constituencies).

The only other party to win any seats was the predominantly Muslim United Sabah National Organization (USNO), another National Front member and the chief opponent to the Sabah United Party in the Sabah Assembly. After the election, charges were levelled that federal government had intervened secretly on behalf of USNO in an attempt to undermine Pairin. Shortly before the elections the federal government had released details of an alleged plot to take Sabah out of the Federation. Pairin denied that any such plot existed, but four people, including one of his close associates, were placed in detention under the Internal Security Act. Relations between the state government and the federal government worsened in October when Pairin pulled the party out of the National Front only five days before the general election. In what was widely regarded as a politically motivated action, Pairin was arrested in early 1991 and charged with corruption. He was released on bail but other members of his staff, including his brother Jeffrey Kitangan, were detained under the National Security Act under suspicion of harbouring anti-federalist designs. A few months later Jeffrey Kitangan was again arrested on charges of involvement in a plot to pull Sabah out of Malaysia.

That month the United Malays National Organization (UMNO), the largest party in the National Front, won a seat in the Sabah State Assembly for the first time, defeating the Sabah United Party in a by-election. In May 1991, UMNO defeated the party in a State Assembly by-election. It was the first time the party had competed outside of peninsula Malaysia.

United Pasok Nunukragang National Organization
Pertubuhan Kebangsaan Pasok Nunukragang Bersatu

Address. 5, Tingkat 4, Oh How Teck Place, Jalan Sentosa, Kampong Air, 88000 Kota Kinabalu, Sabah.

Founded. 1978.

History. This small party has no representation in either state or federal legislature.

United Sabah National Organization
Pertubuhan Kebangsaan Sabah Bersatu

Address. 3, Lorong Dewan, PO Box 927, 88716 Kota Kinabalu, Sabah.

Leadership. Tan Sri Sakaran Bin Dandai (acting pres.).

Orientation. Supported largely by the state's Muslim community.

Founded. 1961.

History. The United Sabah National Organization (USNO) was founded by Mustapha Harun and played a leading role in bringing Sabah into the Federation of Malaysia in 1963. The party ruled the state from 1963 until 1975, when it was ousted by Berjaya, a new party created by USNO dissidents. USNO was again comprehensively defeated by Berjaya in the 1981 State Assembly elections. The party was expelled from the ruling federal National Front in 1984 (it had been a founder member, and before that a member of the Alliance) for its criticism of the government during the previous year's constitutional crisis; it was re-admitted to the Front in 1986.

The previous year the party had performed well in State Assembly elections, winning 16 seats, but had failed in an attempt to form a new coalition government with Berjaya. Instead, a Berjaya offshoot, the United Sabah Party (*Parti Bersatu Sabah*—PBS), formed a government and Berjaya joined USNO on the opposition benches.

In 1986 USNO voted to merge with the United Malays National Organization (UMNO), the largest National Front component. However, legal problems over the eventual status of USNO deputies in the Sabah State Assembly stopped the merger. In elections to the State Assembly held in 1990 USNO won 12 seats and the PBS remained in government. In federal elections held a few months later, the party added six seats to the Barisan Nasional's 127 total. In 1991 UMNO announced that it planned to contest state and federal elections in Sabah, the first time the party had offered itself to voters outside of peninsula Malaysia. According to many commentators, the announcement virtually ended USNO's existence as an independent political party. In May 1991 Mustapha Harun, USNO's founder, won a state assembly by-election for UMNO.

Dissident groups in conflict with the government: the **Communist Party of Malaysia** signed a peace treaty with the Malaysian government in 1989.

Sarawak

Parti Buruh Bersatu Sarawak

Address. 132, Tingkat 1, Sarawak House, Sibu, Sarawak.

Leadership. Tan Lung Chiew.

Founded. 1983.

History. This small Sibu-based party is not represented at state or federal level.

Persatuan Rakyat Malaysia Sarawak (Permas)

Address. Tingkat 2, Bangunan Salmas, Lot 271, Jalan Satok, 93400 Kuching, Sarawak.

Leadership. Amar Abang Haj Yusuf Puteh (acting).

Founded. 1987.

History. Founded by Tun Abdul Rahman Yakub, a former Chief Minister of Sarawak and leader of a dissident faction of the ruling PBB. The party contested the 1987 State Assembly elections, winning five seats, but failing to defeat the incumbent ruling coalition headed by the PBB leader, and Abdul Rahman's nephew, Abdul Taib. The party failed to win any seats in the 1991 Assembly elections.

Sarawak Dayak Party

Parti Bansa Dayak Sarawak

Address. 3, Lot 1526, Batu 3.5, Jalan Penrissen, 93250 Kuching, Sarawak.

Leadership. Leo Moggie Anak Irok (pres.); Daniel Tajem (vice-pres.).

Orientation. Dayak-based party; member of the ruling federal National Front.

Founded. 1983.

History. The party was founded by a breakaway group from the Dayak-based Sarawak National Party (SNAP), following a crisis within the party in mid-1983.

The Sarawak Dayak Party quickly joined the ruling federal National Front and formed a coalition state government with the SNAP, Sarawak United People's Party and United Traditional Bumiputra Party after performing well in state elections held in late 1983.

The Sarawak Dayak Party was dismissed from the ruling state coalition in 1987 following a rebellion in the Assembly. An election was called and, although the new three-member coalition (Front of Three or *Barisan Tiga*) was returned to power, the Sarawak Dayak Party emerged as the largest single party with 15 seats. The result prompted commentators to talk of the emergence of Dayak nationalism as a new dimension in the politics of Sarawak. Ethnic Dayaks (the largest Dayak group being the Iban) constituted some 45 per cent of Sarawak's population, but economic and political power (largely determined by the ability to control timber concessions) nonetheless rested with the Malay-Melanau minority.

In the 1990 federal elections the party won four seats for the National Front coalition. Party president Leo Moggie was appointed as Minister of Works in the new Cabinet created after the elections. In September 1991 elections were held to the State Assembly. The Front of Three were again returned to power, winning 49 of the 56 seats. The result represented a resounding defeat for the party, which had campaigned against the Front for the rights of the Dayak, Iban, Bidayuh and Orang Ulu ethnic minorities.

Sarawak National Party

Address. Lot 304-305, Tingkat 1, Bangunan Mei Jun, Jalan Getah, 93400 Kuching, Sarawak.

Leadership. James Wong Kim Min (pres.); Peter Gani Ak Kiai (gen. sec.).

Orientation. Dayak-based party, with heavy support among the Iban; member of the ruling federal National

Front and ruling state Front of Three coalitions.

Founded. 1961.

History. The Sarawak National Party (SNAP) was formed by Stephen Kalong Ningkan and others and was a member of the coalition that ruled Sarawak when the state joined the Federation of Malaysia. Ningkan served as Chief Minister from 1963-66, but with his fall the party went into opposition. In 1976 SNAP rejoined the ruling state and federal level coalitions, after winning a credible number of seats in elections held in 1974.

In the 1990 federal elections the party won three seats for the National Front. In state assembly elections held in September 1991 the ruling Front of Three was returned to power, with SNAP winning six seats.

Membership. 137,000.

Sarawak State People's Party

Parti Negara Rakyat Sarawak

Address. 30-0, Tingkat 1, Jalan Tabuan, PO Box 1073, 93722 Kuching, Sarawak.

Leadership. Mohamad Adam Shah Anuar.

Founded. 1974.

History. This small party is not represented at state or federal level.

Sarawak United Democrats

Sarawak Demokratik Bersatu

Address. 180-30G, Jalan Tabuan, Tingkat 1, 93100 Kuching, Sarawak.

Founded. 1978.

History. This small party is not represented at state or federal level.

Sarawak United People's Party (SUPP)

Parti Rakyat Bersatu Sarawak

Address. 7, Central Road West, 93000 Kuching, Sarawak.

Leadership. Wong Soon Kai (pres.); Datuk George Chan Hong Nam (sec.-gen.).

Orientation. Centre-left, Chinese-based party; a member of the federal ruling National Front and the state-level ruling Front of Three.

Founded. 1959.

History. Founded by Ong Kee Hui and Stephen Yong, the SUPP has played a leading role in state's politics. The party draws its support mainly from Sarawak's Chinese community, who constitute almost 30 per cent of the state's population and are often regarded as the determining factor in any election. SUPP came to an "understanding" with the ruling federal Alliance Party in 1970 and formally joined the National Front in 1976. In the 1990 federal election the party gained five seats for the National Front.

In the September 1991 state elections it managed to retain the traditional Chinese strongholds for the ruling Front of Three coalition. SUPP won 16 of the Group's total 49 seats and the coalition was returned to power.

United Traditional Bumiputra Party

Parti Pesaka Bumiputera Bersatu

Address. 153, Jalan Satok, PO Box 1053, 93722 Kuching, Sarawak.

Leadership. Abdul Taib Mahmoud (pres.); Alfred Jabu Ak Numpang (deputy pres.).

Orientation. Largely Malay-Melanau; member of ruling federal National front and ruling state Front of Three coalitions.

Founded. 1973.

History. Formed as the result of the merger of elements of the *Parti Pesaka* (a Dayak and Malay party), *Parti Bumiputra* (a mixed ethnic party), and the Sarwak Chinese Association. The United Traditional Bumiputra Party has played the leading role in Sarawak politics with its leaders, Abdul Rahman Yakub and Abdul Taib Mahmoud serving as Chief Minister between 1970-81 and since 1981, respectively.

In the 1990 federal elections the party won nine seats for the ruling National Front. State Assembly elections were held in September 1991 and the party was returned to power as the dominant member of the self-styled Front of Three which altogether won 49 of the 56 seats (the United Traditional Bumiputra Party winning 27 seats). Following the election Abdul Taib Mahmoud was re-appointed for another five year term as Chief Minister.

Maldives

Capital: Malé

Population: 214,139 (1990)

The Maldives became a British protectorate in 1887, and the Sultan was forced to accept a constitution in 1932. In 1953 the sultanate became a presidential republic. It gained independence in 1965, and after a referendum in 1968 became a republic. It has been a full member of the Commonwealth since June 1985.

There are no political parties or organisations, and no organised dissidence, although in recent years there has been a more questioning tendency among the younger, less traditional members of the *Majlis* (People's Council). Ex-President Ibrahim Nasir, who left the country after his resignation in 1978, was charged with corruption, and was implicated in a coup attempt in 1980, though pardoned in 1990 in recognition of his role in gaining national independence. President Maumoun Abdul Gayoom's family has also come under increasing criticism for corruption and nepotism over recent years. The main source of burgeoning dissent is from foreign-educated young Maldivians (around 60 per cent of the population is under 24 years).

In November 1988 the Maldives received worldwide attention when Tamil mercenaries from Sri Lanka sailed into the harbour of Malé and attempted to take the President hostage. With the aid of India and Sri Lanka, and the support of 300 Indian paratroopers, the coup was crushed.

The brother-in-law of Gayoom, Illyas Ibrahim, Minister of Trade and Industry, Deputy Defence Minister and Head of the National Security Service, fled the country in May 1990 during the investigation of corruption charges levelled at him. He returned in August willing to answer questions about the State Trading Organisation which was under his control.

Constitutional structure

The Constitution of 1968, amended in 1970 and 1975, proclaims the Maldives to be an Islamic republic with an executive President elected every five years by popular vote. Islam is the state religion and Muslim law the dominant legal system. Maldivian citizenship is confined to Muslims, although non-Muslims are permitted permanent residence and the right to do business there. The formation of political parties and associations is granted by the Constitution, although none exist to date.

Electoral system

The President is head of state, elected by universal adult suffrage for a five-year term. He appoints and presides over the Cabinet. The unicameral *Majlis* (People's Council) consists of 48 members, 40 of whom are popularly elected for five years and the other eight are appointed by the President. Of the elected members, eight are from the capital and each of 19 electoral districts (groups of atolls) elect two

Recent elections

Nasir, Prime Minister and subsequently President after the declaration of the republic, unexpectedly announced his resignation in 1978, when Gayoom, the sole candidate, was elected President. In 1983 he was re-elected unopposed by a reported 96 per cent vote. Again on Sept. 23, 1988, he was re-elected by referendum with an overwhelming majority, having been nominated by the *Majlis* in early August as the sole presidential candidate. Elections to the *Majlis* were held on Nov. 24, 1989.

each. The members of Cabinet, appointed by the President, are individually responsible to the *Majlis*.

Evolution of the suffrage

There is universal adult suffrage from the age of 21. Women are allowed to vote, but not to stand for office.

PARTY BY PARTY DATA

There are no political parties.

Marshall Islands

Capital: Dalap-Uliga-Darrit Municipality on Majuro Atoll.   **Population: 43,355 (1989).**

As part of the UN Trust Territory of the Pacific, established in 1947, the Marshall Islands were administered by the US government. Between 1946 and 1962 the USA conducted 66 atomic and hydrogen bomb tests on Bikini and Enewetak Atolls, and built a large missile range at Kwajalein. In 1982 the government of the Marshall Islands signed a compact of free association, implemented in 1986, under which the US granted internal sovereignty and aid in return for continuing US control of defence and foreign policy, and continued use of its military sites. In December 1990 the UN Security Council approved the termination of the trusteeship in relation to the Marshall Islands and the country joined the UN in September 1991.

Constitutional structure

Under the 1979 Constitution the Marshall Islands has a 12-member Council of Chiefs (*Iroij*), composed of traditional leaders with consultative authority on matters relating to land and custom. Legislative power resides in a 33-member legislature (*Nitijela*), which is elected for four years and which chooses a President from among its members. The President is both head of state and head of government and appoints a Cabinet. Each of the country's 24 inhabited atolls has a local government.

Electoral system

Members of the *Nitijela* are elected by popular vote from 25 districts.

Evolution of the suffrage

Under the 1979 Constitution, universal adult suffrage was adopted as the basis for the country's elections.

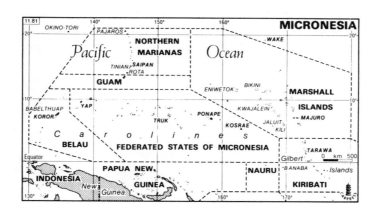

Recent elections

The country's fourth national elections were held in November 1991, with supporters of incumbent President Amata Kabua emerging victorious. All 10 members of the Cabinet were returned to office, although six incumbents lost their seats and, in all, there were eight new members elected. In January 1992 the *Nitijela* met and re-elected Kabua for a further term.

PARTY BY PARTY DATA

Ralik Ratak Democratic Party
Address. c/o *Nitijela*, Majuro, Marshall Islands.
Leadership. Tony DeBrum.
Orientation. Opposition.
Founded. 1991.
History. The Ralik Ratak Democratic Party was founded in June 1991 by Tony DeBrum, a former protégé of Kabua and Foreign Minister, with the aim of co-ordinating opposition to the Kabua government.

Major guerrilla groups

There are no guerrilla groups operating in the Marshall Islands.

Mongolia

Capital: Ulan Bator   **Population: 2,200,000 (1990 UNFPA est.)**

From the 17th century, Mongolia was ruled by the Chinese Manchu Emperors as the province of Outer Mongolia. In 1911, on the fall of the Manchu dynasty, Outer Mongolia became a feudal Buddhist monarchy, achieving independence from China with the help of Tsarist Russia. Although legally under Chinese suzerainty from 1915, Mongolia was effectively a Russian protectorate and, after the Russian Revolution of 1917, Mongolian nationalists received Soviet help in their resistance to encroaching Chinese control. Mongolia's independence was proclaimed on July 11, 1921. The Mongolian People's Republic was proclaimed as the world's second socialist state in 1924 after the Mongolian People's Revolutionary Party established control over the country.

Constitutional structure

The State of Mongolia was, until January 1992, called the Mongolian People's Republic (MPR). This state, described as "a sovereign democratic state of working people", was established in 1924. With effect from Feb. 12, 1992, Mongolia altered its Constitution. The new Constitution renounced socialism and established a parliamentary republic with a directly elected President. Henceforth, according to the Constitution, Mongolia would seek neutrality in foreign policy and would encourage a mixed economy. Constitutional changes in May 1990 had legally established a multiparty system, thus breaking the one-party system in force since the foundation of the MPR.

Electoral system

The new 76-seat People's Great *Hural* (PGH) is directly elected and serves for a six-year term. Elections to it in June 1992 replaced the bi-cameral system of a 430-seat PGH, and the standing parliament—the 53-seat Little *Hural* (including the Chair and two vice-chairs). The Little *Hural* had been abolished in 1950 and reinstated in July 1990. The President is directly elected and serves for four years. Popular presidential elections are scheduled to be held in 1993. Punsalmaagiyn Ochirbat was elected as Mongolia's first President by the PGH on Sept. 4, 1990.

Evolution of the suffrage

All citizens over 25 are eligible to vote.

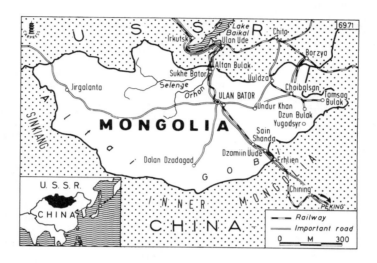

Recent elections

Legislative elections, 1986

The electorate, whose turnout was officially given as 99.99 per cent, voted for a list of candidates nominated by the ruling MPRP. Of those elected to the 370 seats in the PGH 346 were members or candidate members of the MPRH.

Legislative elections, July 29, 1990

The July 1990 elections were Mongolia's first multiparty elections. The turnout was officially estimated as 91.9 per cent.

Party	Seats in PGH	Seats in Little Hural
MPRP	357	31
MDP	16	13
MRYL*	9	—
MNPP	6	3
MSDP	4	3
Independent	39	—

*Mongolian Revolutionary Youth League—Pro-MPRP body.

Legislative elections, June 28, 1992

The elections to the new 76-seat unicameral People's Great *Hural* resulted in victory for the MPRP and a humiliating defeat for the opposition coalition. The turnout was reported as 95.6 per cent.

Party	Seats	Percentage of vote
MPRP	70	56.9
Democratic Coalition	4	17.5
MSDP	1	10.1
Others	1	15.5

PARTY BY PARTY DATA

Free Labour Party

Address. Negdsen Undestnii gudamj 11, Ulan Bator.

Leadership. Choijil Dul (ch.).

Orientation. Liberal.

Founded. March 28, 1990.

History. The party's first leader was H. Maam. The Free Labour Party is the political wing of the Free Labour Movement.

Structure. Eight-member General Political Council, led by the party chair.

Membership. 3,500.

Publications. Chuluut Hudulmur newspaper, published every 10 days.

Mongolian Democratic Party

Address. Erhuugiin gudamj 5, Ulan Bator.

Leadership. Erdene Baat-Uul (ch.); Tsagaandari Enhtuvshin (head of secretariat).

Orientation. Liberal conservative.

Founded. Feb. 17, 1990.

History. The Mongolian Democratic Party (MDP) was the first opposition party in Mongolia, established on the basis of the Mongolian Democratic Union, then the largest political organization outside the ruling Mongolian People's Revolutionary Party (MPRP). The MDP's first congress was held on April 8-9, 1990 in Ulan Bator and was attended by about 865 delegates representing Mongolia's 17 provinces and three municipalities. They approved a programme including the creation of a market economy, the revival of Mongolia's culture (suppressed under Soviet influence), and neutrality in foreign policy. The MDP was a member of the opposition Democratic Coalition which fought the 1992 general elections.

Structure. The ruling body is a National Committee.

Membership. 28,000.

Publications. Shine ue (New Generation) newspaper, published every 10 days; *Ardchilal* (Democracy) daily, circulation 70,000.

Mongolian Democratic Union

Leadership. Sanjaasurengiyn Dzorig (ch.).

Orientation. Democratic.

Founded. December 1989.

History. On its formation, the Mongolian Democratic Union (MDU) was the largest political body outside the Mongolian People's Revolutionary Party and was responsible for organizing many of the opposition demonstrations in 1989-90 which forced democratic constitutional changes. It was accorded official recognition on Dec. 22, 1989, by the People's Great *Hural.* It adopted a party constitution at a conference on June 11-13, 1991, attended by 508 delegates. The conference elected Dzorig as party chair. A university lecturer, he had previously been the MDU's chief co-ordinator. The conference called for the establishment of democracy in Mongolia by all non-violent means. However, 89 delegates walked out of the meeting in disagreement over the new constitution.

Membership. 36,000.

Mongolian National Progress Party

Address. Enhtaivny gudamj, PO Box 099, Ulan Bator.

Leadership. Davaadorj Ganbold (ch.).

Orientation. National liberal.

Founded. March 11, 1990.

History. The Mongolian National Progress Party's (MNPP) inaugural congress was held in May 1990. MNPP Chairman Davaadorj Ganbold was appointed Deputy Prime Minister of the new government in November 1990. The MNPP was a member of the opposition Democratic Coalition in the 1992 elections.

Membership. 69,000 (including members and supporters).

Publications. Undesniy devshil (National Progress) newspaper, published every 10 days.

Mongolian People's Revolutionary Party

Mongol Ardyn Khuv'salt Nam

Address Central Committee of the Mongolian People's Revolutionary Party, Ulan Bator.

Leadership. Budragchaagiyn Dash-Yondon (ch.).

Orientation. Populist-democratic. The Mongolian People's Revolutionary Party (MPRP) abandoned its role as the ruling party in March 1990 and in February 1992 altered the core of its ideology from socialism to the Confucian Golden Mean.

Founded. March 21, 1921.

History. The MPRP took its name in 1924 having grown out of the Mongolia People's Party—a broad coalition of forces formed by Damdiny Sukhbaatar in 1921, which achieved Mongolian independence that same year. The restoration of Chinese sovereignty over Outer Mongolia in 1919 had jeopardized the establishment of an independent Mongolia and independence was finally achieved with the assistance of the Soviet Union. The corollary to this, however, was that between 1924 and 1934, MPRP members in favour of greater independence from the Soviet Union were purged while the MPRP consolidated power over Mongolia and enforced collectivised agriculture. The MPRP became a pro-Soviet communist party, to the extent that Mongolia was sometimes called the "16th republic" of the Soviet Union. Mongolia, for example, supported the Soviet side throughout the Sino-Soviet dispute of the 1960s. Its policy also frequently followed that of the Soviet Communist Party. For example, at the 19th MPRP Congress in May 1986, a campaign was launched against corruption, illegal currency dealing and alcoholism, thus mirroring the policy implemented in the Soviet Union under Yuri Andropov and Mikhail Gorbachev.

Marshal Horloogiyn Choibalsan, who had survived the purges of the 1920s, served as party leader from 1936 until his death in 1952. Choibalsan, who had also been Prime Minister since 1939, was succeeded in both posts by Yumjaagyin Tsedenbal who became MPRP leader in 1958. In 1962-63, Tsedenbal expelled his opponents from the MPRP, and in 1974 he became head of state. At the 18th MPRP Congress in May 1981, the title of party leader was changed from First Secretary of the Central Committee to General Secretary. Tsedenbal was succeeded in 1984 as both General Secretary and as head of state by Jambyn Batmonh (Prime Minister since 1974).

Influenced by the collapse of Eastern Europe communist regimes and the extraordinary reforms in the Soviet Union, as well as by domestic opposition movements, the MPRP held its first extraordinary Congress on April 10-13, 1990, and called on the party to break with the past. Prior to this, in November 1988, the MPRP Politburo had admitted setbacks in Mongolia's economic reforms because of the need for concurrent social reforms, and had proposed changes to the election procedure to party and state office. Shortly before the extraordinary Congress, opposition-led disturbances in Ulan Bator between December 1989 and March 1990 had provoked the resignation of General Secretary Batmonh, as well as the seven-member Politburo and most of the Central Committee (CC) at a CC Plenum on March 12. Gombojavyn Ochirbat was made General Secretary, but negotiations with the opposition collapsed by mid-March and at the People's Great *Hural* (PGH) on March 21, Batmonh resigned as head of state to be replaced by the Minister of Foreign Economic Relations and Supply, Punsalmaagiyn Ochirbat. In addition, the PGH voted with 324 in favour and 10 abstentions to remove Article 82 from the Constitution. Similar to Article 6 in the Soviet

Constitution, which was also removed in March 1990, Article 82 had guaranteed the MPRP's leading role in the government of Mongolia. A new electoral law was passed, but came under criticism from opposition parties for effectively barring non-socialist parties from participation in elections.

After the upheavals of the March session of the PGH, the extraordinary MPRP Congress in April approved policies intended to separate the powers of state and party and to initiate profound changes in the government of Mongolia. These included, for example, the provision that the chair of the presidium of the PGH (the head of state) should not be a member of MPRP ruling bodies. Further proposals endorsed at the congress included: (i) a multiparty system to guarantee respect for human rights; (ii) a mixed economy to replace the centrally-planned system, including private ownership, reformed taxes, social protection, increased wages and modernized agriculture; and (iii) an independent, non-aligned foreign policy. Changes in the MPRP itself included draft rules intended to promote internal party democracy. However, despite calls for changes to its membership, most of the 91-member CC was re-elected, and although the Politburo was replaced by a party presidium, the five men elected to the Politburo after the disturbances in March continued in office by forming the membership of the new presidium. The changes to the Constitution, approved by the MPRP at its congress, were later enshrined in law by the PGH on May 10-11. In addition to a multiparty system, these included the formation of a standing parliament, (the Little *Hural*) and the post of Mongolian President, elected by the PGH.

In the July 1990 multiparty elections to the new PGH and the Little *Hural*, the MPRP won over 60 per cent of the vote, but MPRP leader Ochirbat had only narrowly defeated National Progress Party leader, Davaadorj Ganbold. On July 31, the MPRP offered to discuss arrangements for a coalition government with opposition parties.

During the immediate post-election period, the MPRP's efforts further to distance itself from its past were seen at a plenum on June 29, 1990, when the policies of former leader Tsedenbal were criticised as being responsible for Mongolia's current economic plight, and seven former politburo members were expelled from the MPRP for violation of party discipline. Tsedenbal, who had lived in virtual exile in the Soviet Union since his retirement, had visited Mongolia in August 1988. Opposition groups had been demanding his trial, and at the March 1990 MPRP plenum he had been expelled in disgrace from the party and stripped of his titles. He was accused by some of having planned to take Mongolia into the Soviet Union before Stalin's death (1953). Other investigations into the MPRP's history included the discovery in October 1991 of the mass grave of 5,000 monks, apparently shot on Stalin's orders under the Choibalsan regime. Furthermore, in August 1991, 12 former high MPRP officials, including Jambyn Batmonh, were charged with using state funds for individual purposes between 1977 and 1990.

The 20th MPRP congress, on Feb. 25-28, 1991, was attended by 409 delegates and by representatives of other Mongolian political parties as well as by the traditional delegations from the Soviet and Chinese Communist Parties. An amended party platform adopted at the congress confirmed the decisions of the April 1990 extraordinary congress. A new leadership was elected, including Budragchaagiyn Dash-Yondon as chair of the CC to replace Gombojavyn Ochirbat, who, as outgoing leader, delivered the key report to the congress. The new 99-member CC elected an enlarged seven-member (later eight-member) presidium, which included only one member of the previous presidium.

Ideological changes to the MPRP's programme followed the organizational and constitutional changes. At its 21st congress held in Ulan Bator on Feb. 26-29, 1992, the MPRP adopted a new programme, which replaced socialism and communism by the Confucian doctrine of the Golden Mean. For the first time, delegations from foreign fraternal parties were absent from a MPRP congress. The 600 delegates present represented about 80,000 party members—a drop in membership of approximately 20,000 since the 20th congress in 1991. However, the MPRP's resounding victory at the June 1992 general election showed that it had retained its position as Mongolia's ruling party. Nevertheless, Ochirbat declared after the elections that he wished to offer Cabinet posts to opposition party members.

Structure. The 147-member Central Committee (CC) is elected at the Party Congress held at least every five years. Other leadership structures include a nine-member Central Presidium, a three-member secretariat and a 33-member Control Commission.

Membership. 93,000.

Publications. Unen (Truth) party newspaper, three times weekly, circulation 75,000; *Bodlyn Solbiltsol* weekly newspaper; *Bodrol Byasalgal* and *Yariltsaya* (Dialogue) twice quarterly journals; *Manay Inder* (Our Platform) monthly journal.

Mongolian Social Democratic Party

Address PO Box 578, Ulan Bator 11.

Leadership. Bat-Erdene Batbayar (ch.).

Orientation. Social-democratic.

Founded. March 2, 1990.

History. The Mongolian Social Democratic Party's (MSDP) first congress was held on March 31, 1990. The party pledged itself to promote a mixed economy and neutrality in foreign affairs. The MSDP's influence was demonstrated when a leading member, Radnaasumbereliyn Gonchigdorj, was elected Vice-President and ex officio Chair of the Little *Hural* on Sept. 7, 1990. However, in the 1992 elections, the MSDP won about 10 per cent of the vote and a single seat in the People's Great *Hural*.

Membership. 10,000.

Publications. Ug (The Word) weekly newspaper.

International affiliations. Socialist International.

Minor parties

Mongolian Greens Party; PO Box 1089, Ulan Bator. Munkhtuvshin Ganbat's party held its inaugural congress in May 1990, having been founded on March 9. It is the political wing of the Alliance of Greens and aims for the "harmony of nature and society". With a membership estimated at 3,000, the party publishes a newspaper, *Yertunts*, every 10 days.

Mongolian Party of Herdsmen and Farmers was founded and is chaired by a herdsman, Gansuh, from Hubsugul province. The first congress was held on Dec. 7, 1991, when the party's membership numbered 712.

Religious Democratic Party; Gandantechilen Church, Ulan Bator. Tseren Bayarsuren's party, with a membership estimated at 10,000, was founded in 1990 and registered on June 28, 1991. It is centred on Buddist philosophy and publishes a twice monthly newspaper, *Arga Bilig* (Yin and Yang).

Revival Party of Mongolia was founded by Zardykhaan's wing of the Mongolian People's Revolutionary Party (MPRP) on Nov. 30, 1991, and aims to embody the "continuation of traditions and renewal of the MPRP". Its political influence appears to be weak.

Major guerrilla groups

There are no significant guerrilla groups in Mongolia.

Myanma

Capital: Yangon (Rangoon)   **Population: 41,700,000 (1990 UNFPA est.)**

Myanma (in 1989 the country's name was officially changed from Burma to the Union of Myanma—*Myanma Naing-naga*) became an independent state in 1948. The first Constitution of the new state created a parliamentary system of government, but a military coup in 1962 brought the country's democratic experiment to an end. The ruling military junta (the Revolutionary Council), under the leadership of Gen. Ne Win, established the Burma Socialist Programme Party (BSPP) as the country's sole, legal, political organization.

Following a further military coup in 1988, all state organs and institutions were abolished by the new ruling junta, the State Law and Order Restoration Council (SLORC), and the country was placed under martial law. The SLORC announced that it had taken control of the country "in order to save the general, deteriorating situation in the whole country". However, the ruling junta immediately announced that political organizations other than the BSPP would be permitted to function. Accordingly, multiparty elections were held in 1990, but as of mid-1992 the country remained under total military control.

Constitutional structure

The current Constitution came into force in January 1974 following a national referendum held in December 1973. The Constitution provides for a socialist republican form of government under the one-party rule of the (BSPP). The 451-member People's Assembly (*Pyithu Hluttaw*) was the highest organ of state power. The Assembly convened at least twice a year and when not in session its powers were exercised by a Council of State. The chair of the Council of State, elected by the members of the Council subject to the Assembly's approval, served as President and Head of State. Executive power was vested in the Council of Ministers headed by a Prime Minister.

On Sept. 18, 1985 the SLORC dissolved the following state organs, although the Constitution formally remained in place: the People's Assembly; the Council of State; the Council of Ministers; the Council of People's Justices; the Council of People's Attorneys; the Council of People's Inspectors; Executive Councils of each state, division, township, ward, and village-tract People's Council. A Constituent Assembly was elected in May 1990 to draft and promulgate a new constitution. However, as of mid-1992 the SLORC had effectively prevented the Assembly from convening.

Electoral system

Under the 1974 Constitution the People's Assembly is elected directly by secret ballot for a four-year term. In 1981 the Constitution was amended to extend the term of the Assembly indefinitely. In addition, People's Councils at various local levels are also elected directly by citizens having the right to vote in the area concerned. According to the Constitution the BSPP submits lists of candidates for all elections.

Evolution of the suffrage

Under the 1974 Constitution all citizens over 18 years of age are entitled to vote. Members of religious orders and others disqualified by law are prohibited from voting or standing for election.

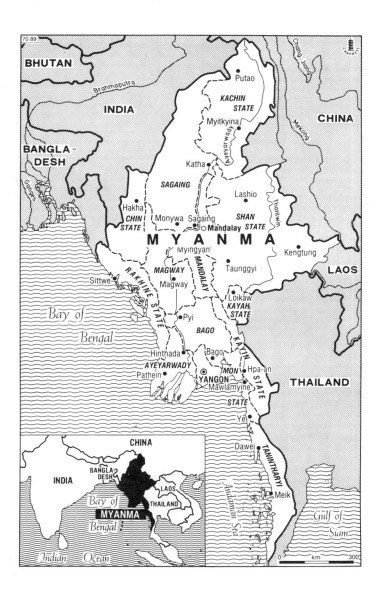

Recent elections

A general election was held on May 27, 1990, and was contested by 93 political parties. It was announced after the election by the SLORC that the newly elected body was to serve as a Constituent Assembly, responsible solely for the drafting of a new constitution. The Assembly would have no legislative power.

Constituent Assembly elections, May 27, 1990

Party	Seats*
National League for Democracy	392
Shan Nationalities League for Democracy	23
Rakhine Democracy League	11
National Unity Party	10
Mon National Democratic Front	5
National Democratic Party for Human Rights	4
Chin National League for Democracy	3
Kachin State National Congress for Democracy	3
Party for National Democracy	3
Union Pa-Oh National Organizations	3
Others	19

*Results were only announced for 476 constituencies, although 485 were actually contested.

PARTY BY PARTY DATA

Immediatly prior to the 1962 military coup which brought Gen. Ne Win to power, the principal political parties in Burma were the ruling Union Party, led by Prime Minister U Nu; the opposition Anti-Fascist People's Freedom League; and the pro-communist National Unity Party and its affiliate, the Burmese Workers' Party. Following Ne Win's coup, the ruling junta, the Revolutionary Council, formed its own political party, the Burma Socialist Programme Party (BSPP). All parties other than the BSPP were banned in 1964. Following the 1988 military coup the State Law and Order Restoration Council (SLORC) rescinded the ban on political parties. By early 1989 over 230 parties had registered. The SLORC subsequently announced that all parties wishing to contest the general election in May 1990 would be required to present at least three candidates each. By the closing date in December, 117 parties had officially registered with the electoral commission. A total of 93 parties contested the general election.

In the period following the election, a large number of political parties had their registration annulled by the electoral commission. These parties included: United League of Democratic Parties; Party for National Democracy: League for Democracy and Peace; Democratic Party for New Society; Democracy Party; Graduates and Old Students Democratic Association; United Nationalities League for Democracy; Patriotic Old Comrades League; Democratic Front for National Reconstruction, Union of Burma; People's Power Party; Patriotic Youth Organization; Union Nationals Democracy Party; National Democratic Party for Human Rights; Anti-Fascist People's Freedom League; Kamans National League for Democracy; Democratic Organization for Kayan National Unity; Zomi National Congress; Mara People's Party; Mon National Democratic Front; Chin National League for Democracy; Naga Hills Regional Progressive Party; Kayah State National Congress for Democracy; Ta-ang Palaung National League for Democracy; Union Danu League for Democracy; and the Lishu National Solidarity Party.

In a broadcast in mid-March 1992 the SLORC announced that "at present there remain only 19 legal political parties under the Political Parties Registration Law". The broadcast went on to say that the Elections Commission had scrutinized the organizational standing, organizational progress, party membership and party strength of registered political parties. The report went on: "In scrutinizing political parties, it has been found that some have been unable to either send or present specific reports listing party branches, organizational situations. It has been found that some political parties were unable to clearly present their parties' political lines, ideologies and policies, while officials of some political parties were found to have shortcomings in observing existing laws, bylaws, rules and regulations. Some political parties have been found to have negelected their organizational activities because they thought their parties' standing was based on representatives being elected. The commission is of the opinion that, in implementing a compact and stable democratic system, such political parties should not be allowed to continue to exist".

In another broadcast in May the SLORC announced that only seven political parties (all listed below) had been invited to attend a meeting in late June to discuss a planned "national convention" to draft a fresh constitution.

Khami National Solidarity Organization
Orientation. Represents the interests of the Khami hill tribe in Arakan province.
Founded. In the aftermath of the 1988 military coup.
History. The Khami National Solidarity Organization (KNSO) was one of the few remaining legal political parties as of mid-1992. As such, one party representative took part in a preliminary meeting with the SLORC authorities in June 1992 aimed at arranging a "national convention" to draft a new constitution.

La-Hu National Development Party
Orientation. Represents the interests of the La-Hu ethnic minority based in the south-east of Shan state.
Founded. In the aftermath of the 1988 military coup.
History. The La-Hu National Development Party (LNDP) was one of the few remaining legal political parties as of mid-1992. As such one party representative took part in a preliminary meeting with the SLORC authorities in June aimed at arranging a "national convention" to draft a new constitution.

National League for Democracy

Address. 97B West Shwegondine Rd, Bahan Township, Yangon.

Leadership. U Aung Shwe (ch.); U Lwin, (sec.-gen.).

Orientation. Pro-democratic movement.

Founded. 1988.

History. Three of Myanma's most prominent opposition figures (Brig.-Gen. Aung Gyi, a former high-ranking figure in the army, "strongman" Ne Win's most potent critic, Gen. Tin U, a former Chief of Staff and Defence Minister, and Aung San Suu Kyi, daughter of Aung San, the country's independence hero) announced the formation of the National League for Democracy (NLD) as a broad-based coalition to unite the country's various anti-government factions on Sept. 24, 1988, a matter of days after the military had taken control of the country. They announced their objective to be "to achieve a genuinely democratic government". The party held its inaugural meeting on Sept. 27 at which Aung Gyi was elected party chair, Tin U vice-chair and Aung San Suu Kyi general secretary. In December 1988, after disagreements over policy with Aung San Suu Kyi, Aung Gyi was expelled from the NLD. Tin U replaced Aung Gyi as chair.

Following increasing tension after student-led, anti-SLORC demonstrations in Yangon in early July 1989, the SLORC announced in the middle of the month that Aung San Suu Kyi and Tin U had been placed under house arrest for up to one year because "they had carried out activities to create conditions which could endanger the state". Aung San Suu Kyi responded to her arrest by going on a hunger strike, which she ended in August. In December, Tin U was sentenced to three years' imprisonment with hard labour for his role in the 1988 anti-government uprising. As part of a general SLORC crackdown on opposition political activity, Aung San Suu Kyi was banned in January 1990 from taking part in a general election scheduled by the junta for May 1990. Officials justified the ban on the grounds of her marriage to a British academic (Michael Aris), her long residence in the UK, and her alleged links with insurgent groups. Nevertheless, the NLD won a massive victory at the general election, taking 392 out of the 485 seats contested. However, the SLORC announced in July that the aim of the poll had not been to elect a new People's Assembly, but rather a Constituent Assembly, whose only function would be to draft a new Constitution along guidelines set down by the military. The announcement prompted an outcry from the newly elected NLD deputies who quickly convened and issued a denunciation of the "shameful" delay in the transfer of power.

NLD-inspired demonstrations to mark the second anniversary of the beginning of the 1988 anti-government protest began peacefully in early August, but resulted in violent clashes between students, monks and police. The following month Kyi Maung, acting secretary-general of the NLD, and Chit Khaing, party secretary, were arrested "for passing state evidence that they should have kept to themselves to an unconcerned person". By early November only four of the 16 NLD central executive committee members were at liberty and a further 50 senior party figures were under arrest. Later that month the remaining leaders reluctantly signed an endorsement pledging allegiance to a SLORC decree which required the new Constitution to be drawn up and submitted to a referendum, a process likely to take at least two years. By this action the NLD abandoned their demand for an immediate transfer of power and effectively nullified their election victory.

A group of candidates elected in the May elections announced in mid-December the establishment of a "parallel government" at Manerplaw on the border with Thailand. The so-called National Coalition Government of the Union of Burma claimed to have the support of the Democratic Alliance of Burma, a rebel and dissident coalition grouping. Most of the eight members of the "government" were from the NLD, and all were subsequently expelled from the party in punishment for their action.

In April 1991 the SLORC announced that the NLD's executive committee had been "invalidated", thus technically removing Aung San Suu Kyi, Tin U and other leading figures from the party. The newly "restructured" party was led by U Aung Shwe (a former army brigadier and ambassador to Australia) as chair and U Lwin as secretary-general. The next month it was reported that 34 NLD members—all but nine of whom had been elected to the Constinuent Assembly in May 1990—had been sentenced, some in absentia, to prison terms of up to 25 years after being found guilty of high treason. The SLORC amended the country's election law in July, adding to the grounds on which an Assembly member could be disqualified or banned from standing for future election. The amendment was widely regarded as simply another means of removing NLD Assembly members from their seats.

Aung San Suu Kyi, still living under house arrest in Yangon, was awarded the Sakharov Prize for freedom by the European Parliament in July and the Nobel

Peace Prize in October. The Nobel committee cited "her non-violent struggle for democracy and human rights". In December, the NLD, by now largely subdued by the SLORC, expelled Aung San Suu Kyi from the party claiming that she was "indirectly receiving support from an organization from a foreign country".

During late 1991 and early 1992 large numbers of NLD Assembly members had their status annulled, actions which coincided with the abolition of large numbers of opposition parties. In April 1992, Saw Maung was removed as SLORC chair and the junta used the opportunity to launch a series of political initiatives, apparently aimed at improving its poor international image. A number of political prisoners were released (including NLD people) and in May Aung San Suu Kyi was permitted a visit by her husband and children. Speaking after his visit, Aris said that his wife was "resolved to continue her endeavour to bring peace and happiness to her country".

The NLD was one of only seven political parties which attended a meeting in late June 1992 to discuss a planned "national convention" to draft a fresh constitution. Of the 28 party representatives at the meeting, 15 were NLD members.
Structure. 16-member executive committee.

National Unity Party
Taingyintha Silonenyinyutye
Address. 93c Windermere Rd, Kamayut, Yangon.
Leadership. U Tha Kyaw (ch.); U Tun Yi (gen. sec.); U Than Tin (gen. sec.).
Orientation. Pro-government.
Founded. 1962 as the Burma Socialist Programme Party.
History. The National Unity Party (NUP) was the new name given to the Burma Socialist Programme Party (BSSP, *Myanma Hsoshelit Lanzin Pati*) in the aftermath of the 1988 military coup.

The BSPP was founded in the immediate aftermath of the 1962 military coup which brought Gen. Ne Win to power. The ruling junta, the Revolutionary Council, created the BSPP in an effort to amalgamate all the existing political movements into one national party. Hence, in 1964 all parties which had refused to join the BSPP were declared illegal. The party's unique ideology, which attempted to synthesise Buddhism and Marxism, was formulated in a series of statements, namely the Revolutionary Council's *Burmese Road to Socialism*, the party's own *System of the Correlation of Man and His Environment*, and *Characteristics of the Burma Socialist Programme Party*. In 1974 the Ne

Win regime disbanded the Revolutionary Council and promulgated a new Constitution which vested power in new state organs, controlled by the BSPP. Under the terms of the Constitution the BSPP was defined as the country's "only political party leading the state".

Following the 1988 military coup the BSPP was officially dissolved, but in reality the party simply altered its name to the National Unity Party (NUP). However, unlike the BSPP, NUP membership was apparently not open to members of the armed forces. In the May 1990 elections the NUP was easily defeated by the opposition National League for Democracy, winning only 21 per cent of the vote and 10 seats. The NUP was one of only seven political parties which in late June 1992 attended a meeting, at which it was allowed three representatives, to discuss a planned "national convention" to draft a fresh constitution.
Structure. 15-member executive committee and 280-member central committee.

Shan Nationalities League for Democracy
Orientation. Represents the interests of the Shan ethnic minority.
Founded. In the aftermath of the 1988 military coup.
History. In the May 1990 elections the Shan Nationalities League for Democracy (SNLD) won the second largest number of seats (23) behind the National League for Democracy. Unlike the majority of the proliferation of ethnic-based parties, the SNLD's legal existence was approved by the Election Commission during its subsequent campaign of inspection and scrutiny. Six SNLD representatives took part in a preliminary meeting with the SLORC authorities in June 1992 aimed at arranging a "national convention" to draft a new constitution.

Shan State Kokang Democratic Party
Orientation. Represents the interests of the Kokang Chinese ethnic minority from Shan state.
Founded. In the aftermath of the 1988 military coup.
History. The Shan State Kokang Democratic Party (SSKDP) was one of the few remaining legal political parties as of mid-1992. As such, one representative of the party took part in a preliminary meeting with the SLORC authorities in June aimed at arranging a "national convention" to draft a new constitution.

Union Pa-O National Organization
Orientation. Represents the interests of the Pa-O ethnic minority in southern hills of Shan state.
Founded. In the aftermath of the 1988 military coup.

History. The Union Pa-O National Organization (UPNO) won three seats in the May 1990 general election. In 1991 the Pa-O National Organization, a small guerrilla organization which had fought against the army, signed a ceasefire agreement with the government making the UPNO the principal representative of the Pa-O.

Unlike the majority of the proliferation of ethnic-based parties, its legal existence was approved by the Election Commission during its subsequent campaign of inspection and scrutiny. A party representative took part in a preliminary meeting with the SLORC authorities in June 1992 aimed at arranging a "national convention" to draft a new constitution.

Dissident groups

The National Democratic Front (NDF), a coalition of organizations and their armed wings representing ethnic minority groups, was formed in 1975 with the aim of establishing a federal union based on national self determination. The NDF is divided into a northern, central and southern command. As of mid-1992, the northern command was composed solely of the **Kachin Independence Organization**, two other members (the **Palaung State Liberation Organization** and the **Shan State Progressive Party**) having signed peace treaties with the SLORC. The central command was composed of the **Karenni National Progressive Party**, the **Chin National Front** and the **Wa National Organization** (the **Pa-O National Organization**, formerly a member of the central command had also signed a peace agreement with the SLORC). The southern command was composed of the **Karen National Union**, the **Arakan Liberation Party**, the **Lahu National Army** and the **New Mon State Party**.

Another dissident coalition grouping was the **Democratic Alliance of Burma** (DAB). The DAB was established at Manerplaw in 1988 in opposition to the SLORC regime. It comprised 21 groups, including National Democratic Front members, dissident student organizations, monks and expatriates.

The Burmese Communist Party (the so-called "White Flag" Party), which had waged armed opposition to the government since the 1950s, was effectively destroyed by a major internal rebellion carried out by Wa hill tribesmen and Kotang Chinese in 1988.

Other dissident groupings included those operated by drug warlords, notably Khun Sa's Shan United Army.

Nauru

Capital: No official capital

Population: 9,000,000 (1989)

Nauru was discovered by Europeans in the late 18th century and, in the late 19th century, was colonized by Germany. It was then administered jointly by the UK, Australia and New Zealand until the creation of the independent Republic of Nauru in January 1968, when the country became an associate member of the Commonwealth. Nauru has amassed a considerable amount of wealth from the royalties derived from phosphate mining, although this activity has left 80 per cent of the island uninhabitable.

Nauru's first President, Hammer DeRoburt, who dominated the political structure of the island since independence, was forced to resign in August 1989 after a vote of no confidence. Since the election of December 1989 the Presidency has been in the hands of Bernard Dowiyogo.

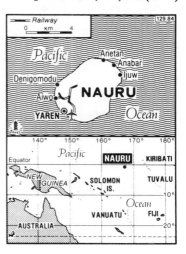

Constitutional structure

Legislative power is vested in an 18-member unicameral Parliament, elected for up to three years, which elects a President from amongst its members. The President, who is the head of government and de facto head of state, governs with the assistance of an appointed Cabinet. The country also has a powerful and well-funded tier of local government in the Nauru Local Government Council, an elected body of nine members which elects one of its number to the prestigious office of Head Chief.

Electoral system

The country is divided into electoral districts, most of which return two members to the legislature. After each general election, the new Parliament meets and elects a President from within its membership on the basis of a simple majority. Although some loose party groupings have evolved, one of which is currently operating, the country's democracy is not based upon political parties and all legislators are traditionally elected as independents.

Evolution of the suffrage

Nauru was established on the basis of universal adult suffrage. Voting is compulsory for all citizens aged 20 years and over.

Recent elections

Elections have been held regularly since 1968. Apart from the period December 1976 to May 1978, and for a few months in 1986 and a few days in 1987, Hammer DeRoburt held the presidency from independence in 1968 until his defeat in a vote of confidence in August 1989. He was succeeded as President by Kenas Aroi who resigned in December 1989 due to ill-health and, following a general election on Dec. 9, Bernard Dowiyogo was chosen as President on Dec. 12 by 10 votes to six.

Date of legislative elections	Presidential candidate subsequently elected
December 1983	Hammer DeRoburt
December 1986	Kennan Adeang*
January 1987	Hammer DeRoburt*
December 1989	Bernard Dowiyogo

*Did not complete full term in office.

PARTY BY PARTY DATA

Democratic Party of Nauru

Address. Parliament building, Nauru.

Leadership. Kennan Adeang.

Orientation. Opposition to the government of Hammer DeRoburt and his successors. The party seeks greater power for the legislature at the expense of the executive.

Founded. January 1987.

History. The Democratic Party of Nauru (DPN) was founded by Adeang as an attempt to provide a loose structure for the opponents of the country's veteran leader, Hammer DeRoburt. Adeang was successful in fomenting sufficient discontent amongst his parliamentary colleagues to oust DeRoburt from the Presidency in September 1986. In the subsequent Presidential elections he defeated his arch rival by nine votes to eight. He held office for only 14 days before his opponents brought him down through a vote of no-confidence and replaced him with DeRoburt. Following the December 1986 election Adeang gained the Presidency, but was once again defeated within a matter of days. He was replaced by DeRoburt who called a second election and was subsequently re-elected President.

Defunct parties

The Nauru Party; founded in the mid-1970s by opponents of Hammer DeRoburt, the Nauru Party's leader, Bernard Dowiyogo, was elected President following the general election of 1976. He remained in office until April 19, 1978, when he was forced to resign. He was replaced briefly by Lagumot Harris, but his government fell in a matter of weeks and opened the way for a return of DeRoburt. In December 1978 the Nauru Party effectively ceased to exist when its senior members, including Adeang, joined the DeRoburt government.

Major guerrilla groups

There are no guerrilla groups operating in Nauru.

Nepal

Capital: Katmandu   **Population: 19,100,000**

The Kingdom of Nepal was ruled by the Rana family, who held the hereditary office of Prime Minister, from 1846 to 1950, when they were overthrown by a popular revolt and the King resumed an active political role. The country's first Constitution was promulgated in 1959 and a Parliament elected the same year. In December 1960, however, King Mahendra dissolved Parliament, arrested most of its members and dismissed the government. All political parties were banned in January 1961. There then followed a 30-year period of absolute rule by the monarchy, although a "basic democracy" system was introduced under a new Constitution in 1962. This was a multi-tiered system revolving around village and town councils (*panchayats*).

In February 1990 a series of peaceful demonstrations demanding the restoration of democracy and human rights escalated into full-scale confrontation with the government after the police fired on demonstrators. In April 1990 the ban on political parties was lifted, restrictions on the press lifted and constitutional reform promised. A new Constitution guaranteeing parliamentary government and a constitutional monarchy was proclaimed in November 1990. The first multiparty general election was held in May 1991 and resulted in a victory for the Nepali Congress.

Constitutional structure

Under the provisions of the 1990 Constitution, Nepal is a Constitutional Monarchy. The King is described in the Constitution as "the symbol of Nepalese nationality and of unity of the people of Nepal".

Although the January 1961 ban on political parties was lifted in April 1990, their activities were widely tolerated from 1979. The 1990 Constitution specifies that no law may be adopted which bans, or imposes restrictions on, political parties.

Electoral system

The 1990 Constitution provides for a bicameral legislature comprising a popularly elected 205-member House of Representatives (*Pratinidhi Sabha*), and a 60-member National Council (*Rashtriya Sabha*), of whom 10 are nominees of the King, 35 (including three women) are elected by the House of Representatives and 15 are elected by an electoral college.

Evolution of the suffrage

Universal suffrage for all adults over 21 was first introduced in the 1959 Constitution.

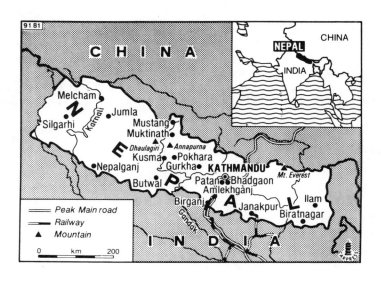

Recent elections

The first multiparty elections, held in February 1959, were dominated by the Nepali Congress Party (NCP), which won 74 of the 109 seats in the lower house of the legislature, in spite of polling only 37.2 per cent of the vote.

In 1980 King Birendra, Mahendra's son and successor, responded to popular protests by holding a referendum which gave voters the choice between a reformed *panchayat* system or a return to multiparty politics. The result was close, with 54.8 per cent of voters supporting the King and the *panchayat* system.

Under a reformed Constitution direct (non-party) elections to a National Council were held in May 1981 and May 1986. Despite a boycott by the NCP, turnout in both elections was relatively high, with 60 per cent of those eligible voting in 1986. Final results of the 1986 elections showed that 69 new members had been elected and 39 sitting or former members were also returned.

A general election, involving candidates from some 20 parties and over 200 independents, was held in May 1991 under the terms of the 1990 Constitution. It resulted in an overwhelming victory for the NCP.

May 1991 elections

Party	Seats
Nepali Congress Party	110
United Nepal Communist Party	69
United People's Front	9
Nepal *Sadbhavava Parishad* Party	6
National Democratic Party (Chand)	3
Nepal *Mazdoor Kisan* Party	2
Communist Party of Nepal (Democratic Manandhar)	2
National Democratic Party (Thapa)	1
Independents	3
Total elected seats	205

PARTY BY PARTY DATA

Communist Party of Nepal (Democratic Manandhar)

Address. Katmandu.

Leadership. Bahdur Manandhar (l.).

Founded. 1949 as the Communist Party of Nepal.

History. The party split in recent years and in January 1991, when the Marxist—Leninist and Marxist factions of the party merged to form the United Nepal Communist Party (UNCP), the Manandhar faction chose to continue on its own. The party won two seats in the May 1991 elections.

National Democratic Party (Chand)

Address. Katmandu.

Leadership. Lokendra Bahadur Chand (l.).

Orientation. Centre-right.

History. Chand was appointed Prime Minister in April 1990 in a move to placate the pro-democracy demonstrators. However, the situation was beyond his control and he was very quickly replaced. The party won three seats in the subsequent elections.

National Democratic Party (Thapa)

Address. Katmandu.

Leadership. Surya Bahadur Thapa (l.).

Orientation. Centre-right; advocates strong bilateral ties with India.

History. Won a single seat in the May 1991 elections.

Nepali Congress

Address. Katmandu.

Leadership. Krishna Prasad Bhattarai (pres.); Girija Prasad Koirala (sec.-gen.); Ganesh Man Singh (l.).

Orientation. Nationalist, although originally espousing socialism, the party has more recently advocated a mixed economy.

Founded. 1946.

History. Founded as the Nepali wing of the Indian National Congress, the Nepali Congress (NCP) in May 1959 formed the country's first popularly-elected government having won three-quarters of the parliamentary seats in the February 1959 elections. In December 1960, however, this government was dismissed by King Mahendra, who the following month banned all political parties. Over the following two decades many NCP activists were detained or restricted, while the exiled leadership under Koirala campaigned for the restoration of democracy.

From 1979, under the leadership of Bhattarai, the party was more or less officially tolerated and in December 1982 it held a national conference in Katmandu which was attended by some 500 delegates.

The NCP refused to participate in elections to the National Council in May 1986 after its demands for the release of political prisoners and dropping of obligation of candidates to be members of one of six *panchayat* class organizations, were not met.

In February 1990 the Movement for the Restoration of Democracy (MRD), which the NCP and seven communist factions had formed, launched a peaceful pro-democracy demonstration. Inspired by events in Eastern Europe and popularly known as the "stir", the MRD sought the ending of the *panchayat* system and the reintroduction of multiparty politics. The launching of the "stir" on Feb. 18 was marked by demonstrations and a mass meeting in the capital Katmandu. According to a government spokesman, three people were killed and 175 arrested in ensuing violent confrontations with the police. Indian press reports, however, indicated a higher total of casualties as well as the arrest of over 350 people including Bhattarai, Koirala and Singh.

The protests continued and in April, in an effort to contain the mounting unrest, King Birendra dismissed the Prime Minister Marich Man Singh Shrestha and appointed the moderate Lokendra Bahadur Chand. However, the situation worsened considerably, culminating with the police opening fire on 200,000 protestors. The killings exacerbated the discontent and the King was forced to act; he quickly lifted the ban on political parties, dissolved parliament and met with the MRD leaders for talks. In the middle of the month he appointed a new multiparty Cabinet headed by NCP president Bhattarai. The following month the King formally delegated the powers of Parliament to the Bhattarai Cabinet and announced a general amnesty for all political prisoners.

In the general election in May 1991, which followed the proclamation of a new multiparty Constitution the previous November, the NCP won an overwhelming majority in the House of Representatives. Koirala was sworn in as the new Prime Minister on May 26, Bhattarai having lost his seat in the election.

Membership. 10,000.

Nepal Party

Mazdoor Kisan

Address. Katmandu.

History. Won two seats in the May 1991 elections.

Nepal Party
Sadbhavava Parishad
Address. Katmandu.
Leadership. Gakendra Narayan Singh (pres.).
Orientation. Promotes the rights of the Terai-based *Madhesiya* community, who are Indian in origin; demands the recognition of Hindi as an official language, that constituencies in Terai be allocated on the basis of population and the granting of citizenship to those who settled in Nepal before April 1990.
History. Won six seats in the May 1991 elections.

United Nepal Communist Party
Address. Katmandu.
Leadership. Man Mohan Adhikari (l.).
Orientation. Independent Marxist.
Founded. January 1991.
History. The United Nepal Communist Party (UNCP) was formed by the merger of the Marxist and Marxist—Leninist factions of the Communist Party of Nepal (CPN). The CPN was founded in Calcutta in 1949 by a group of Nepalese exiles led by Pushpa Lal. After the revolution of 1950 it operated openly in Nepal, but was banned in 1952 for alleged complicity in an attempted left-wing coup in Katmandu. It nevertheless enjoyed considerable support, receiving over half the votes in the Katmandu municipal elections in the following year, winning five of the 18 seats. Legalized in 1956, it obtained 7.5 per cent of the vote and four of the 109 seats in the 1959 parliamentary elections.

After the royal coup of 1960 and the subsequent banning of political parties, the party split with one section, led by Pushpa Lal, adopting a pro-Chinese attitude, and another, led by Keshar Jung Raimajhi, adopting a pro-Soviet attitude. Over the next 25 years the party suffered a series of splits. In 1986 two factions abandoned their pro-Chinese line and adopted a more independent attitude to form the Nepali Communist Party—Marxist.

The Marxist—Leninist faction, an offshoot of the Indian Naxalite movement, was founded in the early 1970s, when it launched a "class annihilation" movement against landowners in eastern Nepal. It abandoned violent revolution in favour of working through the *panchayat* system in the mid-1980s.

The newly-formed UNCP took 69 seats in the May 1991 elections and performed extremely well in the capital, winning four of the five seats. Adhikari, as leader of the party's parliamentary group, became the official leader of the opposition.

United People's Front
Address. Katmandu.
Leadership Tanka Prasad Acharya (l.); Dilli Raman Regmi (l.).
Founded February 1991.
History. Founded by the merger of the Nepal *Praja Parishad* and the Nepali National Congress. Won nine seats in the May 1991 elections.

Other parties

United Left Front (ULF) (Katmandu); Sahana Pradhan (l.). Founded in 1990 by the merger of six factions from the Communist Party of Nepal (CPN) which then, in alliance with the Nepali Congress Party (NCP), formed the Movement for the Restoration of Democracy (MRD) [see Nepali Congress entry for details of MRD activity]. In December 1990 four of the factions left the front.

National People's Liberation Forum (Katmandu); M. S. Thapa (ch.). Left-wing party which considers the 1990 Constitution to be reactionary; boycotted the May 1991 elections.

Guerrilla groups

In 1985 anti-government guerrilla campaigns were launched by two groups, the **United Liberation Torch Bearers** (*Samyukta Mukti Bahini*) and the **Democratic Front** (*Janawadi Morcha*—Ram Raja Prasad Singh (l.)). Both groups are banned.

New Zealand

Capital: Wellington   **Population: 3,345,000**

New Zealand became a British colony in 1840, achieved self-government in 1852, and full independence in 1947. Since independence it has had a stable, two-party system, with periods of government alternating between the social democratic Labour Party and the conservative National Party. The country also has numerous smaller parties.

The social democratic Labour Party came to power in 1984 and, while preserving the country's advanced welfare system, also presided over a period of massive economic restructuring and deregulation. Although re-elected in 1987, the party suffered a decisive defeat at the hands of the conservative Nationalist Party in the election of 1990. The new government maintained the economic policies of its predecessor, but began making deep cuts in the welfare state.

Constitutional structure

New Zealand is a unitarian parliamentary democracy. As an independent member of the Commonwealth, its head of state is the British sovereign, represented by a Governor General. Legislative authority in New Zealand is vested in a unicameral House of Representatives, which consists of 97 members elected for up to three years. (The legislature had originally been bicameral, but the Legislative Council, the upper chamber, was abolished in 1950.) The Prime Minister and Cabinet are responsible to the legislature and are appointed by the Governor General acting upon its advice.

Political parties are not subsidized by the state, although the Broadcasting Corporation of New Zealand (the statutory authority which controls radio and television) allocates free broadcasting time to the various parties in accordance with their respective electoral strengths. Additional time can be purchased by the parties in accordance with their individual campaign strategies and resources.

Electoral system

The number of representatives to be elected and the boundaries of their constituencies are adjusted after every quinquennial census. All members of the legislature are elected as representatives of single-member constituencies, elected upon the basis of simple plurality whereby the candidate with the greatest number of votes wins the seat.

Since 1867 there has been special provision for the representation in Parliament of the country's indigenous Maori population in the form of four large constituencies (which together cover the whole country), each of which returns a Maori member. Since 1975 citizens of Maori descent have been entitled to register on either the Maori or the general role.

Evolution of the suffrage

Universal suffrage for men (over 21 years of age) was introduced in 1879, and for women in 1883. In 1969 the age qualification was lowered to 20 years and in 1974 those over 18 were given the vote. Voter registration is mandatory, but voting is voluntary.

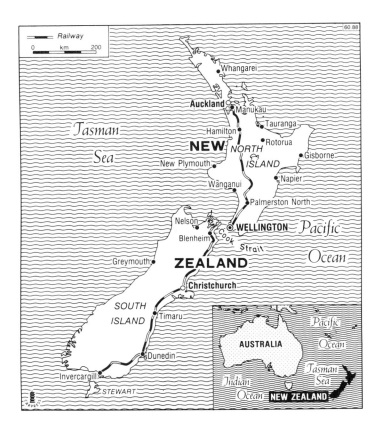

Recent elections

Date	Winning party
1946	Labour Party
1949	National Party
1951	National Party
1954	National Party
1957	Labour Party,
1960	National Party
1963	National Party
1966	National Party
1969	National Party
1972	Labour Party
November 1975	National Party
November 1978	National Party
Nov. 28, 1981	National Party
July 14, 1984	Labour Party
Aug. 15, 1987	Labour Party
Oct. 27, 1990	National Party

General election, Aug. 15, 1987

	Percentage of vote	Seats won
Labour Party	47	58
National Party	45	39
Others	8	—

General election, Oct. 27, 1990

	Percentage of vote	Seats won
Labour Party	35	27
National Party	48	67
New Labour Party	5	1
Others	12	—

PARTY BY PARTY DATA

Democratic Party (also known as New Zealand Democratic Party, NZDP)

Address. PO Box 9967, Newmarket, Auckland, New Zealand.

Leadership. Garry Knapp (l.); Chris Leitch (pres.).

Orientation. Right-wing. The party has largely abandoned its original position of advocating the social credit monetary theories of Maj. C. H. Douglas, although it retains its belief in "a property-owning democracy, a nation of self-employed, owner-operators, co-operative ventures and worker shareholders", with decentralization of power. Since 1982 the party has espoused "armed neutrality" and a non-nuclear defence policy.

Founded. 1953 (as New Zealand Social Credit Political League).

History. The party, which was formed as the New Zealand Social Credit Political League by W. B. Owen and other advocates of the monetary theories of Maj. C. H. Douglas, became the Social Credit Political Party in 1982, and adopted its current name on July 1, 1985. Having repeatedly won significant shares of the vote, the party gained its first parliamentary representatives in 1966 when it won 14.4 per cent and its leader since 1963, Vernon Cracknell, was elected to the House of Representatives. The seat was lost in 1969, however, and the party split in 1972 (its leader J. B. O'Brien, forming a short-lived New Democratic Party).

The Democratic Party leader, Bruce Craig Beetham won a by-election in 1978, and retained the seat in the general election later that year. The party increased its representation to two members at a by-election in 1981. The seats were retained in the general election of 1981 when the party polled 372,056 votes, over 20 per cent of the total. The discrepancy between its share of the vote and the seats won fuelled a public debate over the fairness of the country's first-past-the-post electoral system and was one factor in a 1987 Royal Commission's recommendation for proportional representation.

The party retained its two seats in 1984, although its vote fell to 136,774, 7.6 per cent of the total. Its decline was primarily due to it having been eclipsed by the New Zealand Party as the repository of the "protest vote" within the two-party system. The party's share of the vote continued to decline, and in the 1987 general election it lost its parliamentary representation. The party won no seats in the 1990 general election.

Structure. The party has eight national officers (leader, deputy leader, president, four vice-presidents and a dominion secretary) and a 20-member dominion council. Branches throughout the country send delegates to the annual conference, which determines policy and elects officers.

Membership. 32,000 (1986 est).

Publications. Guardian (monthly).

Green Party of Aotearoa (The Greens)

Address. 20 Fort Street, Auckland, New Zealand.

Leadership. Chris Thomas and Wendy Lynch (conveners).

Orientation. Socialist-ecologist. The party advocates peace, disarmament, decentralization, civil rights, and a community-based co-operative economy.

Founded. May 1972 (as New Zealand Values Party).

History. The party stood candidates in around one half of the country's constituencies in the 1972 election, polling 2 per cent of the vote. In the 1975 contest, the party polled 5.2 per cent of the vote, although this figure dropped in 1978 to 2.5 per cent. Its votes continued to decline in subsequent elections, although the party claims credit for forcing environmental concerns onto the agendas of the two main parties, particularly the Labour Party.

Structure. Policy is determined by the party conference and is implemented by a national council elected by delegates and office-holders. Local branches are co-ordinated by regional committees.

Publications. Linkletter (monthly).

International affiliations. The party has extensive links with Green movements in other countries.

Labour Party

Address. PO Box 784, Wellington, New Zealand.

Leadership. Michael K. Moore (parl. l.); Ruth Dyson (pres.); Anthony Timms (gen. sec.).

Orientation. Democratic socialist. The party was originally founded with a commitment to "the socialization of the means of production, distribution and exchange", although throughout much of its history it advocated a mixed economy based on private enterprise and state regulation. It was also a staunch defender of New Zealand's highly-developed welfare state. From the mid-1980s, in response to the interventionist stance of the Muldoon government and to the country's increasing economic problems, the Labour Party moved towards an economic approach based on deregulation and laissez-faire capitalism. This policy became synonymous with Finance Minister Roger Douglas. The party is also opposed to nuclear weapons and nuclear energy and, when in government, legislated against the use of New Zealand ports and waters by nuclear warships.

Founded. July 1916 (as the New Zealand Labour Party, NZLP).

History. The party was preceded by the Political Labour League (1905-08), the first New Zealand Labour Party (1910-12), the revolutionary syndicalist United Labour Party (1912-13) and the Socialist Democratic Party (1913-16), and also drew on the reformist tradition within the Liberal Party (the rump of which merged into the National Party in 1936). The second NZLP grew from 11,000 members (and 72 affiliated unions) in 1918, to almost 46,000 in 1925.

Having shed much of its early doctrinaire programme and been boosted by the Great Depression, the party first came to power in 1935, after winning 54 of the 76 seats in the lower house of the then bicameral legislature. The Labour government laid the foundations of New Zealand's highly-developed welfare state system. Following the death of Labour's legendary leader, M. J. Savage, in 1940, support for the party steadily declined in the face of bitter factional conflicts. In 1946 its majority was reduced to four. By 1949 the party was associated with prolonged wartime controls and shortages and growing industrial unrest, and was ousted from office. It returned to government in 1957 (under W. Walsh) with a tiny majority, undertook harsh and unpopular budgetary measures, and was defeated once more in the 1960 election.

Labour remained in opposition until 1972, when its leader since 1964, Norman Kirk, became Prime Minister. He died in 1974 and was succeeded by Wallace E. (Bill) Rowling. The party lost the election of 1975, winning 35 of the 87 seats. In 1978 it increased its number of seats to 41 (out of 92), and actually secured a greater share of the vote than the victorious National Party. In the election of 1981 the party lost again, with its share of the vote falling from 40.4 per cent to 38.8 per cent, although its number of seats rose to 43. After the 1981 defeat the clamour for a change of leader became irresistible and Rowling resigned.

In 1983 David Lange was elected leader of the party and immediately proved himself to be a shrewd political operator with an ability to communicate and to project himself convincingly as a man of the people. In the premature election called by Sir Robert Muldoon, in July 1984, Labour increased its vote by 50,000 to 755,551 (41.7 per cent) and won 56 of the 95 seats.

The Lange government became associated with two particular areas of policy. The first was its popular non-nuclear defence policy, which included the banning of nuclear-powered or nuclear-armed vessels from New Zealand's ports and waters. While popular with the New Zealand public, the ban led to freezing of relations with the USA and the suspension of New Zealand from the ANZUS Pact, the 1951 Pacific Security Treaty between New Zealand, Australia and the USA. The second hallmark of the Labour government was its deregulatory economic policy, known as "Rogernomics" after Finance Minister Roger Douglas. This anti-inflationary strategy—which included the removal of credit and money supply controls—attracted acclaim from international commentators and produced some spectacular levels of economic growth in the mid-1980s, fuelled by credit-powered consumption. Towards the end of the decade, however, "Rogernomics" became associated with economic stagnation, growing inflation and, consequently, high interest rates, cuts in the welfare state and growing income disparities arising from tax cuts for the highest paid. In the 1987 election campaign Lange appealed to the electorate to "have the guts to stick with" his government's economic strategy, promising that they would place the country's economy on a much-improved footing and thereby enable the provision of greater welfare benefits in the future. The party was re-elected for a second term (the first time for more than 40 years), increasing its number of seats in the enlarged 97-member House to 58.

Following Labour's re-election, the differences between Lange and Douglas over the latter's zealous commitment to laissez-faire capitalism developed into a bitter feud as the government embarked on a programme of increased privatisation, determined to sell a number of loss-making state enterprises with the intent of cutting public debt by one third by 1993. The privatisation programme was dogged by opposition charges—supported by many economists—that it was poorly handled and that many of the assets were being sold at prices well below their market value. The programme was accompanied by continuing tight monetary policies and further deregulation.

At the beginning of 1988 Lange curbed some of Douglas's authority, and intervened to prevent a reform of the tax system which would have entailed large tax reductions for the wealthy and the introduction of a flat rate of income tax for all, irrespective of income. Relations between the two men deteriorated further and, in December 1988, Douglas was dismissed from the Cabinet. Thereafter he made two unsuccessful attempts to wrest the party leadership away from Lange. Notwithstanding the departure of Douglas, the government maintained the central thrust of its economic strategy and, despite the unpopularity of the privatization programme, in January 1989 it restated its commitment to use asset sales as a means of reducing domestic and foreign debt.

Lange unexpectedly announced his resignation as Prime Minister on Aug. 7, 1989. The timing of his decision was determined by the re-election of Douglas to the Cabinet on Aug 3. Labour MPs chose Douglas and one of his close supporters to fill two Cabinet vacancies, after the former Finance Minister had promised to desist in his criticism of Lange. In his press conference to announce his decision to resign, Lange cited his poor health—he had suffered a heart attack in 1988—and to a past suggestion that he did not intend to lead the Labour Party into a third election campaign. He also referred to the "extraordinary, extremist, ideological convictions" of Douglas which, he warned the party, constituted "flirtations with lunacy . . . a recipe for disaster". On Aug. 8, a caucus of the Labour Party's MPs elected Geoffrey Palmer as leader in preference to Michael Moore. Douglas withdrew his candidature shortly before the vote and chose instead to contest the post of Deputy Prime Minister, where he was defeated narrowly by Helen Clarke.

Palmer, a former law professor who had assisted both the New Zealand and Australian governments in reforming accident compensation law, had a reputation for austere diligence. He entered Parliament at a by-election in 1979, and was elected deputy leader of the Labour Party in 1983. Although adequate, Palmer lacked the personal authority to restore Labour's popularity. As a general election became imminent, Labour continued to trail poorly behind the National Party in the opinion polls. The polls also showed widespread dissatisfaction with Palmer's leadership, his bland and unassertive personal style being compared unfavourably with Lange. Palmer eventually called a general election for Oct. 27, 1990, the latest possible date under the country's constitution.

The approaching election provided the impetus for Palmer's resignation as Labour MPs sought to avert electoral disaster by calling for him to step down in favour of Moore, whom the opinion polls showed to be considerably more popular. As late as Sept. 3, Palmer insisted that he would lead the party into the election but, at a caucus of Labour MPs on the follow-

ing day, he resigned after it became clear that many of those present—including a sizable portion of the Cabinet—had withdrawn their support. The meeting immediately elected Moore, an instinctive populist and one of the few members of the Cabinet with genuinely working class credentials, to lead the party and to attempt to restore those areas of traditional Labour support eroded by the policies of Douglas.

Moore, who had served as Minister of External Affairs and Trade under Palmer, was largely self-educated. As a child he suffered a physical disability and, following the death of his father, was institutionalized at the age of eight in a school for the destitute. He left school at 15, worked as a labourer and then a printer and became active in trade union and Labour Party politics. In 1972, at the age of 23, he was elected to Parliament. After losing his Auckland seat in 1975 he moved to Christchurch and, after a series of manual jobs, trained as a psychiatric nurse. He was re-elected to Parliament in 1978, and then survived a long struggle against cancer.

One of Moore's first acts after his elevation to the leadership was to reverse the government's laissez-faire economic policy by compacting a pay restraint agreement with the trade union movement. The deal formed the centre of a new economic package which aimed to cut the budget deficit, not by reducing public expenditure, but by stimulating economic growth through a reduction of interest rates. Although during his two months as Labour leader and Prime Minister Moore was successful in closing the gap between the two parties, the opinion polls continued to point to a decisive forthcoming National Party victory. This was confirmed on Oct. 27, 1990. Although Moore retained his seat, eight members of his Cabinet were defeated, as was the parliamentary Speaker, his deputy, and two government whips. Reduced to 29, Labour's parliamentary caucus was smaller than at any time since 1931, before the first Labour government had ever been elected.

Structure. The party has individual membership through local branches based in the constituencies, and a system of affiliation by trade unions. Both sections send delegates to the annual conference which elects a New Zealand council, a policy committee and an executive. It liaises with the Federation of Labour through a joint council.

Membership. The party claimed to have 240,000 members in 1987, although only a small proportion of these are active.

International affiliations. Socialist International; Asia-

Pacific Socialist Organization.

New Labour Party (NLP)

Address. PO Box 12-324, Thorndon, Wellington, New Zealand.

Leadership. Jim Anderton (l.); Dave Alton (nat. organizer).

Orientation. The NLP is committed to traditional social democratic principles, including state regulation of the economy. Like many on the left of the Labour Party, Anderton was opposed to the policies of economic deregulation and laissez-faire capitalism associated with Finance Minister Roger Douglas.

Founded. April 1989.

History. The New Labour Party (NLP) was established by Jim Anderton, a Labour MP who was expelled from the parliamentary party in December 1988 for refusing to support government legislation to sell the state-owned Bank of New Zealand. The Labour Party's council ruled that the expulsion was unconstitutional but was overruled in April 1989 by the caucus, a move which led to Anderton's formal resignation from the party on April 18 and his creation of the NLP. Anderton retained his seat in the 1990 general election, with the NLP winning 5 per cent of the total vote.

New Zealand National Party

Address. National Party Centre, Willbank House, 57 Willis Street, PO Box 1155, Wellington, New Zealand.

Leadership. James G. (Jim) Bolger (l.); John G. Collinge (pres.); Cindy Flook (sec.-gen.).

Orientation. Conservative. The National Party stands for private enterprise, a property-owning democracy and personal freedom. Although traditionally the party has accepted the principle of an extensive welfare state, the National Party government which came to power in 1990 has begun to make wholesale cuts in the welfare system [see below]. The party's economic philosophy, after going through a phase of support for a high-level of state intervention during the Muldoon era, is currently based upon the principles of deregulation, privatisation and laissez-faire capitalism. The party has traditionally drawn support from rural areas and from the urban middle class.

Founded. May 1936.

History. The party was formed from a merger of the Reform and Liberal Parties—two principal opposition groups to the Labour Party. Under its second leader, S. G. Holland, it won the general elections of 1949 and 1951 and remained in office until 1957 when it was ousted by Labour. It returned to power in 1960, under

Keith J. Holyoake, and remained in office until Labour was returned in 1972. In the general election of 1975 it won 47.2 per cent of the vote and took 55 of the 87 seats in the House. Although its support declined to 39.8 per cent in the election of 1978, it retained an overall majority by winning 50 of the 92 seats. In the election of 1981 the party actually polled 4,000 votes fewer than Labour, but managed to remain in office by winning 47 of the 92 seats.

During this period the party was led by Sir Robert Muldoon (leader 1974-84 and Prime Minister 1975-84), and was associated with highly interventionist economic policies. These included protectionism, farm subsidies, price and wages freezes and legislation to hold down interest rates. The party's advocacy of economic policies more usually associated with social democracy, together with its acceptance of New Zealand's extensive welfare state, meant that there was very little significant difference between the two main parties during this period. This was reflected in 1983 by the foundation of the New Zealand Party, created by millionaire Bob Jones and other National Party members in response to the National Party's "socialistic" tendencies. The new party advocated cuts in taxation, government spending, together with economic deregulation and the rule of market forces. At the 1984 general election it displaced Social Credit as the country's third party by winning 11.9 per cent of the vote. Despite contesting every constituency, however, it failed to win any seats. In 1986, following the replacement of Muldoon, the membership of the New Zealand Party voted to rejoin the National Party.

The convergence between the two main parties began breaking down in the early 1980s when the Labour Party increasingly adopted a economic stance—in reaction to the Muldoon era—based on economic deregulation and free market principles. Another key difference between the two parties was Labour's promise to prohibit nuclear-powered or nuclear-armed ships from entering New Zealand waters or ports, a policy which had particular implications for New Zealand's participation in the ANZUS Pact. In the general election of July 1984 the National Party government was ejected from office after winning only 35 per cent of the vote and 37 seats, and in November of that year Muldoon lost the leadership to his deputy Jim McLay and the party began moving away from the concept of economic interventionism. Muldoon continued to command a significant degree of support within the parliamentary caucus, however, and this faction sought to undermine McLay.

In March 1986 McLay was replaced as leader by his deputy Jim Bolger, a Catholic farmer without a university education, who was descended from Irish immigrant parents. His unflamboyent political style, his physical appearance, and his representation of a remote North Island rural constituency, earned him the nickname "Potato Head". Despite this, Bolger possessed considerable managerial skills and political experience, having served for six years in Muldoon's Cabinet. The 1987 election was fought primarily over the issues of Labour's non-interventionist economic policies and the issue of the prohibition of nuclear ships which had resulted in a radical deterioration in relations with the US and in New Zealand's suspension from ANZUS. Although the party fought an impressive campaign and achieved a favourable swing of 3 per cent, it failed to dislodge Labour from office. The National Party's share of the vote increased from 36 to 45 per cent and the number of seats won in the newly expanded 97-member House rose from 37 to 39.

Following the party's second consecutive election defeat, it revised several of its policies. Muldoon was immediately removed from the Shadow Cabinet and the party totally abandoned the concept of economic intervention. Ruth Richardson, appointed as the spokesperson on finance, was an outspoken proponent of the laissez-faire policies being pursued by the Labour government. In 1990 the National Party also adopted Labour's popular ban on nuclear vessels. On Oct. 27, 1990, a general election was held against a background of economic difficulties, rising unemployment and divisions within the Labour Party. As had been predicted by the opinion polls, the National Party achieved a crushing victory, winning 47.8 per cent of the vote and securing 67 of the 97 seats in the House.

On April 1, 1991, the National Party government reneged on its election campaign pledges by announcing deep cuts within the welfare state. Bolger and Richardson (the new Finance Minister) justified the move on the grounds that it was essential to cut the budget deficit by reducing public expenditure. The cuts affected areas such as pensions and eligibility for unemployment, sickness, and child benefits. The policy resulted in nationwide protests involving up to 100,000 people, the largest demonstrations since those in 1981 against the South African rugby tour. Effigies of Bolger and Richardson were burned in Auckland.

Undeterred, the government unveiled a highly controversial budget on July 30 which severely curtailed the country's welfare state by designating about one half of the population as rich enough to pay for its health, education, housing and retirement needs. Richardson justified the move on the grounds that the country could no longer afford to fund one of the most comprehensive welfare systems in the world, and that it was necessary to replace it with "a true enterprise society living within its means".

The budget slashed government spending—aiming to reduce it from 42.9 per cent of GDP in 1990-91 to 37 per cent in 1992-93—and announced ambitious targets for debt reduction and the cutting of the budget deficit from NZ$1,739 million in 1990-91 to NZ$528 million by 1993-94. Apart from those deemed to be in genuine need, the budget required patients to pay for all or part of the cost of their medical treatment. A new means tested superannuation scheme was announced to replace the existing guaranteed retirement income—thereby reneging upon a specific National Party election pledge—with the age of entitlement lifted progressively from 60 to 65 years. Rents for state housing were to be increased to market levels, students in higher education were to pay part of their fees, and there would be further privatization of state assets. The budget also sharply raised rates of duty on alcohol and tobacco, and increased the price of petrol.

Rumoured discontent within the ruling National Party became public on Aug. 15 when two backbench MPs resigned from the party. The two, Gilbert Myles and Hamish MacIntyre, were known as opponents of the government's economic policies and were particularly opposed to the budget. In announcing their resignations the two men stated their intention to remain in Parliament and to found a new party "that brings honesty back into New Zealand politics". Bolger dismissed the resignations as "predictable". The party was also subject to factional discord arising from supporters of Muldoon, who remained a critical voice on the backbenches, having turned down several minor Cabinet posts which had been offered to him. Bolger also faced increasing opposition from Winston Peters who had been subject to a shadow Cabinet demotion in 1989 for criticizing party policy. Despite being appointed Minister of Maori Affairs following the 1990 general election victory, he continued to defy collective responsibility in his outspoken criticism of the government's economic policies, particularly the social impact of economic deregulation. Opinion polls consistently showed that Peters—who had degrees in politics and law, and who possessed considerable charm, verbal dexterity and political charisma—was substantially more popular than Bolger. Most commentators believed that, at some point, Peters would challenge Bolger for the party leadership.

Structure. The National Party has a loosely organized structure. There are branches in every constituency, the size of which reflect the party's level of support on a constituency-by-constituency basis. In many constituencies there are also separate women's and youth groups. There are further organizational tiers at divisional (regional) and national level. The annual Dominion Conference elects national officers and is the final arbiter of policy decisions.

Membership. The registered membership varies between 80,000 and 150,000 (higher in election years); although only a small proportion of these are active.

International affiliations. International Democrat Union (since 1982); Pacific Democrat Union (since 1983).

New Zealand Self-Government Party
Manu Motuhake o Aotearoa

Address. 49 Erima Avenue, Point England, Panmure, Auckland, New Zealand.

Leadership. Peter Campbell (gen. sec.); Matia Rata.

Orientation. The party seeks greater political and economic autonomy for the country's 400,000 indigenous Maori population.

Founded. 1979.

History. The *Manu Motuhake* (the English translation given above is never used by party representatives) was formed after the resignation from the Labour Party of Matia Rata, who had served as Minister of Maori Affairs in 1972-75. Although since 1975 four seats in the legislature have been reserved for those of Maori descent [see above], the party has failed to win parliamentary representation.

Minor parties

Christian Democratic Union Party (CDUP); 24 Seccombes Road, Epsom, Auckland 3; Henry Lynch (pres.), Thomas Weal (sec.-gen.). The CDUP is a Catholic party which has not been active in New Zealand politics in the last few years, preferring to concentrate on exerting its influence within the Christian Democrat International.

Communist Party of Aotearoa (CPA); 37 St Kevin's Arcade, Box 1785, Greenlane, Auckland, New Zealand); Harold Crook (gen. sec.). Founded in 1921 as the Communist Party of New Zealand, the CPA became pro-Maoist during the 1960s estrangement between the Soviet Union and China, and is currently pro-Albanian. It publishes *People' Voice* (fortnightly).

People's Alliance; Jim Delahunty and Sue Bradford (spokespersons). Founded in 1988 as a left-wing alternative to the Labour Party, the People's Alliance has never secured legislative representation.

Socialist Action League (SAL); Russell Johnson (nat. sec.). The party is a small Trotskyist organization founded in 1969.

World Socialist Party (New Zealand) (WSPNZ); PO Box 1929, Auckland, New Zealand. Founded in 1931 as Socialist Party of New Zealand (SPNZ), as an offshoot of the Socialist Party of Great Britain. It is opposed to capitalism and to the "class collaborationist" parties of the left. It is part of the World Socialist Movement.

Socialist Unity Party (SUP); 161, Willis Street, Wellington, New Zealand; George E. Jackson (pres.), Marilyn Tucker (gen. sec.). Founded in 1966 by pro-Soviet members of the CPNZ who were opposed to the Maoist policies espoused by the party at that time.

Workers Communist League (WCL); Graeme Clark. The WCL is a pro-Chinese group founded in 1980 by the merger of two splinters from the Communist Party of New Zealand.

Defunct parties

Liberal Party. From 1890 to 1912 the party dominated the country's political system, but was subject to strains between the pro-Labour urban elements and the more conservative middle class and rural components, which also dominated the leadership. The party fell from power following the general election of 1911 and disintegrated in the 1930s.

New Zealand Democratic Party [see Democratic Party].

New Zealand Party, founded in 1983 by members of the National Party who were critical of Sir Robert Muldoon's authoritarian style of leadership and the party's adoption of interventionist policies in place of those of laissez-faire capitalism. In 1986 its membership voted to reintegrate with the National Party.

New Zealand Values Party, an ecological party

founded in 1972; became the Green Party of Aotearoa in 1990 [see separate entry].

Reform Party. The party evolved from the opposition to the Liberal Party in the late-19th century and held office between 1912 and 1928. In 1931 it allied itself with the United Party, and this alliance eventually formed the impetus for the creation of the New Zealand National Party [see separate entry].

Social Credit Political Party, founded in 1953 as the Social Credit Political League, based upon the monetary reform theories of Maj. C. H. Douglas. Increasingly it came to occupy the middle ground of New Zealand's political spectrum, and eventually evolved into the New Zealand Democratic Party in 1985 [see separate entry].

Major guerrilla groups

There are no guerrilla groups operating in New Zealand.

New Zealand Associated Territories

Cook Islands

Capital: Avarua, on Rarotonga Island   **Population: 17,185 (1985 census)**

Discovered by Europeans in the 18th century, the Cook Islands became a British protectorate in the late 19th century, and were annexed to New Zealand in 1901. Since 1965 the 15 Cook Islands have been a self-governing territory in free association with New Zealand, which in addition to providing economic assistance, has responsibility for the territory's defence and foreign policy.

Constitutional structure

Executive power is vested in the British monarch as sovereign of New Zealand. On a day-to-day basis this power is exercised by a Premier and an appointed six-member Cabinet, who are responsible to the country's Parliament. The legislature comprises 24 members elected for up to five years, and chooses the Premier from among its numbers. There is also a resident New Zealand Representative whose responsibility it is to liaise between the Niue and New Zealand governments.

There is also a House of Ariki, a chamber of traditional chiefs, which has no legislative powers but serves as an advisory forum to the Parliament.

Electoral system

Members of the legislature are elected for single-member constituencies, nine of which are located on the main island of Rarotonga, and 14 on other islands. Since 1981 a single member has been elected by the many Cook Islanders resident in New Zealand.

Evolution of the suffrage

The first elected federal legislature, covering the southern islands, was created in the 19th century. In 1946 a Legislative Council was established followed, in 1957, by a Legislative Assembly. Elections are held on the basis of universal adult suffrage.

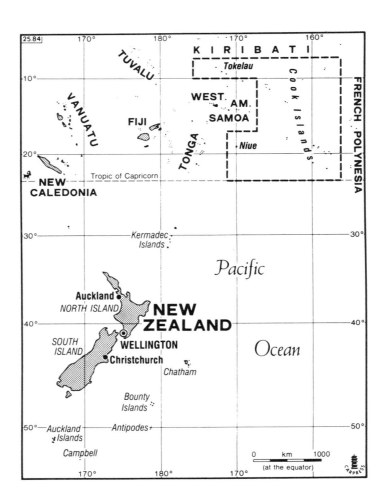

Recent elections

Election date	Winning party
March 1978	Cook Islands Party (CIP)*
March 1983	CIP
November 1983	Democratic Party
March 1985	Democratic Party
January 1989	CIP

*Removed from office in 1979.

Legislative elections, Jan. 19, 1989

Party	Seats won
CIP	12
Democratic Party	9
Democratic Tumu Party	2
Independents	1

PARTY BY PARTY DATA

Cook Islands Party (CIP)

Address. Avarua, Rarotonga.

Leadership. Geoffrey Henry (l.).

Orientation. The Cook Islands Party (CIP), like other Cook Islands parties, has no clear ideological position, being generally based on kinship and regional loyalties. The party seeks to protect the country's Polynesian identity and to maintain its ties with New Zealand.

Founded. 1964.

History. The CIP was the first formally constituted political grouping within the country, although it was predated by a spiritual predecessor, the Cook Islands Progressive Association (CIPA) which had been active in the post-war era, and had sought a greater degree of self-government and economic development. The party won power in the elections of 1965, and remained in government—under the leadership of Albert R. Henry—until 1978. Although the party won a fifth successive election victory on March 30, 1978, it was removed from power in July 1979 when the Chief Justice of the High Court, ruling that the election had been distorted by serious malpractice, awarded eight disputed seats to the opposition. The decision reduced the CIP's share of seats in the 22-member Parliament to seven. Henry and seven of his CIP colleagues were arraigned on corruption charges which resulted in a temporary ban from political activities.

Henry died in 1981 and was succeeded as CIP leader by his cousin, Geoffrey Henry. At the 1983 election the party won a narrow victory, securing 13 of the 24 seats, and Henry became Prime Minister. Henry's small majority was rapidly eroded and fresh elections were held in November 1983 which saw the CIP forced back into opposition. In 1984 the party entered a coalition with the Democratic Party, with Henry serving as Deputy Prime Minister. This broke down in mid-1985 but, although Henry and the majority of the party withdrew support from the Democratic Party administration, four CIP members defied the party leadership by continuing to support the government.

In the election of January 1989 the CIP won 12 seats and, with the support of the two Democratic Tumu Party (DTP) members, formed a stable administration. By the beginning of 1991 the number of seats held by the CIP had increased to 14—one member of the Democratic Party having defected and the sole independent member having joined the CIP—thereby giving the party, in alliance with the DTP, the two-thirds majority required to enact constitutional changes. Al-though Henry was in favour of such reform—including an increase in the size of the Cabinet and a greater recognition of the role of political parties—he denied suggestions that his eventual aim was to achieve complete independence from New Zealand. By the middle of 1991 a combination of defections and by-elections had increased the government's strength to 17 seats.

Democratic Party

Address. PO Box 492, Rarotonga.

Leadership. Terepai Maoate (l.).

Orientation. The Democratic Party was formed as a progressive force with the specific intention of opposing the personal rule of Albert Henry, the leader of the Cook Islands Party (CIP).

Founded. 1971.

History. The Democratic Party, created by Thomas Davis as a new opposition force to challenge the dominance of the CIP, absorbed the previous opposition grouping of the United Cook Islanders' Party. The party remained in opposition, however, until 1978 when a legal ruling overturned the result of the 1977 elections and gave the Democratic Party its first overall majority in Parliament. At the 1983 election the party won 11 sets but was defeated by the CIP. Incumbent Prime Minister Davis and several members of his Cabinet failed to retain their seats. With the CIP unable to hold onto its small majority, fresh elections were held in November 1983. The Democratic Party, still led by Davis, was returned to office in a coalition government which included Henry as Deputy Prime Minister. The coalition lasted for about a year, before most of the CIP withdrew its support.

Although the Davis administration struggled on, and survived the 1985 election, he was increasingly unpopular within his own party because of his authoritarian style of leadership, alleged misuse of disaster funds, and vehement opposition to the New Zealand government's anti-nuclear stance. Bereft of support amongst his colleagues, Davis was defeated by 23 votes to 0 in a vote of confidence on July 29, 1987. He was succeeded as Prime Minister and party leader by Pupeke Robati.

At the general election of January 1989 the Democratic Party, weakened by the defection of some of its members who had left the party to create the Democratic Tumu Party (DTP), won nine seats, and lost power to the CIP. With an election not required until early 1994, the dominant position of the CIP (which increased its number of seat in 1990-91 as a result of recruiting a Democratic Party member and an independent), had the effect of increasing divisions within the opposition. At the annual conference of the Democratic Party in August 1990, Robati managed to avoid a challenge to his position by Norman George, a former Foreign Minister. The issue was deferred until a special convention in October at which Robati resigned and backed Terepai Maoate, a former member of the CIP, who, in the election which followed, narrowly defeated George for the leadership.

Minor parties

Democratic Tumu Party (DTP); PO Box 492, Rarotonga; Vincent Ingram (l.). The DTP was founded in 1985 by a group of defectors from the Democratic Party. At the 1989 general election it won two seats and, thereafter, has supported the Cook Islands Party government.

Cook Islands Labour Party (CILP); founded in 1988 as an anti-nuclear party, it is currently led by Rena Ariki Jonassen.

Cook Islands Party Alliance (CIPA); Rarotonga; founded in 1983 by Tupui Henry, son of the late Albert Henry, the CIPA is opposed to the Cook Islands Party leadership of Geoffrey Henry and, therefore, is closely allied to the Democratic Party.

Defunct parties

United Cook Islanders' Party [see under Democratic Party].

Unity Party; founded in 1978, the Unity Party opposed party politics; it withered away in the mid-1980s having failed to win any legislative representation.

Major guerrilla groups

There are no guerrilla groups operating in the Cook Islands.

Niue

Capital: Alofi. **Population: 2,300 (1989—a further 10,000 of Niue's population live in New Zealand)**

The coral island of Niue was discovered by Europeans in the late 18th century, and became a British possession in 1900. In 1901 it was annexed to New Zealand as part of the Cook Islands, but in 1904 it was made a separate administration with its own resident commissioner. Since 1974 it has been a self-governing territory in free association with New Zealand, which in addition to providing economic assistance, has responsibility for the territory's defence and foreign policy.

Constitutional structure

Under the Niue Constitution Act of 1974, executive power is vested in the British monarch as sovereign of New Zealand. On a day-to-day basis this power is exercised by a Premier and an appointed three-member Cabinet, who are responsible to the Niue Assembly. The legislature comprises 20 members and chooses the Premier from among its numbers. There is also a resident New Zealand Representative whose responsibility it is to liaise between the Niue and New Zealand governments.

Electoral system

Of the 20 legislators in the Assembly, 14 are elected as village representatives and six are elected on a common roll.

Evolution of the suffrage

The first legislature was established in 1960 consisting of an elected representative from each of the 13 villages, operating under the presidency of the commissioner. Further powers were delegated over the years, until self-government was achieved in 1974. Elections are held on the basis of universal adult suffrage.

Recent elections

Elections have been held regularly since 1960. In the April 8, 1990 election Sir Robert Rex, the Prime Minister since 1974, was returned to power.

PARTY BY PARTY DATA

Niue People's Action Party (NPAP)
Address. c/o Niue Assembly, Alofi, Niue.
Leadership. Young Vivian (l.).
Orientation. Opposition.
Founded. 1986.
History. The Niue People's Action Party (NPAP) was founded by Sani Lakatani as an opposition movement to the Rex government. It won a single seat in the 1986 election, although Lakatani failed to secure election to the Assembly. Despite the party's poor election showing, it was revitalized under the leadership Young Vivian. In the 1990 general election, together with its sympathizers, it won 12 of the 20 seats in the legislature. The party's attempts to take control of the gov-

ernment were foiled, however, when Sir Robert Rex, using all of his political experience and powers of patronage, induced four opposition legislators to defect to the government benches.

In September 1990 Rex dismissed two of his three Cabinet colleagues for joining opposition calls for a change of Premier, but he once again preserved his majority by appointing Young Vivian and another opposition member to the Cabinet. When the legislature convened in October 1990, one of the those dismissed moved a vote of no confidence which was defeated by 15 votes to five. Despite vociferous opposition criticism of the Premier's tactics for remaining in office, the government survived throughout 1991 and appeared stable enough to carry Rex through to the next election.

Major guerrilla groups

There are no guerrilla groups operating on Niue.

Tokelau

Capital: Each of Tokelau's three atolls has its own administrative centre

Population: 1,690 (1986—there are also 2,316 Tokelauans resident in New Zealand)

The Tokelau islands are a non-self-governing territory under New Zealand administration. Originally discovered by Europeans in the 18th century, they became a British protectorate in 1877. Administrative control was transferred to New Zealand in 1926, and sovereignty was transferred in 1949. In 1976 the territory was officially redesignated Tokelau.

Constitutional structure

All executive and administrative authority is vested in an appointed Administrator, who is responsible to New Zealand's Minister of Foreign Affairs. In practice, most powers are delegated to the Official Secretary who heads the Office of Tokelau Affairs, which is based in Apia, Western Samoa.

Tokelau has a General Fono, where 15 representatives from each of the three atolls meet about twice a year to discuss matters of territorial importance. The Fono is jointly chaired by the heads of the territory's three atolls, the *Faipule*. The delegations also include *pulenuku* (mayors) of each atoll and town.

Electoral system

The *Faipule* and *pulenuku* are elected for three-year terms.

Evolution of the suffrage

Elections take place on the basis of universal adult suffrage.

Recent elections

Elections for *Faipule* were held in January 1990.

PARTY BY PARTY DATA

There are no political parties in Tokelau.

Major guerrilla groups

There are no guerrilla groups operating in Tokelau.

Ross Dependency

The Ross Dependency, a non-self-governing territory under New Zealand administration, comprises eastern Antarctica and its associated islands. It includes a land area of 400,000 sq km and an ice-shelf of 330,000 sq km. Apart from scientific personnel, it is uninhabited and has no political parties or guerrilla groups.

Pakistan

Capital: Islamabad   **Population: 122,600,000 (1990)**

The Islamic Republic of Pakistan was proclaimed in March 1956, Pakistan having gained independence as a British dominion following the partition of India in August 1947. A federal parliamentary system operated until 1958 when Gen. Ayub Khan seized power in a military coup. The overthrow of Gen. Ayub Khan in 1970 led to the country's first direct general election later that year. Although Zulfikar Ali Bhutto's Pakistan People's Party (PPP) won a majority of seats in West Pakistan (later Pakistan), Sheikh Mujibur Rahman's Awami League won an overall majority, taking almost all seats in East Pakistan (later Bangladesh).

The Awami League's success and the reluctance of West Pakistan to accept an East Pakistan-led national government precipitated a civil war, military confrontation with India, and the creation of the new state of Bangladesh within the borders of East Pakistan in 1971. In the West, Bhutto ruled until his overthrow by Gen. Mohammad Zia ul-Haq in 1977. Zia promised a swift return to civilian rule, but postponed elections twice before his assassination in 1988. Following the elections in November 1988, Bhutto's daughter, Benazir, by then leader of the PPP, became Prime Minister. The PPP government was dismissed by President Ghulam Ishaq Khan in August 1990. Fresh elections in October led to the formation of a coalition government under Nawaz Sharif, leader of the Islamic Democratic Alliance.

Constitutional structure

Under the terms of the (amended) 1973 Constitution, the Islamic Republic of Pakistan is governed by an executive President who appoints an executive Prime Minister. There is a bicameral legislature consisting of a National Assembly and a Senate. Each of Pakistan's four provinces (Punjab, North-West Frontier, Sind and Baluchistan) has its own executive government, headed by a presidentially appointed Governor.

Electoral system

The 1973 Constitution provides for a parliamentary system and a bicameral Federal Legislature. The National Assembly is elected by universal adult suffrage for a five-year term; of the 237 members, 10 are elected to represent the country's non-Muslim minorities and an additional 20 women members are nominated by the four provincial assemblies. The 87 members of the Senate, elected by the National and provincial assemblies, each serve a six-year term, with one-third of their number relinquishing their seats at two-yearly intervals.

The President is elected at a joint sitting of the two chambers of the Federal Legislature for a renewable five-year term.

Evolution of the suffrage

There is universal adult suffrage for all citizens aged 21 and over.

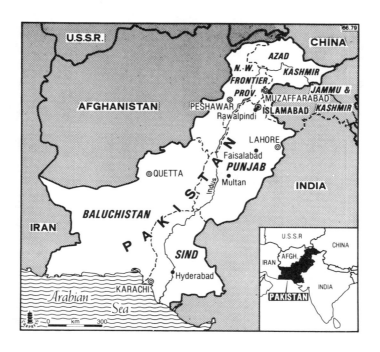

Recent elections

1988 and 1990 National Assembly elections

	Elective seats	
	1988	*1990*
Awami National Party	—	6
Islamic Democratic Alliance	54	105
Jamiat Ulema-i-Islam	8	6
Jamhoori Watan Party	—	2
Muhajir Qaumi Mahaz	13	15
Pakistan People's Party	93	45
Others	22	17
Independents	27	21
Total	217	217

PARTY BY PARTY DATA

Awami National Party (ANP)

Leadership. Khan Abdul Wali Khan (pres.); Ghulam Ahmed Bilour (l.); H. B. Naarejo (vice-pres.).

Address. 16/11 Khayabbane Shujat, Karachi, 755 00.

Orientation. Left-wing; power-base in North West Frontier Province; supported the Soviet-backed government in Afghanistan and has called for the removal of "all vestiges of imperialist domination" in Pakistan.

Founded. July 1986.

History. The ANP was formed by a merger of four regional left-wing parties within the Movement for the Restoration of Democracy (MRD): the National Democratic Party (NDP), the Workers' and Peasants' Party, People's Movement (*Awami Tehrik*) and the Pakistan National Party (PNP). Soon after its formation, the ANP moved to distance itself from the Pakistan People's Party, the leading component of the MRD.

The party's senior vice-president, Fazil Rahu, who had been detained without trial from August 1983 until June 1986, was killed in early 1987; while the police claimed that the murder was part of a long-standing family feud, the ANP maintained that the national intelligence service had been responsible.

The ANP fought the 1990 general election in alliance with the victorious Islamic Democratic Alliance, the ANP winning six seats, and Bilour was given a ministerial appointment in Nawaz Sharif's government.

Conference of Ulema of Islam

Jamiat-i-Ulema-i-Islam (JUI, also known as the Association of Islamic Religious Scholars)

Leadership. Maulana Fazlur Rahman (pres.); Maulana Mufti Mahmud (l.).

Orientation. Islamic fundamentalist, favouring a full restoration of democracy and the establishment of an Islamic state with a constitution based on Sunni Islamic principles.

Founded. 1945.

History. Formerly allied with the National Awami Party (which was banned in 1975), the JUI was a founder member of the Pakistan National Alliance (PNA) formed in January 1977 to contest the March 1977 general elections against the then ruling Pakistan People's Party, the JUI leader becoming president of the PNA. Following the military takeover of July 1977, the party accepted representation in President Zia's government in 1979 but continued to press for an early end to martial law and the holding of democratic elections.

The JUI subsequently became associated with the Movement for the Restoration of Democracy (MRD), and sought to act as a bridge between the opposition and the government. In August 1987 party president Maulana Fazlur Rahman presided over an "all parties conference" of opposition formations held in Lahore, but a prior meeting between him and leading government figures caused some parties to boycott the conference (which nevertheless adopted a joint declaration calling for President Zia's resignation and the holding of democratic elections). In the elections held shortly after Zia's assassination in 1988 the JUI won eight seats. The party opposed the Pakistan People's Party (PPP) government formed as a result of the elections, allying itself instead with the Islamic Democratic Alliance (IDA). The party won six seats in the 1990 elections.

Conference of Ulema of Pakistan (JUP)

Jamaat-i-Ulema-i-Pakistan (also known as the Association of Pakistani Religious Scholars)

Address. Burns Road, Karachi.

Leadership. Maulana Shah Ahmad Noorani (pres.); Maulana Abdul Sattar Khan Niazi (sec.-gen.).

Orientation. Sunni Muslim, progressive Islamic fundamentalist.

Founded. 1968.

History. Established by left-wing *mullahs* (clerics), the JUP gained seven seats in the 1970 National Assembly elections. In 1977 it became one of the original members of the Pakistan National Alliance (PNA) opposed to the then ruling Pakistan People's Party (PPP), but broke away the following year. The party was a founder member of the Movement for the Restoration of Democracy (MRD) in 1981, but withdrew from the alliance after a few months. The party boycotted the 1984 referendum on the government's Islamization programme, the 1985 "none-party" elections and the 1987 "all parties conference" of opposition groups.

Following the 1990 general election the JUP joined the Islamic Democratic Alliance government. Party secretary-general Maulana Niazi resigned from Nawaz Sharif's government in March 1991 over the government's Gulf War policy, but was reappointed six months later.

Islamic Assembly (Pakistan)

Jamaat-i-Islami (Pakistan) (JIP)

Address. Mansoorah, Multan Road, Lahore.

Leadership. Mian Tufail Mohammad (pres.); Qazi Hussain Ahmad (l.); Muhammad Aslam Saleemi (sec.-gen.).

Orientation. Sunni Muslim, right-wing ultra-orthodox Islamic fundamentalist party; support base in the lower middle class.

Founded. 1941.

History. Initially opposed to the creation of Pakistan on the grounds that its creation did not presuppose an Islamic state, the JIP has consistently advocated increased Islamization.

It won four seats in the 1970 general election and contested the 1977 election as part of the Pakistan National Alliance (PNA) in opposition to the ruling Pakistan People's Party (PPP). The party was expelled from the PNA in 1979 after accepting representation in President Zia's government and it went on to provide broad support to the Zia regime. However, in mid-1987 the party boycotted the National Assembly in protest against what it regarded as official hesitation in implementing the Islamization programme approved by referendum in 1984.

The JIP joined the Islamic Democratic Alliance in 1988 and in the 1990 elections won eight National Assembly seats, making it the second-strongest party within the government. In May 1992 the party withdrew from the Alliance, ostensibly in response to Nawaz Sharif's refusal to back the extremist *mujaheddin* faction of Gulbuddin Hekmatyar in Afghanistan. However, the party had also criticized Nawaz Sharif for failing to implement the process of Islamization.

Structure. The party has a militant student organization, *Jamiat-i-Talaba* (JIT), members of which have been involved in clashes with rival groups at universities.

Publications. The party organ is *Jasarat*.

Islamic Democratic Alliance (IDA)

Islami Jumhuri Ittehad

Leadership. Mian Nawaz Sharif (ch.).

Orientation. Right-wing; favours the systematic introduction of Islamic law (*Sharia*).

Founded. 1988.

History. An alliance formed to represent nine right-wing and Islamic parties in the elections of 1988, the IDA opposed the Pakistan People's Party (PPP)-led Movement for the Restoration of Democracy (MRD). It gained 54 seats in the 1988 elections, compared with 93 for the PPP. With the removal of Benazir Bhutto's PPP government in 1990, the IDA triumphed in the general election held later that year, gaining 105 seats. After the elections the IDA became the dominant partner in the country's ruling coalition and its chair, Nawaz Sharif, was appointed Prime Minister. It further increased its power with substantial gains in the May 1991 elections to the Senate.

The parties making up the IDA include: the Conference of *Ulema* of Islam; the Conference of *Ulema* of Pakistan; the Muslim League (Chatta and Pagaro factions); the Islamic People of the Traditions; the System of the Prophet; and the Society of Religious Elders.

The Islamic Assembly withdrew from the Alliance in May 1991 and the Holy War Movement and the National People's Party (NPP) were expelled in September 1991 and March 1992, respectively.

Movement for the Restoration of Democracy (MRD)

Address. c/o PPP, 70 Clifton Road, Karachi.

Leadership. Collective, with the Pakistan People's Party (PPP) acting as convener.

Orientation. The MRD is the umbrella organization of mainly left-wing parties who were opposed to the government of President Zia and seek a return to full democracy on the basis of the 1973 Constitution.

Founded. February 1981.

History. The MRD was launched on Feb. 5-6, 1981, when the leaders of nine opposition parties signed a declaration calling for President Zia's resignation and the holding of free and fair elections within three months. The nine original components were the PPP, the Solidarity Party of Pakistan (*Tehrik-i-Istiqlal-i-Pakistan*), the National Democratic Party (NDP), the Pakistan Republican Party (PRP), the Conference of Ulema of Pakistan (JUP), the anti-Zia faction of the Pakistan Muslim League (PML), the Kashmir Muslim Conference (KMC), the Nation Liberation Front (NLF) and the Workers' and Peasants' Party (*Mazdoor Kisan* Party).

Over succeeding years the composition of the MRD underwent various changes, including (i) the withdrawal of the JUP in late 1981; (ii) membership of the Conference of Ulema of Islam (iii) membership of the Pakistan National Party (PNP) in 1983; (iv) membership of the People's Movement in 1984; and (v) the withdrawal of the Solidarity Party of Pakistan in October 1986. Meanwhile, the NDP, the Workers' and Peasants' Party, the PNP and the People's Movement had in July 1986 formed the Awami National Party (ANP) as a left-wing bloc of regional parties within the MRD, while in May 1987 an application for membership was reportedly submitted by the Communist Party of Pakistan (banned since 1954).

The appointment in late 1981 of a Federal Advisory Council to act as a bridge between the martial law administration and a future Islamic democratic government was described by MRD leaders as an attempt to "hoodwink the national and the outside world" into believing that the military regime was committed to the restoration of democracy. In the course of 1982 the MRD also condemned President Zia's proposal of May 6 calling for the creation of a "Higher Command Council" where the armed forces would have a permanent role in decision-making, as well as a scheme to hold non-party elections. At the same time it pressed for the release of political detainees, claiming in a statement issued in June 1982 that 5,000 political workers were in detention and that 300 had been tortured.

A civil disobedience campaign, launched by the MRD in August 1983 in protest against the continuation of martial law, was intended to be nationwide but in fact gained substantial support only in Sind province, where President Zia deployed troops after rejecting the MRD's demand for collective discussions between the government and the political parties. In the ensuing violence more than 5,000 opposition leaders (mostly from the PPP) were arrested and the death toll by the end of September 1983 was estimated at between 60 and 160. Nearly all those arrested were released by the end of January 1984.

The MRD called for a boycott of the December 1984 referendum in which President Zia secured overwhelming endorsement for his Islamization programme (in a turnout officially given as 62 per cent). It also urged a boycott of the non-party parliamentary elections held in February 1985, during which period over 2,000 MRD activists were detained. Following the lifting of martial law on Jan. 1, 1986, the MRD staged further mass demonstrations calling for full democratization, the campaign being given fresh impetus in April 1984 by the return from exile in London of Benazir Bhutto, who along with her mother, Nusrat Bhutto assumed joint leadership of the PPP.

The partial return to civilian rule and the passage of legislation in December 1985 enabling parties to apply for legal registration created divisions within the MRD from February 1986. Whereas the PPP and other component parties refused to register on grounds that it

would legitimize military rule, the Solidarity Party of Pakistan favoured registration (and later left the MRD). At the same time, some sections of the MRD objected to the high profile assumed by Benazir Bhutto, who was described as "extremely arrogant" by Khwaja Khairuddin (leader of the anti-Zia PML) who became secretary-general of the MRD in July 1986.

Disunity in the MRD resurfaced followed the creation in July 1986 of a left-wing regional alliance, the Awami National Party (ANP), which declined to participate in further national protest actions called by the MRD in August and September 1986. An "all parties conference" held in Lahore in February 1987 failed to overcome emerging differences within the MRD.

Further dissension arose in November 1987 when the PPP contested local council elections, in contravention of the established MRD strategy of boycotting all elections while President Zia remained in power. A degree of unity was restored after a meeting of the MRD's executive committee agreed in Rawalpindi in January 1988 that the movement would continue as an alliance of independent parties. The restoration of parliamentary democracy following general elections in November 1988, effectively signalled the decline of the MRD and its reason for being.

Muhajir Qaumi Movement (MQM)

Leadership. Altaf Hussain (ch.); Azim Ahmed Tarq (gen. sec.).

Founded. 1986.

Orientation. Represents the interests of Urdu-speaking Muslim migrants and calls for the recognition of Muhajirs (Urdu-speaking immigrants from India) as the fifth nationality of Pakistan, on the premise that they have been exploited by the Pathans and the Punjabis and subject to discrimination in employment and education.

History. In Jan. 1987, the MQM called for a strike in protest against the murder of a Mohajir man and his two daughters, provoking clashes with the police in Karachi and Hyderabad. Part of the Muslim League, the MQM won 13 seats in the 1988 elections. After a brief period of co-operation with the victorious PPP-led ruling coalition, the MQM withdrew from the Bhutto government in 1990, severely weakening its position.

In the October 1990 general elections the MQM won 15 out of 217 National Assembly seats and made substantial inroads into the PPP's traditional constituency in Sind where it gained 47 out of 100 seats (the PPP winning only 43). The increased standing of the

MQM at the national and provincial level enabled it to command important ministerial posts in Sind and control up to two portfolios in the national Cabinet. Although allied to the ruling coalition, the MQM did not form a component part of the Islamic Democratic Alliance (IDA) and it abstained from voting on the *Sharia* Bill in May 1991.

By early 1992 relations between the MQM and the IDA-led ruling coalition had deteriorated, in part as a result of the breakdown in law and order in Sind, much of which was attributed to armed gangs loyal to the MQM. In June 1992 the Sharif government authorized large-scale military intervention in Sind which led to the arrest of hundreds of MQM supporters. On June 27 the MQM announced its decision to leave the ruling coalition alleging "victimization" by the army. Meanwhile, there were unconfirmed reports that two MQM federal ministers had also resigned. The resignation of eight MQM deputies in the National Assembly and 10 in the Sind assembly was officially confirmed in July.

National Liberation Front (NLF)
Qaumi Mahaz Azadi
Leadership. Miraj Mohammed Khan (pres.).
Orientation. The NLF supports full democracy, "the rights of the downtrodden", and the maximum possible regional autonomy.
Founded. October 1977.
History. The NLF was launched following the 1977 military coup and welcomed the overthrow of Zulfikar Ali Bhutto (of the Pakistan People's Party) while demanding that elections should be held as soon as possible. The party subsequently joined the Movement of the Restoration of Democracy (MRD) founded in February 1981. Its president (who had been a junior minister in the pre-1977 Bhutto government) was detained in the August 1983 civil disturbances, allegedly tortured and released in June 1985.

National People's Party (NPP)
Leadership. Ghulam Mustafa Jatoi (chair.); S. M. Zafar (chief organizer).
Orientation. Centrist, calls for democracy.
Founded. August 1986.
History. The NPP was founded by Ghulam Mustafa Jatoi, who had left the Pakistan People's Party (PPP)—of which he had been Sind provincial chairman—after disagreement with its leader, Benazir Bhutto. The NPP aimed to be a centrist party, willing to negotiate with the government. While still a member of the PPP, Jatoi had reportedly twice been offered the country's pre-

miership (in December 1984 and January 1985) but had declined, ostensibly because of doubts centring on the regime's commitment to democracy. Jatoi was appointed acting Prime Minister in August 1990 following the dismissal of Benazir Bhutto. He was succeeded in November 1990 by Nawaz Sharif, chairman of the coalition Islamic Democratic Alliance which won a majority of seats in the general elections held in October.

The NPP, which formed one of nine parties of the IDA in 1988, was expelled from the ruling coalition in March 1992 for allegedly co-operating with the PPP against the government.

Pakistan Muslim League (Chatta Group) (PML—Chatta))
Leadership. Khwaja Khairuddin (pres.); Malik Mohammed Qasim (sec.-gen.).
Orientation. This faction of the historic Muslim League opposed the regime of President Zia.
Founded. August 1978.
History. The PML (Chatta) was formed by League dissidents led by Chowhury Mohammed Hussein Chatta who rejected the party's decision to accept government posts under President Zia (the pro-Zia faction becoming known as the PML-Pagaro). The breakaway group immediately experienced internal division, from which Khwaja Khairuddin emerged as leader. As a senior vice-president of the League before the 1978 split, Khairuddin had publicly criticized the Pakistan People's Party (PPP) government of Zulfikar Ali Bhutto. In February 1981 Khairuddin allied with the PPP (now led by Nusrat Bhutto) and seven other opposition parties to launch the Movement for the Restoration of Democracy (MRD), of which he later became secretary-general.

From early 1986 the PML (Chatta) was increasingly involved in internal divisions within the MRD, which were exacerbated by the return to Pakistan in April 1986 of Bhutto's daughter Benazir, who assumed joint leadership of the PPP. In July 1986 Khairuddin resigned as MRD secretary-general after questioning Benazir Bhutto's political experience and high public profile. The PML (Chatta) nevertheless remained a component party of the MRD playing an active part in its campaign to secure the resignation of Gen Zia.

The Chatta and Pagaro factions of the Muslim League together contested the 1988 elections, and in 1988 both joined the Islamic Democratic Alliance coalition which subsequently formed the ruling coalition in November 1990.

Pakistan Muslim League (Pagaro Group) (PML—Pagaro)

Address. Muslim League House, 33 Davis Street, Karachi.

Leadership. Mohammad Khan Junejo (pres.); Iqbal Ahmed Khan (sec. gen.).

Orientation. Conservative, traditionally supported by landowners and larger farmers.

Founded. 1962.

History. The PML (Pagaro) derives from the division into three main factions in 1962 of the historic Muslim League of Muhammad Ali Jinnah. The dominant formation was led by President Ayub Khan. Largely eclipsed under the government of Zulfikar Ali Bhutto, the PML adopted a conciliatory posture towards the military regime led by Gen. Zia, accepting government post for its representatives in July 1987. The move triggered a split which led to the formation of a breakaway progressive faction, the PML (Chatta), leaving the conservative group under the religious leadership of the Pir of Pagaro to continue its co-operation with the government.

Although the February 1985 National Assembly elections were conducted on a non-party basis, over three-quarters of the successful candidates were in fact associated with the PML (Pagaro) formation, whose political leader, Mohammad Khan Junejo, was appointed Prime Minister the following month. Shortly after the lifting of martial law on Jan. 1, 1986, Junejo was elected president of the existing formation, which in February 1986 became the first major party to register with the Election Commission under the latest Political Parties Act (adopted in December 1985).

The new status of the PML (Pagaro) as the official ruling party was confirmed in May 1986 when the Speaker of the National Assembly, an independent, was replaced by a government nominee, after he had agreed to refer to the Chief Electoral Commissioner an objection raised by some members that the Prime Minister and other members of his party should be disqualified from the Assembly because they had declared their membership of a political party before that party had been legally registered. At the same time, President Zia issued an ordinance suspending the relevant disqualification clause of the Political Parties Act, which if applied would have entailed by-elections for some 170 seats held by the Prime Minister's party.

From mid-1987 the ruling party was left virtually without opposition in the Assembly, whose non-PML members began boycotting proceedings in protest, principally, against government economic policy. In countrywide local elections held in November 1987 the ruling PML registered major successes, largely at the expense of the opposition Pakistan People's Party.

The two factions contested the 1988 elections together, and in 1988 both joined the Islamic Democratic Alliance coalition which was elected to power in 1990.

Pakistan People's Party (PPP)

Address. 70 Clifton Road, Karachi.

Leadership. Benazir Bhutto (co-ch.); Begum Nusrat Bhutto (co-ch.); Sheikh Rafiq Ahmad (gen. sec.); Makhdoom Mohammed Zaman Talib-ul-Maula (sr. vice-pres.).

Orientation. At its foundation the PPP described its policy as one of Islamic socialism, democracy and independence in foreign affairs; since the 1977 military coup it has led the opposition campaign for a full restoration of democracy.

Founded. Dec. 1, 1967.

History. The PPP was founded by Zulfikar Ali Bhutto, who had held various ministerial appointments since 1958, including the foreign affairs portfolio in 1963-66, In June 1966 he resigned from the government of President Ayub Khan and denounced it as "a dictatorship with the label of democracy". The East Pakistan branch of the PPP was dissolved on March 3, 1969, after Bhutto had failed to support East Pakistan's demand for full autonomy. In the first general election held in Pakistan under universal suffrage on Dec. 17, 1970, the PPP gained 181 of the 291 contested seats in the National Assembly (all but one in the Punjab and Sind provinces), and became the strongest party in West Pakistan.

Following the secession of East Pakistan (subsequently Bangladesh) in December 1971, Bhutto succeeded Gen. Yahya Khan as President of (West) Pakistan and appointed a Cabinet in which he and other PPP members predominated. Martial law was maintained until April 1972 during which the PPP government introduced numerous reforms in the social, educational and economic fields.

In October 1972 the PPP reached agreement with other major political parties on a new Constitution providing for a federal, parliamentary government, which was adopted by the National Assembly in April 1973 (with all-party support). Under the new Constitution Bhutto relinquished the office of President on Aug. 13, 1973, after being elected Prime Minister by the National Assembly on the previous day. In the Senate elected in July 1973, the PPP held 35 of the 45 seats.

In a Cabinet reshuffle in October 1974 Bhutto remained Prime Minister and retained the Foreign Affairs and Defence portfolios. In 1975 the PPP was weakened by the defection of a number of its leading members; among them, Ghulam Mustafa Khar, former Governor and Chief Minister of the Punjab, who resigned from the PPP in September 1975, accusing Bhutto of imposing a dictatorship. In the general election held on March 7, 1977, the PPP gained 155 of the 200 general seats in the National Assembly amid allegations by opposition parties of widespread vote-rigging. Khar later rejoined the PPP and, in June 1977, was appointed political adviser to Bhutto.

The PPP government was overthrown in July 1977 following a bloodless military coup led by Army Chief of Staff Gen. Mohammad Zia ul-Haq. By August 1977, several leading PPP members had withdrawn their support from Bhutto, among them Mir Taj Mohammad Khan Jamali (former Minister of Health), who announced on Aug. 13 that he would form an independent group which would contest the general election (scheduled for October but later postponed) in co-operation with the Pakistan National Alliance (PNA).

On Sept. 3, 1977, Bhutto was arrested on charges of conspiracy to murder; he was found guilty and sentenced to death on March 18, 1978, amid widespread popular demonstrations in his favour, particularly in Punjab and Sind. On Oct. 1, 1978, Zia postponed the proposed elections indefinitely on the grounds that the election campaign had resulted in "a state of confrontation . . . between the political parties".

Meanwhile, mounting international criticism of the death sentence imposed on Bhutto failed to win a reprieve or secure a presidential pardon. On Feb. 6, 1979 the Supreme Court dismissed Bhutto's appeal against his sentence by a narrow majority, although a subsequent judgement delivered on March 4, 1979, implicitly ruled against the death sentence. Bhutto's execution by hanging, announced on April 4, 1979, fuelled reports attributed to his daughter, Benazir who claimed that her father had died in a struggle with officers after refusing to accept voluntary exile from Pakistan sign in return for clemency.

The period following Bhutto's execution heralded the start of an uneasy modus vivendi between the Zia regime and the PPP, now under Bhutto's widow, Begum Nusrat Bhutto.

Meanwhile, in non-party elections to municipal and district councils held between Sept. 20 and 27, 1979, in all four provinces resulted in a victory for candidates backed by the PPP who were reported to have won between 60 and 80 per cent of the seats in Punjab and the NWFP, with many returned unopposed in Sind. In Rawalpindi, 31 of the 50 seats were won by PPP-supported candidates, most of whom had been imprisoned or flogged under President Zia's regime.

The PPP was one of four major parties (the others being the Pakistan National Alliance, the National Democratic Party and the Pakistan National Party) which refused to seek registration under an amended Political Parties Act in force in September 1979. On Oct. 16, 1979, the President announced that the rescheduled general elections had been postponed indefinitely, and that all political parties stood dissolved. The announcement was followed by the arrest of numerous political leaders (officially stated on Oct. 21 to number 372) and the banning of the PPP newspapers *Musawat* and *Sadaqat*.

In February 1981 the PPP joined with eight other opposition parties to launch the Movement for the Restoration of Democracy (MRD). A petition by the PPP calling for the restoration of democracy was dismissed by the Supreme Court on April 27, 1981. Meanwhile, Begum Bhutto and her daughter, who had been placed in detention in mid-March 1981, were released and placed under house arrest in July and December respectively. In late 1981 the government initiated legal proceedings against the Bhutto family for the recovery of assets allegedly misappropriated by Zulfikar Ali Bhutto for personal and party use during his period of office.

In November 1982 Begum Bhutto left Pakistan for Europe to seek medical treatment; Benazir was released from house arrest in January 1984 to go to London. She returned to Pakistan on July 18, 1985, to bury her brother Shahnawaz (an alleged member of the militant pro-PPP *Al Zulfiqar* movement), and was placed under house arrest in Aug. 29. Bhutto returned to England on Nov. 4, but went back to Pakistan on April 10, 1986, to be elected co-chairman of the party along with Nusrat Bhutto. Within the party she replaced some longstanding officials, notably Ghulam Mustafa Jatoi, then president of the Sind branch of the PPP, who left the party in August to form the National People's Party).

While remaining committed to participation in the MRD, in 1986-87 the PPP became increasingly involved in conflict between the constituent parties over policy and strategy. This intensified when Benazir Bhutto (by now effectively the sole leader of the party, her mother having retired from active politics) unilaterally decided that the PPP would participate in the November 1987 local council elections, notwithstanding established MRD policy that all elections would be boycotted until President Zia resigned. Moreover, the PPP's poor showing in these elections strengthened opposition within the party to her style of leadership and her alleged abandonment of the party's socialist principles.

In the general election held after the death of Zia in 1988 the PPP won a majority in all four provinces. Bhutto became Pakistan's first woman Prime Minister, thus incurring the opposition of Islamic parties. In early 1989 a group of Islamic religious leaders issued a ruling (*fatwa*) to the PPP to dismiss Bhutto and elect a male Prime Minister.

By mid-1990 the popularity of Bhutto's government had declined considerably due to allegations of corruption, economic mismanagement and a steady breakdown in law and order. On Aug. 6, President Ghulam Ishaq Khan dismissed the Bhutto government, claiming that he had acted within his constitutional rights. The general election held in October 1990 resulted in a defeat for the PPP which accused the interim government of vote-rigging and "massive fraud across the country".

Before the elections seven charges had been filed against Bhutto, mostly for improper use of public funds and resources. Her husband and many former ministers were also charged with fraud and other financial irregularities. Allegations against the government of carrying out a political vendetta against the PPP and its allies gained momentum in December 1991 when the son-in-law of President Ghulam Ishaq Khan was implicated in the gang rape of a close friend of Benazir Bhutto. By mid-1992 the PPP had regained the political initiative, encouraged by internal divisions in the ruling coalition and the army crackdown against the Mohajir Qaumi Mahaz (MQM), the PPP's chief political rival in Sind.

Publications. Musawat and *Sadaqat*.

Solidarity Party of Pakistan
Tehrik-i-Istiqlal-i-Pakistan (TIP)
Leadership. Air Marshal Asghar Khan (pres.); Ashaf Vardag (acting pres.); Musheer Ahmad Pesh Imam (sec.-gen.).
Orientation. Seeking to maintain both Islamic and secular values.
Founded. 1968.
History. The TIP was one of the three major parties

which registered with the Election Commission by Sept. 30, 1979. Previously it had been a constituent party of the Pakistan National Alliance (PNA) formed in January 1977 but had withdrawn from it in November of that year.

Although, like all other parties, the TIP was banned in October 1979, its central working committee met in Lahore on April 5-6, 1980, and demanded the immediate ending of martial law, elections to the National and Provincial Assemblies and the release of political prisoners. Air Marshal Asghar Khan was released from house arrest on April 18, but was again placed under house arrest on May 29 after making speeches denouncing the martial law regime. On Aug. 8, 1980, Ashaf Vardag called for a *jihad* (holy war) against the government and said that the only way to end the martial law regime was by co-operation between all parties opposed to it, including the Pakistan People's Party.

In February 1981 the TIP joined with eight other parties in the Movement for the Restoration of Democracy (MRD) to campaign for an end to martial law and a return to parliamentary democracy. Following President Zia's creation at the end of 1981 of an appointed Federal Advisory Council to act as a bridge between the martial law administration and a future Islamic democratic government, Mian Manzoor Ahmed Watoo (a leading member of the TIP) said that the formation of the Council was "a bogus stunt devoid of all meaning and content" and that only an elected assembly could have a mandate for constitutional change.

Unlike other members of the MRD, the party favoured registration under the new Political Parties Act of December 1985. It subsequently refused to join anti-government protest actions in mid-1986 and formally seceded from the MRD on Oct. 12, 1986.

Prior to the elections of 1988, the party allied with the Conference of *Ulema* of Pakistan to form the People's Alliance of Pakistan. Later it became part of the ruling coalition Islamic Democratic Alliance.

Minor parties

Baluchistan National Alliance; leadership: Nawab Mohammad Akbar Bugti (l.). Small regionally based party.

Democratic National Party (*Jamhoori Watan* Party); leadership: Nawab Akbar Bugti. This party won two seats in the 1990 general election.

Pakistan Force of the Companions of the Prophet (*Sipah-i-Sahabah-i-Pakistan*); militant Sunni Muslim organization. Its leader, Muhammad Ghiassudin, was reportedly assassinated in May 1992 during sectarian clashes with Shia militants .

Holy War (*Hizbe Jihad*); leadership: Murtaza Pooya. Small Shia grouping that originally formed part of the Islamic Democratic Alliance. It was expelled from the ruling coalition in September 1991 for allegedly co-operating with opposition parties.

Islamic People of the Traditions (*Islamic Ahle Hadith*); leadership: Maulana Moinuddin LakviMaulana Moinuddin (chief spokesman). Rooted in the conservative Indo-Muslim reform movement, the party was formed in the 1970s in reaction to Shia activism. It is currently a member of the ruling Islamic Democratic Alliance.

Kashmir Muslim Conference (KMC); leadership: Chowdhury Noor Hussein (pres.). Represents the interests of the people of the disputed region of Azad Kashmir.

Movement for the Implementation of the Shia Code (*Tehrik-i-Nifaz-i-Fiqah-i-Jafria*); leadership: Hamid Ali Shah Mousavi. Founded in 1979, registered as a political party, 1987. A Shia grouping formed to oppose the allegedly Sunni bias of Zia's Islamization programme. In 1990, the Movement joined the Pakistan Democratic Alliance, the loose coalition led by the Pakistan People's Party.

Pakistani Democratic Alliance (PDA). Founded in 1990. A loose grouping including the Pakistan People's Party and the Movement for the Implementation of the Shia Code formed in response to the Islamic Democratic Alliance.

Pakistan Democratic Party (PDP); leadership: Nawabzada Nasrullah Khan (l.); Sheikh Nasim Hasan (sec.-gen.). A moderate Islamic and democratic party. Founded in June 1969. The PDP was formed by a merger of four previous right-wing parties: the Justice Party, the National Democratic Front, *Nizam-i-Islami* and the West Pakistan Awami League. In the 1970 elections it gained only one seat in the National Assembly (in East Pakistan). In 1977 it joined the Pakistan National Alliance. Nawabzada Nasrullah Khan, the PDP leader, was one of the three opposition leaders

arrested on Feb. 16, 1981, in a move by the authorities to prevent exploitation of student riots then in progress throughout Pakistan. Following the resumption of qualified civilian rule in 1985-86, the PDP was largely eclipsed by the emergent Pakistan Muslim League led by the new Prime Minister, Mohammed Khan Junejo.

Pakistan Khaksar Party; leadership: Mohammad Ashraf Khan (pres.). Founded during period of British rule. An militant Islamic party. which was dissolved in 1947, but revived later.

Sind-Baluchistan Patriotic Front (SBFP); leadership: Mumtaz Ali Bhutto. Founded in 1986. Advocates independence for young Sindhis. The Front was criticized in Dec. 1986 by Prime Minister Junejo for openly propagating "parochial ideologies".

Sind National Alliance; leadership: G. M. Syed (ch.). Founded in 1988.

Society for the Expansion of the Majority (*Sawaad-i Azam*); leadership: Maulana Azam Asvandyar. Sectarian Sunni (Hanafi) organization established in the late 1970s to counter growing Shia assertiveness which is active among Urdu-speakers in Karachi. It favours a Sunni-based Islamic constitution for Pakistan which would affirm and expand the rights of the Sunni majority against the Shia minority.

Students' Society (*Jamiat-i-Talaba*); leadership: Shabbir Ahmed. The Youth Wing of the *Jamiat-i-Islami*. A rigidly orthodox right-wing fundamentalist organization strongly opposed to the emancipation of women and to Western influences in education. Gen. Zia's ban on student organizations imposed in February 1984 sparked off two months of student protest, and three student leaders were sentenced to 15 lashes and one year's imprisonment after disrupting a meeting addressed by Zia on March 12 in Peshawar.

System of the Prophet (*Nizam-i-Mustapha*); leadership: Maulana Abdul Sattar Khan Niazi (also leader of the Conference of Ulema of Pakistan). Joined the Islamic Democratic Alliance in 1988 which won the October 1990 general election to form the country's ruling coalition.

Principal illegal organizations

There are no major illegal organizations in Pakistan;

the Bhuttoist **Al Zulfiqar** carried out subversive operations against the Zia regime, but has been dormant since Zia's death. With the creation of Bangladesh in 1971, the banned **Communist Party of Pakistan** was left with no support base and has since had little impact on politics in Pakistan.

Papua New Guinea

Capital: Port Moresby   **Population: 3,900,000 (1990)**

Discovered by Europeans in the 16th century, the western half of the island of New Guinea (now Irian Jaya) was later colonized by the Dutch, whilst the eastern portion, which later became the state of Papua New Guinea, was divided between Germany and Britain. The territory of Papua New Guinea was created after the Pacific War, and independence was granted in September 1975.

The combination of weak political parties and rapidly shifting alliances has meant that, since independence, no government has served a full term in office. As a result of the general election of June 1982, Michael Somare became Prime Minister but was defeated in a parliamentary vote of confidence in November 1985 and was replaced by Paias Wingti. A general election was held in June 1987 which resulted in the return of Wingti's coalition government, but this was subsequently defeated in a parliamentary vote of no confidence on July 4, 1988, and was replaced by a new coalition led by Rabbie Namaliu. After the 1992 election a new coalition was formed by Wingti.

Constitutional structure

The head of state of Papua New Guinea, an independent member of the Commonwealth, is the British sovereign, represented by a Governor-General. Legislative power is vested in a unicameral National Parliament, the 109 members of which are elected for up to five years by universal adult suffrage. Executive power is exercised by a Prime Minister and a National Executive Council (Cabinet) who are responsible to Parliament and are appointed to office by the Governor-General, acting upon its advice. A government which loses a vote of confidence is obliged to resign. Each new government is immune to votes of no-confidence during its initial six months in office.

Although political parties have played an important role in the country since independence, they remain loosely-organized and tend to be founded upon individuals rather than any clear ideological perspective. Outside the National Parliament they are weak and, between elections, tend only to function as mechanisms for the distribution of patronage. This, together with the tradition of multiparty coalitions in both government and opposition, means that parties are highly prone to splits and defections, particularly in the immediate aftermath of an election when senior politicians are attempting to construct an overall majority amongst the new legislators. This is exacerbated by the fact that many successful candidates for the legislature are independents who hope to profit from inducements offered by those seeking to construct an overall majority. It is usual for several weeks to pass following an election before a new administration emerges.

Electoral system

At the 1977 election the National Parliament was increased in size to 109 members, 20 of whom represent provincial seats. Each of the country's 19 provinces elects a single legislator regardless of its size or population, as does the National Capital District in which Port Moresby is located. The remaining 89 legislators represent single member constituencies which often cut across provincial boundaries. Each elector casts one vote in provincial and one vote in the open elections. Since 1977 a system of simple plurality has been used for all elections and, as each seat is frequently contested by many candidates—the

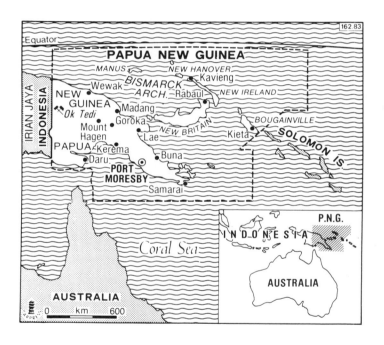

Recent elections

During the transition to independence the legislature elected in 1972 remained in office until mid-1977. At the 1977 elections the National Parliament was enlarged to 109 members.

Legislative elections

Date	Winning Party	Prime Minister
June-July 1977	Pangu-led coalition	Michael Somare*
June 1982	Pangu-led coalition	Michael Somare*
June-July 1987	PDM-led coalition	Paias Wingti*
June 1992	PDM-led coalition	Paias Wingti

*Defeated by vote of no confidence prior to serving a full parliamentary term.

Legislative elections, June 13-July 4, 1987

Party	Percentage of vote	Seats
Pangu Pati	14.7	26
People's Democratic Movement (PDM)	10.8	18
People's Progress Party (PPP)	6.1	5
Melanesian Alliance	5.6	7
National Party	5.1	12
League of National Advancement (LNA)	4.9	3
People's Action Party (PAP)	3.2	6
United Party (UP)	3.2	1
Morobe Independence Group (MIG)	2.2	4
Papua Party	1.3	3
Other parties	1.7	—
Independents	41.2	21
Vacant*	—	3

Legislative elections, June 13-27, 1992

Party	Seats
Pangu Pati	22
People's Democratic Movement (PDM)	15
People's Action Party (PAP)	13
People's Progress Party (PPP)	10
Melanesian Alliance	9
League of National Advancement (LNA)	5
National Party	2
Melanesian United Front	1
Others	1
Independents	30
Vacant*	1

*Seats left vacant because voting was delayed in these constituencies by deaths of candidates.

NB. The number of seats won by various parties tends to change almost immediately as a result of defections during the post-election negotiations over the formation of a coalition government.

largest number for a single seat in the 1992 contest was 48—a winning candidate is usually elected with only a relatively small proportion of the total votes.

Voting is by secret ballot, but because a large proportion of the population is illiterate, election officials are permitted to accept "whispered votes", whereby a voter whispers his preference to the official who then marks his ballot paper accordingly. Practices such as this, together with the tradition of gift-giving by a candidate to the electorate—a custom which is often tantamount to vote-buying—has meant frequent allegations of corruption.

Evolution of the suffrage

Since independence Papua New Guinea has operated a system of universal adult suffrage for all citizens aged 18 years or over.

PARTY BY PARTY DATA

League for National Advancement

Address. PO Box Wards Strip, Waigani, Papua New Guinea.

Leadership. Karl Stack (l.).

Orientation. Left of centre.

Founded. May 1986.

History. The League for National Advancement (LNA) was founded by Sir Barry Holloway and Tony Siaguru, together with a handful of other *Pangu Pati* legislators. The party polled 4.9 per cent of the vote in the 1987 election, but finished with only three seats in the new legislature. Both of its founders were defeated and so the leadership was assumed by Karl Stack who, like them, was a former *Pangu Pati* government minister. The party joined the bloc of parties in opposition to the government of Paias Wingti.

When the Wingti government was defeated in 1988 the LNA joined the Pangu-dominated coalition administration led by Rabbie Namaliu. Stack joined the new government as Minister of the Interior. At the election of 1992 the LNA won five seats, a figure which rose to seven in the post-election period. The party transferred its allegiance from Pangu to the People's Democratic Movement (PDM), thereby enabling it to join a coalition government under Wingti.

Melanesian Alliance

Address. PO Box 193, Rabaul, Papua New Guinea.

Leadership. Fr John Momis (ch.).

Orientation. Socialist-nationalist, with a strong regional base.

Founded. February 1980.

History. The Melanesian Alliance was formed by John R. Kaputin and Fr John Momis, a Catholic priest who, as chairman of the pre-independence Constitutional Planning Committee, had sought a decentralized system of provincial governments. When independence was granted in 1975 on the basis of a unitarian constitution, Momis led a movement which declared an "Independent Republic of the North Solomons" on the island of Bougainville. In August 1976, however, a constitutional amendment creating provincial governments met the movement's principal aims, and the Melanesian Alliance recognised Bougainville as a part of Papua New Guinea.

Upon creating the Alliance, both Kaputin and Momis resigned from the Pangu government in which they had held ministerial office since October 1978 and August 1977 respectively. They accused the party of abandoning its nationalist ideals and joined an opposition vote of no-confidence which brought down the government on March 11, 1980. They then joined the new coalition government as, respectively, the Minister of Finance and the Minister of Decentralization.

At the 1982 elections the Alliance won 8.6 per cent of the vote and eight seats, and joined the opposition to the *Pangu Pati* coalition government. In 1985, however, as Pangu was shaken by a serious split, the party joined the Somare government with Momis becoming Deputy Prime Minister.

The government fell in November 1985 and the Alliance returned to opposition. At the 1987 election it won 5.6 per cent of the vote and six of its 45 candidates won seats, an increase of two over the number of seats held at the dissolution. Its parliamentary strength later increased to seven as it recruited an independent MP. It joined the opposition bloc but

Kaputin, who had left the party and been elected as an independent, was reappointed as Minister for Minerals and Energy, a post which he had originally been given in December 1986.

When the Wingti administration fell in July 1988 the Melanesian Alliance returned to government as a member of the Pangu-dominated coalition. Momis was appointed Minister of Provincial Affairs. At the election of 1992 the party won nine seats.

National Party

Address. PO Box 136, Kundiawa, Chimbu Province, Papua New Guinea.

Leadership. Michael Mel (l.).

Orientation. Centrist. The party emphasises federalism, stable government, and law and order. In recent years its economic nationalism has been tempered by a growing acceptance of the need for foreign investment.

Founded. 1980.

History. The original National Party, formed by students and led by Thomas Kavali, won 10 seats in the pre-independence House of Assembly in 1972. It supported the *Pangu Pati*, but split in the mid-1970s and won only three seats in the 1977 elections. Two of the three, including Kavali, joined the Pangu coalition as independents leaving the party with just one legislator—Iambakey Okuk, a Highlander with a large personal following. In 1978 Okuk allied himself with dissident elements of the United Party to form the People's United Front opposition party.

In early 1980 Okuk, who was by then serving as Leader of the Opposition, reorganized the National Party, and formed an alliance with the People's Progress Party, the bulk of the United Party, the Melanesian Alliance and Papua Besena. This alliance brought down the Somare government and, on March 13, formed a coalition government with People's Progress Party's leader Sir Julius Chan as Prime Minister and Okuk as his Deputy.

In the election of 1982 the National Party won 10 per cent of the vote and 14 seats, and joined the opposition to the new Somare administration. Okuk lost his seat in the election and was succeeded as party leader by Ted Diro. The addition of Diro's supporters brought the parliamentary strength of the party up to 25 seats, making it the second-largest within the legislature. Okuk returned to Parliament at a by-election in 1983 and resumed the party leadership. (He was unseated by a legal challenge in 1984, but regained his

seat in 1985.) Following the political crisis of March 1985 the party joined the Somare government, but withdrew its support in August of that year. It returned to government in November as part of the Wingti coalition, with Okuk serving as Industry Minister. Okuk died in November 1986 and was succeeded as leader by Defence Minister Stephen Tago.

In the 1987 election, 13 of the party's 56 candidates were elected, almost all of whom represented constituencies in the Highlands. The party joined the opposition bloc and Tago, having lost his seat, was succeeded as leader by Michael Mel, a coffee magnate who had been party president since 1978. The party then split as a minority of its legislators were induced to join the Wingti government in return for Cabinet posts. Following the creation of the Namaliu government the party remained divided, with a majority under Mel choosing to remain in opposition, whilst a minority, led by Paul Pora, joined the new administration. Pora became Minister of Finance and Planning.

At the 1992 election the party won only two seats, with Pora choosing to stand successfully as an independent candidate.

Pangu Pati

Address. PO Box 444, Boroko, Papua New Guinea.

Leadership. Rabbie Namaliu (l.).

Orientation. Centre-left. The party advocates a more equitable distribution of wealth, decentralization and the development of the co-operative, village-based agricultural sector.

Founded. 1967.

History. The *Pangu Pati* (founded under the name Papua New Guinea Union Party—Pangu) was created by Michael Somare as the main vehicle for anti-colonial sentiment in the Australian-administered territory of Papua New Guinea. It won 11 of the 84 elected seats in the House of Assembly in the 1968 elections. In 1972 it became the second-largest party, winning 31 of the 100 elected seats and Somare became the territory's first Chief Minister, at the head of a coalition government which included the People's Progress Party (PPP).

In 1977 Pangu increased its representation to 38 of the 109 members in the National Parliament, becoming the largest single party. Somare continued his coalition government, but in March 1980 he was defeated in a vote of no-confidence initiated by the Leader of the Opposition Iambakey Okuk. Somare resigned and became Leader of the Opposition. He returned to government in August 1982 when the *Pangu Pati* won 34 per cent of the vote and secured around 52 seats in the July election, and formed a coalition with the United Party. Personal differences led to a serious split within the ruling party, however, in 1985. Deputy Prime Minister Paias Wingti and a number of other party members defected to form the People's Democratic Movement (PDM), whilst other Pangu members established the League for National Advancement (LNA). Weakened by the splits, the Somare government was ousted in November 1985 and Wingti became Prime Minister at the head of a multiparty coalition.

Following the 1987 election the government of Wingti retained power, with the *Pangu Pati*'s representation falling to around 26 members (14.7 per cent of the vote). After the usual post-election defections and realignments the party finished with 22 representatives, making it second in size to the People's Democratic Movement which emerged from the post-election period with 23 seats. It won most of its support in the northern coastal area, and polled badly in the other two regions, Papua and the Highlands.

Discontent over Somare's leadership grew within the party following his inability to create a viable coalition in the aftermath of the election and his widely perceived failure to exploit the difficulties of the Wingti government. By early 1988 there were persistent rumours that a group of Pangu members were preparing to defect to the government. In a bid to preserve party unity Somare resigned on May 20, and was replaced as leader by Rabbie Namaliu.

In July 1988 Namaliu was successful in mobilizing sufficient opposition support to oust Wingti. He formed a new coalition—consisting of *Pangu Pati*, the Melanesian Alliance, the People's Action Party, the Papua Party, the LNA, and elements of the National Party—which remained in power for the remainder of the parliamentary term.

At the 1992 elections the *Pangu Pati* won 22 seats, making it the single largest party at the beginning of the traditional post-election inter-party negotiations. However, Namaliu only narrowly secured re-election, winning his Kokopo constituency by a margin of 358 votes. Opposition leaders called for an investigation when it was revealed that he had been trailing 1,600 votes behind rival candidate Oscar Tammur at an early stage of the count, but then secured victory following an unexplained power blackout whilst the final ballot boxes were being processed. Following the defection

from the government coalition by the LNA in the immediate post-election period, the *Pangu Pati* was forced into opposition by a new PDM-led coalition government under Paias Wingti.

People's Action Party

Address. PO Box 165, Konedobu, Papua New Guinea.

Leadership. Akoka Doi (l.).

Orientation. Conservative and based almost entirely on the region of Papua.

Founded. December 1986.

History. The People's Action Party (PAP) grew out of the personal following of Ted Diro who resigned as Commander of the National Defence Force in 1981, and was elected to the National Parliament in 1982. He and 10 supporters—mainly businessmen and retired civil servants—formed a bloc of MPs known as the "Diro independents". The group joined the National Party, which Diro led for a short time [see separate entry].

Diro created the PAP in 1986, with the support of two other MPs. In 1987 six of its 33 candidates were elected and, following the post-election negotiations, its strength increased to eight. The party joined the Wingti coalition, with Diro appointed as Minister Without Portfolio, but was increasingly damaged by persistent allegations of corruption against its leader relating to his period as Forestry Minister. A judicial commission of inquiry was established to investigate the charges and, as the scandal grew, Diro was forced to resign from the government on Nov. 8, 1987. In early 1988 the Wingti coalition began to show serious signs of instability as Diro's supporters lobbied intensively for his return to the Cabinet. In order to prevent defeat by a no-confidence motion, Diro was reinstated in April.

The Wingti government fell in May 1988, but Diro remained in the Cabinet by successfully transferring his party's allegiance to the new administration of Rabbie Namaliu. The judicial commission which had investigated Diro's conduct had recommended charges against him, but these were obstructed by further legal challenges. Eventually, in the face of overwhelming evidence of corruption, Diro was suspended from government duty in April 1991. In September an investigating tribunal recommended that he be dismissed from Parliament and banned from holding public office for three years. The Governor-General, Sir Vincent Serei Eri, a former president of the PAP, attempted to reinstate him and was himself forced to resign on Oct. 1 in the face of moves by both government and opposition blocs to petition Queen Elizabeth II for his dismissal.

In the subsequent leadership contest to succeed Diro, Akoka Doi defeated Aruru Matiabe, whereupon the latter left the party. In the 1992 election the PAP won 13 seats, making it the third-largest party as it entered the post-election negotiations.

People's Democratic Movement

Address. PO Box 1828, Port Moresby, Papua New Guinea.

Leadership. Paias Wingti (l.).

Orientation. Centre-right. The party believes in the virtue of private enterprise and balanced budgets. It is nationalist in that it is committed to the preservation of the country's cultures and traditions, and advocates a non-aligned foreign policy with a reduction of the country's reliance on Australia.

Founded. March 1985.

History. The People's Democratic Movement (PDM) was formed by Paias Wingti, a leading member of the *Pangu Pati* and the Deputy Prime Minister in the government of Michael Somare in 1984-85. In March 1985, Wingti and 15 other members of the party defected from the government. Although they failed to bring down the government immediately—Somare realigned his coalition in order to defeat a vote of no-confidence [see above]—the new party became the largest single opposition grouping and Wingti became Leader of the Opposition. When the National Party withdrew from the Somare coalition in the latter half of 1985, the PDM seized the initiative and successfully passed a no-confidence motion on Nov. 21 by 57 votes to 52. Wingti became Prime Minister at the head of a coalition government which included the PDM, the National Party, the People's Progress Party (PPP), the Papua Besena, and elements of the United Party.

At the 1987 election the government was returned with Wingti being re-elected Prime Minister on Aug. 9 by three votes. The PDM won 10.8 per cent of the vote, but only 16 of its 77 candidates were successful in securing election. Following defections, however, its number of seats eventually rose to 23. Nevertheless, the new coalition had a very precarious majority (it controlled 55 seats compared with 52 for the Opposition) and relied on the support of the PPP, People's Action Party (PAP), the Papua Party, the United Party and 12 Independents.

Having campaigned vigorously on an anti-corrup-

tion platform, life was made particularly difficult for Wingti by the serious scandal which enveloped People's Action Party (PAP) leader Ted Diro [see separate entry]. In an attempt to reduce his dependence on the PAP and its scandal-tainted leader, Wingti approached the *Pangu Pati* in mid-1988 in an effort to create a government of national unity. Negotiations initially failed, but then an agreement was signed on May 25 after Rabbie Namaliu replaced Somare as Pangu leader. The agreement broke down on June 1, however, over the allocation of portfolios. On July 4 the Wingti administration fell from power following its defeat by 58 votes to 50 on a vote of no-confidence.

At the 1992 elections, the party finished second to Pangu with 15 seats. Following the defection from the government coalition by the League for National Advancement in the immediate post-election period, however, Wingti formed a PDM-led coalition government. When the new legislature assembled in July Wingti defeated Namaliu in a contest for the premiership by a single vote, the casting vote coming from the Speaker. Subsequent defections to his government, however, appeared to give Wingti a workable majority with the support of around 60 members of the Assembly.

People's Progress Party

Address. PO Box 6030, Boroko, Papua New Guinea.

Leadership. Sir Julius Chan (l.).

Orientation. Conservative.

Founded. November 1970.

History. The People's Progress Party (PPP), formed by Chan and other north-coast conservatives, won 10 of the 100 elected seats in the 1972 House of Assembly elections, and played a key role in determining the economic policies of subsequent *Pangu Pati*-dominated coalition governments. It won 18 seats in the elections to the new Parliament in 1977 and, in November 1978, it went over to the opposition on the grounds that it was being excluded from the policy formation.

When the Somare government was defeated in March 1980 the PPP joined the Melanesian Alliance, Papua Besena, the National Party and part of the United Party in new governing coalition, with Chan serving as Prime Minister. Following the 1982 elections, in which the PPP won 10 seats, the party returned to opposition. It returned to government in November 1985 when it joined the People's Democratic Movement (PDM)-led coalition, with Chan becoming a member of the government and second in status only to PDM leader Paias Wingti.

In the 1987 election, the party's share of the vote fell from 10 per cent to 6.1 per cent and only six of its 89 candidates secured election. Nevertheless, it remained an important component of the Wingti coalition and Chan was reappointed Deputy Prime Minister. It returned to opposition when the government was defeated in July 1988. At the 1992 elections the party won 10 seats and joined the PDM-led coalition, with Chan returning to the post of Deputy Prime Minister in the new Wingti Cabinet.

Minor parties

Melanesian United Front (MUF); Boroko, Papua New Guinea; Utula Samana (l.). Prior to 1988 the MUF was known as the Morobe Independence Group (MIG), a left-of-centre regionalist party which had been established in the early 1980s. At the 1987 election the MIG won 2.2 per cent of the vote and ended up with four seats. It joined the opposition bloc and worked particularly closely with the League of National Advancement. It joined the Namaliu coalition in 1988, and Samana became Minister of Education. Of the party's candidates in the 1992 election, only Tukape Masani was successful in securing election.

People's Solidarity Party (PSP); led by Kala Swokin, formerly a member of the People's Action Party, the PSP joined the Namaliu coalition and Swokin became Minister of Lands. In the 1992 election the party won no seats.

Papua Party (PP); c/o National Parliament, Port Moresby NCD, Papua New Guinea. The PP, a centrist party based in the central and western provinces, was founded in 1987 by former Papua Besena members Galeva Kwarara and Joseph Aoae. In the election of that year it won 1.3 per cent of the vote and three of its 18 candidates won seats in Parliament. It joined the Wingti coalition but, following its fall in July 1988, transferred its allegiance to the Namaliu administration, in which Kwarara served as Minister of Health. In the 1992 election the party won no seats.

United Party (UP); PO Box 1156, Port Moresby NCD, Papua New Guinea; Masket Iangalio (l.). The conservative Highland-based UP was founded in 1968 as the Independent Members' Group. It opposed early independence and favoured continued Australian administration. In 1970 it became the Combined Political Association (Compass) but was subject to severe splits. It adopted its current name in 1971. In 1972 it became the largest party in the House of Assembly, winning 40 of the 100 elected seats and formed the core of the opposition to the *Pangu Pati* ruling coalition. The UP declined to 27 seats in the 1977 elections and, in March 1978, suffered a serious split as a sizeable group of members left to form the People's United Front (PUF) which, in 1980, became the National Party. In November 1978 much of the UP joined the Pangu-led coalition government, but a significant faction of the party remained in opposition. When the coalition was replaced in March 1980 by a People's Progress Party's-dominated government, the position of the two UP factions was reversed. In February 1981 the two factions reunited and supported the government. Under the leadership of Raphael Doa, the UP won six seats in the 1982 election, and joined the Pangu-led government. In 1984 Paul Torato succeeded Doa, and in November 1985 the party transferred its allegiance to the new People's Democratic Movement (PDM)-led coalition government. Torato resigned from the Cabinet in August 1986 because of allegations of corruption, but rejoined the government in the following December.

In the 1987 election the UP vote fell from 7.2 to 3.2 per cent and 25 of the party's 26 candidates (including Torato) failed to win a seat. The party's only successful candidate, Billy Kepi, was later joined by an independent, Masket Iangalio, who became the new leader. They joined the new Wingti government, with Iangalio serving as Minister of Labour. Following the fall of the Wingti government in July 1988, the UP moved into opposition. In the 1992 elections the party failed to win any seats.

Papua Besena (People of Papua); PO Box 596, Port Moresby NCD, Papua New Guinea. Founded in 1973, Papua Besena was formed by Josephine Abaijah who, in 1972, had become the first woman to secure election to the House of Assembly. Abaijah was a Papuan secessionist who refused to co-operate with either government or opposition. In 1975 the Papua Besena attempted unsuccessfully to establish Papua as a separate state, independent of the rest of the country. In 1977 the party won five seats in Parliament, and in March 1980 it overcame fierce opposition from its radical separatist wing and joined the People's Progress Party-led government. Its significance declined,however, with the party winning only three seats in the election of 1982. Following the defection of leading members to the new Papua Party, all 10 of Papua Besena's candidates in the 1987 election, including Abaijah, were defeated.

Wantok; formed in 1986 by Roy Evara, a Minister in the Somare government (1982-85), the party stood 26 candidates in the 1987 but failed to win any seats.

Defunct parties

Morobe Independent Group [see Melanesian United Front].

People's United Front (PUF); formed in March 1978 by members of the United Party, in 1980 it was reorganised as the National Party.

Papuan Action Party; founded in 1982 by two former members of the *Pangu Pati*, the party ceased to exist following its poor showing at the 1982 election.

Papua National Alliance (Panal); founded in 1980, the party supported the 1980-82 Chan government. It ceased to exist in the mid-1980s.

Major guerrilla groups

Bougainville Revolutionary Army (BRA); Francis Ona (l.). The BRA was formed in 1988 by Ona, a former mining surveyor, when the government rejected compensation claims for the despoliation of local land caused by the giant Panguna copper mine on the island of Bougainville. Initially the movement waged a campaign of sabotage against mining property which eventually forced the indefinite closure of the mine in May 1989. Increasingly the BRA came to be a vehicle for the secessionist aspirations of the people of the population of Bougainville, many of whom identified ethnically with the neighbouring Solomon Islanders and who had tried to secede from Papua New Guinea in 1975, prior to the achievement of independence. After an unsuccessful campaign to subdue the rebels, the government evacuated its forces from the island in March 1990 and imposed an air and sea blockade. On May 17, the BRA declared an independent "Republic of Bougainville". Lacking outside

recognition, beleaguered by the blockade, and reportedly unable to establish effective control over the island, the BRA entered into peace talks with the Port Moresby government in mid-1990. Although the "Endeavour Accord" was signed on Aug. 5 as an interim agreement designed to defer the implementation of the independence declaration in return for a lifting of the government blockade, it broke down almost immediately and the two sides remained unable to reach a long-term agreement. In September the government used troops to recapture Buka Island (north of Bougainville), allegedly in response to requests for assistance from the islanders themselves. In the resulting fighting with the BRA, at least 23 people were reported killed. Further negotiations were held in January 1991 in Honiara, the capital of the neighbouring Solomon Islands. In late January the Honiara Accord was signed whereby the government agreed not to station security forces on Bougainville on condition that the BRA disbanded itself and surrendered its weapons and prisoners to an international peace-keeping force. The immediate impetus for the agreement was the need to relax the blockade, which was causing immense hardship to the island's 120,000 population and which, according to some estimates, had resulted in the deaths of as many as 3,000 people. Although the accord meant that essential medical and fuel supplies began reaching the island in mid-February, the agreement's failure to address the central issue of Bougainville's future status ensured that it could not provide a final solution to the conflict. In April the government landed troops in the north of Bougainville, which led to increased clashes with the BRA and further obstructed the prospect of any new dialogue between the warring parties. This was exacerbated by the view held by some members of the Namaliu government that there could be a military solution to the problem.

Papua Independent Organization (*Organisasi Papua Merdeka*—OPM). This guerrilla movement was founded by Papuans in 1963, when Irian Jaya (formerly Dutch New Guinea) was incorporated into Indonesia. In 1971 it established that Provisional Revolutionary Government of West Papua New Guinea. Although the OPM frequently operates from inside Papua New Guinea, the official position of both the Indonesian and Port Moresby governments is that it is an Indonesian internal matter .

Philippines

Capital: Manila

Population: 62,400,000 (1990 est.)

Colonized by Spain in the 16th century, the Philippines declared independence on June 12, 1898, during the Spanish-American War, but following Spain's defeat the territory was ceded to the USA. Internal self-government was granted in 1935, with independence following 10 years later. After Japanese occupation during the Pacific War, the Republic of the Philippines became independent in July 1946.

In 1965 Ferdinand Marcos became President and retained power thereafter through the increasing use of political corruption and coercion. In an attempt to rally domestic support and to placate the US government (upon which his regime was heavily dependent), Marcos agreed to hold a presidential election in February 1986. He was opposed by Corazon Aquino (the widow of the country's most prominent opponent of the Marcos regime until his murder in 1983) and, although Marcos claimed victory, it was generally believed that Aquino had secured a greater number of votes. In the face of huge popular demonstrations in favour of Aquino and a growing mutiny within the armed forces, Marcos fled the country on Feb. 25 and Aquino was declared President. In May 1992 Fidel Ramos was elected President in succession to Aquino.

Constitutional structure

A new Constitution was approved by referendum in February 1987. Under its provisions executive power is in the hands of a President, directly elected for a single six-year term, and an appointed Cabinet. The President, with the consent of the Commission on Appointments, also appoints ambassadors, officers in the armed forces and heads of executive departments. Legislative authority is vested in a bicameral, popularly-elected Congress consisting of a 200-member House of Representatives (elected for three years) and a 24-member Senate (elected for six years). The Constitution also provides the President with the power to appoint 50 members to the House to represent indigenous minority groups for three consecutive terms following the ratification of the Constitution.

Electoral system

All elections are conducted on the basis of universal adult suffrage. Candidates for the House must be at least 25 years of age and may serve no more than three consecutive terms, while those for the Senate must be 35 years or older and may serve no more than two consecutive terms. Candidates for the presidency must be 40 years of age or over. For electoral purposes the country is divided into 165,000 precincts, each of which contains around 300 voters. A 1991 law prohibits political advertisements in the media which, by limiting the scope of non-office-holders to make their names known to voters, has inadvertently strengthened the position of incumbents seeking re-election.

While the normal term for the House of Representatives was three years, a transitionary provision of the 1987 Constitution stipulated that those elected in 1987 could remain in office until June 30, 1992, at the latest. The 1992 elections for the Senate were held on a two-tier basis: the 12 most successful candidates (measured by the total number of votes obtained) were elected for six years, while the remaining 12 successful candidates were elected for three years. The move was designed to enable the Senate to renew one half of its membership every three years.

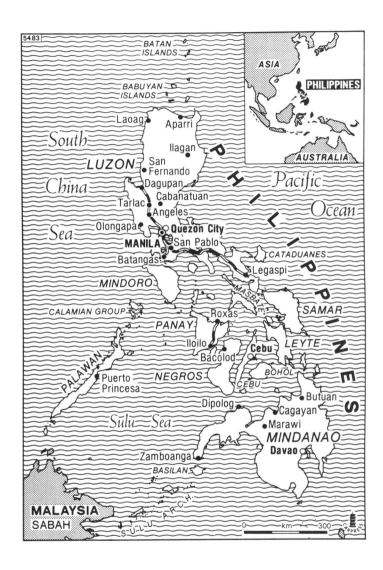

Recent elections

From independence until 1972 the political system was dominated by the Liberal and Nationalist Parties, the former winning the presidential elections of 1946, 1949 and 1961, and the latter winning in 1953, 1957, 1965 and 1969. In September 1972 President Marcos imposed martial law and banned all political parties. A new constitution was approved in January 1973 by a show of hands among the newly formed *barangays*—local groups of citizens aged 15 years and over. Further plebiscites were used by Marcos to legitimize his authoritarian rule. In 1978 political parties were permitted to operate, but with the proviso that they had been certified by the military as non-subversive. Elections were then held to the Interim National Assembly (IBP), with Marcos's newly formed New Society Movement (KBL) winning 152 of the 166 elected seats. On Jan. 17, 1981, martial law was lifted and presidential elections were held in the following June. Boycotted by the opposition, the elections were won by Marcos who claimed 88.8 per cent of the vote. In legislative elections in May 1984 the KBL won 110 of the 183 elected seats in the IBP.

Presidential elections were held on Feb. 7, 1986. Marcos once again claimed victory but it was generally believed that his opponent, Corazon Aquino, had won more votes. A combination of popular protests and an army mutiny forced Marcos from office and Aquino became President. In legislative elections on May 11, 1987, candidates endorsed by the President won a decisive majority in the new Congress. Aquino's chosen successor, Fidel Ramos, candidate of the *Lakas ng Edsa*-National Union of Christian Democrats (*Lakas*-NUCD) coalition, won the presidential elections on May 11, 1992, although the largest party in both houses of the new legislature was the *Laban ng Demokratikong Pilipino* (LDP).

Legislative elections, May 11, 1987

| Party | Seats won | |
	House of Representatives	Senate
Lakas ng Byan	180	22
Grand Alliance for Democracy	20	2

Legislative elections, May 11, 1992

Senate

Party	Seats won
LDP	16
Nationalist People's Coalition	5
Lakas-NUCD	2
Liberal Party-PDP-Laban	1

House of Representatives

As many candidates appeared on the ballot papers representing several different parties (sometimes as many as four), the precise composition of the new House of Assembly was unclear at time of publication. The largest party was the LDP, with more than 70 winning candidates representing it alone. It was followed by the Lakas-NUCD coalition which had more than 30 outright winners, and the NPC with 20.

Presidential elections, May 11, 1992

Candidate	Votes	Percentage of vote
Fidel Ramos	5,340,839	23.6
Miriam Defensor Santiago	4,466,184	19.7
Eduardo Cojuangco	4,114,980	18.2
Ramon Mitra	3,316,255	14.6
Imelda Marcos	2,337,417	10.3
Jovito Salonga	2,301,141	10.2
Salvador Laurel	769,935	3.4
Total	22,646,751	100

Evolution of the suffrage

Under a law of 1916, the franchise was extended to all tax-paying, literate men aged 21 years and older. Under the Constitution of 1935 the voting age was reduced to 20, and in 1937 the franchise was extended to include women. After the imposition of martial law in 1972, several plebiscites were approved by a show of hands among the newly-formed *barangays*, local groups of citizens aged 15 and above. After martial law was lifted in 1981, elections were conducted once again by secret ballot and by universal adult suffrage for those aged 15 and over.

PARTY BY PARTY DATA

People's Struggle

Laban ng Bayan

Address. Salcedo Mansions, Tordesillas Street, Salcedo Village, Makati, Metro Manila.

Orientation. Centre-left. Founded to organize support for the candidacy of Corazon Aquino in the 1986 presidential elections.

Founded. 1985.

History. The *Laban ng Bayan* (usually referred to as *Laban*, although not to be confused with *Lakas ng Bayan*, also known as *Laban*, which was founded in 1978 and later merged with the Partido Demokratiko Pilipino-Lakas ng Bayan—see separate entry) was created as a loose coalition on Nov. 17, 1985. Its express purpose was to unite opposition support behind a single anti-Marcos candidate prior to the presidential elections of February 1986. On Dec. 1 1985 it chose as its candidate Corazon Aquino, widow of opposition leader Benigno Aquino who had been assassinated upon his return to the Philippines in August 1983.

Laban was registered as a national political party on Dec. 11, 1985, and immediately reached an agreement with the United Nationalist Democratic Organization (UNIDO—see separate entry) on combined support for Aquino's candidacy, with UNIDO leader Salvador Laurel as her vice-presidential running-mate. With the bulk of the anti-Marcos voters united behind the Aquino-Laurel ticket, Marcos was defeated in the presidential election of February 1986. His crude attempts to manipulate the voting figures, together with his refusal to relinquish power, sparked huge popular demonstrations against him. With his support within the army crumbling, he eventually fled the country and Aquino was sworn in as President on Feb. 25.

Although the disparate individual parties within *Laban* maintained their separate identities, structures and policies, the coalition held itself together. At the 1987 legislative elections, its candidates won decisive majorities in both houses of Congress. Increasingly, however, as the Aquino presidential term progressed, the coalition became less than the sum of its parts. As the 1992 election approached the inter- and intra-party manoeuvring to determine her successor meant that the *Laban ng Bayan* ceased to exist as an effective political grouping. Nevertheless, several candidates who chose to list *Laban* along with other party endorsements were elected in May 1992.

Laban ng Demokratikong Pilipino

Address. 3rd Floor, ASA Building, EDSA corner, P Tuazon Street, Cubao, Quezon City.

Leadership. Neptali A. Gonzales (pres.); Jose Cojuangco (sec.-gen.).

Orientation. Centrist. The party is a very broad coalition and has no central ideological position.

Founded. 1987.

History. Founded in 1987, the *Laban ng Demokratikong Pilipino* (LDP) was reconstituted in 1988 by the inclusion of much of the *Partido Demokratiko Pilipino-Lakas ng Bayan* (PDP-*Laban*—see separate entry) and the *Lakas ng Bansa* (People's Struggle). In its current form the party arose as a vehicle for the pro-Aquino legislators elected in 1987, and was, therefore, driven by organizational rather than ideological considerations. Throughout Aquino's Presidency the party displayed frequent signs of instability, and these were massively accentuated in the run-up to the 1992 elections. There was intense rivalry for the presidential nomination between former Defence Secretary Fidel Ramos (who had joined the party in April 1991), and Speaker of the House Ramon Mitra. Despite poor opinion poll showings and his reputation as an old-style patronage politician, by the end of 1991 Mitra had managed to mobilize sufficient support within the party to guarantee his nomination. Ramos left the LDP and founded the *Lakas ng Edsa*, and Mitra was formally nominated as the LDP presidential candidate at a convention on Jan. 25, 1992. Numerous party members defected to Ramos's new party, a trend which was accentuated by Aquino's endorsement of Ramos as her preferred successor.

Nevertheless, the LDP remains the only truly national political party in the Philippines in that its influence is not confined to any one or more geographical regions, nor is it specifically based upon a single individual. In addition to having the most powerful and extensive political machinery, the party also entered the 1992 elections with the advantage of possessing the greatest number of incumbent office-holders. Its candidates included 10 incumbent Senators, 121 members of the House, 43 of the 73 governors, and some 700 of the 1,538 mayors.

At the presidential elections, Mitra, who had fought a less than effective campaign, finished in fourth place with 3,316,255 votes (14.6 per cent). The party fared better in the legislative contest winning 16 Senate seats, and over 70 seats in House. Although it was the country's largest political party, however, it remained highly unstable following the divisions which had been exposed in the run-up to the elections.

Structure. The party's policy-making body is the 57-member executive committee. This comprises the president, the general secretary, four deputy general secretaries and 47 vice-presidents drawn from provincial governors, city mayors and regional co-ordinators.

Lakas ng Edsa

Address. c/o National Assembly, Metro Manila.

Leadership. Fidel Ramos (l.); Jose de Venecia (sec.-gen.).

Orientation. Centrist.

Founded. 1991.

History. Lakas ng Edsa was founded by Fidel Ramos, who had resigned as Defence Secretary in July 1991 in order to pursue his presidential ambitions. The party underwent several changes of name during the first months of its existence. Its current name refers to Manila's Edsa (Epifanio de los Santos Avenue) highway where the phenomenon of "People Power" manifested itself to protect Ramos and the other members of the military who rebelled against Marcos following the fraudulent 1986 elections.

Ramos left the *Laban ng Demokratikong Pilipino* (LDP) after a straw poll on Nov. 30—which he claimed had been rigged—had chosen Ramon Mitra, the Speaker of the House of Representatives, as the party's presidential candidate. Ramos's candidacy received a boost on Jan. 25, 1992, when President Co-

razon Aquino announced her support for him. Aquino's endorsement effectively anointed Ramos as the legitimate heir to the "People Power" revolt which had provided the impetus for the overthrow of President Ferdinand Marcos and had installed Aquino in office in February 1986. As acting Chief of Staff of the Armed Forces under Marcos, Ramos had led a military mutiny in support of Aquino, and it was this which had finally convinced Marcos that he could no longer continue to cling to office. Thereafter, as Chief of Staff under the new government and then Defence Secretary, the unswerving loyalty of Ramos was the single-most important factor in Aquino's defeat of the numerous coup attempts against her. In accepting Aquino's endorsement of his candidacy, Ramos stated that "her unique moral authority" would greatly assist his campaign and would mean that "we will no longer be voices crying in the wilderness".

Aquino's choice was criticised in some quarters for instigating a possible split in her support—between those who would remain loyal to the LDP and those who would support Ramos—and thereby allowing an opposition candidate to win. The choice of Ramos also ran contrary to the wishes of Cardinal Jaime Sin, the head of the country's Roman Catholic Church and a loyal supporter of Aquino. He was known to have advised against choosing a Protestant for the presidency of a predominantly Catholic country.

Nevertheless, in alliance with the National Union of Christian Democrats (NUCD—see separate entry) Ramos fought a highly effective campaign. After a convoluted counting process, the final tally of returns for the May 11 presidential elections gave him a lead of more than 874,000 votes over his nearest rival, Miriam Defensor Santiago, although his 5,340,839 votes amounted to only 23.5 per cent of the total, the slimmest margin ever attained by a winning presidential candidate. A joint session of the Philippine Congress on June 22 formally proclaimed Ramos as winner of the election and dismissed protests, particularly from Santiago, that the poll should be declared void because of widespread corruption. The vote in the House of Representatives was 106 in favour of proclamation, two against and 21 abstentions; in the Senate it was 15 in favour, two against and one abstention. On the same day the Congress also proclaimed Joseph Estrada as the winner of the vice-presidential contest.

In the legislative elections, held simultaneously with the presidential contest, the *Lakas*-NUCD alliance won only two seats in the Senate. In the House of Representatives it won finished second to the LDP, with more than 30 clear victories, and several other candidates who listed the coalition among several party allegiances.

Liberal Party

Address. 7 First Street, Acacia Lane, Mandaluyong, Metro Manila.

Leadership. Jovito Salonga (pres.); Rauls Daza (sec.-gen.)

Orientation. Centre-left. The party moved towards the left during the Marcos years when it was subject to considerable official persecution.

Founded. 1946.

History. The Liberal Party (not to be confused with the short-lived party of the same name founded in 1901 and which changed its name to *Partido Independista* in December 1902) was formed in 1946 by defectors from the ruling *Nacionalista Party*. Although the defectors came from the liberal wing of the *Nacionalista Party*, the new party, like that from which it had emerged, was a loose coalition of shifting interests without a clear or consistent ideological position. It held the Presidency until 1952, and then again in 1961-65. In 1965 it lost the Presidency to Nacionalista candidate Ferdinand Marcos and, thereafter, remained in opposition. Its secretary-general at this time, until his arrest under martial law regulations in 1972, was Benigno Aquino.

The party boycotted the 1980 provincial and local elections in protest over the continuation of martial law. As part of the United Democratic Organization it also boycotted the 1981 presidential elections. In 1982 it became part of the United Nationalist Democratic Organization (UNIDO—see separate entry).

The Liberal Party was revived as a significant political force by Jovito Salonga, who returned to Manila after almost four years of voluntary exile abroad on Jan. 17, 1985, after subversion charges against him were dropped. Although much of the party supported the candidacy of Corazon Aquino against Marcos in the presidential elections of February 1986, Salonga increasingly accused her of seeking to establish an "Aquino dynasty". In 1988 a section of the party defected to the opposition and aligned itself with the Grand Alliance for Democracy (GAD), and other party members left to found their own groupings or defected to the LDP. Having emerged from the 1987 elections with seven Senators, more than any other party, the Liberals entered the 1992 elections with only two and, prior to the election, the weakness of the party was illustrated by Salonga's deposition as president of the

Senate and his replacement by LDP leader Neptali Gonzales.

As early as March 1991, Salonga engineered his selection as the party's nomination for the presidential elections, but was forced to reopen the nomination process as a result of strong support for the alternative candidacy of former Chief Justice Marcelo Fernan. Fernan eventually lost the nomination to Salonga at a meeting of the party's executive committee in October 1991. During the campaign itself, Salonga was also supported by the left-wing PDP-*Laban* following an announcement on Jan. 3, 1992, that the two parties had formed an alliance. PDP-*Laban* leader, Aquilino Pimentel was selected as Salonga's vice-presidential running mate. Salonga won 2,301,141 votes (10.2 per cent), finishing in sixth place. The alliance also won one seat in the Senate.

Nationalist Party

Nacionalista Party

Address. 1666 Edsa corner Escuela and Guadalupe Street, Makati, Metro Manila.

Leadership. Juan Ponce Enrile (sec.-gen.); Jesus Paredes (deputy sec.-gen.).

Orientation. Conservative.

Founded. 1907 (revived in 1988).

History. The Nationalist Party was founded in 1907 and was the dominant political force in the Philippines until its liberal wing split in 1946 to form the Liberal Party. The party returned to power in 1952 and held the office of President until 1961. In 1965 and 1969 its presidential candidate, Ferdinand Marcos, was elected to the Presidency. In 1978 the party moved into opposition after the founding of the *Kilusan Bangong Lipunan* (KBL—New Society Movement) as a vehicle for the continuation of Marcos's rule. In 1982 the party joined the United Nationalist Democratic Organization (UNIDO).

The Nationalist Party was revived as a political force in 1988 as part of a realignment of the right-wing opposition to the administration of President Aquino. The issue of who to choose as presidential nominee for the 1992 elections caused extreme problems for the party. In November 1991 Salvador Laurel (Aquino's estranged, Vice-President), expelled Eduardo Cojuangco and Juan Ponce Enrile, his two main rivals for the nomination. Four days later Cojuangco—Aquino's cousin, but sworn enemy—held a meeting which he claimed was representative of the "true" Nationalist Party, and at which Laurel was expelled. Enrile also held a party convention at which he announced that he was withdrawing his nomination bid in the interests of party unity and called upon Laurel and Cojuangco to do likewise. The Enrile faction, which included Senator Arturo Tolentino, eventually chose to support the LDP in the election campaign.

Neither Cojuangco nor Laurel complied with Enrile's request, and although the latter eventually secured the nomination, the Cojuangco faction left to join the Nationalist People's Coalition [see separate entry]. Laurel polled a paltry 769,935 votes (3.4 per cent) and finished in seventh position. In the legislative elections, held simultaneously with the presidential contest, the Nationalist Party won 48 seats in the House.

National Union of Christian Democrats

Address. CAP Building, Amorsolo Street, corner Herrera Street, Legaspi Village, Makati, Metro Manila.
Leadership. Raul S. Manglapus (pres.); Jose Rufino (sec.-gen.).
Orientation. Centrist.
History. The National Union of Christian Democrats (NUCD) is a Christian-democratic party which participated in the popular campaign to overthrow Marcos in 1986. In October 1987 the party's president, Raul Manglapus, was appointed as Foreign Secretary in the Aquino government. The party fought the 1992 elections in alliance with the *Lakas ng Edsa* [see separate entry] created by Fidel Ramos. In addition to winning the Presidency, the alliance also won two Senate seats, while in the House of Representatives it finished second to the LDP, with more than 30 clear victories, and several other candidates who listed the coalition among their party allegiances.
International affiliations. The party is affiliated to the Christian Democrat International.

National People's Coalition

Address. c/o National Assembly, Metro Manila.
Leadership. Eduardo Cojuangco.
Orientation. Centre-right.
History. The National People's Coalition was founded as a centre-right coalition shortly before the 1992 election. It was based upon that faction of the Nationalist Party which supported Eduardo Cojuangco, and was primarily conceived as a vehicle for his presidential ambitions. Cojuangco, who was also supported by elements of the Liberal Party, fought a highly effective campaign which utilised his enormous wealth and the huge network of patronage which he had established in the Marcos years. He finished in third place among the seven candidates with 4,114,980 votes (18.2 per

cent of the total). His running mate Joseph Estrada won the Vice-Presidency. The party also won five Senate seats and won 21 clear victories in the elections for the House, while a further 18 candidates listed the National People's Coalition among their party affiliations.

Pilipino Democratic Party-People's Power Movement

Partido ng Demokratikong Pilipino-Laban
Address. Room 6-A, Maya Building, Cubao, Esda, Quezon City.
Leadership. Aquilino Pimentel (pres.); Augusto Sanchez (sec.-gen.).
Orientation. Centre-left.
Founded. February 1983.
History. The Pilipino Democratic Party-People's Power Movement (referred to exclusively in its abbreviated form of PDP-*Laban*) was created from a merger of (i) the Pilipino Democratic Party which had been established on Feb. 7, 1982, under the leadership of Lorenzo Tanada (and had then claimed to represent about 80 per cent of the country's opposition forces); and (ii) *Laban* (Lakas ng Bayan—People's Power Movement, which had been formed in 1978 and led by Benigno Aquino (husband of Corazon Aquino) until his assassination in August 1983. Another leading member of the party was its current leader Aquilino Pimentel, Mayor of Cagayan de Oro (Mindanao), who had been active in a Mindanao Alliance in 1978-81 and had joined the Social Democratic Party (itself formed in 1981 under the leadership of Mariano Logarta, Francisco Tatad and Reuben Canoy.

For the 1984 elections the PDP-*Laban* allied itself with the United Nationalist Democratic Organization (UNIDO—see separate entry) to run a unified opposition campaign in 183 districts and was soon thereafter part of a broad alliance of opposition forces which worked to bring down President Marcos in February 1986. On Nov. 17, 1987, the PDP-*Laban* merged with the *Lakas ng Bansa* (Power of the Nation) but retained its name. The party was formally dissolved in September 1988, following the foundation of the *Laban ng Demokratikong Pilipino* (LDP—see separate entry), but some of its members, led by Pimentel, continued to operate as an independent political force. The PDP-*Laban* continued to support President Aquino and co-operated closely with the LDP, the Liberal Party and others as part of the *Lakas ng Bayan* coalition which provided her with an overall majority in the National Assembly.

255

On Jan. 3, 1992, it was announced that the PDP-*Laban* had formed an alliance with the Liberal Party. The alliance's presidential nominee was Liberal Party president Jovito Salonga, with PDP-*Laban* leader, Aquilino Pimentel, as his vice-presidential running mate. At the election, Salonga polled 2,301,141 votes (10.2 per cent) and finished in sixth place, while Pimentel polled 2,022,319 votes and finished fifth. In the simultaneous legislative elections, the alliance won one seat in the Senate. In the elections for the House, the alliance won at least four seats outright, and several other successful candidates listed either PDP-*Laban* or Liberal among other party affiliations.

Minor parties

Bagong Alyansang Makabayan (Bayan); FMS Building, 1823 E. Rodriguez Street, Metro Manila; Lorenzo M. Tanada (ch.); registered April 1987.

Democratic Nationalist Alliance (DNA); Room 411, Unlad Condominium Taft Avenue, corner Malvar Street, Malate, Metro Manila; Reynaldo T. Fajardo (nat. ch.); registered March 1987.

Farmers' Party of the Philippines; Room 300, Dela Merced Delta Building, West Avenue, Quezon City; Marcelo de Guzman (pres.); registered August 1987.

Federal Party of the Philippines; 3434 Magsaysay Blvd., Sta Mesa, Metro Manila.

Grand Alliance for Democracy (GAD); 1509-J Princeton Street Mandaluyong, Metro Manila; Francisco Tatad (ch.), Wilson Gamboa (sec.-gen.). The GAD was created in 1986 as an opposition alliance to the Aquino government and included elements of the Liberal Party, the Mindanao Alliance, the Nationalist Party, the Social Democratic Party and the *Kilusan Bagong Lipunan*. Among its leading members were Juan Ponce Enrile and Arturo Tolentino. The former was a Marcos loyalist who, as Defence Minister, had defected to Aquino and, thereby, had played a crucial role in Marcos's overthrow. Although given the equivalent post in Aquino's first Cabinet, Enrile's close association with right-wing military dissidents intent upon staging an army coup led to a rapid estrangement between him and Aquino and he was dismissed from the Cabinet in November 1986. Thereafter he became a focus for right-wing opposition to Aquino. Tolentino was a former Foreign Minister and vice-presidential running mate of Marcos who also had extensive contacts among the military, and who had been deeply implicated in the July 1986 coup attempt against Aquino. The GAD registered as a party on April 20, 1987, and constituted the main opposition force in the legislative elections of May 11, 1987. Although decisively defeated, the party did secure a number of seats and Enrile was successful in his bid to gain election to the Senate. Since the election, the grouping has been largely ineffective and has been eclipsed as a vehicle for anti-Aquino opposition by the newly revived Nationalist Party.

Kilusan Bagong Lipunan (KBL—New Society Movement); KBL Headquarters, Room 309, 3rd Floor Jovan Condominium Shaw Building, corner Samat Street, Mandaluyong, Metro Manila; Nicanor E. Ynigue (l.). The KBL was established in 1978. As a vehicle for the continued personal rule of President Marcos, the organization also served as a distributive network for Marcos's extensive system of patronage and corruption. The official results of the 1978 elections to an interim national assembly, of provincial and municipal elections held in 1980, and of further municipal elections held in 1982 gave the KBL overwhelming majorities in all cases. The overthrow of Marcos in February 1986 meant that the party was thoroughly discredited, and many of its members aligned themselves with other right-wing organizations which opposed the Aquino administration. The party continued to exist and remained influential in some areas, particularly in Marcos's home province of Ilocos Norte. The revival of the Nationalist party in 1988, however, meant that it failed to achieve its ambition of functioning as the co-ordinating mechanism for those opposed to the liberalism associated with the Aquino government. In the 1992 presidential election the party supported the candidacy of Imelda Marcos, widow of the former President, who polled 2,337,417 votes (10.3 per cent), finishing in fifth place.

Lapiang Manggagwaw (LM—Worker's Party); 304 Dona Amparo Building, Espana, Metro Manila; Jacinto Tamayo (l.).

Muslim Federal Party, 7 Stella Street, Del-Air Village III, Metro Manila; Ahmad Domacao Alonto (ch.); registered in April 1987.

National Democratic Front (NDF). The communist-dominated NDF was created in August 1986 in order to conduct talks with the Aquino government on the possibility of ending the 17 year-old insurgency campaign by the New People's Army (NPA). After protracted negotiations, a 60-day truce was signed on Nov. 27, 1986. No permanent solution was negotiated, however, and the ceasefire ended on Feb. 8, 1987 [see under New People's Army]. The party did not formally participate in the 1992 elections, although it did support some candidates on a local basis.

Partido Komunista ng Pilipinas (PKP—Communist Party of the Philippines). The PKP was founded in 1930 and, within a year of it was declared illegal and its leaders were imprisoned. During the Pacific War it organized the *Hukbo ng Bayan Laban sa Hapon* (*Hukbalahap*—Anti-Japanese People's Army), groups of which continued to fight a guerilla campaign against the government into the 1970s. In 1968 the party split between pro-Soviet and pro-Chinese factions. Whereas the Maoist faction (the Communist Party of the Philippines—Marxist-Leninist—CPP-ML) intensified the guerilla war through its military wing, the New People's Army [see under guerrilla groups], the pro-Soviet PKP faction, pursued a more reformist and constitutional approach. In 1974 the PKP leaders were amnestied and the party, while still illegal, was permitted to operate with little interference. Although the party participated in the popular movement to oust Marcos in February 1986, it has little political influence and, as the country's primary vehicle for communist ideology, has been eclipsed by the CPP-ML.

Partido Nasyonalista ng Pilipinas (PNP—Nationalist Party of the Philippines); 3rd Floor, Gemini Building, 215 Gil Puyat Avenue, Makati, Metro Manila. Founded by Blas F. Ople (a former member of Marcos's Cabinet), the PNP formally registered itself on March 5, 1987. With the *Kilusan Bagong Lipunan* (KBL—New Society Movement, see separate entry) thoroughly discredited following the fall of Marcos, the PNP served as a politically respectable point of focus for right-wing opponents of President Aquino. The revival of the Nationalist Party in 1988, however, largely eclipsed the PNP.

Partido ng Bayan (PNB—People's Party); 89 West Avenue, Quezon City; Alan Jasminez (sec.-gen.), Nelia Sancho (ch.). The PNB was founded in May 1986 upon the explicitly left-wing platform of demanding the removal of the US military bases from the Philippines and the ending of the country's continued dominance on multinational corporations. At its opening congress on Aug. 30-31, 1986, the presiding figures included (i) Jose Maria Sison (the party's chairman) who was a leading figure in the illegal Communist Party of the Philippines—Marxist-Leninist [see separate entry]; and (ii) Bernabe Buscayno (known as Comandante Dante) a senior figure within the guerilla New People's Army. Party representatives denied, however, that the PNB was merely a legal front for these two illegal organizations. Having registered as a political party on Feb. 24, 1987, the PNB took part in the May 11, 1987 legislative elections as the leading element within the Alliance for New Politics, which advocated objectives—including land reform—which were almost identical to those of the PNB. However, the Alliance polled negligibly and obtained no more than two seats in the House of Representatives. In the 1992 election the party refrained from endorsing any candidates at national level, but supported numerous candidates at mayoral, municipal and district councillor level.

Partido ng Masang Pilipino (PMP); Room 405 San Buena Building, EDSA corner Shaw Blvd., Mandaluyong, Metro Manila; Joseph Estrada (pres.), Tony Garcia de Escano (sec.-gen.). This centre-right party is led by Joseph Estrada who had been elected to the Senate in 1987, and who won the election fro Vice-President in 1992, polling 6,737,215 votes.

Partido Pilipino; 76 A Scout Lumbaga Street, Quezon City; Fernando T. Barbican (pres.).

Philippine Christian Nationalist Party (PCNP); 5 University Valley, Tandang Sora Avenue, Old Balara, Quezon City; Andres V. Genito (pres.); registered in December 1985.

Philippine Labor Party; 1429 A. Rizal Avenue, Sta. Cruz, Metro Manila; Salvador A. Purisma (l.).

Philippine Republic Reformist Party (PRR); Room 305-306, Medalla First Div Building, EDSA and McArthur Highway, Cubao, Quezon City; Nemesia P. Diaz (pres.).

Pilipinas '92 (Political Movement); Room 509, Ermita Centre, 1350 Roxas Blvd., Metro Manila; John H. Osmena (ch.); publishes a bi-monthly newsletter called the *Philippine Progress Reporter*.

People's Reform Party (PRP); 25 EDSA, Makati, Metro Manila; Ambrosio Padilla (pres.); Miriam Defensor Santiago (sec.-gen.). The PRP is a centre-right party which provided support for Miriam Defensor Santiago's attempt to win the 1992 presidential election. The scale of the party was tiny, operating upon a maximum of 12 full-time staff, including Santiago's six brothers and husband. Stressing discipline and anti-corruption, the party took as its logo a clenched fist clutching a bolt of lightning. Despite the limited resources available to her, Santiago fought a very effective campaign, portraying herself as an "outsider" who was untainted by the corruption endemic to the country's political system. She finished in second place behind Fidel Ramos, but claimed that the election had been invalidated by corrupt practices. Initially she attempted to stop Ramos taking office through legal action and promised to lead a campaign of massive civil disobedience. Eventually, however, she accepted the results and conceded defeat.

Republican Socialist Party; 310 Calvo Building, Escolta, Metro Manila; Ponciano Subido (pres.); registered in February 1987.

Social Democratic Party (SDP); 376 Trece de Abril Street, Cebu City; Andrea N. Corominas (l.).

Union for Progress (UP); 2/F Corporate Business Centre, 151 Paseo de Roxas, Makati, Metro Manila. The party is led by ex-Chief Justice Marcelo Fernan, who was the vice-presidential running mate of LDP candidate Ramon Mitra in the 1992 elections. Fernan polled 4,437,364 votes and finished in second place.

Defunct parties

United Nationalist Democratic Organization (UNIDO); centrist organization founded in 1982 as an alliance of anti-Marcos groups, including the United Democratic Opposition (an eight-party opposition coalition established in 1980), the Nationalist Party, the Philippine Democratic Party, *Laban*, and the Liberal Party. It provided a considerable degree of opposition unity during the 1984 legislative election campaign and, in 1985, it reached an agreement with *Laban ng Bayan* to run a joint presidential campaign, with Corazon Aquino nominated for President and Salvador Laurel, UNIDO's president, as the nominee for Vice-President. The UNIDO-*Laban* candidates defeated Marcos in the election of February 1986 and

subsequently took office, although relations between Laurel and Aquino rapidly deteriorated. In 1989 UNIDO was absorbed into the revived Nationalist Party, although some elements of the party have continued to use the UNIDO name.

Kabisig (Linking Arms Movement). This organization, which is not strictly a political party, was founded by President Aquino in June 1991 in an attempt to revive the "people power" which had propelled her into office in 1986. The movement had little real political impact, other than souring Aquino's relationship with the *Laban ng Democratikong Pilipino* (LDP).

Major guerrilla groups

Bangsa Moro National Liberation Front (BMNLF); Dimas Pundato (l.). Also known as MNLF-Reformist Group, like the Muslim Islamic Liberation Front (MILF) the BMNLF developed within the Moro National Liberation Front (MNLF) [see below] in the early 1980s, and by the end of 1982 had a distinct identity. Unlike the MILF, however, it retained close links to the MNLF despite developing a high degree of autonomy. Supported by Saudi Arabia, the BMNLF has always been the smallest of the three Muslim secessionist movements. It includes the Bangsa Moro Islamic Party faction.

Communist Party of the Philippines—Marxist-Leninist (CPP-ML); Benito Tiamzon (ch.); Saturnino Ocampo (gen. sec.). The CPP-ML is an illegal organization which split from the pro-Soviet PKP in 1968. Since 1968 the party's military wing, the New People's Army (NPA), has been waging a guerrilla war in pursuit of the Maoist strategy of building a rural revolutionary movement. At the time of the collapse of the Marcos regime the NPA was estimated to number around 20,000 fighters. Although it has probably declined since then, it remains one of the most significant guerrillas movements in Asia.

Muslim Islamic Liberation Front (MILF); Hashim Salamat (ch.). The MILF developed from within the Moro National Liberation Front (MNLF) in the early 1980s, and by late 1982 had a distinct identity. Whereas the MNLF was supported by Libya and Iran, the MILF drew its international support from Egypt. The bulk of its membership is concentrated in Lanao del Sur. In early 1988 there was heavy fighting between the MILF and the MNLF.

Moro National Liberation Front (MNLF); Nur Misuari (chair and president of central committee). The MNLF is a militant Muslim organization founded in 1968 to co-ordinate armed struggle against the Manila government through its military wing, the *Bangsa Moro* Army. Its aims include the achievement of independence for the traditionally Muslim provinces of the south through armed struggle. At times, however, it has taken a reformist position by demanding increased resources for the country's Muslim population together with greater autonomy for the southern provinces. In 1977 Misuari defined the MNLF as "a Muslim nationalist movement trying to free a Muslim country from the Philippine colonial yoke".

New People's Army [see under Communist Party of the Philippines—Marxist-Leninist].

Various dissident groups within the armed forces. There are an unknown number of shadowy organizations within the armed forces. The most prominent of these are **Reform the Armed Forces Movement** (RAM) and the **Young Officers Union** (YOU), both of which were involved in coup attempts against the Aquino government.

Singapore

Capital: Singapore City

Population: 2,700,000 (1990 UNFPA est.)

Singapore achieved internal self-rule from the United Kingdom in 1959, and four years later joined with the Federation of Malaysia, Sabah and Sarawak to form the Federation of Malaysia. Singapore was excluded from the federation in 1965 and it adopted a republican form of government. The People's Action Party, under the leadership of Lee Kuan Yew, has been the country's ruling party since 1959.

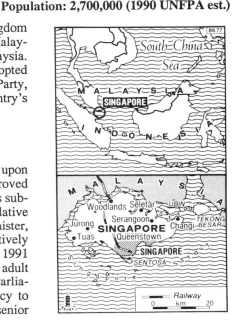

Constitutional structure

Singapore's Constitution consists of the basic form adopted upon the achievement of self rule in 1959, with amendments approved during its temporary Malaysian affiliation (1963-65) and its subsequent adoption of republican status in 1965. The legislative organ is an 81-member unicameral Parliament. A Prime Minister, appointed by the President, heads a Cabinet that is collectively responsible to Parliament. The Constitution was amended in 1991 to provide for the election of a President by universal adult suffrage (the President previously having been elected by Parliament), and to extend the responsibilities of the Presidency to include reserve veto powers over financial provisions and senior public service appointments.

Electoral system

Parliament is elected by universal adult suffrage for a five-year term. A Constitutional amendment approved by Parliament in 1984 provided for up to three "non-constituency" parliamentary seats for the opposition (with restricted voting rights) if none were won in a general election. In 1988 legislation was passed introducing group representation constituencies (GRCs), whereby 39 constituencies were arranged into 13 groups of three to be contested by teams of three candidates, one of which had to be of minority (i.e. non-Chinese) origin; this was designed to secure a minimum 15 per cent ethnic minority representation in Parliament. In 1991 the Constitution was further amended, stipulating that the number of candidates contesting GRCs should be a minimum of three and a maximum of four.

Under a 1991 Constitutional amendment, the President would henceforth be elected by universal adult suffrage for a four-year term.

Evolution of the suffrage

All Singaporean citizens resident in the country and at least 21 years of age are entitled to vote. Voting is compulsory, failure to vote resulting in the offender's name being erased from the electoral register.

Recent elections

	Seats won		Share of total valid votes cast (%)	
	1988	1991	1988	1991
People's Action Party	80	77	63.2	61.0
Workers' Party	0	1	16.7	14.3
Singapore Democratic Party	1	3	11.8	12.0
Others	0	0	8.3	12.7
Total	81	81	100.0	100.0

PARTY BY PARTY DATA

Islamic Movement

Angkatan Islam
Address. Singapore.
Leadership. Mohamad Bin Omar (pres.); Ibrahim Bin Abdul Ghani (sec.-gen.).
Orientation. Moderate Islamic.
Founded. 1958.
History. As in the case of the other smaller parties in Singapore, the Islamic Movement has contested a small number of seats at successive general elections without any success. The party did not contest any seats in the 1991 election.

National Solidarity Party

Address. Singapore.
Leadership. Kum Teng Hock (pres.); Rasiah Thiaga-rajah (sec.-gen.).
Orientation. Centrist.
Founded. 1986.
History. The National Solidarity Party (NSP) was established by former members of the Singapore Democratic Party (SDP) with the aim of attracting the votes of young professionals. The party contested eight constituencies in 1988 winning 3.8 per cent of total votes cast but failed to secure parliamentary representation. The party again contested eight constituencies in 1991 and again failed to win a parliamentary seat; however, it almost doubled its share of total valid votes cast to 7.3 per cent.

People's Action Party

Address. 510 Thomson Rd, 07-02, Singapore 1129.
Leadership. Lee Kuan Yew (gen. sec.); Goh Chok Tong (first asst. sec.-gen.); Lee Hsien Loong (second asst. sec.-gen.); Ong Teng Cheong (ch.); Tony Tan (vice ch.).
Orientation. Originally a democratic socialist party, the People's Action Party (PAP) has in recent years combined strong anti-communism with pragmatism, promoting the development of Singapore on the basis of a strongly free-market economy and at the same time continuing to place emphasis on social welfare. In 1982 the PAP altered its constitution, redefining its objectives as being to defend the independence and territorial integrity of Singapore, to safeguard freedom and well-being through representative and democratic government, to build a multiracial society tolerant to all and with commitment to Singapore, to create a disciplined and self-reliant society with compassion for the aged, sick and handicapped as well as the less fortunate, and to achieve optimum economic development, social and cultural fulfilment in harmonious and co-operative social relationships.
Founded. 1954.
History. The PAP was formed by a group of trade unionists and intellectuals around Lee Kuan Yew, who in 1955 defined the party's aim as "immediate independence for a free, democratic and non-communist Malaya" and "the destruction of the colonial system by methods of non-violence". Having won only three out of 30 seats in its first election in 1955, in elections held in 1959 to the 51-member Legislative Assembly (under the 1957 Constitution conferring home rule on Singapore) the PAP gained an absolute majority of 43 seats and thereupon formed a government. In 1961, however, the party's effective majority was reduced to 26 out of 51 members of the Assembly as a result of defections and the formation of the radical offshoot Socialist Front (*Barisan Sosialis*—BS, see Workers' Party entry). With the formation of the *Barisan Sosialis*, the PAP leadership effectively transformed the party from a radical socialist party into a moderate, anti-communist organization which emphasized, above all else, Singapore's economic development. In elections held to the Singapore Legislative Assembly shortly after the incorporation of Singapore in the newly established Federation of Malaysia in 1963, the PAP gained 37 seats against the *Barisan Sosialis'* 13 (the latter standing on a anti-federation platform).

In 1965 Singapore seceded from the Federation of Malaysia, and since December of that year the PAP has been in government as the ruling party of the independent Republic of Singapore. In the 1968 elections the PAP took all 58 seats in the Legislative Assembly (51 of its candidates being returned unopposed). The party won all of the parliamentary seats in general elections held in 1972, 1976 and 1980.

The PAP was returned for its seventh consecutive term of office in 1984; however, for the first time since 1963, it failed to win all the (79) seats in Parliament, and its share of the overall vote fell by some 13 per cent compared with 1980. The seats not taken by the PAP went to J. B. Jeyaretnam, secretary-general of the Workers' Party, who retained the Anson seat which he had won at a by-election in 1981, and Chiam See Tong, secretary-general of the Singapore Democratic Party [see separate entry], who won the Potang Pasir constituency. Concern over the drop of support for the party at the 1984 elections led to increased efforts by the party's youth movement (headed by Lee Kuan Yew's son Lee Hsien Loong) to improve lines of communication with the public. Nevertheless, "old guard" PAP leaders made it clear that the party had no intention of purposely attenuating its grip on power. In the 1988 elections the PAP won all but one of the 81 elected seats (the remaining seat being retained by Chiam See Tong), but received under 63.2 per cent of the total popular vote, the lowest figure since the party came to power in 1959.

Lee Kuan Yew resigned as Prime Minister in 1990 in favour of Goh Chok Tong, but remained as party secretary-general. Goh called an early general election in August 1991 in an attempt to win a mandate for his more liberal, participative style of government. In the event the PAP lost four of the 81 seats contested (three to the Singapore Democratic Party and one to the Workers' Party) and its share of total valid votes fell to 61 per cent. The party entered the elections with an assured majority after the opposition had agreed not to oppose PAP candidates in 41 seats. Nevertheless, the result constituted the opposition's biggest success since the 1960s and was a serious blow for Goh and his new government. According to many commentators the election results strengthened the position of Lee Hsien Loong, Goh's designated successor and leader of the party's conservative wing.

Structure. Since the mid-1950s, when communists made an attempt to take over the party from within, the PAP has operated a cadre system under which only selected members can elect or be elected to higher party bodies. The highest party organ is a 14-member central executive committee, last elected in 1986.

Membership. 8,000-10,000.

Publications. Petir (official organ).

International affiliations. Following criticism of the alleged repressive nature of the Singapore government expressed by many West European member parties of the Socialist International (of which the PAP had been a member since 1966), the PAP withdrew from that organization in 1976.

Singapore Democratic Party

Address. Blk 108, 01-496, Potong Pasir Av. 1, Singapore 1335.

Leadership. Chiam See Tong (gen.-sec.); Ling How Doong (ch.).

Orientation. Main opposition party; liberal and centrist.

Founded. 1980.

History. The Singapore Democratic Party (SDP) was founded by Chiam See Tong, a lawyer and political activist, in an attempt to create a liberal opposition to the ruling People's Action Party (PAP). The party has failed to establish itself as a credible opposition, but nevertheless it has pressured, from inside and outside parliament, for a free press and freedom of speech and has staunchly opposed government legislation on housing, employment and industrial relations. In the 1980 elections the SDP contested three seats, but gained only 1.77 per cent of the national vote and no seats. The party contested four seats in the 1984 election and Chiam won the Potang Pasir constituency. However, Chiam's victory was one of only two defeats for the PAP. Chiam retained Potang Pasir in 1988 with a marginally increased majority. The party contested a total of 18 seats and increased its share of total valid votes cast from 3.7 per cent to 11.8 per cent. In the 1991 election the party contested nine seats and Chiam again retained the seat and increased his support from 63.1 per cent to 69.6 per cent. The SDP won a total of three seats in the 1991 election and again increased its share of the total valid votes cast to 12 per cent. Ling How Doong, the party's chair and, like Chiam, a lawyer by profession, narrowly defeated Seet Ai Mee (Minister of State for Community Development) in Bukit Gombak. Cheo Chai Chen, a businessman, narrowly defeated senior PAP figure Ng Pock Too in Nee Soon Central. Commenting on the SDP success in the 1991 elections, Chiam conceded that "the voters want to keep the PAP in power" but claimed that "they also want a strong opposition in parliament to keep an eye on the government". The election result, he said, was "a sign that Singapore's democracy is growing up".

Publications. Demokrat (in late 1989 Chiam was acquitted of charges that he had published *Demokrat* without government approval).

Singapore Justice Party

Address. Singapore.

Leadership. A. R. Suib (pres.); Muthusamy Ramasamy (sec.-gen.).

Founded. 1972.

History. The Singapore Justice Party (SJP) presents a small number of candidates in each general election, but has yet to win a seat. In the 1991 election the party gained 1.9 per cent of the vote.

Singapore Malays National Organization

Pertubuhan Kebangsaan Melayu Singapura

Address. 218F, Changi Rd, PKM Bldg, Fourth Floor,

Singapore 1440.

Leadership. Sahid Sahooman (pres.); Mohammed Aziz Ibrahim (sec.-gen.).

Orientation. Seeks to advance the rights of Malays in Singapore.

Founded. 1954.

History. The Singapore Malays National Organization (more commonly known as the PKMS) was founded as an affiliate of the United Malays National Organization in Malaysia and has been in opposition to the government since its inception. It was re-organized as the PKMS in 1967. It fields a small number of candidates in general elections, but always fails to muster the necessary votes to win a seat. In the 1991 elections the PKMS gained 1.6 per cent of the total vote.

United People's Front

Address. 715, 7th Floor, Colombo Court, Singapore 0617, Singapore.

Leadership. Ang Bee Lian (ch.); Harbans Singh (sec.-gen.).

Orientation. Opposes the "authoritarian and repressive" People's Action Party regime.

Founded. 1975.

History. The United People's Front (UPF) was founded as an alliance of factions from five opposition groups—the United National Front, the Singapore Malays National Organization (SMNO), the Singapore Chinese Party, the Justice Party, and the United Malays National Organization of Singapore—together with some former members of the Socialist Front and the United Front. However, the SMNO dissociated itself from the UPF shortly after its formation. The party unsuccessfully contested a small number of constituencies in the 1976, 1980, 1984 and 1988 elections. In the 1988 elections it won only 18 per cent of the vote in the five constituencies in which it challenged. The party did not contest any constituencies in the 1991 election.

Workers' Party

Address. 237A Silat Rd, Singapore 0316.

Leadership. J. B. Jeyaretnam (sec.-gen.); Gan Eng Guan (ch.).

Orientation. Seeks establishment of democratic socialist government.

Founded. 1957.

History. The Workers' Party (WP) was originally founded in 1957 by David Marshall (who had been Singapore's first Chief Minister in 1955-56), and it was revived in 1971 by J. B. Jeyaretnam, its present secretary-general. Its 22 candidates contesting the 1976 general elections were all unsuccessful, and so were its eight candidates in the 1980 elections. However, Jeyaretnam won a by-election held in the Anson constituency in October 1981, thus becoming the first opposition member of Parliament since 1968.

Jeyaretnam retained his Anson seat in the 1984 elections, after which the WP refused an additional "non-constituency" seat. In highly controversial circumstances Jeyaretnam was fined and imprisoned for one month in late 1986 having been found guilty of making a false declaration about his party's finances in the early 1980s. The fine meant that Jeyaretnam was forced to forfeit his Anson seat under legislation prohibiting a person serving in parliament if penalized over US$2,000 for a criminal action. Jeyaretnam and the WP leadership characterized the whole episode as a PAP plot to undermine the party.

Before the 1988 election, the Socialist Front (*Barisan Sosialis*—BS) and the Singapore United Front (*Barisan Bersatu Singapura*—BBS) merged with the WP. The left-wing BS had been established in 1961 by People's Action Party militants under the leadership of Lim Chin Siong. The BS immediately gained a strong position in parliament and was the official opposition to the PAP. However, the party refused to accept Singapore's secession from the Federation of Malaysia in 1965, and the following year its members resigned from parliament, some of them going underground. The party boycotted the 1968 elections, but unsuccessfully contested a small number of seats in the 1972, 1976, 1980 and 1984 elections. The BBS, formed in 1973, contested the 1976, 1980 and 1984 elections. In the latter the party contested 13 constituencies, but won no parliamentary seats.

In the 1988 elections the WP contested 32 constituencies and gained 16.7 per cent of the total valid votes cast, making it the second most popular party. The party failed to win a seat, but following the elections Francis Seow, a former Solicitor-General, and Lee Siew Choh, former BS chair, were awarded non-constituency seats. Seow was subsequently indicted on income tax-related charges and fled into exile. In the 1991 election the WP contested 13 seats, won one and gained 14.3 per cent of the total valid votes cast. The party's victory occurred in Hougang, where businessman Low Thia Khiang defeated a PAP candidate.

Minor parties

Other small political parties registered in Singapore

(none of which have ever achieved parliamentary representation) are: Alliance Party Singapore; National Party of Singapore; *Partai Kesatuan Ra'ayat*; *Partai Rakyat*; People's Front; People's Republican Party; *Persatuan Melayu Singapura*; Singapore Chinese Party; Singapore Indian Congress; United National Front; United People's Party.

Dissident groups

There are no dissident groups in conflict with the government.

Solomon Islands

Capital: Honiara (island of Guadalcanal)   **Population: 314,707 (1990 est.)**

Discovered by Europeans in the 16th century, the northern Solomon islands became a German protectorate in 1885, and the southern Solomons a British protectorate in 1893. The territory was unified under British rule at the turn of the century, and became an independent member of the Commonwealth in July 1978. Solomon Mamaloni became Prime Minister in March 1989 following the election victory of his People's Alliance Party. He resigned as party leader in October 1990, but remained as Prime Minister at the head of a coalition government of "national unity".

Constitutional structure

The head of state of the Solomon Islands is the British sovereign represented by a Governor-General, appointed for up to five years on the advice of the legislature. Legislative authority is vested in a unicameral National Parliament, the 38 members of which are popularly elected for up to four years. The Prime Minister (who is elected by MPs from among their number) and an appointed Cabinet (which many number up to 15 members including the Prime Minister) exercise executive power and are responsible to Parliament.

Electoral system

Voting in parliamentary elections is conducted in single-member constituencies on the basis of simple plurality.

By tradition, political parties are based upon individuals and issues of kinship rather than ideologies and, therefore, tend to be subject to defections and divisions. As in neighbouring Papua New Guinea, an election is followed by an intensive period of negotiations during which the many independents are induced into supporting a prospective coalition government, and those in existing parties are encouraged to switch their allegiance. This political culture was reinforced by Mamaloni's creation of a "national unity" government because, by splitting both the ruling party and the opposition, it weakened further the existing party structures.

Evolution of the suffrage

Since independence, the country has operated on the basis of universal adult suffrage. In 1976 the voting age was reduced from 21 to 18 years.

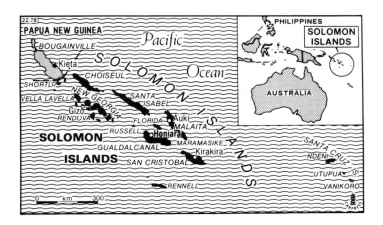

Recent elections

Date	Winning Party
June 1980	Solomon Islands United Party-led coalition*
October 1984	Solomon Islands United Party-led coalition
February 1989	People's Alliance Party

*Ousted from office in August 1981.

General election, Feb. 22, 1989

Party	Seats won
People's Alliance Party (PAP)	11
Solomon Islands United Party (SIUP)	4
Nationalist Front for Progress (NFP)	4
Solomon Islands Liberal Party (SILP)	3
Solomon Islands Labour Party(SLP)	2
Independents	14
Total	38

PARTY BY PARTY DATA

Nationalist Front for Progress

Address. PO Box 821, Honiara, Solomon Islands.

Leadership. Andrew Nori (l.).

Orientation. Melanesian-nationalist. The party emphasises the importance of preserving traditional Melanesian social structures.

Founded. October 1985.

History. Following its formation by three incumbent legislators in 1985, the Nationalist Front for Progress (NFP) joined the Solomon Islands United Party (SIUP)-led coalition government under Prime Minister Sir Peter Kenilorea in July 1986. Its ministers resigned in November 1986 in protest over the cyclone aid scandal [see under Solomon Islands United Party entry], but rejoined the government following the resignation of Kenilorea in December.

The disastrous showing of the SIUP in the 1989 election resulted in the NFP winning an equal number of seats. Under the able leadership of Nori, who became Leader of the Opposition in 1989, the NFP gradually eclipsed the SIUP to become the leading component of the opposition to the Mamaloni government. Following the decision of Mamaloni to form a non-party government of national unity, the NFP appeared to be the least damaged of the three main parties and provided a solid core around which the anti-Mamaloni forces could unite. However, despite widespread contempt for Mamaloni's manoeuvre, the opposition remained divided, not least over the issue of who should be elected as Prime Minister in place of Mamaloni. In the face of this indecision, Nori resigned as Leader of the Opposition on Nov. 1, 1991, and was replaced by Labour Party leader Joses Tuhanuku.

People's Alliance Party

Address. PO Box 722, Honiara, Solomon Islands.

Leadership. David Kausimae (acting pres.).

Orientation. Centre-left, federalist. The party advocates the devolution of executive powers and administrative resources to the provinces. It supports a non-aligned foreign policy, and a strengthening of relations with other Melanesian countries including Papua New Guinea and Vanuatu.

Founded. 1979.

History. The People's Alliance Party (PAP) arose from a merger of the People's Progressive Party (PPP) and the Rural Alliance Party (RAP). The PPP, formed in 1973, was in government in 1974-75 and in a coalition with the (now-defunct) United Solomon Islands Party (USIP) in 1975-76. PPP's leader, Solomon Mamaloni, was first Chief Minister of the British Solomon Islands Protectorate in 1974-75 and, after 1976, of the Solomon Islands. He resigned from the then Legislative Assembly in 1977 after failing to secure re-election as Chief Minister. The RAP (founded in 1976 as the Solomon Islands Rural Party) was created by David Kausimae who, in 1971-72, had led the left-wing Solomon Islands United Party (SIUP). Following the creation of the PAP in 1979, Kausimae was its leader and only parliamentary representative.

In the election of 1980 the new party won 10 seats. Kausimae was defeated, but Mamaloni returned to the legislature and immediately became leader of the PAP and Leader of the Opposition. On Aug. 31, 1981, the SIUP government fell and Mamaloni became Prime Minister, with a Cabinet which included eight PAP members, two members of the National Democratic Party, and four independents. His government pursued its aim of devolving power to the provinces and sought to champion an anti-nuclear foreign policy. It also came into conflict with the USA over the seizure of an unlicensed US fishing vessel. In the 1984 election the PAP won 23 per cent of the vote and 12 seats. It was forced back into opposition, however, by a new coalition led by the SIUP.

The PAP fought the election of February 1989 on a platform of transforming the country into a federal republic. It was returned to government, winning 11 seats. This figure soon increased as a result of the traditional post-election negotiations. In March Mamaloni defeated Bartholomew (Bart) Ulufa'alu, leader of the Solomon Islands Liberal Party, in the election for Prime Minister. Although the new government included several independents, including several former member of the dissolved *Solomons Ano Sagufenua* (SAS), it was widely hailed as a new departure in that it provided the first instance of single-party government since independence in 1978. Nevertheless, Mamaloni came under increasing pressure both from opposition leader Andrew Nori and from growing dissatisfaction from within the PAP. Although Mamaloni successfully defeated a motion of no confidence in May 1990, a second vote was scheduled when the legislature reconvened in October. A week before it was due, Mamaloni resigned as leader of PAP and announced that he would continue in office as the head of a government of national unity. He dismissed five of his ministers (including Deputy Prime Minister

Danny Philip) and replaced them with four members of the opposition and one PAP backbencher.

In February 1991, those members of PAP who remained in Mamaloni's national government in defiance of the party's instructions were expelled from the party. Although many observers doubted that Mamaloni could command a legislative government, he was successful in staving off the prospect of an opposition vote of no-confidence. He used a strike by 4,000 government workers and civil servants as a pretext for postponing the reconvening of Parliament, scheduled for May. He was also assisted by deep divisions within the opposition. When the legislature did eventually meet, a no-confidence motion was tabled in early August, but was withdrawn without a vote after the opposition failed to agree upon a successor to Mamaloni. Nori resigned as Leader of the Opposition (effective from Nov. 1), and was replaced by Labour Party leader Joses Tuhanuku. In early November the Solomon Islands Council of Trade Unions gave Mamaloni an ultimatum to resign as Prime Minister or else to face countrywide industrial unrest.

Solomon Islands United Party

Address. c/o National Parliament, Honiara, Solomon Islands.

Leadership. Ezekiel Alebua (l.).

Orientation. Centre-right and pro-western. When in power, the party has tended to proceed on a pragmatic basis, seeking strong central government and the creation of a single national identity to embrace the country's diverse linguistic and cultural traditions.

Founded. 1979.

History. The Solomon Islands United Party (SIUP), also known as the United Party, was formed by Peter Kenilorea who, as leader of the loosely-organized United Democratic Action Group (UDAG) and with the support of some People's Progressive Party (PPP) members and a group of independents, had become Chief Minister following the 1976 election. He subsequently became the country's first Prime Minister following the granting of independence in 1978 and, in the following year, attempted to solidify the basis of his support through the creation of the SIUP. The party was the dominant partner in the Kenilorea-led coalition government which emerged from the 1980 election. However, the coalition was heavily dependent on the support of a bloc of independents led by Deputy Prime Minister Francis Billy Hilly. When this bloc withdrew its support in August 1981, the Kenilorea government was ousted by the opposition.

In the 1984 election the SIUP won 22 per cent of the vote and 13 seats, and Kenilorea was elected Prime Minister with 21 of the 33 valid votes. The SIUP-led coalition also included the newly-formed *Solomone Ano Sagufenua* and three independents. In accordance with the SIUP's belief in strong central government, many of the devolutionary measures enacted by Mamaloni were rescinded. The government survived several narrow no-confidence votes and, after the withdrawal of the SAS from the coalition in mid-1986, bolstered Kenilorea's position by securing the support of the newly-formed Nationalist Front for Progress (NFP).

In 1986 the country was severely damaged by a typhoon which left about one-third of the population homeless. Gradually it emerged that Kenilorea had accepted a large French aid donation and had spent it almost entirely on his home village. In November 1986, three members of the Cabinet resigned in protest over the scandal, and Kenilorea himself was forced to resign in December.

Kenilorea was succeeded by Ezekiel Alebua, an independent member of the Mamaloni government of 1981-83, who had become Deputy Prime Minister after joining the SIUP in 1984. Kenilorea remained an influential figure within the party, however, serving as Deputy Prime Minister within the new administration. Damaged by the scandal, the SIUP was soundly defeated at the 1989 election and retained only four seats. Thereafter it was increasingly eclipsed as the primary source of opposition to the Mamaloni government by the Nationalist Front for Progress. Some members of the SIUP, including Kenilorea, joined the new government of national unity formed by Mamaloni in November 1989 following his break with the PAP.

Minor parties

Coalition for National Unity (CNU); founded in 1989 as a loose parliamentary structure to co-ordinate the activities of the independents within Parliament.

Solomon Islands Labour Party (SLP); c/o National Parliament, Honaria, Solomon Islands. The SLP was founded in 1988 as a social democratic alternative to the Solomon Islands Liberal Party. Led by Joses Tuhanuku, it won two seats in the 1989 election. Following the divisions which beset the opposition after the formation of Mamaloni's government of national unity in late 1989, Tuhanuku succeeded Andrew Nori as Leader of the Opposition in November 1991.

Solomon Islands Liberal Party (SILP); c/o National Parliament, Honaria, Solomon Islands. The party was founded in 1975 as the political wing of the General Workers' Union, led by Bartholomew (Bart) Ulufa'alu, and advocated social-democratic policies. Originally called the Nationalist Party, it contested the 1976 elections under the name of the National Democratic party (Nadepa) when it won five seats. It led a loose Coalition Opposition Group (COG) which broke up in early 1977, leaving Nadepa as the largest single opposition grouping. The party retained two seats in the 1980 elections and, in September 1981, it joined a coalition government led by the People's Alliance Party with Ulufa'alu serving as Finance Minister. In the 1984 elections the party retained only a single seat, with Ulufa'alu failing to win re-election. It changed its name to the SILP in 1986, and in 1989 it won three seats, a figure which rose to four following the post-election negotiations.

Defunct parties

People's Progressive Party (PPP) [see under entry for People's Alliance Party].

Solomons Ano Sagufenua (SAS); founded in 1984 by Seth Lekelau, the SAS won four seats in the 1984 election and joined the Solomon Islands United Party coalition led by Kenilorea. The party disintegrated in the late 1980s, although several of its former members retained seats in Parliament, and at least one joined the People's Alliance Party government of Mamaloni.

United Democratic Action Group (UDAG); emerged among the pro-government members of the legislature elected in 1976 and formed the core component of the SIUP, created by Sir Peter Kenilorea.

United Solomon Islands Party (USIP); established in 1973 by members of the Governing Council who had formerly been civil servants. It lost power at the election of 1974 and its leader, Benedict Kinika was replaced by Philip Funifaka who became leader of the opposition. In early 1975 Funifaka joined the Mamaloni government, and was followed by a number of colleagues. By the end of the year the USIP had broken up, with its members sitting as independents.

Major guerrilla groups

There are no guerrilla groups operating in the Solomon Islands.

Sri Lanka

Capital: Colombo

Ceylon gained its independence from the United Kingdom in 1948, and in 1972 it became a republic and changed its name to Sri Lanka. The country has been ruled since 1977 by the United National Party. From 1983 onwards the conflict between the Sinhalese majority of the south and the northern Tamil minority came to dominate Sri Lankan politics.

Constitutional structure

Under its 1978 Constitution, Sri Lanka has an executive President, who is head of state and President of the government and appoints (or dismisses) the Prime Minister and members of the Cabinet. The President is also empowered to dissolve the unicameral Parliament.

Electoral system

Under the 1978 Constitution the President is directly elected by universal adult suffrage for a six-year term. The legislature is a unicameral Parliament with 225 members directly elected for a period of six years, subject to dissolution by the President.

Evolution of the suffrage

Citizens aged 18 years or over are entitled to vote.

Population: 17,200,000 (1990)

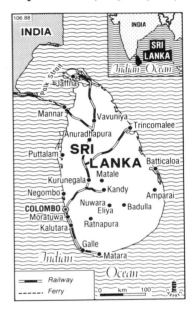

Recent elections

1977 and 1989 general elections

	Elective seats	
	1977	*1989*
United National Party	140	125
Sri Lanka Freedom Party	8	67
Tamil United Liberation Front	18	10
Sri Lanka Moslem Congress	—	3
People's United Front	—	3
*United Socialist Alliance	—	3
+Independent Tamils	—	14
Independent	2	—
Total	168	225

*Alliance of the Lanka Equal Society Party, the Communist Party of Sri Lanka, the Sri Lanka People's Party and the New Equal Society Party.

+All but one of the 14 sponsored by the Eelavar Democratic Front.

PARTY BY PARTY DATA

Bahejana Nidahas Pakshaya

Address. Colombo.

Leadership. Chandrika Kumaranatunge (l.).

Orientation. Left wing.

Founded. 1991.

History. This small party was created by Chandrika Kumaranatunge, widow of Vijaya Kumaranatunge, the assassinated founder of the Sri Lanka People's Party, and daughter of Sirimavo Bandaranaike, leader of the Sri Lanka Freedom Party (SLFP). The party allied itself with the SLFP, the Lanka Equal Society Party, the New Equal Society Party and the Communist Party for the May 1991 local elections, but the alliance was easily defeated by the ruling United National Party.

Ceylon Workers' Congress

Address. 72 Ananda Coomaraswamy Mawatha, Colombo 7.

Leadership. Savumyamoorthy Thondaman (pres.); Muthu Sangaralingam Sellasamy (sec.).

Orientation. Represents the interests of Tamil workers of Indian origin on tea plantations in Sri Lanka (many of them still British-owned).

Founded. 1940.

History. The Ceylon Workers' Congress (CWC) was allied with the moderate Tamil United Liberation Front (TULF) during the 1970s and much of the 1980s. Following the 1989 general elections, the party entered into coalition with the ruling United National Party (UNP). The CWC has no parliamentary representation, but in local elections held in May 1991 the party won two council seats, compared to 191 won by the UNP.

Publications. *Congress News* (fortnightly, in English); *Congress* (fortnightly, in Tamil).

Communist Party of Sri Lanka

Address. 91 Cotta Road, Colombo 8.

Leadership. Pieter Keuneman (proc.), Kattorge P. Silva (gen. sec.).

Orientation. Formerly pro-Soviet, the party has called for the nationalization of banks, estates and factories, and for the use of national languages (rather than English).

Founded. 1940.

History. The Communist Party of Sri Lanka (CPSL) was formed as the (Stalinist) United Socialist Party, which broke away from the *Lanka Sama Samaja Party* (LSSP—Lanka Equal Society Party). Because of its support for the war effort after 1941, it was legalized in 1943 when it adopted the name of Communist Party. It obtained three seats in the 1947, 1952 and March 1960 parliamentary elections, and four in July 1960 and in 1965.

The party contested the 1970 elections in alliance with the Sri Lanka Freedom Party and the LSSP, gaining six seats. The Communist ministers resigned in 1977, and the party fought the elections in the following July in alliance with the LSSP but lost all its seats. However, it gained one seat in a by-election in 1981. In the October 1982 presidential elections, it supported the candidature of Hector Kobbekaduwa of the Sri Lanka Freedom Party. The party was briefly proscribed under the state of emergency imposed in May 1983 as a result of intercommunal violence.

The party initially took part in the all-party talks on the Tamil issue which began in 1984, but soon withdrew, claiming that the government was seeking a military rather than a political solution to the problem. It was one of the four parties which formed the United Socialist Alliance in 1988. The Alliance gained only three seats in elections held the following year.

Structure. The party's primary organizations are based on places of work or residence, and in addition there are area and district committees. The party's supreme authority is its national congress (to be convened every two years), which elects a president, a general secretary, a central committee, a central control commission and a central auditing commission. The central committee elects a political bureau, a secretariat, and other bureaux and office-bearers.

Publications. *Aththa* (Truth, daily, in Sinhala); *Mawhima* (Homeland, weekly, in Sinhala); *Deshabimani* (Patriot, Tamil weekly); *Forward* (weekly, in English).

Democratic United National Front

Address. Colombo.

Leadership. Lalith Athulathudali (l.); Gemini Dassanayake (l.).

Founded. 1991.

History. The Democratic United National Front (DUNF) was formed by dissidents from the ruling United National Party, who made an unsuccessful attempt to impeach President Premadasa in September 1991.

Democratic Workers' Congress

Address. P.O. Box 1009, Colombo 10.

Leadership. Abdul Aziz (pres.); Vythilingam Palanisamy (sec.).

Orientation. Left wing.

Founded. December 1978.

History. Although politically active as a trade union since the 1930s, the Congress was not registered as a political party until 1978. It currently has no parliamentary representation.

Membership. 229,470 (1986 claim).

Publications. Jananayaga Thozhilali (Democratic worker, fortnightly, in Tamil).

International affiliations. World Federation of Trade Unions.

Eelavar Democratic Front

Leadership. V. Balakumar.

Orientation. Supports the creation of a separate Tamil homeland (Eelam) in north-eastern Sri Lanka.

Founded. 1988.

History. The Eelavar Democratic Front (EDF) was formed by members of the Eelam Revolutionary Organization of Students (EROS), a Tamil militant group allied with the Liberation Tigers of Tamil Eelam. In a largely unexpected result, 13 independents sponsored by the EDF won North-Eastern Province seats in the 1989 general election. The EDF-sponsored MPs—the third largest grouping in the Sri Lankan parliament—boycotted the opening session in protest at the sixth amendment to the Constitution which required them to sign an oath of allegiance to the unitary state before taking up their seats.

Lanka Equal Society Party

Lanka Sama Samaja Party

Address. 457 Union Place, Colombo 2.

Leadership. Bernard Soysa (gen. sec.); Athuada Seneviratne (deputy gen. sec.).

Orientation. Socialist.

Founded. 1935.

History. Because of its anti-war policy, the avowed Trotskyist *Lanka Sama Samaja* Party (LSSP) was banned during World War II and its leaders were detained. However, it was active as an underground organization and sought to build organizational links with Trotskyist groups in India. The re-legalized LSSP took part in parliamentary elections in 1947, when it gained 19 seats; five others were won by a Bolshevik-Leninist breakaway grouping, which rejoined the LSSP in 1950. In subsequent elections the LSSP ob-

tained nine seats in 1952, 14 in 1956, 10 in March 1960 and 12 in July 1960.

In 1964 the LSSP formed a coalition government with the Sri Lanka Freedom Party (SLFP) and was subsequently expelled from the Fourth International. The coalition was defeated in elections held in 1965, when the LSSP retained 10 seats in Parliament. It contested the 1970 elections in alliance with the SLFP and the Communist Party: it won 19 seats and subsequently entered a United Front government with three ministers. However, as a result of differences with the SLFP leadership, these ministers were dropped from the government in 1975. In elections held in 1977, which the party fought in alliance with the Communist Party, the LSSP failed to win any seats. For the 1982 presidential elections, it nominated Colvin de Silva as its candidate, but he obtained only 0.2 per cent of the vote. In 1988 the LSSP joined the four-party United Socialist Alliance and in the 1989 general election, its deputy general secretary, Athuada Seneviratne, gained a parliamentary seat, the first for the party since 1975.

Structure. The party's highest authority is vested in a congress of delegates and, between congress sessions, in a central committee elected by the congress. The central committee elects officers, among them a general secretary, and appoints a political and an organizational bureau.

Publications. Samasamajaya (Equal Society), *Samadharmam* (Tamil Weekly), and *Samasamajist* (English Weekly) (all weeklies, in Sinhala, Tamil and English respectively).

Liberal Party

Address. 88/1 Rosmead Place, Colombo 7.

Leadership. Chanaka Amaratunga (l.); Rajiva Wijesinha (pres.); Rohan Ed Risinha (deputy sec. gen.).

Orientation. Liberal, centrist, anti-nationalist and non-socialist.

Founded. 1987.

History. The Liberal Party was an offshoot of the Council for Liberal Democracy, which had been formed in 1981. It has strongly opposed violations of human rights, the state's excessive control of the Sri Lankan economy and the growth of racism. In particular, it has campaigned against the extension of the current term of the Sri Lankan parliament by six years, against deprivation of civic rights (of Sirimavo Bandaranaike, the former Prime Minister, and others), and against the effective expulsion from Parliament of the Tamil United Liberation Front members in 1983. The party has advocated the adoption of a federal constitution for Sri Lanka and the constitutional recognition of Sinhala, Tamil and English as official languages. It co-operates closely with the Sri Lanka Freedom Party (SLFP, the principal opposition party) and has supported SLFP candidates at several by-elections.

Structure. The party has an annual congress (at which every party member is entitled to attend and to vote), a national committee elected by the annual congress and special committees appointed by the national committee, as well as regional and constituency committees.

Membership. Approx. 5,000.

Publications. The Liberal Review (Monthly, in English); *Liberal Nidahasa* (weekly, in Sinhala).

International affiliations. Liberal International.

New Equal Society Party

Nava Sama Samaja Party

Leadership. Vasudeva Nanayakkara (gen. sec.)

Founded. 1979.

Orientation. Trotskyist.

History. The *Nava Sama Samaja Party* (NSSP) was formed by a breakaway left-wing faction of the *Lanka Sama Samaja G54*Party (LSSP—Lanka Equal Society Party). Its candidate in the October 1982 presidential election, Vasudeva Nanayakkara, obtained only 0.3 per cent of the vote. It is one of the four parties which, in February 1988, formed the United Socialist Alliance, for which it won one of its three seats in the 1989 election.

People's United Front

Mahajana Eksath Peramuna

Address. 75, Gothami Road, Borella, Colombo.

Leadership. Dinesh P. R. Gunawardene (gen. sec.).

Orientation. Left wing; strongly Sinhalese and Buddhist.

Founded. 1956.

History. The *Mahajana Eksath Peramuna* (MEP) was formed by Philip Gunawardene, effectively as a united front organization for the Sri Lanka Freedom Party (SLFP). It won a sweeping majority in the 1956 elections and introduced far-reaching economic, political and cultural reforms. The SLFP split from the MEP in 1959, and in the two elections held the following year the party managed to secure only three seats. It won two seats in 1965, after which it supported the United National Party government until 1970. In a by-election held in 1983, it re-gained a seat in Parliament, and it was one of the parties which took part in a preliminary

conference held later that year to discuss the Tamil issue. Recently it has fared better, winning three seats in the 1989 general elections.

Sri Lanka Freedom Party

Sri Lanka Nidahas Pakshaya

Address. 301 T.B. Jayh Road (Darley Road), Colombo 10.

Leadership. Sirimavo R. D. Bandaranaike (pres.); S. Dassanayake (sec.); Anura Bandaranaike (nat. org.).

Orientation. Campaigned vigorously for Sri Lanka's attainment of republican status (achieved in 1972); stands for a non-aligned foreign policy, for the progressive nationalization of industry and for Sinhalese as the official language (with certain safeguards for ethnic minorities).

Founded. 1951.

History. Founded by Solomon Bandaranaike upon his resignation from the United National Party (UNP) in 1951, the Sri Lanka Freedom Party (SLFP) first came to power in 1956 as a partner in the *Mahajana Eksath Peramuna* (MEP—People's United Front). Following a split in the MEP in June 1959, it held office as the sole government party until March 1960. Meanwhile, the assassination of Solomon Bandaranaike in September 1959 and the succession of his widow, Sirimavo Bandaranaike, had precipitated a split in the SLFP—its right wing subsequently forming the Ceylon Democratic Party (which gained only four seats in the March 1960 general elections and two in the July 1960 elections). The SLFP was again in power from July 1960 to 1965 and in 1970-77, in coalition with the Lanka Equal Society Party in 1964-68 and 1970-75. The SLFP lost power as a result of its heavy defeat in the July 1977 elections, when it won only eight seats (out of 168) as against 91 (out of 151) in 1970.

In 1980 Sirimavo Bandaranaike was deprived of her civil rights for seven years on the grounds of abuse of power while she had been Prime Minister (in 1970-77), a government resolution to this effect being opposed only by the SLFP and Tamil United Liberation Front (TULF) members of Parliament. For the 1982 presidential elections, the SLFP presented as its candidate Hector Kobbekaduwa (who had been a Cabinet minister in 1970-77), and he obtained 39.1 per cent of the vote (against 52.9 per cent for President J. R. Jayawardene of the United National Party).

In by-elections held in 1983, the party increased its parliamentary representation to nine, and after the exclusion of the TULF members from the House in October 1983 it became the official opposition.

The SLFP attended inter-party talks on the Tamil issue held in late 1983 and early 1984, but refused to take part in a further inter-party conference in 1986. Upon the restoration of her civil rights in 1988, Bandaranaike declared that she favoured a political settlement of Sri Lanka's ethnic problem, but that she would not work with President Jayawardene to that end.

Bandaranaike was only narrowly defeated by the UNP's Ranasinghe Premadasa in the presidential election held in early 1989. She gained almost 45 per cent of the vote, against just over 50 per cent for Premadasa. The party won 67 seats in the 1989 general election, but was easily defeated by the United National Party. In 1991 the party suffered a serious defeat at the hands of the UNP in local elections.

Publications. Dianya (daily); *Sathiya* (weekly).

Sri Lanka Moslem Congress

Leadership. H. M. H. Ashraff (pres.).

Founded. 1980; has operated as a political party since 1986.

History. The Sri Lanka Moslem Congress (SLMC) was created to defend the rights of Moslems in the Tamil-dominated Eastern provinces. It gained three out of 225 seats in the 1989 general election.

Sri Lanka People's Party

Sri Lanka Mahajana Party

Address. 82 Sri Wajiragnana, Mawatha, Colombo 9.

Leadership. Ossie Abeygoonasekara (l.).

Orientation. Left wing.

Founded. 1984.

History. The *Sri Lanka Mahajana Party* (SLMP) was created as a breakaway faction of the Sri Lanka Freedom Party (SLFP) by Vijaya Kumaranatunge, the son-in-law of the SLFP leader, Sirimavo Bandaranaike. In 1988 the SLMP formed, with three other left-wing parties, the United Socialist Alliance. Having been the moving spirit behind the formation of the Alliance, Kumaranatunge was shortly afterwards assassinated by Sinhalese extremists. His wife, Chandrika Kumaranatunge, briefly took over the leadership before it passed to Abeygoonasekara. In the 1989 presidential elections, Abeygoonasekara gained just under 5 per cent of the vote. In the general elections held shortly afterwards, the Alliance gained only three seats.

Tamil United Liberation Front

Address. 238 Main Street, Jaffna.

Leadership: K. Padmanhabha (gen. sec.); Vardharaja Perumal (l.).

Orientation. The Tamil United Liberation Front's (TULF) aim is the peaceful creation of an independent Tamil homeland (Eelam) in north-eastern Sri Lanka.

Founded. May 1976.

History. The TULF was initially organized as the Tamil Liberation Front (*Tamil Vimukthi Peramuna—* TVP), which included the Federal Party (*Illankai Tamil Arasu Kadchi—*ITAK), the National Liberation Front (*Jatika Vimukthi Peramuna—*JVP), the All Ceylon Tamil Congress (ACTC), the Muslim United Front and the Ceylon Workers' Congress. It succeeded an earlier Tamil Liberation Front formed before the 1970 elections by the Federal Party and the Tamil Congress.

It contested the 1977 general elections in 24 constituencies in the predominantly Tamil Northern and Eastern provinces, and as a result of the elections it became the largest opposition group in Parliament. However, the TULF consistently refused to take part in the affairs of parliament in protest at the lack of progress towards the realization of Tamil aspirations. The party boycotted the 1982 presidential elections, although the ACTC, one of its components, fielded a candidate.

After the extension of Parliament for another six years in 1892, the TULF announced in November of that year that its members would resign their seats. The party nevertheless participated in local elections held in May 1983 (despite a boycott call issued by separatist guerrillas) and gained majorities on several councils in the predominantly Tamil areas. However, in July 1983, a TULF convention agreed to renounce the parliamentary path towards the establishment of a separate Tamil state and to boycott a round-table conference on the Tamil question called by President Jayawardene.

In the wake of widespread inter-communal violence in 1983, Parliament in August unanimously passed constitutional amendments under which parties advocating separatism were to be banned and members of Parliament were obliged to take an oath forswearing separatist aspirations. The TULF members thereupon refused to take this oath and absented themselves from Parliament, with the result that from late October they were declared to have forfeited their seats.

During 1984 the TULF rejected various government proposals involving the creation of committees to examine methods of devolution for areas inhabited by Tamils. In July-August 1985 the TULF, together with other Tamil separatist groups, was engaged in secret talks with a Sri Lankan government delegation in Bhutan, but these talks broke down when the Tamil delegations withdrew as further killings of Tamils were reported from north-eastern Sri Lanka. Further talks held in Bhutan in 1986 also proved inconclusive.

The TULF was not invited to take part in further inter-party talks which began in July 1986. However, talks between the TULF and President Jayawardene in July and August of that year were followed by a first meeting, held in December 1986, between a delegation of the ruling United National Party and Tamil separatists (including the Tamil Tigers).

In the 1989 elections, the TULF (which now included the Eelam People's Revolutionary Liberation Front) won 10 seats, compared with 14 won by Tamil independents backed by groups broadly sympathetic to the militant Tamil Tigers.

United National Party

Address. 532 Galle Road, Colombo 3.

Leadership. Ranasinghe Premadasa (pres.); Sirisena Corray (gen. sec.).

Orientation. The United National Party (UNP) adopted a democratic socialist programme in 1958, but its policies in government since 1977 have reflected its strong support in conservative landowning, business and professional circles. It advocates a neutralist, non-aligned foreign policy and supported the status of Sinhala as the country's official language until the Tamil emergency elicited concessions on this front.

Founded. 1947.

History. The UNP was in power from the achievement of independence in 1947 until 1956, from March to July 1960 and in 1965-70. In opposition in 1970-77, the party supported the 1972 Constitution (under which Sri Lanka became a republic) introduced by the government led by Sirimavo Bandaranaike.

The UNP returned to power as a result of its landslide victory in the July 1977 general elections. The administration moved the following year to introduce a presidential form of government, with J. R. Jayawardene vacating the premiership to become President. On the basis of the popular mandate given to President Jayawardene in the presidential election of October 1982 (when he received 52.9 per cent of the votes cast), the UNP government subsequently introduced a Constitutional amendment extending the life of the 1977 Parliament for a further six years.

The UNP played a leading role in the preliminary all-party conferences and the negotiations which led to the conclusion of the Indo-Sri Lanka agreement on ending the Tamil-Sinhalese conflict in July 1987. A number of leading members of the UNP criticized the agreement, among them Prime Minister Premadasa. A number of leading UNP members subsequently fell victims to acts of violence committed by militant Sinhalese opposed to the agreement. In particular, Harsha Abeywardene, elected party chairman in December 1987, was assassinated after a few days in office.

Jayawardene announced in September 1988 that he would not stand in the 1989 presidential election, whereupon Premadasa was nominated as the party's new candidate, and went on to win the election. In the general elections held shortly afterwards, Premadasa led the party to a far-from-convincing victory, winning 125 out of 225 seats. However, in May 1991 the party won a sweeping victory in local elections. Later that year Premadasa successfully withstood a challenge from a dissident faction within the party who attempted to impeach him.

Publications. The Journal (weekly, in Sinhala and English).

United Socialist Alliance

Leadership. Vasudeva Nanyakkara (l.).

Orientation. In a declaration issued at its foundation, the United Socialist Alliance (USA) defined its main aim as to ensure the implementation of the Indo-Sri Lankan agreement of July 29, 1987, which provided an "initial and viable" basis for a political solution of Sri Lanka's separatist problem, which (the declaration said) could halt the efforts of "US imperialism and its allies to extend their political and military tentacles over Sri Lanka".

Founded. 1988.

History. The USA was formed by four left-wing parties (the Sri Lanka People's Party (SLMP); the Communist Party of Sri Lanka; the *Lanka Sama Samaja Party (LSSP—Lanka Equal Society Party); and the Nava Sama Samaja Party* (NSSP—New Equal Society Party. Its aim was to increase support for the divided left. The founding leader was Chandrika Kumaranatunge, the widow of Vijava Kumaranatunge who, as leader of the SLMP, had been the moving spirit behind the formation of the USA but who was assassinated by Sinhalese extremists in early 1988. The Alliance had little success in the 1989 general election, winning only three seats.

Major guerrilla organizations

The **Liberation Tigers of Tamil Eelam** (LTTE or Tamil Tigers); Velupillai Prabhakaran (l.). The main Tamil separatist guerrilla group. Rival militant Tamil groups were effectively relegated to exile politics from early 1990.

The (nominally left-wing) Sinhala guerrilla group, the **Janatha Vimukti Peramuna** (JVP—People's Liberation Front) was effectively wiped out as a serious threat by ruthless army action in its southern heartlands in late 1989 and early 1990.

Taiwan

Capital: Taipei

Population: 20,359,403 (May 31, 1991 official est.)

China ceded the offshore island of Taiwan (also known as Formosa), together with the surrounding minor islands, to Japan in 1895. In 1945, on Japan's defeat in the Second World War, Taiwan reverted to Chinese rule, becoming a province of the Republic of China, then under *Kuomintang* (KMT) rule. The present government of Taiwan is derived from the KMT government which fled China in 1949 after the communist victory there, and continues to claim to be the rightful government of mainland China.

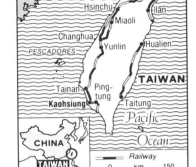

Constitutional structure

Under the 1947 Constitution, legislative authority is vested in the National Assembly (*Kuo-Min Ta-Hui*), which receives legislative proposals from the partially elected Legislative *Yuan* (*Li-Fa Yuan*). Elections to a new 405-member National Assembly in December 1991 were preceded by constitutional changes, effected in April 1991, which provided for the retirement of all 469 remaining "senior parliamentarians". These had been elected on mainland China in 1947-48 and granted life terms upon the formation of the Taiwanese government in 1949. Prior to the 1991 National Assembly elections, 81 "senior members" of the Legislative *Yuan* and 15 "senior members" of the Control *Yuan* had also retired. Elections to these two bodies were scheduled for 1992 and 1993.

The Executive *Yuan* is responsible to the Legislative *Yuan* and is the highest executive body. There are also Control, Judicial and Examination *Yuan*. A party requires a minimum of 20 seats in the Legislative *Yuan* to be able to introduce legislation. An Executive President is elected for a six-year term by the National Assembly.

Martial law, imposed in 1949, was lifted on July 24, 1987, opening the way to the formation of political parties. Martial law on the islands of Chinmen (Quemoy) and Matsu, however, was lifted only in September 1991, because of their proximity to the mainland.

Electoral system

In the new National Assembly, 225 seats were directly contested and 100 allocated proportionally among the parties according to votes won, with a 5 per cent threshold. These allocated seats included 20 seats reserved for presidential nominations from overseas Chinese. The remaining 80 seats were held by incumbents elected in 1986. Partial elections to the Legislative *Yuan* to supplement the life-members are held every three years, and were last held in 1989. In 1991 the Legislative *Yuan* consisted of 213 seats.

Recent elections

Supplementary elections to the National Assembly, 1969-1986

	1969	1972	1980	1986
Percentage turnout	54.75	68.52	66.43	65.43
Available seats	15	53	76	84
KMT	15	43	61	68
YCP	—	—	—	—
CDSP	—	—	1	1
DPP*				11
Independent	—	10	14	4

*Formed in 1986.

Supplementary elections to the Legislative Yuan 1969-1989

	1969	1972	1975	1980	1983	1986	1989
Percentage turnout	55.00	68.18	75.97	66.36	63.17	65.38	75.17
Available seats	11	51	52	97	98	100	101
KMT	8	41	42	79	83	79	72
YCP	—	1	1	2	2	2	—
CDSP	—	—	—	—	1	1	—
DPP*						12	21
Independents	3	9	9	16	12	6	8

*Formed in 1986.

National Assembly elections, Dec. 21, 1991

Party	Elected seats	Allocated seats	Percentage
KMT	179	75*	71.17
DPP	41	25·	23.93
National Democratic Independent Political Alliance	3	0	2.27
Others	2	0	2.63

*60 national representatives, 15 overseas Chinese.

·20 national representatives, five overseas Chinese.

The seats were contested by 667 candidates proposed by 17 political parties.

Evolution of the suffrage

All citizens over 20 are eligible to vote.

PARTY BY PARTY DATA

China Democratic Socialist Party

Address. 6 Lane 357, Ho-ping East Road, Sec. 2, Taipei.

Leadership. Wang Shih-hsien (ch.); Wong Hou-sen (sec.-gen.).

Orientation. Allied since its formation with the ruling *Kuomintang* (KMT), the China Democratic Socialist Party's (CDSP) platform consists of promoting democracy in keeping with Chinese traditional culture, raising the standard of living through industrialization and agricultural development, and narrowing the gap between rich and poor.

Founded. 1932.

History. The National Socialist Party and the Democratic Constitutionalists, both of them KMT supporters in China's dispute with Japan, merged in 1932 to form the CDSP. The Nationalist Socialist Party was organized in 1932 as a political scholars' association; the Democratic Constitutionalists, based in San Francisco, promoted the idea of constitutional government in China. In 1946, the CDSP sent delegates to the Chinese Constituent Assembly and participated in the elections for the National Assembly, Legislative *Yuan* and Control *Yuan.* The CDSP signed a joint political platform with the KMT, the Young China Party [see separate entry] and non-party members on April 13, 1947, and in 1948 held 212 seats in the (Taiwanese) National Assembly and 29 in the Legislative *Yuan.* However, the CDSP's subsequent loss of influence was demonstrated by the election results to the National Assembly in 1986, when the CDSP obtained only one seat.

Structure. The party has a five-member presidium, a standing central committee, a central control committee, a secretariat, and specialized departments and committees.

Membership. 30,000.

Publications. Renaissance and *Universe* (both Taipei monthlies); *Liberty* (Hong Kong, monthly).

Democratic Progressive Party (DPP)

Address. 115 Chien Kuo North Road, 7th Floor, Sec. 2, Taipei.

Leadership. Hsu Hsin-liang (ch.); Chang Chun-hung (sec. gen.).

Orientation. Supports an independent, sovereign Taiwan which would abandon the claim to mainland China; calls for direct presidential elections and fully-elected legislative authorities.

Founded. Sept. 28, 1986.

History. The Democratic Progressive Party (DPP) was formed while the restrictions of martial law still applied (in 1987 these were lifted to allow the formation of political parties, provided these did not advocate communism or "the division of national territory" ie. advocate Taiwanese sovereignty thus contradicting the *Kuomintang* (KMT) claim to mainland China). The DPP was formed by 135 members of a loose opposition movement, *Tangwai,* meaning "outside the party", which was set up in 1983 to promote a multiparty democracy. Although still technically illegal, the DPP contested the December 1986 elections, gaining seats on the legislative bodies [see Constitutional structure].

The DPP held its first annual conference on Nov. 10, 1986, attended by 165 delegates. At the second conference in 1987, a resolution claimed the right to advocate Taiwanese independence for Taiwanese citizens, although it was denied that this was official DPP policy. At the third conference, the former secretary-general, Huang Huang-hsiung, replaced the DPP's first Chair, Yao Chia-wen, who had been imprisoned in 1980-1987 for inciting a riot. The DPP applied for registration with the Interior Ministry in April 1989, despite its objections to the January 1989 laws on the registration of political parties. These required political organizations which pledged to obey the Constitution and eschew communism to register with the Interior Ministry and enforced the restrictions on political activity which had been enacted on the lifting of martial law in July 1987.

Yao Chia-wen, DPP Chair in 1987-88, came from the radical New Movement faction in the DPP which advocated extra-parliamentary means of protest. The DPP's tactics have largely consisted of occasionally violent disruption of the National Assembly meetings. For example, DPP members were barred at the National Assembly plenum in February 1990, convened to elect the President, for trying to swear loyalty to "Taiwan" rather than to the "Republic of China". The

DPP's intransigence over political reform caused prominent mainland-born politicians, Lin Chang-chieh and Fei Hsi-ping, both members of the Legislative *Yuan*, to leave the party. Lin left the DPP on June 2, 1991 over disagreements about Taiwanese independence as advocated by the DPP, and Fei resigned in December 1988 in protest at the DPP's uncompromising stand on the issue of the retirement of mainland-born politicians.

An alternative draft constitution for "Taiwan" was adopted by the DPP in August 1991. As the KMT acceded to more of the DPP's demands for political reforms, such as the lifting of martial law and electoral reform, the DPP's programme was forced to centre on the issue of Taiwanese self-determination, in effect independence. The New Movement faction, a strong advocate of independence, suffered however from the suppression of China's pro-democracy movement in the Beijing Tiananmen Square massacre of 1989. The KMT used the incident to spread warnings of the potential danger to Taiwan of a People's Republic of China (PRC)-led repression of any open declaration of Taiwanese independence.

In the 1991 elections to the National Assembly, the DPP had campaigned largely on a "Taiwanese independence" ticket, despite the legal restrictions against this. The DPP failed however to gain enough seats to be able to influence the political and constitutional reform programme, which the new National Assembly was expected to draft. The DPP's poor showing was variously attributed to fears of possible PRC repression, whipped up largely by the KMT; to low exposure for the DPP and poor financing; and to the party's factional nature.

Structure. An annual National Congress elects a chair and members of an Executive Committee, which in turn elects a Standing Committee. The Chair appoints a secretary-general and two deputies for the Secretariat, which manages five to six specialized departments.

Membership. 20,000.

Publications. Minchu Chinpu Choukan, a weekly political magazine.

Labour Party

Kungtang

Address. 300, Roosevelt Road, 5th Floor, Sec. 3, Taipei.

Leadership. Wang Yi-hsiung (ch.); Wang Yau-nan (sec.-gen.).

Orientation. Labour rights. The *Kungtang* (KT) aims to become the leading political movment of the industrial workforce of Taiwan.

Founded. Nov. 1, 1987.

History. Wang Yi-hsiung, a member of the Legislative *Yuan*, left the Democratic People's Party (DPP) to form the KT, stating his intention to complement but not compete with the main opposition party. The KT thus grew out of the DPP's internal debate over whether or not to adopt a class-based political approach. The platform of the KT, the first workers' party in Taiwan, included improved conditions for women and native Taiwanese in addition to foregrounding the issues of health and safety at work. Its first congress was held on Dec. 5, 1987, when Wang was elected Chair and Su Chin-li secretary-general. A splinter group in 1989 formed a more radical party, the Workers' Party [see separate entry], while the KT continued its gradualist approach and parliamentary campaigns to achieve legal improvements for the workforce.

Membership. 4,500.

Nationalist Party of China

Kuomintang

Address. 11 Chungshan South Road, Taipei.

Leadership. Lee Teng-hui (ch.); James Soong (sec.-gen.).

Orientation. The ruling party, it aims to supplant communism in mainland China, of which it sees itself as the legitimate government. Its ideology is based upon that of its founder Sun Yat-sen, who espoused the Three Principles of the People: nationalism, democracy, and social well-being.

Founded. 1894.

History. The *Kuomintang* (KMT) gained its name in October 1919, having grown out of revolutionary groups, including the *Hsing Chung Hui* (Society for Regenerating China) founded by Sun Yat-sen in 1894 in Hawaii. The KMT played an important role in the defeat of China's Manchu emperors and their warlord successors. In this it was helped by the Soviet Union, whose leadership believed that the KMT embodied the "bourgeois nationalist" stage of revolution. The KMT's Reorganization Conference in January 1924 established the party's structure along the lines of Leninist democratic-centralism. Initially, members of the Chinese Communist Party (CCP) were allowed to join the KMT as individuals, during a brief period of co-operation between the two parties. However, Gen. Chiang Kai-shek, Commander of the KMT forces which defeated the northern Chinese generals in 1926-

28, succeeded Sun Yat-sen as KMT Chairman on the latter's death in 1925 and purged the KMT of communists at the KMT's second National Congress in January 1926, when one third of the delegates were CCP members. A new Constitution for China, incorporating Sun Yat-sen's Three Principles of the People, was promulgated on Dec. 25, 1946, and did allow a limited role for other parties, because KMT control was relaxed during the Japanese invasion of 1937-45. However, the victory of the CCP in the Chinese civil war in 1949 forced the KMT government to flee China for the offshore island of Taiwan (Formosa), while on the mainland, the People's Republic of China (PRC) was proclaimed on Oct. 1, 1949.

With the proclamation in Taipei of the Republic of China in 1949, the fundamental theme of Taiwan's KMT government was openly declared: that the KMT was the legitimate government of mainland China. In April 1948 the KMT had pronounced the "Temporary Provisions effective during the Period of Communist Rebellion", which extended the terms of the newly-elected delegates to the National Assembly until "free and fair elections" could be held in mainland China. Meanwhile, the KMT's dubious claim to politically represent mainland China rested on the election of 3,045 National Assembly deputies in Nov. 21-23, 1947, and of 180 Control *Yuan* and 773 Legislative *Yuan* delegates in May 1948 by only about 20 million of China's 540 million population.

In Taiwan, after 1949, the KMT established a complex administrative structure, in which every level of local and national government was shadowed by a corresponding party organization. Although at first mainlanders dominated the KMT, in the 1950s more native Taiwanese candidates began to be proposed for the local elections as they were expected to receive the popular vote rather than mainland Chinese candidates. Mortality among the mainland politicians later forced the holding of the first supplementary elections to the three main legislative bodies in 1969, following a constitutional amendment of 1966.

Taiwan's economic success and consequent opening to the outside world brought demands for a broader political structure. The transfer of international recognition from Taiwan to the People's Republic of China in the 1970s, and the death of Chiang in April 1975, also forced the debate over Taiwan's political future. Chiang was replaced as Chair of the KMT by his son, Gen. Chiang Ching-kuo, who in May 1978 also became President. Meanwhile, in 1977 the first protests against KMT rule took place, when the ruling party was accused of manipulating local elections which had been contested by the dissident Hsu Hsin-liang, later to become leader of the Democratic Progressive Party (DPP) [see separate].

A KMT Central Committee plenum in March 1986 raised the sensitive issues which had to be tackled if reform of the moribund system were to take place. They included new political parties; lifting martial law; improving provincial representation and the rejuvenation of the legislature. In May 1986, Chiang instructed the KMT to open talks with the *Tangwai* (non-KMT political activists). The December 1986 elections were then, for the first time, contested by an opposition party in the form of the DPP. Although Chiang died in January 1988, to be succeeded by Vice-President, Lee Teng-hui for the remaining two years of the presidential term, in February 1988, the KMT Central Standing Committee approved measures initiated by Chiang gradually to reduce the quota of life-members in the National Assembly and to increase Taiwanese representation at the expense of seats reserved for mainland constituencies. Lee was confirmed as KMT Chair at the 13th KMT National Congress in July 1988, having been acting Chair since January, and thus became the first native Taiwanese to hold the posts of KMT Chair and Taiwanese President. In 1989, James Soong became KMT secretary-general, succeeding the moderate Lee Huan who had held the post since 1987 and had been appointed Prime Minister.

The 13th KMT Congress also reformed the party itself. Taiwan-born second generation mainlanders in the KMT were demanding faster changes to the National Assembly membership, although they did not advocate its dissolution and fresh elections as demanded by the DPP, as this would have cast doubt over the legitimacy of the KMT claim to mainland China. The Central Committee was expanded from 150 to 180 seats and for the first time elected rather than appointed. About half of the 360 candidates were nominated by the KMT Chair, and 33 of them failed to be elected. Twelve seats were replaced on the Central Standing Committee, which thus for the first time had a majority of Taiwan-born politicians (16 out of 31). The average age of the Central Committee dropped from 68 to 59. The charter and platform of the KMT were also revised, with the Secretariat now divided into three sections: policy co-ordination, organization and administration. Despite these important changes, the emphasis of the main speeches to the Congress was on continuity and stability.

The results of the December 1991 National Assembly elections gave the KMT over the three-quarters majority which it needed to control the course of the constitutional changes scheduled for debate during 1992 and 1993. The election result was no doubt partly due to the KMT's highly centralized nature, its domination of the national electronic media and the revenue provided by its ownership of 18 businesses.

Structure. A National Congress convenes at least every four years to elect the Central Committee and the KMT Chair. The Central Committee, which holds an annual plenary session, elects a 31-member Central Standing Committee (which meets weekly). The Central Secretariat, under the secretary-general and three deputies, manages 12 specialist departments.

Membership. 2,400,000 (about one-third of adult males in Taiwan are KMT members).

Publications. *Chungyang Jih Pao* (Central Daily News), circulation 530,000; *Chungkuo Shih Pao* (China Times), circulation 725,000.

Young China Party

Ching-nien Tang

Address. 256 King Hwa Street, Taipei.

Leadership. Li Huang (ch.).

Orientation. The Young China Party (YCP), like the *Kuomintang* (KMT), aims to recover sovereignty over mainland China, to promote relations with the non-communist world and to safeguard democracy and the Constitution.

Founded. 1923.

History. The YCP participated in the elections for the National Assembly, Legislative *Yuan* and Control *Yuan* in 1946, when relaxation of political control by the KMT during the Japanese invasion allowed other parties' activity. The YCP, however, is pro-KMT and has always supported the government. In mid-1990 it held seven seats in the Legislative *Yuan*.

Minor parties

China Socialist Democratic Party (CSDP); 2F-1, 4 Ching Dao East Road, Taipei. The party was formed in 1991 as a breakaway faction from the Democratic Progressive Party [see separate entry] by Ju Gao-jeng, who had resigned from the parent party and remains the CSDP leader.

Chinese Freedom Party; founded on July 11, 1987, when over 300 delegates attended the inaugural meeting. The party advocates direct parliamentary elections, détente and the liberalization of relations with the People's Republic of China and anti-corruption measures.

Democratic Liberal Party (DLP); Hung Chao-nan, a former member of the National Assembly, announced the formation of the DLP on Sept. 6, 1987. The DLP aims to promote political democracy and economic liberty.

Workers' Party; 181 Fu-hsing South Road, 2nd Floor, Sec. 2, Taipei. The party was formed in 1989 by a faction of the Labour Party [see separate entry] when 200 members left the parent party in support of textile worker Lou Meiwen's demands for workers' rights and improved conditions. Lou criticised the leadership of the Labour Party as opportunist and too moderate. The party demands labour rights for Taiwan's workforce, to be achieved by extra legal action if necessary.

Major guerrilla organizations

There are no guerrilla organizations in Taiwan.

Tajikistan

Capital: Dushanbe **Population: 5,358,000 (official est. as of Jan. 1, 1991)**

The Republic of Tajikistan was formed on Oct. 16, 1929 as a constituent union republic of the Soviet Union. It declared sovereignty on Aug. 25, 1990 and independence on Sept. 8, 1991. It became a founder member of the Commonwealth of Independent States (CIS), which was constituted on Dec. 21, 1991 on the collapse of the Soviet Union. Riots in Dushanbe in March-May 1992 forced the President Rakhmon Nabiyev to agree to a coalition government including representatives of opposition parties.

Constitutional structure

Following the spring 1992 disturbances, an 80-seat *Majlis* took over the legislative role of the 230-seat Supreme Soviet. The *Majlis* would temporarily consist of Supreme Soviet deputies and representatives of political parties, and would sit until fresh elections scheduled for Dec. 6, 1992. A directly-elected Presidency was instituted in November 1991; previously the de facto President had been elected by the Supreme Soviet as its Chair.

Electoral system

Contested elections for the Supreme Soviet were introduced in 1990. Voting went to a second round if a candidate failed to win at least 50 per cent of the vote. Following demonstrations in September 1991 in protest at the continued leading role of the Communist Party, national presidential elections were held.

Evolution of the suffrage

Adults over 18 can vote unless in prison or in psychiatric institutions, or declared incapable by a court.

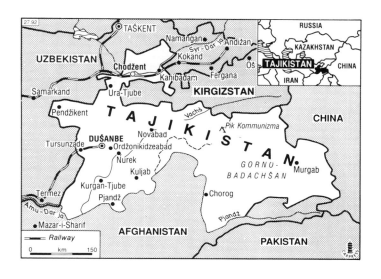

Recent elections

Legislative elections, Feb. 25, 1990

The elections were not contested on a party basis, but each seat was contested by between two and 17 candidates.

Presidential elections, Nov. 24, 1991

Candidate	Percentage of vote
Rakhmon Nabiyev	58
Davlat Khudonazarov	30

PARTY BY PARTY DATA

Communist Party

Kommunisticheskaya partiya Tadzhikistana

Leadership. Kakhar Makhkamov (first sec.).

Orientation. Communist.

Founded. 1929.

History. The Tajik Communist Party (CP), originally the republican branch of the Communist Party of the Soviet Union (CPSU) was declared independent from the CPSU and its property nationalised on Aug. 28, 1991. It was banned and re-legalized in Tajikistan by the Supreme Soviet several times during the crisis of government in September and October 1991, and was renamed as the Socialist Party on Sept. 21. On Jan. 20, 1992 it regained its original name.

Structure. A Central Committee and ruling Presidium and Politburo.

Publications. *Narodnaya Gazeta* (People's Newspaper), formerly *Kommunist Tadzhikistana*.

Democratic Party

Demokraticheskaya partiya

Leadership. Shodmon Yusupov (ch.).

Orientation. Multi-ethnic; recognises Islam, but in a secular state.

Founded. Aug. 10, 1990.

History. The Democratic Party (DP) grew from the Democratic Platform within the Communist Party of the Soviet Union (CPSU), many of whose members left the CPSU after nationalist rioting in Dushanbe in February 1990 and, together with some *Rastokhez* [see below] activists, formed the DP. The founders were mainly members of the intelligentsia, including presidential candidate, Davlat Khudonazarov, a cinematographer. In November 1990 the DP organized a hunger strike demanding (unsuccessfully) national presidential elections. The first congress held on Dec. 1-2, 1990 and Jan. 5-6, 1991 elected the leadership. The second congress on Sept. 22, 1991 unsuccessfully attempted to create a United Democratic Party with the Russian and Turkmen DPs.

Structure. 42-member governing body.

Membership. 15,000, including four Supreme Soviet members.

Publications. Fortnightly newspaper *Adolat* (Justice) in Tajik and Russian. Circulation 10,000-15,000.

Affiliations. Democratic Congress.

Islamic Renaissance Party

Islamskaya partiya vozrozhdeniya

Leadership. Mukhammad Sharif Khimmatov (ch.).

Orientation. To create the conditions for believers to be able to practice their faith.

Founded. Oct. 6, 1990.

History. The Tajik branch of the Islamic Renaissance Party (IRP) was formed together with the national (ex-Soviet) party in June 1990. Although banned by the authorities, the IRP, co-operating with the Democratic Party [see above], was at the forefront of anti-communist demonstrations in Dushanbe after the failure of the August 1991 coup in Moscow. The ban on the IRP was lifted on Oct. 7, 1991 and the founding congress of the IRP of Tajikistan was held on Oct. 26. It lent support to Davlat Khudonazarov's candidature in the November 1991 presidential elections. The IRP is especially influential in the south of Tajikistan. With the formation of a coalition government in May 1992, IRP deputy chair, Davlat Usmanov, became Deputy Prime Minister.

Structure. Council of 18 *ulema*.

Membership. 20,000.

Ruby of Badakhshan

Lali Badakhshon

Leadership. Amirbek Azobekov (ch. of Presidium).

Orientation. Demands status of an autonomous republic for the Gorno Badakhshan region.

Founded. March 1991.

History. The movement began in the autumn of 1989 as an informal group and has become the main political organization of the Pamir region in Tajikistan. The Pamir region, which is home to many small nationalities, demanded greater economic autonomy from the Tajik authorities, organizing petitions and meetings to press their demands. The party's official registration, which occurred on May 30, 1991, meant that a founding congress had to be held (March 1991). The Tajik authorities, however, have not yet reached a decision on altering the status of the region. *Lali Badakhshon* co-operates with other Tajik opposition organizations.

Structure. 22-member ruling body, with 9-member Presidium and chair.

Membership. 1,000.

Renaissance Organization
Organizatsiya Rastokhez

Leadership. Takhir Abdujaborov.

Orientation. Demands economic and political reform.

Founded. Sept. 14, 1989.

History. Until the nationalist protests of February 1990, *Rastokhez*, which grew out of an informal discussion group, worked in step with the government. After February 1990, it went over to the opposition, although declaring itself still prepared to co-operate with the Tajik authorities. Abdujaborov was elected to the Supreme Soviet in the March 1990 elections. The first congress in January 1991 affirmed the programme and leadership of the movement. There is little input from the ethnic Russian population of Tajikistan, although some members of the Uzbek ethnic group have joined.

Structure. 66-member Great Council, elected at Congress, with 15-member Presidium.

Membership. 25,000.

Publications. *Tunyo* (Peace) newspaper, issued irregularly, circulation 10,000-20,000.

Thailand

Capital: Bangkok

Population: 55,700,000 (1990)

The Kingdom of Thailand is the only Southeast Asian country not to have been colonized by a European power. Modern Thailand came into being in 1932 when a civilian-military group carried out a coup (commonly referred to as a "revolution") which removed the country's absolute monarchical system in favour of a system modelled on the European constitutional monarchies. However, shortly after the 1932 "revolution", the military took power and the army has since been the most potent force in Thai politics. The 1991 coup was the 17th succesful intervention by the military since 1932. Military rule has been interspersed with short periods of democratic government, most notably in the mid-1970s and late 1980s.

Constitutional structure

Following the military coup of Feb. 23, 1991, the ruling military junta, the National Peace-Keeping Assembly, abrogated the country's 1978 Constitution and dissolved the leading political organs. A new Constitution, the country's 15th, came into effect on Dec. 9, 1991, after its signature by King Bhumibol Adulyadej. The Constitution provided for the creation of a legislative body, the National Assembly, comprising an elected House of Representatives and an appointed Senate, and a Cabinet headed by a Prime Minister. Following elections to the new House of Representatives in March 1992 a pro-military government was formed headed by the junta leader, Gen. Suchinda Kraprayoon. Demonstrations opposing Suchinda's premiership were brutally suppressed by the army and Suchinda was forced to resign in late May. Shortly afterwards the House of Representatives approved a number of amendments to the Constitution, the chief of which, intended to reduce the role of the military, stipulated that a future Prime Minister had to be an elected member of the House.

Electoral system

The 360-member House of Representatives is elected for a four-year term by universal adult suffrage. In elections held in March 1992 pro-military parties secured enough seats to form a government. The government fell in the aftermath of the army's violent suppression of pro-democracy demonstrations in May and fresh elections were scheduled for September 1992. The 270 members of the Senate were appointed by the ruling junta under a provisional clause of the 1991 Constitution.

Evolution of the suffrage

Every person of Thai nationality not less than 20 years of age as of Jan. 1 of an election year is entitled to vote.

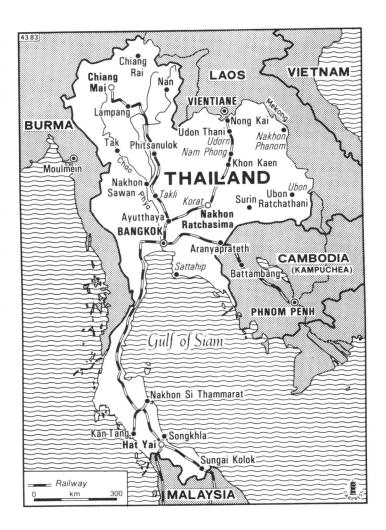

Recent elections

House of Representatives 1986-92

Party	Year		
	1986	1988	1992
Democrat Party	100	48	44
Chart Thai	63	87	74
Social Action Party	51	54	31
United Democrat Party	38	5	—
Prachakon Thai	24	31	7
*Ruam Thai	19	35	
Rassadorn	18	21	4
*Community Action Party	15	9	
*Progressive Party	9	8	
Muan Chon	3	5	—
Liberal Party	1	3	—
*Prachachon	—	19	
Puangchon Chao Thai	1	17	1
Palang Dharma	—	14	41
Sammakhi Tham	—	—	79
New Aspiration Party	—	—	72
*Ekkarparb			6
Others	5	1	0
Total	347	357	360

*Merged as Ekkarparb in 1989.

PARTY BY PARTY DATA

Chart Thai *see* Thai Nation

Citizens' Party
Rassadorn
Address. House of Representatives, Bangkok.
Leadership. Gen. Mana Rattanakoset (sec.-gen.)
Orientation. Conservative; pro-military.
Founded. 1986.
History. Founded by Gen. Tienchai Sirisamphan, a former Deputy Army Commander, the party immediatly attracted the support of a large number of military personnel. It gained 18 seats in elections held in 1986 and joined the Democrat-led coalition under Prem Tinsulanonda. Tienchai was appointed as a Deputy Prime Minister. *Rassadorn* increased its representation to 21 seats in the 1988 election and joined the new *Chart Thai*-led government. Tienchai resigned as party leader in the aftermath of the February 1991 coup after military leaders accused him of corruption. The party performed poorly in the 1992 election winning only four seats. Nevertheless, the party joined the new pro-military coalition led by *Samakkhi Tham*.

Democrat Party
Pak Prachatipat
Address. House of Representatives, Bangkok.
Leadership. Chuan Leekpai (l.); Maj.-Gen. Sanan Khachonpraset (sec.-gen.).
Orientation. Moderate liberal, conservative and monarchist.
Founded. 1946.
History. Founded by Khuang Aphaiwong, with the support of Kukrit and Seni Pramoj, the Democrat Party is Thailand's principal party of opposition. Although it is the country's oldest party, it managed to form only two governments during its first 30 years (the first under in 1947-48 and the second under Seni in 1978) and on both occasions the military launched coups after a matter of months. In the 1986 election the Democrats won by far the largest number of seats and entered into coalition with the Social Action Party and *Chart Thai*, under the premiership of Gen. Prem Tinsulanonda. Factional in-fighting led to a split in the party in 1988 and the House of Representatives was dissolved early. In the resultant elections the party's representation was cut from 100 to 48. However, the party managed to maintain its traditional support base in the southern regions. The Democrats joined the Chatichai coalition, but withdrew into opposition in

late 1990. In the post-coup elections of 1992, the Democrats again maintained their southern support, winning 44 seats. Subsequently, the party joined the pro-democracy alliance which opposed continued military involvement in politics.

Democratic Labour Party
Raeng Ngan Pracha Tippatai
Address. Bangkok.
Leadership. Prasert Sapsunthorn (l.); Yongyut Watanavikorn (sec.-gen.).
Orientation. Centre-left.
Founded. 1988.
History. Secured one seat in the 1988 election, but did not contest the 1992 election.

Force of Spiritual Righteousness
Palang Dharma
Address. House of Representatives, Bangkok.
Leadership. Maj.-Gen. Chamlong Sirimaung (l.); Chinuut Soonthorn (sec.-gen.).
Orientation. Centre-left, anti-military and pro-democracy.
Founded. 1988.
History. *Palang Dharma* was formed by Chamlong Sirimaung, the popular, charismatic and ascetic governor of Bangkok. The Bangkok-based party projected a "clean image", stressing in its literature the virtues of discipline and self-sacrifice. In the 1988 elections, the party performed poorly against the pro-military *Prachakorn Thai* in Bangkok, winning only 14 seats. Chamlong's outspoken criticism of the 1991 military coup increased support for *Palang Dharma* and the party won 41 seats in the March 1992 general election, including 32 of the capital's 35 seats. After the election Chamlong became the major spokesman for the so-called pro-democracy alliance which opposed continued military involvement in national politics.

Kaset Seri
History. This small party contested the 1992 election, but did not win any seats.

Liberal Party
Seriniyom
Address. Bangkok.
Leadership. Col. Narong Kittikachorn (l.); Surasak Chavewongse (sec.-gen.).
Orientation. Pro-business.

Founded. 1981.

History. The Liberal Party won one seat in 1986 and three in 1988, but did not contest the 1992 election.

Mass
Muan Chon

Address. House of Representatives, Bangkok.

Leadership. Police Capt. Chalerm Yubamrung (l.); Sophon Petchsavang (sec.-gen.).

Orientation. Right-wing.

Founded. 1985.

History. *Muan Chon* was formed in 1985 by a group of MPs from various government and opposition parties. In its first election in 1986 the party won three seats and the number was increased to five in 1988. After the 1988 election, party leader Chalerm took the party into the ruling coalition headed by Chatichai Choonhaven's *Chart Thai*. Chalerm entered the government as a Minister attached to the Prime Minister's Office. In 1990 the outspoken Chalerm was at the centre of a major political controversy when he effectively accused the new Defence Minister, Gen. Chaovalit Yongchaiyut, of corruption. Chaovalit resigned from the government and the powerful military establishment began pressuring Chatichai to dismiss Chalerm. Chatichai resisted the pressure until November, when he demoted Chalerm and the next month *Muan Chon* pulled out of the ruling coalition. Following the February 1991 coup, Chalerm fled Bangkok to avoid arrest. In the May 1992 elections, *Muan Chon* managed to win only one seat.

New Aspiration Party
Pak Kuam Vuang Mai

Address. House of Representatives, Bangkok.

Leadership. Gen. Chaovalit Yongchaiyut (l.); Prani Mi-Udon (sec.-gen.).

Orientation. Centre, pro-democratic.

Founded. 1990.

History. The New Aspirations Party (NAP) was formed as a vehicle for the political ambitions of former Army Chief and self-styled "soldier for democracy", Gen. Chaovalit Yonchaiyut. Chaovalit had resigned as Army Commander earlier in the year in order to enter Gen. Chatichai Choonhavan's Cabinet as a (non-party) Defence Minister and Deputy Prime Minister. He resigned from the Cabinet after only three months in office following a public dispute with another Cabinet member, *Muan Chon* leader Chalerm Yubamrung. After his resignation, Chaovalit was courted by a number of established political parties,

but he chose to form his own organization. Internal wrangling within the NAP led to the resignation of Chaovalit's deputy, Squadron Leader Prasong Soonsiri, and his faction in January 1992.

Nevertheless, the NAP won 72 seats in a general election held two months later, reflecting, in part, heavy pre-election spending in the poor Isarn (northeast) district. Following the election, Chaovalit went on to play a major role in the so-called pro-democracy coalition which opposed continued military involvement in national politics.

Pracha Dhamma Party

Address. Bangkok.

Leadership. Kriengkamol Laohapairojn (co-ordinator).

Orientation. Left-wing, anti-military.

Founded. 1991.

History. The party was formed in 1991 by a group of left-wing political activists, most of whom had been involved in the pro-democracy student movement of the 1970s. The party is opposed to military involvement in politics.

Ruam Phalang Mai

History. This party contested the 1992 election but did not win any seats.

Saha Prachathipatai

History. This party contested the 1992 election but did not win any seats.

Social Action Party
Pak Kit Sangkhom

Address. House of Representatives, Bangkok.

Leadership. Montri Phongpanit (l.); Prayut Siriphanit (sec.-gen.).

Orientation. Moderate conservative.

Founded. 1974.

History. The party emerged as a conservative outgrowth from the Democrat Party. It obtained a majority in the 1979 elections and was again the leading party in 1983, serving as the core of the coalition government under Gen. Prem Tinsulanonda. Internal divisions within the party led to the resignation of long-time leader Kukrit Pramoj in 1985 and his replacement by Air Chief Marshal Siddhi Savetsila. It was runner up to the Democrats in the 1988 elections and entered the *Chart Thai*-led government headed by Gen. Chatichai Choonhaven. Siddhi Savetsila was removed as party leader in mid-1990 and was replaced, on a temporary basis, by Kukrit. A year later Montri Phongpanit was elected as the new leader, with Prayut Siriphanit as the new secretary-general.

Prior to the leadership elections, in late 1990, the party had withdrawn its support from the Chatichai coalition. In the 1992 post-coup election the party won 31 seats, a considerable reduction on the 54 it had won in 1988. The party subsequently joined the *Samakkhi Tham*-led coalition under the premiership of Gen. Suchinda Kraprayoon.

Social Democratic Force
Palang Prachathipat Sangkhom
Address. Bangkok.
Leadership. Chatchawal Chompudaeng (l.); Insorn Buakiew (sec.-gen.).
Orientation. Left of centre.
Founded. 1974.
History. Founded as the New Force (*Palang Mai*) in 1974 by a group of intellectuals opposed to the military regime. It supported the Prem Tinsulanonda government after the 1983 elections, but failed to win representation. It won one seat in 1986 and retained it in 1988. The group was renamed as the Social Democratic Force in 1988, but did not contest the 1992 election.

Solidarity
Ekkaparb
Address. House of Representatives, Bangkok.
Leadership. Bunchu Rotanasathian (l.); Uthai Phimchaichon (sec.-gen.).
Orientation. Centrist, latterly pro-democratic.
Founded. 1989.
History. Ekkaparb was formed by the merger of four opposition parties (*Ruam Thai, Prachachon*, Community Action Party and the Progressive Party) in an attempt to strengthen the opposition to Gen. Chatichai's *Chart Thai*-led coalition. Originally the party had 71 seats, but its strength was reduced considerably when nine members of the *Prachachon* faction defected to *Chart Thai*. At the time of its foundation the party was led by veteran politician, Narong Wongwan. In late 1990 *Ekkaparb* was persuded to enter the beleagured Chatichai coalition. In the aftermath of the 1991 coup, the party virtually disintegrated. Narong soon left to join the newly formed *Samakkhi Tham* [see separate entry]. In the post-coup elections of 1992, *Ekkaparb* won only six seats. The party subsequently lent its diminished weight to the anti-military pro-democracy alliance.

Thai Citizens' Party
Prachakorn Thai
Address. House of Representatives, Bangkok.
Leadership. Samak Sundaravej (l.); Kosol Kraiverk (sec.-gen.).
Orientation. Right-wing, pro-military.
Founded. 1979.
History. The *Prachakorn Thai* was founded by Samak Sundaravej, a right-wing, populist Democrat dissident and former Interior Minister. The party performed extremely well in its first general election in 1979, capturing 29 out of 32 seats in Bangkok (where the Democrats had won all the seats in 1976). Samak did not take the party into government until after the 1983 election, when the dominance of the party in the capital lessened.

This trend continued in 1986, but two years later the party managed to gain 20 seats in Bangkok (four more than in 1986), largely at the expense of the Democrats and the Social Action Party. Following the 1988 election, Samak took the party into opposition (he had supported Prem Tinsulanonda's 1986-88 government from outside), but the party joined Chatichai Choonhaven's faltering *Chart Thai*-led coalition in late 1990, a matter of months before the military moved against the government. Following the coup, Samak was one of a number of high-ranking politicians placed under investigation for corruption by the military. *Palang Dharma* decimated *Prachakorn Thai's* hold on the capital in the March 1992 elections. The party, with only seven seats, lent its diminished support to the pro-military coalition formed after the election.

Thai Nation
Chart Thai
Address. House of Representatives, Bangkok.
Leadership. Air Marshal Sombun Rahong (l.); Banharn Silpa-archa (sec.-gen.).
Orientation. Right-wing, pro-business.
Founded. 1975.
History. Three generals, Chatichai Choonhavan, Pramarn Adireksan and Siri Siriyothin, founded *Chart Thai* in order to contest the 1975 general election. All three had been active in politics in the 1950s, serving in various capacities during the so-called Phin-Phao military dictatorship. However, with the acsension of Marshall Sarit Thanarat in 1958, the three were effectively excluded from national politics. The "democratic revolution" of 1973 paved the way for their political re-emergence. In the 1975 election *Chart Thai*, heavily backed by big business and various mili-

tary factions, won 28 seats in the House of Representatives and subsequently joined Kukrit Pramoj's coalition government. *Chart Thai* increased its representation to 56 seats (second only to the Democrats) in the 1976 elections and entered the new, short-lived coalition which was toppled in a military coup.

Elections held in 1979 confirmed *Chart Thai* as one of the country's leading political parties and its leaders again chose to enter the ruling coalition. The party withdrew from the coalition in 1983, but after winning 63 seats in the 1986 elections, joined the Democrat-led government under Gen. Prem Tinsulanonda. In the 1988 elections *Chart Thai* won the most seats and Gen. Chatichai, the party leader, formed a coalition government. *Chart Thai's* victory reflected the massive financial support provided by the country's increasingly powerful big business community.

After a period of conflict between the government and the military, and also between various contending military factions, the army launched a successful coup in early 1991 and Chatichai's government was replaced by a military junta. The coup left the party in some disarray, especially after the military placed Chatichai under investigation for corruption. In late 1991 the party elected Air Chief Marshal Somboon Rahong, hitherto governor of the Thai Airport Authority, to replace Chatichai.

Chart Thai won 74 seats in general election held in March 1992, performing strongly in the central regions where it won 42 out of 83 seats. The party entered into coalition with *Samakkhi Tham* and other pro-military parties. However, following the military's massacre of pro-democracy demonstrators in May, the new government was replaced in June by a Cabinet of politically non-aligned technocrats ahead of fresh elections in September.

Thai People or Thai Mass
Puangchon Chao Thai
Address. House of Representatives, Bangkok.
Leadership. Maj.-Gen. Boonyoong Watthanapong (sec.-gen.).
Orientation. Centre-right.
Founded. 1981.
History. Puangchon Chao Thai had no success in the 1983 election and gained only one seat in 1986. Prior to the 1988 election, party leader Maj.-Gen. Ravi Wanpen was replaced by former army strongman Gen. Arthit Kamlang-Ek. The party campaigned against Prime Minister Prem Tinsulanonda and, after spending lavishly in the poor Isarn district (the north-east) man-

aged to win 17 seats. Arthit took the party into Chatichai Choonhaven's ruling coalition in mid-1990 when he entered the government as a Deputy Prime Minister, a move which caused a measure of apprehension within leading military circles. Following the 1991 coup Arthit was arrested, although he was later released. In January 1992 Arthit resigned as party leader in order to join *Samakkhi Tham*. The party contested the 1992 election without Arthit, but gained only one seat.

Thongthin Kaona
History. This small party contested the 1992 election but did not win any seat.

United Democratic Party
Pak Saha Prachathipatai
Address. Bangkok.
Leadership. Col. Phol Roengprasertvit (l.); Tamchai Kamphato (sec.-gen.).
Orientation. Conservative and pro-business.
Founded. 1986.
History. Organized by the Social Action Party and *Chart Thai* dissidents who opposed Prem Tinsulanonda prior to the 1986 elections. In the election it won 38 seats. However, in 1988 its support collapsed and it won only five seats after a faction led by Boontheng Thongsawasd withdrew in favour of *Chart Thai*. The party did not contest the 1992 elections.

United in Virtue
Samakkhi Tham
Address. House of Representatives, Bangkok.
Leadership. Narong Wongwan (l.); Buntheng Thongsawat (l.); Sqadron Leader Thiti Nakhonthap (l.).
Orientation. Pro-military.
Founded. 1991.
History. Founded while the country was under military rule, *Samakkhi Tham* was widely regarded as a party under the patronage of the Air Force and its Commander-in-Chief (and Armed Forces Supreme Commander), Air Chief Marshal Kaset Rojanani. In the March 1992 gemeral election the party won the largest number of seats (79), partly as a result of lavish pre-election spending in the Isarn district (the poor north-eastern region). Party leader Narong Wongwan (who had left *Ekkaparb* to take the leadership) moved to take the premiership, but his effort was obstructed when the US State Department leaked allegations that he was involved in drug trafficking. A new government, with *Samakkhi Tham* as the dominant coalition partner, was

subsequently formed under the premiership of Army Commander-in-Chief and architect of the 1991 coup, Gen. Suchinda Kraprayoon.

Demonstrations opposing Suchinda's premiership began in mid-April and a month later troops opened fire on crowds of demonstrators in Bangkok. Following mediation by King Bhumipol, Suchinda resigned in late May and in June a new, non-party Cabinet was formed ahead of fresh elections in September 1992. Following the collapse of the Suchinda government, *Samakkhi Tham* virtually disintegrated.

Dissident groups in conflict with the government

Communist Party of Thailand, hitherto the country's main insurgent grouping; has not posed a significant security threat since the mid-1980s.

Communist Party of Malaya once had operational bases in southern Thailand, but in 1989 it officially abandoned its campaign.

Tonga

Capital: Nuku'alofa   **Population: 98,000**

The kingdom of Tonga, consisting of three main islands and many smaller ones, is an independent constitutional monarchy within the Commonwealth. Discovered by Europeans in the early 17th century, Tonga was a British Protected State for 70 years before achieving full independence in 1970.

Constitutional structure

The basis of the current kingdom is derived from a Constitution which became effective on Nov. 4, 1875. It guarantees the freedom of the individual, and protects rights of property and worship, but does so within a feudal context. The Tongan sovereign is head of state and exercises executive power in conjunction with an appointed Privy Council consisting of 10 ministers (including the Prime Minister), together with the Governors of Ha'apai and Vava'u. When not presided over by the King, the Privy Council functions as a Cabinet and is presided over by the Prime Minister. All land is owned by the Crown, and the monarch grants estates to nobles who, in turn, lease land to commoners.

Electoral system

The 30-member unicameral Legislative Assembly consists of the Privy Council, nine hereditary nobles and nine popularly elected representatives. Elected representatives hold office for three years.

Evolution of the suffrage

Those nobles who serve in the legislature are elected by the country's 33 noble families. Commoners are popularly elected by Tongan citizens aged 21 years and over.

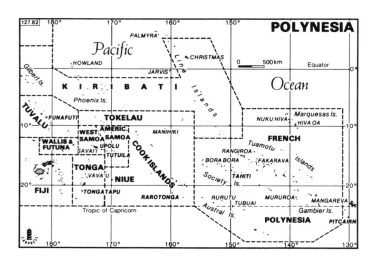

Recent elections

Although general elections are held regularly as all Ministers are appointed by the Crown and the bulk of the legislature is not subject to popular election, they have little bearing on the composition or policies of the government. Elections were held on Feb. 18-19, 1987, and Feb. 15, 1990.

PARTY BY PARTY DATA

Although there were no official parties in mid-1992, an unofficial opposition grouping known as the **People's Party**, led by Akalisi Pohiva, emerged strongly in the 1980s. Despite official disapproval, Pohiva has led a vigorous campaign in favour of constitutional reform with the specific aim of achieving fully democratic and accountable government. Following the 1990 general election, around six of the commoner MPs were associated with the Pohiva's pro-democracy movement.

Major guerrilla groups

There are no guerrilla organizations in Tonga.

Turkmenistan

Capital: Ashkhabad   **Population: 3,714,000 (official estimate at Jan. 1, 1991)**

Turkmenistan was formed as a constituent union republic of the Soviet Union on Oct. 27, 1924. Having declared sovereignty on Aug. 22, 1990, it declared independence on Oct. 27, 1991, following a referendum which gave 94.1 per cent support for an independent republic. Opposition to republican President, former Communist Party First Secretary Saparmurad Niyazov, grew slowly in comparison with the other Soviet Central Asian states and the opposition still suffers a certain amount of political repression—political parties being officially permitted only since Dec. 1, 1991.

Constitutional structure

A new Constitution, adopted on May 18, 1992, made the directly-elected President both head of state and head of government. The legislature, the 50-seat *Majlis*, is elected by district constituencies for a five-year term. The *Khalk Maslakhty* (People's Council), under the President, is the supreme representative body, consisting of the *Majlis* deputies and 50 separately-elected seats, together with legal officials. The 175-seat Supreme Soviet will carry out the duties of the *Majlis* and the People's Council until elections to these bodies.

Electoral system

The President is elected nationally. Elections to the Supreme Soviet were held on a constituency basis. In the 1990 Supreme Soviet elections, voting went to a second round if a candidate failed to win at least 50 per cent of the vote.

Evolution of the suffrage

Adults over 18 are entitled to vote, unless in prison or in a psychiatric institution, or declared to be incapable by a court.

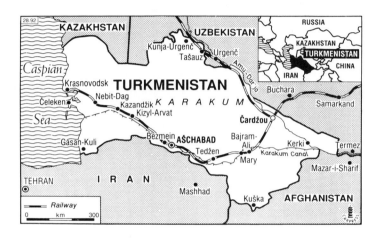

Recent elections

Supreme Soviet elections, Jan. 7, 1990

All 175 seats were contested, with none reserved for social organizations, as in Kazakhstan for example. However, given the republican leadership's reluctance to allow opposition activity, the "open election" posed no danger to the established order.

Presidential elections, Oct. 27, 1990

Candidate	Percentage of vote
Saparmurad Niyazov	98.3

Presidential elections, June 21, 1992

Candidate	Percentage of vote
Saparmurad Niyazov	99.5

PARTY BY PARTY DATA

Akzybirlik (Unity) Movement

Dvizhenie Akzybirlik

Leadership. Nurberdy Nurmamedov (ch.).

Orientation. Turkmen nationalist, basing attitude to Islam on Turkey (ie. a secular state in an Islamic country).

Founded. Sept. 1, 1989.

History. Akzybirlik developed during the period of the elections to the USSR Congress of People's Deputies in 1989. *Akzybirlik* was banned as a political organization on Jan. 15, 1990 after having organized the commemoration of a 19th century Russian conquest of a Turkmen fortress, and since then has functioned as an informal movement. It objected to the official sanctioning of equal rights for the Russian and Turkmen languages and was prepared to co-operate with the government only after the independence declaration of October 1991 and the change in the republic's name to Turkmenistan from the russianized Turkmenia. It was unable to hold a founding congress because of pressure from the authorities.

Structure. 21-strong governing body.

Publications. Co-operates with *samizdat* (self-published) newspaper *Dayang* (Support), issued irregularly with a 30,000 circulation.

Democratic Party

Demokraticheskaya partiya

Leadership. Saparmurad Niyazov (ch.).

Orientation. The ruling party, following a policy of strengthened Turkmen independence.

Founded. Nov. 19, 1991.

History. The Turkmen Communist Party (CP) was renamed the Democratic Party (DP) at a Central Committee plenum in November 1991, despite the existence of a party with that name [see below]. The intention to dissolve the CP into a "People's Democratic Party", following the example of Uzbekistan, was announced on Aug. 26, 1991 after the failed Moscow coup. The re-registration of CP members into the DP began in February 1992. The DP officially inherited the CP's role at the latter's 25th Congress on Dec. 16, 1991.

Structure. Equivalent to that of the defunct CP—workplace cells, with local branches structured to mirror the divisions of the territorial administration. The supreme body, a Congress, meets at least every five years. The ruling Political Council is under the party Chair, who may combine this post with that of republican President.

Democratic Party

Demokraticheskaya partiya

Leadership. Durdymurat Khoja-Mukhammedov.

Orientation. Liberal economic reformist.

Founded. Dec. 22, 1990 [for November 1991 renaming of Communist Party as Democratic Party see above].

History. The Democratic Party (DP) grew out of the *Akzybirlik* movement. Its first congress, in Moscow because of a ban by the Turkmen authorities, was held on Oct. 20, 1991. Its leadership structure, drawing together the local regions of Turkmenistan, reflects the fear of internal ethnic/tribal conflict, but its youth wing, *Nazaret* (View), is more nationalistically oriented.

Structure. Five co-chairs representing five regions of Turkmenistan.

Publications. As *Akzybirlik* [see above].

Affiliations. Democratic Congress.

Tuvalu

Capital: Funafuti atoll   **Population: 8,229**

Tuvalu, formerly part of the Gilbert and Ellice Islands, consists of nine atolls, eight of which are permanently inhabited. The territory was a British colony until Oct. 1, 1978, when it was granted independence as a "special member" of the Commonwealth. Although the country lacks political parties and is heavily dependent on overseas aid, since independence it has maintained a system of stable parliamentary democracy. Tomasi Puapua, who became Prime Minister following the general election of September 1981, was returned to office in September 1985. Following a general election in September 1989, he was defeated by Bikenibou Paeniu.

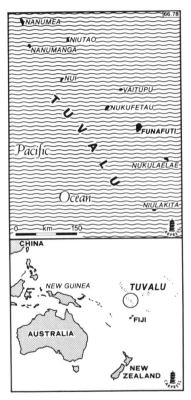

Constitutional structure

Tuvalu is a parliamentary democracy. As a member of the Commonwealth its head of state is the British sovereign, represented by a Governor General. Legislative authority is vested in a unicameral 12-member Parliament, which is popularly elected for up to four years. Four islands (Nanumea, Niultao, Vaitupu and Funafuti) each return two members, whilst the other four inhabited atolls return one member each. Executive power is exercised by a Prime Minister and a Cabinet.

Electoral system

The first general election was held in August 1977. Voting is on a common roll, with all citizens of Tuvalu aged 18 years and over entitled to participate. A candidate for Parliament must be 21 years or over. The Prime Minister is elected by Parliament from amongst its members. This occurs after each general election, and may be necessary during the lifetime of a Parliament if the Prime Minister resigns or dies in office.

Evolution of the suffrage

Since independence, Tuvalu has maintained a system of universal adult suffrage.

Recent elections

Date	Subsequent Prime Minister*
Aug. 29, 1977	Toalipi Lauti
Sept. 8, 1981	Tomasi Puapua
Sept. 12, 1985	Tomasi Puapua
Sept. 27, 1989	Bikenibeu Paeniu

*Prior to independence the head of government was a Chief Minister rather than a Prime Minister.

PARTY BY PARTY DATA

Tuvalu has no formal political parties. Although the Parliament contains a government and an opposition, these groupings are loose in construction and informal in nature. The opposition consists of those MPs who were supporters of the candidate or candidates defeated in the election for Prime Minister.

Major guerrilla groups

There are no guerrilla organizations in Tuvalu.

United Kingdom Dependent Territories in Pacific

Pitcairn

Capital: Adamstown   **Population: 49**

The British Dependency of the Pitcairn Islands, consisting of Pitcairn and three uninhabited neighbouring territories, was settled in the late-18th century by mutineers from the British warship HMS *Bounty*, together with some of the native inhabitants of Tahiti. The territory was formally colonized by Britain in the 19th century.

Constitutional structure

Under the 1940 Constitution, executive authority is in the hands of a Governor, who represents the British monarch. (Since 1970 the British High Commissioner in New Zealand has acted as Governor of Pitcairn). He governs in consultation with an Island Council. The Council is presided over by the Island Magistrate, who is elected triennially. The Council is composed of four members elected annually, five members who are appointed by the Governor (three upon the advice of the elected members and two at his own discretion), and the Island Secretary who is an ex-officio member. Liaison between the Governor and the Council is through a Commissioner, who is usually based in the Office of the British Consulate-General in New Zealand.

Electoral system

Elections to the Island Council take place annually in December, and are conducted on the basis of universal adult suffrage.

Evolution of the suffrage

Universal adult suffrage was included as part of the territory's first Constitution, drawn up in the early 19th century, and has been a feature of the island's political system ever since.

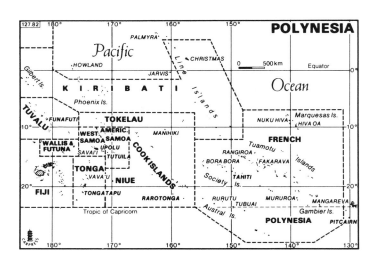

Recent elections

The most recent election for the post of Island Magistrate resulted in the election of Brian Young.

PARTY BY PARTY DATA

There are no political parties in Pitcairn.

Major guerrilla groups

There are no guerrilla groups operating in Pitcairn.

United Nations Trust Territory of the Pacific

Belau (Palau)

Capital: Koror, on Koror Island   **Population: 15,105 (1990)**

The Republic of Belau is the last of the four components of the UN Trust Territory of the Pacific which was set up in 1947 and administered by the USA. The three other components (the Federated States of Micronesia, the Marshall Islands and the Northern Mariana Islands) adopted revised constitutional relationships between 1978 and 1991. Although a compact of free association was signed in 1982 between Belau and the USA, it could not be implemented until the territory altered its Constitution (which required a 75 per cent vote in favour in a referendum) to rescind the clauses which banned the entry, storage or disposal of nuclear, chemical or biological weapons. Repeated referendums were held between 1983 and 1990 in an attempt to achieve this end, but each failed to secure the necessary 75 per cent approval level.

Constitutional structure

Since 1987, the remaining responsibilities of the trusteeship have been discharged by the US Department of the Interior, with administrative authority being exercised by the Assistant Secretary (Office of Territorial and International Affairs). In 1990 the Secretary of the Interior empowered the Assistant Secretary to appoint a resident representative in Belau to assist with communications between the Department of the Interior and the government of Belau.

Under its 1981 Constitution, Belau has a President, elected for a four-year term by popular vote, who functions as both head of state and head of government. The President governs with the assistance of an appointed Cabinet. The legislature (*Olbiil Era Kelulau*) is bicameral, and consists of a House of Delegates comprising one representative from each of the territory's 16 states, and a 14-member Senate. There is also a Council of Chiefs, and each state has its own political institutions.

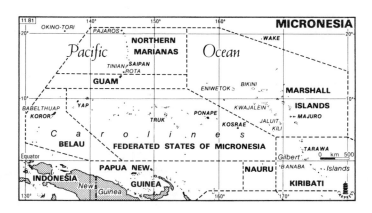

Recent elections

Presidential elections

Date	Winning candidate
1984	Haruo Remiliik (assassinated in June 1985)
September 1985	Lazarus Salii (committed suicide in August 1988)
November 1988	Ngiratkel Etpison

Presidential elections November 1988

Candidate	Votes received
Ngiratkel Etpison	2,383
Roman Tmetuchl	2,344
Thomas Remengesau	1,761
John O. Ngiraked	764
Ibedel Yutaka Gibbons	729
Moses Uludong	588
Santos Olikong	475

Electoral system

Elections are held on the basis of universal adult suffrage. Most state governors are elected, but some are chosen on the basis of traditional status.

Evolution of the suffrage

Since its foundation in 1981, the Republic of Belau has operated a system of universal adult suffrage.

PARTY BY PARTY DATA

Although Belau does not have formal political parties, the fierce and protracted debate over the compact of free association has led to the evolution of loose political groupings by those who support and those who oppose the Compact. These are the **Coalition for Open Honest and Just Government** which opposes the compact, and the **Ta Belau Party** which supports it. The current President is a supporter of the compact, as was his predecessor.

Major guerrilla groups

There are no guerrilla groups operating in Belau.

United States Pacific Territories

American Samoa

Capital: Pago Pago

Population: 38,2003 (1989 est.)

Discovered by Europeans in the 18th century, the chiefs of the eastern Samoan islands ceded their territory to the United States of America in 1904. The islands became an official unincorporated territory of the USA in 1922.

Constitutional structure

American Samoa is an unincorporated territory of the USA and is not, therefore, covered by all provisions of the US Constitution. Under the 1967 Constitution, executive authority is vested in a Governor, who is popularly elected for a four-year term. The legislature (*Fono*) consists of an 18-member Senate elected for four years by *Matai* (traditional clan leaders), and a popularly elected 20-member House of Representatives elected for two years. In addition to the 20 voting representatives in the House, the Constitution also provides for the election of one non-voting delegate from Swain's Island, elected at a meeting of the island's adult permanent residents.

The territory also elects one (non-voting) delegate to the US House of Representatives. In 1986 a constitutional convention comprehensively revised the territory's Constitution, but the changes have yet to be ratified by the US Congress.

Electoral system

The Senate is elected from, and by, the *Matai*, from 12 Senate districts, while the members of the House are drawn from 17 House districts.

Evolution of the suffrage

Until 1978 the Governor was appointed by the US government. Since then, the post has been, like membership of the House, determined by elections on the basis of universal adult suffrage.

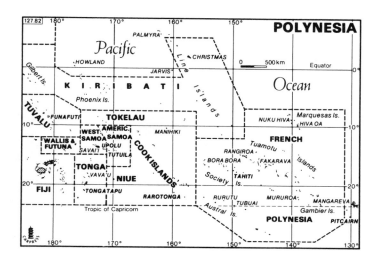

Recent elections

Gubernatorial contests

Date	Winning candidate
November 1977	Peter Coleman
November 1980*	Peter Coleman
November 1984	A. P. Lutali
November 1988	Peter Coleman

*Election held one year early in order to synchronize the election cycle with that of the USA.

PARTY BY PARTY DATA

There are no political parties in American Samoa.

Major guerrilla groups

There are no guerrilla groups operating in American Samoa.

Guam

Capital: Agana   **Population: 132,726 (1990 est.)**

Guam, the southern-most and largest of the Mariana Islands, was discovered by Europeans in the 16th century, and colonized by Spain. It was ceded to the United States of America after the Spanish-American War of 1898, and became an unincorporated US territory in 1950. In a referendum in September 1976 the island's population voted to maintain close links with the USA, but to seek an improvement in the current status of the territory. A further referendum in 1982, in which only 38 per cent of voters participated, suggested that the most popular option was the status of a commonwealth in association with the USA, although subsequent negotiations failed to agree upon a new constitutional package.

The main obstacles to an agreement appeared to be the desire of the Guam government to retain veto powers over the application within the territory of US federal legislation, and the issue of self-determination for the indigenous *Chamorros*, who constituted some 45 per cent of the population. A further problem arose in the form of opinion polls which consistently showed that commonwealth status was desired only by a small, and shrinking, minority of the population. The fact that the majority had apparently come to support a continuation of Guam's current status was interpreted as a product of the protracted nature of the negotiations following the referendum, and the territory's recent high levels of economic growth.

Constitutional structure

As an unincorporated territory of the USA, Guam is not covered by all provisions of the US constitution. Under the Organic Act of Guam (1950), which gave the territory internal self-government, executive authority is vested in a Governor who, since 1970, has been popularly elected for a four-year term. The Guam Legislature consists of 21 members (Senators) who are popularly elected for two years. The territory elects one (non-voting) delegate to the US House of Representatives.

Political activity mirrors that on the US mainland, and is therefore dominated by the Democratic Party and the Republican Party.

Electoral system

Members of the legislature are elected from four legislative districts.

Evolution of the suffrage

Since 1970 the officer of Governor has, like that of Senator, been filled on the basis of universal adult suffrage for those aged 18 years and over.

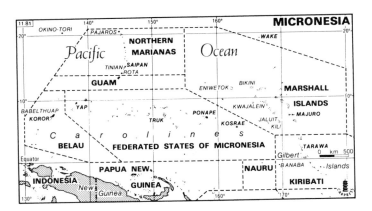

Recent elections

Gubernatorial elections

Date	Winning candidate
November 1982	Ricardo J. Bordallo (Dem.)
November 1986	Joseph F. Ada (Rep.)
November 1990	Joseph F. Ada (Rep.)

Congressional elections

Date	Winning party
November 1980	Republican Party
November 1982	Republican Party
November 1984	Republican Party
November 1986	Democratic Party
November 1988	Democratic Party
November 1990	Democratic Party

Distribution of seats in Guam Legislature following 1990 elections

	Seats
Democratic Party	11
Republican Party	10

PARTY BY PARTY DATA

Democratic Party

Address. c/o of Guam Legislature, Agana, Guam.
Orientation. Centrist; aligned with the US Democratic Party.
Founded. 1950 (as the Popular Party).
History. The first legislative elections under the 1950 Organic Act of Guam returned a 21-member populist bloc, which became the Popular Party. In 1964 it formally affiliated to the US Democratic Party, adopting its current name. Throughout its existence the party has dominated Guam's political system, holding a majority in the legislature from 1950-80 with the exception of the period 1964-66. It narrowly lost the 1980 election, but re-established its position as the natural party of government in the latter part of the decade.

Republican Party

Address. c/o of Guam Legislature, Agana, Guam.
Orientation. Conservative; aligned with the US Republican Party.
Founded. 1955 (as the Territorial Party).
History. The Republican Party was directly descended from the Territorial Party which was created in 1955 as a result of the defection of the conservative wing of the Popular Party. In 1967 the party adopted its current name and affiliated to the US Republican Party. Apart from 1964-66, the party spent the 1960s and 1970s in opposition, but narrowly won the election of 1980. It retained its control of the legislature in the early 1980s but, towards the end of the decade, was once more forced into opposition. In the election of November 1990 it won 10 seats in the legislature compared with the 11 won by the Democratic Party. The Republican Party did, however, win the 1990 gubernatorial election, thereby retaining the office it had won in 1986.

Major guerrilla groups

There are no guerrilla groups operating in Guam.

Northern Mariana Islands

Capital: Saipan   **Population: 31,563 (1987 est.)**

Originally part of the UN Trust Territory of the Pacific administered by the United States of America, the Northern Mariana Islands voted to become a US Commonwealth Territory in 1975, and a new Constitution became operational in 1978. One of two US Commonwealth Territories (Puerto Rico is the other), its inhabitants have US citizenship. Technically, however, the territory's new status was not internationally recognized until the formal termination of the UN's Trusteeship in December 1990.

Constitutional structure

Executive authority is vested in a Governor, popularly elected for a four-year term, who is assisted by the Northern Marianas Commonwealth Legislature. The legislature consists of a nine-member Senate and a 18-member House of Representatives; its members are elected for two-year terms.

Political activity mirrors that on the US mainland, and is, therefore, dominated by the Democratic Party and the Republican Party.

Electoral system

Three senators are elected for each of the territory's three Senatorial Districts: Rota; Tinian and Aguijan; and Saipan and the northern islands.

Evolution of the suffrage

All elections are conducted on the basis of universal adult suffrage.

Recent elections

Gubernatorial elections

Date	Winning Candidate
November 1985	Pedro P. Tenorio (Dem.)
November 1989	Lorenzo (Larry) De Leon Guerrero (Rep).

Congressional elections

Election date	Winning party	
	House of Representatives	Senate
November 1987	Republican Party	Republican Party
November 1989	Republican Party	Democratic Party
November 1991	Republican Party	Republican Party

Distribution of seats in Commonwealth Legislature following 1991 elections

	House of Representatives	Senate
Republican Party	10	8
Democratic Party	6	1
Independents	2	—

PARTY BY PARTY DATA

Democratic Party
Address. c/o of Commonwealth Legislature, Capitol Hill, Saipan, MP 96950.
Leadership. Felicidad Ogumoro (l.).
Orientation. Centrist. The party is aligned with the US Democratic Party, and seeks greater economic self-sufficiency for the islands.
Founded. 1963 (as the Popular Party).
History. The Democratic Party draws strong, but not exclusive, support from the majority *Chamorro* population (descendants of Micronesians, Spanish and Filipinos). The party campaigned in the 1960s against the possible unification of the Northern Marianas with Guam. After Guam finally rejected unification in 1969, the Popular Party switched its main energies to advocating separation of the islands from the rest of the UN Trust Territory, with a view to creating a separate and closer relationship with the USA.

With separation achieved in 1975 and a closer relationship in association with the USA accomplished in 1977, both the racial basis of the party, and its platform, became increasingly difficult to distinguish from its major opponent, the Territorial Party. Partly as an attempt to redefine its image, the Popular Party increasingly identified with the US Democratic Party, and adopted its name at around the time of the first elections to the new Commonwealth Legislature in 1977. The party lost the legislative elections, but won the simultaneous gubernatorial contest. In 1979 it won control of the House of Representatives, only to lose it, together with elections for the Senate and the Governorship in 1981. It won the Governorship in 1985, but lost it again in 1989. It also lost the elections for both houses of the legislature in 1987 and 1991, although it briefly held control of the House of Representatives in 1989-91.

Republican Party
Address. c/o of Commonwealth Legislature, Capitol Hill, Saipan, MP 96950.
Leadership. Alonnzo Igisomar (l.).
Orientation. Conservative. Aligned with (but independent of) the US Republican Party, it is committed to continued commonwealth status for the islands.
Founded. 1962 (as the Territorial Party).
History. The Republican Party was directly descended from the Territorial Party which, in the 1960s, had campaigned for unification of the Northern Marianas with Guam. After this proposal was finally laid to rest in 1969, the party campaigned for union with the rest of Micronesia in opposition to the separatist position taken by the Popular Party. During this period the Territorial Party drew the bulk of its support from the minority Carolinians and Rotanese. Although it lost the struggle over union, the party increased its level of support after commonwealth status was achieved in 1977. It lost the gubernatorial contest of that year, but won control of both houses of the newly-established Commonwealth Legislature.

After Ronald Reagan's victory in the 1980 US presidential elections, the party changed its name to the Republican Party, although unlike the Democratic Party, it did not establish any formal links with the political structure of the mainland USA. It retained control over both houses of the legislature, except for the periods 1979-81 and 1989-91 when it was in a minority in the House of Representatives. It won the Governorship in 1981, lost it in 1985, but regained it in 1989 with the election of Lorenzo (Larry) De Leon Guerrero.

Major guerrilla groups

There are no guerrilla groups operating in the Northern Mariana Islands.

Other US Pacific Territories

There are several Pacific territories which are administered by the US Department of Defence. These include **Wake Island** and the neighbouring **Wilkes and Peale Islands**, comprising an area of 8 sq km and a population of 1,600. **Johnston Atoll**, with a population of 327 (1980), **Midway Island,** with a population of 2,200 (1983), and the uninhabited **Kingman Reef** are each designated a Naval Defence Sea Area to which unauthorized access is forbidden. None of these territories has any political parties.

Uzbekistan

Capital: Tashkent   **Population: 20,708,000 (official est. at Jan. 1, 1991)**

The Republic of Uzbekistan was formed as a constituent union republic of the Soviet Union on Oct. 27, 1924. It declared sovereignty on June 20, 1990. The independence declaration of Aug. 24, 1991 was confirmed by 98.2 per cent in favour in a referendum on Dec. 29, 1991. The first direct presidential elections were also held on Dec. 29.

Constitutional structure

The Constitution is still that of the ex-Soviet republic, with the addition of a directly elected Presidency. The 500-seat Supreme Soviet is the highest legislature and is elected on a constituency basis.

Electoral system

In the 1990 Supreme Soviet elections, voting went to a second round if a candidate failed to win at least 50 per cent of the vote, even when the seat was uncontested.

Evolution of the suffrage

Adults over 18 are eligible to vote, provided they are not in psychiatric institutions, prison or declared incapable by a court.

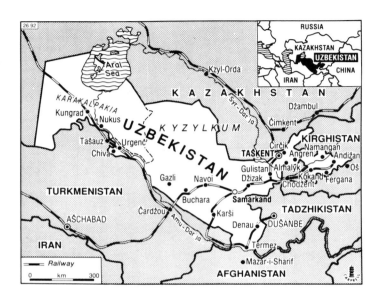

Recent elections

Supreme Soviet elections, Feb. 18, 1990

Of the 500 seats 179 were contested by a single candidate, mostly Communist Party officials; 39 seats were contested by more than five candidates and 111 seats were contested by between three and five candidates. In the first round, of the 368 seats which were decided 348 were won by Communist Party members.

Presidential elections, Dec. 29, 1991

Candidate	Percentage of vote
Islam Karimov	85.9
Mukhammad Solikh	12.45

PARTY BY PARTY DATA

Democratic Reform Movement
Dvizheniye demokraticheskikh reform
Leadership. Faizulla Iskhakov (ch.).
Orientation. Democratic reform to be achieved by constitutional means.
Founded. Dec. 7, 1991.
History. Discussions on forming an Uzbek branch of the Democratic Reform Movement (DRM), a former Soviet reformist movement founded in July 1991 by leading communist and non-communist reformers, began in August 1991, and were initiated by Iskhakov. The Organizing Committee met on Sept. 10, and negotiated with the Unity Party (*Birlik*) [see Unity Party entry], the Islamic Renaissance Party (IRP) [see separate entry] and leading members of the local intelligentsia. The DRM has thus united a part of the *Birlik* Movement with other small Uzbek political movements.

Freedom Democratic Party
Demokraticheskaya partiya Erk
Leadership. Mukhammad Solikh (ch.).
Orientation. Uzbek independence; a mixed economy with strong state sector.
Founded. Apr. 27, 1990.
History. The Freedom (*Erk*) Democratic Party was formed as a split from the *Birlik* Movement in 1989. Disagreeing with *Birlik's* [see Unity Party entry] policy of demonstrations and extra-parliamentary opposition, *Erk's* future leaders (then part of *Birlik*) preferred to work for change within the political system. *Erk* was registered on Sept. 5, 1991. Solikh, the permanent chair and an Uzbek People's Deputy, was a candidate in the presidential elections. The Third Congress on Aug. 25, 1991 elected the ruling bodies.
Structure. Central Committee with 35 members and Central Ruling Body of 17.
Membership. 10,000. Eight Supreme Soviet members.
Publications. Once- or twice-monthly *Erk* newspaper with a circulation of 30,000.

Free Party
Svobodnaya dekhanskaya partiya
Leadership. Mirzaali Mukhammejanov (ch.).
Orientation. The promotion of private farming, with consequent gradual dissolution of collective farming. Recognises the right of all citizens of Uzbekistan (not just Uzbeks) to land.
Founded. Dec. 14, 1991.
History. The constituent congress brought together representatives of existing peasants' organizations. The Free (*Dekhan*) Party unites private, co-operative and collective farmers, and is politically close to *Erk* [see Freedom Democratic Party entry]. Mukhammejanov was a member of the Communist Party until it became the People's Democratic Party [see separate entry].
Structure. 50-member Council; 11-member Executive Committee.

Greens' Party
Partiya zelyonikh
Leadership. Pirmat Shermukhammedov (ch.).
Orientation. Ecological issues in Uzbekistan.
Founded. Nov. 20, 1991.
History. The Greens' Party grew out of the ecological movement set up in defence of the Aral Sea, which was also the cradle of *Birlik* [see Unity Party entry].
Structure. Ruling body with 37 members.
Membership. 3,000.
Publications. There are plans for a newspaper, *Trevozhny mir* (Troubled World).

Islamic Renaissance Party
Islamskaya partiya vozrozhdenie
Leadership. Abdullo Utayev.
Orientation. The Islamic Renaissance Party (IRP) agitates for legislation allowing believers to live according to Islamic law. It opposes officially-sanctioned Islam (the headquarters of the leader of Islam in the former Soviet Union are in Tashkent).
Founded. Jan. 26, 1991.
History. The constituent congress was dispersed by the authorities, causing an influx of new members. The IRP is especially strong in the areas of Tashkent, Namangan and Kokand. The IRP has faced repression from the authorities, and co-ordinates opposition activities with *Birlik* [see Unity Party entry].
Structure. Council of Ulemas. The Uzbek IRP is part of the inter-republican IRP [see also Tajikistan].
Membership. 20,000.
Publications. Irregularly published newspaper *Da'vat* (Homily) in Uzbek, with circulation of up to 10,000.
International affiliations. IRP.

People's Democratic Party
Narodno-demokraticheskaya partiya
Leadership. Islam Karimov.

Orientation. Uzbek independence, strong presidential power, "order and work".

Founded. Nov. 1, 1991.

History. The People's Democratic Party (PDP) is the transformed Uzbek Communist Party (UzCP). Karimov, the UzCP First Secretary, announced immediately after the failure of the attempted Soviet coup of August 1991 that the UzCP would become independent of the Communist Party of the Soviet Union (CPSU) and would change its name. The UzCP was dissolved at an extraordinary congress on Sept. 14, 1991. The PDP membership includes people who were not previously members of the UzCP, and its programme excludes communist ideology. It remains Uzbekistan's ruling party.

Structure. 150-member Central Council and 12-member Political Executive Committee.

Membership. 351,000.

Publications. Uzbekiston Ovozdi (The Voice of Uzbekistan), formerly the Uzbek-language paper of the UzCP.

Unity Party

Partiya Birlik

Address. c/o Union of Writers of Uzbekistan, 700000 Tashkent, ul. Pushkina 1.

Leadership. Abdurakhim Pulatov (ch.).

Orientation. Uzbek independence and liberal economic reform.

Founded. June 17, 1990.

History. Originally named the Democratic Party of Uzbekistan, it took the name Unity (*Birlik*) at its second congress on Oct. 27, 1991. It is the political wing of the *Birlik* Movement, the leading opposition movement in Uzbekistan (400,000 members), which in turn had developed in 1988 out of the ecological movement. Initially pressing for Uzbek language rights and protection for Uzbeks in the Soviet Army, *Birlik* began agitating for economic reforms at its third congress in May 1990. After initial repression by the authorities, the Movement was registered on Nov. 11, 1991, but was still not allowed to put forward a candidate for Republican President. *Birlik* has two former USSR People's Deputies among its leading members.

Membership. 10,000. One Supreme Soviet deputy.

Publications. Birlik, weekly paper in Uzbek, 2,000-4,000 circulation. Periodically issued in Russian.

International affiliations. Democratic Congress.

Vanuatu

Capital: Port Vila   **Population: 157,000**

Formerly known as the New Hebrides, the Republic of Vanuatu became an independent member of the Commonwealth in July 1980. The move brought to an end a period of 65 years of joint British and French administration. The country's administration as an Anglo-French Condominion left it deeply divided between English and French-speaking communities which account, respectively, for around 60 and 40 per cent of the population. Opposition to independence by members of the French-speaking community led to an attempt at secession in 1980 by Espiritu Santo (the country's main island) led by Jimmy Stevens. The rebellion was crushed in August 1980 when the newly independent government called upon the assistance of troops from Papua New Guinea.

From independence until 1991 the country was governed by the Anglophone *Vanua'aku Pati*. At the election of December 1991, however, a coalition government came to power consisting of the Francophone Union of Moderate Parties and the smaller, Anglophone, National United Party.

Constitutional structure

The country's head of state is an elected President. Executive power is exercised by a Prime Minister who governs with the assistance of a Council of Ministers (Cabinet), which consists of MPs appointed by the Prime Minister and which must not exceed 25 per cent of the size of the legislature. Legislative authority is vested in a unicameral Parliament, the 46 members of which are elected for four years.

A considerable degree of power is devolved to 11 island-government councils; the large towns of Vila and Luganville also have municipal councils led by mayors. There is also a National Council of Chiefs composed of representatives elected from a number of District Councils of Chiefs. The Council, which elects its own president, meets at lest once per year and advises the government on issues concerning the country's traditions and languages.

Electoral system

The President is elected for five years by an electoral college, composed of the Parliament and the Presidents of the island-government councils. The President can be removed for gross misconduct or gross incapacity by a motion introduced by at least one-third of the electoral college and supported by two-thirds of its members. The Prime Minister is elected by Parliament from among its members by secret ballot.

Evolution of the suffrage

Since independence the country has operated on the basis of universal adult suffrage. Prior to 1975 there was an Advisory Council (established by the colonial authorities in 1957), a minority of whose members were determined by election. This was replaced by a Representative Assembly elected on the basis of universal adult suffrage, but which included special seats reserved for members of the Chamber of Commerce. After pressure from the *Vanua'aku Pati*, elections were held in 1979 upon the basis of universal adult suffrage.

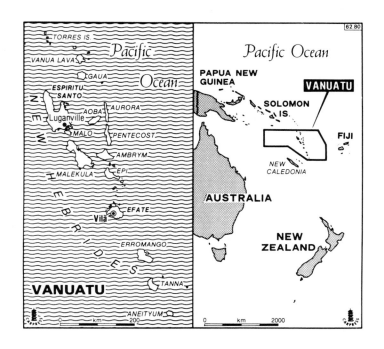

Recent elections

Date	Winning Party
Nov. 2, 1983	*Vanua'aku Pati*
Nov. 30, 1987	Vanua'aku Pati
Dec. 2, 1991	Union of Moderate Parties and National United Party

General election, Dec. 2, 1991

Party	Seats won
Union of Moderate Parties	19
National United Party	10
Vanua'aku Pati	10
Melanesian Progressive Party	4
Fren-Melanesian Party	1
Independents	2
Total	46

PARTY BY PARTY DATA

Melanesian Progressive Party

Address. PO Box 22, Port Vila, Vanuatu.

Leadership. Barak Sope (ch.).

Orientation. Socialist-nationalist.

Founded. 1988.

History. The Melanesian Progressive Party (MPP) was founded as a breakaway group from the *Vanua'aku Pati* [see separate entry] following a prolonged period of tension between its founder, Barak Sope, and the *Vanua'aku Pati* leader, Walter Lini. The tension culminated in Sope's dismissal from the Cabinet in May 1988 after a riot in Port Vila, allegedly fomented by his supporters. In addition to personal factors, the conflict between Sope and Lini reflected underlying ethnic and regional divisions within the country. While Sope's Francophone supporters were based largely around Efate atoll (the location of Port Vila), Lini and the other Anglophone leaders were from the northern and outer islands.

In the 1991 elections, the MPP won four seats and entered into talks with the Union of Moderate Parties (UMP) over the possibility of forming a coalition government. The talks collapsed, allegedly because the MPP demanded several key portfolios, including the Premiership, in return for entering into a partnership.

National United Party

Address. Port Vila, Vanuatu.

Leadership. Fr. Walter Lini (pres.).

Orientation. Socialist-nationalist.

Founded. 1991.

History. The National United Party (NUP), also known as the Vanuatu National United Party, was founded in August 1991 following Fr. Walter Lini's loss of control of the *Vanua'aku Pati* [see separate entry]. Although Lini managed to induce a significant number of *Vanua'aku Pati* members to join his new organization, the new party lacked an overall majority in the legislature. Lini attempted to postpone the recall of parliament in order to evade being ousted by a motion of no-confidence, but eventually the opposition managed to summon Parliament and Lini's government was defeated on Sept. 6. He immediately resigned and led his new party into opposition.

In the election of December 1991 the NUP won 10 of the 46 seats in Parliament. The party subsequently joined a coalition government as the junior partner to the Union of Moderate Parties [see separate entry].

Union of Moderate Parties

Address. PO Box 922, Port Vila, Vanuatu.

Leadership. Maxime Carlot.

Orientation. Conservative coalition representing the Francophone community.

Founded. 1979.

History. The Union of Moderate Parties (UMP) was founded in 1979 as a loose coalition of Francophone groups which opposed the *Vanua'aku Pati*'s drive for independence. Although it quickly became the primary party for the French-speaking community, it was badly damaged in 1980 by its association with the ill-fated secessionist revolt on Espiritu Santo, led by Jimmy Stevens.

In the election of 1983 the party won 33 per cent of the vote and secured 12 of the 39 seats in the legislature. In the mid-1980s the UMP accused the *Vanua'aku Pati* administration of increasing authoritarianism and constitutional abuse. This led to a boycott of Parliament by the UMP in 1986 in protest over the alleged partisan behaviour of the Parliamentary Speaker, Fred Timakata. In the 1987 election the UMP won 42 per cent of the vote and increased its number of seats in the 46-member Parliament to 20.

The splintering of the *Vanua'aku Pati* in 1991 enabled the UMP to make further electoral gains and it emerged from the December election as the single largest party, winning 42 per cent of the vote and 19 of the seats in the 49-member Parliament. After intensive inter-party negotiations, the UMP formed an alliance with National United Party (NUP), and Carlot was elected as Prime Minister when the new legislature convened on Dec. 16. Seven of the 11-member Cabinet were members of the UMP, and four (among whom NUP leader Walter Lini was not included) were members of the NUP.

Vanua'aku Pati

Address. PO Box 472, Port Vila, Vanuatu.

Leadership. Donald Kalpokas (pres.); Sela Molisa (sec.-gen.).

Orientation. Socialist-nationalist. The *Vanua'aku Pati* developed a particular brand of "Melanesian socialism" which placed great emphasis on developing a non-aligned foreign policy and which vehemently opposed nuclear weapons and testing in the Pacific.

Founded. 1971.

History. The Vanua'aku Pati (English translation: Our Land) was founded as the New Hebrides National

Party in 1971. Associated with the Anglophone urban community, it aimed to replace the *Na-Griamel* movement as the vehicle for nationalist sentiment. It advocated full independence, the nationalization of foreign-owned land, and the establishment of an elected legislature. In 1977 the party changed its name to the *Vanua'aku Pati*.

In 1975 the party won 17 of the 29 elected seats in the newly established Representative Assembly and, following intensive pressure, it succeeded in forcing the British and French authorities to consent to the establishment of a wholly elected legislature in preparation for independence. At the subsequent 1979 election, the *Vanua'aku Pati* won 63 per cent of the vote and took 26 of the 39 seats. Under its leader, Anglican priest Fr. Walter Lini, the party led the country to independence. In July 1982 several members of the party, including two former Cabinet members, resigned to found the Vanuatu Independence Alliance Party. In the 1983 election the party's share of the vote fell to 56 per cent, but the party retained a comfortable majority in Parliament, winning 24 seats.

In 1986 Lini established diplomatic relations with the Soviet Union and Libya, neither of which had until then managed to gain a foothold in the Pacific. This was followed by the negotiation of a fishing deal with the Soviet Union. Lini was also a leading figure in the campaign against French nuclear testing and a vociferous supporter of the Kanak struggle for independence in the French territory of New Caledonia.

Divisions within the ruling party remained, however, and there were further splits in 1986. The roots of this internecine situation lay in the increasing reservations concerning Lini's leadership, particularly the charge that he was becoming too authoritarian. His position was further undermined by his growing ill-health, after suffering a cerebral haemorrhage in February 1987. Nevertheless, he was re-elected to a further four-year term as party president in mid-1987. In legislative elections at the end of the year, the party polled 47 per cent and secured 26 seats in the 46-member Parliament. Immediately after the November election Lini was challenged for the leadership by Barak Sope. Although Lini fought off the challenge and, in the interests of "party unity", Sope agreed to remain in the Cabinet, relations between the two men continued to deteriorate. Sope was eventually dismissed in May 1988, and Lini then used his majority to expel Sope and several of his supporters from Parliament. The Union of Moderate Parties began a boycott of Parliament to protest against the expulsions, and Lini then declared the party's seats to be vacant and held by-elections to fill them. The by-elections were also boycotted by the opposition and voter turnout was low, leading to increased charges that the Prime Minister was becoming a dictator.

Matters came to a head on Dec. 16, 1988, when the country's President, George Ati Sokomanu, attempted to dissolve Parliament and to appoint Sope, who was also his nephew, as caretaker Prime Minister. A brief power struggle followed but, following the Supreme Court's decision that Sokomanu had exceeded his constitutional authority, both he and Sope were arrested. Sokomanu was formally dismissed from office on Jan. 12, 1988, and on Jan. 30 the electoral college chose Fred Timakata as his successor.

Despite retaining power, the authority of Lini was seriously undermined by the affair and the party remained racked by internal feuding. Increasingly insecure, Lini sacked an ever-growing number of colleagues and civil servants. Between February and August 1991 he dismissed eight Ministers and at least 50 ministerial aides, political appointees and civil servants. In many cases they were replaced by friends and relations of Lini, whom he considered to be more loyal. In May Lini suffered a heart attack. After receiving treatment in Australia, he returned to work on June 14 and, on June 27, dismissed four Ministers who had refused to take a loyalty pledge to him. These included Donald Kalpokas, the party's general secretary, who was sacked as Minister of Education and Foreign Affairs.

Lini's opponents within the *Vanua'aku Pati* summoned an extraordinary party congress at Mele Village, outside Port Vila, on Aug. 7, at which they voted to remove him from the Presidency. He was replaced by Kalpokas. Lini responded by creating the National United Party (NUP). In September the *Vanua'aku Pati* joined the opposition and passed a vote of no-confidence in Lini's administration. Lini resigned and the party returned to government under Kalpokas. Parliament was dissolved on Oct. 14, and a general election was held on Dec. 2 at which the *Vanua'aku Pati* lost power, winning only 10 seats.

Structure. The annual national congress is the ultimate source of authority within the party, although an extraordinary congress may also be summoned. Between meetings of the congress, power is in the hands of an executive, headed by the party president, which is elected by congress.

Minor parties

Fren Melanesian Party (Luganville, Santo, Vanuatu); founded in 1982 by a group of defectors from the Union of Moderate Parties. In the December 1991 elections the party won one seat in the legislature.

Na-Griamel (Luganville, Santo, Vanuatu). The party's name is derived from the names of two local plants (*nagria* and *namele*). It was first used by a rural movement founded in the 1960s, under the leadership of Jimmy Stevens, which was organized as a vehicle for rural discontent and the protection of tribal customs. In the early 1970s the group developed links with groups representing the interests of European business and French planters. This unlikely coalition was the basis of the Santo secessionist movement which led to the abortive 1980 rebellion by Stevens.

National Democratic Party (NDP); founded in 1986 as a result of a split from the *Vanua'aku Pati*, the NDP advocates closer links with both Britain and France.

New People's Party (NPP), founded in 1986 as a result of a split from the *Vanua'aku Pati*.

Tan Union; founded in 1977 as a coalition of Francophone groups. In 1979 its role as chief opposition group to the *Vanua'aku Pati* was taken over by the New Hebrides Federal Party, which later became the Union of Moderate Parties [see separate entry]. Following the loss of all seats by the Melanesian Progressive Party and the Union of Moderate Parties in 1988—the seats were declared vacant after an opposition boycott of Parliament, and the subsequent by-elections were also boycotted—the Tan Union won six seats and its leader, Vincent Boulekone, became Leader of the Opposition. At the 1991 election, the party failed to retain any of its seats.

Vanuatu Independence Alliance Party (VIAP); founded in July 1982 by defectors from the *Vanua'aku Pati*, the VIAP supports free enterprise. It lost all three of its parliamentary seats in the 1983 election and, thereafter, became an insignificant political force.

Defunct parties

Mouvement Autonomiste des Nouvelles-Hebrides (MAHN); founded in 1973. The MAHN was a conservative francophone party which drew its support primarily from the French planter community on Espiritu Santo. In the late 1970s it faded out of existence and its supporters aligned themselves with other francophone groups.

New Hebrides National Party [see under *Vanua'aku Pati*].

Union de la Population des Nouvelles-Hebrides; formed in 1971 by conservative European business interests and French planters as a response to the emergence of the New Hebrides National Party. Opposed to independence, the party faded away in the mid-1970s.

Union des Communautes des Nouvelles-Hebrides; a planter-based party which broke away from the *Union de la Population des Nouvelles-Hebrides* in 1974. In 1977 it was one of the pro-French groups which formed the Tan Union.

Major guerrilla groups

There are no guerilla organizations in Vanuatu.

Vietnam

Capital: Hanoi

Population: 66,700,000

The Socialist Republic of Vietnam (SRV) was proclaimed on July 2, 1976, after North Vietnam-backed communist insurgents had effectively reunified the country in April 1975 by overthrowing the US-supported government of South Vietnam. The SRV succeeded both the Democratic Republic of Vietnam (DRV), which had been founded in 1945 and had governed North Vietnam since 1954, and the Provisional Revolutionary Government, established in 1969, which had taken over responsibility for the government of South Vietnam in 1975. Effective political power in the SRV is exercised by the Communist Party of Vietnam (CPV). The party permeates the entire political structure, including the National Assembly, the Council of Ministers and the People's Army of Vietnam.

Constitutional structure

The 1980 Constitution proclaims that the SRV is "a state of proletarian dictatorship" in which the CPV is "the only force leading the State and Society". Under the terms of the Constitution the National Assembly is the highest representative authority and the highest state authority. It has the power to draw up and amend the Constitution, make and amend laws, and elect and remove members of other leading organs. Elected for five years, the Assembly meets at least twice every year. The Council of State, the republic's collective Presidency, is elected by the Assembly from among its members. It performs many of the Assembly's tasks when the latter is not in session. The Council chair commands the armed forces and acts as chair of the country's National Defence Council. A Council of Ministers, headed by a Chair, is also elected by the National Assembly, to which it is responsible

Electoral system

Under an electoral law adopted in December 1980, in each constituency the Vietnam Fatherland Front (the CPV-controlled body embracing the country's various mass organizations) nominates candidates "on the basis of consultations with the local collective of the working people and with political parties and mass organizations". Those candidates receiving more than half the valid votes cast are declared elected. If several candidates receive the same number of votes, the senior in age is elected. If a sufficient number of candidates is not elected, a by-election is held within 15 days to enable the voters to choose between the unsuccessful candidates. If less than half the electorate vote, a new election is held within 15 days. If the central or local committee of the Fatherland Front demand a deputy's recall, a referendum is held in the constituency, and if a majority of the electorate then vote for the recall, the deputy is deprived of his seat.

Recent elections

Elections were held to a National Assembly representing both North and South Vietnam in April 1976. Elections to the SRV National Assembly were subsequently held in April 1981 and April 1987.

Evolution of the suffrage

Under the 1980 Constitution, all Vietnamese citizens have the right to vote if over 18 and to stand for election if over 21, except the insane or people deprived of such rights by law. In the most recent nationwide elections (1987) the turnout of eligible voters was recorded as averaging 98.44 per cent in the major cities.

PARTY BY PARTY DATA

Communist Party of Vietnam
Dang Cong San Viet-Nam

Address. 10 Hoang Van Thu Street, Hanoi, Vietnam.

Leadership. Do Muoi (sec.-gen.); Do Muoi, Le Duc Anh, Vo Van Kiet, Dao Duy Tung, Doan Khue, Vu Oanh, Le Phuoc Tho, Pham Van Kai, Bui Thien Ngo, Nong Duc Manh, Pham The Duyet, Nguyen Duc Binh, Vo Tran Chi (members of political bureau); Do Muoi, Le Duc Anh, Dao Duy Tung, Le Phuoc Tho, Nguyen Ha Phan, Hong Ha, Nguyen Dinh Tu, Trong My Hoa, Do Quang Thang (members of secretariat).

Orientation. Since its sixth congress in December 1986, the Communist Party of Vietnam (CPV) has been engaged in its own version of economic and political reform known as *doi moi*. The launch of the reform programme reflected Vietnam's desperate economic predicament. At the same time it seemed to be an acknowledgement that the party leadership had taken note of the example set by other communist parties (including the Communist Party of the Soviet Union) which had pioneered the path of economic and political renovation. Considerable progress was made during the mid- and late-1980s in renovating the Vietnamese economy, especially in the encouragement of private enterprise.

However, in 1989 *doi moi* was called into question when the party leadership responded to events in China, the Soviet Union and Eastern Europe by rejecting any further political reform. The party general secretary and architect of *doi moi*, Nguyen Van Linh, rejected calls for political pluralism, warned the country's media against criticizing the party and attacked the profound changes under way within most of the communist world. The party again rejected political reforms at its seventh congress held in June 1991. In his political report to the congress, Linh stated that the adoption of a multi-party system would only create the conditions for internal and foreign reactionary forces to grow. However, Linh pledged that the party would continue to press ahead with economic reforms. The appointment of Do Muoi (a conservative who had supported Linh's general reformist line) as Linh's successor at the congress appeared to reflect the party's desire to balance the requirements of political stability and economic reform.

Founded. February 1930.

History. The CPV is descended from the Indo-Chinese Communist Party (ICP), founded in 1930 by Ho Chi Minh, with which it claims full continuity. In 1931 the ICP was recognized as an autonomous section of the Third (Communist) International (or Comintern) and in 1935 it held its "first" congress. Ho formally dissolved the ICP into an Association of Marxist Studies in late 1945. There is little doubt that the disbanding of the ICP was a largely cosmetic exercise, and that the party continued to function and thrive. It was publicly revived in February–March 1951, when the Vietnamese Workers' (*Lao Dong*) Party held its "second" congress. A separate Cambodian communist party emerged later that year and a separate Lao party was created in 1955. The *Lao Dong* retained its name until the fourth congress in 1976, when it became the Communist Party of Vietnam.

Following the formation of the ICP, a peasant revolt against French rule broke out in Vietnam with communist backing and, after its suppression, Ho Chi Minh was sentenced to death in absentia by the French authorities. After the failure of a further ICP-led uprising in 1940, Ho joined other Vietnamese exiles in China where he established the *Viet Minh* as an alliance of communist and nationalist organizations. *Viet Minh* bands carried on a guerrilla resistance to the Japanese forces which had occupied Vietnam in 1940.

After the surrender of Japan in August 1945 the *Viet Minh* set up a provisional government and on Sept. 2, 1945, the Democratic Republic of Vietnam (DRV) was proclaimed in Hanoi with Ho as president. Various attempts to reach a compromise settlement with the re-established French authorities broke down and from late 1946 Ho's *Viet Minh* guerrillas engaged in bitter hostilities with the French forces, which culminated in the decisive defeat of the latter at Dien Bien Phu in

May 1954.

Under the 1954 Geneva agreements, Vietnam was temporarily divided at the 17th parallel and Ho became both President and Premier of North Vietnam; he retained the Presidency and party chair until his death in 1969. In 1959 the party decided to resume the armed struggle in South Vietnam (by this stage a US-backed republic led by Ngo Dinh Diem), which had been pursued under the ostensible leadership of a non-communist National Liberation Front (NLF). A separate People's Revolutionary Party of South Vietnam was created in 1961. However, actual party control below the 17th parallel was held by the *Lao Dong's* own southern office (the Central Office for South Vietnam, COSVN) which directed the war in accordance with the line established at the party's third congress in 1960 and with subsequent politburo directives. Protracted negotiations involving ceasefire and peace proposals by both sides led to the 1973 Paris Peace Agreements, but in fact the war ended only with the fall of the southern regime and the de facto reunification of the country on Apr. 30, 1975.

The party had organized a massive programme of land reform and agricultural co-operativization in the North during the 1950s. The completion of agricultural transformation led the party leadership to start planning "socialist construction" in the early 1960s. Hence, the party's first five-year plan (1961–65) aimed at rapid industrialization on the basis of centralized planning. However, US bombing of the North during 1965–68 rendered the plan futile. The Vietnam War resulted not only in the destruction of much of the Northern infrastructure, but also necessitated a decentralization of economic planning and production. The political re-unification of Vietnam in 1976 could not disguise the economic disparity between the North and the South. A year after reunification the party moved to rapidly increase "socialist transformation" in the South, stepping up co-operativization and abolishing "bourgeois" trading activity. The move failed and added sharply to the number of "boat people" fleeing southern Vietnam during the late 1970s.

From the early 1960s, the party encountered the dilemma of how to respond to the growing dissension between the Chinese Communist Party (CCP) and the Communist Party of the Soviet Union (CPSU). During the 1960s the party leaders assiduously avoided confrontation with China. At the same time they declined to imitate the radical Maoism of the Great Leap Forward or the Cultural Revolution. The Vietnamese refused to follow the CCP into open revolt against the

Soviet Union and the position was made clear in 1966 when Le Duan (the party's first secretary who was subsequently noted for his pro-Moscow line) chose to attend the 23rd CPSU congress. After Vietnamese reunification in 1976, the CPV shifted much closer to the CPSU, a process which culminated in an open break with the CCP and the signing of a Vietnamese-Soviet Friendship Treaty in 1978. It was at this point that western reports of a CPV leadership divided between pro-Beijing and pro-Moscow factions was shown to be erroneous. In 1979 Vietnam and China fought a brief, but bloody, border war.

The collapse of communism in Eastern Europe in 1989 induced major changes in the CPV's relations with the Soviet Union and China. The Soviet Union began reducing its massive aid programme to Vietnam, prompting the Hanoi leadership to boost its efforts to improve relations with China. In September 1990 CPV secretary-general, Nguyen Van Linh, made a secret visit to China, setting in motion a train of events that culminated in an official visit to Beijing by the Vietnamese Foreign Minister, Nguyen Manh Cam, in September 1991.

The party has always placed great emphasis on its relations with the Lao and Cambodian communist movements. Relations with the Lao movement have always been close. However, relations with the Cambodian communists deteriorated in the 1960s with the ascendancy of an ultra-nationalist and pro-Chinese faction led by Pol Pot. Vietnam overthrew the Pol Pot regime in 1979 and established in its place a regime led by pro-Vietnamese communists.

In the early 1980s, party leaders in South Vietnam, including Nguyen Van Linh, then party chief in Ho Chi Minh City, began experimenting with private trading enterprises. The so-called Southern "reformers" received a set-back at the sixth party congress in 1982 when the experiments were criticized and Linh was removed from the politburo. However, the "reformers" continued to press ahead with their experiments, and in 1985 the politburo approved a major package of wage and subsidy reforms.

Le Duan, the leader of the Communist Party of Vietnam (CPV) since Ho Chi Minh's death in 1969, died in mid-1986. He was replaced by Linh, at the party's sixth congress held in December, who immediately launched his programme of renovation (*doi moi*) aimed at reforming the economy.

Linh's efforts to reconstruct Vietnam's war-shattered economy and increase the general efficiency of governmental control were seriously undermined in the late 1980s by events in the Soviet Union and Eastern Europe. Party leaders reacted with distinct unease at the collapse of communism in Eastern Europe. During 1990 the imprisonment of prominent reformists in the South, curbs on press freedoms, and a decision to limit the number of Vietnamese studying in Eastern Europe and the Soviet Union were all interpreted as attempts to reduce the pressure for political reform. At the party's eighth central committee plenum in March, the outspoken reformist Tran Xuan Bach was removed from the politburo, a move regarded as a victory for the party's 'conservative' wing. At the 10th plenum in December, the party finalized details of its Draft Platform on Socialist Construction for the Transitional Period. The Draft constituted the party's second political platform, the first having been adopted at the time of the founding of the ICP in 1930. Commentators were unclear whether the document indicated a continuation of economic reform policies or advocated a return to more centralized planning.

The Draft Platform, along with a 10-year socioeconomic plan, was eventually approved at the party's seventh congress held in June 1991. The congress had originally been scheduled to take place earlier, but intense debate within the party over economic and political policy had forced a postponement. In the event, the congress avoided discussion of the more controversial policy details relating to the reform process, while approving widespread leadership changes. Do Muoi, the 74-year-old Premier, replaced Nguyen Van Linh as CPV general secretary. Muoi, widely regarded as a conservative force at the time of his appointment as Premier in 1988, had tended to confound his critics by generally supporting Linh's reformist line. Nevertheless, Muoi was widely regarded as a cautious leader who would be unlikely to speed up the pace of reform. Six others were removed from the politburo, namely Vo Chi Cong, Nguyen Duc Tam (head of the central committee's powerful organization committee), Nguyen Co Thach (the Foreign Minister), Mai Chi Tho (the Interior Minister), and Dong Sy Nguyen and Nguyen Thanh Binh. Commentators suggested that Tho, Tam and Thach had been removed because of their close association with Le Duc Tho, the veteran CPV leader and brother of Mai Chi Tho who had died in October 1990. In the case of Thach, his removal also reflected deep divisions within the

leadership over foreign policy. Thach had long been in a minority within the party leadership because of his implacable opposition towards normalization of relations with China. His removal, therefore, was regarded as an important step in the normalization process.

Structure. The party's supreme organ is its congress. It has a central committee (146 full members), whose political bureau has 13 full members. The party's secretariat has nine members. There are over 100,000 party cells. Mass organizations are the Ho Chi Minh Communist Youth Union and the Vietnamese Women's Union.

Membership. More than 2,000,000.

Publications. Nhan Dan (The People), daily national official organ; *Tap Chi Cong San* (Communist Review), monthly; Vietnam Courier, monthly.

Minor parties

The Communist Party of Vietnam is the sole legal political party in Vietnam.

Defunct parties

The **Vietnam Democratic Party** (VDP) and the **Vietnam Socialist Party** (VSP) both ended their activities in October 1988. Both parties had represented sections of the middle classes and intelligentsia since the mid-1940s. Immediately prior to their dissolution, the Gold Star Order had been accorded to both parties by the Council of State to mark awareness of the "great contributions to the national revolutionary struggle" made by them.

Principal illegal organizations

National United Front for the Liberation of Vietnam; the largest and best organized anti-communist resistance group operating in Vietnam.

United Front for the Struggle of the Oppressed Races (*Front unifié de la lutte des races opprimées*); an illegal organization established by the tribal people of the central highlands of Vietnam (whom the French collectively termed Montagnards) in pursuance of their demand for autonomy for the 12 northern provinces of southern Vietnam.

Western Samoa

Capital: Apia   **Population: 159,862 (1992)**

Discovered by Europeans in the early 18th century, Western Samoa became a German colony in 1899. From 1918 to 1962 the country was administered by New Zealand. In 1962 Western Samoa became the first Pacific country to become independent. In 1970 it joined the Commonwealth and, in 1976, the United Nations. Full democracy was implemented in December 1990, although the right to stand for election to the legislature remains restricted to clan leaders.

Constitutional structure

Western Samoa is a constitutional monarchy with the head of state, the *O le Ao O le Malo*, possessing the power to dissolve the unicameral, 49-member *Fono* (the legislative assembly) and to appoint a Prime Minister upon its recommendation. The constitution provides for the *O le Ao O le Malo* to be elected by the *Fono* for a term of five years, but in the first instance it was decided that two High Chiefs, Tupua Tamasese and Malietoa Tanumafili II, should become joint heads of state for the duration of their lives unless they resigned or were removed by the assembly. On Apr. 5, 1963, Tupua Tamasese died, leaving Malietoa Tanumafili II as sole head of state.

Executive power is in the hands of a Prime Minister and Cabinet, who are responsible to the unicameral, 49-member legislature, the *Fono*. The Constitution also provides for a Council of Deputies (the membership of which cannot overlap with that of the *Fono*) to undertake ceremonial duties and to act as a head of state if the *O le Ao O le Malo* is incapacitated or unavailable for duty.

Electoral system

The *Fono* is elected by universal suffrage for up to three years. Upon assembling, the new *Fono*, using a secret ballot, expresses support for one of its members for the post of Prime Minister, and he is then appointed to the post by the head of state.

Evolution of the suffrage

The first instance of universal adult suffrage was a UN-supervised plebescite on May 9, 1961, which approved the proposed Constitution and expressed support for independence. The Constitution under which the country became independent, however, provided for 45 of the 47 members of the *Fono* to be elected by the country's several thousand *Matai*, the traditional male heads of extended family groups. The two others were elected by those of European origin. On Oct. 29, 1990, a referendum of the whole electorate voted in favour of adopting a system of universal adult suffrage for those aged 21 and over, although the right to stand for election remains in most instances confined to members of the *Matai*.

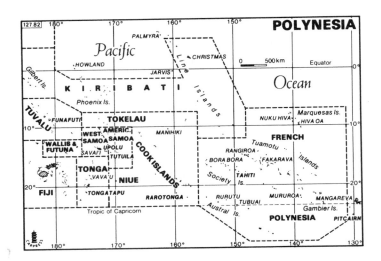

Recent elections

Although elections were held regularly following independence, the first political party did not appear until 1979. Parties remain organized around individuals rather than ideological issues.

Date of Election	Winning Party
February 1982	Human Rights Protection Party
February 1985	Human Rights Protection Party
February 1988	Human Rights Protection Party
April 5, 1991	Human Rights Protection Party

PARTY BY PARTY DATA

Human Rights Protection Party

Address. PO Box 3898, Apia.
Leadership. Tofilau Eti Alesana (l.).
Orientation. Centrist.
Founded. 1979.
History. The Human Rights Protection Party (HRPP) was formed in 1979 as a means of uniting those opposed to the government of Tupuola Taisi Efi, the incumbent Prime Minister. The party lost the 1979 election, but won the election of February 1982 with 24 of the 47 seats in the *Fono.* The party's leader, Va'ai Kalone, was appointed Prime Minister, but was removed from office in September after his majority was eroded by a judicial investigation into electoral irregularities. Tupuola Taisi Efi returned to power but, resigned in December after the defeat of his budget. The HRPP then returned to government under its new leader Tofilau Eti Alesana.

The party reinforced its slender majority in the *Fono* at the 1985 election, winning 31 of the 47 seats. A number of HRPP members defected to the opposition, however, and in December Tofilau Eti Alesana resigned after a *Fono* defeat and was replaced as Prime Minister by Va'ai Kalone. The Kalone government was supported by 12 HRPP members and 15 members of the Christian Democratic Party (CDP).

At the election of 1987, the HRPP and the CDP each won 23 seats, with the remaining constituency being tied. Although the seat was eventually awarded to the CDP, before it could form a government the HRPP induced a CDP member to defect, and in April Tofilau Eti Alesana was elected as Prime Minister. The party retained power at the 1991 election, initially winning 26 seats. By the time that the new *Fono* convened in early May, the traditional political manoeuvring had increased the HRPP's legislative strength to 30 seats, and Tofilau Eti Alesana was re-elected Prime Minister for what, he later stated, would be his final term in office.

Samoan National Development Party

Address. Apia, Western Samoa.
Leadership. Tupua Tamasese Efi and Va'ai Kalone.
Orientation. Centrist.
Founded. 1988.
History. The Samoan National Development Party (SNDP) was founded in 1988 as an alliance between the Christian Democratic Party (CDP) led by former Prime Minister Tupuola Taisi Efi, and elements of the Human Rights Protection Party (HRPP) who supported Va'ai Kalone rather than Tofilau Eti Alesana. Following a defeat for Prime Minister Tofilau Eti Alesana in December 1985, the CDP formed a government with the support of a number of HRPP legislators. Led by Va'ai Kalone and then by Tupuola Taisi Efi, the alliance coalesced into a new party.

In the 1991 general election, the SNDP won 18 seats, although by the time that the new *Fono* convened in early May, the traditional political manoeuvring had decreased this figure to 16. Among those defeated at the election was opposition leader Tupua Tamasese Efi. After legal challenges concerning the validity of the election in Tupua Tamasese Efi's constituency, the seat was declared vacant, and Tupua Tamasese Efi won the subsequent by-election in August after polling 58 per cent of the votes cast.

Defunct parties

Christian Democratic Party (CDP); founded shortly before the 1985 election to oppose the Human Rights Protection Party (HRPP), the CDP was the forerunner of the Samoan National Development Party (SNDP). In the 1985 election it won 16 seats, but formed a government in January 1986 with elements of the HRPP. This alliance was the basis for the foundation of the SNDP in 1988.

Major guerrilla groups

There are no guerrilla groups operating in Western Samoa.

Index of personal names

H

I

J

Index of parties

D